JUBB, KENNEDY, and PALMER'S

Pathology of DOMESTIC ANIMALS

SEVENTH EDITION Volume 2

JUBB, KENNEDY, and PALMER'S

Pathology of DOMESTIC ANIMALS

SEVENTH EDITION Volume 2

Edited By:

M. GRANT MAXIE, DVM, PhD, DIPLOMATE ACVP

Co-Executive Director (Retired), Laboratory Service Division
Director (Retired), Animal Health Laboratory
University of Guelph
Guelph, Ontario
Canada

ELSEVIER

Elsevier
3251 Riverport Lane
St. Louis, Missouri 63043

JUBB, KENNEDY, AND PALMER'S PATHOLOGY OF DOMESTIC ANIMALS, SEVENTH EDITION

ISBN: 978-0-4432-7911-9 (3 VOLUME SET)
978-0-4431-2071-8 (VOLUME 1)
978-0-4431-2072-5 (VOLUME 2)
978-0-4431-2073-2 (VOLUME 3)

Executive Content Strategist: Lauren Willis
Content Development Specialist: Laura Fisher
Publishing Services Manager: Deepthi Unni
Senior Project Manager: Beula Christopher
Designer: Brian Salisbury

Printed in India

Last digit is the print number: 9 8 7 6 5 4 3 2 1

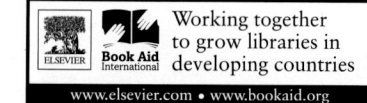

Contributors

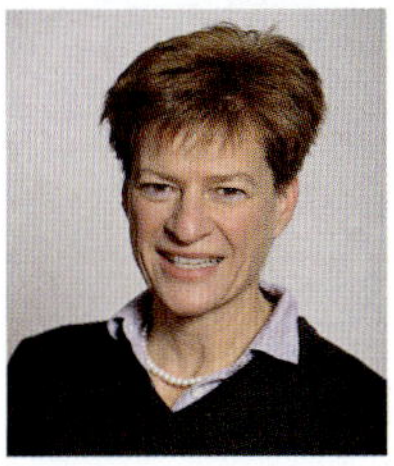

Dorothee Bienzle, DVM, PhD, Diplomate ACVP
Professor
Department of Pathobiology
Ontario Veterinary College
University of Guelph
Guelph, Ontario, Canada
Hematolymphoid system

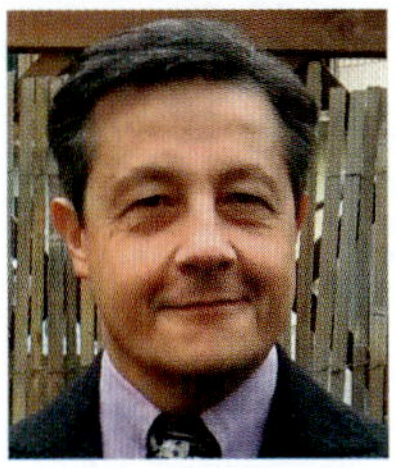

Carlo Cantile, DVM, PhD
Full Professor of Anatomic Pathology
Department of Veterinary Science
University of Pisa
Pisa, Italy
Nervous system

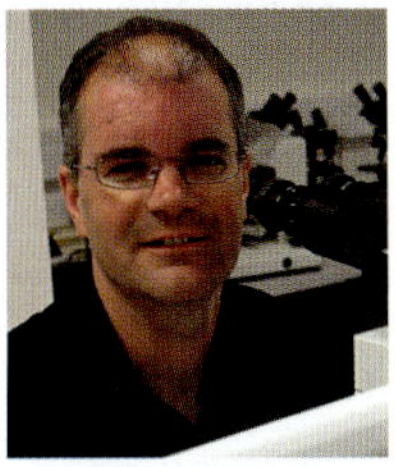

Jeff L. Caswell, DVM, DVSc, PhD, Diplomate ACVP
Professor
Department of Pathobiology
Ontario Veterinary College
University of Guelph
Guelph, Ontario, Canada
Respiratory system

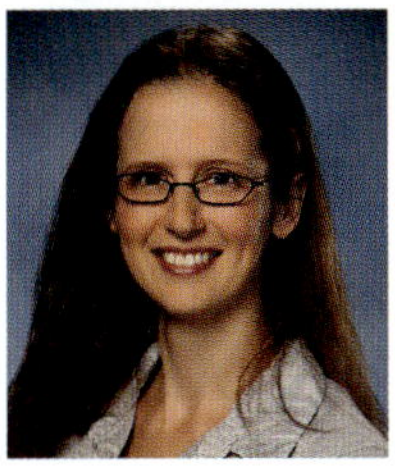

Rachel E. Cianciolo, VMD, PhD, Diplomate ACVP
Anatomic Pathologist
Zoetis Reference Labs
Zoetis
Comparative Nephropathologist
Niche Diagnostics, LLC
Columbus, Ohio, USA
Urinary system

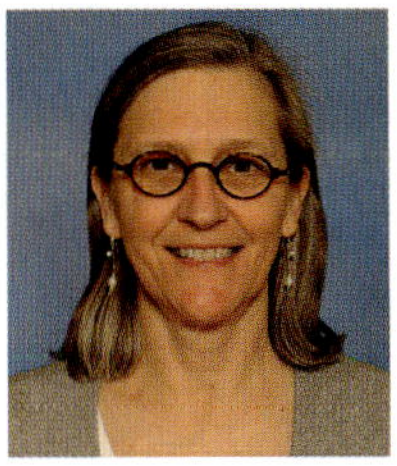

Linden E. Craig, DVM, PhD, Diplomate ACVP
Clinical Professor
Department of Biomedical and Diagnostic Sciences
University of Tennessee College of Veterinary Medicine
Knoxville, Tennessee, USA
Bones and joints

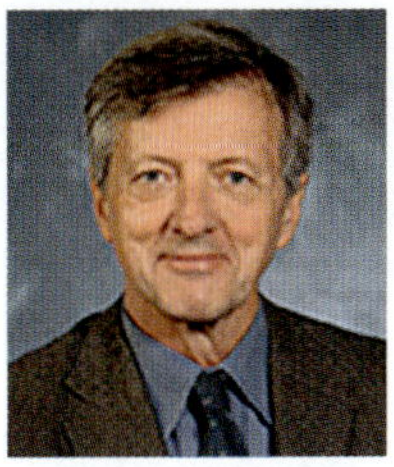

John M. Cullen, VMD, PhD, Diplomate ACVP
Professor Emeritus
Department of Population Health and Pathobiology
College of Veterinary Medicine
North Carolina State University
Raleigh, North Carolina, USA
Liver and biliary system

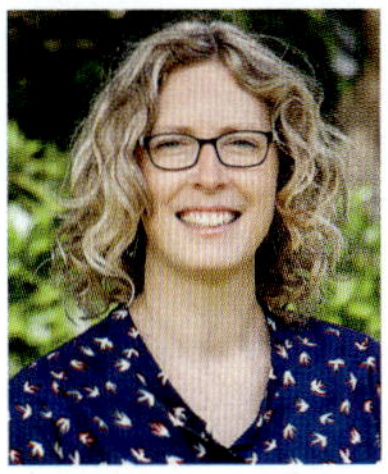

Keren E. Dittmer, BVSc, PhD, Diplomate ACVP, FHEA
Professor
Pathobiology and Infectious Disease Group
School of Veterinary Science
Massey University
Palmerston North, Manawatū, New Zealand
Bones and joints

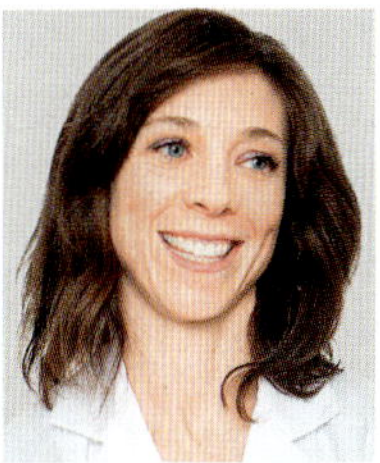

Taryn A. Donovan, DVM, Diplomate ACVP
Department of Anatomic Pathology
Schwarzman Animal Medical Center
New York, New York, USA
Cardiovascular system

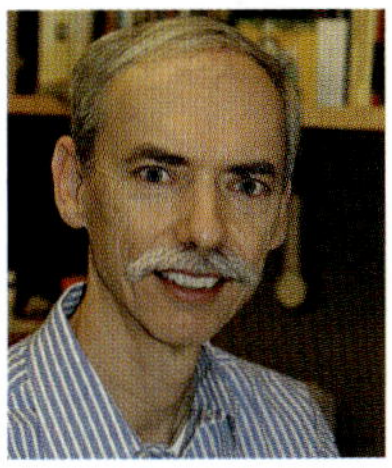

Robert A. Foster, BVSc, PhD, MANZVCS, Diplomate ACVP
Professor
Department of Pathobiology
Ontario Veterinary College
University of Guelph
Guelph, Ontario, Canada
Female genital system
Male genital system

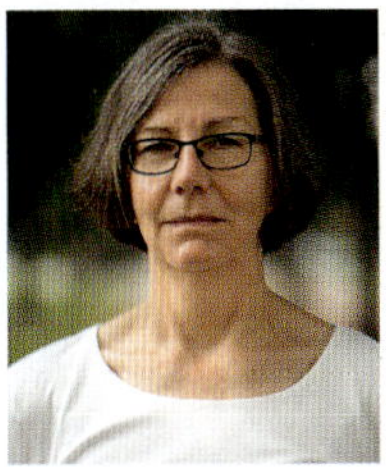

Andrea Gröne, DVM, PhD, Diplomate ACVP, Diplomate ECVP
Professor
Division of Pathology
Faculty of Veterinary Medicine
Utrecht University
Utrecht, The Netherlands
Endocrine glands

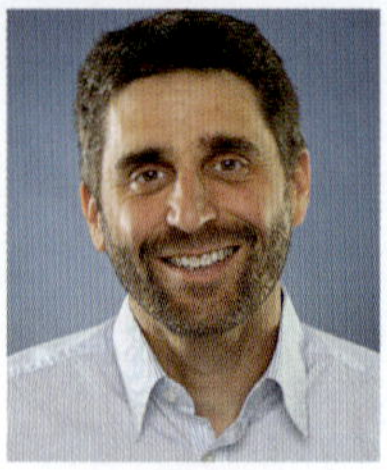

Stefan M. Keller, DVM, Dr. Med. Vet., PhD, Diplomate ECVP
Associate Professor
Department of Pathology, Microbiology, Immunology
School of Veterinary Medicine
University of California, Davis
Davis, California, USA
Hematolymphoid system

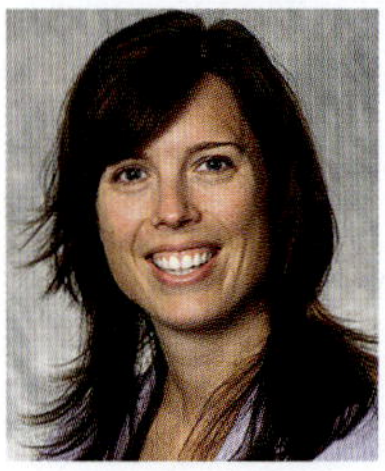

Kathleen M. Kelly, DVM, PhD, Diplomate ACVP
Veterinary Pathologist II
Pathology/Safety Assessment
Charles River Laboratories
Ashland, Ohio, USA
Cardiovascular system

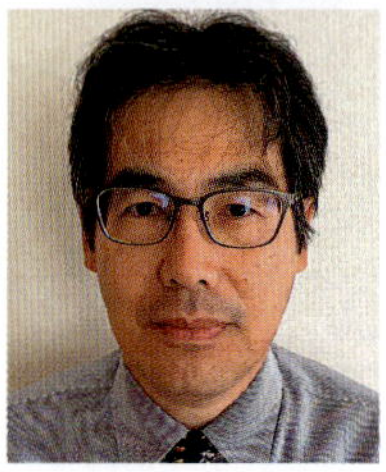

Yoshiyasu Kobayashi, DVM, PhD, Diplomate JCVP
Professor
Laboratory of Veterinary Pathology
Department of Veterinary Medicine
Obihiro University of Agriculture and Veterinary Medicine
Obihiro, Hokkaido, Japan
Muscle and tendon

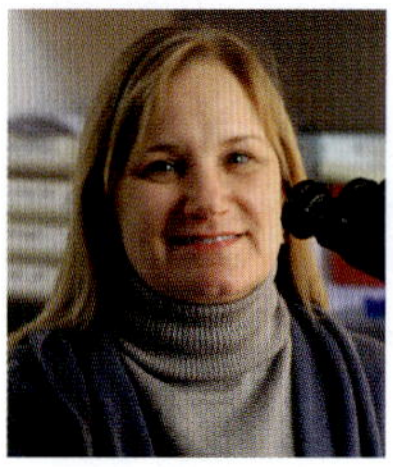

Elizabeth A. Mauldin, DVM, Diplomate ACVP, Diplomate ACVD
Professor
Department of Pathobiology
School of Veterinary Medicine
University of Pennsylvania
Philadelphia, Pennsylvania, USA
Integumentary system

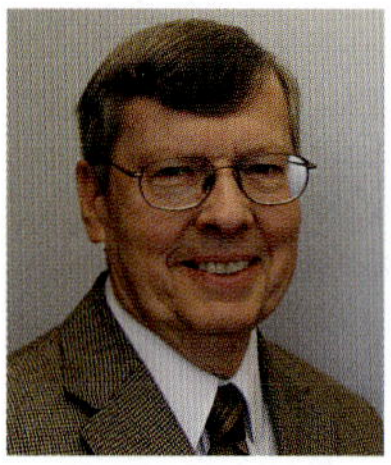

M. Grant Maxie, DVM, PhD, Diplomate ACVP
Co-Executive Director (Retired), Laboratory Services Division
Director (Retired), Animal Health Laboratory
University of Guelph
Guelph, Ontario, Canada
Editor
Introduction to the diagnostic process

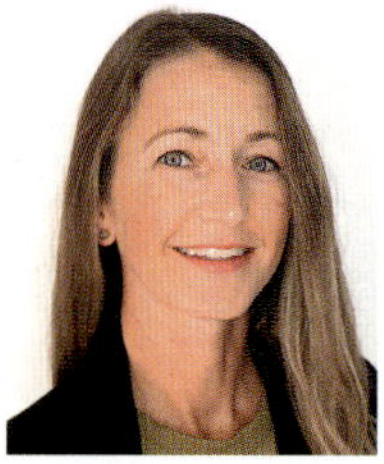

Shannon M. McLeland, DVM, PhD, Diplomate ACVP
Pathologist
Pathology
International Veterinary Renal Pathology Service (IVRPS)
Hugo, Minnesota, USA
Urinary system

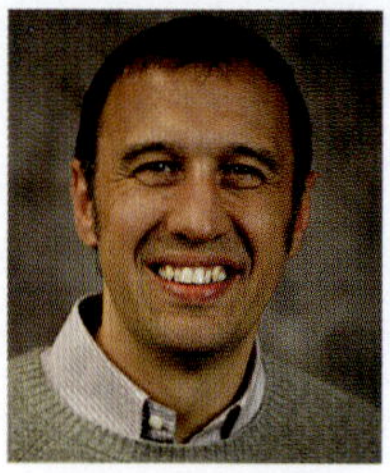

Andrew D. Miller, DVM, Diplomate ACVP
Associate Professor
Population Medicine and Diagnostic Sciences, Section of Anatomic Pathology
Cornell University College of Veterinary Medicine
Ithaca, New York, USA
Nervous system

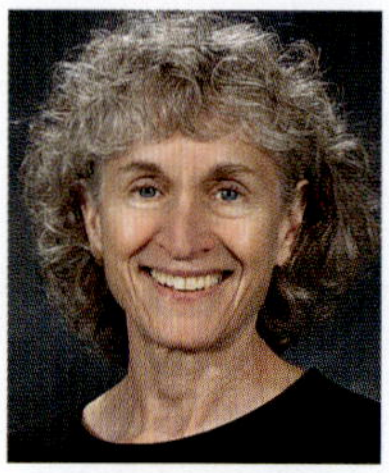

Margaret A. Miller, DVM, PhD, Diplomate ACVP
Professor Emerita
Department of Comparative Pathobiology
Purdue University
West Lafayette, Indiana, USA
Introduction to the diagnostic process

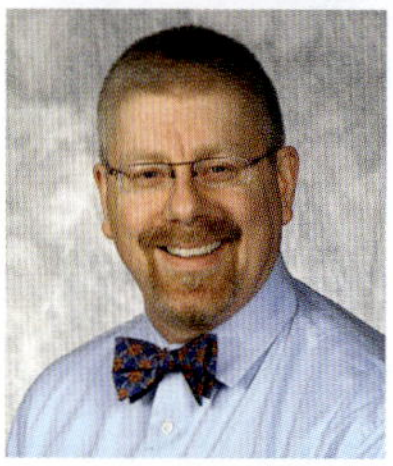

Bradley L. Njaa, DVM, MVSc, Diplomate ACVP
Senior Pathologist
Anatomic Pathology
Greenfield Pathology Services, Inc.
Greenfield, Indiana, USA
Special senses

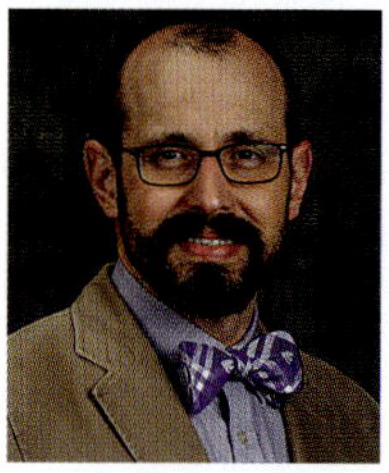

Brandon L. Plattner, DVM, PhD, Diplomate ACVP
Professor
Diagnostic Medicine and Pathobiology
Kansas Veterinary Diagnostic Laboratory
Kansas State University
Manhattan, Kansas, USA
Alimentary system

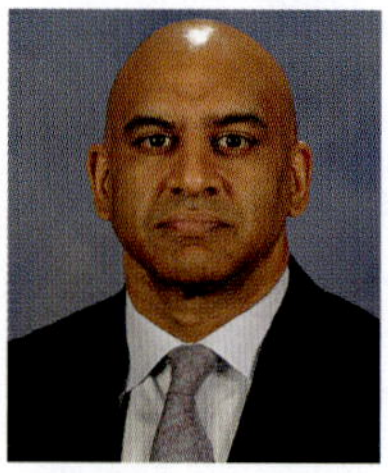

Christopher Premanandan, DVM, PhD, Diplomate ACVP, Diplomate ACT
Professor Clinical
Department of Veterinary Biosciences
College of Veterinary Medicine
The Ohio State University
Columbus, Ohio, USA
Female genital system
Male genital system

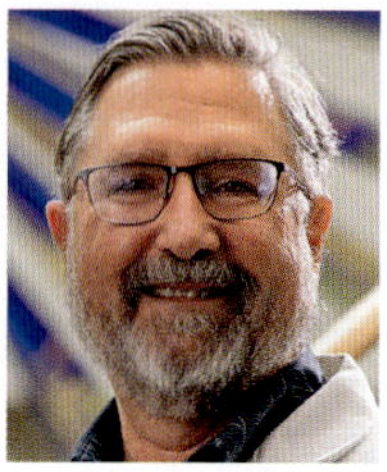

Thomas J. Rosol, DVM, PhD, MBA, Diplomate ACVP
Professor
Biomedical Sciences
Heritage College of Osteopathic Medicine
Athens, Ohio, USA
Endocrine glands

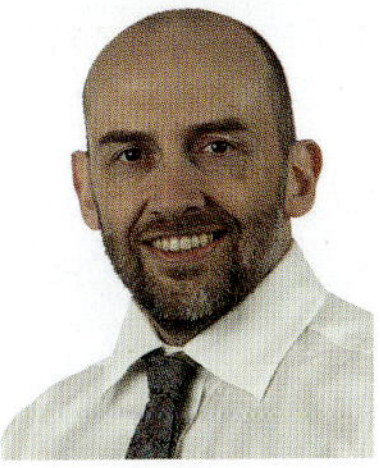

Andrew W. Stent, BVSc, MANZCVS, PhD, Diplomate ACVP
Veterinary Pathologist
Gribbles Veterinary Pathology
Melbourne, Victoria, Australia
Pancreas

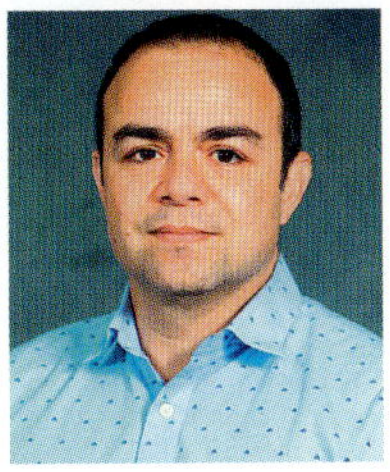

Leandro B.C. Teixeira, DVM, MSc, Diplomate ACVP
Associate Professor
Pathobiological Sciences
Director
Comparative Ocular Pathology Laboratory of Wisconsin—COPLOW
University of Wisconsin-Madison
Madison, Wisconsin, USA
Special senses

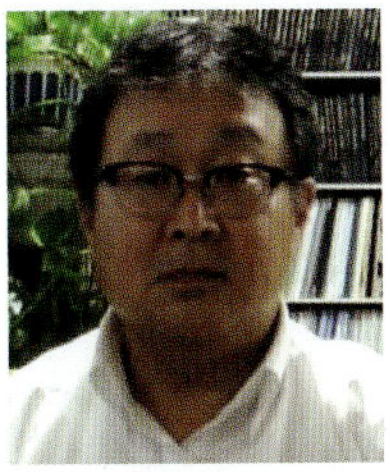

Kazuyuki Uchida, DVM, PhD, Diplomate JCVP
Professor
Veterinary Pathology
The University of Tokyo
Tokyo, Japan
Muscle and tendon

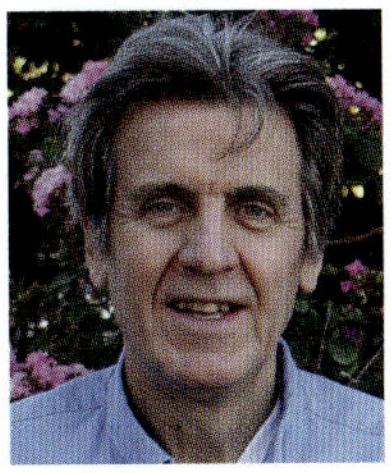

Francisco A. Uzal, DVM, FRVC, MSc, PhD, Diplomate ACVP
Distinguished Professor and Branch Chief
California Animal Health and Food Safety, San Bernardino Branch
University of California, Davis
San Bernardino, California, USA
Images Editor
Alimentary system

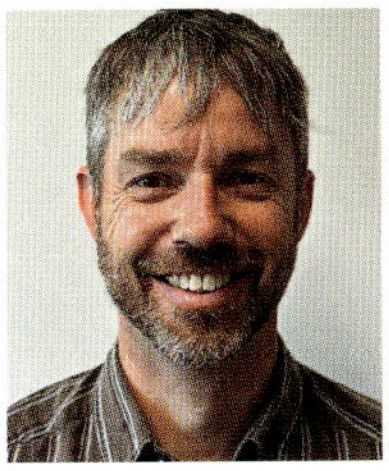

Arnaud J. Van Wettere, DVM, MS, PhD, Diplomate ACVP
Professor
Department of Veterinary Clinical and Life Sciences
College of Veterinary Medicine
Utah State University
Logan, Utah, USA
Liver and biliary system

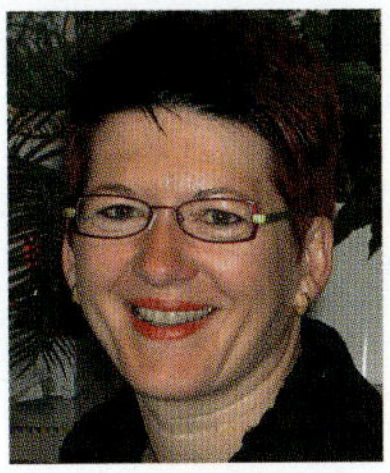

Monika M. Welle, Dr Med Vet, Diplomate ECVP
Associate Professor, Head of Biopsy Service (Retired)
Department of Infectious Diseases and Pathobiology
Institute of Animal Pathology
Bern, Switzerland
Integumentary system

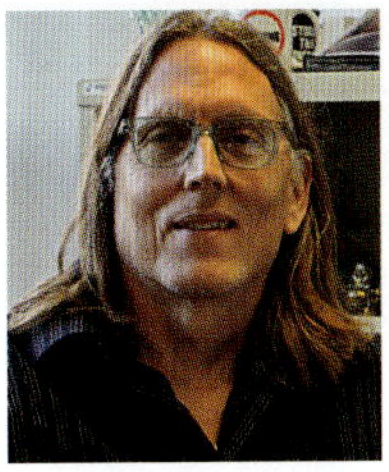

Kurt J. Williams, DVM, PhD, Diplomate ACVP
Director, Oregon Veterinary Diagnostic Laboratory
Professor, Biomedical Sciences
Carlson College of Veterinary Medicine
Oregon State University
Corvallis, Oregon, USA
Respiratory system

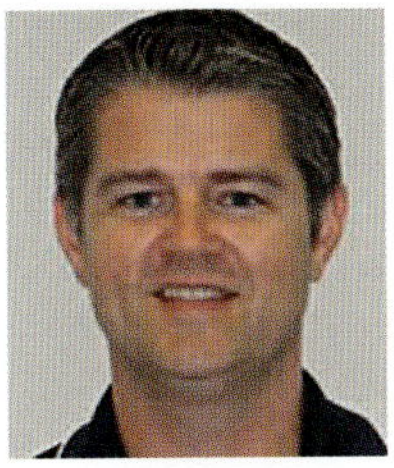

R. Darren Wood, DVM, DVSc, Diplomate ACVP
Professor
Department of Pathobiology
Ontario Veterinary College
University of Guelph
Guelph, Ontario, Canada
Hematolymphoid system

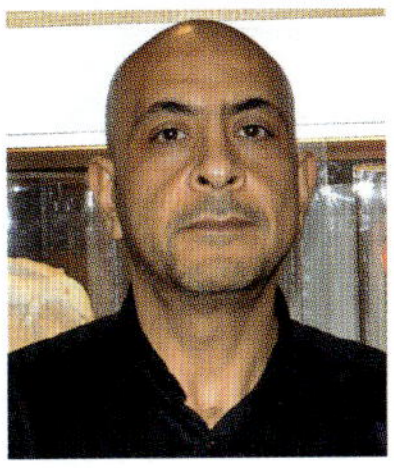

Sameh Youssef, BVSc, PhD, DVSc, Diplomate ACVP
Director
Pathology
J&J Innovative Medicine
Beerse, Belgium
Nervous system

Preface

My thanks to the contributors to this seventh edition of *Pathology of Domestic Animals* for their rigorous perusal of the literature in their areas of interest, for their addition of insightful information to their chapters, and for their inclusion of many new figures. True to the spirit of the first edition, this text is designed to explain the pathogenesis of common and not-so-common diseases, define the distinguishing features of a wide variety of conditions, and put them in a context relevant to both students and working pathologists. I hope that we have captured significant changes and have synthesized this new knowledge to provide a balanced overview of all topics covered.

In this time of advanced imaging, whole genome metagenomic sequencing, and artificial intelligence, is there a role for the veterinary diagnostic anatomic pathologist? Angst has been expressed, but I believe that the future is bright. We have a wealth of new information to work with in the diagnostic investigation of infectious disease cases, to the point of sorting out a range of competing etiologies. New infectious agents or mutated old ones appear. Toxic events continue to occur. The pathologist is in a position to sort out lesions from nonlesions or background. In addition, the ongoing advantage of the pathologist is the ability to detect agents within lesions through tools such as immunohistochemistry or in situ hybridization and hence establish causation. The wealth of tumor markers and the availability of PARR greatly assist in the definition of subtypes of tumors through immunohistochemistry and immunocytochemistry, to the benefit of patients and individualized therapy. Integration of the ancillary -ologies and -omics in case diagnoses and interpretations typically falls to the pathologist. I see this role being augmented and not disappearing and trust that these volumes will provide excellent support for diagnostic pathologists.

Full-color **images** were included throughout the sixth edition, and many of these have been retained; some, called out in the text as "**eFigs**," have been moved online. New images have been added to clearly depict the diagnostic features of many conditions. The complete index is again printed in each volume as an aid to readers. "**Further reading**" reference lists have been pruned, updated, and moved online to save space.

Since my time as editor-in-chief of the *Canadian Veterinary Journal* (1986-1991), and in my current role as editor-in-chief of the *Journal of Veterinary Diagnostic Investigation* (2015-present), I have railed against misuse of words and praised simplification and the exact use of words.[2–5] This crusade has continued throughout these volumes.

- We have followed the KISS principle ("keep it super simple") in eliminating *double vowels* (i.e., ae, oe, ou; hence, anemia, edema, tumor, rather than anaemia, oedema, tumour) and *excess syllables* (e.g., the more direct dilation, vacuolation, euthanasia, rather than dilatation, vacuolization, euthanatization).
- *Redundant words* have been removed, especially "multifocal," a word grossly overused by pathologists (*multifocal* is a redundant modifier of lesions that are inherently *multi* and *focal*, including abscesses, aggregates, ecchymoses, foci, masses, nodules, petechiae). Similarly, other unnecessary terms have been deleted: "fibrovascular" stroma, lesions are "characterized by"…, due to "the presence of"…
- In keeping with the distinction between *parasitosis* (the parasite is pathogenic and harms its host) and *parasitiasis* (the parasite is potentially pathogenic but does not harm its host),[2] the reader will find that a few traditional names have been updated (e.g., trypanosomosis in preference to trypanosomiasis, especially with respect to the pathogenic African trypanosomes).
- We have anglicized nomenclature where possible, based on the Nomina Histologica Veterinaria, 1st ed., 2017 (https://www.wava-amav.org/downloads/NHV_2017.pdf) (lists English equivalents) and the Nomina Anatomica Veterinaria, 6th ed., 2017 (unfortunately still lists Latin terms only; the peer-reviewed scientific literature and Wikipedia have alternatives). Plus, we have replaced eponymic names with names that are more useful descriptors of conditions.[6,8]

ANGLICIZED OR ENGLISH EQUIVALENTS	EPONYMIC OR LATIN TERMS
aggregated lymphoid nodules	Peyer patch
ameba, amebic, amebiasis	amoeba, amoebic, amoebiasis
American trypanosomosis	Chagas disease
basal, spinous, granular, (clear), corneal layers	stratum basale, spinosum, granulosum, (lucidum), corneum
celom, celomic	coelom, coelomic
cerebral arterial circle	circle of Willis
ciliary margin	ora ciliaris
cochlear duct	scala media
connecting duct	reuniens duct
dorsal nucleus	Clarke column, column of Clarke, nucleus dorsalis of Clarke
equine neorickettsiosis or equine monocytic ehrlichiosis	Potomac horse fever
equine serum hepatitis	Theiler disease
fascicular or fasciculate zone—adrenal	zona fasciculata
glomerular capsules, urinary spaces	Bowman capsule and spaces

ANGLICIZED OR ENGLISH EQUIVALENTS	EPONYMIC OR LATIN TERMS
glomerular zone—adrenal	zona glomerulosa (multiformis, arcuate)
greater vestibular glands	Bartholin glands
hemorrhagic purpura	purpura hemorrhagica
hippocampus proper	Ammon horn
hyperadrenocorticism, hypercortisolism	Cushing disease/syndrome
hyposegmentation of granulocytes	Pelger-Huët anomaly
indolent corneal ulcer	Boxer ulcer
inner tunnel	tunnel of Corti
intestinal crypts	crypts of Lieberkühn
intrahepatic bile ductule	canal of Hering
iridial granules	granula iridica or corpora nigra
lamellar corpuscles	Pacinian corpuscles
mesencephalic aqueduct	aqueduct of Sylvius
mesonephric ducts	Gartner ducts
mesonephric tubules and ducts	Wolffian tubules and ducts
myelin-sheath gaps	nodes of Ranvier
myenteric plexus	Auerbach plexus
nests of residual glia	islands of Calleja
neuroblastic rosette	Homer-Wright rosette
osteonic canal	Haversian canal
osteons	Haversian systems
otolith	otoconium
outer phalangeal cells	Deiters cells
paramesonephric duct	Müllerian duct
paratuberculosis	Johne disease
perforating canals	Volkmann canals
perforating fibers	Sharpey fibers
perilenticular vascular tunic	tunica vasculosa lentis
periportal space	space of Mall
perisinusoidal space	space of Disse
perivascular space	Virchow-Robin space
pseudorabies	Aujeszky disease
resorption lacunae	Howship lacunae
reticulate zone—adrenal	zona reticularis
retinal rosette	Flexner-Wintersteiner rosette
reverse Horner syndrome	Pourfour du Petit syndrome
sellar diaphragm	diaphragma sellae
spiral organ	organ of Corti
submucosal plexus	Meissner plexus
terminal ridge	crista terminalis
terminal sulcus	sulcus terminalis
terminal thread	filum terminale
testicular sustentacular cell	Sertoli cell
thymic corpuscles	Hassall corpuscles
tympanic duct	scala tympani
utricle	utriculus
uveodermatologic syndrome	Vogt-Koyanagi-Harada-like syndrome
vestibular duct	scala vestibuli
vestibular membrane	Reissner membrane

Keeping pace with evolving agents and their changing impacts is a never-ending challenge. We have used current microbial terminology, based on internationally accepted reference sources. As a result of intensive genetic analyses of closely related organisms, taxonomic changes seem to be never ending. We have tried to stay current, and give former names for clarity. A few examples follow:

FORMER NAME	CURRENT ACCEPTED NAME
Arcanobacterium pyogenes	*Trueperella pyogenes*
Clostridium difficile	*Clostridioides difficile*
Clostridium spiroforme	*Thomasclavelia spiroformis*
Mycoplasma bovis	*Mycoplasmopsis bovis*

As noted by the authors documenting the renaming of *Mycoplasma bovis* to *Mycoplasmopsis bovis*[7]: "The inclusion of a name on this list is not to be construed as taxonomic acceptance of the taxon to which the name is applied. Indeed, some of these names may, in time, be shown to be synonyms, or the organisms may be transferred to another genus, thus necessitating the creation of a new combination." Even after due consideration by learned bodies, taxonomic changes do not occur without debate.[1] For example, in response to concerns raised over the renaming of *Mollicutes* species, the authors state that: "…the proposed name changes rectify numerous taxonomic anomalies that have long plagued the classification of *Mollicutes* species, leading to a better understanding of their evolutionary relationships and bringing their nomenclature in conformity with the Code."[1]

A level of complexity was recently added to **viral names**. Binomial viral taxonomy was updated in the 2022 ICTV release, ratified March 2023: https://ictv.global/taxonomy/taxondetails?taxnode_id=202201440. We've depended on the Report Chapters of the International Committee on Taxonomy of Viruses (https://ictv.global/report) for clarity. For example, the former bovine herpesvirus 1 (BoHV1, infectious bovine rhinotracheitis virus, IBRV; family *Herpesviridae*, species *Bovine alhpaherpesvirus1*) became family *Orthoherpesviridae*, species *Varicellovirus bovinealpha1*. Our standard format for text entries is: bovine alphaherpesvirus 1 (BoAHV1; *Orthoherpesviridae*, *Varicellovirus bovinealpha1*). Despite our best efforts at updating viral nomenclature, viral taxonomy will no doubt continue to evolve. The tool I find very useful in the ICTV toolbox is Find the Species (https://ictv.global/taxonomy/find_the_species), which links to the latest release.

I trust that users of the seventh edition will find the text to be very readable and easily comprehended. Feedback is always welcome.

ACKNOWLEDGMENTS

My thanks to Elsevier for their help and support throughout this project, specifically Kristin Wilhelm, content director; Lauren Willis, executive content strategist; Ellen Wurm-Cutter, director, content development; Laura Fisher, content development specialist; Sakthi Mahalingam and Oviya Balamurugan, project managers; and the entire behind-the-scenes production team. My thanks also to Dr. Francisco (Paco) Uzal as images editor of the 7th edition, and to all contributors of both old and new images. We have attempted to contact all contributors of figures from previous editions and apologize to any that we were unable to contact or who were overlooked.

Grant Maxie
Guelph, Ontario, 2025

REFERENCES

1. Gupta RS, Oren A. Necessity and rationale for the proposed name changes in the classification of Mollicutes species. Reply to: 'Recommended rejection of the names Malacoplasma gen. nov., Mesomycoplasma gen. nov., Metamycoplasma gen. nov., Metamycoplasmataceae fam. nov., Mycoplasmoidaceae fam. nov., Mycoplasmoidales ord. nov., Mycoplasmoides gen. nov., Mycoplasmopsis gen. nov. [Gupta, Sawnani, Adeolu, Alnajar and Oren 2018] and all proposed species comb. nov. placed therein', by M. Balish et al. (Int J Syst Evol Microbiol, 2019;69:3650-3653). Int J Syst Evol Microbiol 2020;70:1431–8.
2. Kassai T, et al. Standardized nomenclature of animal parasitic diseases (SNOAPAD). Vet Parasitol 1988;29:299–326.
3. Maxie G. Pleura, pleurae, plural - in praise of exactitude. Can Vet J 1990;31:155–7.
4. Maxie G. Autopsy/necropsy, diagnosis/detection what's in a word? J Vet Diagn Invest 2016;28:87.
5. Maxie G. Guest editorial. Clarity of expression in scientific writing. The Davis-Thompson Foundation Newsletter 2022;52:4–6. https://davisthompsonfoundation.org/clarity-of-expression-in-scientific-writing/
6. Maxie G. Response to "Eponyms in science: a proposal to minimize their use". Vet Pathol 2024;61:849.
7. Oren A, Garrity GM. List of new names and new combinations previously effectively, but not validly, published. Int J Syst Evol Microbiol 2018;68:3379–93.
8. Schulman YF, Rissi DR. Eponyms in science: A proposal to minimize their use. Vet Pathol 2024;61:846–8.

These volumes are dedicated to Drs. Kenneth V.F. Jubb (1928–2013), Peter C. Kennedy (1923–2006), and Nigel C. Palmer, (1938–2019), and to my family—Laura, Kevin, and Andrea.

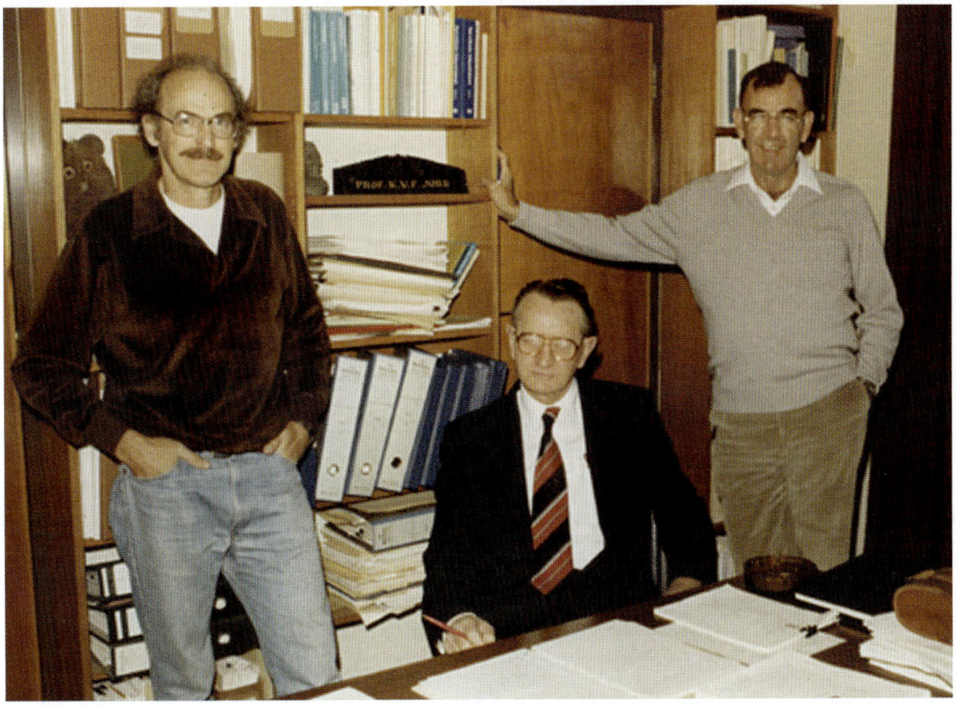

Drs. Palmer, Jubb, and Kennedy while working on the third edition in Melbourne, 1983. (Courtesy University of Melbourne.)

Contents

CHAPTER 1

Alimentary System

Francisco A. Uzal • Brandon L. Plattner

ACKNOWLEDGMENTS

We gratefully acknowledge the contributions of all previous authors of this chapter, including Drs. Ken Jubb, Peter Kennedy, Nigel Palmer, Ian Barker, Tony van Dreumel, Corrie Brown, Dale Baker, and Jesse Hostetter. We also acknowledge the following colleagues for critical review (or other significant input) for several sections of this 7th edition: Drs. Gustavo Delhon, Donal O'Toole, Heather Fritz, Jorge Garcia, Renato de Lima Santo, Karen Shapiro, Cindy Bell, and Brian Murphy.

The alimentary system is an elongated and complex tube-like organ with various anatomic arrangements and specific functions in animal species; it is composed of oral cavity, tonsils, salivary glands, esophagus, forestomachs/stomach, and intestine. Several ancient manuscripts provide accounts of various maladies affecting the bowels including Babylonian and Mesopotamian writings such as the Code of Hammurabi (1772 BC), the biblical text (2 Chronicles 21, 550-450 BC), and commentaries of the Greek physician Hippocrates (460-370 BC). In Greek and Roman culture and medicine, Galen (129-216 AD) recognized the importance of diet in various diseases, including anger, anxiety, and several feverish illnesses, and viewed the stomach as a storehouse of nutrition that sorted the wheat from the chaff. Ancient and medieval scientists produced astonishingly accurate anatomic and physiologic knowledge of the alimentary tract and understood the significance of a healthy gastrointestinal (GI) tract for maintaining health and balance in the body. Although modern scientists more fully understand the importance of GI microbes for digestion and nutrition, this emerging area of research continues to reveal how a healthy GI microbiome contributes to a wide variety of chronic mental and physical health conditions, including infections, neoplasms, immune-mediated diseases, or chronic conditions of integumentary, nervous, cardiovascular, genitourinary, endocrine, musculoskeletal, and hepatobiliary systems. As the major portal for taking into the body and processing nutrients for sustaining life, the alimentary tract from the oral cavity to the anus is truly a window to whole-body health and vitality of living organisms.

ORAL CAVITY

General considerations

Ingested materials are masticated in the stratified squamous epithelium-lined oral cavity, mixed and lubricated with saliva containing digestive enzymes, and delivered to the oropharynx. Normal oral mucous membranes are shiny, moist, and pink, which indicates adequate hydration and perfusion. Examination of the oral cavity is a standard procedure during the postmortem examination. To obtain a clear view of the mucous membranes of the buccal and oral cavity, teeth, tongue, gingiva, and tonsils, it is necessary to split the mandibular symphysis and separate the mandibles. A thorough examination of all structures will reveal local lesions and, in some cases, lesions associated with systemic disease. Lesions identified here may be indicative of congenital anomalies; physical or chemical trauma; bacterial, mycotic, viral, or parasitic infections; metabolic anomalies; various toxicities; immune-mediated conditions; and dysplastic or neoplastic disease. Poor physical condition of an animal may be related to oral lesions that result in difficulties of prehension, mastication, or swallowing of food.

Melanotic pigmentation of mucous membranes in the oral cavity may have physiologic and protective roles, and altered pigmentation (although difficult to detect reliably during autopsy) can be an important indicator of disease. Oral pigmentation can be irregular or diffuse but is normal and common in most breeds of animals; it may increase with age. Diffuse yellow oral mucosal discoloration is seen with icterus. **Mucous membrane pallor** indicates anemia; muddy brown discoloration suggests methemoglobinemia; cyanosis occurs during endotoxemia, sepsis, shock, or other circulatory diseases. Ulceration (along with congestion and cyanosis) is common in dogs and sometimes in cats with chronic uremia. Hemorrhage may accompany local inflammation, trauma, or hemorrhagic diathesis; for example, petechiae on the ventral surface of the tongue and frenulum in horses are consistent with equine infectious anemia, or other thrombocytopenic or purpuric conditions.

Congenital anomalies of the oral cavity

Congenital anomalies of the oral cavity occur as heritable or nongenetic factors, including toxicity and infectious agents. The development of normal face, jaws, and the oral cavity requires the integration of many embryonic processes, most importantly the frontonasal, maxillary, and mandibular processes. The complexity and duration of these processes during fetal development may lead to a great variety of aberrations. These are usually expressed in the newborn in the form of *clefts resulting from failures of integrated growth and fusion of these processes*. A common failure of fusion is that of the maxillary processes to the frontonasal process, which may leave facial fissures, cleft lip (harelip, cheiloschisis), and unilateral or bilateral primary cleft palate involving the area rostral to the incisive papilla.

Facial clefts may involve the skin only, or the deeper tissues as well. They are rare and variably located, with some not obviously associated with normal lines of fusion. The most common is a complete cleft from one angle of the mouth to the ear of that side. This results from failure of fusion of the lateral portions of the maxillary and mandibular processes. A defect extending from a cleft lip to the eye results from failure of fusion of the maxillary and frontonasal processes, which may be a superficial defect with failure of closure of the nasolacrimal duct.

Primary cleft palate (harelip, cheiloschisis) includes anomalies of the upper lip rostral to the nasal septum, columella, and premaxilla. They may be unilateral or bilateral, and superficial or extend deep into the nostril. The defect arises from incomplete fusion of the frontonasal and maxillary processes.

Secondary cleft palate (cleft palate, palatoschisis) (Fig. 1-1) is often associated with primary cleft palate. Except for a small rostral portion from the frontonasal process, the normal hard palate is formed by bilateral ingrowth of the lateral palatine shelves from the maxillary processes to the midline, where they fuse and undergo intramembranous ossification, except in their caudal part, which becomes the soft palate. Inadequate growth of the palatine shelves leaves a central defect in either or both hard and soft palate, which results in direct communication between the oral and nasal cavities. Other manifestations of disordered palatogenesis include unilateral defects

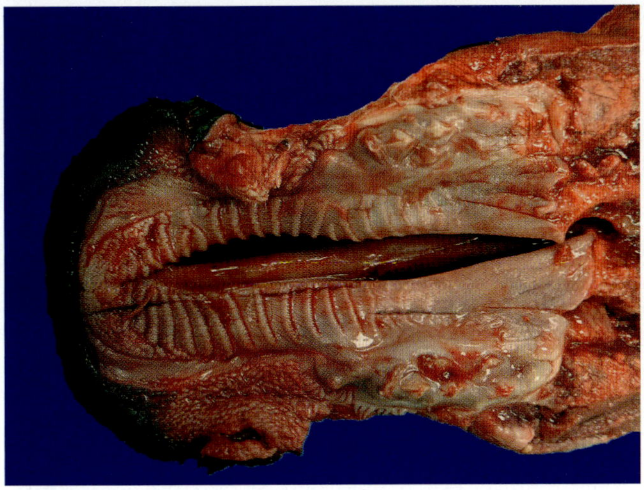

Figure 1-1 **Secondary cleft palate** exposing the nasal cavity in a calf. (Courtesy J. Caswell.)

in the soft palate; bilateral hypoplasia of the soft palate; or dorsal displacement of the soft palate with excess soft tissue on the caudal portion. Affected animals have difficulty sucking, may have nasal regurgitation, and usually die within the first few days of life from aspiration pneumonia. In dogs, malformation of the soft palate has also been associated with alterations in the tympanic bulla and middle ear dysfunction.

Cleft palates have been reported in most species of domestic animals. In one extensive survey of Thoroughbred foals, 4% of congenital defects were secondary cleft palates. Most of these foals had a complete hard palate cleft; a few had clefts of the soft palate only. Cleft palate is one of the most common anomalies in calves but is very uncommon in sheep. Primary cleft palate is less common than secondary cleft palate in swine, although both often occur together.

The *etiology* of cleft palate is usually unknown, but *hereditary causes*, maternal ingestion of certain *drugs*, or maternal consumption of *teratogenic plants* during pregnancy have been demonstrated. Secondary cleft palate and arthrogryposis frequently occur together in Charolais and Hereford calves, and are likely inherited as simple autosomal recessive traits. Cleft palate in lambs may be genetic or associated with the ingestion of *Veratrum californicum*. Secondary cleft palates have been induced experimentally in newborn piglets by feeding seeds or plants of poison hemlock (*Conium maculatum*) to gilts during gestational days 30-45. Tree tobacco (*Nicotiana glauca*) in the western United States and tobacco stalks (*Nicotiana tabacum*) when fed to gilts early in pregnancy can induce a high incidence of cleft palate and arthrogryposis in newborn piglets. Piperidine alkaloids (coniine, coniceine, anabasine) in hemlock and tobacco plants are responsible for the teratogenic effects of these plants. Lupines (*Lupinus formosus, L. arbustus*) produce piperidine alkaloids, including the teratogen ammodendrine, which can cause cleft palate and arthrogryposis in calves (crooked-calf disease) born of dams fed the lupine at days 40-50 of gestation. Palatoschisis in piglets has also been associated with consumption of feed contaminated with *Crotalaria retusa* seed by sows during gestation. Primary and secondary cleft palate of German Boxer dogs appear to be hereditary, probably because of a single autosomal recessive gene. A single autosomal recessive gene has been associated with cleft palate in Pyrenean Shepherd dogs. Secondary cleft palate occurs in Siamese and Abyssinian cats and is also likely hereditary. Griseofulvin treatment of pregnant female cats or mares may result in palatoschisis in the offspring. The defect has also been reported in both portions of the face in diprosopus cats.

Anomalies in the growth of jaws are quite common. **Brachygnathia superior**, *shortness of the maxillae*, is an inherited breed characteristic in some dogs and swine. Depending on the severity, this can result in malapposition of teeth, which interferes with prehension and mastication. In swine, brachygnathia superior may be confused with atrophic rhinitis. In Angus and Jersey cattle, brachygnathia superior occurs as a hereditary trait. In any species, it may be associated with chondrodysplasia and is described simultaneously with other facial defects.

Brachygnathia inferior or micrognathia is defined as *shortness of the mandibles*, may vary from a mild-to-lethal defect in cattle and sheep, and is a breed characteristic of long-nosed dogs. Brachygnathia inferior is a common defect in calves where it is inherited, probably as a simple autosomal recessive trait with higher incidence in males. This condition has been associated with cerebellar hypoplasia and osteopetrosis in Aberdeen Angus and other breeds (see Vol. 1, Bones and Joints). In Merino sheep, brachygnathia is associated with a cardiomegaly and renal hypoplasia syndrome that has an autosomal recessive inheritance pattern. Transplacental infection with Schmallenberg virus (SBV; *Peribunyaviridae, Orthobunyavirus schmallenbergense*) will lead to brachygnathia and other congenital malformations in lambs and calves. Mild brachygnathia inferior is termed *parrot mouth and* is a common conformational defect in horses, with limited functional deficits.

Prognathism refers to *abnormal prolongation of the mandibles* and is rather common, especially in sheep where it may develop with recovery from calcium deficiency (see Vol. 1, Bones and Joints). It is difficult in some cases to determine whether the jaw is absolutely elongated or merely apparently so, relative to mild brachygnathia superior.

Agnathia is a mandibulofacial malformation of the *absence of the mandibles*, which is caused by failure of development of the first branchial arch and associated structures. The defect is one of the most common anomalies in lambs but is rare in cattle. Associated malformations in lambs may include ateloprosopia (incomplete development of the face), microglossia or aglossia, atresia of the oropharynx, or anomalies affecting other body systems.

A lethal glossopharyngeal hereditary defect known as **bird tongue** has been reported in dogs, associated with an autosomal recessive gene defect. Affected pups have a narrow tongue, especially the rostral half, where the margins are folded medially onto the dorsal surface. The pups are unable to swallow, although muscle fibers of the affected tongues are normal histologically. A congenital defect called **ankyloglossia** is reported in dogs, which is associated with a thickened or notched and shortened lingual frenulum; the lesion may be most pronounced at the rostral tongue. **Hypertrophy of the tongue** occurs as a congenital anomaly in pigs.

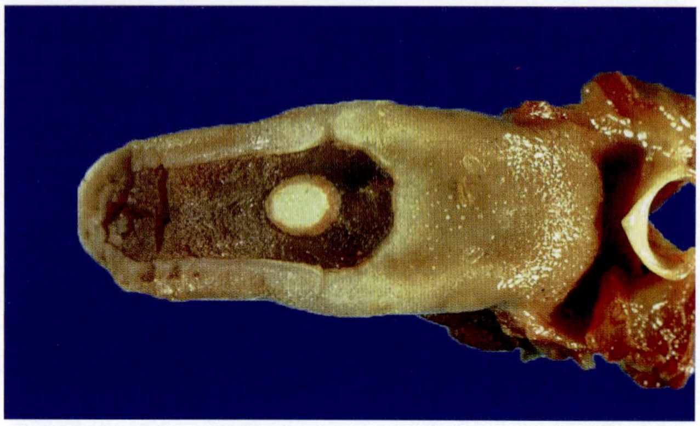

Figure 1-2 **Epitheliogenesis imperfecta** of the tongue of a pig. (Courtesy Noah's Arkives.)

Epitheliogenesis imperfecta is an anomaly that causes *widespread defects in cutaneous epithelium and affects the epithelial lining of the oral cavity, especially the tongue* (Fig. 1-2) (see Vol. 1, Integumentary System). Irregular well-demarcated red areas occur, from which the epithelium of the oral mucosa is absent. There is abrupt absence of gingival epithelium with inflammation of the exposed gingival stroma. The anomaly has been described in most species and is inherited as a simple autosomal recessive trait in cattle, horses, and pigs; the mode of inheritance is unknown in other species. Several hereditary skin conditions in animals have minor involvement of the lips and oral mucosa (see Vol. 1, Integumentary System), including epidermolysis bullosa simplex in Collie dogs, ovine epidermolysis bullosa in Suffolk and South Dorset Down sheep, and familial acantholysis in Aberdeen Angus calves.

Structure, function, and response to injury

Teeth are a critical mechanical organ for biting, tearing (incisors, canines), grinding (premolars, molars), and mixing of prehended food. Dental disease is common and often limits the useful lifespan of an animal, so understanding the basics of dental development is important.

The process of odontogenesis is the result of the complex interplay between odontogenic epithelium and ectomesenchymal cells that arise from the neural crest; the process is described in detail in the primary literature and summarized here. Teeth develop from a linear band of ectoderm known as the *dental laminae* deep to the gingival epithelium. In the initial stage of tooth development, neural crest cells beneath the dental laminae induce nodular thickenings called *tooth buds*. Epithelial cells then form a cap-like structure overlying aggregated ectomesenchymal cells, before proliferating downward to form a bell-shaped structure collectively known as the *enamel organ*, which gives rise to enamel-producing *ameloblasts*. The ectomesenchyme below the enamel organ develops into the *dental papilla*, which gives rise to dentin-producing *odontoblasts* and tooth pulp. Ectomesenchymal cells around the periphery of the enamel organ form a limiting sac called the *dental follicle* or *dental sac*, which ultimately gives rise to cementum-producing *cementoblasts*, the periodontal ligament, and alveolar bone.

The cells of the enamel organ differentiate into 3 layers: outer enamel epithelium, stellate reticulum, and inner enamel epithelium, the progenitor cells of enamel-producing *ameloblasts*. The *cervical loop* forms where the outer and inner epithelium of the enamel organ join. As the enamel organ develops, the dental lamina begins to disintegrate, leaving the tooth separate from the overlying oral epithelium. Remnants of dental lamina can persist and eventually give rise to dental cysts or neoplasms.

Dentin and enamel are then deposited on the developing tooth. Odontoblasts produce *dentin*, which in turn induces differentiation of ameloblasts from the inner enamel epithelium, leading to enamel formation. Formation of dentin is thus essential for the formation of enamel. Reciprocal inductive interactions between epithelium and ectomesenchyme are important not only in tooth development but also in the histodifferentiation of proliferative lesions of dental tissues.

The tooth crown is ultimately shaped by enamel produced by ameloblasts; the shape of tooth root is determined at the level of the cervical loop through epithelial extensions of the enamel organ called the *Hertwig epithelial root sheath* (HERS). HERS guides the formation of the developing root by inducing differentiation of odontoblasts from the dental papilla and cementoblasts from the dental follicle. Typically, HERS then fragments and disintegrates, although remnants of HERS can persist in the periodontal ligament, where they are called *epithelial rests of Malassez*. They are thought to be important in maintenance and repair of the periodontal ligament, although they may give rise to odontogenic tumors or cysts.

The tooth will begin eruption while the roots are still developing, although the mechanisms of tooth eruption are not fully understood. It is likely that the dental follicle plays a critical role in alveolar bone resorption and remodeling necessary to facilitate tooth eruption. The epithelial cells of the enamel organ form the *reduced enamel epithelium*, which protects enamel of the formed tooth before eruption. The reduced enamel epithelium fuses with the gingival epithelium as the tooth erupts and partially persists along the gingival margin of the tooth as *junctional epithelium*. The process of tooth development is similar for permanent teeth as for *deciduous* teeth, although permanent tooth germ is held dormant until later in life when the deciduous teeth are lost, and the permanent teeth develop.

There are important differences between **brachydont teeth** of humans, carnivores, and swine, in which the enamel is restricted to the tooth crown, and **hypsodont teeth** of herbivores, in which the enamel extends deep along the roots and is invaginated into the dentin forming *infundibula*. Hypsodont teeth of herbivores (except mandibular premolars of ruminants) are covered by cementum, which fills the infundibula. Exceptions are observed in hypsodont boar tusks, which are not covered by cementum, and in brachydont ruminant incisors, which have enamel covering part of the root dentin and cementum covering the root enamel.

The 3 hard matrices of teeth are dentin, enamel, and cementum. **Dentin** is grossly light-yellow and comprises most of the tooth. It consists of ~35% organic matter, including type I collagen, and ~65% mineral and is thus of similar composition to bone. Dentin is first produced from cytoplasmic extensions (visible as dentinal tubules in histologic sections of tooth) of the *odontoblasts* as unmineralized *predentin*, which becomes dentin as it is mineralized. As dentin matrix is deposited, odontoblasts move away from the dentin-enamel junction, gradually encroaching on and narrowing the pulp cavity and root canal of the tooth and leaving behind small remnant fragments of epithelium known as *rests of Serres*. Like *rests of Malassez*, these can be associated with the development of odontogenic cysts or tumors.

There are 3 types of dentin. *Primary dentin* is produced by odontoblasts before tooth eruption. *Secondary dentin* is produced by odontoblasts that remain active throughout life, but much slower than primary dentin, and only after root formation is complete. *Tertiary dentin* is produced rapidly and irregularly in response to injury of the tooth and may resemble bone or *osteodentin*.

Normal dentin contains incremental *imbrication lines of von Ebner*, fine basophilic lines oriented at right angles to the dentinal tubules, which represent normal variations in structure and mineralization of dentin. Sublethal injury caused by certain infections, metabolic stresses, or toxins may injure the odontoblasts, which then produce accentuated incremental lines known as the *contour lines of Owen*. Irregular zones of unmineralized or poorly mineralized dentin forming between foci of normal mineralization are called *interglobular dentin*, which may be indicative of hypophosphatemia or hypovitaminosis D.

Enamel has ~5% organic matter and ~95% mineral and is produced by *ameloblasts*; formation ends before tooth eruption. Enamel is produced in the form of prisms or rods cemented together by a matrix and is mineralized as soon as it is formed. Enamel is hard, dense, brittle, translucent, and white. Mature enamel is not evident in demineralized tissue sections, although immature enamel matrix may be visible near ameloblasts of developing teeth.

Normal enamel contains *incremental lines of Retzius*, which are analogous to the incremental lines of von Ebner in dentin, and altered lines reflect variations in structure and mineralization. Ameloblasts are sensitive to environmental changes, and the incremental lines are accentuated during periods of metabolic stress. Severe injury such has fluorosis or viral infections can result in *enamel hypoplasia or aplasia*.

Cementum is an avascular bonelike substance produced by *cementoblasts*; it contains ~55% organic and ~45% inorganic matter. Cementum covers the dentin of brachydont teeth wherever dentin is not covered by enamel and is formed along with the dentin formation in the root, following degeneration of the HERS. Some layers of cementum are acellular; in other layers, *cementocytes* are enclosed in lacunae. Sharpey fibers from alveolar bone embedded in the cementum facilitate tooth attachment and act as a buffer medium against stress. Cementum is more resistant to resorption than bone and is not normally resorbed and replaced as it ages. New cementum is occasionally deposited overlying older cementum, including in some pathologic conditions in which cementum is resorbed. **Hypercementosis** is abnormal thickening of cementum and may involve part or all of one or many teeth; this can occur as a reactive response to improve the functional properties of teeth or associated with chronic inflammation. Deficiency of cementum is called *hypoplasia*, occurs mostly in the infundibulum or equid cheek teeth, is considered a developmental malformation caused by insufficient blood supply, and is regarded as a major predisposing factor for impaction and infundibular necrosis (discussed below).

The **periodontium** consists of the periodontal ligament, gingival fibrous stroma, cementum, and alveolar bone. The periodontal ligament is derived from the dental follicle and is composed of fibroblasts, cementoblasts, undifferentiated mesenchymal cells, and epithelial cells supported by type I collagen fibers with complex orientation. *Epithelial rests of Malassez* are also present in the periodontal ligament and are particularly numerous in the incisor region of sheep. In all species, these rests may proliferate and become cystic, especially when there is inflammation or injury of the periodontium. The periodontal ligament supports the tooth and adjusts to its movement during growth. It is well supplied with nerves, blood vessels, and lymphatic vessels that drain into alveolar bone. The ligament is normally visible in radiographs as a radiolucent line between the tooth and the adjacent alveolar bone. When alveolar bone is resorbed and the ligament is no longer visualized radiographically, this change is referred to as *loss of the lamina dura*.

Diseases of teeth and dental tissues

Developmental anomalies of teeth

Anodontia is the absence of teeth and is inherited in male calves as a sex-linked recessive trait and commonly is linked to skin defects. **Hypodontia** or **oligodontia** refers to reduced numbers of teeth, which occurs sporadically in domestic species and is considered normal in some species and breeds of dog, such as brachycephalic and toy breeds (cheek teeth and incisors, respectively). **Pseudo-oligodontia** and **pseudoanodontia** result from failed or delayed eruption, documented in Lhasa Apso and Shih Tzu dogs. *X-linked hypohidrotic ectodermal dysplasia* is a heritable condition described in dogs, humans, mice, and cattle, with alopecia and hypodontia or oligodontia in both deciduous and permanent dentition.

Polyodontia is the presence of additional teeth and mostly involves incisors of brachycephalic dogs; it is probably genetic. Polyodontia due to an extra maxillary premolar is described in dogs, and in horses and cats with additional incisors, molars, or premolars. **Pseudopolyodontia** is defined as retention of deciduous teeth after eruption of the permanent dentition and occurs in horses, cats, and dogs. Retention of deciduous teeth occurs mostly in miniature breeds and can lead to malocclusion.

Heterotopic polyodontia, which is described in horses, cattle, dogs, pigs, and sheep, refers to an extra tooth or teeth outside the dental arcades. The best-known example is the *ear tooth or temporal teratoma* of horses, which develops within a branchiogenic dentigerous cyst in the temporal region, probably following premature closure of the first branchial cleft and misplaced tooth germ during embryological development. Cysts are lined by stratified squamous epithelium with mucus-producing goblet cells and may contain one or more teeth, either loosely attached in the cyst wall or embedded in the temporal bone. The cysts typically form in the parotid region near the ear, can be bilateral, and may fistulate to the exterior, or even form as a pedunculated skin-covered mass.

Anomalous tooth shape is more likely from dysplastic development instead of primary enamel or dentin disorders; this is classified as **geminous** or dichotomous when there is a single root and partially or completely separate crowns; **fused** when the dentin of 2 teeth is confluent; **concrescent** when the dentin is separate, but the roots are joined by cementum; **dilacerated** when there is curvature of the tooth root; and **deflected** when there is deviation from the normal eruption pattern due to a retained deciduous tooth. *Malformation or malposition of teeth* may accompany abnormalities of the maxillae or mandibles. Aberdeen Angus and Hereford calves with congenital osteopetrosis have brachygnathia inferior, malformed mandibles, and impacted cheek teeth; the latter is also described in Shorthorns, although not linked explicitly to osteopetrosis.

Odontogenic cysts are epithelium-lined cysts that arise during odontogenesis from within tooth-bearing regions of the jaw, typically originating from epithelial remnants including rests of Malassez, Serres, dental laminae, reduced enamel epithelium, or malformed enamel organs. **Dentigerous cysts** are the most common odontogenic cyst in animals, and by definition they contain part or all of a tooth. They are usually associated with permanent teeth and are thought to occur when normal eruption fails due to odontodystrophy or when tooth eruption is interrupted by trauma, including mandibular or maxillary fractures. The cyst forms over a developing tooth and encloses at least the crown of the tooth, often prior to tooth eruption, which occurs within the preformed cysts. All odontogenic cysts then are potentially dentigerous, except those derived from cell rests of Malassez, which are more likely to result in periodontal cyst development. The most common forms of dentigerous cysts in animals are those involving the *vestigial wolf teeth* of horses and the *vestigial canines*, especially of mares. Smaller cysts appear as tumors of gingiva; some larger cysts may cause swelling of the mandible or adjacent maxillary sinus. Dentigerous cysts most commonly affect the premolar teeth of brachycephalic dogs and can be bilateral. Dentigerous cysts of animals are less destructive compared with humans, in which they are regarded as the most common benign destructive skeletal lesion. A cyst resembling *odontogenic keratocyst* of humans has been reported in a dog, with a high rate of recurrence after removal.

Other odontogenic cysts occur along the lateral surface of a tooth, gingival, radicular (periapical), or at the root apex, and can be associated with endodontic disease and inflammation. Although these features do not reliably distinguish various types of cysts, common histologic features of odontogenic cysts include the following: 1) nonkeratinizing stratified squamous epithelial lining; 2) a cyst wall composed of fibrous connective tissue, often with embedded metaplastic bone; or 3) evidence of chronic hemorrhage as hemosiderin or cholesterol clefts. Odontogenic cysts are often expansile and can be locally destructive, especially when they occur in mandibular or maxillary bone. Accurate classification requires clear communication to correlate clinical, radiographic, and histologic features of the lesions. It has been hypothesized that various odontogenic cysts can develop and progress into odontogenic neoplasia, and although many odontogenic neoplasms have cystic aspects, there is no definitive evidence that cysts progress toward neoplasia with any regular frequency.

Cystic dental inclusions involving vestigial supernumerary teeth are described in juxtamolar positions in cattle, and may be dentigerous, but also may represent primordial cysts developed prior to enamel formation and lack mineralized tooth structures; these are insignificant but may give rise to ameloblastomas.

A high incidence of dentigerous cysts involving incisors occurring in some sheep flocks in Scotland, Australia, and New Zealand has been reported; the cause remains unclear. A congenital disease involving jaws and teeth of calves in Germany (*odontodysplasia cystica congenita*) with massive fibro-osseous enlargement of the maxillae and horizontal rami of the mandibles occurs, with cystic spaces lined by fibrous tissue or epithelium derived from the enamel organ, and malformed, misshapen, or absent teeth; bone changes are likely primary, and dental lesions are considered secondary. Most affected calves are aborted or stillborn and have ascites and hydrocephalus; an environmental cause is suspected but unproven.

Permanent teeth are unique in that they continue to develop after birth; hence, inflammatory and metabolic diseases of postnatal life, such as canine distemper virus (CDV; *Paramyxoviridae, Morbillivirus canis*) infection (Fig. 1-3A), can produce hypoplasia of enamel or dentin. Enamel hypoplasia in deciduous teeth occurs in calves with intrauterine bovine viral diarrhea virus (BVDV; *Flaviviridae, Pestivirus*) infection (see Fig. 1-3B) and has been described in calves and pigs following irradiation of the dam during gestation. Dentinal and enamel dysplasia of mandibular premolars and molars has been seen in young uremic dogs. Extreme fragility of deciduous teeth is a feature of *bovine osteogenesis imperfecta* (see Vol. 1, Bones and Joints). Dental dysplasia, with normal dentin, absence of

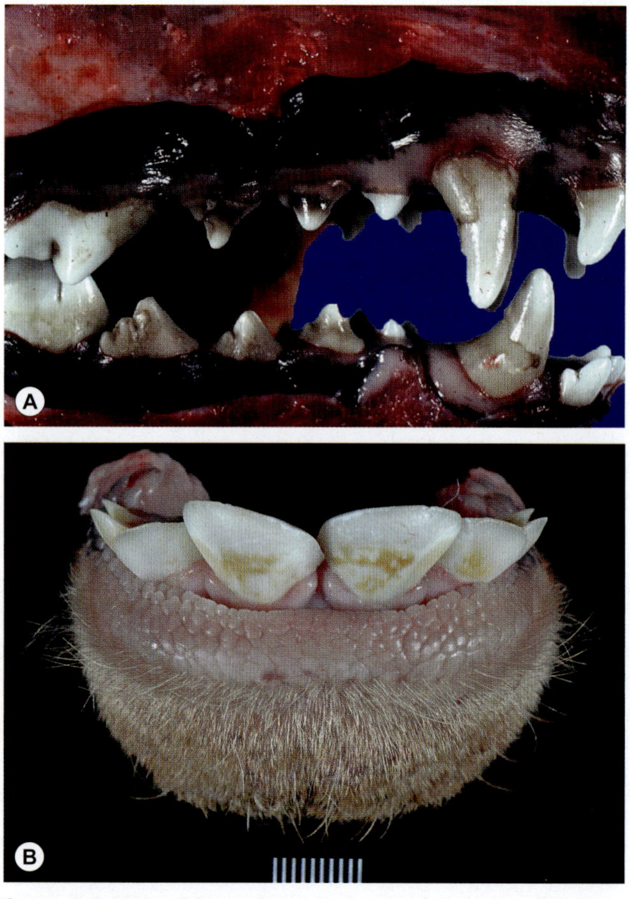

Figure 1-3 Enamel hypoplasia. **A.** A sequel to canine distemper virus infection in a dog. **B.** Subsequent to intrauterine infection by bovine viral diarrhea virus in a calf. (Courtesy Noah's Arkives.)

enamel matrix, and excess irregular cementum, was described in a foal with epitheliogenesis imperfecta involving the oral mucosa.

Degenerative and inflammatory conditions of teeth and dental tissues

Pigmentation of the teeth. Normal enamel is white and shiny; normal cementum is off-white to light-yellow; normal dentin can be variable but is typically darker yellow. Hypoplastic enamel of chronic fluorosis can be discolored yellow, brown, or black. Discoloration of brachydont teeth results from pigmentation of dentin, which is then visible through the semitransparent enamel, or from pigmentation of the cementum of the root. Dentin may be red-brown or gray due to pulp hemorrhage or inflammation, and yellow due to icterus. *Amelogenesis imperfecta* is a hereditary disorder of enamel formation reported in cattle and the Standard Poodle that leads to inadequate mineralization of enamel and usually yellow discoloration of teeth. *Congenital erythropoietic porphyria* of calves, cats, and swine causes red discoloration of dentin in young animals (pink tooth) and dark-brown discoloration of dentin in adults; the discoloration often disappears with aging in swine.

Yellow-to-brown discoloration of teeth often with bright-yellow fluorescence in ultraviolet light is caused by deposition of tetracycline antibiotics in mineralizing dentin, enamel, and cementum, and occurs in all species. Tetracycline therapy of the pregnant dam may cause staining of deciduous teeth in the offspring. Tetracyclines are toxic to ameloblasts and cause enamel hypoplasia at high dosages. Dark-black discoloration of ruminant cheek teeth is extremely common and is caused by ingestion of herbage containing chlorophyll and porphyrin pigments.

Dental attrition is mastication-associated loss of tooth structure. Mature conformation of teeth is largely the outcome of opposed growth and wear, and the degree of wear and attrition thus depends on the type of tooth, species of animal, and material chewed. Irregularities of wear are a common dental abnormality, especially in herbivores (Fig. 1-4); this is a very frequent lesion in horses. With normal occlusion and use, the extra-alveolar length of the tooth remains constant; this is maintained initially by growth and eventually by both hypertrophy of root cementum/dentin, and proliferation of alveolar bone. Senile atrophy of alveolar bone and gingival recession may cause increased length of the tooth crown. Cementum hypertrophy and alveolar atrophy with subnormal wear in aging animals may result in loss of teeth or in abnormally elongated teeth. Normal wear of premolars and molars of horses and cattle causes smoothing of the occlusal surfaces. When loss of enamel exposes the dentin (which is softer and wears more rapidly), secondary or tertiary dentin is deposited to protect the underlying pulp, although with time dentin may fill the pulp cavity and cause death of the tooth. Excessive wear of deciduous and permanent central incisors occurs in certain sheep flocks in New Zealand and may be severe enough to expose the pulp cavity. The cause of excessive wear is unknown but may be secondary to delayed eruption of adjacent teeth.

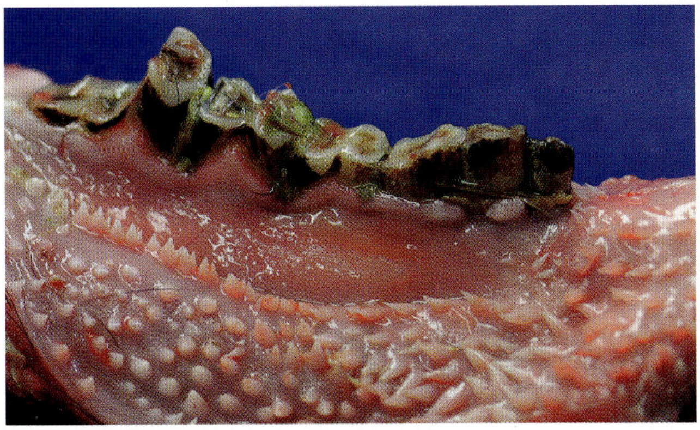

Figure 1-4 **Irregular wear** of the teeth of a sheep.

Subnormal wear results in abnormal lengthening of teeth and is caused by loss of the opposing tooth, oligodontia, abnormal spacing of adjacent teeth, and acquired loss of teeth. Such elongated teeth may grow against the opposing gingiva or into the cheek or lip.

Abnormal wear resulting from abnormal chewing or subnormal wear with incomplete loss of antagonism is caused by voluntary or mechanical impairment of jaw movement. Incomplete longitudinal alignment of the molar arcades allows irregular wear and hook formation on the first and last cheek teeth. Lateral movements of the jaws without the normal rotary grinding movements allow the ridges of the teeth of herbivores to become accentuated. Unilateral or bilateral angulation of the occlusal surfaces results from inadequate lateral movement of the jaws, leading to the formation of sharp edges on the buccal aspect of the maxillary teeth and the lingual aspect of the mandibular teeth. Affected teeth wear progressively sharper and result in the teeth passing each other like shear blades; hence, the term **shear mouth**. Subnormal resistance to wear of the molar teeth results in **wave (weave) mouth** or **step mouth**, in which successive teeth within an arcade wear at different rates. Opposing teeth of the upper and lower jaws do not develop simultaneously, so discontinuous nutritional deficiencies may result in abnormal wear. Vices such as crib biting also produce abnormal wear. Severe wearing of ruminant incisors may reveal a central black core of secondary dentin deposited in the pulp cavity; it is important to recognize this simply as secondary dentin and not dental caries.

Odontodystrophies are diseases of teeth caused by nutritional, metabolic, or toxic insults. They are manifest by changes in the dental matrices and supporting structures of teeth, and often occur during tooth development. Because of their close anatomic association with the bones of the jaws, teeth are very susceptible to disruption in the harmony of growth. This harmonious arrangement is often disturbed in odontodystrophies and osteodystrophies, which may lead to malocclusion, anomalous development of teeth, and tooth loss. Lesions of enamel and dentin are emphasized here; the most prominent effects of odontodystrophies appear in enamel, and lesions of enamel are most significant because they are irreparable.

Formation of enamel begins at the occlusal surface and progresses toward the root; mineral maturation occurs in the same sequence, beginning at the dentin-enamel junction and moving toward the ameloblasts. Deleterious influences have their most severe effects on ameloblasts as they form and mineralize enamel. Depending on the severity of the insult, ameloblasts may produce no enamel, minimal enamel, or poorly mineralized enamel. Removal of the insult permits inactive ameloblasts to make enamel, so enamel defects vary in severity from isolated opaque spots or pits on the surface to deep and irregular horizontal indentations. These defects are most clearly seen on incisors and canine teeth and are usually bilaterally symmetrical. As previously discussed, lesions similar to odontodystrophies are also produced by injury to ameloblasts by infectious agents such as CDV and BVDV (see Fig. 1-3). Odontoblasts are susceptible to many of the same influences as ameloblasts, but injured or lost odontoblasts are replenished from undifferentiated stem cells of the dental pulp, so lesions of dentin formation by injured odontoblasts may be repaired, whereas lesions in enamel are permanent. Several nutritional and toxic conditions cause odontodystrophy.

Fluorine poisoning is exemplary (see Vol. 1, Bones and Joints). **Vitamin A deficiency** is linked to a lack of normal differentiation of ameloblasts and odontoblasts via reciprocal inductive interactions discussed previously, which ultimately results in development of enamel hypoplasia and hypomineralization, vascularized dentin (osteodentin), and delay or failure of tooth eruption.

Calcium deficiency delays tooth eruption and causes enamel and mild dentinal hypoplasia. Teeth formed during the period of deficiency are very susceptible to abnormal wear. Prolonged calcium deficiency in sheep results in malocclusion caused by prognathia inferior, which may also reflect inadequate maxillary repair during the recovery phase.

Phosphorus deficiency, combined with vitamin D deficiency in sheep, depresses dentin formation but has virtually no effect on enamel. Malocclusion and abnormalities of bite in rachitic sheep occur secondary to mandibular deformity. Severe experimental **malnutrition** causes malocclusion that is not corrected by recovery; the lesions usually include misshapen and malformed teeth, as well as oligodontia and polyodontia. A syndrome of dental abnormalities of sheep in New Zealand includes excessive wear of deciduous teeth, maleruption and excessive wear of permanent teeth, periodontal disease involving permanent teeth, development of dentigerous cysts involving permanent incisors, and mandibular osteopathy. This is hypothesized to be associated with deficiencies of calcium and copper, and perhaps other nutrients such as protein and energy. This syndrome is typical of naturally occurring odontodystrophies with a complex pathogenesis and association with osteodystrophy. Although dental lesions are not described, tooth loss caused by periosteal dysplasia and osteopenia occurs in Salers cattle afflicted with hereditary hemochromatosis.

Bacterial diseases involving tooth surfaces are caused by the development of supragingival and subgingival **plaque**. *Supragingival plaque* is located on the exposed crown of the tooth and causes dental caries. *Subgingival plaque* is found in the crevicular groove and causes periodontal disease. Tooth enamel is covered by a translucent *enamel pellicle* consisting of selective complex salivary proteins and other macromolecules including immunoglobulins. Adhesion of bacterial *biofilm* with the pellicle forms dental plaque, which is initially reversible but can transition to a permanent form. Plaque alone is insufficient to cause oral disease, but the presence and involvement of various plaque-associated bacteria predispose to periodontal disease and formation of mineralized plaque, dental calculus, and caries. Reduction of salivary flow or regions of teeth where flow is reduced (interproximal regions and areas of pits or fissures) increases the prevalence of caries in some species.

The bacteria in supragingival plaque are members of the indigenous oral flora and are usually gram-positive aerobes. Most are streptococci and *Actinomyces* spp., which form an organized array on the tooth surface that becomes larger and more complex over time, facilitated by bacteria or host-generated extracellular polymers or other bacteria including anerobic gram-negative organisms. *Supragingival plaque* is metabolically active and utilizes dietary carbohydrates to produce adhesive polymers and acids necessary to demineralize enamel and drive inflammation. Extensive deposits of supragingival plaque are virtually invisible grossly; plaque is also difficult to see histologically due to loss of enamel during processing unless the plaque biofilm remains adhered to bone surfaces after processing. *Subgingival plaque* is less organized than supragingival plaque, and many of the organisms involved are likely asaccharolytic, weakly adherent, and motile gram-negative anaerobes that derive their nutrients from the crevicular fluid. The flora of subgingival plaque is less well characterized than that of supragingival plaque by culture, although next-generation sequencing data suggest that the most abundant microbes of supragingival and subgingival plaque in dogs from various geographic regions are similar in health and during early periodontitis.

Dental calculus (*tartar*) *is mineralized supragingival or subgingival plaque* formed by the deposition of mineral (predominantly calcium carbonate in horses and dogs) from saliva or crevicular fluid. Calculus is frequent in geriatric dogs and cats, occasional in horses and sheep, and rare in other species. The distribution is often uneven, but it is *often most abundant next to the orifices of salivary ducts*. Equine dental calculus is chalky and easily removed; in dogs it is hard, firmly attached, and often discolored. Red-brown to black calculus with a metallic sheen develops in pastured sheep and goats and usually involves incisors. Deposits occur principally on the neck of buccal tooth surfaces, although minor calculus is seen along the gingiva-tooth junction of molars, and occasional larger hard black concretions protrude from between opposed surfaces of premolars. Calculus formation may be affected by diet; a high prevalence of calcium-, magnesium-, and phosphorus-rich calculus mostly involving the premolars of sheep on the Scottish island of North Ronaldsay was related to their seaweed-rich diet.

Materia alba is a mixture of salivary proteins, desquamated epithelial cells, disintegrating leukocytes, and bacteria adhered to teeth. Materia alba is easily removed; it is distinct from dental plaque and food debris, which also accumulates between uncleaned teeth.

Dental caries is the loss of the hard dental matrices; *demineralization of the inorganic portion and enzymatic degradation of the organic portion* of the tooth occurs. **Erosions** of teeth occur with removal of hard tissues. Caries is common in horses and sheep, but rare in dogs.

Two major types of caries are recognized: 1) **pit or fissure caries** develop in irregularities or indentations usually on occlusal surfaces of teeth. Plaque is not essential for initiation of this form of caries; *infundibular necrosis of horses* is an example. 2) **Smooth surface caries** occurs mostly on proximal (adjacent) surfaces of teeth, often at contact points or around the neck, and requires dental plaque for its initiation. Organic acids that initiate demineralization are produced by bacterial fermentation of dietary carbohydrates or leukocytes within plaque. Progression of lesions depends on various factors such as salivary pH, hardness, and resistance to demineralization of enamel, and frequency of access to carbohydrate. Demineralization of enamel often occurs in the subsurface enamel but progresses to caries with prolonged exposure to acid; infrequent acid exposure allows remineralization of enamel between meals. Carious enamel loses its sheen and becomes dull, white, and pitted; once dentin is exposed, the lesions become brown or black. Dentin is softer and more readily demineralized than enamel, and a pinpoint loss of enamel may lead to a large defect when the carious process reaches the dentin. Enamel loss to caries is permanent; odontoblasts at the pulp-dentin junction can generate tertiary dentin in response to dentinal damage and loss. Nerve endings have not been identified at the enamel-dentin junction, so the pain of caries is likely caused by chemical or pressure changes in dentinal tubules. Neuropeptides, including substance P, are generated in the pulp and may enhance pain during caries. Spread of infection along the dentinal tubules to the pulp cavity may result in the formation of reparative dentin, pulpitis, or periapical inflammation and tooth loss.

Infundibular necrosis of horses is common and develops most often on the occlusal surface of the maxillary first molar. Enamel invaginations or infundibula of equid cheek teeth are normally filled with cementum prior to tooth eruption; however, when filling is not completed before eruption, the blood supply is cut off resulting in ischemic necrosis of residual cementogenic tissue in the infundibula (Fig. 1-5A). Teeth with incompletely filled infundibula may accumulate food material and bacteria, which can lead to bacterial fermentation, lactic acid production, and demineralization (see Fig. 1-5B). In some animals, the cavitated demineralized area expands to involve cementum as well as adjacent enamel and dentin, which may result in coalescence of adjacent infundibula and creation of a large defect in the occlusal surface, and to fracture of teeth, root abscess, and/or empyema of adjacent paranasal sinuses. The incidence of infundibular necrosis increases with age, and although 80-100% of horses >12-years-old may have the lesion, they typically lack clinical signs and do not progress. Inflammation of the dental pulp (pulpitis) in horses and in other species may result from direct expansion of caries from penetration of bacteria and bacterial degradation products along the dentinal tubules. Production of reparative dentin in the pulp cavity is expected. Horses also develop *peripheral caries* outside the infundibulum. This typically occurs in the caudal cheek teeth and leads to the loss of cementum that may contribute to irregular wear and periodontal disease.

Equine odontoclastic tooth resorption and hypercementosis (EOTRH) refers to a specific syndrome in which tooth resorption and proliferation of mineralized matrix of the tooth (likely cementum) occurs. EOTRH typically affects roots of incisors, canines, or cheek teeth of horses. Characteristic histologic features include odontoclastic resorption of dental matrices along with deposition of irregular cementum as a reparative non-neoplastic change resulting in bulbous expansion of the intraalveolar portion of the tooth that also may be accompanied by periodontitis.

Nodular hypercementosis (historically called *cementoma*, although this name is incorrect and should not be used) of

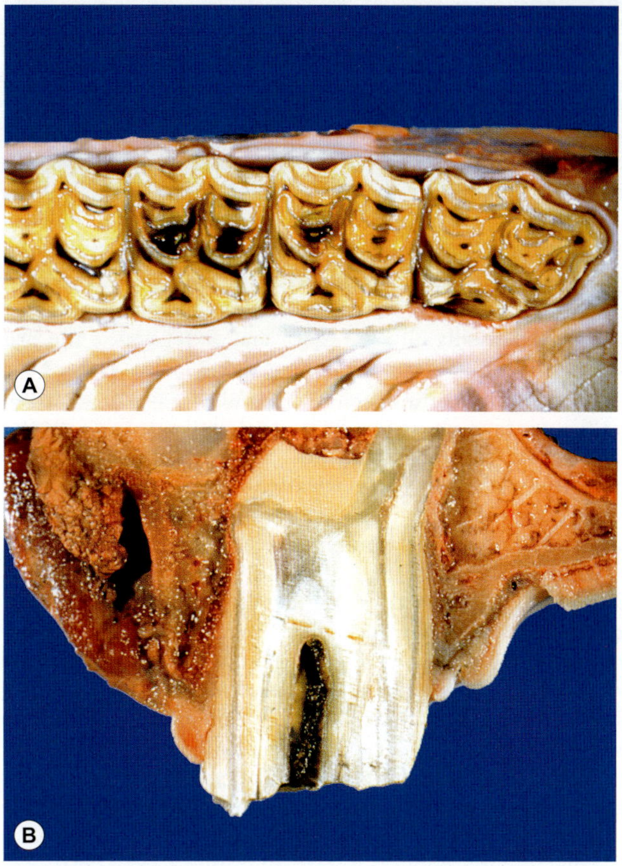

Figure 1-5 **A. Infundibular necrosis** of the maxillary molars in a horse. **B.** Section through (A) showing black discoloration of infundibulum.

horses is a multifocal tooth root-associated reactive or hyperplastic lesion that occurs as a nodular accumulation or concretion of cementum in the cheek teeth of horses and other herbivores. These can be confused with proliferative cementum of EOTRH (above), so may require the study of the radiographic features to make a distinction.

In **sheep**, the proximal surfaces of mandibular teeth are usually affected by caries, which is commonly accompanied by periodontitis and erosion of the neck region of deciduous teeth.

Cattle develop loss of dentin just below the crown of incisor teeth at increasing frequency with age. This usually follows recession of the gingiva and is not considered to be a form of caries, but proteolytic digestion of dentin in an alkaline pH.

In **dogs and cats**, caries mediated by acidic bacterial metabolites are uncommon, and mostly affect geriatric animals. In contrast to caries, **tooth resorption** defined as physiologic or pathologic loss of dental matrices mediated by odontoblasts is common in cats and dogs (these were formerly called *odontoclastic resorptive lesions*). Two main patterns are recognized: *inflammatory tooth resorption* occurs as a localized disease secondary to periodontitis and inflammatory mediators such that resorbed tooth is replaced by granulation tissue; *replacement tooth resorption* occurs when resorbed tooth is replaced by bone or cementum-like matrix, although the pathogenesis remains unclear.

Tooth resorption in cats is common, and less common in dogs; the prevalence increases with age. Lesions initially involve the subgingival neck or upper root near the cementoenamel junction of cheek teeth. This can occur as a more generalized disorder along with other dental diseases, such as periodontal ligament degeneration or **alveolar bone expansion and osteomyelitis of the jaws of cats**, although the pathogenesis remains poorly understood. Odontoclasts are recruited or form at the tooth where they resorb the hard dental matrices of the tooth. A reddened swollen and painful area of gingiva or granulation tissue lies over the lesion, often on the labial or buccal aspect of the tooth, and resorptive lesions progress from the cementum into the underlying dentin and eventually into the root canal. Extension of the process coronally undermines the enamel, which is resorbed or breaks off causing destruction or loss of the crown. Extension of the dentinal resorptive lesion apically leads to resorption of the root, although remnants of the root may persist, but are often overgrown by gingiva following loss of the crown. Destruction of the root may result in obliteration of the periodontal ligament, resorption of adjacent alveolar bone, and odontoalveolar ankylosis by reparative hard tissues, all with retention of the crown in the dental arcade. In some cases, retained roots can become a nidus of inflammation, persistent osteomyelitis, and granulation tissue until the root remnant is removed and the alveolus debrided. The prevalence of tooth resorptive lesions has increased markedly in the past 60 years, suggesting an association with dietary changes, but the lesion remains idiopathic with no clear relationship to periodontitis, mechanical trauma, viral infections, nutritional, or metabolic disturbances. Several specific factors have been proposed to be involved with feline tooth resorptive lesions, including increased local inflammatory mediators, altered local pH, and increased vitamin D intake.

Pulpitis is inflammation of dental pulp, which is a loose syncytium of stellate fibroblasts containing histiocytes and undifferentiated mesenchymal cells, which are odontoblastic precursors. Pulp is derived from the dental papilla and surrounded by odontoblasts and dentin except at the apical foramen, through which vessels and nerves pass.

The apical foramen is narrow, which predisposes to vascular occlusion (by reparative dentin or inflammation) and ischemic necrosis of the pulp. Pulpitis is usually secondary to bacterial infection, but can also be sterile and initiated by mechanical, thermal, or chemical trauma. Mild pulpitis may heal but usually results in tooth necrosis, periapical abscessation, fistula formation, or osteomyelitis if inflammation of the pulp extends to the periodontium and the jaws.

Periapical abscess and osteomyelitis of the jaws are complications of pulpitis that may follow clipping of the deciduous third incisors and canine teeth (needle teeth) of piglets. Trimming of the incisor teeth of sheep to avoid the effects of broken mouth often exposes the pulp cavity, although the exposed pulp canal is healed in 30-50 days by deposition of reparative and secondary dentin. Maxillary (malar) abscess of dogs involves the periapical tissues usually of the carnassial tooth and may cause a discharging sinus ventral to the eye. Chronic pulpitis may become slowly expansive spherical granulomas involving the root apex (root granulomas). Occasionally, these granulomas are enclosed by an epithelial cyst (periodontal cyst) derived from cell rests of Malassez.

Periodontal disease is the *most common dental disease of dogs and sheep* and an important problem in other ruminants, horses, and cats. Although there are minor differences among species, periodontal disease in general begins as *gingivitis* associated with subgingival plaque and may progress to gingival recession, loss of alveolar bone, chronic *periodontitis*, and possibly complete tooth loss.

The gingival sulcus (crevice) is an invagination formed by the gingiva as it joins with the tooth surface at the time of eruption. Clinically normal animals have a few lymphocytes, plasma cells, and macrophages beneath the crevicular gingival epithelium that lines the crevice and opposes the adjacent tooth enamel.

Gingivitis is inflammation of the oral soft tissues surrounding the tooth; **periodontitis** implies inflammation of the gingiva as well as the periodontal ligament, cementum, and alveolar bone. Gingivitis precedes but does not necessarily progress to periodontitis. Clinical gingivitis is usually initiated by accumulation of plaque in the crevice but may be associated with impaction of feed material between teeth. Gingivitis is initially seen as increased numbers of leukocytes and fluid in the gingival crevice, and then by accumulation of neutrophils, plasma cells, lymphocytes, and macrophages in the marginal gingiva. As the disease progresses, marked loss of gingival collagen fibers can occur in a few days. This is probably related to the activity of prostaglandins and matrix metalloproteinases generated in inflamed tissue, or possibly enzymes from plaque bacteria such as *Porphyromonas gingivalis*, which also produce enzymes (gingipains) thought to damage junctional epithelium. Grossly, the gingiva is red and swollen because of the hyperemia and edema of inflammation. Acute gingivitis may become quiescent, with lymphocyte aggregations beneath the junctional epithelium.

Continuation of gingivitis will lead to periodontitis, including inflammation of the ligament, apical recession of the tooth-gingiva junction, and possibly to resorption of alveolar bone, which is a major part of chronic periodontal disease (Fig. 1-6). This modifies the attachment site of the periodontal ligament, leads to the formation of periodontal pockets of inflammation lined by epithelium, and contributes to exposure of tooth roots, destruction of the

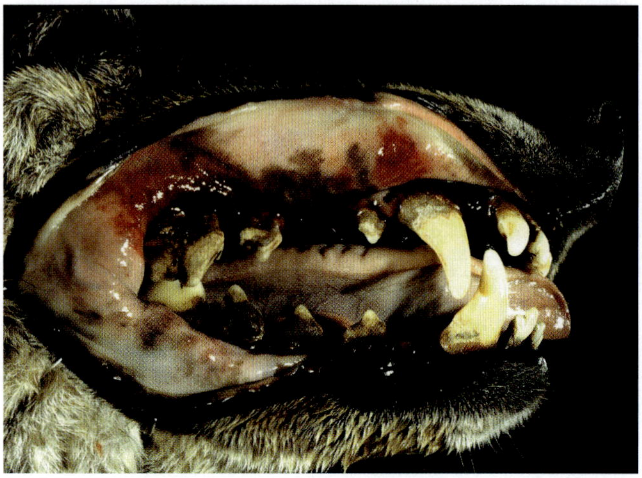

Figure 1-6 Marked gingival recession with exposure of roots of the molar teeth in advanced **periodontal disease** in a dog.

periodontium and periodontal ligament, resorption of alveolar bone, cementum, root dentin, and eventually *progresses to loss of teeth*.

Gingivitis is common in **dogs**, and gingival fibrous and epithelial tissues are often replaced by collagen-poor, highly vascular granulation tissue, which appears as a red, rolled edge next to the tooth. Alveolar bone loss in dogs is often more severe at the bifurcation of 2-rooted teeth than in interproximal areas. In dogs, the premolars and to a lesser extent the first molars and central incisors are most severely affected, especially in toy and smaller breed dogs; the second molars and mandibular canines appear to be more resistant.

Gingivitis is also common in **cats** and generally resembles that in dogs. In cats, periodontitis of the canine teeth, premolars, or molars can progress to **feline alveolar bone expansion and osteomyelitis**, formerly known as *peripheral or alveolar osteitis*, or *peripheral buttressing*. There is smooth expansion of the buccal surface of alveolar bone, due to deposition of abundant loose myxomatous-to-fibrous stroma, variable mixed inflammation (which is subtle in many cases), and irregular woven bone. Feline gingivitis is addressed more thoroughly as feline chronic gingivostomatitis (FCGS), in the following sections.

In **sheep**, periodontal disease may involve all teeth and is a major cause of premature loss of teeth. Sheep develop acute gingivitis during tooth eruption that can be most severe on incisors; as in other species, inflammation is mostly associated with the accumulation of subgingival plaque.

Cara inchada (swollen face) is an epidemic periodontitis of **cattle**, formerly common in the west-central part of Brazil. Animals 2-14-months-old were mostly affected, and herd prevalence of >50% is reported. Progressive cara inchada contributes to the loss of teeth and eventually malnutrition. It is associated with dental eruption, and ingestion of forage thought to contain low levels of antibiotics derived from soil actinomycetes that permit colonization of the periodontal space by a variety of gram-negative bacteria, including *Prevotella melaninogenica*. Severe periodontitis and tooth loss are an important part of the syndrome associated with *bovine leukocyte adhesion deficiency*.

Sequelae of neutrophilic periodontitis have many variations but typically involve *osteomyelitis*. Osteomyelitis of actinomycosis is discussed in Vol. 1, Bones and Joints. If the mandible is involved, a fistula can develop along the ventral margin. If the maxillary molars are involved, fistulation may occur into the maxillary sinus. If the premolars are involved, fistulas may develop into the nasal cavity or externally.

Degenerative and inflammatory diseases of the buccal cavity and mucosa

Foreign bodies in the oral cavity

Food material in the mouth of a cadaver is abnormal except in ruminants, which may eructate feed into the caudal pharynx at or near death. It is often attributable to disease that results in paralysis of deglutition or semiconsciousness, such as encephalitis, encephalomalacia, or hepatic encephalopathy. The food in such cases is usually poorly masticated and readily differentiated from postmortem reflux. Bones or other large foreign bodies lodged in the pharynx of cattle may suggest pica of phosphorus deficiency; these may cause asphyxiation or pressure necrosis in the wall of the pharynx. Dogs often have bones and sticks that wedged across the palate behind the carnassial teeth.

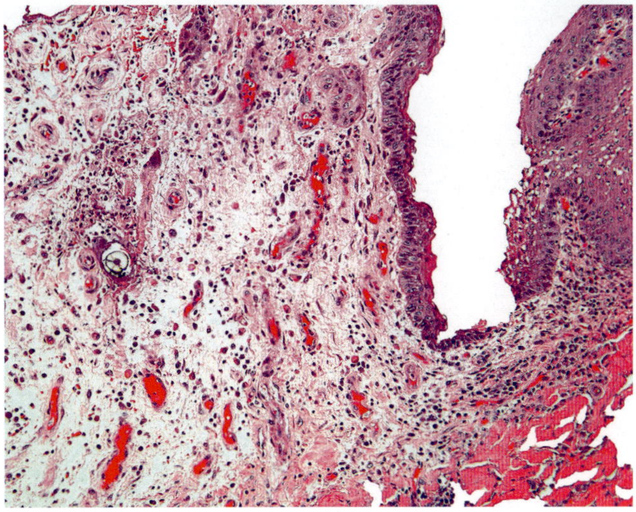

Figure 1-7 Granulomatous reaction to plant material and hair in the tongue of a dog; **foreign-body glossitis**.

Foreign-body stomatitis occurs in dogs caused by plant fibers, burrs, or quills (Fig. 1-7). Long-haired dogs are especially prone to develop this type of lesion when they attempt to remove plant material that is trapped in their hair coat. Lesions typically start in the gingiva of incisors and canine teeth, and small papules, vesicles, or shallow ulcers may be evident on the tongue; plant fibers may protrude from the lesions. Chronic cases are have *exuberant gingival granulation and inflammation*, often associated with ulceration, and must be differentiated from neoplasms.

Grass seeds and awns frequently impact between retracted gingival margins and teeth in periodontitis of ruminants and exacerbate the local initial lesion, and possibly predispose to the development of osteomyelitis. Metallic objects such as wire may lacerate the oral mucosa. Horses or ruminants fed brittle feedstuffs may develop severe oral ulceration with numerous awns embedded in the ulcers. The 1-mm to 5-cm ulcers are mainly located at the junction of the labial and gingival mucosa adjacent to the upper corner incisors, the lingual frenulum, the sublingual folds, the base of the dorsum of the tongue, and the soft palate. Similar lesions in horses have been associated with foxtail migration.

Swine have a diverticulum of the pharynx in the caudal wall immediately above the esophagus, where barley awns or other rough plant fibers lodge before penetrating the pharynx. This occurs also in young pigs, and death can occur following pharyngeal cellulitis. Similar lesions in this location occur in ruminants following improper use of drenching equipment, such as hoses or balling guns.

Inflammation of the oral cavity

Stomatitis is inflammation of the oral cavity; lesions may be focal or diffuse and may predominantly affect certain regions to produce pharyngitis (pharynx), glossitis (tongue), gingivitis (gingiva), tonsillitis (tonsils), or angina bullosa (soft palate) (Fig. 1-8). Lesions can be limited to the superficial mucosa of the oral cavity or become seated into the deeper connective tissues of the mouth, which tend to be a sequel to superficial lesions. Stomatitis has many causes, and inflammatory lesions of the tissues of the mouth are often biopsied because they appear in many cases grossly similar and

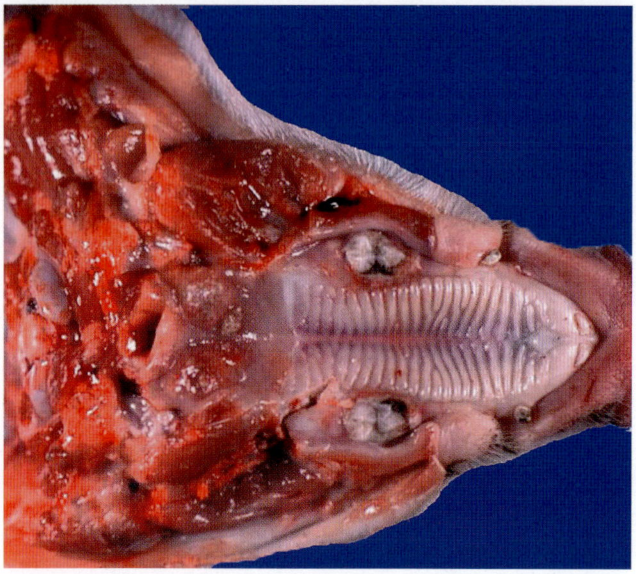

Figure 1-8 Necrotic palatine **tonsillitis** in a pig. (Courtesy Noah's Arkives and A. Doster.)

must be distinguished from hyperplastic, neoplastic, or other diseases of the oral cavity that may indicate systemic disease. Additional specific clinical information including radiographic evaluation of underlying hard tissues is often critical for definitive diagnosis.

Stomatitis is common, although the pathogenesis and etiology often remain unknown; clinical disease likely involves chronic antigenic stimulation (such as dental plaque, discussed previously) and dysregulated host immune response. Inflammation is often caused by oral microbes including anaerobes such as *Actinomyces*, *Fusobacterium*, or spirochetes that normally exist in balance with each other and in harmony with the host. Healthy oral mucosa is quite resistant to microbial invasion for several reasons, including the microbiota itself, the squamous epithelial lining, antibacterial constituents of saliva such as lysozyme, immunoglobulin (especially immunoglobulin A) in oral secretions, inflammatory cells, and a rich submucosal vasculature. Factors such as bacterial, viral, or fungal pathogens, systemic disease, stress, or nutritional and hormonal imbalances are known to alter the oral microbial population, although the mechanisms remain poorly understood. The integrity of the oral epithelium depends on a high rate of epithelial regeneration to balance loss resulting from a high rate of abrasion and desquamation. Rapid epithelial replication promotes quick healing of superficial lesions. The subepithelial connective tissue of the oral cavity is well vascularized, but generally dense and relatively inelastic. For this reason, there is little distension of lymphatics and tissue spaces with fluid exudates, and except for the gingival margins, swelling resulting from edema is not a significant part of stomatitis involving hard palate and gums.

Feline chronic gingivostomatitis (FCGS) is a progressive stomatitis that occurs mostly in cats with periodontal disease, gingivitis, or tooth resorption; clinical signs range from drooling and reduced appetite to severe oral pain and enlarged lymph nodes. Although most common in cats, a similar disease is described in dogs and is discussed below. The cause remains unknown, but studies have evaluated potential viral involvement, including feline calicivirus (FCV; *Caliciviridae*; *Vesivirus*), felid alphaherpesvirus 1 (FeAHV1; *Orthoherpesviridae*; *Varicellovirus felidalpha1*), feline immunodeficiency virus (FIV; *Retroviridae*, *Feline immunodeficiency virus*), or feline leukemia virus (FeLV; *Retroviridae*, *Feline leukemia virus*); however, no definitive causal link has been demonstrated. FCGS occurs most commonly in cats from multi-cat households, supporting the hypothesis that the disease has an infectious etiology or that stress significantly exacerbates disease in affected cats. FCGS typically begins at the palatoglossal arches (the caudal fauces), but often extends to adjacent mucosae including gingiva, palate, and tongue. Several terms have historically been used to describe this clinical entity, including *lymphoplasmacytic stomatitis* and *plasma cell gingivitis-stomatitis-pharyngitis*; it is likely that they represent a continuum of disease processes. Various treatment options are available, but the long-term prognosis continues to be quite poor; partial or complete remission rates as low as 30% or as high as 70-80% are reported with full-mouth tooth extractions.

Microscopically, there is chronic and often diffuse plasmacytic, lymphocytic, and neutrophilic inflammation (and scattered mast cells in many cases) of the oral mucosa and submucosal connective tissue (including muscles and salivary glands in severe cases), often with surface erosion and occasional ulceration. Moderate-to-severe cases are dominated by many mature plasma cells with fewer Mott cells. When ulcerated, significant surface inflammation and granulation tissue can further complicate interpretation. In the oral cavity, irregular and prominent gingival epithelial hyperplasia can be difficult to distinguish from squamous cell carcinoma (SCC), especially in small biopsies that are difficult to orient properly.

Early-onset gingivitis (EOG) and aggressive periodontitis (juvenile gingivitis) occur in young cats, often first recognized at 6-8 months of age. Similar to FCGS, the etiology of EOG remains unknown, but severe gingival inflammation and erythema often extend to involve deeper tissues, such as the periodontal ligament, and can lead to gingival recession and early tooth loss. Some cases of EOG have been reported to resolve at sexual maturity, while others progress to the more widespread and extensive FCGS. Affected cats have moderate-to-severe neutrophilic-to-lymphoplasmacytic inflammation with erosions and ulcers, as well as gingival epithelial and fibrous hyperplasia, bone loss, and loss of teeth. The lesions of EOG are histologically similar to FCGS, although EOG tends to be seen in younger cats and has a more restricted distribution in the oral cavity.

Canine chronic ulcerative gingivostomatitis (CCUS) is the canine version of FCGS, and the clinical and pathologic features overlap significantly. Some breeds may be predisposed, including Greyhounds, Cavalier King Charles Spaniels, and Maltese. The most prevalent form of stomatitis in dogs is contact-associated inflammation known as **chronic ulcerative paradental stomatitis** (CUPS), which occurs due to gingival contact along tooth surfaces with significant periodontal disease and surface plaque formation. CCUS probably progresses from CUPS and typically involves the oral cavity in a more widespread distribution including (as in cats) the soft and hard palates, tongue, and deep connective tissues of the mouth. Similar to FCGS in cats, oral inflammation is progressive and painful, with a poorly understood pathogenesis and a limited response to therapeutic attempts. There is infiltration of many plasma cells and lymphocytes, and the evidence of regulatory T lymphocytes and T helper 17 cells in high numbers of these lesions supports the hypothesis of an immune-mediated pathogenesis.

The histologic features of CCUS in dogs are typically mixed and superficial inflammation of the oral cavity soft tissues, although 3 distinct histologic subtypes described include *granulomatous stomatitis*, with mostly histiocytes within the submucosa; *lichenoid stomatitis*, with interface lymphocyte and plasma cell infiltrates; and *deep stomatitis*, with lymphocytes and plasma cells extending into the deeper connective tissues of the mouth including deep buccal mucosa and skeletal muscle of the lip. However, no significant correlation has been documented between subtype and clinical severity, response to therapy, or overall prognosis.

Granulomatous stomatitis in dogs and cats can be caused by several mechanisms or pathogens, including chronic bacterial or fungal infection, foreign bodies including migrating plant material, or even allergic or hypersensitivity response. Diagnosis is straightforward if the cause is identified histologically with the help of special stains, or by bacteriologic or molecular testing. Granulomatosis with polyangiitis (Wegener granulomatosis) is an autoimmune vasculitis that occurs in dogs, and although usually a systemic disease, oral cavity involvement is described. Diagnosis of this disease requires elimination of other causes of chronic inflammation, and an appropriate response to immunosuppression therapy.

Eosinophilic stomatitis (eosinophilic ulcerative stomatitis), common in cats and less common in dogs, is part of the eosinophilic granuloma complex (collagenolytic granuloma, linear granuloma, eosinophilic ulcer, labial ulcer, rodent ulcer), which represents several variations of chronic superficial ulcerative inflammatory lesions involving mucocutaneous junctions of the lips or oral mucosa and skin (see Vol. 1, Integumentary System for discussion of cutaneous eosinophilic granuloma complex lesions). The cause is unknown, although their morphology and response to corticosteroid therapy suggest that these arise from an allergic or type 1 hypersensitivity reaction following exposure to unknown environmental, parasitic, or other antigens. Primary eosinophil dysfunction has also been proposed as a cause for this inflammatory complex, but this remains unproven. The lesions may respond to corticosteroids, oral progestogens, cryosurgery, or radiation therapy, although recurrences are common. Well-demarcated red-brown shallow ulcers often with elevated margins occur on the upper lip on either side of the midline, tongue, or palate of cats. They are usually a few millimeters wide and can be up to several centimeters long. Occasional ulcers are present elsewhere in the mouth, such as on the gingiva, palate, pharynx, or tongue. Skin lesions are located in areas that are frequently licked, such as the neck, lumbar region, or abdominal body wall. Microscopically, the squamous epithelium is ulcerated with large areas of necrosis of the underlying connective tissues, which is accompanied by large numbers of eosinophils, neutrophils, and other mixed inflammatory cells on a variably well-organized layer of collagen, plump fibroblasts, and granulation tissue. A key diagnostic feature of eosinophilic granuloma complex lesions is dense granulomatous-to-eosinophilic inflammation with multinucleate giant cells centered on aggregates of extracellular hypereosinophilic degenerated collagen and degranulated eosinophil-associated proteins, including major basic protein 1. Eosinophils and macrophages may be less prominent, especially in chronic stages of the lesion.

Oral eosinophilic granuloma or stomatitis (collagenolytic granuloma) of dogs occurs as a familial disease in young Siberian Huskies; sporadic cases have also been reported in other breeds, especially Cavalier King Charles Spaniels—suggesting a strong hereditary tendency in these breeds. Affected dogs have single-or-multiple, firm, raised oval-to-circular plaques or ulcers covered by yellow-brown exudate that, in contrast to cats, occur most commonly on the palate and less frequently on the tongue (especially in smaller dogs). Eosinophilic oral inflammatory lesions in up to 70% of subclinical dogs resolved without medication or with allergen therapy alone, so most subclinical dogs respond well to conservative management.

Oral eosinophilic granuloma must be differentiated from oral mast cell tumors (MCTs), which also affect the tongue of dogs. Degeneration of collagen fibers can be a feature of MCTs; however, in MCTs a mixture of mast cells and eosinophils infiltrates the tongue and connective tissues more diffusely. The mast cells may be in various stages of degranulation, and secondary inflammation is minimal or absent in MCTs, unless they are ulcerated.

Horses with **eosinophilic epitheliotropic disease** (see Vol. 1, Integumentary System and the Eosinophilic Enteritis in Cats and Horses sections later in this chapter) may also have eosinophilic stomatitis and lingual ulceration.

Vesicular stomatitis (VS) is the formation of oral vesicles and occurs in most species of domestic animals. The vesicles develop as accumulations of serous fluid within the epithelium or between the epithelium and the subgingival fibrous stroma. These may coalesce to form *bullae*, and the elevated epithelium is easily rubbed off during chewing, which leaves raw erosions and ulcers with fragments of adherent epithelium. The transition from vesicle to erosion occurs rapidly, so true vesicles in individual animals may not be evident in some cases. This is especially common in dogs and cats because the oral epithelium is very thin. Because the basal epithelium or basement membrane often remains intact, regeneration and healing of the epithelial defects are complete in a few days unless the local lesions are deeper into the underlying stroma, or complicated by bacterial or mycotic infections.

Historically, vesicular stomatitides in animals were associated with *viral infections*, and these are still important causes. VS, foot-and-mouth disease (FMD), and more recently senecavirus A (SVA)–associated disease are all associated initially with vesicle formation; however, bovine viral diarrhea (BVD) and malignant catarrhal fever (MCF) produce sharply demarcated erosive-to-ulcerative lesions without initial vesicle formation. *Oral erosions and ulcers in horses, ruminants, and swine should be regarded as indicating one of the vesicular diseases to which the species is susceptible, until proven otherwise* (see the Infectious and Parasitic Diseases of the Alimentary Tract section, later in this chapter). Sunburn, photoirritation associated with grazing on celery and related crops, or parvoviral infection in swine may cause lesions of the snout resembling vesicular diseases. Animals exposed to irritant chemicals in feed or bedding may develop vesicles and erosions of the face and oral cavity, as can exposure of horses and dogs to irritant quassinoids found in wood shavings derived from *Simaroubaceae* species.

Erosive and ulcerative forms of stomatitis are seen as local epithelial defects of the oral and nasolabial epithelium and are usually associated with acute diffuse stomatitis and pharyngitis. *Erosions* are circumscribed areas of loss of epithelium, which leave the stratum germinativum and basement membrane intact, and they are usually associated with acute inflammation in the underlying propria. The erosions vary in size and shape. Although they are often a nonspecific development in a wide variety of conditions, they are also observed during several important diseases. They heal cleanly and quickly, but if secondarily infected or complicated, may develop into ulcers.

In contrast to erosions, ulcers are deeper deficiencies that extend deep to the basement membrane into the underlying gingival fibrous stroma. They too can vary greatly in size and shape; the margins tend to be elevated and ragged, and they tend to heal with scar formation.

Causes of ulcerative stomatitis are in general those of erosive stomatitis; however, some recognized syndromes and specific diseases are described in which the predominant change is ulceration. Phenylbutazone intoxication in horses may cause oral ulcers in concert with ulcers of the stomach, intestine, and colon; the syndrome is discussed with ischemic diseases of the GI tract.

Feline viral rhinotracheitis is a common upper respiratory tract infection of cats, caused by FeAHV1 (see Vol. 2, Respiratory System). This virus may cause oral ulceration especially on the tongue, although oral and skin ulcers rarely occur without evidence of concurrent respiratory tract infection. Microscopic foci of squamous epithelial cytoplasmic vacuolation evolve into areas of necrosis and ulceration, which are often covered by a layer of fibrinocellular exudate. Intranuclear eosinophilic herpetic inclusions may be present in epithelial cells at the periphery of the ulcers.

Feline calicivirus (FCV) mainly causes respiratory tract infection in cats. The disease is often accompanied by *lingual and oropharyngeal ulcers* that typically start out as vesicles. They are 5-10 mm in diameter, smooth, and well demarcated from the surrounding normal mucosa. Vesicles and ulcers occur mainly on the rostrodorsal and lateral surfaces of the tongue and each side of the midline on the hard palate. Microscopically, the earliest lesions consist of foci of pyknotic cells in the stratum corneum and superficial stratum spinosum that progress to vesicle formation and then subsequent erosion and ulceration of the mucosa. Regeneration of the oral mucosa in the ulcerated areas generally occurs within 10-12 days. A single layer of squamous epithelial cells extends from the margins of the ulcer beneath a layer of exudate. Viral inclusions have not been observed in oral epithelial cells, although active viral replication takes place in the tonsillar crypt epithelial cells, and virus may be recovered from these areas for weeks postinfection. FCV can be isolated from a high percentage of cats with chronic stomatitis in general, and, as previously mentioned, some have hypothesized that FCGS in cats represents a chronic immune-mediated reaction to this agent, although this has yet to be proven definitively. Concurrent infection with other common agents such as FeAHV1, *Chlamydia felis*, or *Mycoplasmopsis (Mycoplasma) felis* is frequent and may be responsible for more severe oral lesions and respiratory signs. Outbreaks of a highly virulent FCV infection have been seen in many countries; this virus causes severe systemic infection often accompanied by severe oral and digital or cutaneous necrosis and ulceration.

Blistering immune-mediated or autoimmune skin diseases (see also Vol. 1, Integumentary System) target either epithelial cell adhesions (pemphigus) or epithelial-subepidermal connective tissue adhesions [autoimmune subepidermal blistering diseases (AISBDs)], and often occur with oral cavity involvement. Although the gross lesions are nonspecific and mimic many other causes of oral ulcerations, including physical, chemical, infectious, metabolic, or neoplastic diseases, thorough clinical history, signalment, and histologic evaluation is often sufficient for confirmation. Although oral lesions can be detected initially in many cases, most immune-mediated or autoimmune diseases are not restricted to the oral cavity, and affected patients will have lesions elsewhere.

Pemphigus vulgaris (PV) is a severe, acute or chronic, vesiculobullous autoimmune disease mediated by autoantibodies to the desmosome protein desmoglein 3, which is involved in joining adjacent epithelial cells to each other in the deep epithelium of skin; desmoglein 3 is highly expressed in suprabasal oral epithelium. Canine PV follows a similar pathogenesis to that of humans with transcriptional regulation by the proto-oncogene *c-Myc*. PV is most common in dogs and cats, with rare reports in horses. Acantholysis of the basal epidermis leads to the formation of fragile vesicles and bullae, which typically develop into ulcers involving mucocutaneous junctions and oral mucosa, or less commonly haired skin. Clinically affected dogs and cats have erosions and ulcerations of the oral mucosa, which generally precede and are more prominent than skin lesions. Lesions typically occur in a symmetrical pattern, and in the haired skin often involve axillary or inguinal areas. Oral lesions are most dramatic on the dorsal surface of the tongue, although lesions can vary greatly in severity and distribution. Bullae are rarely seen in the oral cavity because they ulcerate rapidly. Clinical differential diagnoses should include other immune-mediated bullous skin diseases, such as mucous membrane pemphigoid (MMP), epidermolysis bullosa acquisita (EBA), or bullous pemphigoid (BP); several biopsies from intact vesicles or from the margins of erosions are necessary to make a definitive diagnosis. Oral PV lesions have rarely been associated with drug reactions or as a paraneoplastic syndrome in dogs and cats.

Microscopically, the earliest PV lesion consists of *suprabasilar acantholysis*, which is followed by the formation of clefts, leading to ulceration of the mucosa. Basal cells of the epidermis remain attached to the basement membrane and form a so-called row of tombstones, and a few neutrophils and eosinophils may infiltrate the epithelium. There is variable lymphocytic and plasmacytic lichenoid infiltration in the subepithelial fibrous stroma of the oral cavity. *Suprabasilar clefts and bullae caused by acantholysis were considered diagnostic for PV*; however, extensive erosion and ulceration of the mucosa and secondary bacterial infections frequently obscure these clefts and bullae.

Autoimmune subepidermal blistering diseases (AISBDs) are grossly similar but target the subepidermal basement membrane instead of the deep epidermal attachment. The most common are bullous pemphigoid (BP), mucous membrane pemphigoid (MMP), and epidermolysis bullosa acquisita (EBA), although several infrequently described diseases in dogs also fit in this category, including junctional EBA, linear IgA dermatosis, mixed AISBD, or type 1 bullous systemic lupus erythematosus. MMP is the most common of these and is the only disease that primarily affects the oral cavity and mucosa; the others generally are seen with lesions also present on haired skin. Similar to pemphigus, the diagnosis of these diseases is best made by histology coupled with signalment and presenting clinical syndrome; however, these diseases are not readily differentiated without additional specialized immunologic testing, which is not routinely available or performed, unfortunately leaving specific AISBDs unconfirmed.

Mucous membrane pemphigoid (MMP) is the most common AISBD of small animals, causing about half of all cases. Adults are predominantly affected, and among dogs, German Shepherds are overrepresented. The oral mucosa is a common site for lesion development, most cases involve gingiva, palate, and tongue. Subepidermal vesicles in MMP are associated with a relatively sparse inflammatory infiltrate. Subepidermal or submucosal vesicles can vary in size, and rare scattered individual apoptotic keratinocytes can be observed in basal or suprabasal mucosal epithelium. Similar to the human disease, canine MMP apparently targets collagen XVII or, in a low number of cases, laminin 332. Basement membrane–fixed immunoglobulins including IgG, IgM, IgA, and complement C3 have been detected by direct immunofluorescence or immunoperoxidase staining in formalin-fixed paraffin-embedded tissue, although these are not readily available for routine diagnostic use. PAS staining or anti-collagen IHC is described to label the dermal side of the blister to confirm the diagnosis, although these are insensitive tests and are not helpful to distinguish most AISBDs.

Epidermolysis bullosa acquisita (EBA) is a rare disease of dogs and the second most common AISBD, representing ~25% of cases. Affected dogs develop lesions prior to a year of age, and the most common anatomic sites include mucosae, mucocutaneous junctions, and haired skin located at points of friction. EBA has a poor prognosis and often is accompanied by footpad lesions, pain, pruritus, fever, lethargy, lymphadenopathy, and anorexia. Typical lesions are similar to other AISBDs; intact subepidermal vesicles in some cases may contain no inflammatory cells; in other cases, neutrophils or eosinophils accumulate at the basement membrane, and sometimes form subepidermal microabscesses. Autoantibodies are directed against collagen VII, which makes up the anchoring fibrils that join the lamina densa of the basement membrane to the type I collagen of the dermis. As for other AISBDs, diagnosis of EBA is based predominantly on signalment, clinical signs, and compatible histologic lesions. Cutaneous histochemical staining such as PAS, IHC assays for collagen, or serum or immunofluorescent antibody testing can be done, and typically resemble those in BP or MMP; autoantibodies may be recognized binding to the basement membrane.

Bullous pemphigoid (BP) is a term that has been applied generically to superficial autoimmune vesiculobullous or ulcerative disease of mucous membranes (including the oral mucosa) and skin, with subepithelial clefting. BP is the most common AISBD in humans, and although the term was used frequently historically for blistering skin diseases of dogs, it is now recognized that there is a complex of similar diseases that vary in their target antigen, clinical manifestations, and prognosis; thus, true BP is only rare in dogs, although it has also been reported in pigs, horses, and cats. BP is, however, retained as the name for the third most common of the AISBDs in dogs and cats. Lesions mainly occur on haired skin, and a minority of cases involve the mucocutaneous junctions or mucosae including the mouth, which is affected about one-third of the time; the lesions are less severe than other AISBDs in small animals, and footpad lesions or systemic illness is uncommon. Microscopically, a rich neutrophilic and eosinophilic dermal infiltrate is adjacent to and sometimes spilling into variably sized subepidermal bullae. The targets for the autoimmune response are epitopes on canine collagen XVII (also called BP antigen 180 or BPAg180). Collagen XVII is an epithelial transmembrane protein that is a component of the hemidesmosome that joins basal keratinocytes to the lamina densa of the basement membrane. As for other AISBDs, diagnosis of BP is based on suggestive clinical signs including mild blistering skin disease with or without oral mucosal involvement, and compatible histologic lesions. Again, PAS or IHC (collagen) may be supportive of a diagnosis of AISBDs generally, but will not reliably distinguish the different diseases. Immunotesting is not widely available or accessible.

The oral lesions of PV and of the AISBDs must be differentiated from other potentially similar lesions in the oral cavity caused by trauma, vasculitis, erythema multiforme, toxic epidermal necrolysis, Stevens-Johnson syndrome, lupus erythematosus, uveodermatologic syndrome, drug eruptions, chronic uremia, mucocutaneous candidiasis, and epitheliotropic lymphoma involving the mucocutaneous junctions or the oral cavity.

Thrush or **oral candidiasis** occurs most commonly in foals, pigs, and dogs. It involves the proliferation of yeasts and hyphae in the parakeratotic superficial layers of the oral epithelium. It appears grossly as patchy pale-gray pseudomembranous material on the oral mucosa and back of the tongue and probably reflects alterations in epithelial turnover and oral microbiota (see the Infectious and Parasitic Diseases of the Alimentary Tract section, later in this chapter). Mold products of *Stachybotrys alternans* cause catarrhal and necrotizing stomatitis and colitis if feed is contaminated. Gingivitis and ulceration of the oral mucosa may rarely be associated with infection caused by *Nocardia* spp. in dogs.

Uremia associated with chronic renal disease often causes odoriferous *ulcerative stomatitis* in dogs and less commonly in cats. Gray-brown ulcers occur on the gingiva, lateral surfaces and margin of the tongue, and on the inner surface of the lips and cheeks, often adjacent to the openings of salivary ducts. The margins of the ulcers are swollen and hyperemic. The pathogenesis of the oral lesions in uremia is still poorly understood. Elevations in blood and salivary urea in combination with urease-producing bacteria normally present in the oral microflora may generate ammonia from salivary urea. Ammonia has a caustic effect on the oral mucous membranes. Experimental antibody production against urease renders some intestinal bacteria nonpathogenic and prevents uremic colitis, providing evidence of the importance of urease. However, there is poor correlation between the levels of blood urea and the development of uremic stomatitis, suggesting that other important factors are also involved. Uremic vasculitis and impaired microvascular perfusion may contribute to the pathogenesis of uremic stomatitis.

Salivary glucose levels may be elevated in dogs and cats with *diabetes mellitus*, resulting in an imbalance of the oral microflora and predisposing to chronic gingivitis.

Ulcerative glossitis and stomatitis in **swine** can be part of **exudative epidermitis** (greasy pig disease) in preweaning pigs (see Vol. 1, Integumentary System). In addition to the characteristic skin lesions, about a third of the piglets develop ulcers on the dorsum of the tongue, or erosions and ulcers on the hard palate. Microscopically, the squamous mucosa is ulcerated, with coagulative necrosis and vesicle or pustule formation in the superficial epithelium over the rete pegs formed by oral epithelium. A mixed cellular inflammatory reaction is evident in the connective tissue below the ulcers.

Inflammation in the oral cavity can also be associated with ingestion of irritating chemicals, including caustic or toxic compounds such as *paraquat*, a herbicide that may cause severe erosive stomatitis in dogs. Dogs and cats that chew on the plant *Dieffenbachia* may develop oral erosions and ulcers. *Electrical burns* are occasionally seen in puppies or kittens that chew through electrical wires.

Deep stomatitis occurs when inflammation involves the deeper connective tissues of the mouth and is usually preceded by superficial lesions of the oral mucosa that permit entry of pyogenic bacteria (including normal oral flora) into the connective tissues of the oral cavity. Purulent inflammation or cellulitis may develop in the lips, tongue, cheek, soft palate, and pharynx, and abscesses may form that fistulate through the mucosa or skin. Pharyngeal wall abscesses may result from necrosis of retropharyngeal lymph nodes. Necrotic stomatitis with simple necrosis of the epithelium and the subepithelial fibrous stroma may be produced by thermal or chemical agents, but in animals it is usually caused by *Fusobacterium necrophorum* and other anaerobes. *F. necrophorum* is the principal cause of **oral necrobacillosis** or **necrotic stomatitis** in animals and is also associated with coagulative necrotizing lesions in both upper and lower alimentary tract, and liver. Wherever it occurs, it is usually a secondary invader following previous mucosal damage (Fig. 1-9A). The bacterium produces a variety of exotoxins and endotoxins including leukotoxin, the major virulence factor of *F. necrophorum*, which enhances the pathogenicity of the organism by mediating necrosis of tissue while modulating host immune defense response.

The best-known form of necrobacillary stomatitis is **calf diphtheria**, an acute coagulative necrosis of buccal and pharyngeal mucosa; many cases often involve the laryngeal mucosa (**necrotic laryngitis**) or the palatine or pharyngeal tonsils. The predisposing lesions may include trauma or infectious agents including bovine rhinotracheitis or papular stomatitis viruses. The incidence of diphtheria in slaughtered beef cattle may be as high as 1.4%. The same syndrome is rather common in housed lambs as a complication of contagious ecthyma. Infection also may be initiated in the gingiva of erupting teeth in any species, and by the trauma produced in piglets during removal of the needle teeth. In young animals, extension from the oral cavity via the bloodstream to other organs results in a frequently fatal infection, while in adults oral necrobacillosis tends to remain localized to the oral cavity, although infection may spread distally along the alimentary tract.

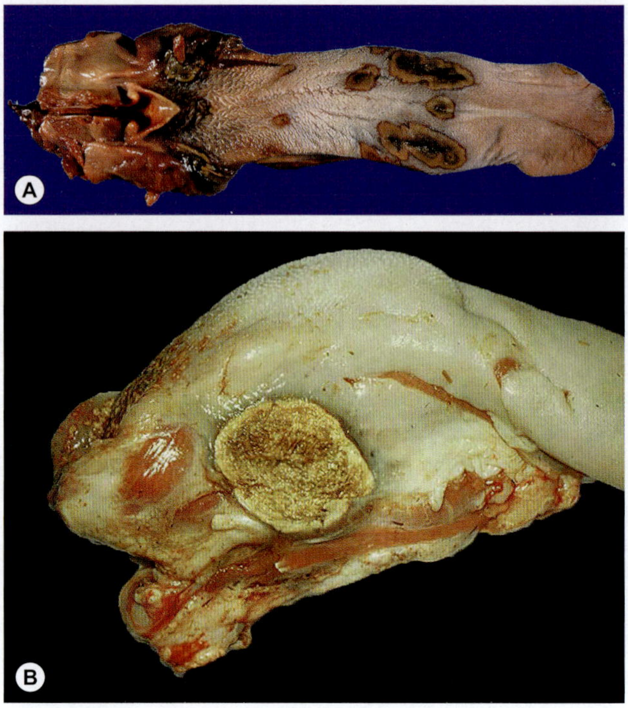

Figure 1-9 A. Necrotic **glossitis and stomatitis** in a dog. B. Oral necrobacillosis in a calf. (Courtesy Noah's Arkives.)

Early lesions are large well-demarcated yellow-gray and dry areas of necrosis surrounded by a zone of hyperemia (see Fig. 1-9B). They are found on the lateral or dorsal groove of the tongue, on the cheeks, gingiva, palate, pharynx, and often in the laryngeal ventricles or in the recesses adjacent to the larynx. Lesions near the larynx often lead to respiratory distress, and death may be associated with asphyxia. The necrotic tissue projects above the mucosal surface and can be friable, or firmly adherent, although surface coagulative necrosis may leave deep ulcers that heal by granulation. Necrotic tissues are surrounded initially by a zone of hyperemia, then by a dense narrow rim of leukocytes, and eventually by thick encapsulating granulation tissue. Bacteria are arranged in long filamentous clusters along the advancing margins of the lesions, and submucosal inflammation and necrosis may extend deep into the underlying soft tissues and bone.

Spread from the oral cavity or larynx occurs distally along the trachea causing aspiration pneumonia, along the esophagus, and/or via blood vessels. Death may occur acutely from septicemia with only various small serosal hemorrhages as evidence, or the spread of bacteria with severe inflammation and suppuration may occur in other tissues. Venous drainage via the vascular sinuses of the meninges may result in development of pituitary and cerebral abscessation. The characteristic gross lesions make diagnosis straightforward in most cases; identification of bacteria may be confirmed by a smear from the margin of the lesion. The organism is difficult to cultivate because it is a *strict anaerobe*.

Fusobacterium equinum is a bacterial opportunist that is closely related to *F. necrophorum*. It is a component of the normal microbiota of the equine GI tract, including the oral, reproductive, and respiratory mucosae. *F. equinum* also produces a leukotoxin that has been associated with necrotizing lesions, including within the oral cavity of horses.

Noma (cancrum oris) is a rapidly spreading *pseudomembranous or gangrenous stomatitis;* it is not caused by a specific pathogen but is associated with tissue invasion by the normal oral flora, particularly fusobacteria and spirochetes with extensive local tissue destruction. The predisposing factors are unknown but are probably nonspecific and associated with mucosal trauma and debility. The disease is occasionally observed in horses, dogs, and monkeys and is in many respects similar to oral necrobacillosis. Spirochetes can typically be found in large numbers at the advancing margins as well as in peripheral viable tissue. Fusiform bacterial organisms are observed in the deeper layers of necrosis, while a variety of other organisms including cocci can be present along the surface. Initial small ulcerations of the cheek or gingiva can spread rapidly. It is often intensely fetid and consists of a necrotic pseudomembrane surrounded by a zone of acute inflammation. The necrotic tissue may slough to leave deep ulcers, and even the cheek may be perforated to leave a gaping necrotic defect.

Actinobacilli can cause stomatitis, glossitis, and lymphadenitis in cattle, sheep, and pigs, and sometimes pyogranulomas in the wall of the forestomachs of ruminants. *Actinobacillus lignieresii* is considered normal oral flora, but after penetration of the oral mucosa in cattle is associated with deep stomatitis. **Actinobacillosis** is typically a sporadic *disease of soft tissue*, spreading as a *lymphangitis* and usually involving the regional lymph nodes; this feature distinguishes actinobacillosis from actinomycosis, which causes mostly bone lesions. The tongue is most often involved in actinobacillosis, and chronic inflammation produces clinical *wooden tongue*, although more widespread lymphatic, cutaneous, or systemic disease has been described. Entry of organisms to soft tissues of oral mucosa and tongue is likely gained by traumatic surface injury from tooth-induced abrasion or injury, or from trapped grass seeds and awns, many of which become embedded within or along the lingual groove.

Pyogranulomatous inflammation is seen histologically and is often centered on large clusters of gram-negative coccobacilli (so-called club colonies) surrounded by radiating eosinophilic material typical of the Splendore-Hoeppli phenomenon, composed of immune complexes, tissue debris, and fibrin (Fig. 1-10). These are surrounded by variable numbers of neutrophils, macrophages or giant cells, lymphocytes, and plasma cells within reactive fibrous granulation tissue. Individual inflammatory foci appear grossly as firm pale nodules from a few millimeters up to 1 cm in diameter with central minute yellow *sulfur granules*.

Lymphogenous spread is common, and affected lymphatics are thickened, often with nodules distributed along their course. This distribution is best seen beneath the mucosa of the dorsal and lateral surfaces of the tongue and often can be traced through to the pharyngeal lymphoid tissue (Fig. 1-11). The most common form of lingual actinobacillosis consists of granulation tissue in which are embedded many variably sized nodular granulomas or abscesses surrounded by a dense connective tissue capsule, beneath an intact or ulcerated epithelial surface. Diffuse sclerosing actinobacillosis of the tongue (*wooden tongue*) is firm because of extensive deposition of connective tissue, which replaces muscle fibers.

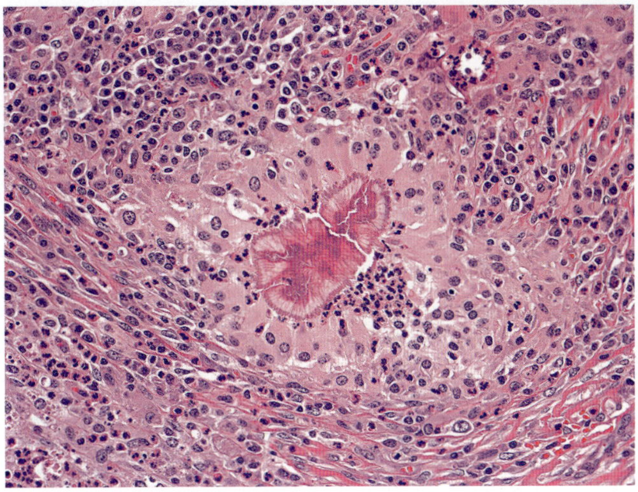

Figure 1-10 Pyogranulomatous inflammation containing a club colony of *Actinobacillus lignieresii* in **actinobacillosis** in a cow.

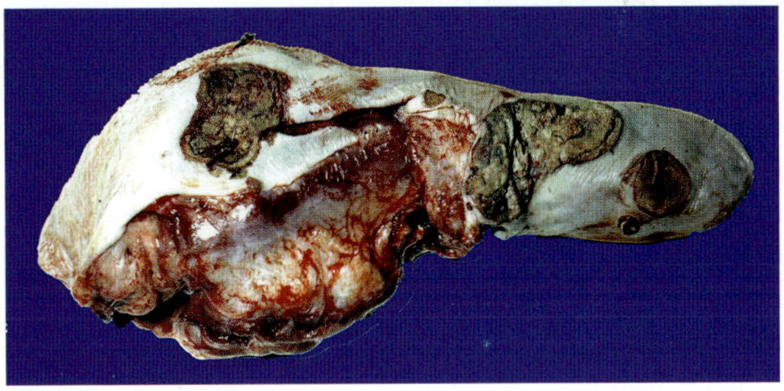

Figure 1-11 **Actinobacillosis** in a cow. Granulomas bulging on lateral surface of the tongue.

Atypical actinobacillosis (involvement of tissue other than the tongue) often is associated with *regional lymphadenitis*. The cut surface of the node reveals small, soft, yellow-or-orange granulomas containing characteristic *sulfur granules* embedded within chronic sclerosing inflammation of the adjacent tissues, which may cause adhesion to overlying skin or mucous membranes. The retropharyngeal and submaxillary nodes are most often affected, as well as the lymphoid tissues of the submucosa of the soft palate and pharynx. Involvement of the pharynx and the retropharyngeal lymph nodes may cause dyspnea and dysphagia.

Oral actinobacillosis in *swine* causes lesions similar to those in cattle, including glossitis. Actinobacillosis may also occur sporadically or as outbreaks in *sheep*, but in this species the tongue seems to be exempt. The characteristic lesions in sheep occur in the subcutaneous tissue of the head, especially of the cheeks, nose, lips, and submaxillary and throat regions, and on the nasal turbinates. They may also occur on the soft palate and pharynx as complications of wounds received at drenching. The organism has rarely been isolated from horses.

Lesions morphologically similar to actinobacillosis may be caused by a variety of organisms. *Trueperella pyogenes* has been isolated from lingual ulcers and granulomas in lambs. Microscopic examination of these lesions reveals well-demarcated submucosal granulomas with plant fibers in the center, surrounded by a marked neutrophilic reaction. The organisms were thought to gain entry after the mucosa was damaged by hard fibrous plant fibers from the weed lambsleaf or lanceleaf sage (*Salvia reflexa*) present in the bedding. *Actinomyces bovis* is a gram-positive filamentous bacterium that causes pyogranulomatous mandibular and maxillary osteomyelitis in cattle and mastitis in sows. *Actinomyces weissii* has been isolated from dogs with stomatitis/gingivitis. Staphylococci may cause pyogranulomatous lesions (botryomycosis) in any species. Less common causes of similar microscopic lesions include *Nocardia* and the various agents associated with mycetomas (see Vol. 1, Integumentary System).

Oral dermatophilosis caused by *Dermatophilus congolensis* has been reported in cattle and cats. *D. congolensis* most commonly causes exudative dermatitis in a wide variety of species (see Vol. 1, Integumentary System). In cattle, oral dermatophilosis has also been associated with *A. bovis* infection. In cats, the organism is uncommonly associated with oral granulomas, especially affecting the tongue and tonsillar crypt. Large numbers of gram-positive filamentous branching organisms with longitudinal and transverse divisions may be demonstrated in the necrotic centers of submucosal granulomas. The organisms probably enter through damaged mucosa. The gross lesion must be differentiated from the more common SCC of the tongue.

Parasitic diseases of the oral cavity are of minor significance. Sarcosporidiosis and cysticercosis occur in the striated muscle of the tongue and produce the same lesions as they do elsewhere (see Vol. 1, Muscle and Tendon). *Trichinella spiralis* may be found in muscles of the tongue and mastication. *Gongylonema* spp. are found in the mucosal lining of the tongue, especially in swine allowed to graze, and are observed less commonly in cattle and sheep. They evoke little or no inflammation of the mucosa, but a mild-to-moderate lymphocytic and eosinophilic reaction may be evident in the underlying lamina propria. Larvae of *Gasterophilus* spp. in the horse and of *Oestrus ovis* in sheep can occasionally be found attached to the pharyngeal mucosa, where they may cause focal ulceration and incite mild inflammation. The larvae of *Gasterophilus nasalis* migrate from the lips, through the gingiva especially of the alveolar processes where they incite purulent or eosinophilic inflammation. *Halicephalobus gingivalis* has been observed in granulomas of the mandibular gingiva as well as bone, skin, kidney, central nervous system (CNS), mammary gland, and eye of horses. Parasitic leeches of the genus *Myxobdella* may infect the oral cavity of cattle and humans, and *Limnatis nilotica* the oral cavity of dogs, leading to minor dysfunction and hemorrhage. Known colloquially as the *tongue worm*, the pentastome *Linguatula serrata* infects the nasal cavity and nasopharynx of dogs and humans. Nodular and ulcerative glossitis can occur in dogs as an unusual manifestation of canine leishmaniosis caused by *Leishmania infantum*, an endemic zoonotic parasite in southern Europe.

Proliferative and neoplastic lesions of the oral cavity

Many of the lumps, bumps, and cysts that develop in and around the oral cavity are malformations, hyperplasias, and neoplasias originating in soft or hard tissues of the oral cavity or jawbones, or in the odontogenic tissues, including tooth germ or teeth. Malformations of dental origin have been considered previously under developmental anomalies of teeth. Gingival masses of various types, many of which are of tooth germ origin, are common in dogs, but occur much less frequently in other species. In this discussion, we follow revisions in the nomenclature of lesions formerly included as various epulides, separating those that are clearly of dental origin from hyperplastic or reactive lesions. Prognostic implications have not changed, despite reclassification and renaming of many of these conditions.

Epulis *is a generic clinical term for tumorlike masses of the gingiva*, and the term has in the past been used to describe developmental, inflammatory, and hyperplastic lesions, as well as several specific neoplastic lesions of tooth germ origin. It has no specific pathology connotation, and *the term should not be used in a morphologic diagnosis*.

The oral and pharyngeal mucosa is a common site of malignant neoplasms in dogs and cats. Malignant oral neoplasms account for ~6% of all canine and ~7% of all feline neoplasms. Large domestic animals have a low prevalence of malignant oral neoplasms, and when they occur in ungulates, they are usually relatively nonaggressive. There are regional geographic differences in the prevalence of certain oral neoplasms, especially in dogs and cattle. Such differences may be related to the distribution of carcinogens in the environment and warrants further investigation from the point of view of comparative oncology.

The most common types of malignant oral neoplasms in dogs and cats are squamous cell carcnioma, fibrosarcoma, and, in dogs only, malignant melanomas. These vary somewhat in their behavior depending on the species in which they occur and the type and specific location of the lesion. Dogs and cats >6-7-years-old are mainly affected. The canine population with fibrosarcomas has a mean age of ~8 years. Melanomas in dogs tend to occur in a notably older age class than the other neoplasms, with the mean of the distribution at ~11-12 years. Typical clinical signs are determined by the location, behavior, and stage of the lesion, but typically include drooling, halitosis, pain, dysphagia, anorexia, weight loss, loose teeth, mandibular fractures, oral bleeding, noisy respiration, coughing, and altered voice.

Boxers, Cocker Spaniels, German Shorthaired Pointers, Weimaraners, and Golden Retrievers apparently have a higher prevalence of malignant oral neoplasms compared with other breeds of dogs, whereas Dachshunds and Beagles apparently have a very low prevalence. The male-to-female ratio has been reported to be as high as 6:1 for melanomas, 3:1 for tonsillar carcinomas, and 2:1 for fibrosarcomas, although the ratios must be interpreted with some caution because they may be partly related to differences in the ratio of males to females in the general population.

All types of malignant oral neoplasms in dogs and cats tend to progress rapidly and, regardless of the type of malignancy, the prognosis is generally poor unless the lesion is completely resected early in its clinical course and before metastasis occurs.

In the following sections, we consider non-neoplastic proliferative lesions of the oral cavity, neoplasms of soft tissues of the oral cavity, neoplasms of odontogenic tissues, and then finally neoplasms of the bones of the jaw. A hearty note of appreciation to Drs Brian G. Murphy, Cynthia M. Bell, and Jason W. Soukup, authors of the excellent work Veterinary Oral and Maxillofacial Pathology (Wiley, 2019), is in order at this point; we highly recommend that text for a more thorough treatment of many of the conditions discussed in the following sections.

Non-neoplastic proliferative and reactive lesions of the oral cavity

There is a broad range of benign reactive or inflammatory lesions that are commonly observed in the oral cavity of animals, particularly of dogs and cats. Importantly, these nodules can appear grossly indistinguishable from more malevolent lesions that also occur here, so biopsy is frequently utilized to reach a definitive diagnosis. Clinical presentation, gross description, photographs, radiographs, and behavior of these lesions often provide significant information for pathologists seeking to establish a definitive diagnosis. Veterinarians should be strongly encouraged to include this information for pathologists with biopsy samples, especially when small incisional biopsies are submitted.

Fibrous or epithelial gingival hyperplasia (formerly part of fibrous or fibromatous epulis, also known as *gingival hypertrophy*) is a common lesion in dogs. This lesion has various causes or inciting factors and can be composed of proliferative gingival epithelium or gingival stroma (including various contributions of each in the same lesion). It may be generalized and diffuse in the oral cavity, or focal and localized to one or more teeth. When focal, it is a discrete tumorlike proliferative mass and whether localized or generalized, the lesion may cover part of the crown of adjacent teeth (Fig. 1-12). A significant clinical challenge is distinguishing focal gingival hyperplasia from fibromatous hyperplasia of the gingival ligament [formerly known as both *fibromatous epulis of periodontal ligament origin* (FEPLO) and *peripheral odontogenic fibroma* (POF)], or from more malevolent neoplasms of the oral cavity, and thus they are frequently biopsied. The nodular lesion occurs due to proliferation of the gingival epithelium and/or the gingival fibrous connective tissue stroma, often with low cellular density. The proliferative gingival fibrous stroma is histologically identical to normal gingival fibrous stroma, whereas the proliferative gingival epithelium can occur either as thickened acanthotic and hyperkeratotic epithelium of the oral surface or as elongated plexiform anastomosing hyperplasia of the sulcus epithelium. Localized masses may be exacerbated by chronic surface trauma, ulceration, granulation tissue, gingival epithelial hyperplasia, and inflammation—often associated with periodontal disease. Frequently there is an accompanying band of mononuclear cells, predominantly plasma cells and lymphocytes, in the superficial gingival fibrous stroma adjacent to the epithelium.

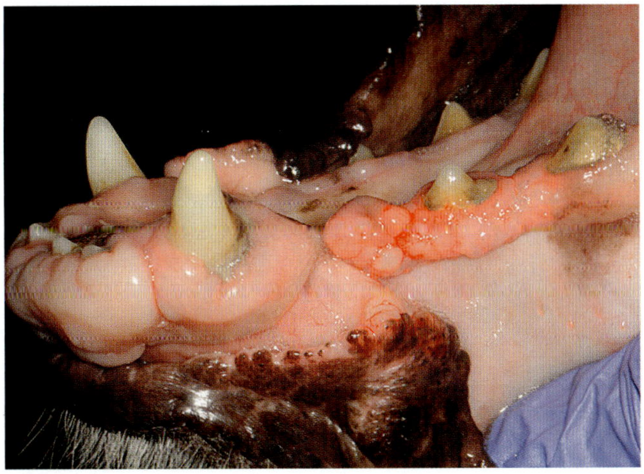

Figure 1-12 **Generalized gingival hyperplasia** in the mandible of a dog. (Courtesy D. Winter.)

Diffuse fibrous hyperplasia is described as a familial condition in Boxer dogs, although in some of these lesions, areas reminiscent of gingival or periodontal ligament hyperplasia are observed. A more severe overgrowth, termed *hyperplastic gingivitis*, occurs as a recessive inherited disease in Swedish silver foxes. In the foxes, both jaws are affected, and the lesion causes displacement and malalignment of teeth, eventually reaching such proportions that the mouth cannot be closed.

Fibromatous hyperplasia of the gingival ligament (formerly FEPLO, POF, or fibromatous epulis) is a very common lesion of dogs that occurs less commonly in other species, including cats, and is *indistinguishable clinically from focal fibrous hyperplasia* and many other proliferative oral nodules. The naming of this lesion has been a debate rooted in controversy regarding both the origin and pathogenesis of this lesion. Although the debate continues, this common entity is an idiopathic, hyperplastic, non-neoplastic, and proliferative lesion arising from the gingival (or peripheral periodontal) ligament of the alveolar crest of the oral cavity. The lesion is not directly comparable to the uncommon human neoplasm known as POF.

Fibromatous hyperplasia of the gingival ligament is most commonly identified in the rostral maxilla adjacent to the carnassial or canine teeth, or the caudal mandible; they usually occur in dogs >3-years-old. These are firm-to-hard gray-pink nodules that often project from between the teeth or hard palate near the teeth; they are often mushroom shaped with a smooth lobulated surface. They are attached to the periosteum and may displace teeth mechanically, but do not invade the underlying bones of the jaw. Fibromatous hyperplasia of the gingival ligament is composed mostly of interwoven bundles of proliferative mesenchymal tissue and collagenous stroma reminiscent of periodontal or gingival ligament. They are distinguished from gingival fibrous hyperplasia, granulation tissue, or neoplastic mesenchymal lesions of the jaw by the mesenchymal stroma, which is composed of densely arranged small stellate-to-fusiform fibroblasts within a dense collagen matrix, with regular often dilated empty vascular spaces (reminiscent of gingival or periodontal ligament). In addition, these lesions often also contain variable amounts of proliferative odontogenic epithelium arranged in thin ribbons or clusters and trabeculae (in dogs they may lack odontogenic epithelium, the human lesion known as POF has the odontogenic epithelium), and variable amounts of often mineralized dental matrix resembling bone, cementum, or osteodentin arranged in islands or lakes surrounded by proliferative collagenous mesenchyme (Fig. 1-13). About 60% of these lesions contain branching cords or islands of odontogenic epithelium, of which the basal layer may display classic features of odontogenic epithelium (antibasilar nuclei, cytoplasmic clearing, palisading, intercellular bridges). Epithelium within fibromatous hyperplasia of the gingival ligament may be continuous with the overlying gingiva or originate in epithelial cell rests of Malassez embedded within the periodontal ligament.

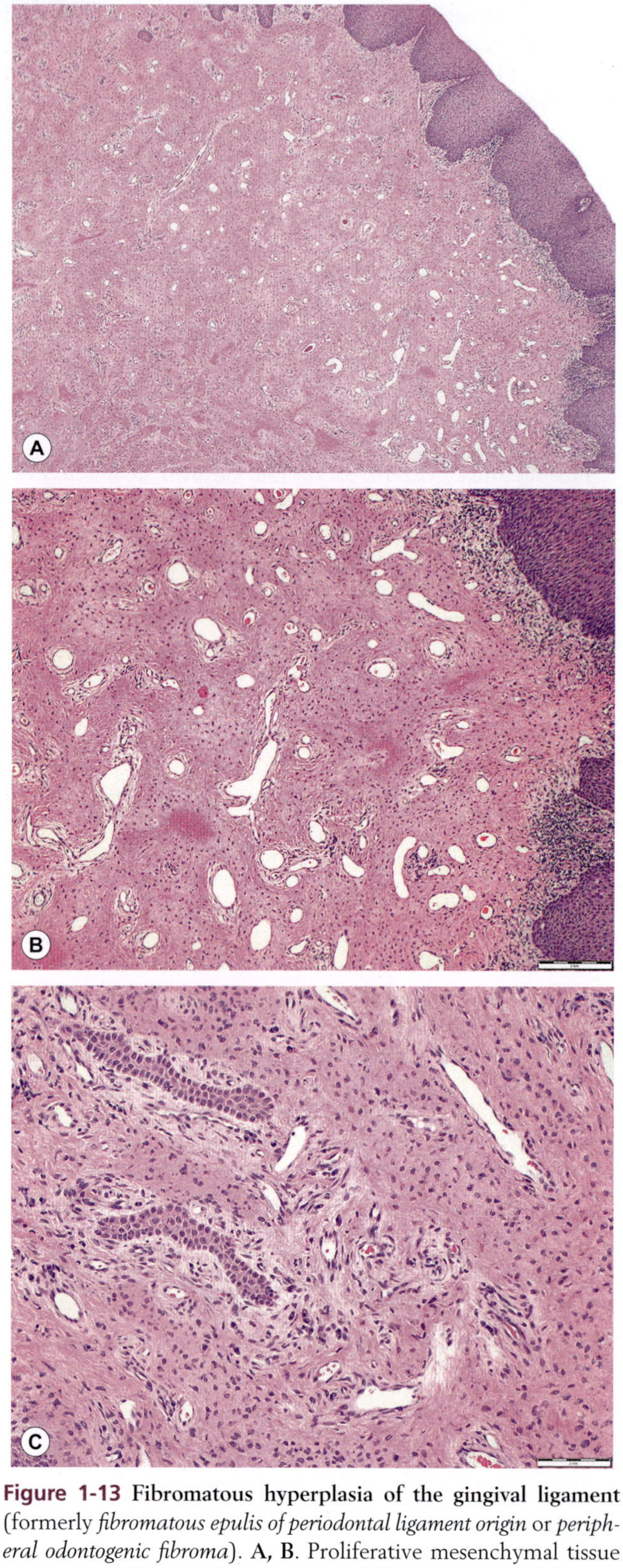

Figure 1-13 **Fibromatous hyperplasia of the gingival ligament** (formerly *fibromatous epulis of periodontal ligament origin* or *peripheral odontogenic fibroma*). **A, B**. Proliferative mesenchymal tissue reminiscent of gingival or periodontal ligament. **C**. Proliferative odontogenic epithelium is arranged in thin ribbons or cords and embedded within the proliferative mesenchymal tissue.

The origin or significance of the islands or lakes of dental matrix is not fully understood but likely has no prognostic significance, even though it can be quite extensive in chronic lesions and should not be confused with invasion of bone of the jaw.

Peripheral giant cell granuloma (formerly *giant cell epulis*) occurs in dogs and cats as red, smooth, and sessile or pedunculated *gingival masses*. Giant cell granuloma is the second most common gingival tumor in cats after fibromatous hyperplasia of the gingival ligament. In dogs, these are categorized as either 1) classic peripheral giant cell granulomas with many multinucleate giant cells admixed with spindle cells and collagenous matrix or 2) collision peripheral giant cell granulomas in which there are many multinucleate giant cells within a population of proliferative mesenchymal tissue with features typically associated with fibromatous hyperplasia of the gingival ligament. These are likely not true granulomas in dogs or cats because the giant cells have been shown by IHC to be osteoclast-like cells. This entity is likely a variant of the fibromatous hyperplasia of the gingival ligament in which extensive ulceration and inflammation induces the osteoclast-like giant cells. They should be regarded as hyperplastic or reactive lesions and have occurred at sites of tooth resorption, loss, or extraction. Similar lesions described as *central giant cell granulomas* may occur more deeply in the jaw. The gingival epithelium is ulcerated or hyperplastic and extends deeply into the underlying mass, which is well vascularized and often contains hemosiderin-laden cells. Characteristic of all forms of this lesion are the numerous multinucleate osteoclast-like giant cells with multiple central nuclei and abundant eosinophilic cytoplasm, which are embedded within a densely cellular stroma. Deposits of matrix (possibly mineralized osteoid or other dental hard matrix) may be present.

Fibrous dysplasia is an unusual lesion among proliferative fibro-osseous lesions of the oral mucosa and jaws, most histologically similar to the neoplasm known as ossifying fibroma. Fibrous dysplasia is included here with non-neoplastic lesions (ossifying fibroma is considered below with neoplastic conditions) because it is currently classified as a *dysplastic* process. Fibrous dysplasia can be locally destructive but is usually a self-limiting lesion that develops within and replaces bone of the mandible or maxilla of young horses, dogs, and cats. The pathogenesis remains unclear in animals, although in humans, fibrous dysplasia is a genetic defect of osteoblasts and part of the polyostotic McCune-Albright syndrome of youth that stabilizes with skeletal maturity. The lesion is composed of sheets and streams of bland proliferative mesenchymal cells with minimal atypia and rare mitotic figures; scattered throughout are individual or clusters of multinucleate giant cells. Within the proliferative fibro-osseous stroma are variably mineralized and haphazardly arranged matrix elements or bone-like trabeculae, but often without obvious transition to mature mineralized bone with embedded osteoblasts. Most but not all fibrous dysplasia lesions lack a palisading rim of osteoblasts (this has historically been considered a distinguishing feature of fibrous dysplasia from ossifying fibroma, in which these are present). Fibrous dysplasia is not as well circumscribed within the bone as ossifying fibroma, so radiographs and clinical behavior are very important to determine a definitive diagnosis. Some authors have proposed that fibrous dysplasia is a less mature stage of ossifying fibroma, but this has not been proven definitively.

Calcinosis circumscripta is an uncommon oral lesion that occurs mostly along lingual surfaces in the oral cavity of dogs. This condition, which also occurs in haired skin mostly of young, large-breed dogs, is most frequently identified in the deep skeletal muscle of the tongue, and while thought to be associated with traumatic injury, calcinosis circumscripta is considered an idiopathic and ectopic dystrophic mineralization with deposition of calcium salts into soft tissues. The histologic lesions are characteristic and composed of distinct well-circumscribed and often multilocular aggregates of crystalline finely basophilic mineral-rich material surrounded by macrophages, multinucleate giant cells, and fibrous connective tissue. This is frequently an incidental lesion with no clinical signs or abnormalities in affected patients. Because this is a non-neoplastic and reactive lesion, surgical excision is the recommended therapeutic approach, and this is usually curative.

Oral traumatic injury (the so-called **oral pyogenic granuloma**) is a bright red or blue smooth nodule on the gingiva of dogs and cats. In cats, the lesion seems to occur commonly in the buccal gingiva near the rostral mandibular molars. It is composed of extremely vascular granulation tissue covered by gingival epithelium, and despite the name is not genuinely a lesion of granulomatous inflammation. The surface is often ulcerated, infiltrated by leukocytes, and bleeds easily. The cause is not completely understood; the lesion is probably an exaggerated response to local trauma including chewing (these have also been called *traumatic or chewing granulomas*), irritation, and/or localized infection. The cause of such lesions is not typically evident in biopsies, but it is important to distinguish these from neoplastic oral lesions. In horses, exuberant granulation tissue of periodontal origin sometimes develops at the site of extracted teeth to produce a tumorlike mass in the dental arcade. Gingival or odontogenic epithelial remnants and proliferative dentinal matrix or bone may be observed within the granulation tissue in such cases.

Oral fibroepithelial polyps are also trauma-induced lesions that occur in the oral cavity of dogs and less frequently cats. They are pedunculated oral lesions arising beneath or lateral to the tongue, and less commonly are found along labial and gingival mucosae, or palate. Fibroepithelial polyps have a dense fibrovascular-to-collagenous stalk covered by hyperplastic and hyperkeratotic squamous gingival epithelium with frequent ulceration and mild mixed inflammation. Distinction between fibroepithelial polyp and pyogenic granuloma can be subtle, but fibroepithelial polyps tend to be comparatively less vascular and less inflamed, they occur more frequently along or ventral to the tongue, and they are observed more frequently in dogs than in cats. Surgical excision is usually curative.

Other lesions due to chewing, rubbing, abrasion, laceration, or even chemical or thermal burns, as well as nodular lymphoid hyperplasia, can occur in the oral cavity, but unless the trauma is severe and ongoing, these usually heal by granulation quickly so that only mild chronic inflammation, fibrosis, or proliferative gingival or mucosal epithelium are present. Sites of contact with teeth due to malocclusion, or lateral and ventral surfaces of the tongue are most commonly affected.

Ectopic sebaceous glands in the oral cavity are a type of choristoma (histologically normal tissue in an abnormal anatomic location) and are usually incidental with no clinical significance. Intra-oral sebaceous gland neoplasia has also been described rarely in dogs, with histologic features similar to the very common sebaceous adenoma and epithelioma of haired skin. In addition, sebaceous glands have been described within canine oral papillomas; presumably, these undergo sebaceous differentiation or arise from ectopic glands in the oral cavity.

Histiocytic foam cell nodules are apparently most common in Miniature Dachshund dogs, although they have been seen in other breeds. The well-demarcated nodules are found mostly on the ventral and lateral surface of the tongue (like fibroepithelial polyps) and are composed of aggregates and clusters of CD204+ and MHC class I+ histiocytes with abundant foamy clear vacuolated cytoplasm and variable numbers of mixed inflammatory cells. They are similar to xanthomas, which are common in the skin of birds and related to abnormal cholesterol or triglyceride levels; however, histiocytic foam cell nodules are negative with Oil Red O, which distinguishes them from classic xanthomas. These nodules are histologically similar to other oral inflammatory processes, and they should be distinguished from oral neoplasms; notably, macrophages of these nodules are described as PAS negative (ruling out granular cell tumor). Some have proposed that these nodules are a type of granulomatous disorder, especially in the Miniature Dachshund breed.

Nodular chondroid hyperplasia is an uncommon idiopathic lesion of the oral cavity described in dogs. This may be a form of tracheobronchopathia osteochondroplastica, a rare degenerative condition of chondrodysplasia that results in mucosal expansive nodules composed of variably mineralized cartilage, fibrous tissue, or bone, all overlying degenerate or necrotic cartilage of laryngeal, epiglottal, or arytenoid cartilages.

Neoplasms of soft tissues of the oral cavity

Neoplasms are common in the oral cavity, especially of dogs and cats; many types of neoplasms arising from various soft tissues of the oral cavity are histologically and behaviorally similar to their counterparts in other anatomic areas; others have unique features in the oral cavity. Given the similarity of many of these neoplasms to more benign processes and nodular proliferative lesions in the oral cavity, differentiation by biopsy is highly significant and frequently requested.

Melanocytic neoplasms *are the most common oral neoplasms in dogs*. Oral melanocytic neoplasms, including those arising from melanocytes in the nonhaired portion of lips or within the oral cavity proper of dogs, have a worse prognosis and shorter overall survival times compared with cutaneous melanocytic neoplasms. However, location alone is not of prognostic significance because a benign and less-aggressive variant known as histologically well-differentiated oral melanocytic neoplasms are well described in the lip and oral cavity. Pigmented basilar epithelial cells are frequently present in superficial areas of the oral soft tissues in a variety of non-neoplastic lesions resulting from irritation to the mucosa, and this should be differentiated from melanocytic neoplasia. Cutaneous melanomas are common in gray horses and certain breeds of swine, but these species have no tendency to develop oral melanomas, although rare cases are reported. Oral melanocytic neoplasms are rare in cattle, sheep, and cats.

Histologically well-differentiated oral melanocytic neoplasms (canine oral melanocytoma or canine oral melanocytic neoplasms of low malignant potential) are the benign version of oral malignant melanoma; these are uncommon in the oral cavity of dogs but occur more often in dogs than in other species. As with oral malignant melanomas, canine benign oral melanocytomas are diagnosed more frequently in some breeds, including Golden Retrievers, Cocker Spaniels, Poodles, Chow Chows, and mixed-breed dogs, and although the literature is variable, they are equally common in males and females. Most oral melanocytic neoplasms are small <1-cm pigmented nodules that appear on the lips or within the oral cavity. The gross appearance can vary, and up to 30% of all melanocytic tumors in dogs are amelanotic, so oral melanocytic neoplasms can appear grossly similar to other oral neoplastic, inflammatory, or reactive nodular lesions. Cytology is an excellent screening tool, but histologic evaluation—often with bleaching—is important to establish a definitive diagnosis and distinguish well-differentiated melanocytic neoplasms from oral malignant melanoma.

Neoplastic cells are arranged in packets, sheets, or bundles, and various morphologic features and arrangements can be observed in the same lesion. The cells comprising well-differentiated melanocytic neoplasms are round-to-polygonal or elongated, uniform in size with a single small round nucleus, a single centrally oriented nucleolus, and a low mitotic count of <4 per 2.37 mm^2 at 400× magnification (reported as 10 high-powered fields in most publications). Nuclear atypia is an important distinguishing diagnostic feature for well-differentiated melanocytic neoplasms, and <30% atypical nuclei are expected. Well-differentiated neoplasms are often heavily pigmented, so bleach is frequently required to facilitate visualization of nuclear morphology and mitotic figures; there is rarely evidence of lymphatic vascular invasion. *Junctional activity* (nests or individualized neoplastic melanocytes in the basal epithelial layer) or *lentiginous or radial growth* (lateral migration or spread of junctional activity) is uncommon. If a definitive diagnosis cannot be established by H&E staining, IHC is often helpful; IHC reactivity of melanocytic tumors is discussed below with oral malignant melanoma. Well-differentiated oral melanocytic neoplasms are benign with extremely low recurrence rates (3.1%) and low metastatic potential; wide surgical excision is typically curative.

Most oral melanomas in **dogs** are malignant and highly aggressive neoplasms, and many have metastasized by the time they are diagnosed. **Oral malignant melanomas** are common and make up over 1/3 of all malignant oral neoplasms in dogs. Males have been overrepresented in some studies but not others. Some data suggest that melanomas are more common in smaller breeds or in those with a dark hair coat and/or pigmented mucous membranes, such as Scottish and Boston Terriers, black Cocker Spaniels, Dachshunds, Miniature Poodles, and Chow Chows, but not all studies have found size or breed associations. *The degree of pigmentation of these tumors varies considerably, and many are at least partially amelanotic, but there appears to be no relationship between the amount of pigment and biological behavior.* Metastases are usually pigmented, but in some cases the primary tumor is pigmented and the metastases are not, and vice versa.

Patients with oral malignant melanoma drool, have dysphagia and/or halitosis, and lesions appear as single or multiple, often pigmented masses on the lips or within the oral cavity. Oral malignant melanoma is usually pigmented gray to red or blue, but because other nodular lesions of the oral cavity can be pigmented, and up to 1/3 of malignant melanomas in dogs are amelanotic, pigmentation alone does not definitively indicate melanoma. Cytology can be helpful, although it is important to remember that amelanotic malignant melanomas may grossly and cytologically resemble other oral sarcomas or carcinomas. Lesions often are large, ~3-4 cm in diameter when discovered. The initial size of the primary tumor is reported to be prognostically significant, and important in staging. They grow rapidly, and necrosis and ulceration are common (Fig. 1-14A), as is invasion of bone by gingival neoplasms. Many oral malignant melanomas

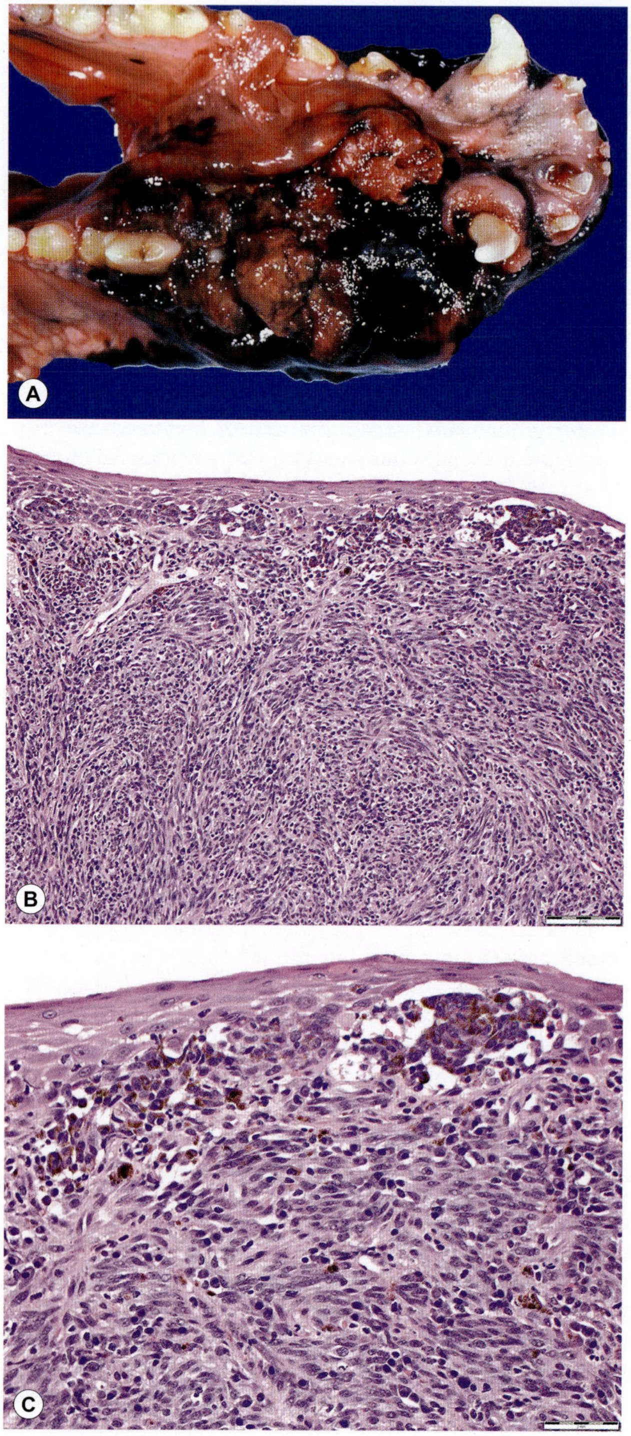

Figure 1-14 Malignant melanoma of the mandible in a dog. **A.** Gross appearance, with invasion, necrosis, and ulceration. **B.** Neoplastic melanocytes arranged in dense sheets. **C.** Junctional activity in the overlying gingival epithelium.

metastasize rapidly to regional lymph nodes, including ipsilateral and contralateral mandibular and medial retropharyngeal nodes. Unfortunately, without thorough serial sectioning of lymph nodes, micrometastases in these nodes are easily and probably often overlooked. About 33% of patients with oral malignant melanoma have multinodal metastasis; 42% have metastasis to contralateral nodes at initial diagnosis. Eventual contralateral dissemination has been shown to occur in 62% of dogs, with ipsilateral dissemination in 92%. They spread via hematogenous and lymphatic routes to more distant sites, especially the lungs, where they may be evident at autopsy, but often are too small to be detected radiographically. The median survival time for untreated dogs with oral malignant melanoma is reported as 65 days, although survival varies between 3 and 18 months, depending on stage of disease and treatment, such as surgical excision, radiation, and/or chemotherapy. The median survival time of dogs with no bone, lymph node, or distant organ metastatic disease detected at diagnosis is ~8 months after surgical resection.

The histologic appearance of melanomas varies greatly, from a well-differentiated heavily pigmented type to a highly anaplastic amelanotic type. The diagnosis of the latter is often difficult and impossible without IHC. However, certain features are evident in most of these tumors. Nuclear atypia, mitotic count (number of mitoses in a field area of 2.37 mm² at 400× magnification), degree of pigmentation, level of infiltration, and vascular invasion are the most useful parameters that predict behavior and prognosis for oral malignant melanomas in dogs. In contrast to well-differentiated oral melanocytic neoplasms, oral malignant melanomas are composed of neoplastic cells with highly variable pigmentation; amelanotic variants are common. Neoplastic cells have highly variable morphology, from elongate spindle cells arranged in interwoven bundles, to epithelial, round, or polygonal cells arranged in nests or sheets (see Fig. 1-14B); various cellular morphologies and arrangement patterns are commonly observed in the same lesion. Multinucleate giant cells may be present, and osteoid and cartilage have been reported in the stroma of a low number of canine oral malignant melanomas.

Various histologic patterns have been shown to be more common than others, although this likely has limited prognostic significance. Anisokaryosis and anisocytosis of oral malignant melanomas are often moderate to marked. Although somewhat subjective, *cellular and nuclear morphology is significant prognostically*, and >30% atypical neoplastic cells is observed in malignant oral melanomas. *Mitotic count is a reliable prognostic indicator* for all oral melanocytic neoplasms, and although interobserver variability can be high, a mitotic count of ≥4 per 2.37 mm² is associated with shorter survival times. Pigmentation can also vary, and whereas well-differentiated oral melanocytic neoplasms are highly pigmented, the degree of pigmentation is a less reliable prognostic indicator in malignant variants. Oral malignant melanomas often are not limited to the superficial tissues alone, but also involve deeper structures of the oral cavity, including submucosa, skeletal muscle, salivary gland, or bone; malignant variants often invade blood or lymphatic vessels. *Malignant melanomas frequently display junctional activity and lentiginous growth*, and it is common to observe atypical neoplastic melanocytes within the epithelium (see Fig. 1-14C). As for well-differentiated oral melanocytic neoplasms, the importance of cytologic features of neoplastic melanocytes in determining the diagnosis and prognosis is highly significant, so bleaching of pigmented lesions is often necessary.

Molecular parameters have been evaluated as prognostic markers. Ki-67 is an IHC stain that identifies a nuclear protein associated with ribosomal RNA transcription and proliferation and thus reflects the growth fraction of a neoplastic cell population by detecting proliferative cells in the cell cycle. Ki-67 has been shown to accurately predict the prognosis of oral melanocytic neoplasms with less interobserver variation and higher reproducibility compared with mitotic counts or other markers. Bleaching of highly pigmented lesions may be necessary prior to Ki-67 evaluation. Ki-67 is assessed as the average number of positive nuclei per area, using a 1 cm² ocular grid reticle at magnification of 400× in the highest labeled area of the neoplasm. For oral melanocytic neoplasms, *a threshold of >19.5 positive nuclei per grid is associated with lower survival times*.

For lesions in which H&E sections are insufficient to establish a definitive diagnosis (particularly for amelanotic spindle-cell melanomas that histomorphologically resemble other oral sarcomas), IHC is an important diagnostic tool. Most melanocytic neoplasms are cytokeratin negative and vimentin positive, but this does not differentiate them from other oral sarcomas. Immunoreactivity for S100, NSE, or SOX10 is also observed in melanomas, but these markers are nonspecific. Immunoreactivity for melan A is considered the most specific IHC marker for melanocytic neoplasms; however, studies have shown that only 92% of canine oral melanomas (a population that included 32% amelanotic neoplasms) were melan A positive; presumably, amelanotic malignant melanomas more frequently lack immunoreactivity for melan A. PNL2 and tyrosinase reactive proteins (TRP) 1 and 2 also are shown to be highly specific markers that target melanocytic antigens, and a melanocytic diagnostic IHC blend containing antibodies targeting melan A, PNL2, TRP1, and TRP2 has been shown to maintain 100% specificity while improving the sensitivity to 94% compared with melan A alone. This is currently the gold standard for diagnosing or confirming oral malignant melanomas in dogs. In oral malignant melanomas, intraepithelial neoplastic melanocytes are most often immunoreactive by IHC, thus it is critical to assess specimens with overlying oral epithelium.

In **cats**, oropharyngeal malignant melanoma is rare and accounts for <1% of all feline oral neoplasms; 22.5% of non-ocular melanocytic neoplasms occur in the lip or oral cavity of cats. The epithelioid variant is the most common histologic pattern, with spindloid, mixed, or balloon-cell variants also described. Most oral neoplasms in cats have ulceration and junctional activity, and <50% display lymphatic or vascular invasion, or intratumoral necrosis. The median survival of cats with oral melanocytic neoplasms is 83 days. When located in the oral cavity, neoplasms with negative prognostic factors including a mitotic count of ≥4 per 2.37 mm² (reported as per 10 hpf), significant cellular atypia, or intratumoral necrosis should be considered high grade. Melan A and PNL2 are highly sensitive markers to confirm feline oral melanocytic neoplasms, including amelanotic lesions.

Oral fibroma/fibrosarcoma (including canine and feline maxillary sarcomas). In **dogs**, fibrosarcoma is the third most common oral malignant tumor (behind melanoma and SCC), comprising ~8-25% of all malignant neoplasms. Oral fibromas are occasionally diagnosed, although they are much less common than their malignant counterpart. These need to be distinguished from proliferative fibro-osseous lesions, including ossifying fibroma, fibrous dysplasia, or fibromatous hyperplasia of the gingival ligament in dogs. Oral fibrosarcoma occurs at a median age of 8 years in dogs; one report indicates that 25% of oral fibrosarcomas occur in dogs <5-years-old. Larger breeds appear to be predisposed, and the Golden Retriever is over-represented. Oral fibrosarcomas occur as firm red nodules, primarily on the gingiva of the maxilla, hard and soft palate, rostral mandible, and less often in the buccal mucosa, lips, and tongue. These are not the same entity as soft tissue sarcomas of other anatomic locations, and oral fibrosarcomas often behave locally more aggressively, with infiltrative growth, ulceration, and possible deformity of the bones of the face; up to 72% of oral fibrosarcomas in dogs invade underlying bone. Overall survival is 270-740 days; up to 57% of masses recur locally, the metastatic rate is 0-23%.

Microscopically, the gingival fibrous stroma is infiltrated by densely cellular sheets and interwoven bundles of pleomorphic fusiform fibroblasts with variable but often relatively small amounts of collagen. The features of poor differentiation of the mesenchymal cells, increased mitotic figures, locally infiltrative growth, and areas of necrosis all aid in differentiation of fibrosarcoma from fibroma. Differential diagnoses should include odontogenic tumors, which usually include odontogenic epithelium, oral osteosarcoma, which produces extracellular osteoid matrix, and the spindle-cell variant of oral malignant melanoma. IHC for melanocytic markers (melan A, PNL2, TRP1, TRP2) is often required to distinguish amelanotic malignant melanoma from oral fibrosarcoma. Fibrosarcomas are expected to be immunonegative for actin, desmin, CD31, factor VIII–related antigen, and CD34.

The **histologically low-grade yet biologically high-grade sarcoma (high-low sarcoma)** of the oral cavity is a unique subtype of oral fibrosarcoma that occurs mostly on the maxilla of dogs. Histologic features, including haphazard proliferation of poorly cellular fibrous connective tissue supported by abundant collagenous stroma, minimal anisokaryosis, and low mitotic rate, all suggest a low-grade well-differentiated sarcoma. However, these aggressively infiltrate into adjacent tissue and are thus poorly demarcated from the adjacent soft tissues; they frequently invade readily into underlying muscle and/or bone. Although initial staging is often negative, metastases of fibrosarcoma to lung or local lymph nodes occurs in up to 20% of cases; the median survival is similar to routine oral fibrosarcomas. Although the histologic appearance is unique and suggests benignancy, this lesion should be strongly considered when observed in the oral cavity or maxilla, because an aggressive approach is warranted to obtain local control.

Oral or maxillary sarcomas in cats include fibrosarcomas and sarcomas with indeterminate histomorphology, but not melanocytic neoplasms. These are a group of aggressive mesenchymal neoplasms that occur mostly in the maxilla, palate, and upper lip of middle-aged to older cats. Oral sarcoma of cats has been considered historically to be the second most common oral neoplasm of cats behind SCC, although categorization has not always been clear. The most common presentation is a solitary nodule on the maxillary gingiva or as a localized irregular thickened and occasionally ulcerated region on the palate, which appear grossly identical to many other common oral lesions of cats (hyperplasia, granulation tissue, inflammation, etc.) and thus can be easily overlooked as possible neoplasia. Microscopic features include a population of highly cellular mesenchymal cells arranged in bundles and sheets with collagenous matrix, an average of 21 mitotic figures per 2.37 mm^2 (reported as ten 400× fields), and variable mixed inflammation or surface ulceration. Most cats experience rapid progressive disease as local recurrence including gingival and maxillary bone invasion, although distant metastasis has not been documented. Oral fibrosarcomas occur rarely in other species and have been described in sheep, cattle, and horses.

Several additional lesions have been grouped as proliferative fibro-osseous lesions of the oral cavity and jaws of animals. **Ossifying fibroma** is included here because it is considered a true neoplasm; the similar lesion known as **fibrous dysplasia** is considered above under the Non-neoplastic Proliferative and Reactive Lesions of the Oral Cavity section, because it is considered a dysplastic process.

Ossifying fibroma is considered a benign and rare neoplasm arising from tooth-bearing regions of the mandible and less often the maxilla, mostly in horses <1-year-old, dogs, and cats, although cases have also been reported in a rabbit, a llama, and a sheep. These intraosseous lesions are radiographically and clinically well-circumscribed masses of mandibular or maxillary bone. In the horse, these are often rapidly growing and can be locally invasive and destructive. They are composed microscopically of bland spindle-shaped neoplastic mesenchymal cells supported by minimal-to-moderate fibrovascular stroma and trabeculae of woven or lamellar bone, or mineralized bone spicules that appears to form intramembranously via osseous metaplasia. Although the trabeculae can vary in number and thickness, they are often covered by a single layer of osteoblasts; osteoclasts and bony trabecular remolding is occasionally observed. Some lesions have mineralized bony structures reminiscent of islands of cementum (cemental spheroids), and their presence suggests a more appropriate diagnosis of **cemento-osseous fibroma** (or cementifying fibroma). In addition, there can be destruction of the adjacent maxillary or mandibular bone along with tooth resorption, although these changes are probably secondary to atrophy. The major differential diagnoses for ossifying fibroma include fibrous dysplasia, low-grade osteosarcoma, fibrous osteodystrophy, osteoma, and fibromatous hyperplasia of the gingival ligament, although clearly the major challenge is distinguishing ossifying fibroma from fibrous dysplasia. Historically, palisading osteoblasts covering bone trabeculae were considered the defining feature of ossifying fibroma, but it is now recognized that this change may also occur in fibrous dysplasia. The bone in ossifying fibroma is usually well differentiated compared with the so-called proto-bone of fibrous dysplasia, which is composed of thinner spicules and poorly defined margins; however, this is not widely accepted as a defining or distinguishing feature. Ossifying fibromas are not invasive or infiltrative compared with fibrous dysplasia, so radiographs are key in determining the definitive diagnosis when histologic features are unclear. Features expected in low-grade osteosarcomas include infiltrative growth into adjacent bone (again, radiographs are often essential), the presence of cartilage, irregular mineralized woven bone, increased nuclear pleomorphism, and increased mitotic count. Osteomas are also well circumscribed but are composed of histologically dense bone with irregularly spaced osteocytes in lacunae, and with intervening medullary spaces containing fibrous connective tissue, and occasional marrow stromal cells.

Oral papilloma (papillomatosis) is a benign exophytic and often papillary epithelial neoplasm (*wart*) in dogs, cats, horses, and cattle, mostly associated with various host-specific papillomaviruses. In **dogs**, the cause is canine papillomavirus 1 (CPV1; *Canis familiaris* oral papillomavirus 1; *Papillomaviridae*, *Lambdapapillomavirus* 2), although canine papillomaviruses are quite diverse, so others may be involved. Lesions occur mainly in young animals, although older dogs in close contact may become infected. Oral papillomas are singular or multicentric, tend to expand progressively as pedunculated or rarely as irregular flattened plaques, and may become traumatized and bleed, but only cause significant concern when the lesions become severe and interfere with chewing, swallowing, or respiration.

Papillomaviruses are site specific, although several specific viruses have tropism for various organs (i.e., skin, oral cavity). Injury to the oral mucosa often precedes viral infection. Infection of basal epithelium of the squamous epithelium stimulates mitosis, and viral genome replication occurs in the differentiating keratinocytes of the spinous and granular layers. The incubation period is generally ~2 months. Spontaneous recovery is mediated by CD4 and CD8 T cells, usually occurs within 4-8 weeks, and is then followed by *enduring antibody-mediated immunity to reinfection*. Rare cases in dogs have been shown to progress from papilloma of the oral cavity to haired skin, or to SCC.

The lesions develop as single smooth papular elevations of the epithelium and then progress to various cauliflower-like pedunculated and exophytic firm white-to-gray squamous epithelial proliferations covering thin fibrovascular connective tissue cores (Fig. 1-15A). They develop on the lips, gingiva, buccal mucosa, tongue, palate, and oropharynx; less frequently, the esophagus and the skin of the muzzle are involved. Persistent and progressive infections, which may also involve haired skin remote from the mouth, are likely attributable to immunocompromise of the host.

The *microscopic structure* of fully developed lesions is typically verrucous, with irregularly thickened and hyperplastic keratinizing squamous epithelium covering thin branching often pedunculated cores of vascularized proprial papillae (see Fig. 1-15B). Epithelial cells of the basal, spinous, and granular layers are proliferative, and typically dysplastic and disorganized; irregularly sized and shaped basophilic keratohyaline granules are evident. Individual or clusters of papillomavirus-infected keratinocytes undergo ballooning degeneration, with expansion of lightly basophilic cytoplasm, and a small eccentric shrunken nucleus surrounded by a clear cytoplasmic halo (koilocytes) (see Fig. 1-15C). Additional viral cytopathic (CP) effects observed include individual swollen cells with abundant finely granular blue-gray cytoplasm, and irregular variably sized or clumped keratohyaline granules within the granular layer. *Basophilic intranuclear viral inclusions* may be found in cells in the outer spinous layers, but they are transient; intracytoplasmic inclusions also may be present (see Fig. 1-15C). Regressing lesions can be infiltrated by moderate numbers of T lymphocytes. Viral antigen can be demonstrated in nuclei of koilocytes or other infected epithelial cells by IHC, or electron microscopy reveals intranuclear 50-55 nm viral particles forming paracrystalline arrays.

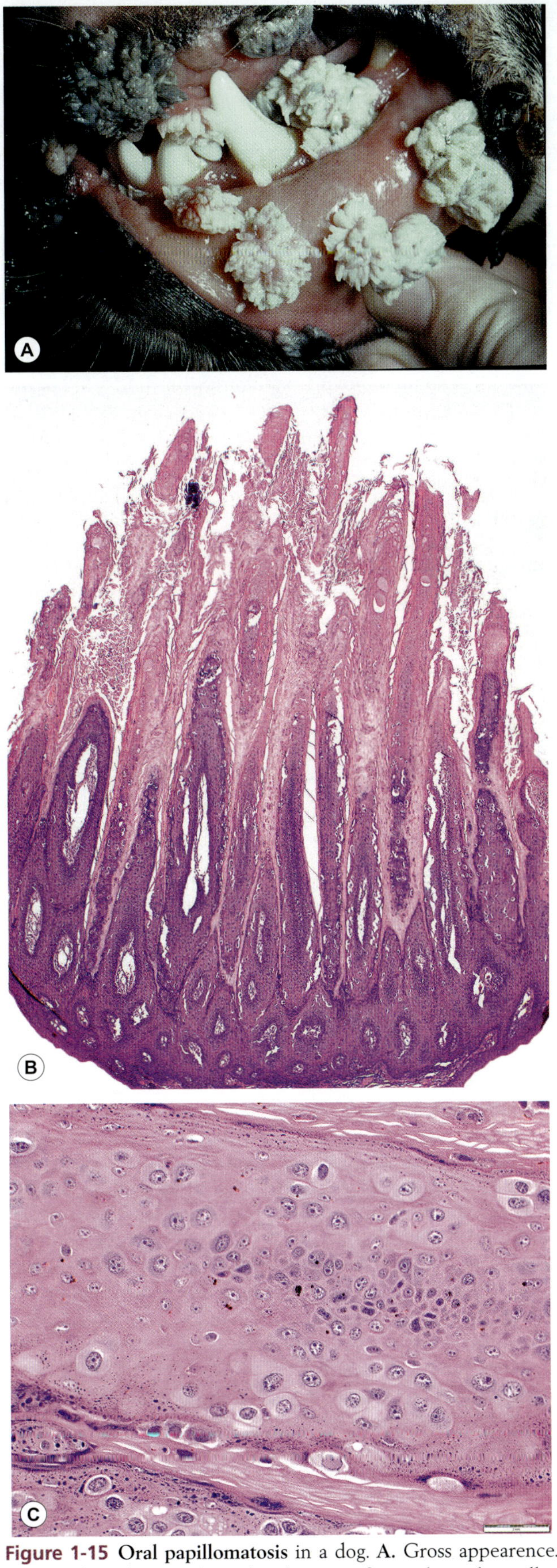

Figure 1-15 Oral papillomatosis in a dog. **A.** Gross appearence. **B.** Thin branching pedunculated cores of vascularized papillae extending from the gingival surface. **C.** Individual cells have viral cytopathic effects including intranuclear inclusion bodies.

In domestic and wild species of **cats**, oral papillomas are very rarely reported. These are likely caused by feline papillomavirus 1 (FcaPV1; *Felis domesticus* papillomavirus 1, *Papillomaviridae, Lambdapapillomavirus 1*) and occur most commonly in clusters on the ventral aspect of the tongue, although they are typically more sessile than verrucous. Histologic features are similar to canine oral papillomas, and they are also thought to regress spontaneously in most cases. Studies have detected FcaPV1 DNA in some oral SCCs and non-neoplastic oral tissue of cats, hence, while evidence shows that feline papillomaviruses infect the oral mucosa of cats, the role of the virus in development of oral papillomas or oral SCC remains unclear.

Oral papillomas in **cattle** caused by bovine papillomavirus 4 (BPV4; a strain of bovine papillomavirus 3, BPV3; *Bos taurus* papillomavirus 3, *Papillomaviridae, Xipapillomavirus 1*) occur in endemic areas. Their morphology and distribution in the oral cavity are similar to papillomas of dogs, but because they infect the esophagus and forestomachs extensively, they are considered more fully later in the section Proliferative and neoplastic lesions of the esophagus and forestomachs. A single report of a laryngeal papilloma in a **horse** was associated with equine papillomavirus 2 (EcPV2; *Equus caballus* papillomavirus 2, *Papillomaviridae, Dyoiotapapillomavirus 1*). A papillomavirus highly homologous with bovine papillomavirus 1 (BPV1; *Bos taurus* papillomavirus 1, *Papillomaviridae, Deltapapillomavirus 4*) has been isolated from a **llama** fibropapilloma.

Squamous cell carcinoma (SCC) is a significant disease in the oral cavity of dogs, and of wild and domestic cats; oral SCCs are also described in horses, ruminants, rodents, and various small mammals. Oral SCC is a malignant neoplasm arising from stratified squamous epithelium lining the oral cavity. This is a locally invasive and destructive neoplasm in all species and readily invades underlying bones of the maxilla or mandible (Fig. 1-16A). There is considerable morphologic variation in oral SCC, and although the proliferative keratinizing stratified squamous epithelium of well-differentiated SCC is readily recognized, neoplastic cells exhibiting poor differentiation, anaplasia, spindle-cell morphology, or those that do not produce keratin can be much more diagnostically challenging.

In **dogs**, SCC is one of the top 3 malignant neoplasms in the oral cavity, along with malignant oral melanoma and oral fibrosarcoma, although the incidence of each varies somewhat by study. Canine oral SCC occurs in slightly younger dogs overall compared with the other malignant neoplasms of the oral cavity (median of 8 years for oral SCC in dogs), and large dogs may be affected more often. Oral SCC has been described in juvenile dogs (<2-years-old), but the long-term prognosis was excellent with wide surgical excision, with no reports of recurrence or metastasis. Oral SCC frequently involves the tonsils and gingiva, although other oral anatomic locations, including buccal epithelium, palate, tonsillar crypts, or tongue, are involved less frequently. Mandibular and maxillary gingival epithelium appear to be equally affected. The etiology is likely multifactorial, including via initial gingival epithelial hyperplasia associated with chronic gingivitis, carcinogens associated with smog and smoke exposure in urban dogs, and, as alluded to previously, canine oral papillomavirus in some cases. Canine oral SCC has a reputation for local tissue destruction, including invasion into the underlying bone; metastasis occurs only later in the course of disease, usually to the regional lymph nodes, lungs, or more distant sites. Tonsillar SCC is less common but has a much higher metastatic rate than other locations. Lesions in the rostral oral cavity have a better prognosis, in large part because they are easier to completely excise surgically. Wide surgical excision continues to be the treatment of choice for oral SCC in general, and in most cases, this will prove to be curative.

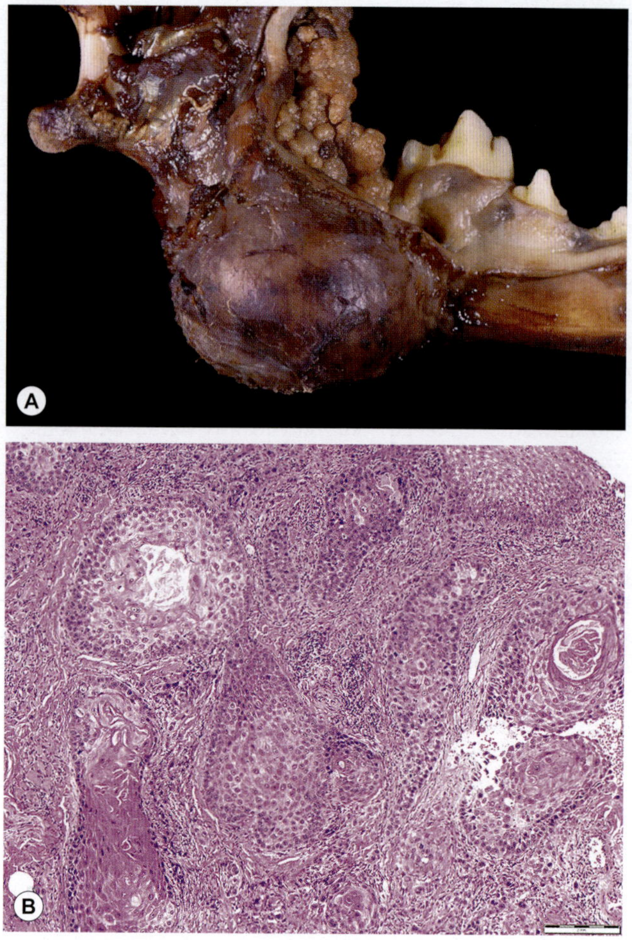

Figure 1-16 Squamous cell carcinoma arising from the gingiva and invading the mandible in a dog. **A.** Gross appearance (Courtesy Noah's Arkives.) **B.** Infiltrative neoplastic squamous epithelial cells form irregular branching trabeculae and islands with irregular maturation and dyskeratosis.

Gross features of oral SCC are quite variable, and these can appear as exophytic, nodular or multinodular, friable oral masses with surface ulceration, or they can appear as thickened, elevated, and firm plaque-like masses with normal overlying squamous epithelium. Thus, definitively distinguishing oral SCC from other proliferative lesions of the oral cavity is often impossible without radiographs and histologic evaluation. For the tonsillar form, lesions are usually unilateral. Early changes include a small slightly elevated granular plaque on the mucosal surface, which can be easily overlooked. In advanced stages, the affected tonsil is replaced by nodular firm neoplastic tissue, and the surface becomes ulcerated. Histologic examination reveals features typical of SCC, including neoplastic squamous epithelial cells forming islands, anastomosing trabeculae, or sheets embedded within dense fibrous stroma (scirrhous tissue). Neoplastic epithelial cell islands are rimmed by a layer of basal epithelial cells that mature centrally into polygonal keratinocytes with variably prominent intercellular bridges (desmosomes), and they form around central aggregates of keratin known as keratin pearls (see Fig. 1-16B). As a carcinoma, neoplastic cells display clear infiltration of the basement membrane and into the subepithelial fibrous stroma of the oral cavity, and these are observed as individual, clusters, or ribbons and cords of rounded, dysplastic, and often dyskeratotic eosinophilic squamous epithelial cells. Osteoid matrix can be produced in some gingival SCCs, so careful distinction should be made between gingival SCC and osteosarcoma. Inflammation is often a prominent feature in oral SCC and is likely exacerbated in neoplasms that undergo keratinization, or those with extensive surface ulceration.

Several histologic subtypes of oral nontonsillar SCC have been described in humans, including well to moderately to poorly differentiated conventional, papillary, basaloid, verrucous, spindle cell, and adenosquamous types. In dogs, most oral SCC are well differentiated and conventional, although there is no definitive evidence that subtype is correlated with prognosis. A critical challenge for pathologists is to distinguish canine oral SCC from the odontogenic neoplasm acanthomatous ameloblastoma (AA), because the 2 neoplasms can share several features. A key to the distinction is that oral SCCs lack the classic features of odontogenic epithelium (discussed below, with odontogenic neoplasms).

Papillary oral SCC is a unique subtype described in dogs that occurs as 1) an exophytic growth of neoplastic squamous epithelium reminiscent of a benign squamous papilloma projecting from the oral mucosal surface, or 2) as an epithelial-lined invasive intraosseous cavitating cyst within the maxillary or mandibular bone. Although they are described as 1 of these 2 distinct patterns, many lesions have features of both. The intraosseous variant can induce significant bone lysis and destruction, but these all appear to have minimal metastatic potential in dogs, and thus wide surgical excision is the treatment of choice. Canine oral papillary SCC may be misdiagnosed as oral papilloma if only superficial aspects of the lesion are evaluated, so it is important to carefully evaluate the margins histologically for evidence of invasive or infiltrative growth.

SCC *is by far the most common oral malignancy of* **cats** and represents ~70% of all malignant oral neoplasms in cats; oral fibrosarcoma and malignant melanoma occur much less frequently in cats than in dogs. Although there is anatomic variation, feline oral SCC is most frequently located on the ventral surface of the tongue, on the midline near the frenulum. The gingiva is the next most common site, and other locations including the tonsils, are generally involved much less frequently. In early stages, gingival SCCs can be easily mistaken for inflammation or other proliferative and ulcerated oral lesions; they are often quite advanced at presentation. *The neoplasm is locally invasive* especially into bone and local soft tissues and has an overall high mortality rate. Feline oral SCC has historically been considered metastatic only late in disease (as in dogs), but up to 36% of oral SCC are metastatic to local lymph nodes at the time of presentation. The cause continues to be debated, but several potential causes have been suggested including feline oral papillomavirus, tobacco smoke, consumption of canned food or tuna, use of flea collars, or chronic oral inflammation of periodontal disease.

Grossly, feline oral SCC are irregular nodular red-gray friable masses, often with an ulcerated surface that bleeds easily. Some are adhered to underlying soft tissue structures and even periosteum or bone; they often invade underlying bone and cause significant local destruction of maxilla, mandible, palatal bone, and nasal turbinates. Microscopically, the neoplasm is a conventional SCC in appearance, with usually well-differentiated squamous epithelial cells in nests, interconnected trabeculae, or sheets embedded within dense fibrous connective tissue. As for canine oral SCC, there is often extensive intratumoral inflammation (especially in ulcerated lesions), and there may be formation of cysts, comedones, or true keratin pearls. Subtypes have not been described in cats (as for dogs), although various subtypes likely occur. Subtype has no apparent significance with respect to behavior or prognosis, and even well-differentiated oral SCC in cats can be highly aggressive and locally destructive. Although bone invasion is common, care must be taken to distinguish this from metaplastic bone. As for dogs, surgical excision with wide margins is the standard of care, although, because local invasive behavior has often occurred by initial presentation, adequate local control is often difficult to achieve and median reported survival is 3-14 months.

In **horses**, SCCs are found rarely on the gingiva, tongue, pharynx, and hard palate, possibly arising in chronically inflamed and hyperplastic alveolar epithelium during chronic periodontitis. There is evidence for involvement of papillomaviruses in the etiology of equine mucosal SCC, although the role of papillomavirus in oral SCC has not been well established. They are slow growing, but are often exceedingly locally destructive, and metastasize late to regional lymph nodes. Such tumors are large when first observed and may project from the palate or gingiva as gray ulcerated masses, or as craterous ulcers. The large ones are extensively necrotic, and the teeth are lost or loosely embedded in the tumor. These tumors of the maxilla rapidly fill the adjacent sinuses and cause bulging of the face, and may extend into the nasal, orbital, and cranial cavities. As is true for other species, the microscopic appearance of oral SCC in horses varies considerably, from well-differentiated lesions with keratinization of individual epithelial cells and formation of keratin pearls, to poorly differentiated lesions with little or no evidence of keratinization.

In **cattle**, oral SCCs are very rare with the exception of a few geographic areas where they are associated with oral papillomatosis and ingestion of bracken fern. A similar association is made in the etiology of SCC of the esophagus and forestomachs in cattle and is considered more fully in the section Proliferative and neoplastic lesions of the stomach and abomasum. There are sporadic reports of oral SCC on the lower lip of **sheep**. Oral SCCs also occur in **camelids**.

Lymphoma occurs in many species, in almost equally impressive and diverse variations and types, and with a wide variety of biologic behaviors. **Oral lymphoma** is described infrequently in dogs and cats and mostly occurs as part of generalized disease. Oral lymphomas may arise in oral-associated lymphoid tissue, such as mucosal-associated lymphoid tissue (MALT) including tonsil (usually of B-cell origin). Localized spread into the oral mucosa from the nearby lip or nasal cavity, or metastatic spread from a distant site also occur. Many cases of oral lymphoma are composed of epitheliotropic T cells, but most epitheliotropic lymphomas are not restricted to the oral cavity and involve haired skin of affected patients.

Rare cases of non-epitheliotropic oral cavity lymphoma are described. Histologic features of lymphoma in the oral cavity are similar to lymphomas occurring in other locations. As one would expect, the prognosis for oral lymphoma is usually guarded, although localized radiation is an effective treatment. Differential diagnoses should include lymphoid hyperplasia, chronic inflammation, or other round-cell neoplasms. Definitive diagnosis or lymphoma can be aided by IHC using T- or B-cell markers. Rare cases of oral lymphoma are also described in horses and ruminants.

Granular cell tumor is an uncommon benign lesion that is described in the oral cavity of dogs and rarely cats, or in the lung of horses. These occur mostly in the tongue of older dogs, some are multifocal and are thought to derive from neuroectodermal precursor cells; possibly they are of neural crest origin. Granular cell tumors are small solid nodules comprising dense sheets, nests, or cords of large polygonal cells with abundant finely eosinophilic granular cytoplasm and are supported by minimal collagenous stroma. The nuclei are small, mitotic figures are rare, and the cytoplasmic granules are usually variably PAS positive, but do not stain by acid fast, toluidine blue, or Giemsa stains. Ultrastructurally, these granules are most consistent with *phagolysosomes*. None of these lesions in dogs have recurred after excision, and there are only rare reports of metastasis to thoracic organs. They are histomorphologically similar to rhabdomyoma and oncocytoma in the oropharyngeal space, so special stains and IHC may prove helpful in definitive diagnosis, although overlap exists in that oncocytomas of salivary gland origin can also stain positive by PAS. There is some debate whether these represent true neoplasms, and some suggest that they are more likely an inflammatory or reactive lesion. **Oral histiocytic foam cell nodules** are described as aggregates of inflammatory or reactive histocytes that are PAS negative and positive for the macrophage receptor CD204; however, there is considerable histomorphologic overlap between foam cell nodules and granular cell tumors. There are a few reports of granular cell tumor in the tonsil, tongue, gingiva, and palate of **cats**. In **horses**, granular cell tumors occur most frequently in the lungs (see Vol. 2, Respiratory System).

Although very common in the skin of dogs, **mast cell tumor (MCT)** occurs only rarely in the oral cavity and even less frequently in cats. Most commonly they are found on the lip of dogs, but they may arise in gingiva or other oral mucosae. MCT is diagnosed using the same criteria as cutaneous MCTs, and *all should be considered potentially malignant*, with metastasis to regional lymph nodes more common than for cutaneous or subcutaneous MCTs. In one study, 55-72% of dogs had evidence of mast cells in draining lymph nodes by cytology (although these were not confirmed histologically) at presentation, and 48% died or were euthanized due to local or regional mast cell disease. Lymph node metastasis was common and appears to be a significant negative prognostic indicator, although distant metastatic disease was rare. Overall, oral MCTs have a more aggressive biologic behavior than their cutaneous variants. Oral tumors with >5 mitotic figures per 2.37 mm^2 (reported as 10 hpf) have significantly reduced time to the progression of disease. MCT should be considered in the differential diagnosis of oral lesions resembling granulation tissue or eosinophilic granuloma in dogs and cats. **Oral MCTs in cats** are very uncommon, and little is known about their behavior. A major differential diagnosis should be oral eosinophilic granuloma, which is more common in the oral cavity of cats. MCTs typically lack significant necrosis, collagenolysis, prominent eosinophilic infiltration, and evidence of degranulation of mast cells.

Extramedullary oral plasma cell tumor accounts for ~5% of all oral neoplasms in dogs, and are very rare in cats. These are aggregates of proliferative monoclonal plasma cells originating in soft tissues including oral cavity (as well as skin and GI tract); they rarely represent metastases from primary bone marrow multicentric myeloma. Historically, oral plasma cell tumors have been considered completely benign, although local recurrence or distant metastasis does occur.

Oral plasma cell tumors occur as red lobulated nodules, usually located on the tongue, gingiva, or lips; lesion location has no prognostic significance. Histologically, the neoplasm is well-circumscribed, nonencapsulated, and the overlying mucosa is usually intact unless it has been traumatized in large tumors. Neoplastic cells are often quite pleomorphic with variable amounts of amphophilic-to-basophilic cytoplasm, a single round-to-oval often-indented nucleus. The cells are densely packed into nests and sheets and divided by scant fibrovascular stroma. Anisokaryosis and karyomegaly, as well as binucleate or prominent large multinucleate cells, are often evident in the center of the neoplasm, with the most well-differentiated plasma cells more prominent along the periphery. Degree of differentiation, cellular pleomorphism, or multinucleation are not correlated with the progression of disease or plasma cell tumor-related death. The mitotic count can vary widely, and although most plasma cell tumors are benign, mitotic count has been shown to be significantly related to biologic behavior or disease progression. Immunoglobulin (especially IgG) can frequently be demonstrated by IHC in the neoplastic cells, and AL (light chain) amyloid is occasionally present among the tumor cells, which can be confirmed by Congo red staining. While historically considered benign, a retrospective study has suggested that recurrence or progression of plasma cell disease occurs in a small percentage of dogs through the development of additional plasma cell tumors in the oral cavity or skin, metastatic disease to the liver or lung, and even progression to multiple myeloma (2 dogs). Although disease progression appears to be quite uncommon, predictive histologic features including high mitotic count (>28 mitotic figures per 2.37 mm^2) and moderate-to-severe nuclear atypia may be associated with more biologically aggressive variants. Complete surgical excision remains the treatment of choice. Rarely in dogs and cats, oral plasma cell tumors can infiltrate underlying maxillary or mandibular bone causing localized osteolysis, but even with evidence of more aggressive behavior, these probably do not metastasize widely, and excision is likely to prove curative in most cases. Differential diagnoses for oral extramedullary plasma cell tumor include other round-cell tumors, such as MCT, lymphoma, histiocytoma, or melanoma; IHC using multiple myeloma 1/interferon regulatory factor 4 (MUM1/IRF4) is a sensitive and specific antibody for confirming plasma cells, although some lymphomas may also express MUM1.

Vascular tumors, including congenital *vascular hamartomas, hemangiomas, and hemangiosarcomas*, have been described in the gingiva of neonatal calves and in the oral cavity of puppies. Benign hamartomas or congenital vascular malformations are focal disorganized overgrowths of mature vascular tissue endogenous to the organ involved. They may have an inflamed or ulcerated surface and resemble trauma-induced granulation tissue. These are mostly located on the rostral mandibular gingiva adjacent to the incisors or tongue. Microscopically, the lesions consist of irregular thin-walled vascular channels containing erythrocytes or proteinaceous material and lined by well-differentiated endothelial cells.

Hemangioma is a benign well-circumscribed noninvasive lesion of proliferative well-differentiated endothelial cells lining vascular channels; this has been described or observed rarely in the oral cavity of mature horses, dogs, and cats. Hemangiosarcomas are malignant endothelial cell neoplasms that probably arise mostly from the tongue of dogs, but have been described in tongue, gingiva, palate, or lips of dogs and cats. Histologic features are similar to hemangiosarcoma in other tissues, can be locally aggressive, and have significant potential for distant metastasis. For less-well-differentiated lesions that lack vascular channels, IHC targeting factor VIII-related antigen, CD31, or claudin 5 may be diagnostically useful. A single hemangiosarcoma in a young calf has been described that involved palate and gingiva, with presumed metastasis to distant sites.

Neuroendocrine carcinomas (carcinoids) originate from the dispersed neuroendocrine system present at a low density throughout the GI tract, mostly these tumors arise from the mucosa of stomach or intestine, and parenchyma of the pancreas or liver in several mammalian species; lesions rarely are reported in the oral cavity of dogs and cats. Carcinoids are considered moderately aggressive and may be endocrinologically active. They have histomorphologic features similar to neuroendocrine carcinomas in other locations, with epithelial cells forming nests and packets supported by fine fibrous and highly vascular stroma. Features that suggest malignancy include cellular atypia, increased mitotic count, local infiltrative growth, or distant metastasis. Oral carcinoids should be differentiated from oral mucosal granular cell tumors and from malignant melanomas; special or immunohistochemical reactions are typically helpful. Carcinoids are PAS negative, although they are positive for argyrophilic granules by Churukian-Schenk staining; they are usually but variably immunoreactive by IHC for synaptophysin, neuron-specific enolase, chromogranin A, cytokeratin, synaptophysin, or somatostatin. Ultrastructurally, the neoplastic cells contain *cytoplasmic secretory granules characteristic of neuroendocrine cells*.

Various additional **miscellaneous** benign or malignant neoplastic lesions in the oral cavity have been reported sporadically. Benign masses in **dogs** include dermoid cysts, histiocytoma, lipoma, lymphangioma, rhabdomyoma, chondrosarcoma, and ganglioneuroma. Malignant neoplasms that have been reported in the oral cavity, mainly in the lip and tongue, include leiomyosarcoma, ectopic thyroid carcinoma, schwannoma or peripheral nerve sheath tumors, osteosarcoma, rhabdomyosarcoma, and malignant undifferentiated tumors. Benign masses in **cats** include fibroxanthoma; malignant neoplasms of cats include malignant oral and tonsillar lymphoma, schwannoma or peripheral nerve sheath tumor, and osteosarcoma. Salivary tumors are described later in the Salivary Glands section.

Neoplasms of odontogenic tissues

Evaluating proliferative lesions of the tooth-bearing regions of the jaws and oral cavity can be particularly confusing because various tissue components are often intermixed, including epithelium, variably mineralized dental matrices, and stromal elements. It is thus important to recall the inductive pattern of tooth development, reviewed beautifully in the text Veterinary Oral and Maxillofacial Pathology, by Murphy et al., 2019. Based on this updated classification system, the best approach to accurate diagnosis of odontogenic neoplasms must begin with consideration of the 4 major odontogenic tissues, including 1) odontogenic epithelium; 2) dental matrices; 3) dental papilla; and 4) dental follicle.

Remnants of **odontogenic epithelium** from tooth embryogenesis persist in the gingiva and periodontium, and nests of odontogenic epithelium are found incidentally in many proliferative lesions of this region. Gingival squamous-type epithelium proliferates in response to irritation and can form complex branching patterns within the subepithelial fibrous stroma that are easily confused with odontogenic-type epithelium. Neoplasms of odontogenic epithelium can arise *centrally* from the periodontium embedded within the alveolar sulci of the bones of the mandible and maxilla, or *peripherally* from the gingival epithelium lining the oral cavity. Correct identification of odontogenic epithelium in proliferative lesions of the oral cavity and jaws is thus critical; it can be at times quite difficult to distinguish from other types of epithelium. Odontogenic epithelial cells often display one or more of the classic histomorphologic features, including 1) reverse polarity of the cells with their nuclei located at the apex of the cell and distal to the basement membrane (antibasilar nuclei); 2) palisading arrangement of the epithelium along the fibrous stroma; 3) distinct basilar cytoplasmic clearing; and 4) prominent intercellular desmosomal bridges between central polygonal odontogenic epithelial cells (reminiscent of stellate reticulum). Odontogenic epithelial cells commonly are arranged as plexiform ribbons, round follicle-like structures, anastomosing trabeculae, and/or unique structures known as ink drops, and although various phenotypes can be observed in a single lesion, they are not specific for odontogenic epithelium. Because the epithelium can also undergo squamous metaplasia, complex lesions can be quite confusing and disorienting. Centralized degeneration and cyst formation are common features of odontogenic epithelium, and recognition of this can be a helpful diagnostic feature.

Dental matrices refer either to enamel generated by ameloblasts, dentin produced by odontoblasts, or to woven bone produced by osteoblasts, but not to cementum produced by cementoblasts (associated with the dental follicle). Dentin is the more commonly observed matrix in proliferative odontogenic lesions of animals, although it is usually atubular osteodentin or tertiary dentin (discussed previously) that lacks recognizable dentinal tubules. Due to the inductive process of odontogenesis that renders ameloblasts incapable of producing enamel without the reciprocal inductive signals from accompanying odontoblasts, the odontoblasts are thus required for lesions featuring odontogenic matrix production. Odontogenic matrix is often rimmed by a row of epithelial cells including ameloblasts or odontoblasts, although the matrix itself can appear histologically similar to other eosinophilic substances, including amyloid, fibrin, or keratin, or it can bear resemblance to the matrices of the dental follicle including cementum and osteoid.

The **dental papilla** is the ectomesenchyme induced by the enamel organ (ameloblasts producing enamel) that eventually becomes the dental pulp of the forming tooth structure.

This appears histologically as a loose aggregate of bland spindle-shaped cells supported by mucinous-to-myxoid stroma, and it must be distinguished from the normal gingival fibrous connective tissue stroma of the oral cavity, and from the periodontal or gingival ligament. This is not always straightforward, so cytokeratin and vimentin IHC can be helpful to confirm odontogenic epithelium and ectomesenchyme-derived pulp tissue, respectively; however, some authors have reported embryonic enamel organ (stellate reticulum and ameloblasts) to express both cytokeratin and vimentin.

The **dental follicle** is the precursor to the periodontal ligament, cementum, and the peripheral rim of alveolar bone; multipotential stem cells of the dental follicle are able to produce cementum (by cementoblasts), osteoid (by osteoblasts), and collagen (by fibroblasts), which collectively anchor the tooth in the alveolar socket of the mandible and maxilla. Given the frequency of fibromatous hyperplasia of the gingival ligament in the oral cavity of dogs, the gingival (or periodontal) ligament should be recognized by classic histomorphologic features including poorly to densely cellular aggregates of fibroblasts and regular empty blood vascular spaces embedded within the fine fibrillar matrix, but they lack robust bundles of collagen indicative of gingival fibrous stroma. Successfully distinguishing the periodontal or gingival ligament-derived connective tissues from gingival fibrous stroma, reactive fibrosis, and neoplastic fibroblasts of the oral cavity is important, and can be surprisingly difficult in some cases.

Because of the process of reciprocal induction of dental tissues during odontogenesis, a common feature in complex odontogenic neoplasms is that of *induction*, which implies an effect on the dental follicular ectomesenchyme by the odontogenic epithelial ameloblasts. In some but not all odontogenic neoplasms, neoplastic epithelial cells induce development of ectomesenchyme derived from the dental papilla, which results in true mixed odontogenic tumors; by definition, these are composed of neoplastic odontogenic epithelium + induced ectomesenchyme (Fig. 1-17).

In summary, proliferative lesions of dental tissues are classified in general based on identification of the 4 specific odontogenic features described above and are typically classified either as *epithelial neoplasms* (with or without odontogenic ectomesenchyme and/or dental matrices) or *ectomesenchymal neoplasms*. True *neoplasms of dental tissues are rare*, except for canine acanthomatous ameloblastomas. Most are *nonmalignant, although some can be quite infiltrative, locally destructive, or expansive*. Their location predetermines destruction of alveolar bone and displacement of teeth, and they can be quite difficult to excise completely.

Conventional ameloblastoma (CA) and **ameloblastic carcinoma** are uncommon in dogs and cats and are similar to their much more common relative, the acanthomatous ameloblastoma (below). The terms *adamantinoma* and *enameloblastoma* were formerly used for this lesion but are now considered obsolete synonyms. This is a slowly progressive and locally invasive neoplasm arising from proliferative odontogenic epithelium (ameloblasts) embedded within the fibrous connective tissue stroma of the oral cavity. These are more common in dogs than in cats and horses and are more common in the mandible than in the maxilla. Neoplasms formerly described as ameloblastomas in young cattle now fit best within the criteria of ameloblastic fibromas (AFs), discussed in the following section. Ameloblastomas originate from transformed odontogenic epithelium arising from the enamel organ, dental lamina, outer enamel epithelium, dental follicle around retained unerupted teeth, or odontogenic cysts of oral or extraoral sites. They are *predominantly intraosseous,*

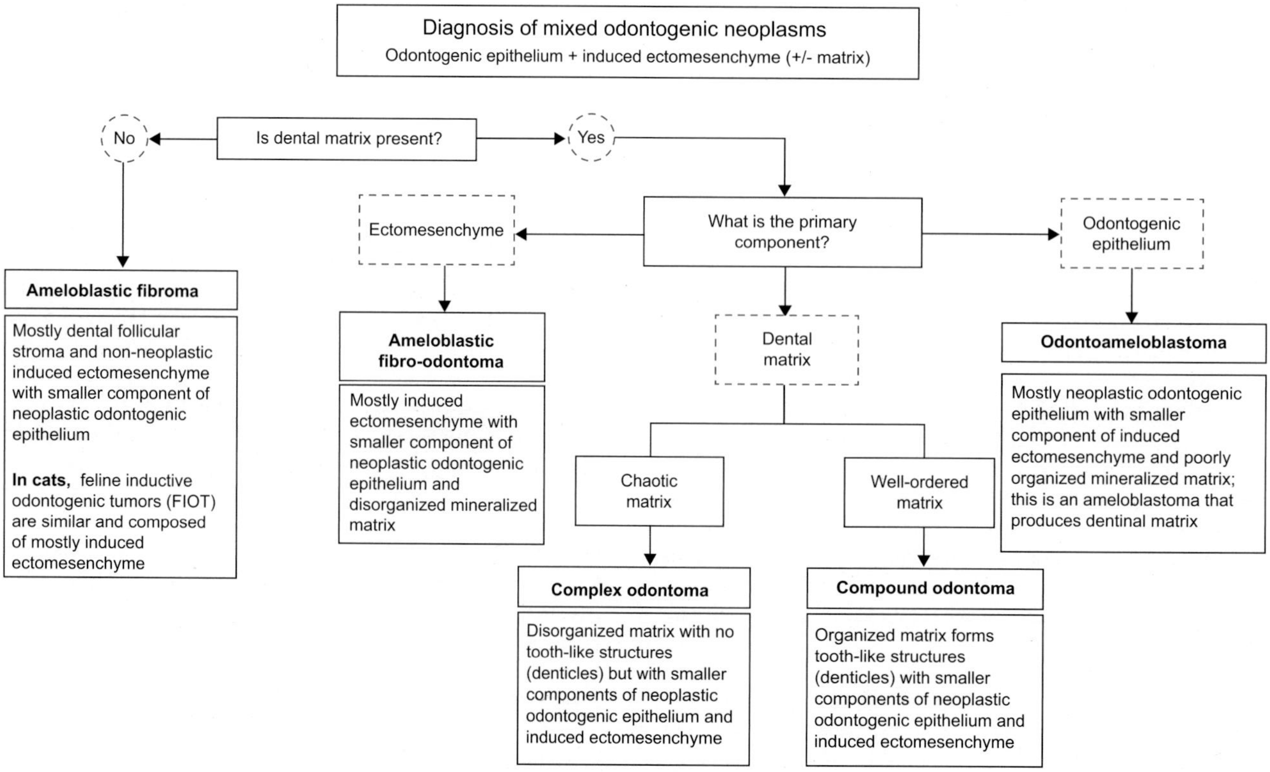

Figure 1-17 Diagnosis of mixed odontogenic neoplasms.

although they also occur as solitary gingival masses. Even though they are considered benign, they may destroy large amounts of bone due simply to their anatomic location, and they may extend into the oral cavity or sinuses; large tumors may undergo central degeneration and become cystic.

Odontogenic epithelium is the sine qua non criterion for diagnosis of ameloblastoma, although the proportions of odontogenic epithelium and peripheral stroma can vary significantly. Neoplastic cells of CA usually display all features of odontogenic epithelium including peripheral palisading basilar epithelium with antibasilar nuclei and basilar clear zone. Importantly, the long prominent intercellular desmosomal bridges between central odontogenic epithelial cells that are reminiscent of stellate reticulum of the enamel organ are usually prominent in CA, although they are not often evident in acanthomatous type ameloblastoma. Odontogenic epithelium of ameloblastoma may appear as any of several patterns, including follicular, plexiform, islands, irregular anastomosing trabeculae or strands, or ink drop structures; many contain several patterns. Odontogenic cysts may develop following central degeneration of odontogenic epithelial islands or from stromal degeneration. Small cysts may coalesce to form grossly evident cavities. Ameloblastomas also may occasionally undergo keratinization (these were formerly termed *keratinizing ameloblastoma*) or mineralization, and although these features lack significant prognostic significance, they can cause confusion during description and histologic diagnosis; CA thus may be confused with SCC or osteosarcoma. CAs are locally invasive (including into bone) but not metastatic (as previously discussed), so local excision is the treatment of choice; surgical excision with relatively narrow margins is usually sufficient to achieve clearance of the ameloblastoma and localized cure.

Ameloblastic carcinoma is the malignant variant of ameloblastoma, and these are uncommonly reported in dogs and a single horse. The histologic features are as expected for neoplasms of odontogenic epithelium, although a diagnosis of carcinoma is warranted when there are additional features of malignancy, including cellular pleomorphism, anisocytosis, or anisokaryosis, increased mitotic count, areas of necrosis, loss of odontogenic features, evidence of overt invasion through the basement membrane by neoplastic odontogenic epithelial cells, or distant metastasis (although the latter 2 features are extraordinarily uncommon). Because this lesion is often poorly differentiated and lacks the classic features of odontogenic epithelium (which are normally present in conventional ameloblastoma), and because they can undergo keratinization, there may be considerable difficulty distinguishing ameloblastic carcinoma from SCC; these are probably impossible to distinguish in some cases. A diagnosis of ameloblastic carcinoma should be considered in cases of odontogenic epithelial neoplasia arising from gingiva or bones of the jaw, in which there are cytologic features of malignancy.

Canine acanthomatous ameloblastoma (AA) is an odontogenic epithelial neoplasm arising from odontogenic rests of ameloblasts located either peripherally within the gingival epithelium or centrally within the periodontal ligament adjacent to alveolar bone and tooth of dogs. These are exceedingly common and unique to the dog; they display affinity to bone, and thus can be locally aggressive and invasive into the underlying bones of the jaw (Fig. 1-18A), causing tooth loss and frequent local recurrence following conservative

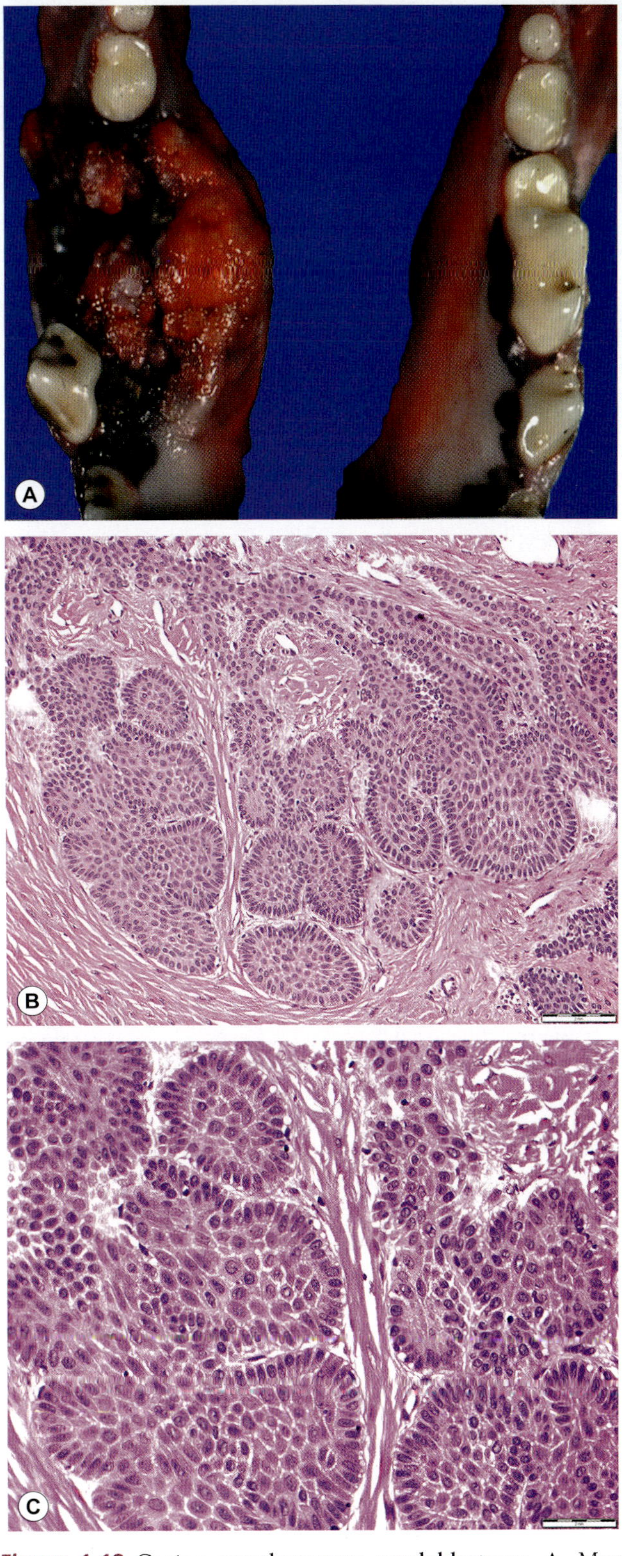

Figure 1-18 Canine **acanthomatous ameloblastoma.** A. Mass invading bone of the mandible and displacing teeth. (Courtesy Noah's Arkives.) B. Neoplastic odontogenic epithelium forming interconnected cords in the subgingival connective tissue. C. Neoplastic cells with features of odontogenic epithelium, including antibasilar nuclei, prominent intercellular desmosomes, and basal vacuoles.

treatment. Because this lesion arises from odontogenic epithelium, it is not considered a mixed or inductive odontogenic neoplasm, although the neoplastic ameloblasts do influence the supportive fibrous connective tissue stroma, which probably arises from the dental follicle and thus often bears considerable resemblance to periodontal ligament. These lesions arise from anywhere on the maxillary or mandibular gingiva (although the rostral mandible is most commonly affected), and they appear initially as small solid sessile-to-irregular and exophytic nodules; it is not possible to distinguish them from other common benign or malignant oral proliferative lesions in dogs. As an ameloblastoma, the neoplastic epithelium displays the characteristic histomorphologic features of odontogenic epithelium outlined above (see Fig. 1-18B); however, instead of the typical elongated arborizing intercellular desmosomes reminiscent of stellate reticulum observed in CAs, the central odontogenic epithelial cells of AA are what gives this lesion its identity and name. Sheets of thorny interlocking eosinophilic epithelial prickle cells are reminiscent of the spinous layer cells of haired skin (see Fig. 1-18C). The surrounding stroma of the AA likely arises from the periodontal ligament, and as such there are frequently islands of variably mineralized dental matrix embedded, which should not be confused with tumor bone (osteoid). These are usually relatively homogeneous lesions with minimal cellular atypia, although increased mitotic figures or cellular pleomorphism is observed in inflamed or ulcerated lesions, making interpretation more difficult. Finally, continuity with the overlying hyperplastic gingival epithelium and/or keratinization are both features of AAs, so care should be taken to avoid misdiagnosis of SCC, which is not expected to display the features of odontogenic epithelium. Like CA, canine AA is often locally invasive, especially into underlying bone, so excision (which often includes partial mandibulectomy or maxillectomy) is typically curative, even in cases in which excision margins are narrow; metastases are not recorded in the literature. SCC, and occasionally fibrosarcoma or osteosarcoma, has been reported from the site of irradiated AAs, several months to many years after treatment.

Amyloid-producing ameloblastoma, formerly known as *amyloid-producing odontogenic tumor* and *calcifying epithelial odontogenic tumor*, is a rare odontogenic neoplasm that occurs as an unencapsulated gingival mass in dogs and cats (and individual reports in a wide variety of species). These arise from odontogenic epithelium within the gingiva of the mandible or maxilla. They can arise from within the bone or from the soft tissues adjacent to the bone (presumably from ectopic ameloblasts); regardless, these are usually locally invasive and destructive, and thus difficult to excise completely. Histologic features of these lesions can be impressively variable. The odontogenic epithelium has histomorphologic features of odontogenic ameloblastic epithelium, as well as frequent cyst formation, resulting from central degeneration as described previously. In some cases, the odontogenic epithelium is poorly differentiated, lacks the classic morphologic features, and resembles proliferative mesenchymal stroma, so IHC using keratin and vimentin to differentiate epithelium from mesenchymal tissue types, or simply careful evaluation of additional sections to definitively identify even small regions of odontogenic differentiation may be warranted. As for other ameloblastomas, the epithelium may undergo keratinization and further complicate the diagnostic process, especially because keratin can appear histomorphologically similar to amyloid. In addition to neoplastic ameloblasts, abundant amyloid or amyloid-like deposits are typically scattered as islands of extracellular eosinophilic material often surrounding individualized or clustered neoplastic epithelial cells. These deposits can be partially mineralized or intermixed with enamel matrix proteins, keratin, dental matrices, osteoid, or pre-existing lamellar bone, all contributing to diagnostic difficulty. Congo red staining and light polarization, thioflavin T, or mass spectrometry–based proteomic analysis indicate that the material is consistent with amyloid or amyloid precursor proteins (ameloblastin, amelogenin, sheathlin) secreted by ameloblasts; however, the material in some cases appears histomorphologically indistinguishable but lacks staining for either Congo red or thioflavin T. Similar to other ameloblastomas, major differential diagnoses include conventional ameloblastoma, SCC, or less likely odontoameloblastoma (OA). Although histologically distinct, these tumors have biologic behavior similar to other ameloblastomas and are considered benign but potentially highly locally invasive odontogenic neoplasms that are still mostly cured with local control via complete surgical excision.

Two specific mixed odontogenic neoplasms are composed of neoplastic odontogenic epithelium (ameloblasts) and *induced* odontogenic ectomesenchyme of the dental papilla but *lack dental matrices*: these include the ameloblastic fibroma and feline inductive odontogenic tumor (FIOT) (see Fig. 1-17).

The **ameloblastic fibroma** (AF) is considered a true mixed odontogenic neoplasm with induction but without dentinal matrices [enamel or dentin, which distinguishes this lesion from the ameloblastic fibro-odontoma (AFO)]; because AF does not produce dentinal matrix, it has been considered a less-differentiated variant of the AFO and possibly the odontoma by some. These are complex neoplasms of odontogenic epithelium that have also been referred to as fibroameloblastoma (it is after all, an epithelial neoplasm with induction of non-neoplastic ectomesenchyme); however, this is mostly considered an antiquated term. AF is a slowly growing and non-infiltrative neoplasm that occurs mostly in young horses, dogs, and cats (these have been mostly recategorized as FIOTs). It is the *most common odontogenic tumor of cattle and* is found most often near the mandibular incisors of calves. This neoplasm often appears as a well-circumscribed lucency in the mandible and may be associated with tooth eruption; in fact, it has been hypothesized to represent a form of dysplasia rather than neoplasia by some authors.

The lesion is composed histologically of neoplastic odontogenic epithelium (ameloblasts) arranged in cords or plexiform ribbons and embedded within the nodular aggregates of poorly differentiated induced non-neoplastic ectomesenchyme of dental papilla origin and fibrous stroma (periodontal ligament) of dental follicle origin, but *without* dentin or enamel matrix production. Based on a few case reports, these generally behave like ameloblastomas, although they are less likely to infiltrate or invade bone. Rare cases of malignancy are reported. Some of these have been diagnosed as ameloblastic (fibro)sarcoma. These should be distinguished from conventional and acanthomatous ameloblastomas, SCCs, and FIOTs. For most AFs, excision of the tumor is sufficient to achieve a cure.

Feline inductive odontogenic tumor (FIOT, *infiltrative inductive AF*, or previously *inductive fibroameloblastoma*) is a rare true mixed-odontogenic tumor that is very similar histologically to the AF. This lesion is specific to cats and occurs almost exclusively in kittens as osteolytic nodules peripherally or centrally in the rostral maxilla (other locations are much less common), causing tooth loss or facial distortion. Aggregates or plexiform ribbons of neoplastic odontogenic epithelium partially envelop spherical or polypoid nodules of variably cellular dental ectomesenchyme that may form structures reminiscent of the early cap stage of tooth development in which odontogenic epithelium invests the dental papilla prior to differentiation of odontoblasts or formation of dentinal matrices dentin or enamel. This likely represents abortive attempts at odontogenesis, and therefore the presence of odontogenic epithelium and odontogenic ectomesenchyme in a young cat warrants a search for histologic evidence of the early cap stage development to confirm the diagnosis, although that feature can be uncommon in some lesions. Some (but not all) can be locally infiltrative, and although limited information has been published for biologic behavior of FIOTs, these are likely slowly growing masses that do not metastasize, and for which complete surgical excision is curative.

Mixed-odontogenic tumors with dental matrices include AFO, OA, and odontoma (see Fig. 1-17). All are mixed-odontogenic neoplasms that share features of neoplastic odontogenic epithelium, induced ectomesenchyme of dental papilla origin, and dental matrix; the major distinction between AFO and OA is that they represent opposite ends of the spectrum with respect to the dominant component tissue; the AFO is primarily composed of ectomesenchyme; the OA is primarily composed of odontogenic epithelium. The odontomas rest between these extremes and typically contain the highest proportion of dental matrices.

The **ameloblastic fibro-odontoma** (AFO) is very similar to the previously described AF, although in addition to those features described for AF, there is also evidence of dental matrix production, usually in the form of dentin or enamel. In essence, the AFO is an AF with dental matrix production and is distinguished from odontoma and odontoameloblastoma by the large proportion of induced ectomesenchyme of the dental papilla (this is the major component in AFO lesions). Most authors consider this to be part of the spectrum of mixed-odontogenic neoplasms, although the AFO has been removed from the World Health Organization classification of head and neck tumors in humans. This is an uncommon lesion that has been described in dogs, horses, and cattle. Grossly, these are distinct cystic and sclerotic lesions in bone of maxilla and mandible. Histologic features include abundant, often primitive, myxoid ectomesenchyme of the dental papilla with less embedded odontogenic epithelium (although the amount of epithelium can vary), typically arranged as follicles or plexiform anastomosing ribbons typical for odontogenic epithelium; the epithelium can be quite minimal and difficult to find, but it is worth the search because *the diagnosis relies specifically on this feature.* The additional required and distinguishing feature for AFO is the *presence of dental matrix*, which though the amount can vary within lesions, it should be less than the ectomesenchyme but may increase over time and with maturity. Dental matrix is often arranged as linear irregular ribbons embedded within the ectomesenchyme but can also interact with ameloblasts and odontoblasts to form more complex structures. AFO should be distinguished from ameloblastoma and odontoma based on the presence or absence and the organization of the produced dental matrix. Making the challenge of diagnosis for AFO (and for that matter odontogenic tumors in general) more difficult and complex is the fact that some have described *complex hybrid lesions* (AF with AFO, odontoma, or other sarcomas).

Odontoameloblastoma (OA) is also a mixed-odontogenic tumor with several notable similarities to both AF and odontoma. OA is also a neoplasm composed of mostly neoplastic odontogenic epithelium (thus ameloblastoma), but also the abundant epithelium is embedded within ectomesenchyme of the dental papilla, as well as mineralized dental matrix. This neoplasm should be considered *essentially an ameloblastoma that is also producing dental matrix*. They occur most often as well-defined focal proliferative intraosseous masses within the mandibular bone, but they can be locally aggressive and expansile with destruction of adjacent bone of the jaw. The infiltrative odontogenic epithelium is arranged in follicles and plexiform anastomosing ribbons embedded in a minimal amount of ectomesenchymal stroma. The epithelium may display features of odontogenic epithelium, but these features are not always obvious in an OA. In addition, the third diagnostic requirement for OA is the presence of dental matrix (enamel or dentin, including tertiary osteodentin), which is usually present as thin wedges or ribbons (some can be somewhat organized and appear like dysplastic teeth) often surrounded on both sides by palisading ameloblasts and aggregates of polygonal odontoblasts, and dental matrix which can be abundant in some cases. The OA is composed of predominantly neoplastic odontogenic epithelium, and *differential diagnoses* including amyloid-producing ameloblastoma (matrix-like material consistent with amyloid), AFO (proliferative induced ectomesenchyme is dominant), and odontoma (higher proportion of variably well-ordered mineralized dental matrices) should all be carefully considered for each of these complex lesions.

Odontomas are usually located in the mandibular or maxillary arch and are rare in animals, although less rare in cattle and horses than in other species. These are also true mixed-odontogenic neoplasms in which fully differentiated dental tissues are represented, and they are classified as 1 of 2 subtypes, complex or compound odontoma, based on how well the components recapitulate odontogenesis, although this distinction is often arbitrary and prognostically inconsequential. Compound odontomas are the most well differentiated and contain recognizable tooth structures; complex odontomas are less well differentiated and contain a seemingly haphazard arrangement of odontogenic tissues. **Complex odontomas** develop mostly during tooth development in the young and are classified as benign neoplasms that display less differentiation of tissues compared with compound odontomas. The lesions are composed of odontogenic epithelium intermixed with dental matrices within fibrovascular stroma that usually lacks the features of dental papilla ectomesenchyme. The matrix is usually dentin, but complex odontomas do not contain well-organized tooth-like structures, and instead, the matrix is arranged haphazardly as ribbons, linear strips, or islands. Odontogenic epithelium is always present but may be minimal and subtle, so cytokeratin IHC is often warranted to demonstrate them as ameloblasts. Compared with OA, the complex odontoma has a much less significant proportion of neoplastic odontogenic epithelium that may or not show classic features of odontogenic epithelium, as well as central degeneration with cyst formation. **Compound odontomas** usually develop also in the young during tooth development (and are considered hamartomas by some), often as discrete well-circumscribed noninfiltrative or invasive lesions of the jaw. In these lesions, well-differentiated malformed tooth-like structures known as denticles often include a central fibrovascular pulp chamber surrounded by mostly well-ordered dental matrices (dentin, possibly with enamel or cementum), all embedded within a fibrous stroma.

Although well characterized in humans, **cementoblastoma** is a rare neoplasm in animals—distinct from the more common *nodular hypercementosis* (formerly known as *cementomas*) of horses, in which neoplastic cementoblasts produce cementum. The lesions, as one would expect, adhere intimately to the tooth root and are histologically composed of a dense mass of cementum along with palisading cementoblasts and scattered osteoclasts. This is a unique lesion with a unique radiographic appearance; the diagnosis is best made in light of the radiographic and gross appearance of the lesion.

Odontogenic myxoma of the mandible or maxilla is a rare locally destructive expansile neoplasm described in young horses and in a few individual dogs. It is unique in that it is thought to arise from odontogenic dental papilla ectomesenchymal cells; however, it *does not contain neoplastic odontogenic epithelium*, so it is not considered a true mixed-odontogenic neoplasm, nor is it inductive. Some have diagnosed these as simply myxomas or myxomatous tumor of the jaw. As for many other lesions of the tooth-bearing regions of the jaw, review of radiographs is often necessary to make a definitive diagnosis. The radiographic appearance of the mandible or maxilla is characteristic—the appearance is uni- or multilocular cystic to moth-eaten. Odontogenic myxoma is soft grossly, and myxomatous or gelatinous on section that is reminiscent histologically of dental papilla or pulp. Because this arises from the tooth-bearing regions of the jaw, causes focal disruption of odontogenesis, and often resembles odontogenic ectomesenchyme of the dental papilla, it is presumed and classified as an odontogenic neoplasm, although this has not been shown definitively. Because they may be confused with myxoma or sarcoma of the jaw or oral mucosa, or histiocytic foam cell nodules, careful evaluation of the lesion is necessary. Limited data are available, but these are presumed to be slow growing and minimally infiltrative, so they respond well to complete surgical excision.

Neoplasms of the bones of the jaw and oral cavity

Maxillofacial osteomas are rare, circumscribed, mineralized, expansile, well-differentiated bone neoplasms that occur in several species. They arise mostly from the craniofacial bones of the skull, but can also originate from the bones of the jaw and thus involve the oral cavity. Osteomas are slowly progressing pedunculated or broad-based lesions that blend subtly with adjacent bone tissue and are composed of well-differentiated and well-organized bone that can range from spicules of woven bone to interconnected trabeculae separated by loose fibrovascular and adipose tissue with hematopoietic cells. They may appear histomorphologically indistinguishable from hyperplastic bone or localized bony exostosis; further, they should be distinguished from ossifying fibroma and fibrous dysplasia, both lesions of the oral mucosa for which there is considerable diagnostic difficulty. However, some pathologists hypothesize that these represent variably well-differentiated versions of proliferative lesions of the bones of the head and that may be a valid interpretation; it is often quite difficult or impossible to distinguish these lesions satisfactorily, especially from small incisional biopsy samples. Osteomas involving the oral cavity have rarely been described in the **cat**.

Maxillofacial osteosarcoma is a tumor of malignant osteoblasts that produces osteoid and is mostly diagnosed in older, large-breed **dogs** and less frequently in **cats**. Of all axial osteosarcomas, ~50% occur in jawbones, hard palate, or craniofacial bones. They arise mostly as central lesions from the medullary cavity, and a few from the periosteum. This is a locally aggressive disease, and ~50% of dogs have local recurrence; the metastatic potential varies by location of the primary neoplasm, with work suggesting rates of metastasis at the time of diagnosis at <10% for osteosarcomas of the canine head (which includes mandible and maxilla), which is lower than for most osteosarcomas.

Production of osteoid matrix is the sine qua non diagnostic feature for osteosarcoma, although the matrix within osteosarcomas has wide variation; in most cases, osteoid appears as eosinophilic homogeneous material arranged in wisps or larger lakes, with embedded malignant osteoblasts; when mineralized, the osteoid can take a dark-purple hue. A significant challenge when attempting to confirm a diagnosis of osteosarcomas arising from the tooth-bearing regions of the jaw is that tumor-associated osteoid matrix appears histologically similar or identical to other eosinophilic matrices, such as amyloid, keratin, collagen, dentin, cementum, chondroid, and hyperplastic or native bone. It is unfortunate that special stains or immunohistochemistry are still unavailable for use by pathologists to positively identify osteoid matrix or osteoblasts in these lesions.

Central maxillofacial osteosarcoma occurs more commonly than periosteal osteosarcoma of the head and is typically an aggressive and malignant neoplasm with histologic appearance and biologic behavior similar to appendicular skeletal osteosarcoma, although they probably metastasize less readily. When they occur in the oral cavity, the most significant effect is usually local, which can result in localized destruction and distortion of bone including maxilla, mandible, palate, zygomatic arch, or even nasal cavity. Histologic features are common to osteosarcomas in other anatomic locations and include neoplastic spindle-shaped cells arranged in interwoven streams or sheets, significant cellular pleomorphism, high mitotic rate, necrosis, and importantly, the presence of tumor-associated osteoid matrix. As for other osteosarcomas, they can be categorized by predominant histologic pattern, which includes poorly differentiated, osteoblastic, chondroblastic, fibroblastic, telangiectatic, and giant cell type, although this likely has minimal prognostic significance. Most osteosarcomas here are of the osteoblastic type, and fibroblastic osteosarcoma has a more favorable prognosis than the telangiectatic type, as for osteosarcomas in other anatomic locations.

An uncommon variant of **low-grade osteosarcoma** of the maxilla or mandible is described, and these also are thought to arise from the central marrow cavity of the bones of the jaw. Although some had histologic features of aggressive or infiltrative growth (increased mitotic rate, cellular pleomorphism and atypia, ill-defined lesion margins, mixed radiographic opacity, and bone lysis), low-grade osteosarcoma appears to have less aggressive localized growth overall, reduced metastatic potential, and is more amenable to wide surgical excision. An important differential diagnosis for low-grade osteosarcoma of the jaw is fibrous dysplasia, although osteosarcoma is expected to have more invasive localized growth; some authors hypothesize that these can transform into conventional central osteosarcoma, although this has not been demonstrated definitively. Importantly, this lesion should be diagnosed only after careful review of the histology, radiographic or other imaging data, and clinical suspicion.

Oral multilobular sarcoma of bone (*multilobular tumor of bone, multilobular osteosarcoma, multilobular chondrosarcoma, multilobular chondroma, multilobular osteoma, chondroma rodens*) is an uncommon but highly unique lesion that has experienced significant confusion, discussion, reclassification, and renaming. This neoplasm has been described mostly arising from the flat bones of the head of **dogs**, and less frequently in cats, horses, or other species. Lesions involve the maxilla (they often occur in the hard palate), mandible, occipital bone, orbit, zygomatic process, or even the tympanic bulla; some authors hypothesize that these arise from suture lines (syndesmoses) of the skull, which may account for the anatomic predilections, and for the various tissue types often observed histologically, including cartilage, bone, and fibrovascular connective tissue. Multilobular sarcoma of bone is a progressively malignant neoplasm and occurs as a uniquely sharply lobulated (a so-called popcorn ball appearance is seen radiographically) appearance, usually with minimal bone lysis. When they arise from the palate and extend into the oral cavity, lesions are often nodular ulcerated lesions that appear similar to any other nodular mass of the gingiva. When sectioned, numerous nodules can be seen embedded within abundant dense fibrous stroma.

Histologic features are unique; these neoplasms are composed of many often contiguous variably sized nodules with a distinct trilaminar appearance due to centers of variably mineralized immature bone and/or cartilage, surrounded by a variably prominent aggregate of neoplastic cells (presumed to be osteoblasts) and variably mature fibrous connective tissue. Lending support to the theory that these arise from syndesmoses, there is often recapitulation of the syndesmosis joint between tumor lobules. In most multilobular sarcomas of bone, there is minimal pleomorphism and a low mitotic rate; these are thought to be slowly progressive lesions, although given sufficient time they often either invade or compress adjacent tissue that results in significant clinical signs (brain, nerves, eyes, nasal, and oral cavity), or they transition into a highly locally aggressive neoplasm that is capable of distant metastasis. Due to their anatomic location, they can be quite difficult to completely excise, and recurrence is described in ~50% of cases. There can be significant histomorphologic variation, with some composed mostly of cartilaginous matrix (and thus they mimic chondrosarcoma) or osseous matrix; others can be poorly differentiated with loss of the distinct nodular architecture, thus making the definitive diagnosis challenging. A thorough histologic search is warranted to find the classic lobular arrangement in many cases, especially of bony proliferative lesions arising from the palate of dogs. A grading system has been proposed which is based on the overall size of the lobules (small or large), invasiveness, organization, mitotic count, pleomorphism, and metastasis; this has been shown to predict time to metastatic disease, recurrence, and overall survival time.

Oral chondroma and chondrosarcoma is described in dogs, cats, ruminants, and rarely horses; chondrosarcomas occur much more commonly in long bones or nasal cavity; oral lesions are much less common. Most oral chondrosarcomas likely result after extension from the nasal cavity or progression of multilobular sarcoma. Chondrosarcoma is (as in other anatomic locations) a malignant neoplasm of spindle cells producing cartilaginous but not osteoid matrix (which if found should result in a diagnosis of osteosarcoma) and is less behaviorally aggressive compared with osteosarcoma. Nonnasal chondrosarcomas (which includes oral chondrosarcomas that are not extensions of nasal chondrosarcomas) are graded based on their histologic criteria, which include cellularity, mitotic count, differentiation, presence and amount of cartilaginous matrix, and invasive or infiltrative growth.

Diseases of the tonsils

The tonsils are normally prominent and protrude slightly from the tonsillar fossa in the dog and cat. In these species, tonsils are compact fusiform structures with a finely stippled pale-pink surface. In swine, tonsillar lymphoid tissue is concentrated in the caudal soft palate where it forms a thickened and pitted mucosal plaque. In horses, tonsillar tissues are dispersed over pharyngeal and epiglottic mucosal surfaces and consist of a series of plaques and nodules in the mucosa. Various sets of tonsils in cattle include palatine, lingual, soft palate, and pharyngeal tonsils; in other ruminants, the tonsils are spread more diffusely. Tonsils are subject to conditions involving other lymphoid tissues, including atrophy, necrosis, inflammation, neoplasia, and hyperplasia, and they commonly undergo progressive atrophy with age.

Tonsils are part of the MALT and are constantly exposed to antigenic stimuli by virtue of their function in immune surveillance in the oropharynx. Many bacteria native to the oropharyngeal mucosa colonize and inhabit the tonsillar crypts, and consequently, the tonsils may serve as portals of entry for various bacterial or viral agents. A significant percentage of swine carry *Erysipelothrix rhusiopathiae*, *Salmonella* spp., and *Streptococcus suis* serotype 2 in their tonsils.

Desquamated epithelium, bacteria, necrotic debris, and neutrophils may normally be present to a moderate degree in *tonsillar crypts*. The immunologic reaction is exaggerated in tonsillar lymphoid tissue and may lead to ulceration and inflammation of involuted tonsillar lymphoid tissue and crypts during antigenic stimulation causing formation of grossly visible yellow nodules during some bacterial infections, including *Pasteurella* in sheep and pigs, *Actinomyces* in swine, and *Fusobacterium* in all species (see Fig. 1-8). Hemorrhagic and necrotizing tonsillitis is reported in pigs infected with *Bacillus anthracis*.

Prion proteins can be identified in tonsillar tissue of infected animals. *Scrapie*-associated prion protein is consistently detected by IHC in the centers of primary and secondary lymphoid follicles of infected sheep with clinical and/or histologic lesions of scrapie, and in cervids with chronic wasting disease, although sensitivity is probably limited in early stages of the disease. The prion protein of bovine spongiform encephalopathy has been shown to accumulate in palatine tonsils of cattle as early as 10 months after experimental infection.

The tonsil is the site of primary viral multiplication in pseudorabies in swine, and necrotizing tonsillitis with intranuclear viral inclusion bodies may be seen in cryptal epithelial cells.

Involution of B-dependent tonsillar lymphoid follicles resulting from virus-induced lymphoid depletion and lymphocytolysis is observed during lymphotropic viral diseases, such as feline panleukopenia, canine parvoviral enteritis, canine distemper, BVD, and swine vesicular disease (SVD). Involuted tonsils following CDV infection are susceptible to secondary bacterial invasion. Compensatory lymphoid hyperplasia occurs during the postviremic phase of parvoviral and distemper viral infections. The tonsil appears to be the preferred organ of viral persistence in subclinical carrier cats infected with FCV. In porcine circovirus 2 (PCV2; *Circoviridae, Circovirus porcine2*) infections, involution of lymphoid tissue and accumulation of macrophages or histiocytes and multinucleate giant cells containing basophilic cytoplasmic circoviral inclusions are often seen, as they are in other lymphoid organs.

Benign proliferative tonsillar polyps occur infrequently in old **dogs**. They are usually unilateral, 1-3-cm-long, flat-to-pedunculated, rubbery masses with a smooth-to-irregular surface arising from the palatine tonsil or the tonsillar sinus. Most affected dogs are subclinical, but some show evidence of oral bleeding, cough, retching, or dyspnea. Histologically, the lesions are composed of mature, sometimes edematous, and highly vascularized connective tissue covered by squamous epithelium. Variably dense aggregates of lymphocytes and plasma cells are scattered throughout the connective tissue. These polyps have been subcategorized based on major histologic features: lymphangiomatous polyps have prominent ectatic lymphatic spaces; angiofibromatous polyps have increased fibrovascular connective tissue; myxomatous polyps are highly edematous with interstitial myxomatous material; and lipomatous polyps have increased mature adipocytes. The subcategorization does not affect the prognosis of affected dogs. Some have argued that these are hamartomatous lesions, but they likely develop as a reaction following chronic recurrent episodes of subclinical tonsillitis; chronic inflammation, hyperplasia, and lymphatic obstruction may also result in mucosal prolapse and polyp formation. Tonsillar polyps are similar to aural inflammatory polyps in many ways, and because they show no evidence of malignant or invasive growth behavior, complete surgical excision is expected to prove curative in most cases.

Primary neoplasms, including lymphoma and SCC, can cause unilateral or bilateral tonsillar enlargement in dogs. The tonsil is an uncommon metastatic site in dogs, mostly from neoplasms originating from the head and neck region, and includes malignant melanoma, salivary carcinoma, adenocarcinoma, basal cell tumor, hemangiosarcoma, fibrosarcoma, malignant histiocytosis, urothelial carcinoma, or undifferentiated or unknown metastatic carcinomas. Bilaterally enlarged and soft pale swollen tonsils are usual with lymphoma, and these may become clinically obvious and cause dyspnea before development of peripheral lymphadenopathy.

SALIVARY GLANDS

Structure, function, and reaction to injury

Salivary glands have crucially important functions for oral health maintenance and during initial digestion phases of ingesta including not only lubrication of the food bolus for mastication and transport, but also provision of bicarbonate as an important buffer, and electrolytes and enzymes, which initiate digestion of the ingested food; these functions are under autonomic nervous system control. Salivary glands are a complex set of exocrine secretory epithelial glands including the large discrete major glands of the head and cranial neck region, and an extensive series of thousands of submucosal minor salivary glands of the oral cavity including the tongue, oropharynx, and larynx. The major glands are compound tubuloacinar glands composed of ducts, tubules, and acini. The minor glands are much smaller and mostly are simple tubuloacinar glands. Salivary glands are divided into lobules composed of terminal acini that either produce mucous or serous secretion, or a mixture of both. Small (intercalated, striated) and larger (interlobular, secretory) salivary ducts empty into the oral cavity at the oral papillae.

Common *acute reactions* to injury include hypersecretion, necrosis, edema, and inflammation; gland atrophy, ductular fibrosis and obstruction, and squamous metaplasia may develop following *chronic injury*. *Oncocytic metaplasia* is a benign *age-related* lesion of salivary duct epithelium in which normal ductal epithelial cells are replaced by swollen eosinophilic granular cells (oncocytes) containing abundant cytoplasmic mitochondria.

Diseases of salivary glands

Degenerative and inflammatory conditions of salivary glands

Many common anomalies of the salivary glands are functional. *Ptyalism* (or sialorrhea) is defined as excessive flow of saliva, which can lead to drooling, and should be differentiated from failure to swallow. Ptyalism occurs in a variety of conditions, including stomatitis, organophosphate, or heavy-metal poisoning, and can be occur secondary to encephalitis. *Aptyalism* is reduced or absent secretion of saliva and is less common but may accompany fever, dehydration, and salivary gland disease, such as inflammation, obstruction, or neoplasia.

Ptyalism in cattle and horses may be observed following mycotoxicosis. *Slafractonia* (formerly *Rhizoctonia*) *leguminicola* has a wide geographic distribution, and infestation of legumes (in particular red clover) resulting in black patch disease is associated with slobbers syndrome, although mycelial growth on well-cured hay is not usually grossly visible. Two biologically active alkaloids—*slaframine* and *swainsonine*—are produced by the fungus. Slaframine causes no specific lesions, but as a parasympathomimetic alkaloid, is associated with drooling, lacrimation, anorexia, diarrhea, frequent urination, bloat, reduced milk production, and weight loss. Guinea pigs are extremely sensitive to the toxin. A presumptive diagnosis may be based on feeding trials in that species if chromatographic analysis for slaframine is not readily accessible.

Ptyalism may be associated with *neurointoxication*, particularly those agents that affect the trigeminal nuclei. Known causes include ingestion of ergotized *Paspalum destichium* (knotgrass) and *Prosopis glandulosa* (honey mesquite), poisoning with cholinergic stimulants, snake envenomation, and neurotropic viruses (especially rabies virus); dogs exposed to the toad *Bufo marinus* experience neurologic abnormalities and ptyalism. Vesicular and ulcerative diseases affecting the oral cavity, such as FMD or BVD, are usually associated with ptyalism.

Foreign bodies such as plant awns or fiber are occasionally present in the ducts; the parotid duct is more often affected than the submaxillary duct. These foreign materials invariably cause some degree of inflammation or secondary infection, and if the duct epithelium is destroyed, saliva leakage leads to localized cellulitis. **Sialolithiasis** (*salivary calculi*) may cause obstruction, inflammation, and possibly rupture and sialocele. Sialoliths are more common in **horses** than other species, and the parotid duct is most commonly affected. Microliths are formed routinely and likely undergo regular turnover; however, prolonged secretory inactivity (anorexia, dehydration, etc.) can cause microliths to expand and lead to the formation of large calculi that are more likely to cause obstruction. Sialolithiasis causes swelling of the affected gland or duct (with or without pain), resulting from partial or complete obstruction of saliva flow. Many lodge at the duct orifice and cause some degree of salivary retention, glandular atrophy, and predisposition to infection and further inflammation. In dogs, the composition varies, but calculi in horses are mostly observed in the proximal parotid duct, and usually are a single hard white laminated structure composed largely of calcium carbonate. Sialolith removal and sialoadenectomy is the treatment of choice; in most cases in dogs, there are low rates of localized recurrence; in horses the rate of local recurrence may be higher (up to 24% reported), which is likely related to incomplete removal of all sialoliths at the time of surgery.

Dilations of salivary ducts are due to stagnation or obstruction of flow resulting from congenital atresia, foreign bodies, calculi, inflammation, or postinflammatory fibrotic stricture. The dilated ducts appear as fluctuating cords, sometimes with local diverticula. **Ranula** *is the term applied to a smooth rounded fluctuant cystic distension of the salivary duct ventral to the tongue in the floor of the mouth.* The lining ductal epithelium may or may not be intact or evident either grossly or in histologic sections, and cyst contents may be serous watery fluid or thick tenacious mucus. Rupture of a duct or a gland to an epithelial surface results in a permanent fistula as the continued flow of saliva prevents normal restoration, and the duct epithelium eventually fuses with the surface.

Salivary mucocele or **sialocele** *is an accumulation of salivary secretions in single or multilocular cavities with or without a secretory epithelial lining* (the epithelium may or may not be visible in histologic sections, these are sometimes referred to as pseudocysts) *in the soft tissues of the mouth or neck.* Sialoceles are often thought to be the result of trauma to the duct, and there may be a history of ductal ectasia, or even of ranula in the mouth. Most sialoceles are subcutaneous and they may be up to 10 cm in diameter and pendulous. They can be located anywhere from the mandibular symphysis to the middle of the neck, but most are located in a more ventrolateral direction along the midline. They occur following a defect in major, or less commonly in minor, salivary gland or ducts, and most commonly from the sublingual salivary gland (eFig. 1-1A); sialoceles in other locations are observed sporadically. Pharyngeal sialoceles may be more common in brachycephalic dogs, usually involve minor salivary glands or ducts in the soft palate, and are uncommon; however, affected dogs may be dyspneic. Zygomatic and palatine sialoceles also occur, can be associated with inflammation, and cause exophthalmos and soft palate swelling, respectively. Small <0.5-cm sialoceles are occasionally observed along the margins of the *bovine tongue*, and presumably result from obstruction and/or rupture of the dorsal sublingual gland ducts.

The wall of the sialocele is soft, pliable, well-vascularized connective tissue with a glistening lining; in chronic cases there can be extensive lining granulation tissue. The sialocele contents are initially mucinous but become progressively inspissated and tenacious. The histologic appearance of sialoceles varies greatly, depending on the stage of development. Centrally, there is abundant amorphous amphophilic material with a mixed inflammatory reaction, which may be very mild. Initially, the wall consists of an outer well-vascularized layer of immature connective tissue and an inner layer of loosely arranged fibroblasts and pockets of foamy mucus or saliva-filled macrophages (see eFig. 1-1B). As the sialocele ages, mature fibrous and often dense connective tissue forms the wall, plasma cells or lymphocytes are the most numerous inflammatory cells, and the material in the center becomes progressively more basophilic. Osseous metaplasia occurs in the sialocele wall of some chronically inflamed cases, and although adding complexity clinically and histologically, this change likely lacks prognostic significance.

Anomalous regression of remnants of the embryologically important pharyngeal pouch or cleft system (these contribute to several adult structures, including the thymus, parathyroid gland, pharyngeal tonsils, as well as middle and external ear) results in **pharyngeal** (formerly called *branchial*) **cysts, sinuses**, or **fistulae**, mostly reported in dogs and cats and rarely in ruminants. These can be confused with sialoceles if not evaluated carefully. The lining of pharyngeal cysts can vary from squamous to pseudostratified and often partially ciliated epithelium that derives from the embryonic pharynx; occasionally more than one type of epithelium is observed. Congenital cervical sinuses, cysts, and fistulae have been reported in veterinary species. Complete surgical excision is typically curative. **Thyroglossal duct cysts** are reported in cats and dogs. These remnants of primordial pharyngeal thyroidal epithelium occur directly along the ventral cervical midline and are readily distinguishable from sialoceles and pharyngeal cysts histologically because they are lined by thyroidogenic epithelium.

Sialoadenitis is defined as *inflammation of the salivary glands*, is an uncommon lesion, but is probably more frequent in dogs and cats than is neoplasia. Extraoral major salivary glands are most commonly affected, and the submandibular gland is usually affected. Due to the anatomic location, inflammation of the zygomatic gland in dogs is a cause of retrobulbar abscessation. The route of infection is usually via the excretory duct, although it also may be hematogenous or secondary to localized trauma. Duct obstruction is due to inflammatory exudate, desquamated epithelial cells, and mucus, which may be expressed digitally from the duct orifice. Partial or complete obstruction of the duct produces secondary atrophic changes in the upstream glands, although there is initial gland enlargement and often pain resulting from the combined effects of partial-to-complete obstruction, retained secretion, and inflammation. Ducts throughout the gland initially become dilated and inflamed. Acini swell and then rupture if the obstruction persists, and this often leads to marked neutrophilic inflammation. In chronic cases, there is marked glandular atrophy and granulation tissue present, with only remnants of atrophic salivary glandular epithelium embedded within inflamed fibrous connective tissue.

Specific causes of inflammation of the salivary glands in domestic animals are few. An example is rabies virus infection, which causes focal lysis of acinar epithelial cells, mononuclear infiltration, and rare Negri bodies in ganglionic neurons. Other examples include strangles in horses, and distemper virus infection in dogs. *Eosinophilic sialoadenitis* may be a component of the eosinophilic epitheliotropic syndrome in horses discussed in the Eosinophilic enteritis in cats and horses section. *Sjögren-like syndrome* has been diagnosed in cats and dogs, and in these species, the swollen salivary glands have significant lymphoplasmacytic sialadenitis histologically. Sialadenitis can also occur *secondary to squamous metaplasia of interlobular salivary ducts*, which is an early lesion of **hypovitaminosis A**. Exposure to highly chlorinated naphthalenes is now rare but can lead to hypovitaminosis A and subsequent squamous metaplasia.

Necrotizing sialometaplasia (salivary gland infarction) is a distinct and rare disease of dogs, cats, and humans; the cause remains unknown. Affected patients usually have acute firm and often severe painful swelling of usually the submandibular or less frequently the parotid glands, although some cases have only swelling of the gland that resolves within several days without treatment. Some have suggested the use of the term *salivary gland infarction* for the relatively benign cases, and *necrotizing sialometaplasia* for cases with more severe clinical signs (and more guarded prognosis); however, the terms are currently used interchangeably. There is characteristic and often severe ischemic necrosis of salivary gland lobules (eFig. 1-2A), and depending on the chronicity, there is secondary mixed inflammation along with extensive often quite bizarre and pleomorphic squamous metaplasia of the ducts, *features easily and often misinterpreted as malignant transformation* (see eFig. 1-2B). These are not salivary or SCC, and the clear demarcation of salivary gland infarcts (not always visible in small sections of tissue), associated with normal adjacent salivary gland parenchyma along with the lack of solid acinar proliferation are key distinguishing histomorphologic features. The cause is thought to be vascular compromise induced by trauma, although immune-mediated destruction of blood vessels, thrombosis, or infection have also been hypothesized. The disease is seen mostly in small-breed dogs, primarily terriers; the submandibular gland is preferentially affected.

Salivary gland lipomatosis is a degenerative change in which salivary gland parenchyma is extensively infiltrated by mature adipocytes; significant atrophy and loss of parenchyma are limited to the salivary gland parenchyma, and a peripheral capsule is lacking. The morphologic features of lipomatosis overlap with salivary gland lipoma (*sialolipoma*), which is a disease mostly of humans. Salivary lipomatosis results in diffuse enlargement of the gland without a discrete neoplastic mass; sialolipoma is histologically similar but forms a discrete expansile and noninfiltrative mass, usually with a distinct peripheral capsule.

Proliferative and neoplastic lesions of salivary glands

Neoplasms of the salivary glands are rare in all species; in dogs, they occur in ~0.015% of cases and 0.03% in cats. They have been reported in cattle, sheep, goats, horses, dogs, and cats, but not swine; only in dogs and cats do salivary tumors occur often enough to make a few general conclusions about their biology and behavior. Salivary neoplasms are usually unilateral and may arise from any salivary gland; the parotid and mandibular glands are most commonly affected. Neoplasms develop mostly in aged animals and are almost exclusively carcinomas. Cats tend to have more aggressive disease at the time of diagnosis, and metastasis to regional nodes and distant sites, especially the lungs, is more common. Cases with metastatic disease involving nodes or beyond at diagnosis have a worse prognosis than those with disease localized to the gland.

The histomorphologic diversity of salivary gland neoplasms mimics the histomorphologic diversity of salivary glands with over 40 histologic subtypes recognized in humans (many of these are also described in animals), so neoplasms are generally subdivided by histomorphologic pattern and whether they are benign or malignant. The vast majority of salivary gland neoplasms are malignant, and these can be graded as low- or high-grade based on histologic features, including mitotic count, cellular pleomorphism, and differentiation; however, because so few individual distinct patterns are published, definitive evidence to link subtype or grade to behavior or prognosis has not been demonstrated. A multicenter study demonstrated local recurrence in 42% of dogs and metastatic disease in 32%; lymph node metastasis at the time of diagnosis was the only significant negative prognostic factor. Because the prognosis for dogs with salivary gland carcinoma treated surgically may be more favorable than previously thought, complete surgical excision should be considered the treatment of choice.

The most frequent benign salivary neoplasm is the **pleomorphic adenoma**, which is described in the dog, cat, cow, and horse. This is a mixed tumor comprising neoplastic epithelial or myoepithelial cells arranged in sheets, trabeculae, and clusters, with occasional ducts or squamous keratinized nests intermixed or surrounded by non-neoplastic proliferative mesenchymal cells. Similar to mixed mammary tumors, chondroid or osseous metaplasia has been described. Complete excision can be difficult, but widely excised lesions are unlikely to recur locally. **Oncocytomas** are rarely described in cats and are composed of large polygonal neoplastic cells arranged in solid nests with occasional ducts or cords. The characteristic feature of oncocytoma is abundant eosinophilic cytoplasm containing dark granules, which stain positively with phosphotungstic acid hematoxylin (PTAH) or PAS stains—the granules are often partially diastase resistant. Presumably, these have low local recurrence or distant metastasis; however, insufficient data have been published to establish prognosis. Several other benign salivary gland neoplasms occur in dogs and cats (most are individual case reports) that include various adenomas with sebocytic, ductal, or canalicular differentiation; cystic variants are also described.

Malignant neoplasms are **salivary adenocarcinomas**, which are by far more common than salivary gland adenomas; various structural patterns or subtypes are recognized, including acinic carcinoma, mucoepidermoid carcinoma, and malignant mixed carcinoma; various subtypes can be observed within the same lesion. When distinct histologic subtypes are not evident in malignant salivary neoplasms, a diagnosis of adenocarcinoma is likely sufficient. Neoplastic cells in adenocarcinomas form acini, ducts, trabeculae, or sheets; some form cysts. They are usually poorly demarcated neoplasms that can efface the native salivary gland parenchyma and infiltrate the adjacent connective tissue. Pleomorphism and mitotic count can be significant, as can necrosis, hemorrhage, and local invasive behavior; these features likely indicate more aggressive growth, studies have not shown grading systems to be prognostically significant in dogs.

Acinic cell carcinomas are described in dogs, but only sporadically in the cat, horse, and sheep. These are composed of well-differentiated salivary epithelial cells arranged in small nests, glands, follicles, or a papillary pattern. Several distinct cell types may be observed that are hypothesized to arise from acinar, intercalated duct, vacuolated, or glandular cells. Large neoplastic cells resemble glandular epithelium with fine basophilic and PAS-positive cytoplasmic granules; smaller cuboidal neoplastic cells with basophilic cytoplasm are arranged in small clusters or nests surrounding small glandular acini that resemble native intercalated ducts. In addition, large heavily vacuolated cells are also frequently observed throughout the neoplasm. There is usually minimal cellular pleomorphism and a low mitotic count. Although acinar carcinomas frequently infiltrate along the margins, these are usually low-grade malignancies, with metastasis described only late in the course of disease.

Mucoepidermoid carcinomas are uncommon in animals, and these are glandular neoplasms with variable mucus production or rarely keratinization. These are composed of a combination of squamous epithelial cells, mucus-producing cells, and intermediate cells (i.e., epidermoid cells with cytoplasmic keratohyaline granules or dyskeratosis) that may also produce mucus; neoplastic cells can be arranged in solid lobules or line mucus-filled cysts. Cyst rupture initiates granulomatous inflammation. Special stains such as PAS, Alcian blue, or mucicarmine may be helpful diagnostically to positively identify mucus. As for other salivary carcinomas, infiltrative peripheral growth pattern, increased cellular atypia, or high mitotic count are more likely to be correlated with local recurrence of the neoplasm after incomplete removal or distant metastasis.

Malignant mixed salivary tumors are composed of malignant epithelial cells along with a population of non-neoplastic proliferative mesenchymal or myoepithelial cells. Variations have also been described in the salivary glands of dogs following from the nomenclature described for mammary neoplasia, which include malignant myoepithelioma (malignant mesenchymal or myoepithelial population with non-neoplastic epithelial cell population), carcinosarcoma (both populations are neoplastic), or carcinoma arising within a benign mixed tumor. Most malignant mixed tumors are thought to develop within pleomorphic benign mixed tumors (i.e., carcinoma ex pleomorphic adenoma).

Additional malignant neoplasms arising from various salivary glands have been described mostly as individual cases or small series, including basal adenocarcinoma, cystadenocarcinoma, SCC, extraskeletal osteosarcoma, and salivary ductal adenocarcinoma. The salivary glands can certainly be a metastatic site for neoplasms originating elsewhere, including lymphoma, SCC, fibrosarcoma, infiltrative lipoma, melanoma, and MCT.

ESOPHAGUS

Structure, function, and response to injury

The esophagus is composed of an inner circular layer and an outer longitudinal layer of skeletal muscle for much or all of its length. In the pig, there is a short segment near the cardia that is composed of smooth muscle, and in horses and cats, smooth muscle is found in the distal third of the esophagus. The esophagus is lined by stratified squamous epithelium with a variable number of submucosal mucous glands, depending on the species and location along the esophagus. Esophageal protection against aggressive insults resides mainly in the squamous epithelium, which forms a permeability barrier, and the mucus and bicarbonate produced by salivary and esophageal submucosal glands.

The esophagus merits particular attention during the examination of animals with inadequate growth rate, cachexia, drooling, dysphagia, regurgitation, vomition, and aspiration pneumonia. In ruminants, tympany may be a sequel to esophageal disease. A *bloat line* in the esophagus at the thoracic inlet may indicate a condition causing increased intra-abdominal pressure, such as gastric dilation or ruminal tympany. The squamous mucosa is frequently eroded or ulcerated in viral diseases that cause similar lesions elsewhere in the upper alimentary tract or when affected by trauma or caustic substances. Conditions of striated muscle, such as nutritional myodegeneration and eosinophilic myositis in the ruminant, or polymyositis, systemic lupus erythematosus, and trypanosomiasis in the dog, involve the esophageal muscle. Envenomation following snake bite may lead to myopathy of the esophageal musculature in dogs. Diseases of the neuromuscular junction, such as myasthenia gravis, and peripheral neuropathies, including giant axonal neuropathy and polyneuritis, result in esophageal disease.

Diseases of the esophagus

Developmental anomalies

Hypertrophy of the smooth muscle of the distal esophagus, most commonly the inner smooth circular layer, occurs in **horses**. It is usually found incidentally at autopsy, and some cases also have concurrent terminal ileal muscular hypertrophy. However, marked caudal hypertrophy of the esophageal musculature associated with megaesophagus has been described in Friesian horses, a breed that is more predisposed to several esophageal disease than others. The lesion is considered idiopathic, but potential factors in the pathogenesis include autonomic imbalances or defects in the smooth muscle pacemaker cells normally found at these sites.

Congenital anomalies of the esophagus are very rarely recorded in domestic animals, and their interpretation can be difficult because similar defects may develop as sequelae of esophageal trauma or inflammation.

Congenital duplication cysts of the esophagus have been reported in horses and dogs. Esophageal cysts are classified as duplication by 3 essential criteria. The cyst must 1) be located within the esophageal wall, 2) be lined by columnar, squamous, cuboidal, ciliated, or pseudostratified epithelium, and 3) have a double muscle layer in the wall. Esophageal duplication cysts may be clinically silent; however, they manifest as space-occupying lesions if they fill with cellular debris and secretion. Potential complications are associated with compression of adjacent structures or cyst rupture.

Rare **segmental aplasia** of the proximal esophagus may be apparent in the neonate. A short blind pouch communicates with the pharynx, and a thin fibrous band connects it to the distal patent esophagus that follows a normal course to the stomach. Esophageal atresia and congenital esophagorespiratory communications result from anomalies occurring when the respiratory primordium buds from the embryonic foregut.

Esophagorespiratory fistulae without esophageal atresia are also rare in animals. Esophageal fistula formation is likely acquired following foreign body perforation of the esophagus; however, in calves and dogs, some are likely congenital. Short fibrous bands with a narrow epithelial-lined lumen connecting an esophagus of normal diameter with the trachea or bronchus are reported, as are small apertures connecting the lining of esophageal diverticula with the respiratory tree. The lining of such defects changes from stratified squamous to columnar respiratory epithelium in the fistula or wall of the diverticulum. Gastric distension by air in calves, and pneumonia resulting from aspiration, have been associated with esophagorespiratory fistulae.

Esophageal diverticula are irregular outpouchings or herniations of the esophageal mucosa through a defect in the esophageal tunica muscularis. They communicate with the esophagus by variously sized, often slit-like, apertures. Most are probably acquired, and they occur most often in the lower cervical esophagus near the thoracic inlet and the distal thoracic esophagus just cranial to the diaphragm. Increased intraluminal pressure associated with foreign bodies, obstruction, or stenosis are potential causes of *pulsion diverticula*, in which the mucosa is forced out through the distended or ruptured muscularis. Such diverticula may be large spherical structures with a narrow neck and are most common in the horse and dog. The rare *traction diverticulum* is the result of contraction of a paraesophageal fibrous adhesion, following perforation and inflammation, drawing with it a pouch of esophageal mucosa that is usually small and inconsequential. In contrast to pulsion diverticula, which have a layer of epithelium lining the inner aspect of a wall of fibrous connective tissue, *traction diverticula* have a wall composed of all layers of the esophagus. Ingesta and foreign bodies may accumulate in diverticula, causing gradual enlargement with the potential for local esophagitis, ulceration, and perforation or formation of a fistula.

Other rare *anomalies* of the esophageal mucosa include epithelial inclusion cysts and distal esophageal papillae in cattle resembling those of the rumen, and gastric heterotopia.

Degenerative and inflammatory conditions of the esophagus

Hyperkeratosis, hyperplasia, and metaplasia of the esophageal epithelium are lesions that may be signs of vitamin A deficiency or chlorinated naphthalene toxicity, which has been described in herbivores. This is accompanied by squamous metaplasia of mucous glands and ducts of the esophagus and throughout the body. Mild hyperkeratosis may be difficult to assess in herbivores because some degree of keratinization is normal, and anorexia or failure to swallow results in loss of the abrasive effect of food passage leading to accumulation of keratinized squames. Parakeratosis and epithelial hyperplasia are indicative of response to epithelial injury. In the distal esophagus of pigs, this lesion is often observed concomitant with ulceration of the gastric pars esophagea. Esophageal parakeratosis can also occur in pigs with cutaneous parakeratosis caused by zinc deficiency.

Dysphagia is defined as difficulty swallowing. Swallowing is a complex and highly coordinated physical act that may be divided into 3 sequential phases: oral, pharyngeal, and esophageal; dysphagia can be classified according to the same 3 phases. Any of the forms of dysphagia is an important risk factor for aspiration pneumonia. **Oral dysphagia** occurs because of painful lesions involving any of the structures within the oral cavity, such as stomatitis, glossitis, and gingivitis, neoplasia, or lesions that impair movement of the tongue or delivery of the bolus to the oropharynx, such as loss of hypoglossal nerve function associated with hydrocephalus, trauma, myasthenia gravis, or botulism. Cleft palate can result in nasal regurgitation. **Pharyngeal dysphagia** may be associated with painful inflammatory or neoplastic lesions involving the pharynx, tonsils, or retropharyngeal region, which may physically intrude on the pharyngeal space required for swallowing. Encephalitis involving the medulla oblongata and nuclei or tracts of the major cranial nerves involved in pharyngeal contraction and lingual function (V, IX, X, XII) should be carefully examined in cases of pharyngeal dysphagia unexplained by other lesions. Rabies and brain abscess in all species, and infectious bovine rhinotracheitis and listeriosis in ruminants, are important central causes of pharyngeal paralysis. Retropharyngeal abscesses or other lesions of the equine guttural pouch may cause peripheral nerve damage and paralysis. Idiopathic myodegeneration, muscular dystrophies, and myasthenia gravis have been reported to impair pharyngeal muscle function. **Esophageal or cricopharyngeal dysphagia** is recognized in dogs as a swallowing disorder of the upper esophageal sphincter with *cricopharyngeal muscle asynchrony or achalasia* (failure of the muscle to relax). The cause is unknown, but this may be a primary muscular disorder because cricopharyngeal myotomy or myectomy is curative.

Megaesophagus, or *esophageal ectasia*, is recognized as dilation of the esophageal lumen, and is the result of atony and flaccidity of the esophageal muscle (Fig. 1-19). This occurs as the result of segmental or diffuse motor dysfunction of the body of the esophagus and results in failure of peristaltic propulsion of the food bolus through the lower esophageal sphincter into the stomach. Ingesta accumulates in the esophageal lumen, which may lead to putrefaction and esophagitis in dilated or dependent areas; undigested food is eventually regurgitated. The volume of the dilated thoracic and cervical esophagus may greatly exceed that of the stomach causing ventral displacement of the intrathoracic trachea and heart. Animals with megaesophagus may have signs of malnutrition, including emaciation, dehydration, and osteopenia as well as rhinitis and aspiration pneumonia resulting from regurgitation.

Congenital idiopathic megaesophagus (CIM) is relatively common in **dogs**; it may improve functionally to some extent with time. CIM has its highest prevalence in Great Danes, German Shepherds, and Irish Setters. In Miniature Schnauzers, the condition has an inheritance pattern of simple autosomal dominant with incomplete (60%) penetrance. With very rare exceptions, it is not secondary to physical obstruction or failure of the lower esophageal sphincter to open. Motor stimulation to the striated esophageal muscle, despite being carried in the vagus, is not autonomic, and seems intact. There is strong evidence that CIM results from a selective defect in the distension-sensitive afferent autonomic arm of the reflex that coordinates esophageal function. Male German Shepherd dogs are twice as likely to be

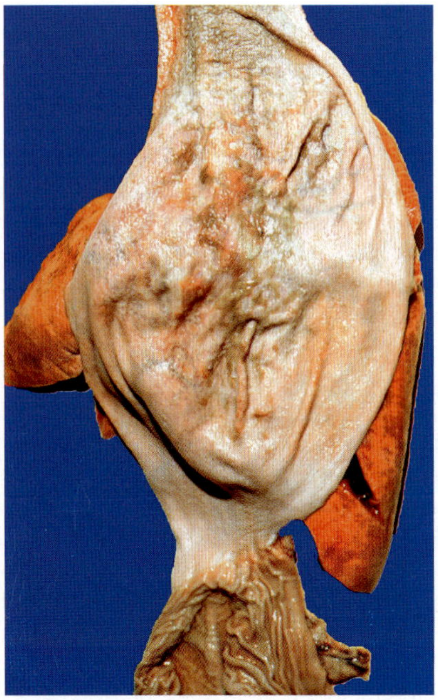

Figure 1-19 Congenital **esophageal dilation** in a dog. The mucosa is eroded, and the capacity of the distal esophagus (top) exceeds that of the stomach (bottom.)

affected as females, regardless of body size; female endogenous factors (e.g., estrogen) may be protective because they promote relaxation of the sphincter between the esophagus and stomach, facilitating food passage. In this breed, CIM is associated with an intronic variable number tandem repeat in melanin-concentrating hormone receptor 2.

Idiopathic megaesophagus can develop in *mature dogs*, and based on some studies, this represents most cases. Most cases of idiopathic megaesophagus in dogs are not comparable with humans, in which *esophageal achalasia* is a significant primary motor disorder.

Megaesophagus may be acquired secondary to glycogen storage disease in Lapland dogs, localized or systemic myasthenia gravis, administration of cholinesterase inhibitors, hypoadrenocorticism, canine giant axonal neuropathy, immune-mediated polymyositis, polyradiculoneuritis, canine distemper, systemic lupus erythematosus, lead poisoning, American trypanosomosis, snake envenomation, and certain foods.

Megaesophagus in the **cat** may be congenital, and it appears most common in the Siamese breed. The pathogenesis is unclear. Neuronal degeneration or neurogenic atrophy of muscle is not recognized in the esophageal wall. Acquired megaesophagus in cats has been associated with functional pyloric stenosis, hiatus hernia, upper respiratory obstruction/nasopharyngeal polyps, and lead poisoning.

Presumed congenital megaesophagus has been reported in **foals**. Histologic examination of the segmentally dilated proximal esophagus revealed no significant lesions of muscle or ganglia. *Aganglionosis* has also been implicated in megaesophagus in foals. Megaesophagus also may be acquired in foals; in such cases, there is usually ulceration of the distal esophagus, as well as the gastric pars esophagea. Friesian horses seem to be overrepresented in cases of megaesophagus.

Megaesophagus in **cattle** has been described as congenital, or more commonly an acquired lesion associated with hiatus hernia, or pharyngeal trauma presumably causing vagus nerve damage. Megaesophagus is rarely reported in small ruminants.

Esophageal obstruction can have *intrinsic* or *extrinsic* causes, and the lesions are generally obvious. The esophagus proximal to the stenotic area may be dilated, contain retained ingesta, or have evidence of erosion, ulceration, or inflammation. *Choke*, or esophageal impaction, is the most common example of *intrinsic obstruction* and occurs when large or inadequately chewed and lubricated foods, masses of grain or fibrous ingesta, or medically administered boluses lodge in the lumen of the esophagus (Fig. 1-20). Predisposed sites are where the esophagus deviates or is slightly restricted normally: the area overlying the larynx, the thoracic inlet, the base of the heart, and just cranial to the diaphragmatic hiatus.

Complications of obstruction include *pressure necrosis and ulceration of the mucosa*, which may progress to perforation or less commonly development of esophageal diverticula or fistulae. Sharp objects, such as bones, are most likely to cause *perforation*. Severe cellulitis of the periesophageal tissue ensues, and depending on the site of perforation, may involve the mediastinum directly or by extension along fascial planes from the cervical region. Perforation of the thoracic esophagus may lead to pleuritis and/or pericarditis. Sharp objects, such as needles, quills, grass seeds, and awns, may penetrate and track from the esophagus through adjacent tissues.

Removal or dissolution of an obstruction may allow healing of the segmentally ulcerated esophagus. As for reflux esophagitis, *fibrosis and scarring* of large ulcers may result in narrowing of the lumen, stricture, or stenosis. Although hypertrophy of internal and external muscle layers is seen occasionally in the distal esophagus of cattle and horses (in which species the distal esophageal muscle is normally relatively thick), this change is usually not clearly the result of obstruction. Stenosis rarely is caused by intramural or intraluminal neoplasia, or more commonly by external compression, which can be due to enlarged thyroid glands, thymus, and cervical or mediastinal lymph nodes.

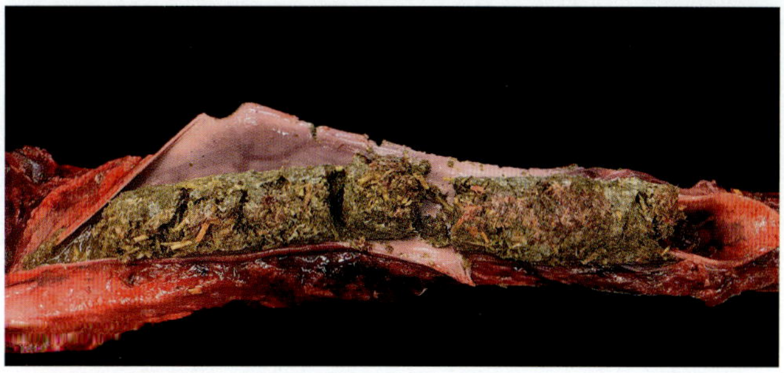

Figure 1-20 **Esophageal impaction** in a sheep. (Courtesy P. Blanchard.)

The most common causes of external compression and constriction of the esophagus are **vascular ring anomalies** seen in dogs, occasionally in cats, and rarely in other species. *Persistence of the right fourth aortic arch* is the most common of these anomalies and occurs when the right aortic arch develops instead of the normal left aortic arch. With this condition, the *ligamentum arteriosum* forms a vascular ring around the esophagus, resulting in entrapment and constriction of the esophagus against the trachea. *Other vascular anomalies* that may constrict the esophagus are reported only in the dog and include persistence of both right and left aortic arches, persistent right ductus arteriosus, aberrant left subclavian artery in association with persistent right aortic arch, and aberrant right subclavian artery arising distal to the left subclavian artery and passing dorsally over the esophagus. The Irish Setter, German Shepherd, German Pinscher, and Boston Terrier are breeds most commonly afflicted with vascular ring anomalies.

Esophagitis can have noninfectious or infectious causes. Caustic or irritant chemicals, ionizing radiation, electrochemical reactions (batteries), or heat may cause mucosal injury, the severity of which depends on the nature of the insult and duration of exposure. Mild acute insult may result in reddening of the mucosa. More severe insult results in liquefactive necrosis associated with alkalis, and coagulative necrosis associated with exposure to acids and toxins (paraquat, oak toxicosis, cantharidin) and may result in deep esophageal ulceration and sloughing of the mucosa. Trauma caused by improper tubing of the esophagus in several animal species is frequently responsible for esophageal ulceration.

Superficial epithelial damage heals uneventfully; repeated insult may cause irregular epithelial hyperplasia. Ulcerated mucosa heals by granulation, and raised islands of surviving proliferative epithelium may be observed on the surface. The inflammatory reaction in ulceration frequently involves tunica muscularis and adventitia. Fibrosis and scarring may cause stricture or stenosis if the original defect involved a significant portion of the esophageal circumference.

Reflux esophagitis occurs because of a loss of functional integrity of the lower esophageal sphincter associated with airway occlusion and increased intra-abdominal pressure, the pharmacologic effects of preanesthetic agents, or abnormality of the hiatus. Esophagitis is due to the action of gastric acid, pepsin, and probably regurgitated bile salts and pancreatic enzymes, on the esophageal mucosa. Reflux esophagitis is most common in dogs and cats as a sequel to surgery involving general anesthesia, although it may follow chronic gastric regurgitation or vomition for any cause (Fig. 1-21). In swine and horses, it may be associated with ulceration of the squamous portion of the stomach. In dogs, it can be associated with hiatus herniation. A high prevalence of apparent gastroesophageal reflux disease in the distal esophagus of premature calves was demonstrated by endoscopy; however, the pathogenesis remains unclear.

Stratified squamous epithelium appears more susceptible to the corrosive effects of gastric secretion than other types of mucosae in the lower GI tract. Relatively short duration of exposure to refluxed gastric content is required to induce epithelial damage, which can be seen as hyperemia, linear erosions, ulcers, or superficial fibrinonecrotic debris. Such damage is most common in the distal esophagus, but in some instances can extend to the pharynx. Epithelial hyperplasia and neutrophilic exocytosis occur in response to mild superficial epithelial necrosis. A consequence of chronic gastroesophageal reflux, well recognized in humans and described in dogs and cats, is columnar and mucous cell metaplasia of the distal esophagus. In humans, the lesion is known as *Barrett esophagus* and is an important risk factor for the development of esophageal adenocarcinoma; this has been described in dogs but has not been clearly demonstrated in other animal species.

Hiatus hernia usually involves sliding herniation of all or part of the abdominal esophagus, cardia, and stomach into the thoracic esophagus, rather than periesophageal herniation. It is generally self-reducing, but usually results in lower esophageal sphincter failure and reflux, rather than gastric herniation and obstruction. *Gastroesophageal intussusception* is a rare event, most reported in puppies of large-breed dogs, and is associated with recurrent vomition that may lead to aspiration pneumonia.

Erosive and ulcerative esophagitis is a common finding associated with viral diseases causing similar lesions in the oropharynx or reticulorumen, such as BVD, bovine papular stomatitis, infectious bovine rhinotracheitis, and feline caliciviral infection. Ulcerative esophagitis was a classical lesion of rinderpest before its eradication. Bacteria such as *F. necrophorum* and *Pseudomonas aeruginosa* can cause ulcerative esophagitis. Epithelial proliferation or granulation tissue during healing of ulcers may result in raised opaque areas at the lesion margin or surface, respectively.

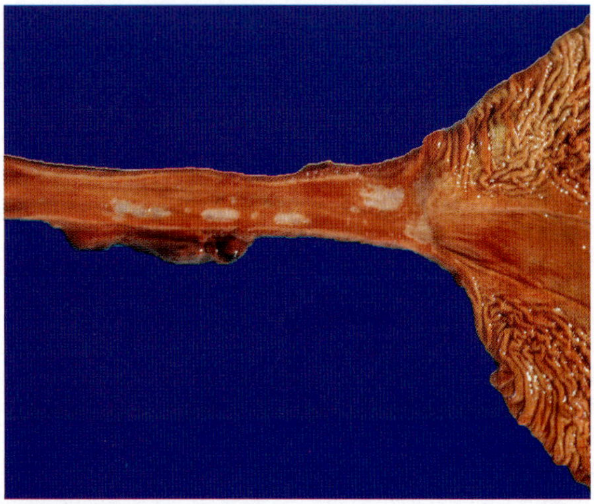

Figure 1-21 Reflux esophagitis of the distal esophagus following chronic vomition in a dog.

Thrush, or mycotic esophagitis caused by *Candida albicans*, is seen in piglets and weaner swine, and may involve the squamous mucosa of the entire upper alimentary canal. *C. albicans* is an opportunist seen secondary to antibiotic therapy, inanition, or esophageal gastric reflux, and is considered more fully in the Mycotic, Oomycotic, and Algal Diseases of the Alimentary Tract section.

Sarcosporidiosis (sarcocystosis) occurs in the striated esophageal muscle of sheep. Esophageal sarcocysts appear as ovoid, white, ~1-cm long, thin-walled nodules projecting from the esophageal muscle. *Sarcocystis gigantea*, the species that produces large esophageal cysts and similar large cysts in the skeletal muscle, is spread by cats. Microscopic sarcocysts of other species also may be encountered in the esophageal striated muscle of a variety of hosts (see the Protistan Diseases section, and Vol. 1, Muscle and Tendon). Sarcocysts in esophageal muscle normally incite little or no local inflammatory reaction and are only of significance in meat inspection. *Eosinophilic myositis* can be observed in the esophageal muscle and, although the cause of this lesion is not certain, it is thought to be associated with rupture of cysts of this parasite.

In horses, ***Gasterophilus*** spp. larvae may be temporarily attached to the caudal pharyngeal, cranial esophageal, or distal esophageal mucosa adjacent to the cardia; ulcers may occur at the sites of attachment.

The larvae of the warble fly ***Hypoderma lineatum*** reside for some time in the submucosa or adventitia of the bovine esophagus before they migrate to the dermis of the back. Here the small 2-4-mm translucent larvae grow up to 6 times before migrating toward the back of the host, but can cause local hemorrhage and inflammation. Death of first-stage larvae in the esophageal wall following systemic insecticide treatment, for example, can lead to severe acute inflammation in the esophageal submucosa and potentially esophageal obstruction, tympany, and perforation.

Spirurid nematodes of the genus ***Gongylonema***, including *Gongylonema pulchrum* and *G. nepalensis*, may be encountered in the stratified squamous mucosa of the upper alimentary tract, including the esophagus, in ruminants, swine, and occasionally other species. These white, 10-15-cm long, threadlike worms burrow in the epithelium or propria of the esophagus and produce white or red, blood-filled, serpentine tracks (Fig. 1-22). Their presence is inconsequential to the host.

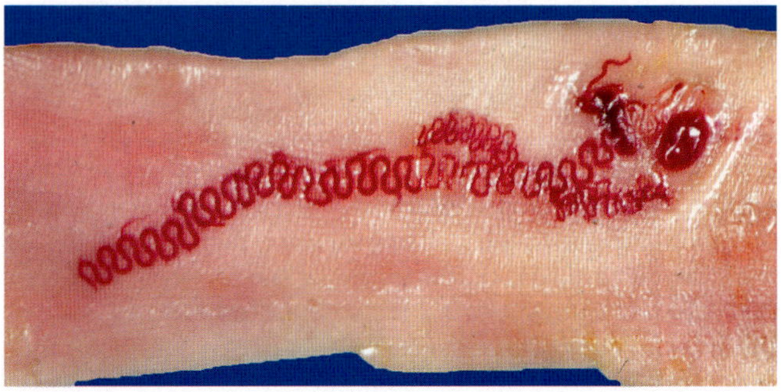

Figure 1-22 Blood-filled tracks and small hematoma in esophageal mucosa caused by ***Gongylonema pulchrum*** **migration** in a cow.

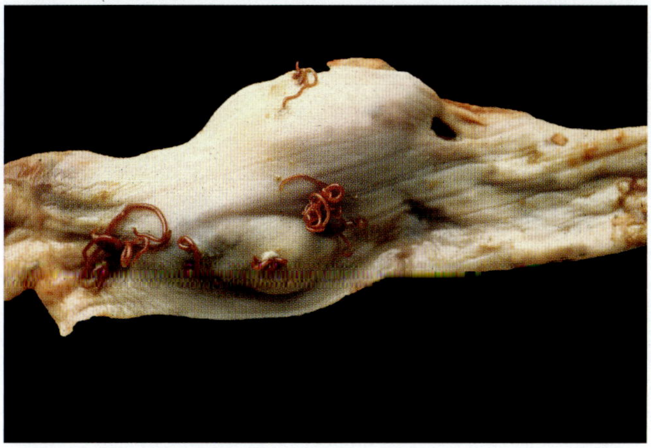

Figure 1-23 ***Spirocerca lupi*** **nodules** in the distal esophagus of a dog. Worms protrude through fistulae into the esophageal lumen. (Courtesy R.G. Thomson.)

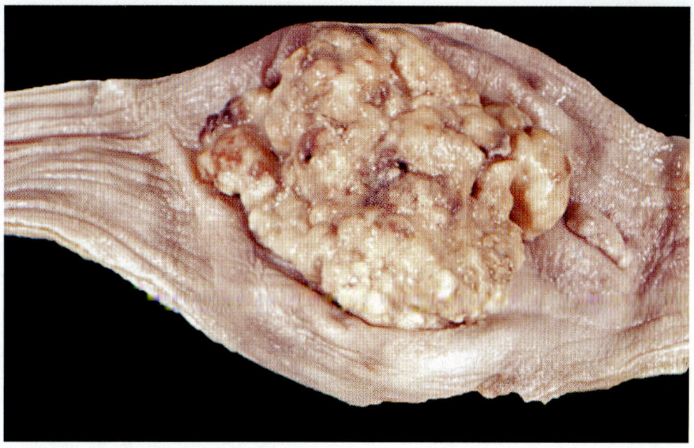

Figure 1-24 Ulcerating **fibrosarcoma** associated with *Spirocerca lupi* granuloma in the distal esophagus of a dog. (Courtesy R.G. Thomson.)

Spirocerca lupi is a spirurid nematode that parasitizes the esophageal wall of *Canidae* and some other carnivores. It is most common in warm climates where dogs ingest third-stage larvae either via the dung beetle intermediate host or one of several insectivorous vertebrate paratenic hosts, such as rodents, chickens, or reptiles. Larvae penetrate the gastric mucosa and migrate along arteries to the aorta, then subintimally to the caudal thoracic area, which they attain within several weeks of infection. Following 2-4 months in a granuloma in the aortic adventitia, worms migrate to the subjacent esophagus where they develop to adulthood. Here the adult nematodes are found within large, thick-walled, cystic granulomas in the submucosa of the distal esophagus or gastric cardia. A fistula leading to the esophageal lumen is usually present, through which the tail of the female worm may protrude, and which provides the outlet for ova to the GI tract (Fig. 1-23). Larvae that adopt aberrant migratory pathways may be found in granulomas in sites, such as the subcutis, bladder, kidney, spinal cord, as well as stomach and intrathoracic locations.

Aortic lesions associated with *Spirocerca* are described in Vol. 3, Cardiovascular System, but include intimal and medial hemorrhage and necrosis with eosinophilic inflammation, intimal roughening with thrombosis, aneurysm with rare aortic rupture, intimal and medial mineralization, and heterotopic bone deposition. Persistent aortic lesions in the dog, even in the absence of esophageal granuloma, are evidence of prior infection with *S. lupi*. Caudal thoracic vertebral body spondylitis occurs in greater than half of cases; exostoses or bony spurs arise from the ends of the vertebral bodies. The pathogenesis is unclear but may by initiated by migrating worms or inflammatory mediators.

In some animals with *S. lupi* infestation, *mesenchymal neoplasms* develop in the wall of the esophageal granuloma (Fig. 1-24); pulmonary fibrosarcoma has been associated with an ectopic worm. The granulomas around *S. lupi* contain highly reactive pleomorphic fibroblasts with large open nuclei and numerous mitotic figures. Neoplasms arising from such lesions have cytologic characteristics typical of fibrosarcoma, osteosarcoma, or chondrosarcoma, with local tissue invasion, and in many cases, pulmonary metastasis. The carcinogenic stimuli associated with the development of these tumors are unknown, although it has been suggested that *S. lupi* proteinaceous secretory/excretory products may play a role in neoplastic transformation. Hypertrophic pulmonary osteopathy is occasionally found in animals with *Spirocerca*-associated sarcoma and, rarely, granuloma.

FORESTOMACHS

Structure, function, and response to injury

The rumen is the central processing unit for ingesta and is critical to the ruminant's well-being. However, because most of this occurs as a chemical process with minimal morphologic correlates, the rumen is an organ that is easily overlooked by pathologists. Examination of ruminal contents may provide critical clues about general metabolic states. Overly dry contents are an excellent indicator of dehydration. Voluminous frothy contents occur with primary bloat. Urea toxicity can be detected by an ammoniacal odor and alkaline pH. An odor of cooked turnips or a pungent insecticidal smell is suggestive of organophosphates. In grain overload, contents have a fermentative odor and pH may be <5.0. However, with putrefaction and release of toxic amines into the rumen, pH in cases of acidosis may return to near-normal levels as the postmortem interval progresses. In animals with subacute ruminal acidosis, the ruminal epithelium remains adherent to the submucosa despite any intervening postmortem changes, and it is an important clue to mucosal disease. Vagus indigestion, often associated with dysfunction of the esophageal groove, leads to accumulation of large volumes of watery fluid within the forestomachs. Recognition of characteristic foliage in rumen content may lead to a diagnosis of poisoning by several different toxic plants, including cyanogenic plants of the genus *Prunus*, oleandrin-containing plants of the genus *Nerium, and* taxine alkaloid-containing plants of the genus *Taxus*. Motor oil, paint flakes, or metallic lead present in the rumen would support a diagnosis of lead poisoning. Several other toxic substances can be identified by visual inspection of the ruminal contents. Whole individuals or parts of the pollen beetle *Astylus atromaculatus* can be found in the rumen content of animals intoxicated by these insects.

Postmortem changes in the forestomach are important to recognize. The ruminal mucosal epithelium usually sloughs within a few hours after death. It separates from the lamina propria in large gray patches, which cover the ingesta when the rumen is opened. *Persistent firm attachment of the ruminal epithelium is abnormal.* This undue adhesion occurs in subacute and chronic rumenitis, especially if caused by fungi, and about scars of healed rumenitis. Adhesion usually does not occur in acute ruminal acidosis.

Hyperplasia and dysplasia of the forestomachs. The ruminal mucosa is unique in that it has a stratified squamous epithelium that functions in absorption as well as protection from the vat of fermenting bacteria contained within. Langerhans cells are distributed within the mucosa throughout all compartments of the ovine rumen. T lymphocytes are found individually, and in aggregates, in both intraepithelial and subepithelial locations, with most in the cranial sac and relatively few dorsally.

Ruminal papillae in newborn calves are rudimentary and their subsequent development is dependent on diet, possibly as a consequence of stimulation by insulin-like growth factor 1. The end products of ruminal carbohydrate fermentation, propionate and butyrate, stimulate papillary growth. Papillae can take a variety of shapes, including long and flat, conical, spade-shaped, or hair-like. High-concentrate rations, which provide abundant propionate and butyrate, tend to produce papillae that are club-shaped, clumped (Fig. 1-25), and may be dark. Microscopically, these papillae are covered with epithelium displaying acanthosis, hyperkeratosis, orthokeratosis, and parakeratosis, and hyperpigmentation. Secondary papillae may be hyperplastic as well, creating the clumped appearance or rosette-like configurations. Rumens in animals fed barley rations have similar changes. Hairs from the rachilla of the barley adhere to the mucosa, especially in the interpapillary areas, giving it a distinct matted appearance. These penetrate the mucosa and lamina propria, where they evoke a leukocytic reaction, often causing microabscesses. A diffuse pleocellular reaction is evident in the thickened fibrotic wall.

Roughage also plays a role. When animals receive adequate levels (~15%) of coarse roughage, propionic and butyric acids decrease, whereas acetic acid levels increase, precluding hyperkeratosis and parakeratosis.

Hyperkeratosis of the ruminal epithelium also occurs in calves deficient in vitamin A.

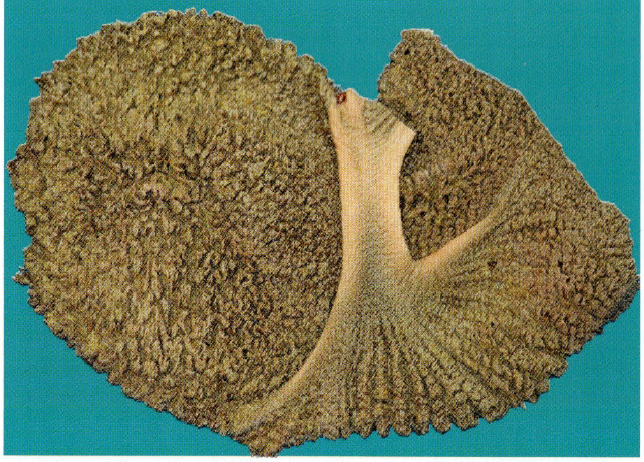

Figure 1-25 Clubbing and adhesion of rumen papillae with parakeratotic epithelium, associated with feeding a high-concentrate ration in a calf. (Courtesy S.S. Diab.)

Diseases of the forestomachs

Degenerative and inflammatory conditions of the forestomachs

Rumen tympany or tympanitic distension of the forestomachs (hoven, bloat) may be acute or chronic and recurrent. In acute or primary tympany of cattle fed legumes or high-concentrate rations, rumen contents foam, which prevents gas from being eructated; in chronic or recurrent (secondary) tympany, the gas is free but retained because of some physical or functional defect of eructation.

Primary tympany is also called *frothy bloat*. Foam production in ruminal contents occurs normally. However, the amount of foam produced is small and unstable. There is apparently a delicate balance between profoaming and antifoaming factors in the rumen. These factors are multiple, and there is considerable controversy as to the extent to which each one influences the production of the foamy, viscous ruminal content so characteristic of frothy bloat, the most common cause of rumen distension.

The formation of foam is dependent on *soluble proteins*, especially fraction I proteins, which are present in high levels (up to 4.5%) in bloat-inducing legumes, such as alfalfa and clover, especially in the prebloom stage of growth. Other legumes, notably sainfoin, trefoil, and cicer milk vetch, are not associated with bloat. Soluble proteins, released from chloroplasts, are degraded by the rumen microflora, and they rise to the surface where they are denatured, become insoluble, and stabilize the foam. The optimal pH (isoelectric point) for foam production by soluble proteins is 5.4-6.0. *Pectins* are considered to increase the viscosity of ruminal fluid and may act as foam-stabilizing agents. Plant lipids may act as antifoaming agents by competing for metal ions with the soluble proteins, thus inhibiting the denaturation of these proteins and resulting in decreased foam production. Development of bloat is associated with increased richness and diversity of ruminal microbiota.

Eructation is a complex series of muscular contractions in which gas is forced from the rumen through the cardia and is released through the esophagus. The eructation sequence is initiated by free gas in the dorsal sac of the rumen. Thus, if ruminal conditions prevent normal contractions from occurring in the reticulorumen, or if movement of free gas through the cardia or esophagus is obstructed, bloat occurs. Excessive foam production causes distension of the rumen because it prevents formation of a free gas cap and the clearing of the cardia, which is essential for normal eructation to take place. When foam enters the esophagus, it stimulates the swallowing reflex, which also interferes with normal eructation. Gassy froth accumulates in the rumen as a consequence.

The variation among animals in their susceptibility to bloat may be determined in part by variations in the amount and composition of *saliva*. Saliva apparently has properties that may promote or prevent foaming in the rumen. When secretion of saliva decreases, the viscosity of ruminal contents increases, which in turn promotes foaming. Cows that have high susceptibility to bloating produce less saliva than cows that have low susceptibility. Succulent and high-concentrate feeds reduce saliva secretion, thus increasing viscosity of rumen contents. The composition of saliva also affects foam production in several ways. Combination of salivary bicarbonate with organic acids such as citric, malonic, and succinic, which are present in high levels in legumes, results in the production of large amounts of *carbon dioxide*, enhancing bubble formation. Carbon dioxide accounts for 40-70% of the total gas produced in the rumen.

High and low susceptibility to bloat can be temporarily transferred between animals by exchange of total reticulorumen contents. The understanding of the full role played by these various factors in bloat is incomplete, and other factors may be involved.

Rations high in concentrate and low in roughage not only reduce saliva secretion but also change the ruminal microflora. They promote the growth of large numbers of encapsulated bacteria, which increase the concentration of polysaccharides, and these, in turn, increase the viscosity, promoting foam. These bacteria are also often mucinolytic and may destroy salivary mucins. Perhaps this explains the more gradual onset of **feedlot bloat** because it takes time for the ruminal flora to change. Particle size of the grains fed may be one factor in feedlot bloat, with smaller particle size predisposing more to bloat.

The *cause of death* in bloat is probably a combination of physical and metabolic effects. Increased intra-abdominal pressure on the diaphragm inhibits respiration and adversely affects cardiac function. Hypoxia may be caused by respiratory embarrassment. Increased intra-abdominal pressure also has a marked effect on the hemodynamics of the abdominal viscera, which are compressed, driving blood out of them. The caudal vena cava is also compressed, decreasing venous return to the heart. Distension also affects mucosal permeability and alters vagosympathetic reflexes.

The bloated animal is often found dead and distended with gas; blood exudes from the orifices, and because of the gaseous distension, the carcass often rolls on its back and assumes a sawhorse posture, with forelegs extended forward and rear legs pointing backward. The blood is dark and clots poorly; both features are indicative of death from anoxia. Subcutaneous hemorrhages are prominent in the cranial extremities, which are congested. There is marked edema, congestion, and hemorrhage of the cervical muscles and of the lymph nodes of the head and neck. An inconsistent but suggestive finding is the so-called *bloat line* in the esophageal mucosa (Fig. 1-26A). This lesion is formed because of congestion with petechial and ecchymotic hemorrhages in the mucosa of the cervical esophagus, which changes abruptly or gradually to a pale mucosa at the level of the thoracic inlet. Although this line is usually considered highly suggestive of bloat, a similar change can apparently be seen in other conditions and some pathologists do not interpret this line as diagnostic for bloat.

The tracheal mucosa is hemorrhagic, especially cranial to the thoracic inlet. Blood clots are frequently seen in the bronchi, and in paranasal and frontal sinuses. The lungs are pale and compressed into the cranial thorax by the bulging diaphragm. There is pressure ischemia of the abdominal viscera, especially the liver, although the extreme margins of the hepatic lobes may be congested. Lymph nodes and the muscles of the hindlimbs are pale.

There may be marked subcutaneous edema, particularly of the vulva, inguinal region, and perineum, and intestines may herniate through the inguinal canals. If the autopsy is done soon after death, the ruminal contents are bulky and foamy (see Fig. 1-26B). The foam gradually disappears after death and is usually absent if the autopsy is delayed for 10-12 hours. Inguinal hernia and diaphragmatic rupture may occur after death.

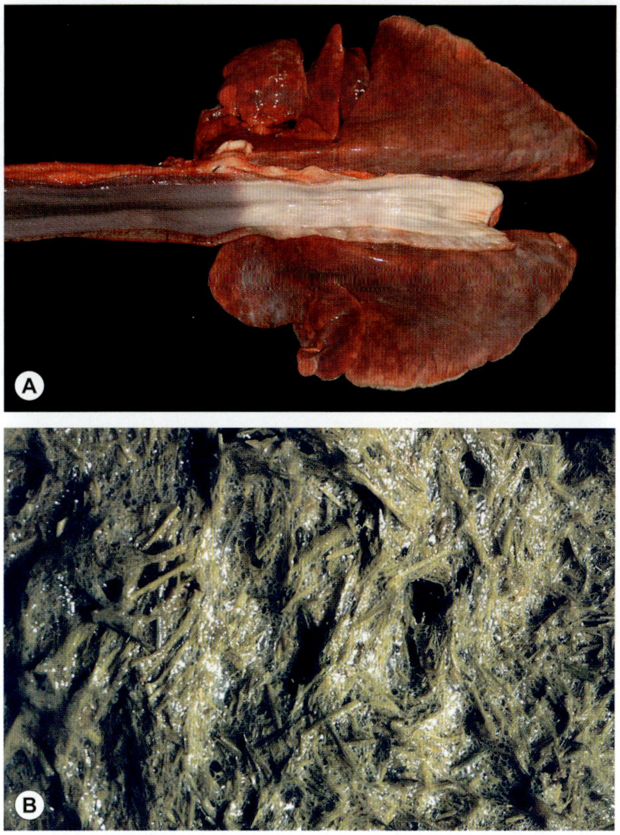

Figure 1-26 **A. Bloat line** in the esophagus of a goat with ruminal tympany. (Courtesy N. Streitenberger.) Congestion of the esophagus and connective tissue cranial to thoracic inlet and blanching of esophagus caudal to thoracic inlet. **B. Frothy bloat** in a cow. Fine bubbles in the rumen content.

Secondary tympany (free gas or secondary bloat) may be acute, but is generally chronic, with periods of acute exacerbation. It is usually the result of a physical or functional *defect in eructation of gas* produced by normal rumen fermentation. The more common physical problems include internal or external obstructions of the esophagus or esophageal groove by tumor, foreign body, or esophageal stenosis of any cause. Reticular adhesions, abscesses, peritonitis, or tumor masses that interfere with contractions of the forestomach can result in bloat. Functional causes of secondary tympany include organophosphate intoxication, and vagal damage caused by adhesions, lymphomatous infiltrates, or right-sided abomasal displacement and volvulus. Secondary tympany is a component of the syndromes collectively termed *vagus indigestion*. Bloat caused by muscular dystrophy of the diaphragmatic muscles has been described in both Meuse-Rhine-Issel and Holstein-Friesian breeds of cattle.

Secondary tympany, which is sometimes fatal, occurs in *bucket-fed calves*. This may be a persistent problem in some veal calves, which are known as *ruminal drinkers*. They ingest large amounts of milk, which escapes the reticular groove when the esophageal groove reflex fails, and flows into the rumen, where it putrefies because of digestion by proteolytic bacteria and transformation of lactose into lactate by lactobacilli causing ruminal and metabolic acidosis. Casein clot formation in the abomasum is partly inhibited. The clinical signs include inappetence, unthriftiness, recurrent tympany, abdominal distension, and clay-like feces. Because of butyric and lactic acid accumulation in the epithelium of the reticulorumen, ruminal drinking leads to hyperkeratotic parakeratosis and severe reticulorumenitis accompanied by epithelial loss, erosions, and necrosis, associated with bacterial and fungal infections.

Animals fed rations that have excess indigestible roughage may have recurrent episodes of bloat. Feed must contain adequate portions of protein, starch, and/or sugars, and cellulose to stimulate growth of the cellulolytic microflora. Indigestible roughage accumulates in the rumen and reticulum when the intake of digestible nutrients (starches and sugars) is inadequate. As a result, the forestomachs become dilated, which in turn inhibits reticuloruminal contractions that are required for clearance of the cardia and subsequent eructation.

A postmortem *diagnosis of secondary bloat* is based on autopsy findings, which are similar to those described in primary bloat, but without frothy rumen content, and with the addition of any physical causes of impaired eructation. Postmortem distension of the rumen must not be mistaken for antemortem tympany.

Foreign bodies. Cattle are notoriously lacking in alimentary finesse, a deficiency that allows an amazing variety of foreign bodies prehended with the food to be deposited in the forestomachs. Although sheep and goats have more selective eating habits, foreign bodies can also be found, albeit less frequently in their rumens. A large proportion of adult cattle, and fewer goats or sheep, have metallic, wood, or plastic foreign bodies in the rumen and reticulum, but rarely in the omasum. Some of these foreign bodies can have a large size that can occupy a significant part of the rumen, reducing the capacity of the rumen to function normally, and occasionally cause blockages.

Spherical masses consisting largely of hair or wool **(trichobezoars)** or plant fibers **(phytobezoars)** may also form in these compartments. Hairballs are most common in younger ruminants, the hair being swallowed after licking, particularly by animals deprived of dietary fiber. They may have some other foreign body as a nucleus and contain a proportion of plant fibers, the whole mass concreted by organic substances and inorganic salts. The same general comments apply to phytobezoars. Being smooth, neither are important unless regurgitated to lodge in the esophagus or passed on to obstruct the reticulo-omasal orifice, the pylorus, or the intestine, which is very infrequent. Otherwise, these bezoars are an incidental finding.

The important foreign bodies are those (such as lead) that cause *intoxication* when dissolved and those that (being abrasive or sharp) *penetrate the mucosa*. In calves on diets low in roughage, ingestion of wood shavings or straw may lead to diffuse transmural inflammation of the forestomachs and sometimes the abomasum. A mixed aerobic and anaerobic bacterial flora is responsible for that inflammation, presumably following mucosal trauma. The sequel to penetration by sharp objects in adult cattle is traumatic reticuloperitonitis.

Traumatic reticuloperitonitis. Perforation of the forestomachs by foreign bodies is virtually always caused by a long, thin, and sharp foreign body, usually a *wire or nail*, penetrating the reticular wall. Incomplete perforation is usually inconsequential, although in some cases focal neutrophilic or granulomatous inflammation develops in the wall of the reticulum, with or without minor overlying peritonitis. There are no adequate answers as to why perforation occurs, but it is probably caused by forceful contraction of the reticulum, and many cases seem to be predisposed by the increased intra-abdominal pressure of late pregnancy and parturition.

The prophylactic use of *magnets* is common in many herds, and this probably has contributed to a marked decrease in fatal cases of traumatic reticuloperitonitis. Magnets are often found incidentally in the reticulum, completely covered by metal foreign bodies, including nails and wires, which might otherwise have penetrated the reticular wall. The replacement of baling wire with twine in many parts of the world is another reason for the decline in the prevalence of this disease.

The outcome of complete perforation is common, but variations in the pattern are frequent. The perforation is usually in the cranioventral direction and is followed immediately by *acute local peritonitis*. If the foreign body is short or bent, it may progress no further, and some foreign bodies are apparently withdrawn with the next reticular movement; in such instances, only *chronic local peritonitis* with adhesions develops. The foreign body may advance to perforate the diaphragm and pericardium, resulting in *traumatic pericarditis*.

A ventral penetration may result in subperitoneal and subcutaneous abscessation near the xiphoid. Rare perforation of one of the larger regional arteries may result in sudden death from hemorrhage, and sudden death may also occur if there is penetration of the myocardium or rupture of a coronary artery. Septicemia is also a possible but uncommon complication. Penetration of the thoracic cavity may occur without perforation of the pericardium, causing pneumonia and pleuritis. Right lateral deviation of the penetrating agent involves the wall of the abomasum. It is unusual for the liver or spleen to be penetrated, but metastatic abscesses in the liver are common.

As soon as the foreign body penetrates the serosa, local fibrinous peritonitis develops, which later leads to dense adhesion of variable extent between the reticulum and adjacent structures. Further progression of the foreign body is ordinarily slow and produces a canal surrounded by chronic granulation tissue and containing, besides the foreign body, ingesta, purulent exudate, and other detritus. The bacteria commonly active in the tract include *T. pyogenes*, *F. necrophorum*, and various other microorganisms. In many cases, a foreign body cannot be found, perhaps because it has rusted away or been withdrawn into the reticulum.

One of the variants in the usual pattern of migration of the foreign body is penetration of the right side of the reticulum, leading to neutrophilic inflammation in the grooves between the reticulum, omasum, and abomasum. The acute local peritonitis causes immediate cessation of ruminal movements; however, persistent ruminal atony or irregular motility with gradual onset of bilateral abdominal distension, inappetence, and decreased milk production may ensue. Clinically, this is referred to as **vagus indigestion**, which also may be a sequel to abomasal displacement. At autopsy, there are very characteristic changes in the stomachs with this syndrome. The rumen is distended with enough fluid to cause sloshing if the carcass is jolted. There is no ruminal fermentation or normal odor, and bits of unmacerated straw and food particles float on the watery fluid; the more normal ingesta has sedimented. The omasum can be very large and impacted with dehydrated ingesta. The abomasum may be distended and impacted with dry ingesta, presumably because of functional pyloric stenosis or abomasal stasis.

The question of the importance of vagal nerve damage in the pathogenesis of vagus indigestion remains unresolved. The consensus is that this syndrome is associated with mechanical or functional impairment of outflow of ingesta from the forestomachs or abomasum, but in some cases the primary defect appears to reside in flaccidity of the reticular groove and in degeneration of its muscle and intramuscular nerve plexus. The rumen and reticulum are dependent on intact vagi for normal movement, and a minority of cases of vagus indigestion appears to be associated with damaged nerves. *Vagal lesions* may be in the pharyngeal and cervical areas, or intrathoracic, such as lymphomatous infiltration, or abdominal. The latter are usually investment of the nerve in adhesions following reticular perforation, or trauma following abomasal volvulus.

In other cases, degeneration of the vagus is not evident. In these, the dysfunction and lesions are more likely to be due to peritonitis and the subsequent abscessation, or adhesions that disrupt the normal tension-receptor activity or cause a pain response that interferes with normal motility of the forestomachs and abomasum.

In **failure of omasal transport** (*type II vagus indigestion*), there is impairment of movement of ingesta from the reticulorumen to the omasum, associated with abscesses adjacent to the reticulo-omasal orifice. There, lesions probably result in mechanical or neural interference to emptying of the reticulorumen.

A *diagnosis* of vagal indigestion at autopsy is ordinarily dependent on evidence of abnormal abomasal, omasal, or reticuloruminal motility, in association with morphologic lesions of the vagus nerves, adhesions, or neoplasms involving the forestomachs and abomasum.

Traumatic pericarditis is a less common sequel now, perhaps because many of the initial penetrations are diagnosed and the foreign body removed surgically; furthermore, as discussed previously, cases of traumatic reticuloperitonitis have decreased. The pericardial reaction is copious and fibrinopurulent. There are usually additional lesions of traumatic pneumonia and pleuritis.

Various *bacterial, viral, parasitic, mycotic, toxic,* and *nutritional diseases* can cause **inflammation of the forestomachs in ruminants**. Bacterial, viral, parasitic, and mycotic rumenitis are described fully in the Infectious and Parasitic Diseases of the Alimentary Tract section, later in this chapter. In neonatal calves, necrosis of ruminal mucosa is an important sequel to bovine alphaherpesvirus 1 infection. *Bovine papular stomatitis* and *contagious ecthyma* may also cause rumen lesions, albeit less frequently. Ruminal erosions and ulcers are present occasionally in cattle with *FMD* or *BVD*. Extensive hemorrhage and ulceration of the reticuloruminal mucosa may be seen in *bluetongue (BT)* in sheep and *epizootic hemorrhagic disease (EHD)* of deer and cattle. Adenoviral infection occasionally causes multifocal fibrinohemorrhagic rumenitis in cattle and deer. *MCF* can also produce erosions and ulcers in the rumen of cattle, bison, and wild ungulates. Primary bacterial or mycotic inflammatory lesions of the rumen are uncommon; they can occur subsequent to chemical rumenitis, primary viral rumenitis, sepsis, or intensive antibiotic treatment.

Mild inflammation of the forestomachs occurs in some young *ruminal drinker* calves fed *milk* from a pail, as discussed previously. A similar problem occurs with feeding by stomach tube. Putrefaction in these compartments leads to mild neutrophilic rumenitis.

Accidental consumption of excessive quantities of *urea*, in the form of nonprotein nitrogen supplement, or fertilizer, in liquid or powder form, results in the production of ammonia in the rumen. The toxic effect is accelerated by urease in soy-based rations and is based on the production of high blood levels of ammonia. Rumen contents smell ammoniacal when the organ is opened; the content is alkaline (pH 7.5-8); and there may be congestion or coagulative necrosis of the cranioventral wall of the rumen. Elevated ruminal and abomasal pH values (7.0), without specific lesions, have been associated with ingestion of *boron* fertilizer by cattle and goats.

Ingestion of toxic levels of *sulfur* results in chemical rumenitis because of the conversion of sulfur to hydrogen sulfide, and possibly sulfurous acid, in the rumen. Large amounts of yellow sulfur particles are usually found in the rumen and abomasum. Eructation and subsequent inhalation of hydrogen sulfide result in acute alveolitis. Absorption of sulfides from the lungs leads to marked depression of the respiratory and cardiovascular centers in the CNS. Affected animals also develop acidosis, probably caused by the absorption of acids, and impaired renal function associated with the direct toxic effects of sulfur metabolites on tubular epithelial cells.

Inflammation of the forestomachs may be associated with certain *plant toxicoses*, mainly in Australia, Africa, and South America. Examples are Kikuyu grass (*Cenchrus clandestinus*, previously *Pennisetum clandestinum*), prickly paddy melon (*Cucumis myriocarpus*), and several species of *Bryophyllum*, *Lupinus*, and *Phytolacca*. The pollen beetle, *A. atromaculatus*, has been associated with rumenitis in cattle and sheep.

Feeding rations deficient in fiber, which is increasingly the case in developed countries, can alter the microflora, predisposing the animals to metabolic disorders or rumenitis. In addition, acute chemical rumenitis develops after overeating on rapidly fermentable carbohydrate, usually grain.

Fusobacterium necrophorum is a normal inhabitant of the anaerobic ruminal environment. This bacterium is commonly responsible for complications of ruminal acidosis, producing characteristic lesions in the forestomachs (Fig. 1-27A) and in the liver. Invasion of the wall of the rumen takes advantage of the foothold provided by the superficial necrosis and inflammation of acidosis. Inflammatory changes favor the adherence of *F. necrophorum* to ruminal epithelium.

Necrobacillary rumenitis is common in feedlot cattle, probably a product of mild acidosis following a too-rapid introduction to a high-concentrate ration. It affects the papillated areas of the ventral sac and occasionally the pillars. On the mucosal surface, the early lesions are visible as various irregular patches 2-15 cm across, in which the papillae are swollen, dark, slightly mushy, and are matted together by fibrinocellular inflammatory exudate. Affected papillae are necrotic, but ulceration may be delayed if there is ruminal atony and stasis. If the animal recovers from the immediate effects of overeating, the necrotic epithelium sloughs, the ulcer contracts, and epithelial regeneration begins from the margins. The regenerated epithelium is flat and white, and the papillae do not return completely. A stellate scar often remains (see Fig. 1-27B), but many of the smaller lesions may disappear completely. Liver abscesses are the main complication of the *F. necrophorum* rumenitis, and the term "*rumenitis-liver abscess complex*" is frequently used to describe this condition. Although the precise mechanism is not fully understood, it is recognized that bacterial emboli are released from the *F. necrophorum*–infected ruminal wall into the portal circulation, followed by bacteria being filtered by the liver, resulting in hepatic infection and abscess formation. *Hepatic lesions* are initially the typical coagulative necrosis of necrobacillosis, but in time they liquefy to

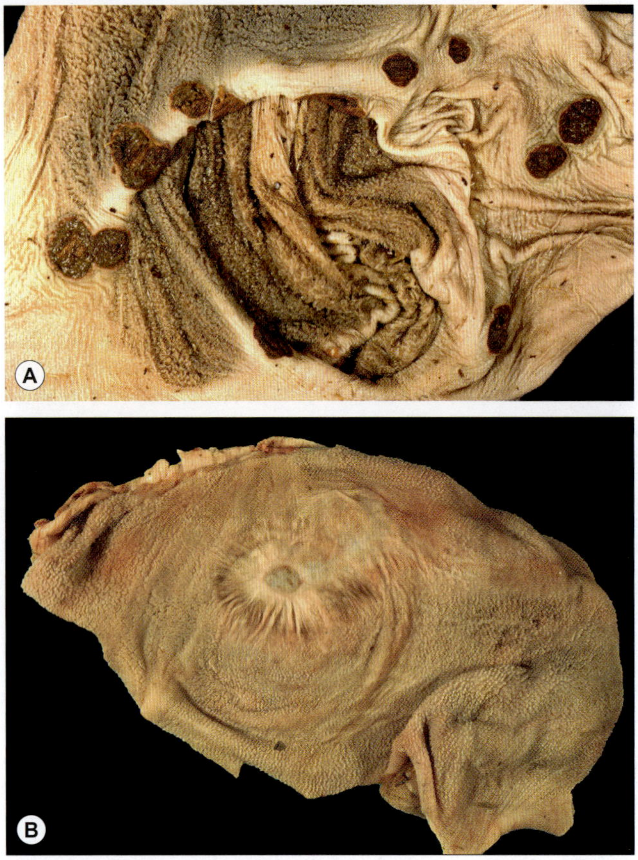

Figure 1-27 **Necrobacillosis** in the rumen of a cow. **A.** Plaques and coalescing areas of necrosis are evident on the mucosa. (Courtesy V. Perez.) **B.** Stellate scarring of incompletely healed ulcer in the rumen mucosa.

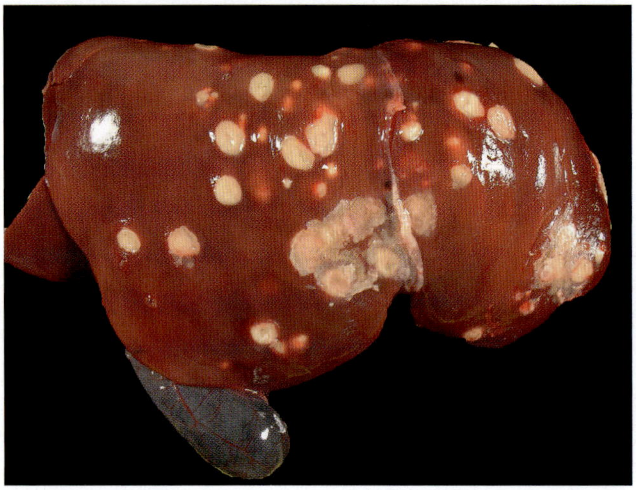

Figure 1-28 Hepatic abscessation in **necrobacillosis** in a lamb. (Courtesy V. Perez.)

form abscesses (Fig. 1-28), and these often persist long after the initial ruminal lesions have cicatrized or disappeared.

It is unusual for ruminal necrobacillosis in cattle to be more than a superficial infection, and although the muscle layers are involved in the inflammation, they are not ordinarily invaded by the organism. However, perforation of the omasal leaves is common. In sheep, the infection is more aggressive, although less frequently observed, than it is in cattle. *Fusobacterium varium* has also been reported to produce liver abscesses associated with rumenitis in sheep. Alimentary necrobacillosis of the gastric compartments has also been described in alpacas, in most of which the condition was considered secondary to neoplasia or other chronic debilitating conditions.

Several **viral diseases** that affect the oral cavity and esophagus can extend to the rumen. These include BVD, BT, contagious ecthyma, EHD, infectious bovine rhinotracheitis, and MCF, among others.

Mycotic infection should be suspected when inflammation in the wall of the forestomachs extends to the serosa and is *hemorrhagic* and *angiocentric*. The fungi, which, like *F. necrophorum*, are opportunists, are usually of the order *Mucorales* (formerly *zygomycetes*), including genera *Rhizopus, Mortierella*, and *Lichtheimia* (formerly *Absidia*), which cannot be differentiated from each other in histologic sections. The disease occurs in cattle, sheep, goats, bison, and other ruminant species.

Mycotic rumenitis is much more severe and extensive than necrobacillary rumenitis and is often fatal. *The basis for the lesion is submucosal venular thrombosis caused by fungal invasion*, causing venous infarction of the tissue field involved. The inflammation extends to the peritoneum, causing hemorrhagic and fibrinous peritonitis that mats the omentum to the rumen. In fatal cases, most of the ventral sac and parts of the reticulum, omasum, and/or abomasum are involved. The lesions are very striking and suggest on initial inspection that the walls have been massively infarcted, which in part they have (Fig. 1-29A). The margins are well demarcated, usually by a narrow zone of congestive swelling. The affected areas are roughly circular, red-to-black, sometimes with a pale central area, thickened to 1 cm or more, firm, and leathery. There is acute fibrinohemorrhagic inflammation of the overlying peritoneum, and blood-stained, inflammatory edema in the grooves beneath. The spleen also may be affected.

On the inner surface of the rumen, the lesions are more hemorrhagic than those of necrobacillosis, and more irregular in outline (see Fig. 1-29B), and the necrotic epithelium is difficult to detach. Histologically, there is transmural hemorrhage of the rumen wall, copious fibrinous exudate, and rather scant leukocytic reaction. *Fungal hyphae* with nonparallel walls are readily visible in the necrotic tissues and the lumina of the thrombosed blood vessels. Granulomatous inflammation occurs in the deeper parts of the mucosal lesion in more chronic cases.

Mycotic rumenitis and omasitis may occur in cows that do not have a history of acidosis. It has been suggested that these cases may be a sequel of sepsis, with reflux of abomasal fluid into the forestomachs, and therapy with broad-spectrum antimicrobials acting as predisposing factors for mycotic infections. It can also be a sequel to ruminal damage in survivors of BVDV infection. Secondary infections sometimes occur in the liver and cause necrotizing thrombophlebitis of the portal radicles visible as small irregular tan areas of infarction surrounded by a deep red margin.

Other conditions that have been associated with ruminal acidosis are *laminitis* and an *encephalopathy*, which morphologically resembles the lesions of early polioencephalomalacia (see Vol. 1, Integumentary System; Vol. 1, Nervous System).

Ruminal acidosis and rumenitis associated with ingestion of excess carbohydrate are problems mainly of *intensive beef and dairy cattle production*. Although ruminal acidosis frequently leads to metabolic acidosis, these are 2 different conditions,

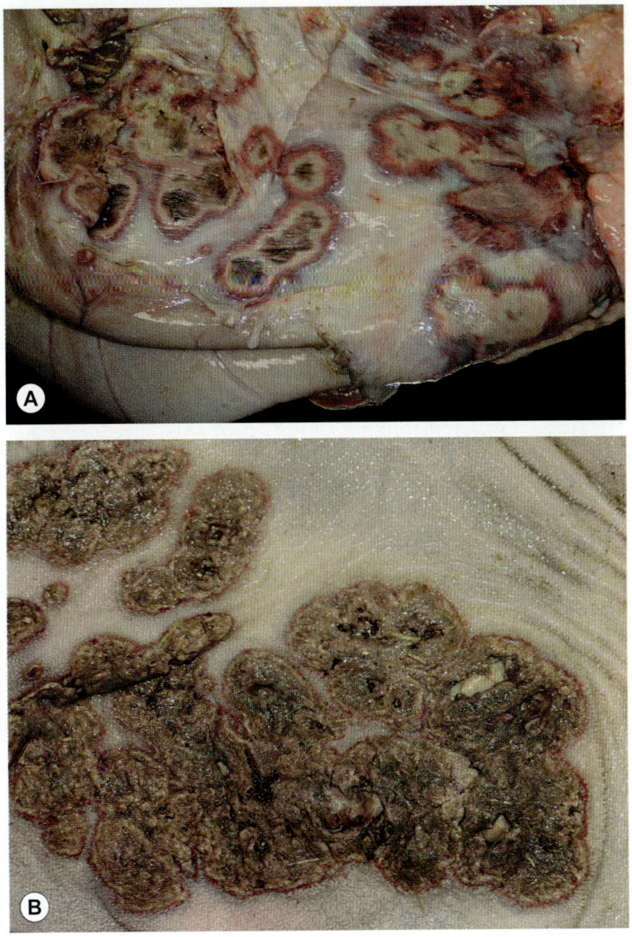

Figure 1-29 **Mycotic rumenitis** (mucormycosis) following acidosis in a reindeer. **A.** Roughly circular and dark areas of infarction, most of them with a pale halo, involving rumen and reticulum. **B.** Appearance of mucosal surface of rumen; large areas of necrosis surrounded by a red halo of hemorrhage and inflammation.

and in this section we will be dealing with the former. Sheep and goats are also susceptible to this problem. Its importance lies partly in loss of production and partly in mortality because of the acute disease, in which rumenitis is of minor significance and lactic acidosis is the major cause of morbidity and mortality. Rumenitis assumes significance in subclinical disease or in survivors of acute episodes, by providing a portal for the entry for fungi and *F. necrophorum*, which cause secondary infections. These complications were discussed earlier. Other complications include coexisting primary tympany (frothy bloat), which may be the fatal partner of grain overload in feedlot cattle.

Ruminal acidosis usually follows the *ingestion of excess carbohydrate* in the form of grain, or other fermentable feedstuffs, such as root crops, bread, waste baked goods, brewers' waste, and apples. There is wide variation in the amount of carbohydrate necessary to kill an animal because tolerance to rations high in starch does develop if they are introduced gradually. Sudden increments in the amount of carbohydrate ingested are of more importance than the actual amount. Sudden changes from concentrates with lower energy values to those with higher values may predispose to acidosis. Extreme environmental temperature changes, either hotter or cooler, may result in temporary reductions in feed consumption, and acidosis may develop once such animals return to full feed.

Shortly after the ingestion of a toxic amount of carbohydrate, ruminal pH begins to fall. The decrease in pH during the first few hours is mainly caused by an increase in dissociated volatile fatty acids, not lactic acid. The production of the latter increases after there has been a marked change in the ruminal flora, which is very responsive to the substrate available for fermentation. *In cattle and sheep, the normal pH of ruminal fluid is 5.5-7.5, depending on the diet fed.* A ruminal content pH of 5.5 or below should be considered indicative of ruminal acidosis.

The gram-negative bacteria that predominate in the normal flora, and the protozoa, are very sensitive to changes in the pH; most die at a pH of 5.0 or less. Once the pH of the ruminal contents starts to fall, streptococci, mainly *Streptococcus bovis*, proliferate rapidly, acting as a major source of lactic acid. When the pH reaches 5.0-4.5, the numbers of streptococci decrease, with a concomitant increase in lactobacilli. The pH of rumen content may fall as low as 4.0-4.5 in fatal cases.

As ruminal pH drops, ruminal atony develops, mainly as the result of an increase in the concentration of the nondissociated volatile fatty acids, lactic, propionic, and butyric. They act on receptors that mediate inhibition of reticuloruminal motility via a vagovagal reflex. Loss of forestomach motility in ruminal acidosis is apparently not dependent on the development of systemic acidosis. There is also cessation of saliva secretion, so that the buffering effect of saliva is absent.

The increase in ruminal organic acids, mainly lactate, causes an increase in ruminal osmotic pressure. This results in movement of fluid from the blood into the rumen, producing bulky and liquid ruminal contents and severe dehydration. Plasma volume is reduced; hemoconcentration, anuria, and circulatory collapse follow. Serum protein levels, urea, inorganic phosphorus, lactate, pyruvate, and liver enzymes are all elevated. The osmotic pressure of the intestinal contents also increases when the ingesta with the high lactate concentrations arrives. Loss of fluid at this level probably contributes further to the dehydration, and it may also play a significant role in the development of the diarrhea that is commonly seen clinically. In addition to the osmotic effects, there is acidosis caused by the absorption of lactate from the rumen, and possibly from the intestine.

The low ruminal pH is lethal to much of the normal flora and fauna. The protozoa appear to be particularly sensitive, but many types of bacteria are also lost. In those animals that survive the acute phase of ruminal acidosis, recovery is not complete until a normal ruminal flora is re-established through contact with other animals or by transplant of ruminal content from healthy animals. Temporary recovery may be followed by what appears clinically to be a relapse in acidosis, but which is a developing mycotic rumenitis. If treatment of the initial fluid imbalance is delayed, death may occur in a week or so from ischemic renal cortical necrosis.

The **gross findings** in this metabolic disease are not specific, and a practical diagnosis requires knowledge of a history of access to fermentable carbohydrate and clinically observed circulatory failure. At autopsy, the eyes are sunken, the blood may be thick and dark because of dehydration and hypoxia, and there is general venous congestion. The appearance of the ruminal contents varies with the time interval between the ingestion of the carbohydrate and the autopsy. In the early stages, there is a copious amount of porridge-like rumen content, which has a distinct fermentative odor. The amount of grain or other source of starch varies considerably and is an unreliable indication of acidosis, and finely ground concentrate may be overlooked. Ruminal pH is only helpful when it is low (<5.5) because it may rise in later stages of the disease or when postmortem putrefaction ensues. Although the ruminal contents may appear relatively normal in more advanced cases of acidosis, intestinal contents tend to remain very watery. The absence of protozoa is consistent with chemical rumenitis but is also influenced by the interval between death and the postmortem examination. In subacute cases of ruminal acidosis there may be no gross changes in the rumen or rest of the body, but histologically, there is superficial neutrophilic rumenitis affecting the ruminal epithelium and submucosa.

The **diagnosis** of ruminal acidosis at autopsy can be difficult. The most suggestive abnormality is the *rumenitis* (Fig. 1-30A). It is probably chemical and dependent on the low pH and is not readily discerned grossly. There may be a slight poorly defined blue discoloration in the ventral sac of the rumen, reticulum, and omasum, visible through the serosa. When the epithelium is detached, the lamina propria may be hyperemic in patches. In some cases, the epithelium appears to have undergone fixation because of low pH and is difficult to peel.

Microscopic examination of the ruminal mucosa is the most reliable way of confirming a diagnosis of subacute or chronic acidosis. The ruminal papillae appear enlarged. There is marked cytoplasmic vacuolation of the epithelial cells, often leading to vesiculation. A mild-to-marked neutrophilic reaction is evident in the mucosa and submucosa, along with variable rumen mucosal parakeratosis (see Fig. 1-30B). In subacute-to-chronic cases, subtle lesions of intraepithelial pustules are evident (see Fig. 1-30C). Focal areas of erosion and ulceration may or may not be present. However, in cases of acute acidosis, there may not be significant microscopic changes in the ruminal mucosa.

Several **parasites** can cause inflammation in the forestomach of ruminants. *Gongylonema* spp. occur in the epithelium of the rumen. They appear as described in the esophagus and are not pathogenic. More important parasites are the conical **rumen flukes** belonging to the family *Paramphistomatidae*. Although several species of *Paramphistomum* have been described, *Paramphistomum cervi* is probably the most widespread species; *Calicophoron daubneyi* is reported to be common in cattle and sheep in Great Britain. *Paramphistomum* parasites are found in cattle and sheep in warm temperate, subtropical, and tropical regions. These red, plump, droplet-shaped flukes are about the size of the papillae between which they reside in the rumen, where they are usually considered to be mostly nonpathogenic (Fig. 1-31A). However, if present in very high numbers, they can cause lymphoplasmacytic rumenoreticulitis, with atrophy of papillae and excessive cornification of the stratum corneum and granulosum (see Fig. 1-31B). Loss of condition has been observed in adult cattle with massive ruminal infestation of *Paramphistomum* spp.

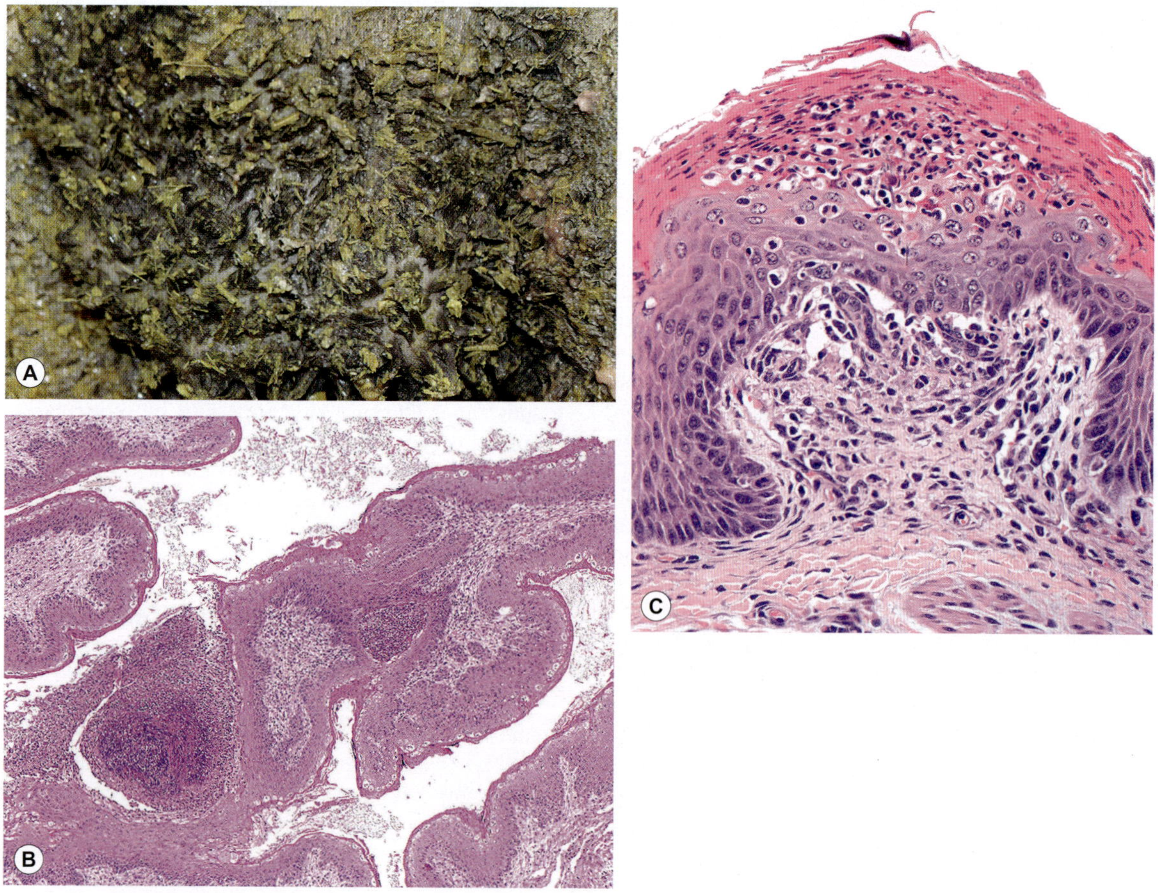

Figure 1-30 Ruminal acidosis and rumenitis. A. Rumen papillae are clumped and adhered to each other. **B**. Parakeratosis and severe neutrophilic inflammation of the mucosa and submucosa of the rumen. **C**. Neutrophilic intraepithelial pustules in subacute-to-chronic chemical rumenitis.

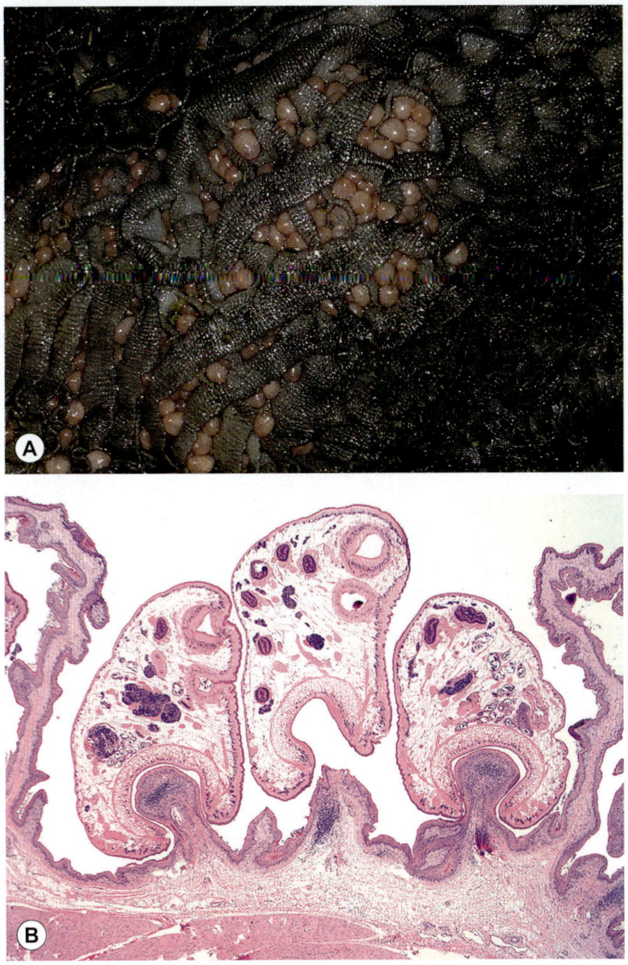

Figure 1-31 ***Paramphistomum*** **spp. flukes** on the mucosa of the reticulum in cattle. **A.** Gross appearance. **B.** *Paramphistomum spp.* flukes associated with lymphoplasmacytic reticulitis.

Larval paramphistomes in the duodenum can cause disease. The biology and pathogenicity of paramphistomes are discussed in detail in the Infectious and Parasitic Diseases of the Alimentary Tract section, later in this chapter.

Myasis of the rumen caused by larvae of the **screwworm fly** *Cochliomyia hominivorax* is occasionally a cause of mortality in young calves in South America. The larvae are presumed to be licked from cutaneous wounds and swallowed. They lodge in, and perforate, the rumen.

Proliferative and neoplastic lesions of the esophagus and forestomachs

Neoplasia of the esophagus and reticulorumen and omasum is, with the exception of papilloma, rare in domestic animals. Because they follow a similar pattern in these organs, they are dealt with together in this section.

Papillomas of the esophagus in dogs are uncommon and may be associated with oral papilloma. In cattle, papillomata of the esophagus and forestomachs are common in some areas. They are caused by bovine papillomavirus 4 (BPV4), which infects only the squamous mucosa of the mouth, pharynx, esophagus, and forestomachs. Bovine alimentary papillomatosis in healthy immunocompetent animals is usually mild with solitary papillomata, although a minority of infected animals may have various lesions. Most are small (<1 cm), broadly pedunculate, tapering masses. They are composed of a number of closely packed fronds of squamous epithelium, each supported by a light core of fibrous stroma, and arising from a common fibrous base. Viral replication and the microscopic changes in infected epithelium are typical, as described earlier for canine oral papillomas, although the characteristic koilocytes and intranuclear inclusions can be sparse. These papillomas are usually rejected by a cell-mediated immune response within ~12 months. However, severe papillomatosis, often accompanied by development of SCCs (see later) in the same location, has been described in the esophagus and forestomachs of bracken fern immunosuppressed, BPV4-infected cattle in Scotland and England.

Fibropapillomas, limited to the esophagus, esophageal groove, and rumen of cattle, are caused mostly by bovine papillomavirus 2 (BPV2), normally associated with cutaneous papillomas and fibropapillomas, but also with BPV4. Alimentary fibropapillomas are smooth pearly white nodules, usually ~0.5-1.0 cm in diameter, but occasionally up to 3.0 cm and plaque-like. They are composed of fibromatous stroma covered by acanthotic epithelium, which occasionally may be ulcerated. No evidence of expression of BPV2 is found in alimentary fibropapillomas, the viral genome being identified by molecular probes. Papillomas and fibropapillomas are normally subclinical, although large lesions of the reticular groove and esophagus may interfere with eructation and deglutition, causing bloating or loss of condition.

Malignant neoplasms of the esophagus and forestomachs in ruminants are ordinarily extremely rare. However, in several localities, **SCC** is relatively common in **cattle**, associated with BPV4-induced papilloma (but not with fibropapilloma because of BPV2). However, BPV4 viral antigens or genome are not detected in these carcinomas. An interaction between papillomavirus and ingestion of carcinogens in bracken fern predisposes to the development of SCCs of the esophagus and forestomachs in Scotland and England. Immunocompromise caused by bracken fern intoxication, which is permissive of severe papillomatosis, is also a cofactor in neoplastic transformation to squamous carcinomas. In Brazil and Bolivia, a similar association is made with carcinomas of the oropharynx and esophagus. A high prevalence of carcinoma of the esophagus and forestomachs has also been reported from the Nasampolai valley in Kenya, in association with papillomata not confirmed as viral, and with a yet undetermined carcinogen apparently ingested with or derived from native forest plants.

Esophageal and ruminal carcinomas are associated with dysphagia or difficult deglutition, ruminal tympany, and apparent abdominal pain with progressive cachexia. Concurrent papillomas, carcinomas, and hemangiomas of the bladder, like those causing enzootic hematuria, but associated with BPV2, are often found in cattle with esophageal or ruminal cancer. In Scotland, intestinal adenomas or adenocarcinoma also occur in many cases.

Esophageal and ruminal carcinoma may be seen developing from recognizable papillomas; as brown irregular roughened hyperplastic epithelium; or as ulcerated or irregular proliferative fungating lesions. Distal esophagus, reticular groove, and the adjacent ruminal wall are the sites most commonly affected with carcinoma. Microscopically, they are typical SCCs, and invade locally, their scirrhous nature causing induration of the wall of the organ. They may metastasize to local lymph nodes, and to distant sites such as the liver and lung.

In **sheep and goats**, alimentary papillomas and SCCs are rare, and little is known of their etiology.

Rarely, SCCs also may be encountered in the esophagus of aged **cats**, where they develop in the mid-thoracic portion, forming proliferative plaques of neoplastic cells that eventually ulcerate and invade the wall of the esophagus and adjacent mediastinum. In **horses**, SCC of the stomach (see Fig. 1-41) may also involve the adjacent terminal esophagus. Rare SCCs, and adenocarcinomas arising from the esophageal glands, are reported in **dogs**. Invasion of, or metastasis to, the canine esophagus by thyroid, respiratory, and gastric carcinomas is also reported.

Mesenchymal tumors of the esophagus, with the exception of the *Spirocerca*-associated fibrosarcomas, osteosarcomas, and chondrosarcomas in dogs, referred to previously in the section on parasitic diseases of the esophagus, are very rare. However, leiomyoma, osteosarcoma, and plasmacytoma have been reported in dogs. Connective tissue tumors of the **ruminant** forestomachs are similarly rare, although fibromas of the reticular groove have been reported. Occasional involvement of the rumen, omasum, and reticulum may occur in cattle with lymphoma, usually also involving the abomasum and more distant sites.

STOMACH AND ABOMASUM

Structure, function, and response to injury

The stomach should be carefully examined in any animals with a history of inappetence, anorexia, cachexia, hypoproteinemia, diarrhea, regurgitation, or vomition. Abdominal distension may be associated with gastric dilation or displacement. Hematemesis, melena, or anemia may indicate gastric bleeding. Many infectious diseases that cause systemic or intestinal tract signs also produce gastric lesions. Systemic diseases such as uremia and endotoxemia cause characteristic gastric lesions in some species.

The stomach has long been considered to lack a native bacterial population (microbiota); however, with the advent of next-generation sequencing technology, numerous and varied bacterial species have been identified in the glandular stomach of normal healthy animals of most domestic species. In fact, the microbiota likely play a significant role in mitigation of gastric disorders and regulation of gastric homeostasis; the significance of microbiota is not limited to *Helicobacter* sp. in the development of gastric neoplasia.

In the horse and pig, the smooth white or yellow **esophageal region** is covered by stratified squamous epithelium, and this region is particularly susceptibility to insult (especially acid) and has reparative capacity like that of the esophagus. The cardiac gland zone is gray and is particularly well developed in the pig where it is situated between the squamous stomach and the fundus, and comprises ~50% the body of the stomach. In the horse, the cardiac glands are also situated along a thin strip between the larger squamous and glandular fundic portions; in the dog, cat, and ruminant abomasum, cardiac glands are limited to a narrow zone along the cardia or omasal opening, respectively. Cardiac glands are branched tubular structures, lined almost exclusively by columnar mucous cells. Chronic inflammation and prominent lymphoid follicular hyperplasia are normally present in the lamina propria and submucosa of the **cardiac gland mucosa** abutting the esophageal region, especially in the pig.

The **fundic (oxyntic) gland acid–secreting mucosa** in the horse and pig is red-brown and slightly irregular but not highly folded. More prominent longitudinally oriented rugae (plicae) are present in the dog and cat, and in the abomasum of ruminants. Gastric secretion undiluted by ingesta in the dog or cat normally should be pH <3.0. Abomasal content should be pH <3.5-4.0.

Tall columnar mucous cells cover the gastric surface and line gastric pits or foveolae. Fundic glands are simple branched glands extending from the base of the gastric pits to the muscularis mucosa. The junction of the base of the foveola and the upper portion of the neck of the fundic gland proper is termed the *isthmus*, and cuboidal or low-columnar pluripotent stem cells located along a narrow zone in this area are mitotically active. Three lineages are identified: 1) pit (foveolar) cells; 2) parietal cells; and 3) zymogen (chief) cells. Daughter cells of the pit cell lineage differentiate terminally into **foveolar or surface mucous cells**, migrating along the glands eventually to the gastric surface, where they are lost in ~4-6 days. Foveolar mucous cells have apical cytoplasm with abundant PAS-positive mucus and project short microvilli into the gastric lumen. Near the neck of the fundic glands below the isthmus are the pyramidal eosinophilic acid and gastric intrinsic factor–producing parietal cells, interspersed with inconspicuous **mucous neck cells** (also with PAS-positive mucus), and various stages in the differentiation of chief, parietal, and scattered endocrine cells. The mature pepsinogen-producing zymogen (chief) cells are concentrated near the base of the fundic glands.

Parietal cells differentiate from stem cells at the isthmus and appear to be relatively long-lived, of the order of weeks to months. A number of long-lived enteroendocrine cells also derived from proliferative stem cells at the isthmus are recognized in the fundic glands; these secrete histamine, serotonin, and somatostatin, among other endocrine/paracrine substances. **Endocrine cells** lack exposure to the gland lumen, and usually abut the basement membrane of the gland and have characteristic basal granules. **Chief cells** are also derived from stem cells at the isthmus and are rather long-lived cells, probably several months. Ultrastructurally, the chief cells have extensive rough endoplasmic reticulum, a prominent Golgi zone, and numerous zymogen granules.

Mitotic figures are not commonly observed in cells at the isthmus of fundic glands and are virtually never seen outside the isthmus, although the fundic mucosa of newborn ruminants and piglets may be relatively poorly differentiated and proliferation may be noted. The active proliferative compartment in the stomach is sensitive to radiomimetic insults, including radiation, cytotoxic agents, and parvoviral infection, the results of which can be observed by necrosis or degeneration of the epithelium lining this portion of the gland.

The **pyloric mucosa** is slightly pitted or irregular and forms the distal portion of the stomach, extending further cranial along the lesser than the greater curvature. The knob-like transverse pyloric fold (torus pyloricus) of the pig is a normal structure that likely functions to delay gastric emptying in this species. The extensively branching tubular glands of the pyloric mucosa open into deep gastric pits that may extend half the thickness of the mucosa. The glands are lined by pale mucous cells with interspersed endocrine elements, mainly G (gastrin) and D (somatostatin) cells, with scattered parietal cells present, especially in glands located nearer the fundus.

The stromal elements of the gastric lamina propria are relatively inconspicuous, and a few lymphocytes, plasma cells, and scattered mast cells are present, mainly deep between glands. Lymphocytic nodules or follicles may be present in the lamina propria, and although they are more common in the pyloric region they can occur anywhere. A variably thick band of hyalinized connective tissue, sometimes termed the *lamina densa*, is present normally between the base of the glands and the muscularis mucosae in the stomach of cats. The cause and significance of this structure are unknown.

Hydrolysis of protein in preparation for subsequent intestinal digestion and absorption is accomplished in the stomach by **acid** and by **pepsin**, activated by autocatalysis from pepsinogen at low pH. *Secretion of acid is the function of the parietal cells*, about one billion of which are present in the stomach of a 20-kg dog. Regulation of the volume and acidity of gastric secretion is physiologically complex and highly integrated, and involves neurocrine, endocrine, and paracrine mechanisms. *Parietal cells secrete hydrochloric acid* in response to stimulation by histamine, acetylcholine, and gastrin. Although all 3 agonists are probably continuously present and involved in basal acid secretion, the effects of acetylcholine and gastrin are largely dependent on concurrent stimulation by histamine. Histamine is a paracrine stimulant secreted by mast cells and enterochromaffin-like cells of the gastric glands. Binding of the H2 histamine receptor causes enhanced generation of cyclic adenosine monophosphate (cAMP), which stimulates protein kinase cascades culminating in translocation of the proton pump to the apical cell membrane, through which hydrochloric acid is secreted.

The neurocrine agonist acetylcholine is released near parietal cells from processes of parasympathetic postganglionic neurons via enhanced vagal activity during central stimulation of the cephalic phase of digestion (the classic Pavlovian response). Gastric distension also stimulates parietal cells via vagovagal and short intramural reflex pathways. Acetylcholine acting on muscarinic M3 receptors elevates intracellular Ca^{2+}, which stimulates acid secretion.

Gastrin is released into the bloodstream by G cells, many of which are in the pyloric antrum. Calcium, amino acids, and peptides in ingesta stimulate gastrin release. Vagal stimulation during the cephalic phase and fundic-pyloric vagovagal reflexes, in concert with local pyloric reflexes initiated by distension, also cause gastrin release. Gastrin acts mainly by a receptor-mediated process to release histamine from the enterochromaffin-like cells. Gastrin is a weak stimulant of acid production but synergizes with histamine and acetylcholine to enhance acid production by parietal cells. Gastrin also has an important trophic effect, increasing the number of endocrine and parietal cells in the fundus, which impacts chief cell differentiation.

Acid production during the gastric phase of secretion is depressed by the negative feedback effect of gastric acid through the inhibitory effect of somatostatin on G cells, at pH<3.0. Acid, fat, and hyperosmolal solutions in the proximal small intestine also inhibit acid secretion, perhaps by the mediation of neural reflexes, secretin, gastric-inhibitory polypeptide, epidermal growth factor, transforming growth factor–α, or other intestinal hormones. Prostaglandin E2 also inhibits acid production by parietal cells. Chief cells are probably susceptible to the same general stimuli for secretion as parietal cells.

Gastric motility is the result of complex interaction between hormonal and neural signals. Neural control is largely from the pacemaker cells of the enteric nervous system, known as the interstitial cells of Cajal, which reside within the GI submucosal and myenteric plexuses in the submucosa and tunica muscularis, respectively. They communicate with enteric neurons and smooth muscle fibers to generate waves of GI motility; these are regulated and mediated by a long list of hormones known to impact gastric and intestinal motility.

The **gastric mucosal barrier** to the acidic luminal environment and autodigestion resides largely in the *single layer of foveolar surface mucous cells and its products*. Tight junctions between epithelial cells are critical for maintenance of barrier function. Integrity of the gastric mucosal barrier implies continuity of the mucosal surface epithelium, so the capacity of these cells to maintain tight junctions, to migrate rapidly to fill defects, and to secrete mucus, bicarbonate, and a hydrophobic phospholipid surface layer, are all central to protecting the gastric mucosa against progressive injury by insults arising in the lumen.

Gastric mucus is freely permeable to hydrogen ions and has little innate buffering capacity, but it resists hydrolysis by intraluminal pepsin, protecting the integrity of the mucosal surface. Unstirred mucus forming a layer immediately over the gastric epithelial cells is the first line of defense from injury and consists of different types of mucin, bicarbonate, and phospholipids. Cardiac, fundic, and pyloric surface mucous cells are stimulated by prostaglandin E2 to secrete bicarbonate in considerable quantities into both the gastric interstitium and the unstirred mucus layer along the surface to buffer acid and prevent back diffusion and are thus resistant to acidic damage.

Prostaglandins, particularly PGE2 and PGI2, have several protective functions in the stomach, including stimulation of bicarbonate and mucus secretion by mucous cells, inhibition of histamine-stimulated acid secretion by parietal cells, reduction of epithelial permeability to reduce acid back-diffusion, and induction of epithelial proliferation, resulting in an increased mass of foveolar mucous epithelium. They may impart greater resistance to water-soluble insults, and they also may neutralize free radicals and other toxic metabolites. Prostaglandins and basal nitric oxide production also cause vasodilation to increase gastric blood flow, which is probably important in maintaining adequate oxygenation of surface and glandular epithelium, buffering the superficial lamina propria against back-diffusion of acid, flushing injurious free radicals from the vicinity of surface epithelium, and regulation of inflammation. Epidermal growth factor and transforming growth factor–α, produced in salivary glands and gastric mucosa, respectively, are also gastroprotective by promoting epithelial proliferation and migration to fill defects and suppress acid production following injury.

Three major **responses of the gastric mucosa to injury** include complete restitution, parietal cell atrophy and loss, and mucous hyperplasia and metaplasia. **Restitution** of acute physical or chemical trauma to the surface epithelium is by rapid migration of wound margin surface and foveolar cells to repair the epithelial injury. This occurs under the initial control of growth factors (transforming growth factor–β, epidermal growth factor) presuming that the progenitor cells are spared; attenuation of epithelial cells and mitotic figures may be observed in the superficial gland epithelium. Sonic Hedgehog protein secreted by parietal cells contributes to gastric epithelial cell differentiation and gastric wound repair in animal models. The epithelial surface is likely protected from significant superficial injuries by mucus, exfoliated epithelium, and fibrin, all of which contribute to effective restitution of the mucosal epithelium. Acute inflammation is observed in more severe lesions, and hemorrhage may be evident on the surface and in adjacent lamina propria. Mucosal blood flow to injured areas of gastric mucosa rapidly increases, which is further protective by dilution and removal of back-diffusing acid and injurious substances from the damaged mucosa.

During the early phases of repair, flattened, cuboidal, or low-columnar cells lining shallow foveolae and covering the surface are basophilic and poorly differentiated. Congestion, edema, hemorrhage, neutrophilic infiltration, and then fibroplasia are seen in the superficial lamina propria. The evolution and repair of gastric ulceration, to which erosion may be antecedent, are discussed later. The multipotential progenitor cells of the fundic mucosa can differentiate to tall-columnar mucus-producing epithelial cells of foveolar or surface type, mucous neck cells, or parietal cells.

Atrophy of parietal cell mass usually occurs associated with chronic inflammation due to *Helicobacter* sp. infection, unidentified environmental factors, or autoimmune disease; this is well characterized in humans but not in animals and is discussed in more detail in the next section. Parietal atrophy *without* extensive mucous cell hyperplasia also occurs in various animal species, mostly secondary to chronic *inappetence*; starvation does not appear to produce comparable lesions. Atrophy may be the result of reduced trophic stimulation of the fundic mucosa, and the change may not be evident grossly. Reduced parietal cells are seen in the upper neck of fundic glands, which can be accompanied by epithelial proliferation, indicated by increased mitotic figures in the isthmus and neck of glands. Mucous neck cells become the predominant cell in the upper gland, and in extreme cases they replace parietal cells and extend to the gland base.

Mucous metaplasia and hyperplasia of glands in the gastric fundus in all species are associated with *persistent injury or chronic inflammation* of the mucosa. Affected mucosa is grossly thickened with an irregular convoluted surface; this is evident especially along the overhanging margin of ulcers, in parasite-induced nodules, or other areas of chronic injury and attempted regeneration. Gastric rugae or plicae are grossly prominent as a result of mucous metaplasia and hyperplasia, as well as submucosal edema. The surface of the stomach is usually pale, although this may be obscured by local congestion or hyperemia; profuse mucus secretion is not usually grossly evident.

Mucous metaplasia can be localized or diffuse, depending on the distribution, severity, and duration of inflammation. Lamina proprial infiltrates of plasma cells and lymphocytes are most common, but neutrophils, eosinophils, and Mott cells are also frequently observed. Intraepithelial lymphocytes (IELs) and globule leukocytes may also be observed. As time progresses, parietal cells are progressively displaced from the surface or isthmus by hyperplastic mucous epithelial cells. Mitotic figures may be numerous in elongated glands. In established lesions, columnar mucous cells with regular nuclear polarity similar to foveolar mucous cells predominate. *Achlorhydria* (discussed further, below) can eventually result as a consequence of parietal cell loss due to widespread persistent injury and damage. Mucous metaplasia and hyperplasia due to persistent chronic injury can be differentiated from fundic atrophy associated with the loss of appetite due to more prominent mucous cell hyperplasia and differentiation, along with evidence of chronic inflammation.

Mucous metaplasia, hyperplasia, and chronic inflammation occur due to a *variety of causes*, especially chronic trauma and inflammation caused by foreign bodies or infectious agents. Gastric parasitism by nematodes such as *Ostertagia* spp., *Teladorsagia* spp., *Trichostrongylus axei*, *Hyostrongylus* spp., and *Ollulanus tricuspis* will cause this change dramatically where the distribution of the lesion is often closely related to the physical presence of nematodes and the interstitial inflammation they incite. The pathogenesis of gastric mucous metaplasia is incompletely characterized, although parietal cells are important for epithelial homeostasis and their loss during chronic inflammation likely contributes to epithelial dysregulation and mucous metaplasia. The loss of parietal cells and hyperplasia of mucous neck cells is presumably partly a response to soluble local immune-mediated stimuli or products of inflammation because it is often localized in the vicinity of glands. The molecular mechanisms of chronic inflammation are complex, especially as related to eventual development of neoplasia in humans; several proinflammatory cytokines including interleukin 1β, tumor necrosis factor, and interferon-γ are likely involved.

Achlorhydria eventually occurs due to persistent chronic gastritis and mucous metaplasia. The pH of gastric secretion approaches or exceeds neutrality as sodium ion replaces hydrogen ion in gastric content and bicarbonate is secreted; diminished gastric acid concentration can lead to progressive microbial colonization of the stomach and upper intestine. The loss of the hydrolytic effects of acid and pepsin during achlorhydria seems to have little effect on digestion of protein and uptake of nitrogen, although inappetence diminishes nutrient intake, and increased mucosal permeability permits protein loss (protein-losing gastropathy); together, these impact the nitrogen economy of the animal to cause reduced productive efficiency and loss of body condition.

Diseases of the stomach and abomasum

Degenerative and inflammatory diseases of the stomach and abomasum

Pyloric stenosis is a functional and occasionally an anatomic anomaly that is relatively uncommon in dogs, and rare in cats and horses; it can be congenital or acquired. Recurrent vomition and poor growth in recently weaned animals may suggest *congenital* pyloric stenosis, and contrast radiographic studies will confirm *delayed gastric emptying*, although there are few publications of confirmed cases of congenital pyloric stenosis in animals. Pyloric stenosis of infancy is recognized in humans, which shares histologic and immunohistochemical features of congenital pyloric stenosis described in brachycephalic breeds of dogs. A leading hypothesis suggests an association with hyperacidity leading to pyloric smooth muscle hypertrophy and obstruction in humans; however, this has not been definitively documented in animals. Hypertrophy of the pyloric smooth muscle and stenosis has been reported in Siamese cats. An association with esophageal dilation has been made in the cat. Congenital pyloric stenosis in a foal was associated with signs of abdominal pain and reluctance to consume solid feed. In all species, the clinical problem is usually abolished by pyloromyotomy.

Several physical causes of acquired pyloric stenosis or outflow obstruction in various species include chronic inflammation or ulceration with granulation, fibrosis and stricture, foreign bodies, polyps, benign or malignant neoplasms, and chronic hypertrophic pyloric gastropathy in dogs.

Chronic hypertrophic pyloric gastropathy is a syndrome of pyloric obstruction in dogs associated with *mucosal hypertrophy (hyperplasia), hypertrophy of circular smooth muscle, or a combination of both*. Mucosal hyperplasia alone is the most common lesion; smooth muscle hypertrophy alone is the least common, although some degree of muscle hypertrophy is seen in about half of cases. Affected dogs are typically middle-aged or older, small-breed males. The pathogenesis remains speculative, and it is unclear whether muscular hypertrophy is primary or whether it occurs secondary to obstruction related to the hyperplastic mucosa. Because mucosal and muscle lesions can be present independently, they may have separate causes. Mucosal dominant hypertrophy has features in common with hypertrophic gastritis, described later. The cardinal presenting sign is *chronic intermittent vomition*, perhaps with weight loss, and with gastric distension in a few cases. Gross examination aided by gastroscopy or gastrotomy, or at autopsy, in most cases reveals *expanded and prominent mucosal folds* obstructing the pyloric outflow tract. The histologic change is irregular-to-papillary hypertrophy and hyperplasia of pyloric foveolar or deeper glands alone, or in combination with cystic dilation of deeper glands and variably severe chronic plasmacytic or sometimes eosinophilic inflammation; small erosions of the mucosal surface may be present. If smooth muscle hypertrophy is a feature of the lesion, this can be observed on the cut surface of the pylorus by irregular firm thickening of the circular muscle. Smooth muscle fibers in affected fascicles are irregularly hypertrophied, although this can be difficult to recognize histologically. Definitive diagnosis is not possible by evaluation of endoscopic biopsies alone and requires additional information including gross lesion appearance, clinical history, and often full-thickness biopsy.

Acquired pyloric stenosis and narrowing is rarely described in cats, and the Siamese breed appears over-represented and may be predisposed. Pyloric stenosis in cats is usually associated with peripyloric fibrosis secondary to chronic inflammation [inflammatory bowel disease (IBD) was diagnosed histologically in most reported cases], pyloric ulceration, foreign bodies including trichobezoars, or benign or malignant neoplasia. In contrast to dogs, anomalies of the pylorus were not detected ultrasonographically, and lesions of the smooth muscle were not described, although only endoscopic biopsies were evaluated.

Gastric dilation in animals is often *secondary* to outflow obstruction of the stomach, small bowel, or to small intestinal ileus. It is also described as part of the syndrome equine dysautonomia (formerly known as *grass sickness*) discussed later in this chapter. Ingestion of *Datura* sp. seeds, which contain a parasympatholytic alkaloid, can also cause ileus leading to gastric dilation. *Primary gastric dilation* in horses is a sequel to consumption of excess fermentable carbohydrate, sudden access to lush pasture, or excessive intake of water. Dilation associated with intake of highly fermentable feedstuffs in horses is likely analogous to grain overload in cattle. Generation of gas and organic acids including lactic acid by bacterial fermentation of carbohydrates occurs in the cranial portion of the stomach. An influx of water follows as the result of increased osmotic pressure in the stomach contributing to increased distension, systemic dehydration, and laminitis in hoofstock.

Gastric rupture may follow *primary* (obstruction due to a lesion within the stomach) or *secondary* (obstruction located aboral to the stomach) dilation of the equine stomach; it may be idiopathic, in that no clear cause is identified at autopsy. Gastric rupture has an estimated prevalence of 1-8% in horses with colic admitted to veterinary hospitals. Rupture usually occurs along the greater curvature of the stomach, parallel to the omental attachment, and releases gastric content into the omental bursa or the abdominal cavity. Frequently, the serosa and tunica muscularis rupture first while the submucosa and mucosa remain intact because these layers are more elastic and resilient (the holding layers) (eFig. 1-3). Death ensues acutely as the result of peritonitis and shock. The margins of the laceration have antemortem hemorrhage, which differentiates the lesion from postmortem rupture of a dilated stomach. There also may be congestion of the cervical esophagus and blanching of the thoracic esophagus, producing a prominent *bloat line*. This, and compression atelectasis of the lungs in some cases, attests to the tremendous increase in intra-abdominal and intrathoracic pressure exerted by the dilated stomach before rupture.

Gastric perforation is distinct from gastric rupture and is rare in the horse and other species, and is mostly associated with gastric ulceration, chronic inflammation, parasitism, neoplasia, or less frequently foreign body trauma to the mucosal surface. Gastric distension or dilation does not necessarily precede gastric perforation.

Gastric dilation and volvulus (Fig. 1-32) occur relatively commonly in dogs and uncommonly in cats. In **dogs**, gastric dilation and volvulus are usually problems associated with eating and probably aerophagia, especially in the *deep-chested breeds* such as Great Danes, Saint Bernards, Irish Setters, Wolfhounds, Borzois, and Bloodhounds. Additional predisposing factors may include increased laxity of the hepatogastric ligament, prior splenectomy, a diet of small food particles, recent kenneling, having a raised food bowl, pre-existing GI diseases including foreign bodies and inflammation, and rarely respiratory conditions that cause increased sneezing or reverse sneezing.

The gas that contributes to the development of dilation is probably the result of aerophagia, and possibly the generation of carbon dioxide by physiologic mechanisms. Inability to relieve accumulated food, fluid, and gas in the stomach causes

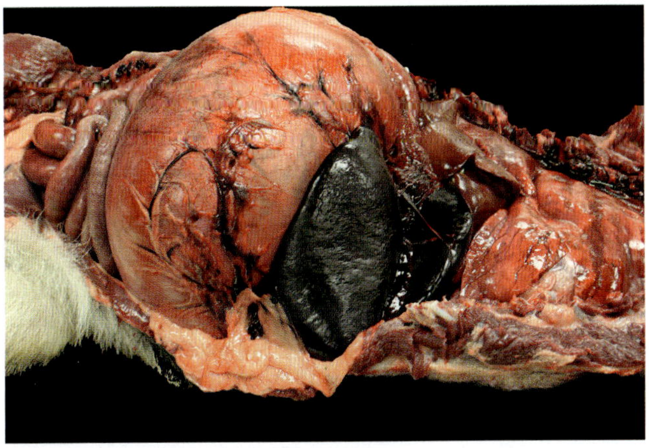

Figure 1-32 Gastric dilation and volvulus in a dog. The stomach is extremely distended and congested. The severely congested spleen is seen on the right side of the abdominal cavity.

the organ to dilate and alter its intra-abdominal position, so that its long axis rotates from a transverse left-right orientation to one paralleling that of the abdomen. In simple dilation, the esophagus is not completely physically occluded, the spleen remains on the left side of the abdomen, and the duodenum is only slightly displaced dorsally and toward the midline. Repeated episodes of gastric dilation probably compromise splenic venous return during periods when the stomach is distended, and eventually lead to episodes of splenic ischemia and segmental infarcts.

For reasons that remain unclear, gastric dilation may progress to gastric volvulus when the stomach rotates in a clockwise direction as viewed from the caudal aspect. The greater curvature of the distended organ moves ventrally and caudally and then rotates dorsally and to the right. This forces the pylorus and terminal duodenum cranially to the right and clockwise around the esophageal axis, where they ultimately become situated to the left of midline and compressed ventrally between the esophagus and the dilated stomach. The *spleen* follows the gastrosplenic ligament and usually is found between the stomach and liver or diaphragm on the right side of the ventral abdomen where it is bent into a V shape by tension on its ligaments, becomes extremely congested, with possible infarction and rupture. The esophagus becomes completely occluded, especially when the rotation is 270-360°. Venous infarction of the gastric mucosa ensues with progressive obstruction of venous outflow of blood from the stomach. The mucosa, and usually the full thickness of the gastric wall, is edematous and dark-red to black, with accumulation of bloody content in the lumen of the stomach. The ischemic mucosa becomes necrotic; a severely distended stomach may rupture. Hemoperitoneum may occur as a result of avulsion of gastric blood vessels.

Obstruction of veins and pressure exerted by the distended stomach result in decreased venous return via the portal vein and caudal vena cava, causing reduced perfusion of intra-abdominal organs, reduced cardiac output, and *circulatory shock*. Increased intra-abdominal pressure impinges on the diaphragm and compromises respiration. Various acid-base and electrolyte abnormalities occur in dogs with gastric dilation and volvulus, contributing to a physiologically precarious state. Cardiac arrhythmias as a sequel to gastric dilation and volvulus have been associated with putative release of *myocardial depressant factor* from an ischemic pancreas, and with myocardial ischemic necrosis. Death is inevitable in dogs with acute gastric volvulus that are not treated early. Rare cases of chronic gastric volvulus are reported, with fixation of the spleen in the right side of the abdomen by omental adhesions.

In **swine**, gastric volvulus is a cause of sudden death in *adult sows*, perhaps following a brief period of anorexia, abdominal distension, or dyspnea. It has historically been associated with excitement in anticipation of feeding among pigs that are fed at regular, often long, intervals, and may be a sequel to rapid ingestion of feed, water, and air. The twist may occur in either direction about the long axis of the stomach, although clockwise volvulus is reported most commonly.

Abomasal displacement and volvulus is a common clinical problem in high-producing, intensively managed dairy **cattle**, particularly around the time of parturition, but it also occurs in animals that are predominantly pasture fed. *The displacement is usually ventral and to the left of the rumen*. Many affected animals have concurrent anomalies including ketosis, hypocalcemia, metritis, and retained placenta. Affected abomasa have decreased sensitivity to acetylcholine, and abomasal atony or altered substance P levels have been implicated as a prerequisite to displacement. Generation of gas in the abomasum is directly related to the amount of highly digestible dietary carbohydrate. Left displacement of the gas-filled abomasum is amenable to treatment and surgical repair, so is rarely encountered at autopsy. Postmortem transportation of a cow with displaced abomasum may self-correct, so autopsy may be unrewarding; other than possible scarring or hemorrhage of the lesser omentum, the abomasum and abdominal contents may be grossly unremarkable. *Abomasal fistulae* draining in the right paramedian abdominal cavity may develop if, during abomasopexy to repair and prevent recurrent displacement, nonabsorbable sutures intended to fix the abomasum to the abdominal wall errantly penetrate the abomasal mucosa.

Simple right displacement accounts for ~15% of abomasal displacements, probably shares a pathogenesis with left displacement; however, right displacement may be complicated in about 20% of right-displaced abomasum cases by progression to abomasal volvulus, which is a clinical emergency. **Abomasal volvulus** is the sequel to 180° to 270° rotation of a loop formed by a distended abomasum and attached omasum and duodenum, and data suggest that progression can occur from left or right displacement of the abomasum. The volvulus occurs in the counterclockwise direction about a transverse axis through the lesser omentum, which causes the cranial duodenum to become entrapped by the distended abomasal body, often medial to the omasum and lateral to the reticulum, when viewed from the right side (Fig. 1-33). Variations of displacement and volvulus have been described historically including cranial and dorsal (relative to the reticulum) displacement, medial displacement, omaso-abomasal volvulus, and reticulo-omaso-abomasal volvulus, although their distinction is subtle and likely clinically inconsequential. Any of these variations are unstable and can shift rapidly into abomasal volvulus. Obstruction of duodenal outflow due to volvulus results in sequestration of chloride in the abomasal content and the development of *metabolic alkalosis*. Severe

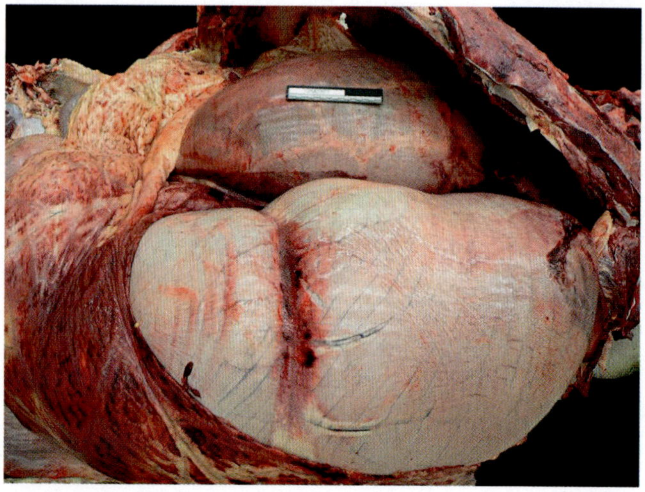

Figure 1-33 Right displacement/volvulus of a bovine abomasum. Distended and hemorrhagic abomasum (with ruler) is dorsal to the distended rumen located along the ventral body wall. (Courtesy M. Yaeger.)

volvulus causes obstruction of blood vessels at the neck of the omasum, as well as trauma to the vagus nerve in the region. The abomasum becomes distended with bloody fluid and gas. Venous infarction of the dilated, deeply congested, and ischemic mucosa may contribute to *abomasal rupture*, often near the omaso-abomasal orifice, and peritonitis. Damage to vagal nerve branches may prohibit return of normal abomasal motility in animals due to vagus indigestion, even in animals in which the displacement and volvulus is successfully repaired. Cases of abomasal volvulus are also occasionally reported in pre-ruminant calves; the cause is not always evident, and these are usually fatal.

Sarcina-like bacteria have been associated with abomasal diseases in **lambs and calves** with various combinations of abomasal bloat, hemorrhage, and ulcers.

Gastroesophageal intussusception, gastroduodenal intussusception, and **pylorogastric intussusception** are uncommon displacements involving the stomach or proximal small intestine of dogs; affected patients have signs of upper alimentary tract obstruction that requires surgical correction.

A fascinating variety of **foreign bodies** may be encountered in the stomach and abomasum. The vast majority are incidental findings, or occasionally, they are associated with vomition, mild acute or chronic gastritis, or ulceration. *Trichobezoars* (hairballs) are often found in the stomach of long-haired cats, and in the rumen, or occasionally abomasum, of calves reared on diets low in roughage. *Phytobezoars* (nondigestable plant material) and *trichophytobezoars* (nondigestible plant material and hair) can cause pyloric obstruction and death in young lambs on pasture and, in some regions, in cattle grazing fibrous plants. *Fine sand* may accumulate in the abomasum in considerable amounts, but usually with no detrimental effect.

Gastric impaction by inspissated feed content in horses and cattle is a type of **primary gastric or abomasal impaction** and is usually related to factors such as consumption of fibrous roughage feed, such as wheat stubble, straw, or persimmons, often coupled with inadequate water intake or poor mastication. It may cause anorexia, mild colic, and loss of body condition; this should be distinguished from other causes of primary gastric impaction and dilation such as foreign bodies, neoplasia, or obstructive inflammatory lesions, and from causes of secondary abomasal impaction. **Secondary abomasal impaction** may follow pyloric stenosis, physical or functional, of any cause. In cattle, it occurs mostly as functional abomasal stasis as a manifestation of *vagus indigestion*. Loss of abomasal motility may be the product of intrathoracic inflammatory or neoplastic vagal lesions including vagal involvement in adhesions following traumatic reticuloperitonitis, vagal trauma in surgically corrected abomasal displacement or volvulus, adhesions of the abomasum and omasum that may physically impair motility; or systemic disease that causes abomasal stasis.

Omasal and ruminal distension are also found in many of these cases due to the accumulation of inspissated digesta and fluid, respectively. Significant metabolic derangements including sequestration of chloride in the rumen following regurgitation from the obstructed abomasum, and hypokalemia resulting from decreased intake in feed in the face of continued normal renal excretion, place these animals in perilous physiologic circumstances. Unresolved abomasal impaction may lead to rupture, which usually is seen along the omasal-abomasal orifice, although it can occur in other locations.

Abomasal dilation and emptying defect occurs in Suffolk and Hampshire **sheep**. The animals develop chronic inappetence and weight loss, and at autopsy they have a markedly distended abomasum containing digesta resembling rumen contents. No morphologic gross or microscopic lesions of the stomach, vagus nerve, or other organs have been consistently observed, except scattered chromatolytic and necrotic neurons in the celiacomesenteric autonomic ganglion. The cause remains unknown, but some studies have shown neuronal degeneration in a significant number of affected sheep, which suggests that this may be an acquired dysautonomia, with toxin exposure or genetics as possible etiology. Rumen chloride levels are usually elevated, presumably secondary to abomasal reflux.

Edema of gastric rugae occurs during hypoproteinemia in any species, in portal hypertension, and in the abomasum of cattle poisoned by arsenic, sheep ingesting tannic acid, and both cattle and sheep with ostertagiosis. Edema collects in the submucosa of the folds and is particularly obvious in the normally thin abomasal spiral folds, or plicae. Edema may contribute to the thickening of rugae seen in gastritis. Submucosal edema of the stomach is a common and important lesion in edema disease of swine, which is considered fully in the Infectious and Parasitic Diseases of the Alimentary Tract section.

Hyperemia of the gastric mucosa occurs following ingestion of chemicals, which usually also cause superficial necrosis of epithelial surface, discussed later under chemical gastritis. Focal hyperemia may be related to local irritation of the mucosa by foreign bodies, or uncommonly due to inflammation secondary to infectious agents. **Congestion** is a nonspecific lesion of the gastric mucosa that can occur in conditions causing portal hypertension, such as cirrhosis in the dog.

Uremic gastritis is seen as severe congestion and hemorrhage of the body of the stomach, usually with hematemesis and melena, is often associated with chronic renal disease in dogs, and occasionally in cats and horses. The mucosa of the stomach is thickened, deep-red-black, and there is often granular material texturally consistent with mineral in the mucosal layer. Gastric ulceration may occur but is not common. Lesions vary in severity, and early milder changes without severe hemorrhage and necrosis can be identified in animals earlier in the course of renal disease.

Microscopically, the gastric lamina propria between glands is edematous in dogs, and there are often increased mast cells. Deposits of basophilic granular mineral are found, especially along the basement membranes of vessels and glands, or on collagen fibrils and in degenerate smooth muscle; these changes occur particularly in the middle and deeper portions of the mucosa. More extensive mineral deposition may also involve parietal cells and the tunica media of submucosal and serosal arterioles; affected vessels may show evidence of endothelial damage, medial necrosis, and, in some cases, thrombosis. In **cats** with uremic gastropathy, ulcerative or erosive and hemorrhagic gastritis is reported as a common change, and this may be accompanied by gastric fibrosis, mineralization, and vascular thrombosis and/or fibrinoid necrosis, although the latter lesions are less common in cats than in dogs.

Uremia is a clinical syndrome associated with renal failure or lower urinary tract disease, which is associated with reduced urinary excretion of metabolites; the etiopathogenesis of various uremia-associated lesions remains incompletely understood. Ischemia is hypothesized to play a significant role, although vascular lesions are not always present. Toxic uremic metabolites or enzymes are also certainly involved, although specific molecules or pathogenesis are not recognized. Mineral deposition is probably the product of altered systemic metabolism of calcium in renal failure, perhaps coupled with metabolic or localized acidosis, inflammatory cytokines, and altered local microenvironment (see Vol. 2, Urinary System, for a discussion of uremia).

Gastric venous infarction is described in swine and occurs even less frequently in ruminants and horses. It is related to endothelial damage and thrombosis of venules secondary to *endotoxemia or other bacterial or toxic damage*. Septicemic salmonellosis and colibacillosis in all species, and in swine, postweaning coliform gastroenteritis, erysipelas, swine dysentery, polyserositis, and porcine dermatopathy and nephropathy syndrome have been associated with the lesion. The fundic mucosa is bright-red or deep-red to black with mucus or fibrin along the mucosal surface; superficial erosion or ulceration can be observed. The lesion is caused by fibrin thrombosis of capillaries and venules in the mucosa and submucosa, which leads to an ischemic zone of superficial coagulative necrosis of the mucosa, hemorrhage, edema, inflammation, and rarely mural injury or perforation.

Gastritis is a term used frequently and generically clinically as a presumptive diagnosis for cases of vomiting thought to arise from gastric irritation; the specific cause is not often identified. In pathology, the term is often used with equal imprecision, referring to a wide range of gastric injury in which histologic criteria of inflammation may not be particularly prominent. Under the broad umbrella of gastritis are usually included several different lesions: gastric mucosal necrosis and erosion or ulceration caused by mechanical, chemical, or ischemic insults (including uremic gastritis, described earlier); true gastritis, in which the lamina propria contains the leukocytic infiltrate and vascular changes characteristic of inflammation; and finally, lesions of gastric mucosal atrophy, fibrosis, and lymphofollicular hyperplasia that are likely the residual lesions of previous active inflammatory disease.

Chemical gastritis or abomasitis causes diffuse gastric congestion, hemorrhage, necrosis, and ulceration; it may be induced by chemicals such as arsenic, thallium, formalin, bronopol, steroidal, and nonsteroidal anti-inflammatory drugs (NSAIDs), phosphatic fertilizers, and by the toxic principle in bitterweed (*Hymenoxys odorata*). **Blister beetle** (*Epicauta* spp.) **intoxication in horses** is induced by the *cantharidin* contained in these insects, may cause necrosis and ulceration of the distal esophagus and pars esophagea, intense hyperemia of the glandular mucosa of the stomach, and in some cases gastric ulceration. In addition to the gastric lesions, cantharidin also is known to cause enterocolitis, nephrosis, urinary bladder hemorrhage, and myocardial hemorrhage and necrosis. **Zinc** toxicosis may cause acute mortality, in which the mucosa of the abomasum and duodenum is necrotic, with an underlying congested and edematous submucosa; radiating crystals are evident microscopically in the necrotic tissue. Subacute or chronic zinc intoxication may cause chronic change in the stomach with the loss of glandular epithelium and reparative proliferation of mucous neck cells, in addition to fibrosing pancreatitis and mild nephrosis. In sheep, type-A trichothecene **mycotoxin** has been associated with rumenitis and abomasal ulceration in acute toxicity. **Mechanical gastritis** is most commonly seen in dogs after ingestion of coarse foreign materials and in cats with trichobezoars; the lesion is discovered as an incidental finding during evaluation or biopsy of the stomach via endoscopy or gastrotomy. Trichobezoars in the abomasum of ruminants are associated with lack of roughage in young animals, but virtually never with disease.

Eosinophilic and mixed inflammatory infiltrates occur in the gastric mucosa of horses with multisystemic eosinophilic epitheliotropic disease (MEED), discussed later with eosinophilic enteritis in horses. **Phlegmonous gastritis** in young horses describes a unique lesion of acute mural necrotizing-to-neutrophilic gastritis with severe submucosal edema but without emphysema (the distinguishing feature of this disease from **emphysematous gastritis** of horses), which has been associated with *Clostridium septicum*. In humans, this is often associated with polymicrobial infections, and this seems to be the case in the equine cases as well. Affected horses also had concurrent intestinal disease, and several pathogens were possibly associated including *Lawsonia intracellularis, Escherichia coli*, and *Clostridium perfringens* type C, although the pathogenesis or association with specific bacteria is tenuous at best.

Most examples of genuine gastritis are seen in dogs and cats with more generalized GI inflammatory disease, such as food allergy or idiopathic IBD, which is discussed further with those topics (see the Inflammatory bowel disease section).

Infectious agents in small animals appear to be minor causes of gastritis, compared with chemical, mechanical, or idiopathic insults. Following the discovery of *Helicobacter pylori* as a major cause of gastric ulceration in humans, a flurry of activity sought to document its significance as a cause of gastritis and/or gastric ulceration in other monogastric species; yet the understanding of ***Helicobacter*-associated infection** continues to evolve. Several species of *Helicobacter* have been described (~50), and many naturally colonize the stomach of dogs, cats, and pigs; these include the human-adapted *H. pylori* and several others including *Helicobacter felis* and *H. heilmannii* within a group of non-*H. pylori* helicobacters (NHPH) in dogs and cats, and *Helicobacter suis* in pigs.

In dogs and cats, *H. pylori* likely is not as pathogenically significant as it is in humans. Almost all dogs and cats are naturally infected, so negative controls are difficult or impossible to find for study; the prevalence of helicobacters in dogs with clinical signs of GI disease or gastritis is similar to or lower than dogs without clinical signs or evidence of gastric inflammation. The improvement or resolution of clinical signs but not resolution of histologic evidence of gastritis in dogs suggests a potential causal role for at least some helicobacters; however, the details remain unknown. More significant inflammation may be present in dogs with a single *Helicobacter* species compared with dogs with mixed *Helicobacter* infection. In **dogs and cats**, *it is quite common to observe spiral organisms* (silver stains often reveal organisms, even if they are not apparent by H&E staining) colonizing the gastric surface and within glands or parietal cell canaliculi of clinically normal animals and in those with gastric inflammation and/or lymphofollicular hyperplasia (eFig. 1-4). These should be reported, especially on biopsy reports, until a better understanding of these agents and associated disease is achieved.

The role of NHPH also remains controversial, and no conclusive evidence has been demonstrated to document association between NHPH and clinical signs or inflammation in dogs or cats. It seems likely that the pathogenicity of helicobacters differ, and possibly within different host species. Given the significance of *H. pylori* and possibly NHPH in humans as a cause of inflammation, ulceration, and mucosal-associated lymphomas or carcinomas (none of these have been definitively linked to helicobacters in domestic animal species), significant effort has also been expended to understand the possible zoonotic potential of these agents. Transfer of these agents from animals to humans (or vice versa) may occur, but many details, including definitive evidence of zoonotic transmission, remain to be shown.

In **pigs**, *H. suis* is known to colonize the stomach and has been associated with gastritis, decreased daily weight gain, hyperkeratosis, and possibly ulceration of the squamous stomach; other helicobacters may also be involved in swine. Similar to dogs and cats, there have been differences in pathogenicity of strains reported, and a clear link between *H. suis* strains and virulence, gastritis, or gastric ulceration has not been documented.

There is convincing evidence for clinically significant gastric *Helicobacter* infection in **ferrets**. Although virtually all adult ferrets have *Helicobacter mustelae* as part of the normal gastric flora, heavily colonized ferrets develop diffuse lymphoplasmacytic gastritis with lymphofollicular hyperplasia and sometimes with mucosal erosions. Progression to neoplasia has not been documented.

Chlamydia have been recognized in surface mucous cells of otherwise normal fundic mucosa in cats with no signs of disease. Experimental infection produced conjunctivitis and respiratory disease, but only mild gastritis.

Chronic hypertrophic gastritis (hypertrophic gastropathy or **giant hypertrophic gastritis)** of dogs, with many similarities to Ménétrier disease in humans, is rare. Vomition and weight loss, and in some cases inappetence or diarrhea, are described in the few cases reported; several cases have been reported in adult Basenji dogs. The characteristic lesion is marked gastric rugal cerebriform hypertrophy and hyperplasia involving part or most of the fundic gland mucosa while usually sparing the antrum and pylorus of the stomach.

Microscopically, there is prominent mucous neck cell and foveolar and glandular epithelial hyperplasia with progressive loss of parietal cells, replacement fibrosis, usually with chronic lymphoplasmacytic-to-neutrophilic inflammation. Cystic dilation of mucous glands may occur, and there is often marked edema, both of which may be evident grossly. Similar to hypertrophic pyloric gastropathy described previously, if the gross appearance of the mucosa in animals with hypertrophic gastritis is not observed by endoscopy or at surgery, biopsies that do not sample the full thickness of the mucosa may be easily misdiagnosed as chronic superficial or diffuse gastritis.

The cause of chronic hypertrophic gastritis is unknown, but may be mediated by immune events in the mucosa. Although few cases have been reported, helicobacters have described in these lesions; whether this represents a secondary or primary infection is unknown. Ménétrier disease in humans causes protein-losing gastropathy and has been linked to the development of gastric cancer; in dogs a link between chronic hypertrophic gastropathy/gastritis and gastric adenocarcinoma or gastric sarcoma has been suggested, but remains unproven. A similar disease has been described in one **cat**.

Braxy, or bradsot, is an acute sporadic abomasitis of sheep and occasionally calves, caused by infection with histotoxic *C. septicum*. The factors initiating bacterial invasion are unknown, although prior local tissue damage in the abomasum is likely necessary. There is an historical association in sheep foraging cold or frozen pastures, so how this alters grazing behavior to increase intake of plant material contributing to local trauma is not specifically understood. Production of the potent pore-forming toxins, including alpha toxin and septicolysin, by *C. septicum* causes epithelial cellular necrosis and hemolysis, necrotizing abomasitis, and death, which usually ensues quickly. A similar gastritis has been associated with *Paraclostridium* (formerly *Clostridium*) *sordellii* infection. At autopsy, there may be blood-tinged abdominal fluid, and the serosa of the abomasum may be congested or fibrin covered (Fig. 1-34A). Abomasal folds are diffusely or regionally thickened, reddened, and often hemorrhagic or necrotic; there is extensive gelatinous edema and emphysema in the submucosa (see Fig. 1-34B), as well as venous thrombosis. These changes may extend into the adjacent mucosa and the tunica muscularis. Gram-positive bacilli are usually evident as individuals or colonies in inflamed and necrotic tissue.

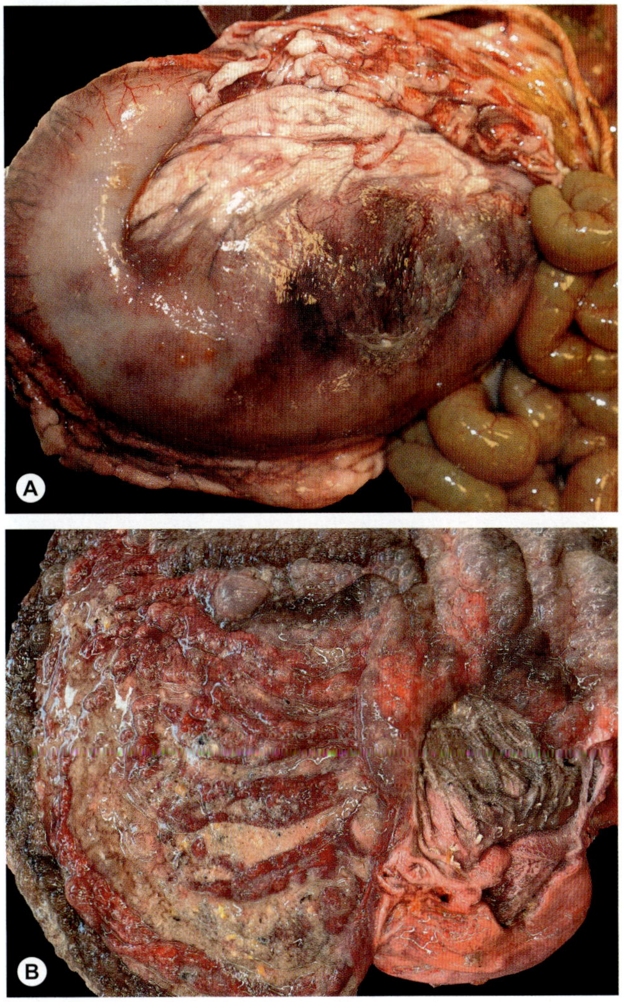

Figure 1-34 **A.** Braxy (*Clostridium septicum*) in a lamb. The serosal surface of the abomasum is hemorrhagic and covered by fibrin. (From Prescott JF, et al. Clostridial abomasitis. In: Uzal FA, et al., eds. Clostridial Diseases of Animals. Wiley, 2016: 205–220.) **B.** Braxy-like clostridial abomasitis in a calf. The abomasal folds are edematous, hemorrhagic, and emphysematous. (Courtesy M. Macias Rioseco.)

Several other agents have been variably linked with clostridial abomasitis, ulceration, and abomasal tympany syndrome in lambs, kids, and calves, including *C. perfringens* type A, *P. (Clostridium) sordellii*, *Clostridium fallax*, and *Sarcina* spp., although the specific role that any of these etiologic agents play in development of disease remains poorly understood.

***C. perfringens* type A** can cause abomasitis in young calves and lambs. Affected animals have abdominal tympany and pain, depression, or may die suddenly. Gross and microscopic changes are similar to diseases caused by histotoxic clostridia, which include congestion, hemorrhage, erosion, and ulceration, usually of the abomasal fundic mucosa; perforating ulcers may develop. Microscopic changes include necrosis of epithelium, submucosal edema, dilation and thrombosis of submucosal lymphatics, and acute inflammation involving mucosa and submucosa; gram-positive bacilli may be observed on the mucosal surface, or in inflamed submucosa. Lesions similar to natural disease have been produced experimentally, but studies have not confirmed the specific toxin(s) associated with disease-causing *C. perfringens* type A, although in addition to α-toxin, the β2-toxin (*cpb2* gene) is often detected. Several additional factors affecting the expression of disease in individual animals include diet, feed texture, colostrum or milk replacer, hygiene, and temperature of milk or colostrum and milk-feeding equipment, as well as alterations of microbiome or gut motility. *C. perfringens* type A is often cultured or identified (and many with β2 toxin production), sometimes in large numbers from abomasa of unaffected animals, so care should be taken when interpreting its significance; it is likely that additional host or environmental factors are critical to development of disease.

P. sordellii or ***C. fallax*** are not found as commonly as *C. perfringens* type A in healthy animals, and both have been identified in cases of abomasitis with gross and microscopic changes described above for *C. septicum* and *C. perfringens* type A. Disease seems to occur mostly in pre-ruminant lambs, calves, and goats; as before, several predisposing factors, including dietary and management factors, are also likely significantly involved.

Sarcina or ***Sarcina*-like bacteria** are linked with abomasal tympany, hemorrhage, and ulceration in pre-ruminant goats and lambs. The disease manifests like other clostridial abomasitides of these species, with severe abdominal pain, tympany, and thickened abomasal wall due to edema, emphysema, hemorrhage, and necrosis. Microscopic lesions include hemorrhage, edema, necrosis of epithelium, neutrophilic inflammation, and vascular thrombosis. Some animals may have acute abomasal bloat and congestion, with limited epithelial necrosis, hemorrhage, or submucosal edema and emphysema. Although bacteria in the classic tetrad morphologic formation are often seen histologically in the abomasal lumen or along the surface adherent to necrotic material, damaged mucosa, or in the surface mucus, the organism has rarely been cultured from affected animals (and occasionally from unaffected animals).

Abomasitis associated with viral infection occurs in a number of the systemic viral diseases affecting the GI tract, including infectious bovine rhinotracheitis in calves and rarely in older animals, herpesviral infections of small ruminants, BVD, MCF, and BT. Abomasal lesions are rarely the sole manifestation of these diseases, but form part of a picture at autopsy that may suggest an etiologic diagnosis. The appearance and pathogenesis of abomasitis in these diseases vary with the conditions (see the Infectious and Parasitic Diseases of the Alimentary Tract section, later in this chapter).

Mycotic gastritis or abomasitis is a sporadic problem almost invariably secondary to insults that cause epithelial damage, necrosis, and ulceration, including acidosis, achlorhydria, or atrophy, generally under conditions that are permissive for mycotic colonization to occur. Immunocompromise associated with endotoxemia, septicemia, endogenous or exogenous steroids, neoplasia, or viral disease also may contribute; altered GI flora due to prolonged antibiotic therapy may further promote development of mycosis. Fungal hyphae reach the submucosa through damaged surface epithelium and mucosa by invading venules and arterioles, causing *thrombosis and hemorrhagic infarction*. The agents involved are usually opportunistic pathogens including *Rhizopus, Mucor, Lichtheimia* (formerly *Absidia*); all are in the phylum *Mucoromycota*, order *Mucorales* (formerly known as *zygomycetes*); rarely, *Aspergillus* may be implicated. There are multifocal, well-demarcated areas of necrosis surrounded by an intensely congested or hemorrhagic periphery; they can range from 1-2-cm in diameter to much larger and more extensive, and involve much of stomach or abomasum (Fig. 1-35A). The affected mucosa is thickened, red or pale in the necrotic zone, with edema and hemorrhage of the submucosa that may extend to the serosa, where it is observed as a

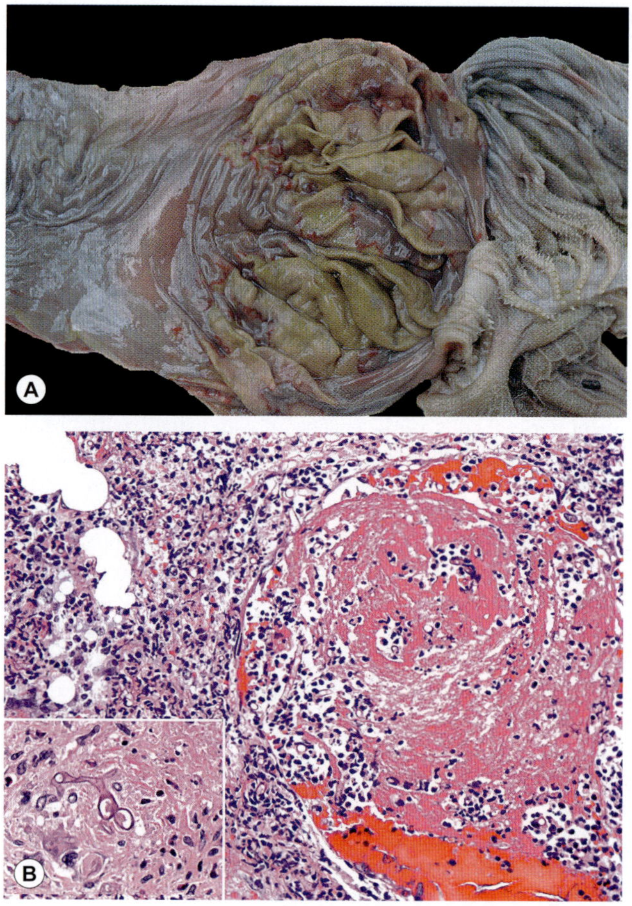

Figure 1-35 Mycotic abomasitis in a sheep. **A.** Multifocal-to-coalescing areas of necrosis surrounded by halos of hemorrhage and inflammation. (Courtesy V. Psychas.) **B.** Thrombosis of a venule in submucosa of abomasum as a result of hyphal invasion (inset).

roughly circular area of hemorrhage. Broad and nonseptate *hyphae* are present in sections of the necrotic mucosa, submucosa, and often within vascular walls or lumens, where they initiate thrombosis (see Fig. 1-35B). *Candidiasis* of the pars esophagea is described in swine, often in association with squamous injury including epithelial hyperplasia and parakeratosis. For an overview of mycosis of the digestive system, and its sequelae, see the Infectious and Parasitic Diseases of the Alimentary Tract section, later in this chapter.

Parasitic gastritis is often subclinical in **dogs and cats;** in a small number of animals with high parasite loads, there can be mucosal injury and vomiting. *Physaloptera* are commonly found in dogs and cats and can cause epithelial injury, although most are incidental. *Gnathostoma* are found in dogs mostly in Africa, Asia, Australia, and southern Europe; the life cycle is complex, but infective larvae are transmitted via ingestion of raw fish, and eventually embed in the gastric wall forming submucosal inflammatory cysts. *Cylicospirura felineus* is a spirurid found mostly in southern Asia and Australia and has been observed occasionally in wild felids of North America; adults are embedded within nodules in the gastric wall, which can mimic neoplasia. *Ollulanus tricuspis* is found on the mucosa of the stomach in cats, where it may cause mild-to-severe chronic gastritis. *Cryptosporidium* infection of the gastric mucosa occurs rarely in cats and dogs, with uncertain significance.

In **horses**, *Draschia megastoma* is found in inflammatory nodules in the mucosa or submucosa, especially along the margo plicatus. The nodules can be several centimeters in diameter and contain necrotic debris and adult parasites. The closely related *Habronema muscae* and *H. majus* are also found in the mucosa and have been associated with mild ulceration, atrophy of mucosal glands, and may predispose to gastric ulcers or colic. *Trichostrongylus axei* may cause chronic gastritis in the horse. Bots of the genus *Gasterophilus* are found attached to small erosions and ulcers in the esophageal and glandular mucosa, which very rarely become complicated or perforate.

In **swine**, several helminths, including *Ascarops* spp., *Physocephalus* spp., and *Simmondsia* spp., are associated with mild gastritis in heavy infections. *Gnathostoma* may be embedded in inflammatory cysts in the submucosa. *O. tricuspis* may be encountered. *Hyostrongylus rubidus* can cause chronic gastritis and wasting in pigs.

In **cattle, sheep**, and **goats**, members of the genera *Haemonchus* and *Mecistocirrus* are large abomasal blood-sucking trichostrongyles, capable of causing severe anemia and hypoproteinemia. In various ruminants, *Ostertagia* spp., *Teladorsagia circumcincta* (formerly *Ostertagia circumcincta*), and related genera, including *Camelostrongylus, Marshallagia*, and *T. axei*, can cause chronic abomasitis with mucous metaplasia, achlorhydria, diarrhea, and hypoproteinemia. *Cryptosporidium andersoni* occasionally causes subclinical abomasitis in cattle, associated with elongation of the gastric glands, hyperplasia of the epithelium in the gland isthmus, attenuation of epithelium lining the neck of fundic glands, and dilation of glands. The small basophilic organisms are present on the surface of epithelium from the base of glands to the mucosal surface.

Globidium (Eimeria) gilruthi is the cause of **abomasal coccidiosis of sheep and goats** and causes a thickened nodular mucosa grossly due to edema, variable lymphocytic-to-eosinophilic inflammation, chronic fundic glandular atrophy, and mucous neck cell hyperplasia associated with numerous, giant embedded 200-300 μm schizonts within the abomasal mucosa. The lesions can appear grossly like those caused by *T. circumcincta*; the taxonomy and life cycle of this parasite remains incomplete. Gastric parasitism is considered more fully in the Infectious and Parasitic Diseases of the Alimentary Tract section, later in this chapter.

The pathogenesis of **gastroduodenal (peptic) ulceration** in animals (and humans) can be summarized as a relative imbalance between the epithelial damaging effects of gastric acid and pepsin on one hand and the ability of the epithelium to maintain its integrity on the other. Impairment of mucosal integrity in the face of normal acid secretion is probably the predominant mechanism, although there are clear instances when hypersecretion of acid is the major cause.

Factors implicated in hypersecretion of acid include stimulated acid secretion (e.g., by histamine or gastrin stimulation), or by abnormally high basal acid secretion possibly associated with an expanded parietal cell mass due to increased trophic stimulation by gastrin.

Mast cell tumor (MCT) or cutaneous mastocytosis in dogs is associated with gastroduodenal ulcer, presumably owing to histamine-stimulated acid hypersecretion and microvascular effects. The tumor (or mastocytosis) does not involve the stomach directly, and ulcers may occur in animals with solitary MCTs in the skin. In one series, single or multiple gastric and duodenal erosions or ulcers were present in 20 of 24 dogs with recurrent or metastatic MCTs. In many cases, the gastroduodenal lesions are clinically silent, and they should be looked for during autopsy in animals with mast cell neoplasia. MCTs have rarely been associated with gastric ulceration in other species, including the cow and cat.

Zollinger-Ellison syndrome is defined as gastroduodenal ulceration caused by acid hypersecretion stimulated by gastrin-producing pancreatic islet cell tumors or gastrinoma and has been reported in a few dogs and fewer cats. The history usually includes inappetence, vomition, weight loss, and possibly diarrhea or melena. Reflux esophagitis and gastric or duodenal ulcer are present in most cases. Small nodules confirmed histologically as islet cell tumors may be found in the pancreas, and metastases to the liver, spleen, or hepatic lymph nodes are often present. Islet cell tumors may be difficult to identify; careful gross and histologic examination is often required to confirm their presence. Definitive diagnosis relies on demonstration of elevated serum gastrin levels by radioimmunoassay or by identification of gastrin-secretion cells in fixed or frozen tumor tissue, usually by IHC.

Ulceration caused by compromise of mucosal protective mechanisms is attributed to NSAIDs, such as aspirin, phenylbutazone, and various others that target one or both isoforms of the cyclooxygenase (COX)1 or COX2 enzymes. NSAIDs are commonly utilized in animals for their analgesic, antipyretic, and anti-inflammatory properties, but they have numerous side effects due to inhibition of both COX1 and COX2 enzymes, which reduce gastroprotective prostaglandins. Although some NSAIDs such as phenylbutazone may also have a direct toxic effect on vascular endothelium in the mucosa, which compromises circulation and predisposes to ischemia-induced ulceration, most deleterious effects of NSAIDs seem to be linked more closely to their inhibition of COX1 and prostaglandin secretion; gastroduodenal toxicity is likely enhanced with COX1–specific or predominant inhibition by NSAIDs such as aspirin. Briefly, COX1 inhibition leads to reduced production of prostaglandin E2 synthesis, which is critical for gastroprotection via maintenance of blood flow, mucus, and bicarbonate production. COX2 selective (or predominant) inhibitors are often considered gastroprotective in the sense that these drugs possess similar anti-inflammatory and analgesic properties but have less deleterious effects on PGE2 synthesis and ultimately on the gastric mucosa.

Reflux of bile salt–rich duodenal contents has been implicated in the induction of gastritis, and gastric or duodenal ulceration, mostly presumed to be secondary mainly due to gastroduodenal dysmotility, is described in humans and rarely in animals. Inflammation is stimulated by reflux contents from the duodenum into the stomach; in particular, bile acids and lysolecithin are primary factors that damage the gastric epithelial barrier, which leads to hyperemia, edema, erosion, and ulceration. In humans, bile reflux–induced gastritis and ulceration are associated with the development of gastric neoplasia (mostly carcinomas); this has not been established in animals.

Glucocorticoids and physiologic stress have been implicated in the genesis of gastroduodenal ulceration, although the role of steroids in the pathogenesis of gastroduodenal ulceration is controversial. Experimentally, gastroduodenal hemorrhage and ulceration occur in some species of animals stressed by restraint, social factors, traumatic injury, and exogenous or endogenous glucocorticoids; however, glucocorticoids have also been shown to have gastroprotective effects in some contexts. The administration of methylprednisolone sodium succinate or immunosuppressive doses of prednisone to dogs was clearly acutely ulcerogenic. It is likely that various factors are involved in the relative ulcerogenic or gastroprotective potential of various glucocorticoids. Reduced mucosal perfusion or ischemia under a number of circumstances may be a principal factor interacting in stress-associated ulceration and likely precedes mucosal hemorrhage, erosion, and eventually ulceration. In combination with the effects of other insults, ischemic damage to surface epithelial cells likely alters mucosal permeability and back-diffusion of acid, while reducing neutralization capacity of acid diffusing into the mucosa. Mucosal ischemia may result from reduction in local prostaglandins (as in NSAID administration) or nitric oxide concentration, thrombosis, as well as local or systemic hypotension. Ischemic damage may be more significant in the fundus compared with the pylorus; this is consistent with the classic description of physiologic stress–induced ulcers of humans, occurring primarily in the fundus.

Whatever the cause, the results of injury to the gastric epithelium have the potential to follow a **common pathway to ulceration** in all species. Acute superficial lesions can be subtle, but are seen as areas of reddening and hemorrhage, especially along the margins of rugae in the fundic mucosa. Acid treatment of hemoglobin gives blood on the surface or in the gastric lumen a red-brown or black color. Melena may be present in the lower intestine, but with minimal gross evidence of hemorrhage or ulceration in the stomach. The microscopic lesion associated with hemorrhage of this type is also subtle and difficult to detect (especially if there is any degree of postmortem autolysis) because bleeding seemingly results from diapedesis with minimal mucosal damage. Superficial erosion and hemorrhage along the surface may be evident though, or healed mild gastric erosion can be suggested by poorly differentiated flattened cuboidal or low-columnar basophilic epithelial cells covering the surface, with mitotic activity in the upper neck of glands.

Progression from the superficial injury of *gastric erosion*, which by definition involves the superficial mucosa only, to *gastric ulceration*, which by definition involves the full thickness of the mucosa and includes a breach of the muscularis mucosa, occurs by progressive *coagulative necrosis of the gastric wall*. Once the superficial portion of the mucosa is destroyed, natural local buffering is lost, and the proliferative compartment of the gland of the isthmus is obliterated, preventing a local epithelial regenerative response. Ulcers that extend into the submucosa may affect arterioles of larger diameter, increasing the risk of significant *gastric hemorrhage*. The ulcer may progress through the tunica muscularis and serosa, eventually resulting in transmural *perforation* of the gastric wall. Severe gastric hemorrhage or perforation are relatively common sequelae of gastroduodenal ulceration in domestic animals.

Perforation is not the inevitable consequence, and ulcers may come into equilibrium with *reparative processes* at any level of the gastric wall; this is most common at the submucosa. Subacute-to-chronic ulcers have a base and sides composed of granulation tissue of variable thickness and maturity, infiltrated by a mixed inflammatory cell population and necrotic debris; this is dependent on the relative balance of reparative processes and progressive damage of the gastric mucosa. Mucous metaplasia and hyperplasia of viable glands occur at the peripheral margins of the ulcer, from which, with time, epithelial cells migrate gradually across and thus heal the defect. *Restitution of mucosal integrity* is a complex process that is promoted by local activity of cytokines and growth factors, secreted as a coordinated response by gastric epithelial and mesenchymal cells. Angiogenesis is also driven by cytokines and growth factors within the healing ulcer and granulation bed and is critical for restoration of the mucosal microvasculature. Localized excessive scarring due to healed ulcers near the pylorus may lead to pyloric obstruction in any species.

Duodenal ulcers, which usually occur proximal to the opening of the pancreatic and bile ducts, resemble gastric ulcers in their microscopic appearance (allowing for their intestinal location), pathogenesis, and sequelae.

Gastric or duodenal ulceration in dogs is common, and although specific mechanisms are not always identified, the most common predisposing factor in dogs is prior treatment with NSAIDs; other mechanisms involving hypersecretion of acid (mastocytoma, gastrinoma), association with systemic disease (uremia, chronic IBD), strenuous exercise, or idiopathic ulceration are also described. Hepatic disease has historically been associated with gastroduodenal ulceration in dogs, and although some data support this hypothesis, the mechanisms remain undescribed, and recent work has found no specific association between various categories of hepatic disease in dogs and gastroduodenal injury. Gastric hemorrhage and gastroduodenal ulceration are occasionally seen in dogs following *trauma or major surgery*. A syndrome of gastric hemorrhage, pancreatitis, and colonic ulceration and perforation is recognized in dogs following *spinal trauma*. The pathogenesis of this is undoubtedly complex and remains obscure.

Clinical signs in dogs include variable loss of appetite, abdominal pain, vomition, melena, and anemia. Ulcers a few millimeters to 3-4 cm in diameter are found most commonly in the pyloric antrum or proximal duodenum. The gross and microscopic appearance of ulcers varies widely; vascular thromboses are often seen and should be sought in the bed of gastric and duodenal lesions associated with anemia or hemorrhage. Perforation of gastric or duodenal ulcers may lead to hemorrhage or release of gastric contents into the abdomen and may initiate pancreatitis. Some ulcers perforate silently, and the serosal lesion heals by granulation and fibroplasia in the omentum, although the irritant nature of gastric contents released in these circumstances often leads to chronic inflammation, granulation, and thickening of the serosa, even when previous perforation can no longer be appreciated. A search for microscopic particles of food material in the serosal inflammatory response confirms perforation in this circumstance. Chronic gastroduodenal ulcers have thickened scirrhous mucosal margins and bases, and these must be differentiated from infiltrative gastric adenocarcinoma in the dog.

Abomasal ulcers in cattle are common (Fig. 1-36A-C); duodenal ulcer is rarely encountered. Acute and variably severe ulcers or erosions are frequently seen in cattle at autopsy (especially in young calves and dairy cows), many are incidental, and the cause is not always identified. Single or multiple ulcers are seen as linear areas of brown or black hemorrhage or erosion along the margins of abomasal rugae, or as punctate hemorrhages and erosions scattered over the mucosa. Ulcers may be present anywhere in the abomasum, but they are common in the pyloric region in cattle, and *especially at the torus pyloricus in young (veal) calves* (see Fig. 1-36A), but they may be found in the mucosa of the fundus as well. Abomasal ulcers occurred in ~34% of feedlot cattle in one study, with about half of the cases subclinical; reports indicate that >6% of slaughtered European dairy cows have evidence of active or previous abomasal ulcers. A very high proportion, often >50%, of veal calves have abomasal ulcers at slaughter.

Gastric ulcers are observed in cattle treated with NSAIDs. Ulcers often seem to occur under physiologically *stressful circumstances*, as in recently weaned and veal calves, postparturient cows, animals with concurrent disease, such as abomasal displacement or mastitis, or after transportation. Lactic acid and histamine entering the abomasum from the forestomachs in animals poorly adapted to high-concentrate rations may contribute to mucosal damage. In veal calves, consumption of straw, shavings, or other roughage has been associated with an increased prevalence of ulcers. Abomasal ulcers can be associated with various infectious diseases, including clostridial abomasitis, BVDV, malignant catarrhal fever virus, or mycotic agents. Mineral deficiencies including copper and selenium, or ingestion of toxins such as arsenic, have also been linked to abomasal ulceration in cattle. Abomasal stasis may play a role in the pathogenesis of ulceration in animals with physical or physiologic abomasal obstruction or displacement. Ulceration of the abomasal mucosa infiltrated by neoplastic lymphocytes is common. In many cases, *various factors and mechanisms contribute simultaneously* to the development of ulceration of the abomasum.

A classification system has been developed for abomasal ulcers in cattle that includes type 1 (nonperforating ulceration, with variably severe subtypes), type 2 (nonperforating bleeding ulceration with intraluminal hemorrhage; see Fig. 1-36B and C), type 3 (perforating ulcer with localized peritonitis), type 4 (perforating ulceration with diffuse peritonitis), and type 5 (perforating ulcer with peritonitis limited to the omental bursa); this classification system mostly represents attempts to improve antemortem diagnosis and clinical management, and is not widely used during autopsy.

The presenting sign in many cases of abomasal ulceration is *melena;* however, hemorrhage causing exsanguination, or

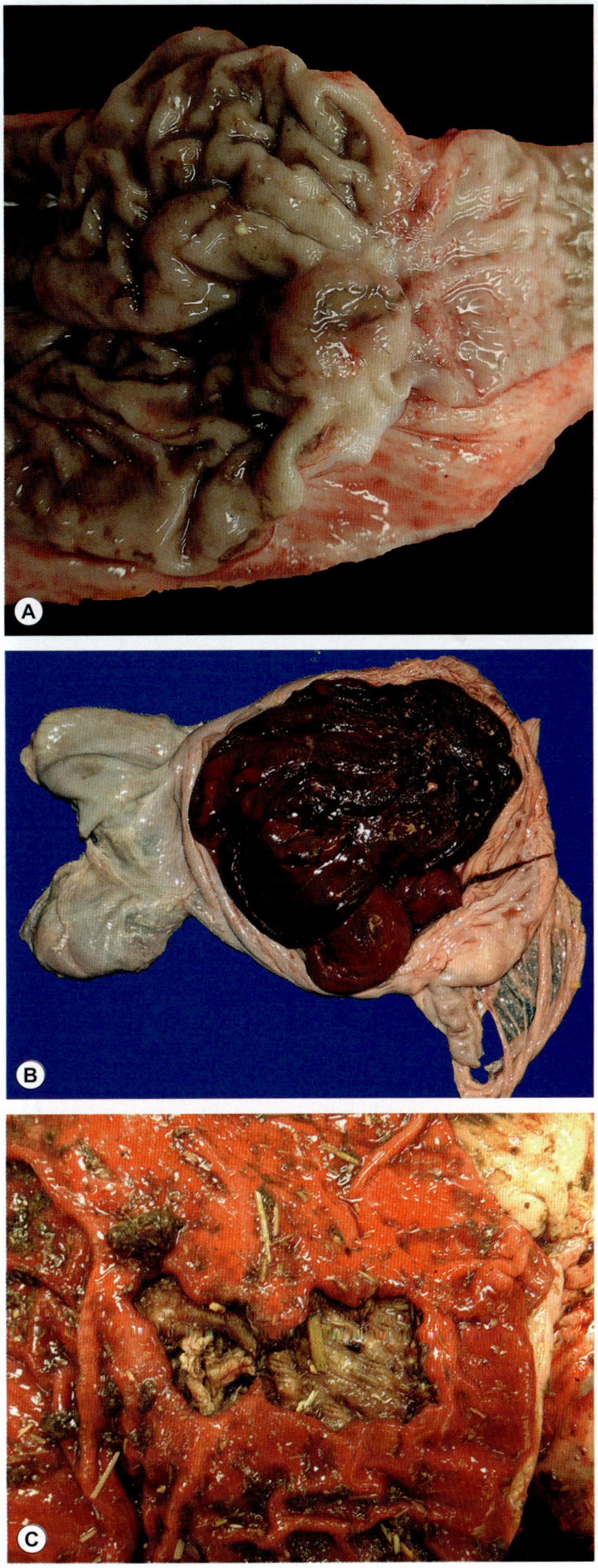

Figure 1-36 Abomasal ulcer in a calf. **A.** Acute ulceration at the torus pyloricus in a calf, due to nonsteroidal anti-inflammatory drug toxicity. (Courtesy S. Fritz.) **B.** Abomasal lumen filled with blood because of a perforating bleeding abomasal ulcer. (Courtesy J. Caswell.) **C.** Deep irregular abomasal ulcer. (Courtesy J. Caswell.)

perforation and septic peritonitis, are not unusual and can result in death as a consequence of abomasal ulcers. Perforation may occur into the omental bursa, localizing contamination and inflammation (omental bursitis is a category 5 lesion), and there can be significant adhesions between the omentum and the abdominal wall.

Gastric ulcers in swine are usually restricted to the *pars esophagea*; in a small proportion of affected pigs, lesions extend into the contiguous esophagus. Rarely are significant ulcers of the cardiac, fundic, or pyloric mucosa encountered in swine. With modern pig husbandry, the prevalence of ulcer and associated abnormalities of the pars esophagea is high, and weaned growers and feeders are commonly affected. Most lesions are subclinical; however, some prove fatal. Pigs die without premonition, or with a short history that may include anemia, weakness, inappetence, vomition, and melena. Other animals can be affected chronically, with signs of anorexia, intermittent melena, and weight loss that may culminate in death or slow recovery with significantly reduced growth rates.

The etiopathogenesis of the ulceration remains controversial. *Finely ground rations have repeatedly been found to be ulcerogenic in swine*, and this may be the single most important predisposing factor. As in other species, physiologically stressful husbandry practices have been considered to contribute to the development of ulcer, although experimental glucocorticoid administration tends to cause lesions of the fundus, not pars esophagea, in pigs. Environment has been identified as a factor, for example, pigs held on slatted floors have a higher incidence of nonglandular ulcers than pigs on solid or straw flooring. Several nutritional factors have been linked to gastric ulcers in pigs: high dietary copper, whey, high-starch and low-protein diets, high unsaturated fatty acids, and microbial production of short-chain fatty acids. An association between *H. suis* (or other less common helicobacters) and gastritis and ulceration has been proposed in pigs, although this has not been definitively substantiated. Other factors that stimulate acid secretion, especially histamine, consistently cause ulcers of the pars esophagea experimentally, suggesting that gastric acidity also plays an important role.

The squamous epithelium has no innate buffering capacity, and it is highly susceptible to injury by gastric acid, pepsin, and refluxed bile. Some evidence suggests altered consistency of feedstuffs or gastric contents (increased water, or finely divided rations, for example) may be significant also, because they alter the ability of the establishment of a declining pH gradient from esophagus to pylorus in stomach ingesta, thus contributing to abnormally low pH at the esophageal end of the stomach. *Lesions of the pars esophagea* may involve only a small part, or the entire gastric squamous mucosa. Early acid-induced damage is seen mostly as parakeratosis, which progresses to fissuring and erosion, and ultimately to full ulceration in severe cases. The parakeratotic epithelium of the pars esophagea appears yellow and is thickened, irregular, roughened, and may flake or peel off readily; *Candida* may also be present over the epithelial surface. Erosion of the epithelium progresses to ulceration with exposure of the submucosa, where small blood vessels are damaged, leading to hemorrhage. A thin rim of squamous epithelium adjacent to the cardiac gland mucosa may be spared (Fig. 1-37A). Depending on stage and severity of the ulcer, there may be a well-developed bed of granulation tissue and inflammation along the margins of the lesion, although *fatal gastric hemorrhage* often occurs.

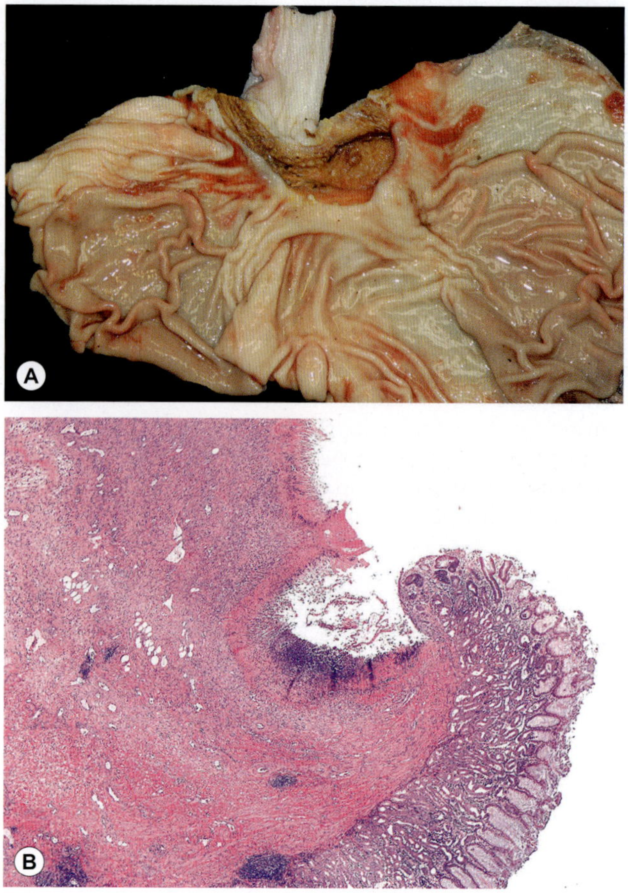

Figure 1-37 Ulceration of the pars esophagea in a pig. **A.** Near complete ulceration of the squamous epithelium. **B.** Remnant cardiac glandular mucosa overhangs the margin of the ulcer.

Fully developed ulceration of the pars esophagea is apparent as a small depressed area with elevated rolled margins, obliterating part or the entire pars esophagea and obscuring the esophageal opening (see Fig. 1-37B). They are easily overlooked, as the floor of the ulcer may be so smooth that it is misinterpreted as normal. If significant hemorrhage is evident, there will be red-brown gastric content, or even massive hemorrhage into the stomach lumen with large blood clots variably adhered to the submucosa at the base of the ulcer. Melenic content will often be present in the intestine, and the colon may contain firm black pelleted feces. The carcasses of animals that exsanguinate with gastric ulcer are very pale. Extensive hemorrhagic contents of the intestine should always be carefully differentiated from similar lesions such as mesenteric volvulus and proliferative hemorrhagic enteropathy associated with *Lawsonia intracellularis* infection. Some pigs with parakeratosis, erosion, and ulceration of the pars esophagea may have esophageal lesions suggestive of gastric reflux. Gastric ulcers in some pigs resolve by granulation, and they may become re-epithelialized. Such lesions usually become scirrhous, puckered, and contracted as the ulcer closes from the periphery, and scarring may be visible from the serosa. In these circumstances, stenotic occlusion of the esophageal opening into the stomach may occur, and pigs with this problem can develop muscle hypertrophy of the distal esophagus.

Two syndromes described in **horses** as **equine gastric ulcer syndrome** are defined based on the anatomic distribution of lesions, specifically whether the ulcers involve the **squamous** or the **glandular** portion of the stomach. The prevalence of gastric ulceration in horses is reported to be quite high, with an incidence of squamous ulceration of ~50% in horses, which may be up to 100% in training racehorses; glandular ulceration has generally lower prevalence of 15-70%. Gastric ulceration causes a syndrome of abdominal pain and is sometimes associated with gastric reflux in foals, and with colic in older horses; however, some affected horses have altered behavior or performance, reduced coat quality, chronic diarrhea, or even no clinical signs.

Gastric squamous ulceration is likely multifactorial, but predisposing factors are mostly management factors associated with elevated or prolonged exposure of the squamous epithelium to gastric acid, including diet (increased carbohydrates, quantity and quality of fiber, fiber size), increased exercise, feed deprivation, and other factors. Squamous ulcers occur as primary disease due to increased exposure of squamous epithelium to acid, or secondary to delayed gastric outflow due either to pyloric stenosis or severe chronic inflammation. In contrast, glandular ulcers occur due to damaged glandular mucosa mostly associated with loss of normal defense mechanisms, such as chronic inflammation, secondary to NSAID usage, or dietary factors (as for squamous disease); glandular ulceration may be a form of gastritis with an immune-mediated component; most cases have significant gastric and intestinal inflammation.

Squamous ulcers are common and readily identified grossly or by endoscopy. They are usually most severe at or adjacent to the margo plicatus, and are often large and irregular in shape. There may be extensive fissuring, erosion, and ulceration of the squamous epithelium of the pars esophagea and esophagus, sometimes extending to the pharynx, especially in foals with severe gastric reflux. Remnant islands of white proliferative squamous epithelium are scattered like plaques on a predominantly ulcerated mucosal surface (Fig. 1-38). Microscopically, there is squamous epithelial hyperplasia with prominent rete pegs and edematous proprial papillae. Parakeratotic hyperkeratosis can be prominent, especially in early lesions; they can then progress through increasing degrees of epithelial erosion to ulceration as described earlier in swine. Glandular metaplasia can be observed in the ulcer bed of chronic lesions.

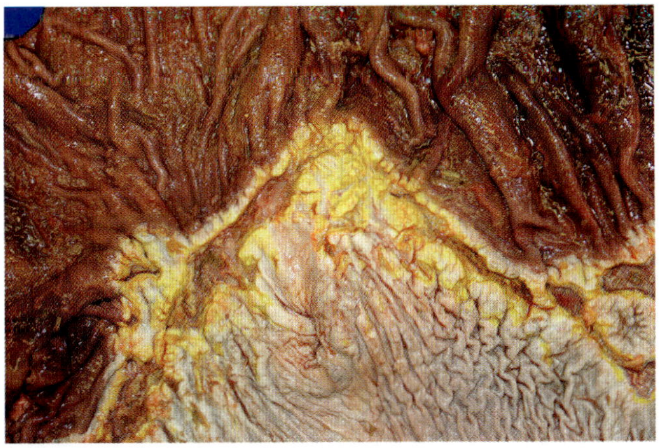

Figure 1-38 Confluent areas of **ulceration of the squamous mucosa** along the margo plicatus in the stomach of a horse.

Glandular ulcers are less common, and much less obvious grossly and endoscopically. These ulcers can be large, multiple, and extensive, although subtle punctate lesions can also occur. Gross and histologic lesions of squamous ulceration are well correlated, but lesions in the glandular stomach have been more difficult to assess; surgical biopsy and histologic evaluation may be necessary to document erosion or ulceration, and inflammation in affected horses. *Perforation* may occur at any site of ulceration, and, in one series, perforation occurred in 1% of 600 autopsies on foals. Some foals may exsanguinate because of bleeding ulcers, and occasionally, clotted blood will fill the stomach.

Pyloric and duodenal stenosis have been associated with healing ulcers in horses. Circumferential ulcerative lesions or those involving the antimesenteric mucosa of the proximal duodenum are more likely to progress to duodenal stricture, seen as a chronic phase of this disease. It is unclear whether the *ulcerative duodenitis* seen in some cases is a product of gastroduodenal ulceration by these mechanisms, or whether it represents a process such as *duodenitis and proximal jejunitis* (DPJ), which in turn results in stricture, gastric reflux, and ulceration. The entity DPJ is discussed in more detail with Clostridial infections, under the *Clostridiodes difficile* section, later in this chapter.

Proliferative and neoplastic lesions of the stomach and abomasum

Neoplasia of the stomach is *uncommon* in all domestic species (Table 1-1). Gastric neoplasms are relatively prevalent among surgical biopsy submissions from dogs and cats, in contrast to their rarity in production animals and horses. Malignant neoplasms are more common than benign lesions, and with the notable exception of lymphoma, *most are carcinomas*.

Gastric epithelial metaplasia or dysplasia are occasionally observed in the stomach of dogs; metaplasia is a potentially reversible change from one fully differentiated cell type to another and is typically considered an adaptive change to environmental injury or trauma. Osseous metaplasia or heterotopic bone formation has been rarely described within hyperplastic polyps and adenocarcinoma of the canine stomach and intestine. The mechanism of heterotopic bone formation is not understood but presumed to be secondary to chronic inflammation and even osteoblastic-type differentiation of the proliferative cells in some cases.

Mucous cell metaplasia has also been described (pseudopyloric metaplasia) in dogs with various forms of gastric atrophy or inflammation and involves metaplastic transformation of usually small regions of fundic mucosa to mucous cell morphology. **Gastric epithelial dysplasia** has also been observed in dogs; little is known about this change in the canine species, so the lesion is presumed similar to the change in humans. There may be architectural (glandular disorganization, budding, irregular branching, dilation) or cytologic (mucin depletion, crowding, pleomorphism, hyperchromatism, increased mitotic activity) anomalies observed in the glands of affected stomachs. In the dog, these are presumed to be reactive or response to injury, and there is no evidence that this is a precursor lesion to neoplasia.

Gastric polypoid hyperplasia (polyps) occurs as focal papillary or papillotubular proliferation of surface gastric epithelium with luminal projections that extend above the mucosal surface. These can be anywhere in the GI tract, although they occur with highest frequency near the colorectal junction of

Table • 1-1

Major primary non-neoplastic and neoplastic proliferative lesions of the lower GI tract of domestic animals

Epithelial	
Benign	Gastric or intestinal epithelial hyperplasia or dysplasia Pyloric hypertrophic gastropathy (canine) Gastric, intestinal, or colorectal papillary adenoma (colorectal polyps of dogs) GI adenoma
Malignant	GI adenocarcinoma Gastric squamous cell carcinoma GI neuroendocrine carcinoma (carcinoid)
Mesenchymal	
Benign	Diffuse GI leiomyomatosis (canine) GI smooth muscle neoplasms (leiomyoma) Intestinal hamartomatous polyps
Malignant	GI smooth muscle neoplasms (leiomyosarcoma) GI stromal tumor Other GI sarcomas (varied subtypes)
Round Cell	
Benign	GI extramedullary plasmacytoma
Malignant	GI lymphoma (lymphoma), various subtypes and presentations GI mast cell tumor
Neoplasms metastatic to the GI tract	

GI = gastrointestinal.

dogs, which are discussed later in this chapter with neoplastic lesions of the intestine. In the stomach (Fig. 1-39), these occur mostly as incidental lesions that only are significant and cause disease if they become obstructive. When they occur in the gastric pylorus, they should be distinguished from chronic hypertrophic pyloric gastropathy. Gastric hyperplastic polyps are most common in older animals, although they have been described rarely in puppies. They usually occur as small lesions in the pylorus; multiple can be present in a single patient. Polyps consist of proliferative glandular epithelial cells covering variably thick fibrous stalks; the cells may occasionally form cystic structures. The epithelial cells can be pleomorphic; some polyps may have epithelial dysplasia, mucous metaplasia, and even surface ulceration or mineralization of the stalk, although usually they are well differentiated with no evidence of infiltrative or invasive growth into or through the basement membrane. The fibrous stalk can be variably inflamed or have prominent lymphoid follicular hyperplasia, but no studies have demonstrated evidence that these represent preneoplastic lesions, making them distinct from the human disease. Some authors subdivide these into inflammatory-type polyps and hyperplastic-type polyps

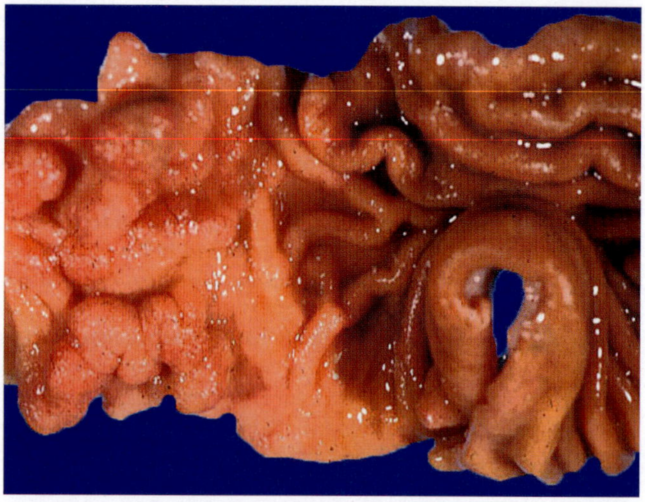

Figure 1-39 Mucosal polypoid proliferation in the pylorus of a dog. (Courtesy Noah's Arkives.)

where, in addition to epithelial proliferation covering polypoid fibroplasia, the inflammatory polyps also have variable but often extensive mixed inflammation and lymphoid follicular hyperplasia in the stroma. There is likely no clinically relevant significant distinction between the two, and both are behaviorally benign. Complete surgical excision of polyps is generally curative.

Neoplasms of epithelial cells. The prevalence and distribution of **gastric adenomas and adenocarcinomas** vary among species. **Gastric adenomas** are uncommon; in a report of gastric lesions in dogs detected by diagnostic imaging, adenomas were diagnosed at a higher prevalence, although these could have included polyps and hypertrophic gastritis in addition to simple adenomas. The histologic features of adenoma are described as well-circumscribed, often polypoid lesions consisting of tubular, villus, or papillary structures covered by a single layer of well-differentiated epithelium; some can include poorly differentiated epithelial cells with altered cellular morphology including cell size and shape; adenomas may have increased mitotic figures but still lack features of a more aggressive carcinoma. Most reports have shown gastric adenomas to be uncommon and incidental, with no evidence that they transform to malignant neoplasia. In contrast, **gastric carcinomas in dogs** are much more common, they comprise 50-90% of all canine gastric malignancies, and are more frequent in the stomach compared with the small intestine and colon.

Reported breed predispositions include the Belgian Tervuren, Bouvier des Flandres, Belgian Sheepdog (Groenendael), Standard Poodle, Norwegian Elkhound, Rough Collie, Chow Chow, and Staffordshire Bull Terrier, but this may be biased by geography and breed popularity. Familial GI adenomatous polyposis has been reported in Jack Russell Terriers with germline *APC* mutations; polyps were diagnosed as adenomas or adenocarcinomas. Clinical signs include vomiting, hematemesis, melena, lethargy, abdominal distension, or abdominal discomfort. The pathogenesis of canine gastric carcinoma remains incompletely understood. Some hypothesize an association with chronic inflammation (including infection with *H. pylori*) or diet; however, this remains unproven in dogs.

Grossly, gastric carcinomas can appear as exophytic lesions that protrude and extend into the gastric lumen, or they can be highly infiltrative and spread along and through the gastric wall without a distinct exophytic mass; this makes them more difficult to detect grossly, and to distinguish from chronic gastric mural fibrosis of other causes (chronic ulceration or other trauma). The antrum and pylorus are common sites for development of gastric adenocarcinoma in the dog. Some carcinomas grossly occur as polypoid growths, but most appear as localized plaque-like thickenings of the gastric wall that obliterate rugae and ulcerate centrally (Fig. 1-40A); some lack prominent ulceration, and occasionally, they merely cause thickening of the wall with no defined mass. Cut sections through the stomach wall invaded by carcinoma reveal edema and pale firm fibrous tissue. Induration or plaque-like masses may be evident on the serosa, where the pale outline of infiltrated lymphatics may be prominent. Widespread gastric mural fibrosis and thickening from desmoplasia induced by the malignant epithelium are common. Gastric carcinomas in dogs are often diagnosed at an advanced stage, which is associated with a poor prognosis and short survival times (median 35 days after diagnosis); ~70-90% of cases have already metastasized at the time of initial diagnosis, often to lymph nodes, omentum, liver, and lung. Metastatic disease is much more likely with non-polypoid or exophytic lesions.

Histologic classification is based on the WHO classification in animals (2003), with several subtypes including *papillary, tubular, signet ring cell, mucinous, squamous*, and *undifferentiated*. Some subtypes described in humans are not included in the WHO classification, but have been observed in dogs, including *poorly cohesive* and *mixed* carcinomas. The various subtypes can also occur together in different regions of the same neoplasm, making classification especially challenging in small endoscopic samples. Most gastric neoplasms are probably of mucinous or signet ring subtypes, although papillary, tubular, squamous, and undifferentiated neoplasms are described. *There is no known prognostic significance linked with various subtypes in dogs*.

In humans, gastric carcinomas are also classified as *intestinal type* if the neoplastic epithelial cells form glands, *diffuse type* if the neoplastic epithelial cells are seen individually or in numerous widely distributed small nests with rare gland formation, or *mixed type* if they have features of both; this system has been applied to canine neoplasms and may give more meaningful prognostic information. In dogs, *most gastric carcinomas are probably of the diffuse type*, with poorly differentiated tubular and glandular epithelial cells, often exhibiting marked infiltrative growth, extensive adjacent fibroplasia, and scirrhous response (see Fig. 1-40B), and in some cases abundant mucus production. In these lesions, clusters or sheets of immature poorly differentiated mucus-producing gastric epithelial cells efface native architecture (see Fig. 1-40C) and can line variably distinct glands or acinar structures; epithelial cells can be suspended in or surrounded by large lakes of mucus and fibroplasia. In cases of sessile carcinoma that lack a definitive mucosal mass, definitive diagnosis is much more challenging. Lakes of mucus or fibroplasia deep to the muscularis mucosa in sections of stomach should warrant a careful search for neoplastic glandular epithelial cells including within draining lymphatic vessels of the submucosa, which can in some cases be few and subtle. If identifiable epithelial glands are present, a diagnosis of carcinoma can be made, although in some cases glandular differentiation can be quite subtle; special stains, including PAS or Alcian blue, may help highlight mucin within the cytoplasm of neoplastic cells.

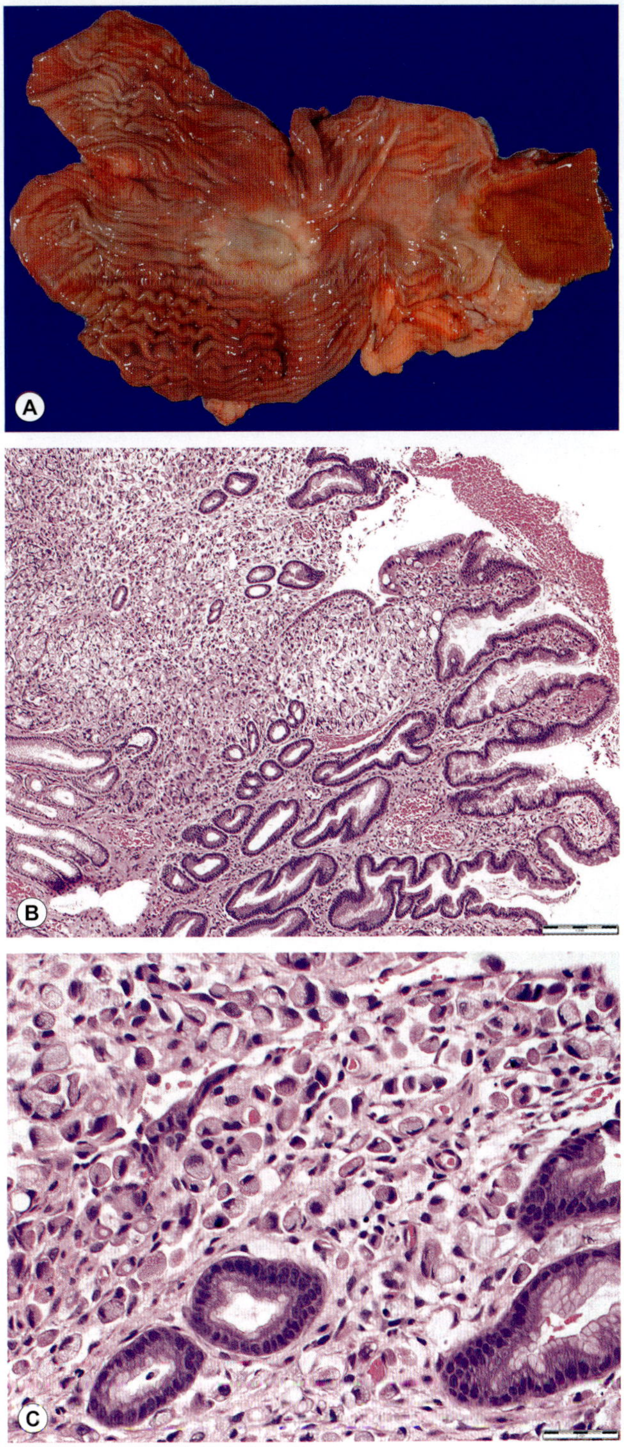

Figure 1-40 **Gastric adenocarcinoma** in a dog. **A**. The gastric wall is focally thickened, with surface ulceration. (Courtesy M. Stalker.) **B**. Neoplastic epithelial cells efface the propria. **C**. Neoplastic epithelial cells are suspended in mucus and proliferative fibrous tissue; cytoplasmic mucus is visible.

Less frequently, canine gastric carcinomas are of the *intestinal type*, with distinct mass formation, and multilobular cohesive masses composed of polarized epithelial cells forming glands. These are more likely to be exophytic lesions with less extensive infiltrative growth, less fibroplasia and desmoplasia, and less mucus production compared with the infiltrative or diffuse carcinomas.

Of note, for lesions in the canine stomach, the histologic diagnosis is best made with a *full-thickness biopsy*. The submucosal and transmural portions of the tumor are routinely larger and more readily identified as malignancy than the mucosal portion of the tumor, which endoscopic biopsies may not capture; caution should be exercised when evaluating endoscopic biopsies if the clinical history or gross appearance suggests that carcinoma is a differential diagnosis. Alternatively, especially when large deep ulcerative lesions are biopsied endoscopically, only the necrosis, inflammation, and fibrosis that accompany neoplastic cells as they infiltrate through the stomach wall may be captured. Misdiagnosis may also be made when attempting to distinguish early gastric carcinoma from the dysplastic repair of recent ulceration; in such cases, a full-thickness biopsy to detect invasion is more reliable than the best endoscopic sample.

IHC may be prognostically useful; specifically, high Ki-67 in neoplastic epithelial cells and vimentin expression in neoplastic epithelial cells and stromal cells may be associated with poor prognosis; more definitive thresholds or specific counts have yet to be established.

Gastric carcinoma in cats is quite uncommon, and some breeds (Siamese and Persian) may be over-represented. Small intestinal and colonic adenocarcinomas are more common in cats compared with gastric carcinomas. Not enough cases are described to know the details of prognosis and behavior, but most appear to be of tubular or diffuse patterns, all are quite highly aggressive with both local infiltration and widespread metastatic disease. Again, full-thickness biopsies are highly preferred because many cases of suspicious proliferative epithelial tissue in cats are due to adenomatous hyperplasia upon further investigation.

Gastric carcinomas of the horse, ruminant, and pig occur in glandular stomach, but are described rarely and all appear to be highly behaviorally aggressive.

Squamous cell carcinoma (SCC) of the stomach is the most common neoplasm of the equine stomach; it is rarely reported in dogs. SCC can appear after an elongated nonspecific course of unexplained anorexia, dysphagia, or weight loss sometimes progressing rapidly to emaciation, or after acute onset of disease. These arise from the squamous epithelium of the equine stomach, and most appear grossly as exophytic vegetative masses that can be quite large with an ulcerated and necrotic surface (Fig. 1-41). Given their infiltrative behavior, they are often recognized quite late in the course of disease and generally have a poor prognosis. There is frequently widespread metastasis at the time of initial diagnosis. At autopsy, there may be peritoneal effusion, and usually, there is evidence of plaques of neoplastic cells and proliferative or scirrhous fibroplasia on the serosa of the stomach and other abdominal organs. Much less frequently, they have been described as diffuse or infiltrative types in which there is thickening and ulceration of the proximal squamous stomach and duodenum without distinct mass formation. The cause has long been assumed to be sporadic or possibly diet related; however, a strong association in some gastric SCCs has been found with *Equus caballus* papillomavirus 2.

Regardless, the microscopic features are characteristic for SCC of other tissues (skin, oral cavity) and are composed of nests and trabeculae of epithelial cells that often have squamous differentiation with frequent formation of keratin pearls; these keratin-producing cells stimulate a dense scirrhous response that can be especially evident along the serosal surface of the stomach and other abdominal organs. Individual neoplastic cells can have significant dysplasia and anaplasia, very high mitotic counts, and frequent extensive necrosis and hemorrhage; the diagnosis is not usually difficult if an appropriate sample is provided for examination. Equine gastric SCCs are usually in late stage at initial diagnosis, due to aggressive infiltration of the stomach wall and trans-abdominal carcinomatosis. Many cases also have evidence of thoracic metastasis, presumably this occurs via the lymphatic or hematogenous routes. Therefore, most horses are euthanized once the definitive diagnosis is established. One case of equine gastric SCC has been reported as a cause of pseudohyperparathyroidism in a horse.

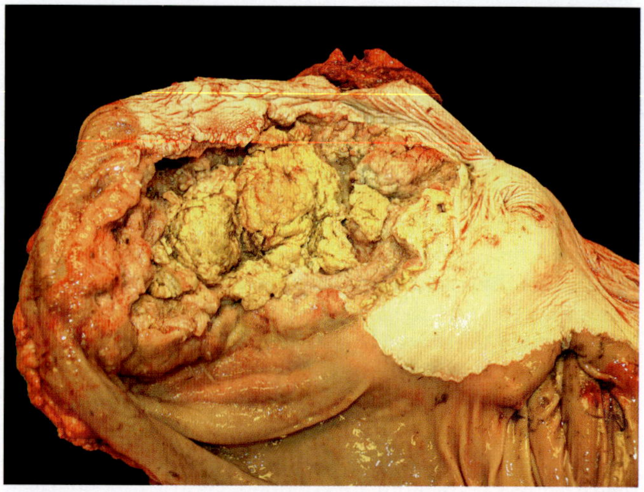

Figure 1-41 **Squamous cell carcinoma** arising from the gastric squamous mucosa of a horse.

Neuroendocrine carcinomas of the stomach (gastric carcinoid) are derived from enteroendocrine cells of the gastric mucosa that are scattered in the mucosa of a wide variety of organs, including the stomach. These cells secrete low–molecular-weight polypeptide hormones, such as secretin, somatostatin, and cholecystokinin, or they are part of the amine precursor uptake decarboxylation (APUD) group, producing compounds such as serotonin (5-hydroxytryptamine). They are very rare in dogs and have not been reported in other species.

Grossly, carcinoids are usually lobulated firm masses that seem to arise from deep within the mucosa of the proximal stomach forming submucosal or subserosal nodules, infiltrating transmurally and into the adjacent mesentery. Carcinoids have a distinct *neuroendocrine appearance* microscopically. Round or oval-to-polyhedral neoplastic cells have abundant finely granular eosinophilic or vacuolated cytoplasm. They form nests, palisading cords, trabeculae, or diffuse sheets and are supported by a fine vascularized fibrous stroma. Amyloid may be observed in intercellular and perivascular spaces. Megalocytes and multinucleate giant cells are described in some cases.

A definitive *diagnosis* of carcinoid is based on the neuroendocrine histologic pattern, cytoplasmic argyrophilic granularity (confirmed by Grimelius staining), and immunohistochemical identification of their specific secreted peptide mediator product, although no gastric carcinoid has been reported to be clinically functional in dogs and cats. They are routinely immunoreactive for neuron-specific enolase and chromogranin A, as are most neuroendocrine tumors. Electron microscopic examination may help differentiate carcinoids from intestinal MCTs; carcinoid cells have dense, round-to-oval, membrane-bound, 75-300-nm, secretory cytoplasmic granules, and abundant rough endoplasmic reticulum. Giemsa and toluidine blue staining are negative and often helpful to rule out gastric MCT. The biologic behavior of intestinal carcinoids in dogs and other domestic species is largely unknown, although most reported cases have been malignant. There may be extensive invasion of the gastric wall and widespread metastatic disease especially to the liver. The few cases that have been described in other domestic species (cat, ferret) have features similar to those described in dogs; several *gastric somastatinomas* are described in bearded dragons.

Neoplasms of mesenchymal cells. In the stomach (and intestine) were once thought to be of exclusively smooth muscle origin as leiomyomas and leiomyosarcomas, but now thanks to immunohistochemical analyses also include gastrointestinal stromal tumors (GISTs), which arise from interstitial cells of Cajal. Together, GI sarcomas represent 10-30% of all neoplasms in the GI tract of dogs.

Leiomyoma and leiomyosarcoma (or benign and malignant smooth muscle tumors) of the stomach arise from smooth muscle cells, either from the muscularis mucosa or from tunica muscularis of the stomach; smooth muscle tumors are common in dogs and usually affect older males. Historically, leiomyoma has been considered much more common than leiomyosarcoma; however, the malignant variant may actually be more common. The gastric cardia and gastroesophageal junction are the regions affected most commonly within the stomach. Leiomyomas are almost always incidental findings, although they can become quite large and cause esophageal or pyloric obstruction. They appear as well-circumscribed, smooth, firm, pale masses beneath an intact mucosa; they may deform the serosal or mucosal profile and eventually become ulcerated. They are composed of swirling interlacing bundles of uniform fusiform cells with abundant eosinophilic cytoplasm and a single central nucleus with blunt rounded ends (cigar shape); usually, no mitotic figures are evident; cellular pleomorphism, many or atypical mitotic figures, or abundant necrosis may suggest a more aggressive variant. By IHC, smooth muscle tumors in general should display positive immunoreactivity for α–smooth muscle actin (α-SMA) and/or desmin but are immunonegative for tyrosine kinase receptor KIT (CD117) and discovered on GIST1 (DOG1) antibodies, which excludes the significant differential diagnosis of GIST. Some reports indicate that smooth muscle tumors of the abdomen (including of the stomach) can be associated with hypoglycemia. This is presumed to represent a paraneoplastic syndrome of smooth muscle tumors from excessive glucose metabolism by neoplastic cells because the hypoglycemia resolves with complete resection of the neoplasm.

Diffuse leiomyomatosis has been described in a single young Dachshund, and this condition is reportedly similar to the human condition of the same name, although the lesions in human cases were much more widespread and severe. This canine patient had circumferential thickening of the gastroesophageal and anorectal junctions, which was histologically composed of proliferative well-differentiated smooth muscle cells without formation of distinct masses. In humans, the condition is considered a benign neoplastic change, mostly because malignant transformation has not been documented.

Leiomyosarcomas (malignant smooth muscle tumors) often resemble leiomyomas grossly, but 2 critically important features distinguish them from leiomyoma: they are locally infiltrative and invasive, and/or they display distant metastasis. The cells resemble the smooth muscle cells of leiomyoma, but there is usually some degree of anisokaryosis and anisocytosis, multiple nucleoli, scattered irregular nuclei, significantly increased mitotic activity, atypical mitotic figures, and often increased necrosis in the mass. Although these criteria of malignancy are not well defined in the veterinary literature, a mitotic count of $\geq$10 per 2.37 mm², local infiltrative growth, and necrosis are suggested as features that warrant a diagnosis of leiomyosarcoma. Leiomyosarcomas in dogs are apparently more common than previously thought and may outnumber leiomyomas significantly. Immunohistochemically, these are similar to leiomyomas. Many neoplasms historically diagnosed as leiomyosarcomas have since been reclassified as GISTs or undifferentiated sarcomas (especially those in the large intestine). Long-term survival may be >20 months, even if there is confirmed metastatic disease, and especially if the primary tumor can be completely excised. In **cats**, gastric smooth muscle tumors are rarely reported, and usually, the details are limited; most smooth muscle tumors in cats affect the intestine. A single report of gastric leiomyosarcoma in a cat had local invasive behavior, but there was no evidence of distant metastatic disease, and complete excision was apparently curative.

GI stromal tumors (GISTs) arise from the pacemaker cells of the intestine, the interstitial cells of Cajal found in the submucosal and myenteric plexuses. They occur most frequently in the intestine and are only rarely reported in the stomach. They are common in dogs, they occur with some frequency in horses, but uncommonly in other species, including cats and guinea pigs. Interstitial cells of Cajal are defined by their expression of CD117 (cKit) and DOG1, which may be more sensitive and specific than CD117. Some may also express α-SMA; they rarely express desmin. IHC expression pattern, and the intensity of CD117 immunoreactivity is important and useful diagnostically and clinically because of differences in behavior, response to therapy, and prognosis for GISTs compared with smooth muscle tumors. Hence, sarcomas of the stomach (and intestine) should be evaluated immunohistochemically to distinguish these from one another.

GISTs are usually well demarcated and grow by expansion, sometimes forming exophytic nodules on the serosal surface, but they may be transmural and invasive. They are histologically indistinguishable from smooth muscle tumors with spindle neoplastic cells arranged in interlacing fascicles, or in a storiform or whorling pattern; neoplastic cells have indistinct borders, a single oval nucleus, and basophilic cytoplasm. There may be nuclear pleomorphism; mitotic figures are usually evident and may be common. Hemorrhage or necrosis may be present within the tumor, and lymphocytic and/or eosinophilic infiltrates can occur. Although GISTs are uncommon in the stomach compared with the intestine, they probably have biologic behavior similar to leiomyosarcomas. Negative prognostic factors for intestinal (and probably gastric) GISTs include localized infiltrative growth, mitotic count >9 per 2.37 mm², incomplete margins, and weak CD117 cytoplasmic immunoreactivity.

In **horses**, tumors of the GI tract have been described that in many cases meet morphologic, ultrastructural, or immunohistochemical criteria for GIST, although these were diagnosed as GIST based on negative immunoreactivity for α-SMA; immunoreactivity to CD117 or DOG1 was not reported.

Most reported GISTs involve the lower intestine (colon, cecum, and rectum), with no cases reported in the equine stomach.

Neoplasms of round cells. Round cell neoplasms in the stomach are mostly **gastric lymphomas**, which occur infrequently in most species including **dogs, cattle**, occasionally **horses**, but are most common in **cats**. Gastric lymphomas can be primary in the stomach or other parts of the intestinal tract, along with intestinal lymphoma, or as part of systemic or multicentric form of the disease (see Vol. 3, Hematolymphoid System). Primary lymphoma of the GI tract includes cases with stomach and/or intestinal lymphoma with possible involvement of the abdominal organs or bone marrow, but lacking lesions in the thorax or peripheral sites (these are considered multicentric lymphomas). Affected animals usually have chronic vomiting, anorexia, and weight loss. They may be mural or transmural lesions and have a gastric mass, or mucosal lesions with more subtle regional or diffuse thickening of the stomach based on endoscopy, ultrasound, or other imaging modalities.

Gastric lymphoma appears grossly as in other locations, as white-to-tan firm nodules or as regional-to-diffuse transmural thickening by white firm tissue; the surface will occasionally be ulcerated. Histologically, there are diffuse transmural dense sheets of neoplastic monomorphic large lymphocytes, often with a single large central vesicular nucleus and multiple nucleoli. Infiltration into the lamina propria is frequent, but there is not usually clear association with pre-existing lymphoid follicles, and in dogs they are not necessarily thought to arise from B lymphocytes in the mucosal lymphoid tissue in the stomach (as in humans and cats). In contrast to cats in which most gastric lymphomas are large B-cell subtype, most cases in dogs are likely associated with intestinal lymphoma, and most appear to be of T-cell phenotype. Lymphomas should be assessed in the stomach as they are in the intestine, by immunophenotype, neoplastic cell nuclear size, grade (mitotic count), and growth pattern, discussed in more detail with the intestine below. Large-cell lymphomas are usually more aggressive; small-cell lymphomas tend to have a low grade indolent course. Definitive diagnosis is usually straight forward, but histochemical stains or IHC may be helpful to rule out other round-cell tumors as possible differential diagnoses, including Giemsa, toluidine blue, or CD117 (MCT), MUM1 (extramedullary plasma cell tumor), and IBA1 or CD18 (histiocytic sarcoma). IHC is valuable for assessing epitheliotropism patterns, and for immunophenotyping gastric lymphomas; several markers are commonly effectively used (CD79a, PAX5, or CD20 for B cells; CD3 for T cells).

In **cows and other ruminants**, abomasal lymphoma is very common. There is a strong association with bovine leukemia virus (BLV; *Retroviridae, Deltaretrovirus bovleu*) infection and abomasal lymphoma in cattle, and most are of the large B-cell phenotype and are rarely isolated to the abomasum. They commonly involve other organs including the heart, uterus, lymph nodes, periocular tissue, or spinal cord. Typical clinical signs include anorexia, weight loss, and possible ataxia or paresis (if the spinal cord is involved). Affected abomasa can have pyloric obstruction leading to abomasal bloat, and many cases have diffuse expansion of the abomasal wall and individual mucosal folds due to thick, firm, white tissue composed of infiltrating neoplastic lymphocytes. Ulceration of the abomasal surface is common, so melena is a frequent presenting sign. Histologic lesions are also similar to lymphoma in other species and consist of dense sheets of monomorphic neoplastic lymphocytes within the mucosa, submucosa, and often the tunica muscularis; many also infiltrate into the adjacent mesenteric adipose tissue.

Diffuse gastric lymphoma also occurs in **swine**. The wall of the stomach is thickened by submucosal lymphocytic infiltrates, which sometimes invade the mucosa locally in many areas, producing nodular elevations that may ulcerate. B-cell lymphomas involving the Peyer patches also have been detected at meat inspection in swine.

Gastric mast cell tumors (MCTs) are uncommon and are often considered with other mucosal MCTs, which are distinct from the much more common cutaneous MCTs of dogs. They occur in aged dogs and occasionally in cats, with clinical signs such as vomition, diarrhea, and melena. It is not always clear if these represent primary MCTs, or metastases from primary cutaneous lesions. Gastric MCTs are seen in biopsies as invasive round-cell tumors that can resemble carcinoid, lymphoma, or extramedullary plasma cell tumor; *definitive diagnosis may require histochemical* (toluidine blue, Giemsa) *and possibly immunohistochemical* (CD117) *confirmation*, especially if the cells are poorly differentiated or lack distinct cytoplasmic granularity. Interestingly, although gastric ulceration is a common occurrence secondary to cutaneous MCTs, ulceration is not often observed with GI MCTs. Primary MCTs of the GI tract likely arise from mucosal mast cells, which differ from connective tissue mast cells such as those found in skin, in that they have few visible granules that often stain poorly in formalin-fixed tissue. MCTs are more common in the intestine than in the stomach.

Gastric extramedullary plasma cell tumors are also *uncommon neoplasms in dogs*, and rare in cats and other species. These are derived from terminally differentiated B cells and arise most frequently in the submucosa of the distal colon and rectum of dogs, where they are associated with signs of large-bowel diarrhea and bleeding. A few cases are described as arising from the stomach, and these have been historically considered to be more biologically and behaviorally aggressive than cutaneous plasma cell tumors, with frequent nodal metastasis described. Monoclonal gammopathy does not seem to be a consistent feature of extracutaneous extramedullary plasma cell tumors in dogs.

Histologically, they usually resemble plasma cell tumors of the skin or oral cavity, although some can be less well-differentiated without typical plasma cell morphologic features. The tumor is formed by solid packets of pleomorphic round cells with various degrees of plasmacytoid maturation, especially at the periphery of the tumor. There can be considerable nuclear pleomorphism, hyperchromasia, multinucleation, and increased mitotic count. The cells are typically arranged in packets or sheets supported by a delicate fibrovascular stroma. Most tumors have a discrete local growth habit amenable to surgical cure, although some will be locally infiltrative. Metastasis of poorly differentiated plasma cell tumor of the stomach to local lymph nodes has been observed, but even these are unlikely to be widely behaviorally aggressive. Some gastric plasma cell tumors have AL amyloid (confirmed by Congo red or thioflavin T histochemical staining) or light-chain immunoglobulin (confirmed by Ig light chain IHC) deposition among the tumor cells. Confirmation of the diagnosis is by IHC for the interferon regulatory factor marker MUM1/IRF4; many of these tumors are also variably immunoreactive for B-cell markers CD79a, CD20, or PAX5. These should not display immunoreactivity for CD3, although a case report in a dog demonstrated aberrant CD3 expression. A **feline** case of primary gastric extramedullary plasma cell tumor is reported.

Primary **gastric histiocytic sarcoma** has been diagnosed in a few dogs, but the stomach may also be involved as a component of disseminated histiocytic sarcoma in dogs. Masses within the gastric submucosa are composed of unencapsulated sheets of densely packed round-to-oval cells with abundant eosinophilic cytoplasm, marked anisocytosis and anisokaryosis, many multinucleate tumor giant cells, with phagocytosis of erythrocytes or other mononuclear cells. Confirmation of the diagnosis is by histomorphologic features of the cells and by exclusion of other round-cell neoplasms by histochemical stains and IHC; in particular other differentials, including large-cell lymphoma, poorly differentiated MCT, extramedullary plasma cell tumor, should be excluded. Positive IHC immunoreactivity for markers of macrophages or dendritic cells (including IBA1, CD18, CD204, MHC, possibly lysozyme, and others) is also often very helpful.

INTESTINE

Structure, function, and response to injury

The microtopography of the **small bowel** is extensively modified to increase its surface area by **villi** that project into the lumen and/or by *spiral mucosal folds* in some species. The villi are projections of lamina propria covered by a single layer of epithelium that expand the absorptive surface of the small bowel 7-14-fold. In most species, villi are tallest in the duodenum and decline somewhat in height distally toward the ileum. The length and shape of villi in normal animals vary with the species, age, diet, intestinal microflora, and immune status. In general, villi in dogs, cats, neonatal piglets, and ruminants tend to be tall and cylindrical; those in horses and in young ruminants tend to be moderately tall and cylindrical; villi in weaned ruminants and swine may be cylindrical, leaf- or tongue-shaped, or rarely ridgelike, with their broad surface at right angles to the long axis of the intestine. Villus length typically decreases after weaning, although this varies by species and anatomic location.

Opening to the mucosal surface around the base of each villus are several *intestinal crypts (crypts of Lieberkühn)*. Depending on the species, anatomic location, and their proliferative status, crypts are perpendicular to the muscularis mucosa or somewhat coiled and lined by a single layer of epithelium. The progenitor compartment of the enteric epithelium resides in the crypts, producing immature epithelial cells that differentiate and move up on to the surface of villi mainly as absorptive enterocytes, ultimately to be extruded as effete cells from the tips of villi into the lumen. The mechanism of this process is probably highly regulated by local immune cells of the intestine (lymphocytes, macrophages) and is considered a form of well-controlled cell death or apoptosis. Disposed cells are either phagocytosed by proprial macrophages, where they likely play a role in development and maintenance of immunologic tolerance in the intestine, or they are extruded into the lumen where they contribute to enzyme content and complexity of the intestinal luminal content.

Stem cells are found at or near the base of the crypts depending on species and the position in the GI tract, and they give rise to rapid-cycling transit-amplifying cells, which eventually differentiate into 1 of *4 main lineages of cells* undergoing continuous cycles of renewal: *Paneth cells, mucous or goblet cells, neuroendocrine cells, and enterocytes*.

Paneth cells are enigmatic cells that turn over slowly (~20 days) in the base of the crypts in the small intestine and are most obvious in horses among the domestic animals. They are not found in dogs, cats, or swine, nor are they prominent in the intestine of ruminants. Conspicuous eosinophilic secretory granules are present in their apical cytoplasm, and these contain a number of *antimicrobial proteins, peptides, and growth factors* including lysozyme, phospholipase, DNAse, ribonuclease, and α-defensins. These molecules are known to be key mediators of host-microbe interactions, innate immune defense, and regulation of intestinal stem cells and regenerative responses of injured intestinal epithelium.

Oligomucous cells are relatively intermediate cells that differentiate eventually into mature **goblet cells**. Both are present in the epithelium of crypts and villi with variable prevalence and distribution at various levels of the intestine and in the different species. They have basal nuclei with distended apical cytoplasm filled with mucin. These cells synthesize and secrete mucin, lubricate mucosal surfaces with a thick mucus covering, act as a frontline host defense against irritants and microbes, facilitate nutrient and antigenic transport from the surface, and thus contribute significantly to tolerogenic local immunity. Mucus also contains a large number of factors and proteins produced by goblet cells and Paneth cells that promote immunoregulation, maintenance of homeostasis, and epithelial restitution after injury. Goblet cell hyperplasia occurs under cytokine control and may contribute to expulsion of invaders, such as parasites; loss of goblet cells due to chronic inflammation has significant negative consequences in the intestine, including failure of the mucus barrier, altered local immune regulation, and reduced ability of repair and regeneration following injury.

Enteroendocrine cells are specialized heterogeneous hormone-secreting cells, representing about 1% of the epithelial cell population. There are at least 8 enteroendocrine subtypes named primarily on their secreted hormones or peptides, although many can secrete various hormones in response to luminal changes. Serotonin, somatostatin, cholecystokinin, peptide YY, glucagon-like peptides, ghrelin, gastrin, histamine, neurotensin, secretin, and others are produced by specialized EC, D, I, L, X, G, N, and S cells in the GI tract, and these molecules are involved in regulation of intestinal motility and peristalsis, secretions, visceral sensations, and appetite. Most enteroendocrine cells exhibit positive IHC immunoreactivity for chromogranin A. Although carcinoid tumors of serotonin-secreting cell origin are described in animals, the overall pathologic implications of these cells are still poorly defined; these cells may have important roles in intestinal dysbiosis and intestinal inflammation.

Poorly differentiated **enterocytes** in the crypts undergo rapid amplification division forming cuboidal or low-columnar epithelial cells before maturing and progressing into the functional compartment of absorptive enterocytes lining the upper crypt and covering the villus. Mature **enterocytes** are tall columnar cells with regular basal nuclear polarity and are responsible for the final digestion and absorption of nutrients, electrolytes, and water; they are by far the predominant epithelial cell type in the intestine. Tight junctions, which are permissive to small molecule and water transport, join the apical margins of adjacent cells, such that the barrier to transepithelial macromolecular movement is maintained even at sites where effete enterocytes are extruded from villar tips. Absorptive epithelial cells lie on the basal lamina, and they are likely involved in communication with the underlying connective and lymphoid tissue. Immediately beneath the basal lamina lies the sheath of syncytial **myofibroblasts** that mediate information flow between the epithelium and lamina propria via growth factors, cytokines, chemokines, prostaglandins, and extracellular matrix molecules that regulate differentiation, growth and tissue repair, tumorigenesis, inflammation, and fibrosis.

The apical surface of normal enterocytes is highly modified into **microvilli**, ~0.5-1.5 µm long and 0.1 µm wide, which are regularly arrayed in close apposition to each other at right angles to the surface of the cell. Visible by conventional microscopy as the *brush border*, microvilli increase the surface area of absorptive epithelium by a factor of ~15-40 times, and they contain many enzyme molecules, including aminopeptidases and disaccharidases involved in terminal digestion of peptides and carbohydrates, which protrude as minute knoblike structures into the mucus coating the microvillar surfaces. The complex of organelles of the absorptive enterocytes is particularly active in handling *absorbed lipid*, which diffuses from micelles at the cell surface through the apical membrane in the form of long-chain fatty acids or monoglycerides. These are then complexed with apoproteins to be excreted through the basolateral cell membrane as *chylomicrons*. Chylomicrons enter the extracellular space and leave the villus via the lacteal.

In neonatal swine and ruminants, vacuolation of the highly absorptive surface enterocytes with nuclear displacement into the apical cytoplasm is normal. In piglets, vacuolation is usually most prominent in the ileum and seems to be a function of cell age. Such vacuolation should be differentiated from the eosinophilic colostrum globules present in cytoplasmic vacuoles of absorptive enterocytes of neonates.

The **lamina propria** supports the epithelium of the small intestinal mucosa. It is composed of loose fibrous tissue within which blood vessels, smooth muscle, inflammatory, and immune cells are interspersed. In addition to functioning in defense against microorganisms, *macrophages* phagocytose inert particulates reaching the lamina propria from the lumen. Bile pigments derived from meconium can be seen within macrophages in villar tips of neonates. Iron homeostasis is regulated in part by lamina proprial macrophages, so apoptotic bodies, ceroid, and hemosiderin are normally observed accumulating within the superficial lamina propria; this can be prominent in horses and should not be mistaken for foci of necrosis.

Lymphocytes, neutrophils, and eosinophils are scattered in the lamina propria of villi and between crypts. Eosinophils are common in the intestine of ruminants and horses, with no specific pathologic connotation; they are highly variable in the intestine of small animals. IELs are frequently observed in villi and less commonly in crypts, and this can vary significantly depending on age, inflammation, and location in the intestinal tract. In general, more IELs are observed in cats compared with dogs (discussed later in the Inflammatory bowel disease section of this chapter); infrequent IELs are expected in the equine intestine; little is known about ruminants. There continues to be some confusion with respect to the unique interepithelial leukocytes with distinct cytoplasmic granules that are observed in the intestine of many species but especially prominent in the distal small intestine of cats and horses. These are often large distinct round-to-polygonal cells within crypts and at the base of villar epithelium with characteristic large eosinophilic cytoplasmic globules. These have been generally, and probably erroneously, referred to as globule (or globular) leukocytes historically; however, in mice these have been shown to be mucosal mast cells based on their histochemical and IHC staining pattern (immunoreactive for mast cell protease, serine esterases, and sometimes granzyme B); in some domestic species and possibly including cats, IHC data suggest that these are consistent with large granular lymphocytes (LGL) due to immunoreactivity for CD3, CD8, and granzyme B. Plasma cells are normally not numerous in villi, but are concentrated in the lamina propria between the upper portions of crypts.

The **vascular supply of the small intestinal mucosa** arrives from submucosal arteries that branch to the fenestrated endothelium-lined capillary plexus supporting the intestinal crypts and the villi. The *lacteal* is the central lymphatic vessel of the villus that is sufficiently permeable to permit the entry of macromolecules and chylomicrons absorbed from the lumen; this is the main route of lipid transport from the villus.

The **cecum and colon** vary widely in anatomy and size among domestic animals, and in particular, variation among species is dependent on the level of hindgut microbial fermentation. Extensive movement of electrolytes and water occurs across the colonic wall, especially in the horse, where a volume of fluid approaching that of the extracellular fluid space may be present within the large bowel lumen; absorption of electrolytes and water is a major function of the colon of dogs and cats, and of the distal colon of herbivores.

The mucosa of the cecum and colon in all domestic mammals lacks villi, although there are ridges or folds on the mucosal surface. **Colonic glands** also house the stem cells of the colon and are straight tubular structures arranged at right angles to the basal lamina and lined by a cell population resembling that of small intestinal crypts, although the cells here have sparse and irregular microvilli compared with the small intestine. *Oligomucous cells*, also derived from basal stem cells, form a second proliferative population in the lower half of the colonic gland. Well-differentiated *goblet cells* are usually present in the upper half of colonic glands and on the surface. Goblet cells are present in variable numbers, depending on the species and a variety of other factors. Significantly fewer subtypes of *enteroendocrine cells* are recognized in the colon. *Paneth cells* are not found in normal colon; in humans, Paneth cell metaplasia is described as a preneoplastic lesion in the development of colonic epithelial neoplasia.

The **lamina propria** of the colon is like that of the small intestine, although overall reduced between the closely packed glands and contains relatively few inflammatory and immune cells in small animals and young herbivores. Older horses may have more numerous superficial proprial inflammatory infiltrates, and macrophages containing phagocytosed debris may be present below the surface epithelium.

The connective tissue of the **submucosa** lies between the mucosa and the **tunica muscularis** of the intestine, which is formed by fascicles of smooth muscle cells arranged as inner circular and outer longitudinal layers. An extensive **enteric nervous system**, with submucosal (Meissner) and myenteric (Auerbach) plexuses containing ganglia, modulates external autonomic neural regulation and coordinates GI motility and function. The neurons of the enteric system equal in number those in the spinal cord, and their ramifications sense and influence epithelial absorption and secretion, local endocrine/paracrine secretion, blood flow, immune events, and motility in the intestine at the level of individual crypts. *Myofibroblastic pacemaker cells of the intestine* (**interstitial cells of Cajal**) are integrated with the extrinsic and enteric nervous system and are distributed throughout the intestinal musculature. Abnormalities including degeneration or inflammation of these cells lead to disorders of motility, and neoplasms of these cells result in GISTs, which are described in dogs, horses, and cats.

Immune elements and the GI barrier. The GI tract is presented continually with antigens in food, allergens, toxins, viruses, commensal and pathogenic bacteria and their products, as well as parasites with their excretions and secretions. The epithelial barrier of the intestine is only a single cell thick and has enormous surface area; the enteric mucosal surface of the average human is estimated to be 300-400 m^2. Therefore, it is not surprising that the epithelium and associated lymphoid and inflammatory cells in the mucosa and submucosa are components of a complex system for excluding, blocking, sampling, tolerating, neutralizing, or eliminating antigens or potential pathogens. Intestinal immune elements are sparse and quiescent at birth; immune activity in the intestine is probably stimulated in response to colonization by normal bacterial flora beginning in the early neonatal period. In the mature animal, *lymphoid tissue is estimated to comprise 25% of the intestinal mucosal mass*, and to exceed that of the spleen in volume.

Elements of GI mucosal defense are diverse and include the volume of fluid secretion and peristalsis for dilution and flushing of contents, respectively, and gastric and bile acids and pancreatic secretions that break down ingested antigens. The indigenous microflora competitively inhibit or actively exclude potential pathogens. Mucins on the luminal surface form the secretory barrier, which includes antibodies and myriad other soluble components of innate resistance. The epithelium also provides a physical barrier, participates in innate resistance by production of proinflammatory cytokines, enables passive immunity by antibody uptake in the neonate, and contributes to active immunity by antigen uptake and presentation. IELs are an important first line of defense against pathogens and play a significant role in epithelial barrier homeostasis. Soluble antibody and complement in plasma and interstitial fluid neutralize antigens penetrating the mucosal barrier. The organized lymphoid tissues of the mucosal immune system, including Peyer patches and regional lymph nodes, are sites for induction of intestinal immune responses, generating antigen-activated B and T cells that ultimately home back to the mucosa where they reside along with populations of macrophages and dendritic cells.

Epithelial cells of neonates are uniquely capable of uptake and transport of macromolecules from the intestinal lumen to the basolateral cell surface. In all species of domestic mammals, **colostral transfer of immunoglobulins** by this route provides the neonate with passive humoral immunity during the early postnatal period. The period of active uptake of macromolecules is short, usually only 24-48 hours in ungulates, after which further bulk transport of macromolecules is precluded. Although bulk transport does not occur in mature animals, nutritionally inconsequential amounts of macromolecules that escape intraluminal hydrolysis and intracellular lysosomal degradation continue to be transferred by enterocytes. Fully differentiated small intestinal absorptive epithelial cells express major histocompatibility complex class II molecules on their basolateral membranes and are capable of presenting antigen directly to T cells. Enterocytes detect commensal and potentially pathogenic bacteria and viruses via *pattern recognition molecules* such as surface toll-like receptors (TLR), for induction of inflammatory responses and promotion of tolerance via production of proinflammatory or immunomodulatory cytokines.

Intestinal intraepithelial T lymphocytes form a large population strategically located between the basolateral surfaces of epithelial cells and may comprise up to 10-20% of the cells within the epithelial layer; they are more numerous in the small intestine than in the large intestine. In domestic animals, they are mostly T cells uniquely expressing the homodimeric form of CD8α; most of these express the $\gamma\delta$ T-cell receptor as opposed to the $\alpha\beta$ T-cell receptor, especially in the small intestine. They function as a front line of defense, as part of the innate immune response to bacterial and plant products such as amylamines, and to damaged enterocytes. They also participate in adaptive immunity as they respond to antigens entering from the lumen, during tumor surveillance, and possibly in enterocyte maintenance and regeneration.

The controversial so-called **globule leukocytes** are visible in H&E-stained tissue sections as *mononuclear cells with large eosinophilic cytoplasmic granules* in the epithelium of the crypt and lower villus, and sometimes in the lamina propria especially of cats. They have been associated with parasitism or hypersensitivity, but their function remains poorly understood. Their origin (and name) also remains uncertain, with some evidence suggesting that they are related to either *mast cells* or *large granular lymphocytes*. Globule leukocytes and neoplasms of globule leukocytes are described historically, and especially in cats, but many of these likely represent granular lymphomas. More complete characterization is needed to clarify their identity, function, and overall significance in the intestine.

The **aggregated lymphoid follicles** are scattered in the mucosa and submucosa of the small intestine; lymphoglandular complexes or solitary proprial lymphoid nodules may be grossly visible throughout the colonic mucosa. **Peyer patches** are present throughout the length of the small intestine in all species, although they tend to be larger and more expansive distally. They are grossly visible usually as oval or elongate structures up to several centimeters wide, thickening the antimesenteric wall of the intestine. They may project slightly above the mucosal surface, or they appear as cupped depressions that must not be mistaken for ulcers, especially in dogs. **Continuous Peyer patches** are found in the distal ileum of calves, lambs, and piglets that develop during late gestation, although they may be poorly developed and not visible grossly. Their role as a primary site of B-cell generation is well established, and they likely play an important role in host defense, especially early in life.

Peyer patches consist of *follicular aggregates of B lymphocytes surrounded by T lymphocytes*, often underlying a discontinuous muscularis mucosae, over which a mixed population of T and B lymphocytes and dendritic cells extend into the lamina propria between villi in rounded mucosal projections known as *subepithelial domes*. Cell populations of Peyer patches in newborns and gnotobiotes of most species tend to be sparser than those in older or bacterially colonized animals, although those in neonatal calves appear relatively well developed.

Membranous or microfold cells (**M cells**) are specialized flattened enterocytes with reduced or absent brush border that are found dispersed within the follicle-associated epithelium overlying subepithelial domes. Within the dome regions are populations of dendritic cells, which play a major role in initiation of mucosal immunity. M cells (and enterocytes to a lesser degree) interact with and transport particulate matter and macromolecules from the lumen to their basolateral membrane pocket where they interact with immune cells including B cells committed to IgA production and T cells, both of which drive mucosal immune responses. Despite, or perhaps because of, its role in adaptive immunity, the M cell is exploited as a portal of entry to the mucosa by certain pathogenic bacteria including *Mycobacterium*, *Salmonella*, *Yersinia*, and *Listeria*, and for some viruses.

Antigen is acquired, processed, and presented to lymphocytes in Peyer patches and mesenteric lymph nodes largely by **dendritic cells** trafficking from the mucosa where they initially acquire antigen. Dendritic cells represent a significant percentage of leukocytes in the lamina propria, and they acquire antigen from enterocytes or M cells, or by direct luminal sampling. **Macrophages** are more common in the lamina propria than in Peyer patches; they are also involved in mucosal protection by phagocytosis of invading pathogenic organisms, scavengers of dead cells or foreign debris, and by antigen processing, presentation, and regulation of ensuing immune responses.

IgA-producing lymphocytes leave MALTs and home to mucosal surfaces, including the intestinal tract, respiratory tract, mammary gland, and salivary glands, where they differentiate into IgA-secreting plasma cells. Dimeric IgA is transported via the polymeric Ig receptor from the basolateral border of columnar crypt epithelial cells onto the apical surface of epithelial cells where it is critical for neutralization of pathogenic threats and maintenance of homeostasis at the luminal surface. IgA-secreting cells are the predominant class of plasma cell in the lamina propria in most species, although **IgM** and **IgG** (especially in cattle) generation is prevalent in young calves, swine, and dogs. IgE is prominent during intestinal parasitism or type I hypersensitivity reactions.

Intestinal mucosal mast cells differ histochemically and physiologically from mast cells in most other tissues. They are less demonstrable using standard metachromatic granule staining techniques following formalin fixation compared with connective tissue mast cells from other tissues. They likely originate from progenitor cells in the blood, then migrate to the intestine where they complete their differentiation process. The role of intestinal mast cells continues to be elucidated; they play a central role in maintenance of epithelial integrity and viability (and thus maintenance of intestinal barrier function), promotion of ion and water secretion, stimulation of innate and adaptive immunity and blood flow, regulation of coagulation, alteration of vascular permeability, promotion of wound healing and fibrosis, facilitation and promotion of peristalsis, and pain perception. These functions are mediated by histamine, serotonin, and other soluble mediators including a unique set of enzymes (compared with other connective tissue mast cells). Intestinal mast cells are recruited and/or activated during inflammatory intestinal diseases, including during GI parasitism and hypersensitivity response.

Intestinal **eosinophils** probably do not differ functionally from eosinophils in other sites as cytotoxic effector cells and modulators of local inflammation, particularly during intestinal parasitism, immune-mediated responses, or hypersensitivity reactions.

Immunoinflammatory events in the large bowel are less well understood than those in the small intestine; similar principles presumably prevail. **Lymphoglandular complexes** consist of submucosal follicular lymphoid aggregates penetrated by glands extending from the mucosa and presumably facilitate contact of surface epithelium of the large bowel with underlying lymphoid tissue. These occur in the cecum and proximal colon of the dog; in the colon of the swine; and at the cecocolic junction, proximal spiral colon, and terminal rectum of ruminants. **Solitary mucosal lymphoid nodules** are generally restricted to the lamina propria and superficial submucosa, and are scattered throughout the cecum and colon in all species.

Electrolyte and water transport in the intestine. ***Water movement in the intestine*** *is passive, following osmotically the transport of electrolyte and nutrient solutes*. The small intestinal mucosa is highly permeable to the passive movement of small ions and water and is therefore considered leaky, despite the presence of tight junctions along the apical margins of absorptive enterocytes to ensure that the content of the small bowel is approximately isosmolar with the interstitial fluid space. The permeability of junctional complexes appears to be sensitive to Starling forces, influenced by intravascular hydrostatic and oncotic pressure, so that fluid and solute actively absorbed may leak back into the lumen, thus modulating *net absorption* by the mucosa. Water is secreted into the GI lumen with digestive juices and is almost entirely resorbed in the small and large intestine; aquaporins, transmembrane water channel proteins, are important in the rapid passage of water across cell membranes. Sodium absorption takes place by several active transcellular mechanisms, which vary in importance at different levels of the intestine, and with the physiologic circumstance. Absorbed solute and water in isotonic proportions thus move into the interstitium of the villus where, within a few micrometers, they encounter a subepithelial capillary or lacteal.

The colon of carnivores, the spiral colon of ruminants and swine, and the small colon of the horse play an important role in reducing the volume of electrolyte and water lost in the feces. In contrast to the small intestine, *the colonic epithelium is relatively restrictive to the free movement of sodium and chloride*, so it normally maintains differences in osmotic pressure, ionic composition, and electrical potential between luminal and proprial surfaces, making it more efficient than the small bowel in absorbing some electrolytes and water.

Solute movement across the intestinal epithelium is regulated by *hormones and neurotransmitters*, which act through intracellular second messengers. Some products of intrinsic and extrinsic neurons, such as vasoactive intestinal polypeptide and acetylcholine, stimulate secretion; others, such as somatostatin and norepinephrine, are absorptive or antisecretory. Local paracrine effects are mediated by the products of enteroendocrine cells, such as somatostatin, neurotensin, and serotonin. Circulating hormones such as aldosterone and glucocorticoids, and mesenchymal elements in the lamina propria, including myofibroblasts, lymphocytes, mast cells, macrophages, and other inflammatory and connective tissue cells, are also involved via production of locally active substances with a direct or indirect effect on epithelial function.

Epithelial renewal in health and disease. The **small intestinal surface** is covered by a population of cells ultimately derived from *stem cells* that are present at or near the base of crypts or glands, but with its proximate source in amplifier populations of undifferentiated columnar or oligomucous cells in the lower half of the crypts. These cells lose their ability to undergo mitosis and differentiate into *goblet cells* and *absorptive enterocytes* as they move from the crypt to the villus. In most species, they are *shed from the tips of villi* in 2-8 days, which is more rapid in the ileum compared with the duodenum; this is related to reduced height of distal small intestinal villi in most species. Apoptosis also contributes to physiologic enterocyte loss. *The mass and topography of the mucosa are quite stable*, the result of a dynamic equilibrium between the rate of movement of cells from crypts to villi, and the rate at which they are lost from villar tips.

In young animals, the intestine grows by generation of new crypts followed by generation of new villi. As the bowel attains mature size, the number of villi and crypts apparently stabilizes; however, some adaptive variation in the ratio of crypts to villi may occur. Adaptive responses to a variety of factors including diet alter the size and rate of turnover of the proliferative and functional epithelial cell populations, and thus the microtopography of the intestine. The appearance of the small intestinal mucosa is essentially a compromise achieved by equilibrium between the rates of cell production and loss. At one extreme is the intestine of germ-free animals with short crypts containing a small proliferative compartment, and tall villi with a low rate of cell loss supporting a large functional absorptive compartment. At the other end of the spectrum is the intestine of an animal with severe intestinal helminthosis with elongated proliferative crypts, shortened stubby villi, few absorptive enterocytes, and a high rate of enterocyte loss into the lumen, reflecting the increased proliferative compartment.

Although quantitative description of epithelial kinetics is possible experimentally, in the diagnostic situation it is often helpful to make a subjective or semiquantitative assessment of the status of the proliferative and functional compartments in tissue sections. The size of the proliferative compartment is reflected in the depth and diameter of the crypts, and in the location of the most superficial mitotic activity. The prevalence of mitotic figures can be assessed subjectively; however, this varies within the intestine during health, so beyond the mitotic count, no definitive inferences can be drawn about the proportion of the crypt cell population that is replicating or the duration of the cell cycle.

The *degree of differentiation* and functional status of enterocytes covering villi can be inferred from their appearance. Cytoplasmic basophilia, loss of regular basal nuclear polarity, low-columnar to cuboidal or squamous morphology, and an ill-defined brush border all indicate a poorly differentiated population of surface enterocytes and suggest increased epithelial turnover. *Fasting* causes atrophy of villi and reduction of mucosal epithelial mass by prolongation of the postmitotic phase of proliferative cells, so that surface enterocytes persist longer and are lost from the villus tips more slowly; fasting-induced atrophy is immediately reversed by refeeding. *Weaning* has similar effects on the microtopography of the intestine, which is observed as marked reduction in height of villi in most species.

Restoration of epithelial integrity is dependent on the degree of damage or injury, and a finely regulated balance of migration, proliferation, and differentiation of adjacent epithelial cells, which are ultimately mediated by growth factors, cytokines, dietary, and other factors present in mucus.

Following minor loss of surface enterocytes, restitution occurs by *lateral migration of adjacent intact epithelial cells* within minutes. If epithelium on villi is obliterated, for instance by transient ischemia or by viral cytolysis, the villus core contracts by myofibroblast activity mediated by the enteric nervous system, and stromal elements rapidly undergo apoptosis. Surviving epithelial cells flatten and migrate laterally across the denuded surface, and proliferation of immature enterocytes occurs such that *regeneration of the mucosal surface* follows in hours to days after injury. Finally, *maturation and differentiation* of epithelial cells occurs to complete *restoration* of the intestinal microtopography within a few days. With more severe mucosal injury or at healing intestinal anastomosis sites after surgery, granulation tissue forms along the base of the injured mucosa, which becomes progressively covered by maturing epithelium, crypts, and eventually full villar mucosal restoration.

Epithelial turnover in **the cecum and colon** is fundamentally similar to that in the small intestine, although villi are not present along the mucosal surface. Epithelial cells arise from the proliferative compartment in the lower part of the glands and differentiate into goblet cells or columnar absorptive cells and mature as they emerge from the gland and migrate along the glands to cover the villar surface. Cells are subsequently lost into the lumen within ~4-8 days of being produced; colonic epithelial cell proliferation and production are influenced by several factors including amount and type of fiber in the diet, and the colonic microbiome; colons of gnotobiotic animals have fewer proliferative cells limited to the lower portion of the glands.

Following insult and exfoliation of surface epithelial cells, restitution of the epithelial integrity in the large bowel resembles that in the small bowel. Within a few minutes of injury, surviving surface epithelial cells emerging from crypts become attenuated and migrate at a rate of several micrometers per minute to cover mucosal defects. Ulcers, surgical incisions, or anastomotic sites in the colon heal by migration of a single layer of epithelium from the periphery of the defect, with gradual differentiation of crypts, and eventual restitution of normal mucosal architecture. Depending on the type of anastomosis, equine epithelial cells have been shown to require >2 weeks to bridge the granulation tissue in large mucosal gaps, and full restoration of mucosal architecture may require ~2 months.

An altered replication rate of colonic epithelium will induce *microscopic lesions in the large bowel*: the number of goblet cells on the surface and in the upper portion of glands is often diminished; epithelial cells appear poorly differentiated and are often of low-columnar, cuboidal, or squamous morphology; the glands become elongated and dilated; glands are lined by increased numbers of proliferating cells with increased cytoplasmic basophilia as well as increased mitotic activity. In some acute or chronic inflammatory conditions of the lamina propria, goblet cell hyperplasia may occur. It is uncertain whether this is caused by primary damage to surface epithelium, or by local cell-mediated immune effects on the proliferative compartment, as occurs in the small intestine in celiac disease of humans.

The *proliferative compartment* in cecal and colonic glands is damaged by the same insults that attack cells in crypts of the small bowel, although the lesions in large bowel tend to be comparatively less severe. This is perhaps because a lower proportion of the proliferative compartment in the colon is mitotically active at the time of maximum exposure to drug or virus. Common agents that damage the proliferative compartment in the colon particularly include bovine and canine coronaviruses, and several species of ruminant coccidia, which develop in the colonic epithelial cells lining glands.

The *evolution and sequelae of lesions* resulting from damage to proliferative epithelial cells in the colon are similar to those in small bowel: dilation of crypts, accumulation of necrotic debris within crypts, and/or attenuation of the lining epithelium. Severe lesions will lead to the loss of glands, erosion, and ulceration of the mucosa; hemorrhage, stricture, and stenosis may ensue. Following milder damage that spares some stem cells in each gland, the mucosa has the potential to recover fully after a period of reparative hyperplasia.

The GI microbiota. A thorough discussion and summary of **the significance of the GI microbiota**, its normal range of variation by anatomic location of various species, and ultimately (for the pathologist), its function and relationship to health and disease in the GI tract and systemically are well beyond the scope of this text. With the advent and increased usage of next-generation and metagenomic sequencing technology in diagnostic contexts, an astonishingly massive amount of data and new literature continues to flow from this enormously significant area of scientific research, and readers and pathologists are encouraged to consult the current literature on this topic. Only a brief general overview is provided here.

After birth, no part of the GI tract is sterile. Myriad species of microorganisms, including mostly anaerobic bacteria but also archaea, eukaryotes, and viruses, many of them unidentified or identified only by metagenomic sequencing approaches, inhabit the stomach and various portions of the intestinal tract, forming an ecosystem of enormous complexity. Now recognized to be important during inflammatory intestinal disease, the microbiota also provide an array of biochemical and metabolic activities important for normal host physiology and maintenance of homeostasis and immunologic tolerance, including metabolism of indigestible compounds; synthesis of essential vitamins; development, maturation, and regulation of intestinal epithelium and the enteric and systemic immune systems; and protection from invasion by opportunistic pathogens. The microbiota thus contribute prominently to homeostasis, regulated inflammation during host defense, and dysregulated inflammation during autoimmunity.

Generally, bacterial populations are least in the stomach and upper small intestine of ruminants and carnivores, being limited by the acid gastric environment and by peristalsis. The anaerobes and facultative anaerobes increase to $\sim 10^7$ per gram of content in the lower small intestine; total bacterial populations $>10^{10}$ or 10^{11} per gram of content are present in the cecum and colon.

The complex ecology of the GI flora imparts considerable stability by which the GI tract is relatively resistant to the intrusion of pathogenic threats. It is no coincidence that bacterial diarrhea occurs most commonly in the neonate with a poorly established flora, or after changes in husbandry, or following antibiotic therapy, all of which disturb the native enteric bacterial population. In addition to the barrier function, short-chain fatty acids generated by microbiota during carbohydrate metabolism are significant energy sources and trophic factors for the maintenance of the health of enterocytes.

The normal flora are important for development of the mucus layer and mucosal lymphoid structures, modulation of immune cell differentiation, and regulation of cytokine and chemokine production in the intestine. *Host factors* influencing gut flora include composition of the diet; peristalsis, which continually flushes the small intestine of a large proportion of its bacterial population; lysozyme; lactoferrin; gastric acidity if unbuffered or undiluted; and, in the abomasum of suckling calves, perhaps a lactoperoxidase-thiocyanide-hydrogen peroxide system. Epithelial maturation is influenced by the microbiota, and it is recognized that germ-free animals have elongated and thinner villi, less-developed proprial vascular network, and shallow crypts with fewer proliferating stem cells, compared with conventional animals.

Mechanisms to enhance and support development and maintenance of microbiota, including the use of oral probiotics or microbial cultures, have been shown to improve body weight gain and decrease diarrhea in newborn calves and pigs, and protect adult animals from colonization with certain pathogens. Numerous systemic health benefits are linked to a healthy and robust GI microbiota in humans and animals, demonstrating that the effects of beneficial GI microbiota extend well beyond improved local GI health and function. In humans, a healthy gut microbiota is linked to a reduced incidence of immune-mediated arthritis, obesity, diabetes, asthma, inflammatory or irritable bowel syndrome, cardiovascular disease, chronic renal disease, and even various mental health disorders and a variety of neoplastic diseases. In veterinary medicine, altered intestinal microbiota is linked to intestinal and systemic inflammation (including idiopathic IBD of dogs and cats) and noninflammatory diseases (including cancer in dogs and cats). Improved production performance secondary to healthy GI microbiota is likely related to improved immune system function in production species, although the mechanisms continue to be explored.

Diseases of the intestine

Pathophysiology of enteric disease

Protein-energy malnutrition caused by inadequate intake of feed or deficiencies in quantity or quality of nutrients is a well-recognized comorbidity factor in many diseases. In its most severe forms, this results in *depletion of fat and muscle mass*, emaciation, and ultimately death by starvation. Importantly, protein-energy malnutrition is a common cause of secondary immune deficiency and is thus associated with increased susceptibility to infections.

Inappetence or **anorexia**, and eventually **cachexia**, are commonly associated with GI diseases. Appetite is modulated by a complex and incompletely understood network of neurologic, neuroendocrine, hormonal, or cytokine signals, and potentially physical impairment, injury, or chronic inflammatory or neoplastic disease affecting the GI tract or other systems that centrally impact satiety. Protein-energy malnutrition must be differentiated from effects of endogenous conditions resulting in malassimilation or protein-loss (enteropathy, nephropathy), from cachexia induced by chronic inflammatory and neoplastic disease, and from other conditions resulting in recumbency and inability to access appropriate food.

Several factors in neonates predispose to death by starvation within the first few weeks of life, including fetal and gestational malnutrition such that the neonate has limited adipose stores at birth; increased energy or metabolic demands associated with extreme temperatures or exposure; and postpartum hyponutrition. Piglets are born with negligible fat reserves and die quickly of hypoglycemia if not fed adequately; neonatal ruminants usually have adipose stores sufficient to compensate for longer periods of inappetence or anorexia (2-4 days for lambs; 6-10 days for calves), although this depends on the quality and quantity of milk, and severity of other external factors (such as cold stress).

In animals that die of inanition, muscle mass is often reduced because of mobilization of amino acids for gluconeogenesis. Adipose tissue in bone marrow, coronary groove, pericardial sac, epicardium, and surrounding the kidneys is completely depleted, or has the gelatinous clear pink appearance of **serous atrophy**. The liver may be atrophied and appear small with sharp margins because of reduced trophic stimuli. A diagnosis of starvation is supported by a history of conditions compatible with reduced quantity or quality of feed, and by ruling out other GI or systemic conditions causing protein loss.

Villus atrophy *is a common pathologic change in the small intestine of domestic animals*. It results in malabsorption of nutrients and fluids and can be associated with loss of plasma protein into the intestinal lumen. Villus atrophy can be categorized histomorphologically into 2 broad types based on injury or damage to crypts, essentially making a distinction between those processes in which the proliferative compartment in the crypts is not directly targeted (intact crypts), and those processes that primarily damage or target the proliferative compartment in the crypts (injured crypts). Categorization aids with recognition of potential causes of lesions, and implications with respect to pathogenesis and prognosis.

Villus atrophy with an intact or proliferative crypt compartment takes 2 primary forms in domestic animals. Villus atrophy can occur due to 1) **injury causing a primary increased rate of loss of surface villar enterocytes**, or 2) **chronic persistent inflammation of the intestine with hyperplasia of crypts**. Histomorphologic distinction may not always be obvious, and severity of lesions can depend on timing between injury and when the intestine is evaluated. Primary increased rate of loss of surface villar epithelium is the major mechanism involved in several important viral infections, including coronavirus and rotavirus; of coccidial infections, which damage surface enterocytes predominantly; of some enteroinvasive bacteria; of transient ischemia, in which the effect is limited to absorptive epithelium; and, in some circumstances, of bacterial-produced toxins released in the lumen of the bowel. The effect is increased loss of surface enterocytes over a relatively short period of time, while sparing the proliferative compartment in crypts. Villi contract and become shortened and blunted, and if the animal survives the metabolic sequelae of malabsorption resulting from damaged or lost surface epithelium, *compensatory expansion of the proliferative compartment in crypts* permits eventual complete recovery. Epithelial cells emerging and differentiating from crypt stem cells result in recovery of normal mucosal topography and full function within a few days; timing of restoration depends on the extent and severity of the initial injury.

The microscopic appearance of the mucosa depends partly on the number of absorptive cells lost, which determines the initial degree of villus atrophy, and partly on the amount of regeneration that has occurred when the intestine is examined. During early phases of injury, damaged epithelial cells are shed into the intestinal lumen and villi are shortened and blunted; alternatively, villi are of normal length but appear misshapen and pointed. Atrophic villi are subsequently covered by poorly differentiated low-columnar to cuboidal or squamous cells and there may be fusion of the lateral surfaces or tips of villi; in severe atrophy there may also be mild erosion if epithelium does not cover the surface. Crypts appear normal early, but within 12-24 hours proliferative activity is noticeably increased and crypts enlarge in diameter and depth to accommodate more mitotic cells. Mitotic cells are poorly differentiated and basophilic, and often quite crowded, with mitotic figures observed close to the epithelial surface. The lamina propria may appear hypercellular, which may be due to contraction of the lamina propria or mononuclear cell infiltration. As regeneration progresses, the length of villi and differentiation of lining epithelial cells increases, and proliferation gradually subsides.

The second form of villus atrophy with intact crypts is associated with **chronic or persistent processes** involving the intestinal mucosa such as chronic nematode parasitism; chronic coccidial infection; giardiasis in some species; response to some dietary components such as soybean protein in calves, kidney bean protein in pigs, and wheat in dogs; idiopathic or specific granulomatous enteritis such as paratuberculosis and histoplasmosis; and chronic IBD. An important distinction is that proliferation of crypts in these conditions *precedes* the development of villus atrophy and *is not a response to it*. These conditions are usually associated with significant infiltration of inflammatory cells into the lamina propria. *Immune and inflammatory reactions in the intestine are associated with increased epithelial cell proliferation*, and although the molecular mechanisms remain uncertain, numerous proinflammatory cytokines and growth factors are likely involved. In most cases, when the cause can be eliminated, the lesion usually resolves within weeks, implying that active host-pathogen interaction is required for its induction and maintenance. Local stimulation of the proliferative crypts is likely mediated by cytokines produced by activated lymphocytes in the intestinal mucosa. Epithelial cells leaving the active crypts usually do not differentiate fully and exfoliate prematurely when they are still near the crypt opening or low on the villus. Epithelial cells that reach the surface also do not differentiate fully, and are rapidly lost into the gut lumen, or undergo mucous metaplasia. Coupled with normal shedding of pre-existing enterocytes, this contributes further to atrophy of villi over a period of several days.

Microscopically, proliferation of crypt epithelium is early, significant, and usually the most prominent change in this lesion. In its milder forms, there may be more prominent elongation and increased depth of crypts and less obvious atrophy of villi. The proliferative compartment is expanded and active, mitotic figures are numerous, and goblet cell hyperplasia may also occur. Elongation of the proliferative crypts may be so extensive that even with severe atrophy of villi, the total mucosal thickness will not be significantly reduced from normal. Careful observation may reveal poorly differentiated enterocytes exfoliating prematurely from ridges along the epithelial surface, or from folds at the base of stubby villi. The lamina propria is usually infiltrated by a prominent population of lymphocytes, plasma cells, and other mixed inflammatory cells; individual IELs (lymphocytic exocytosis) are common. Careful evaluation of the inflamed mucosa should be undertaken for possible etiologic agents or causes using H&E or histochemically stained sections.

However it is induced, atrophy of villi with crypt hyperplasia invariably results in local malabsorption of nutrients and water. Poorly differentiated surface epithelial cells may secrete electrolytes and water, and increased epithelial turnover contributes to enteric loss of endogenous protein. Proprial inflammation and injured or damaged surface epithelium may also contribute to effusion of tissue fluid.

The second broad type of villus atrophy is associated with damage to the proliferative compartment, and this is also commonly seen in domestic animals. This type is the sequel to insults causing necrosis or impairing the mitotic capacity of crypt epithelial cells; agents that cause these lesions usually have a propensity for damaging actively proliferating cells in any tissue. Because ionizing radiation was recognized early as a cause of such lesions, they are generally termed *radiomimetic*. Causes of similar lesions include cytotoxic chemicals and mitotic poisons, such as chemotherapeutic agents, T-2 mycotoxin, and pyrrolizidine alkaloids in large doses; but most commonly, these lesions are associated with viruses that infect actively proliferating cells (particularly the parvoviruses and BVDV). Ischemia of sufficient duration to cause necrosis of some or all cells lining the crypts also causes this lesion.

The microscopic appearance of affected mucosa depends on the severity and extent of the insult, and the interval between the insult and when the intestine is examined. Damage or injury to the proliferative cryptal epithelial cells is the primary lesion, and except in ischemia, microscopic lesions are evident in crypts well before significant atrophy of villi occurs. Individual necrotic epithelial cells and neutrophils may be present in dilated lumens of damaged crypts. With severe damage to crypts, remaining epithelial cells become flattened in an attempt to maintain the integrity of the crypt lining. Following the cryptal epithelial injury, immature epithelial cells with large nuclei, prominent nucleoli, and increased mitotic figures may be observed within crypts as they migrate onto the surface.

Pre-existing surface epithelial cells are shed from villar tips at an apparently normal rate, even though few or no new cells emerge from crypts. Villi thus eventually become atrophic or collapse as the surface cell population is lost without being replaced. If the majority of crypt cells are damaged, crypts are rapidly stripped of epithelium and collapse or drop out and *proprial collapse* occurs, leaving a few scattered epithelial clusters or ectatic crypt remnants in the deeper lamina propria. The overlying surface may appear eroded or partially covered by immature flattened squamous-like epithelial cells derived from surviving crypts. Ulceration of the mucosa eventually leads to granulation tissue deposition, often in the deeper propria; remnant crypts become proliferative within a few days of the original insult, as compensatory and reparative hyperplasia occurs. In viral diseases, the severity of injury and the corresponding gross and/or histologic appearance of the lesion often is segmental within the intestine; this likely corresponds to variable rates and waves of cryptal proliferation and epithelial maintenance within the healthy small intestine. Lesions caused by ischemia tend to be uniform in severity but may be localized depending on the cause; acute or subacute lesions are often hemorrhagic, especially if there has been re-establishment of blood flow.

Extensive crypt cell necrosis, and mucosal erosion or ulceration leads to severe effusion of tissue fluid and hemorrhage, in addition to the severe failure of malabsorption due to villus atrophy. The damaged mucosal barrier is also now highly susceptible to invasion by the enteric flora, sometimes including fungi. Because viral insults damage other proliferative compartments including bone marrow, the overall immune function of affected animals is also diminished, likely contributing to secondary and systemic infection. Small ulcers in areas where a few crypts are damaged or lost will heal as epithelial cells from adjacent crypts migrate to repair the denuded surface; however, crypts may take longer to regenerate, so local villus atrophy will persist accordingly. Local severe ulceration may also contribute to persistent fluid and plasma loss, and if circumferential to eventual stricture formation and stenosis.

Malassimilation. Digestion and assimilation of nutrients have an *intraluminal phase* mediated by biliary and pancreatic secretions, followed by an *epithelial phase* carried out by enzyme systems on the surface and in the cytoplasm of absorptive enterocytes. The final step is delivery of nutrients by enterocytes to the interstitial fluid, for uptake into blood or lymph.

Exocrine pancreatic insufficiency *is the major cause of intraluminal maldigestion* and is usually the result of juvenile pancreatic atrophy in dogs, or of pancreatic fibrosis and atrophy following repeated episodes of pancreatic necrosis (see Vol. 2, Pancreas). It is occasionally seen in cats. This condition may be complicated by bacterial overgrowth in the small intestine. Bile salt deficiency is rarely seen as a cause of intraluminal maldigestion in domestic animals.

The **epithelial phase of assimilation** *is impaired by loss of functional epithelial surface area*, which occurs mostly due to *villus atrophy*, or less commonly in short-bowel syndrome following intestinal resection in which >75-85% of the small bowel has been removed. This phase of assimilation is dependent on complex enzyme systems that generally decline with age; this includes maltase, hydrolase, and sucrase, although specifics vary among domestic animals. Although epithelial malassimilation is often difficult to diagnose definitively without extensive additional metabolic testing, several potential causes and pathogeneses of failure of epithelial assimilation are described. Poorly differentiated surface epithelium on atrophic villi lacks the full complement of enzymes on the brush border and in the cytoplasm necessary for nutrient digestion and assimilation. Lectins present in uncooked beans attach to and damage microvilli on enterocytes, which may explain the malabsorption and diarrhea associated with their use in feeds; lectins also promote bacterial adhesion and overgrowth in the small intestine. A heritable syndrome of *gluten-sensitive enteropathy* is reported in Irish Setter dogs and is characterized microscopically by villus atrophy, increased IELs, and abnormal levels of mucosal microvillar hydrolases. *Cobalamin malabsorption* has been described as a hereditary defect in Beagles, Australian Shepherd dogs, Chinese Shar-Peis, Giant Schnauzers, and Border Collies, resulting in anemia and failure to thrive. Delivery of nutrients (especially lipid) to the circulation may be impaired during intestinal lymphangiectasia. The pathogenesis of malassimilation of the major classes of nutrients will be considered briefly.

Malassimilation of fat can occur in all 3 phases of digestion and absorption. Lipolysis is impaired if insufficient lipase is available, and mostly, this is a result of loss of exocrine pancreatic functional tissue via atrophy or fibrosis; however, it also may be due to failure by immature intestinal epithelial cells to release cholecystokinin, which is necessary to stimulate pancreatic enzyme secretions. Reduced surface area for lipid uptake contributes to malabsorption of fat. The availability of bile salts is reduced during intrahepatic cholestasis, biliary obstruction, or by depletion resulting from reduced ileal absorption following bowel resection or villus atrophy. Poorly differentiated enterocytes may be less able than normal epithelium to re-esterify long-chain fatty acids to triglyceride and to produce chylomicrons for export from the cell. Obstructed lymphatic drainage during lymphangiectasia, granulomatous enteritis, and intestinal lymphoma contributes to reduced flow of chylomicrons to the systemic circulation.

Malabsorption of lipids may cause *steatorrhea* (excess fat in feces) and possibly colonic diarrhea, which is seen in monogastric animals, especially dogs. Severe fat malabsorption may result in deficiencies of fat-soluble vitamins. Malabsorption of calcium, magnesium, and zinc also occurs when these minerals are sequestered in soaps formed by combination with malabsorbed luminal fatty acids. Increased absorption of oxalate predisposing to nephrolithiasis may be a sequel to reduced concentrations of calcium in the lumen because of soap formation.

Maldigestion of polysaccharides occurs if levels of pancreatic amylase are reduced; this is mostly encountered in dogs with severe loss of functional exocrine pancreatic tissue. Ruminants normally have less pancreatic amylase and digest starch poorly in the small intestine. Mucosal oligosaccharidase deficiency occurs in villus atrophy because poorly differentiated enterocytes have a reduced complement of oligosaccharidases, which results in impaired membrane digestion and malabsorption of carbohydrates. The osmotic effect of malabsorbed carbohydrates in the small intestine is an important component of neonatal diarrhea caused by rotavirus and coronavirus, or other conditions in which there is extensive villus atrophy in the small intestine.

Protein maldigestion occurs if pancreatic protease activity is decreased to ~10% of normal, as may occur with exocrine pancreatic insufficiency. Loss of gastric proteolytic activity is of little nutritional significance, but in conditions with villus atrophy, reduced mucosal surface area and poor differentiation of enterocytes result in malabsorption of small peptides and particularly of amino acids by mechanisms similar to those involved in carbohydrate malabsorption.

Diarrhea *is the presence of water in feces in relative excess in proportion to fecal dry matter.* Loss of solute and water in diarrhea may lead to *severe electrolyte depletion, acid-base imbalance, and dehydration*, which are life-threatening if not corrected.

Large volumes of fluid derived from ingesta and from gastric, pancreatic, biliary, and enteric secretions enter the small bowel; in addition, considerable passive movement of water occurs into the upper small bowel from the circulation as an osmotic effect. Overall, the bulk of the fluid entering the small intestine is absorbed by enterocytes, so that the volume leaving the ileum and entering the colon is but a small fraction of the total fluid flux through the small bowel. The large size of this flux implies that relatively small perturbations in unidirectional movement of electrolytes and water in the small intestine may have significant effects on net movement of fluid.

The colon, in addition to its fermentative function, has the ultimate responsibility to minimize fecal water loss by conserving electrolytes and water by absorption from the digesta. It has a finite capacity for absorption, so if this is exceeded by the rate at which content enters from the small bowel, diarrhea occurs. This is important in so-called *small-bowel diarrhea*, in which the lesion is in the small intestine. Given the colon's reserve absorptive capacity, the excess volume entering the colon from the ileum must be considerable for diarrhea to occur. The extraordinary absorptive capacity and fermentative function of the equine colon mitigate to some extent the expression of small-bowel diarrhea in mature horses. *Large-bowel diarrhea*, however, reflects an intrinsically reduced capacity of the colon to handle even normal volumes of fluid and electrolyte presented to it by the small intestine.

Small-bowel diarrhea in general is classified pathogenetically as secretory, malabsorptive, or effusive; however, these mechanisms are not mutually exclusive and are often seen in natural disease as overlapping syndromes. *Infrequent passage of large amounts of fluid feces* is the main feature of small-bowel diarrhea.

Secretory diarrhea is due to an excess of secretion over absorption of fluid, resulting from derangement of normal secretory and absorptive mechanisms. It is best exemplified by the effects of *diarrheagenic bacterial enterotoxins. E. coli* is the most important source of such toxins; some *Salmonella* serotypes, *Yersinia enterocolitica*, and *Shigella* also produce such enterotoxins. Heat-labile *E. coli* enterotoxin acts through the mediation of cAMP to inhibit sodium chloride cotransport at the luminal cell membrane of enterocytes while stimulating chloride secretion, thus reducing passive water absorption and simultaneously enhancing water secretion.

In addition to bacterial enterotoxins, other factors may cause or contribute to secretory diarrhea. Prostaglandins, eicosanoids, histamine, kinins, and various other cytokines directly or indirectly stimulate secretion, often by local stimulation of enteric nervous reflexes, and they thus contribute to diarrhea during IBD. Vasoactive intestinal polypeptide secreted by pancreatic islet cell tumors causes severe diarrhea in humans; a single case has been reported in a dog. This neurotransmitter causes active chloride and bicarbonate secretion mediated by the enteric nervous system. Other circulating agents are directly or indirectly diarrheagenic: calcitonin secreted by thyroid C-cell tumors; serotonin, bradykinin, or substance P secreted by carcinoids; histamine secreted by MCTs; gastrin secreted by gastrinomas. Peptide YY is secreted by enteroendocrine cells of the intestine and is known to inhibit intestinal secretion and promote absorption.

Malabsorptive diarrhea is exemplified by osmotic retention of water in the gut lumen by poorly absorbed magnesium sulfate, used therapeutically as a laxative, and *commonly results from villus atrophy from any cause*. Electrolyte and nutrient solute are malabsorbed as a result of reduced villus and microvillus surface area and are retained in the lumen of the bowel along with water, then ultimately passed into the colon. A secretory component contributes to diarrhea caused by villus atrophy in many cases, at least in transmissible gastroenteritis virus (TGEV) infection of pigs, where fluid secreted by the crypts is not absorbed due to lack of villous absorptive epithelium; poorly differentiated cells emerging from crypts may also retain some secretory capacity. Malabsorptive diarrhea also occurs in *short-bowel syndrome* associated with significantly reduced absorptive surface area.

Increased mucosal permeability may contribute to diarrhea by permitting increased retrograde movement of solute and fluid from the *lateral intercellular spaces* to the lumen, or by facilitating transudation of tissue fluid. In **filtration secretion**, increased protein-rich fluid movement occurs via the *paracellular route* across the mucosa into the intestinal lumen, which is driven by alterations in the interstitial and vascular pressure gradients. Elevated hydrostatic pressure or decreased plasma oncotic pressure in the villus alters Starling forces, permitting leakage of interstitial fluid and large protein molecules. Portal hypertension, right-sided heart failure, hypoalbuminemia, and expansion of plasma volume establish such conditions. Effusion also may be associated with lymphangiectasia, inflammation or edema of the lamina propria, increased vascular permeability, and enteric plasma protein loss. Increased rate of epithelial loss and transient microerosions may provide further potential sites for effusion of interstitial fluid. Extensive epithelial necrosis and mucosal vascular damage cause malabsorption and effusion of tissue fluid and blood, which may be evident grossly as fibrin and hemorrhage in the lumen.

Large-bowel diarrhea *is due to a reduction in the innate capability of the colon to absorb the solute and fluid presented by the more proximal bowel*. A reduction in net absorption by the colon that is relatively small in absolute terms may be sufficient to cause diarrhea. *Frequent passage of small amounts of fluid feces* occurs in large-bowel diarrhea, perhaps with mucus and blood. The colonic mucosa is not as leaky as the small intestinal mucosa because of the nature of the tight junctions between epithelial cells. The colon is thus relatively resistant to alterations in permeability owing to increased hydrostatic pressure in the propria, compared with the small intestine.

When normal enterohepatic circulation of bile acids is interrupted by ileal damage or resection, *excess bile acids* enter the colon where they stimulate colonic epithelial cells to secrete fluid and electrolytes through calcium and cAMP-dependent mechanisms, resulting in diarrhea. *Fatty acids* enter the colon in increased quantities in steatorrhea resulting from bile salt depletion, where they cause diarrhea by altering mucosal permeability and stimulating fluid secretion from colonic epithelium. This is also the mode of action of some laxatives such as castor oil, which contains the hydroxy fatty acid ricinoleic acid.

Although colonic water secretion stimulated by bacterial enterotoxin is not clearly implicated in diarrhea, damage to colonic epithelium by bacterial toxins such as the TcdB toxin of *Clostridioides difficile* (formerly *Clostridium difficile*), or alterations in the colonic microbiome may be detrimental to normal function or epithelial repair after injury. Short-chain fatty acids produced by bacterial fermentation in the lumen regulate colonic epithelial cell growth and differentiation and are linked to electrolyte and fluid absorption in the colon. Reduced production or absorption of short-chain fatty acids secondary to *imbalance of the bacterial flora* in the cecum and colon may explain some instances of wasting and diarrhea in horses in which no morphologic abnormality of the mucosa can be found.

Osmotic overload of the colon results from the delivery of a large volume of fermentable substrate from the small intestine. This is usually caused by malabsorption in the small intestine but may result from excessive intake. Carbohydrate is the only nutrient of significance in initiating *colonic osmotic overload*, as bacterial fermentation of carbohydrate results in the generation of excess short-chain fatty acids. This is rapidly absorbed and buffered in the colon under normal circumstances; however, a heavy carbohydrate load may overwhelm the colonic buffering capacity and cause reduced pH. The result is an *altered intestinal microbiome* in which there is overgrowth of organisms producing lactic acid, further contributing to acidification and increased mucosal permeability. Loss of water and solute into the lumen along the osmotic gradient generated by lactic acid in the lumen contributes to diarrhea.

Increased intestinal motility probably does not have a primary role in the pathogenesis of diarrhea in domestic animals. Often the small intestine of animals with diarrhea is flaccid and fluid-filled, rather than hypermotile. Increased colonic motor activity is often segmental and antiperistaltic, and probably unrelated to increased transit. Hypermotility, if it does occur, may be in response to, rather than a cause of, increased volumes of fluid in the gut.

Protein metabolism in enteric disease. Disorders of protein metabolism attributable to enteric disease are responsible for significant economic loss in the form of reduced weight gain, wool growth, and milk production. Severe derangement resulting in negative nitrogen balance in any species may lead to cachexia, hypoproteinemia, and death.

Decreased protein intake is the most obvious threat to the nitrogen economy, and it is probably the most important in many chronic GI diseases. Subclinical inefficiency in production, reduced growth, and emaciation may be products of various degrees of inappetence, or difficulty in prehension, mastication, swallowing, or recurrent regurgitation. Low-feed quality compounds the effect of reduced feed intake.

Anorexia is *a sharp decline in appetite*, and a common sign of indigestion, obstruction, or systemic disease. In ruminants, loss of appetite to various degrees is an especially important component of the pathogenicity of GI parasites, including those infecting the abomasum (*Ostertagia* or *Teladorsagia*), small intestine (*Trichostrongylus*), and large bowel (*Oesophagostomum*). Complex signaling pathways including cytokines, growth factors, parasympathetic efferent and afferent reflexes, and systemic or GI hormones (e.g., cholecystokinin, leptin) mediate satiety; however, the many details of their mechanisms in health and disease remain unclear.

Malabsorption of peptides and amino acids occurs locally in the small intestine with significant *villus atrophy*; unless the lesion is widespread or distal in the small bowel, net absorption of nitrogen over the length of the small intestine will likely not be reduced given the profound compensatory absorptive capacity of the distal intestine. The contribution of protein malabsorption to disordered nitrogen metabolism is minor in most situations.

Protein-losing gastroenteropathy is defined as increased catabolism and loss of endogenous nitrogen via the GI tract and is important in many diseases. Excess endogenous protein entering the intestine is derived mainly from *effusion of plasma protein into the lumen of the bowel* but can also be associated with *increased turnover of cells lining the intestine*. Protein-losing enteropathies (PLE) can be divided into 3 categories of mucosal injury leading to protein loss: mucosal ulcerations or erosions leading to secondary protein exudation; nonulcerated intact mucosa with abnormal permeability; and lymphatic disruption with leakage of protein-rich lymph (see Lymphangiectasia).

Plasma protein loss may result from the blood-sucking activity of nematodes such as *Haemonchus, Ancylostoma*, and *Bunostomum*, or hemorrhage from sites of trauma in the mucosa caused by the feeding activity of worms such as *Oesophagostomum, Chabertia*, and *Strongylus*. Considerable loss of erythrocytes and plasma protein leads to fibrinohemorrhagic enteritis and occurs secondary to mucosal erosions or ulcerations caused by ischemia, direct enterocyte necrosis, or inflammation associated with bacteria, viruses, and coccidia. Plasma protein can also be lost through transient gaps, or leaks in the mucosa that develop during increased exfoliation of enterocytes into the lumen, because the immature epithelial cells fail to maintain integrity of the surface barrier.

The permeability of tight junctions between epithelial cells may be sufficiently altered to permit transit of plasma protein molecules. **Filtration secretion** occurs when the hydrostatic pressure in the proprial interstitium is elevated, for example, during congestive heart failure or portal hypertension; by decreased plasma oncotic pressure; by increased vascular or paracellular epithelial permeability associated with cytokines during acute or chronic inflammation; and in lymphatic obstruction or lymphangiectasia.

Plasma protein loss into the gut is generally considered nonselective because albumin, immunoglobulins, clotting factors, and a variety of transport or carrier proteins such as transferrin or ceruloplasmin are lost equally. Physiologic consequences of PLE may be observed with increased loss of any of these molecules but are most frequently related to albumin turnover.

The progression and clinical manifestation of PLE vary with the rate of onset of plasma loss and the **fractional catabolic rate** (loss of plasma protein via the enteric system is expressed as a percentage of the total body protein pool). A sudden onset of severe plasma protein loss may occur before there is time for compensatory protein synthesis. If the progression of disease and the rate of protein loss is more gradual or only slightly increased, compensatory protein production occurs and the albumin pool is maintained in equilibrium at only a marginally reduced state (perhaps near or within the reference interval), in which subclinical protein loss occurs.

Endogenous protein derived from exfoliated cells of the stomach or upper small intestine during villus atrophy may be digested and absorbed in the lower small intestine. This is dependent on luminal proteolysis by pancreatic enzymes, digestion, and absorption that may compensate for any malabsorption caused by the more proximal lesions. The efficiency of protein digestion and absorption is not 100%, so a proportion of this increased endogenous protein is added to the protein that escapes digestion in the small bowel and enters the large intestine. Here, most of this protein may be converted to ammonia by the colonic flora and absorbed. The loss of significant protein from stomach or small intestine may thus be accompanied by little or no increase in fecal nitrogen excretion, although much of the protein loss from lesions in the colon is ultimately lost in the feces. Ammonia nitrogen absorbed from the colon is converted in the liver mainly to urea, so animals with increased endogenous protein loss into the stomach or small intestine may have slightly raised levels of plasma urea, and elevated urinary urea excretion.

Elevated hepatic synthesis of albumin resulting from increased turnover of the plasma albumin pool, and increased enteric protein synthesis in support of elevated epithelial turnover in conditions with chronic villus atrophy, is at the expense of anabolic processes elsewhere. Dietary amino acid is diverted preferentially to synthesis of plasma and enteric protein. If protein intake is poor due to inappetence or a low-quality ration, or if the rate of protein loss is high, the animal moves into **negative nitrogen balance**. Catabolism of peripheral protein then assumes an increasingly important role in maintaining the pool of amino acids available for plasma and intestinal protein synthesis. This explains in part the reduced growth rate, decreased muscle mass, and reduced bone matrix in ruminants with subclinical or mild parasitism, as well as cachexia and osteopenia associated with severe parasitism. These principles probably hold for all syndromes causing enteric loss of endogenous protein in any species.

Loss of enteric protein, and especially plasma, should be suspected in cachectic or hypoproteinemic animals, although diarrhea is not invariably present. *The 2 major routes of occult plasma protein loss are GI disease and glomerular disease (particularly glomerular amyloidosis)*; exudative skin lesions are a less common source. Anemia and hypoproteinemia may be due to hemorrhage externally or into the GI tract. Advanced liver disease causes hypoalbuminemia, although concurrent signs of hepatic failure will likely be observed (see Vol. 2, Liver and Biliary System). Inability or reluctance to eat, inadequate nutrition, or starvation also cause emaciation, usually without profound hypoalbuminemia; these should be distinguished from cachexia of malignancy.

When adequately hydrated, the hypoalbuminemic animal has subcutaneous, mesenteric, or gastric submucosal edema, perhaps with hydrothorax or ascites. Wasting of muscle mass may be marked if the protein loss has been severe and chronic. Unlike starvation, protein-losing gastroenteropathy may be associated with adequate internal adipose stores because assimilation of energy is not necessarily severely impaired.

Anemia can be caused by blood loss of any origin *into the GI tract*, including that caused by hematophagous parasites. Erythroid hyperplasia in bone marrow or in extramedullary sites may not compensate for the continued erythrocyte loss. Resolution of the hemorrhage results in eventual restoration of normal red cell numbers and an ultimate decline in erythrocyte production. Chronic blood loss may culminate in depletion of iron stores and development of a nonresponsive hypochromic microcytic anemia.

Intestinal ischemia and infarction

Intestinal ischemia and infarction due to inadequate or interrupted circulation of blood to the gut is a common problem, particularly in the horse. Obstruction of the efferent veins, blockage of afferent arteries, and reduced flow through an open circulation cause hypoxic damage to the intestine. Whatever the initiating cause, the effect of hypoxia at the level of the mucosa is similar.

In the **small intestine**, within 5-10 minutes of the onset of ischemia, changes are observed at the tips of villi in tissue sections examined under the light microscope, and lesions are well advanced by 30 minutes. Separation of the epithelium from the basement membrane, beginning at the tip of the villus and progressing toward the base, causes the formation of the so-called Gruenhagen space. Epithelial cells appear relatively normal and may separate from the villus in sheets. The core of the villus contracts toward the base. Within 1-3 hours, the villus is almost completely denuded of epithelium, and the mesenchymal core is disintegrating or collapsed and stumpy, with hemorrhage from capillaries. Superficial epithelium may persist for several hours in the intestinal crypts.

That this lesion is largely a function of hypoxia is indicated by the mitigating effects of intraluminal perfusion of oxygenated saline demonstrated experimentally in dogs and cats. The putative countercurrent exchange of oxygen between the afferent arteriole and efferent venules in the villus, and an associated progressive decline in oxygen tension distally in the villus, may render the tip prone to early damage in hypoxia. Villus smooth muscle contraction, exacerbating the epithelial exfoliation on the distal villus, may be mediated by sympathetic stimulation in ischemia.

Dissociation and necrosis of cells in the intestinal crypts begin ~2-4 hours after the initiation of ischemia, and within 4-5 hours the epithelium appears completely necrotic or has sloughed, leaving a mesenchymal ghost of the mucosa. The muscularis mucosa may undergo necrosis, but the muscularis externa remains viable for 6-7 hours. During acute ischemia, there is initial hyperexcitability of muscle in the affected areas, followed by progressive loss of contractility, which will fail to recover if ischemia persists beyond 4-6 hours. Mesothelial cells on the serosa undergo necrosis within 30-60 minutes of ischemia and exfoliate; there is a local acute inflammatory response, which may predispose to the development of adhesions. *This speed with which lesions develop in hypoxia emphasizes the significance of rapid fixation of intestinal mucosa if artifact is to be avoided.* Differentiation between postmortem autolysis and necrosis can be particularly challenging in the intestine. A few useful hints to help determining autolysis versus necrosis include hemolysis of red blood cells, large numbers of bacterial rods within blood vessels and tissues not associated with inflammation (postmortem bacterial overgrowth), gas bubbles in the tissues, and desquamation of slabs of epithelial cells. The lack of an inflammatory reaction is also suggestive, although not confirmatory, of autolysis.

The **colon** of the dog and horse seems less sensitive to short-term ischemia than the small intestine. Mild morphologic damage, including mild edema, and separation and exfoliation of surface epithelium between crypts, is found after 1 hour. However, by 3-4 hours, crypt epithelium is becoming necrotic, dissociating, and exfoliating, and from that point events progress as in the small intestine.

Reperfusion injury superimposed on the effects of ischemia alone may enhance the severity of the lesion, if hypoxia is only partial or ischemia is transient, and reflow of blood raises the tissue oxygen tension. Reperfusion injury implies that the effects of the hypoxic episode have not progressed to complete necrosis of the mucosa and that further damage is possible because of oxygen free radicals and/or cytokines. Hence, there is a relatively short duration of hypoxia, and a concomitant mild-to-intermediate degree of mucosal damage, permissive of this phenomenon. In cases of enteric ischemic disease encountered in veterinary medicine, this threshold may frequently have been crossed by the time that the animal is presented for therapy. In addition, there is evidence that in swine and in horses, where intestinal ischemic events are most common, reperfusion injury is less likely to occur than in other species. Because reperfusion injury may cause necrosis and/or apoptosis, it is almost impossible to differentiate morphologically the changes produced by ischemia from those of reperfusion injury.

Reperfusion injury is the result of the interplay among free radical–mediated damage to the microvasculature and probably stromal elements and epithelium; neutrophil margination and diapedesis into tissue; complement activation; and release of proinflammatory proteins and cytokines, some of which may have systemic effects. *Free radicals* in reperfusion injury are largely generated through xanthine oxidase mechanisms in the intestinal mucosa, and through NADPH oxidase mechanisms in leukocytes, mainly neutrophils, already resident in or recruited to the damaged tissue. Hypoxia stimulates the conversion of xanthine dehydrogenase to xanthine oxidase in epithelial cells. In the presence of xanthine oxidase, hypoxanthine accumulating from adenosine triphosphate degradation in hypoxia is converted to xanthine, and molecular oxygen is reduced, generating hydrogen peroxide, superoxide radical, and hydroxyl radical intermediates, which inhibit the accumulation of protective nitric oxide. The hydroxyl radical is likely most significant in damaging proteins and initiating a cascade of lipid peroxidation, resulting in metabolic and structural lesions, and culminating in cell death.

The acute inflammatory response that accompanies reperfusion results in production of free radicals by the respiratory burst from neutrophils, release of proteolytic enzymes, and physical impairment of the microcirculation. Reduction in tissue nitric oxide permits dismutation of oxygen free radicals to H_2O_2, which promotes activation of phospholipase, accumulation of proinflammatory mediators, production of cytokines (tumor necrosis factor, lymphotoxin-α, ILs) and adhesion molecules by endothelium. Complement activation is mediated by adhesion molecules, promoting inflammatory events and release of cytokines, such as tumor necrosis factor and IL1, as well as other cytokines that increase during reperfusion.

Sequelae of ischemia vary with duration and severity of insult. Short-term ischemia (maximally, ~3-4 hours), with preservation of at least the base of the intestinal crypts, will permit repair, as *cells proliferating in the crypts re-epithelialize the mucosal surface within 1-3 days*. Normal architecture is re-established after up to 1-2 weeks, although necrotic muscularis mucosa is not replaced. Effusion of tissue fluid and acute inflammatory cells prevails until epithelium extends to cover the eroded surface fully. Partial damage to

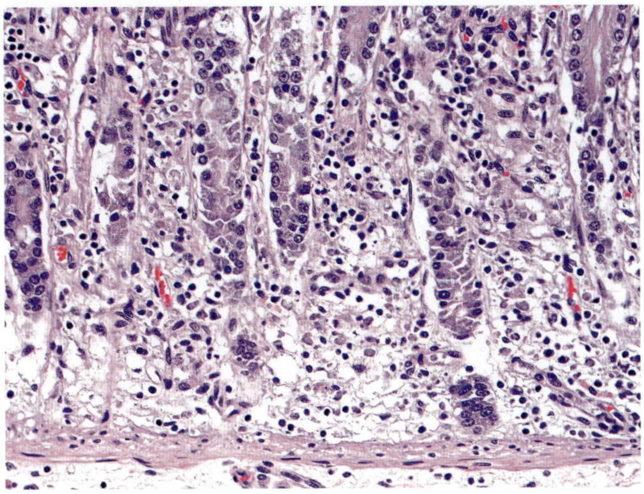

Figure 1-42 Small intestine, sequel to **transient ischemia**. Hyperplastic basophilic cells populate surviving crypts. A few crypts have degenerate and necrotic epithelium. Inflammatory cells, mostly neutrophils, are infiltrating the lamina propria and crypt lumen.

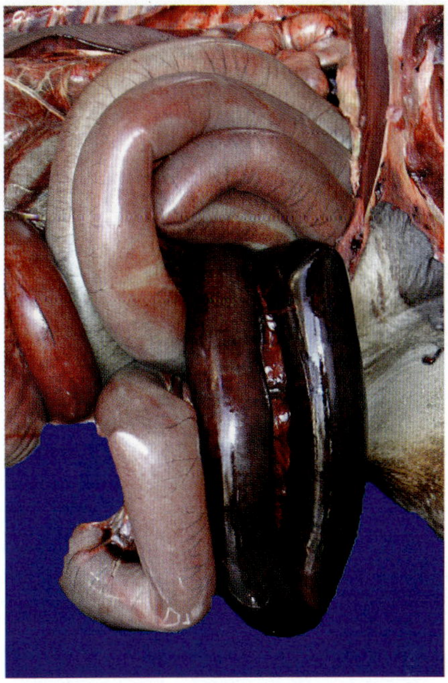

Figure 1-43 **Venous infarction** of a segment of the equine small intestine that has undergone volvulus.

the proliferative compartment initially results in dilation of crypts, which are lined by flattened epithelium resembling that seen after radiation injury. If the amplifier population of progenitor cells can be regenerated, hyperplastic basophilic cells will populate crypts until the mucosal architecture is reconstituted (Fig. 1-42).

Ischemic necrosis of the full thickness of the mucosa will be bounded by an acute inflammatory reaction in the submucosa, which under favorable conditions evolves into a granulating ulcerated surface. Focal ulcerative lesions may ultimately heal by epithelial migration over the bed of granulation tissue from surviving crypts within the lesion and around the periphery.

Extensive *mucosal ulcers* that form following severe ischemia have little chance of resolution because of their large surface area. Chronic ischemic ulcers in the small bowel tend to develop a depressed clean granulating surface, occasionally with some surface fibrinous exudate.

Ischemic ulcers in the large bowel, especially of horses, develop a dirty yellow-gray fibrinonecrotic surface. If the animal does not succumb to the effects of malabsorption and protein loss from the defect, or to transmural bacterial invasion, scarring and stricture may occur. The sequelae of ischemia with reflow are mainly seen in strangulated segments of the intestine that have been reduced without resection, or with inadequate resection, and in some cases of presumed thromboembolic infarction of the equine colon. Persistent ischemia results in necrosis involving all mural elements. The full thickness of the bowel wall ultimately becomes necrotic, green-brown or black, flaccid, and friable.

The *consequences of ischemic lesions* are partly a function of the species, and of the level of bowel affected. Strangulation, volvulus, and similar lesions cause physical obstruction at the site, and ileus proximal to it. Reduced arterial perfusion or thromboembolism causes functional obstruction and ileus. Loss of mucosal integrity results in cessation of electrolyte and water absorption, and ultimately in effusion of tissue fluid and blood into the lumen. Proliferation of anaerobes occurs in the lumen of the stagnant ischemic area, with accumulation of gas, and extreme distension of the closed loop in strangulation obstruction. Toxin production by anaerobes, particularly clostridia, plays a significant role in the development of gangrene and eventual rupture of ischemic bowel, as well as having systemic effects. Absorption of endotoxins and exotoxins from the lumen may occur through devitalized mucosa via the portal flow, lymphatic return, or peritoneum. Toxins have a severe detrimental effect on cardiovascular function, contributing to circulatory failure. If death from some other cause does not supervene, transmural invasion by enteric bacteria or perforation of the devitalized wall results in septic peritonitis that is ultimately fatal.

Venous infarction *due to obstruction of efferent veins is by far the most common cause of intestinal ischemia.* This is a sequel to **incarceration** of herniated loops of bowel; **strangulation** by pedunculated masses, such as lipomas in older horses; **torsion** (twist about the long axis of the viscus); **volvulus** (twist of the intestine on its mesenteric axis); and **intussusception**. In these circumstances, compression of thin-walled veins tends to occur before the influx of arterial blood is obstructed because arteries have thicker walls and higher blood pressure. In venous infarction, the affected tissue field, which often includes involved mesentery, becomes intensely edematous, congested, and hemorrhagic, so that the hypoxic bowel wall is thickened and eventually assumes a deep red-black appearance (Fig. 1-43). It has been estimated that 40 L of fluid may accumulate in the wall of a horse colon that has undergone torsion. Bloody fluid content and gas distend the lumen of the infarcted segment. As gangrene of the intestinal wall proceeds, the tissue becomes green-black, and septic peritonitis and general sepsis eventually ensue, with or without perforation of the bowel. Advanced venous infarction involves the full thickness of the intestinal wall, and the initiating intestinal accident is commonly evident, except in cases subjected to surgery. Even if a displacement has been reduced, the limits of the infarcted segment are usually relatively sharply demarcated, and the affected bowel remains edematous and hemorrhagic. Sharp demarcation of the area of necrosis is telltale of a vascular accident. Microscopically, severe transmural edema, congestion, distension of veins, sometimes venous thrombosis, and hemorrhage are present, initially most severe in the mucosa and submucosa. With time, the full thickness of the mucosa becomes necrotic, and the deeper layers of the muscular wall are also devitalized, with invading enteric flora present throughout. Lesions that have advanced to significant necrosis including effacement of the crypt epithelium are usually fatal unless timely resection occurs. Death is usually associated with hypovolemic and/or septic shock if correction of the strangulation or resection is not done promptly.

Displacements of intestine that may progress to incarceration or volvulus with strangulation and infarction are discussed later in this chapter. They are a common cause of colic and mortality in horses.

Arterial infarction and subsequent ischemia of the gut caused by arterial thrombosis and embolism is rare in domestic animals other than the horse. Mucosal and occasionally transmural focal or segmental infarctive lesions are seen in *Pasteurella* septicemia in lambs and in *Histophilus somni* bacteremia in cattle (eFig. 1-5). Most cases of embolic disease are associated with bacterial infections that cause softening and lysis of thrombi and facilitate the formation of emboli. This is particularly true for the lesions associated with strongyle migrations in horses, in which lesions remain localized unless thrombi induced by the parasite become secondarily infected.

In **horses** infarction is associated with **endoarteritis**, mainly at the root of the cranial mesenteric artery, caused by migrating larvae of *Strongylus vulgaris* (see Vol. 3, Cardiovascular System). Effective nematode control programs have rendered this condition increasingly rare, although it still occurs at least periodically.

Candidates for a diagnosis of nonstrangulating infarction are animals in which the anatomic distribution of an ischemic lesion is incompatible with volvulus or other strangulation, or physical evidence for incarceration or strangulation obstruction is not present in the surgical history or at autopsy, and there is evidence of verminous arteritis. Careful consideration should be given to the fact that verminous arteritis can be present in horses without embolic intestinal lesions. Therefore, the presence of the former does not definitely prove that intestinal infarction was produced by verminous arteritis. Typically, ischemic lesions of this type are limited to the "watersheds" at the periphery of the colic and cecal arterial circulatory fields—the pelvic flexure and the distal cecum—because collateral circulation within these circulatory fields is extensive.

Lesions limited essentially to the mucosa usually are subacute, result from ischemia of relatively short duration, and are ulcerative or fibrinonecrotic, usually with a hyperemic margin. Transmural lesions represent ischemia of longer duration. Devitalized gray-brown intestine of normal thickness is interpreted to represent arterial obstruction without significant reflow, except along the boundary with viable tissue. Large edematous, congested, or hemorrhagic, full-thickness lesions, physically or anatomically inconsistent with strangulation, are interpreted as severe arterial obstruction, with subsequent reflow either by relief of the obstruction or by way of collaterals. Ischemic damage to vessels of the mucosa, submucosa, and perhaps deeper structures results in hemorrhage and edema when blood flow returns (Fig. 1-44A). Ulcerative or fibrinonecrotic mucosal lesions are probably the result of transient ischemia with subsequent reflow (see Fig. 1-44B). Similar lesions may occur after relief of strangulation of short duration, and in NSAID drug toxicosis, salmonellosis, and infections by C. *difficile* or C. *perfringens* type C, all of which involve, in part, mucosal microthrombosis.

Ischemia caused by reduced perfusion of the intestinal vascular bed is a *difficult and uncommon diagnosis*. Circumstances in which it may be expected to occur include severe

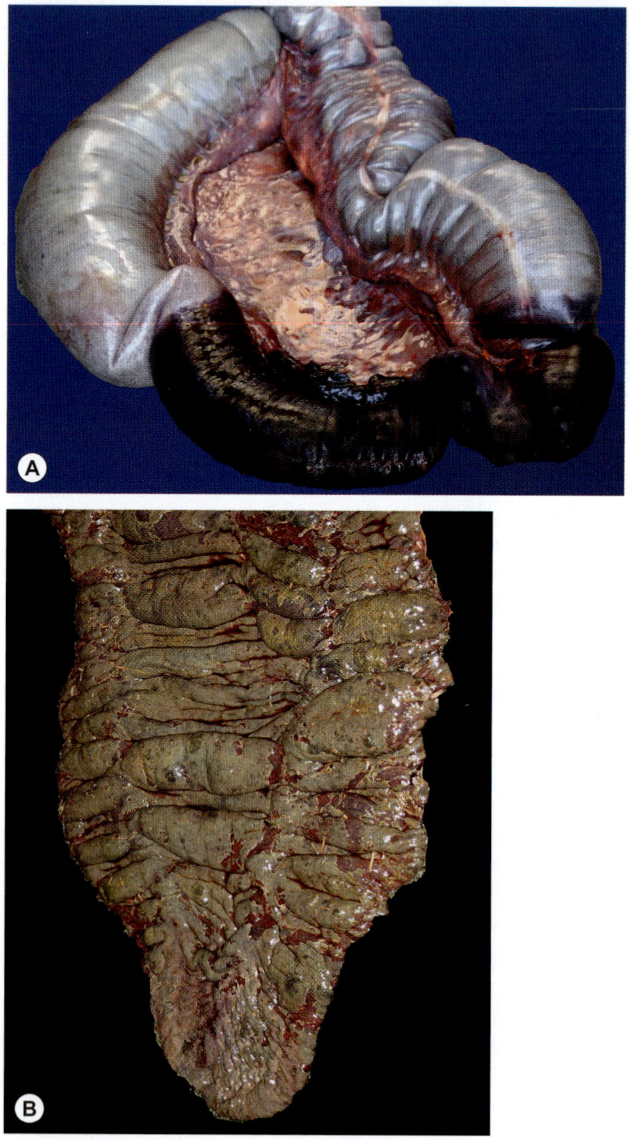

Figure 1-44 A. **Infarction of pelvic flexure** of the large colon of a horse. Hemorrhage and edema of the serosa suggest that arterial thrombosis and infarction have been followed by reperfusion, with extravasation of blood from damaged vessels in the affected tissue. (Courtesy S.S. Diab.) **B**. The mucosa of an equine cecum that has undergone ischemic necrosis resulting from reduced arterial perfusion. Subsequent reflow has occurred and the infarcted mucosa is covered with fibrinonecrotic exudate. Irregular ulcers and exudation are present throughout the mucosa.

hypovolemic states, such as *hemorrhagic shock* in the dog, cat, and possibly other species; in animals, particularly dogs, with *disseminated intravascular coagulation* (DIC); in dogs with hepatic disease and *portal hypertension;* in *hypotensive shock* caused by heart failure; and in animals with reduced mesenteric arterial perfusion, mainly horses with severe *verminous endoarteritis*.

The so-called **shock gut** of dogs, and rarely other species, occurs in association with terminal heart failure, hemorrhage, hypovolemia, and DIC; part or all of the small intestinal mucosa is deeply congested, and the content is hemorrhagic. The pathogenesis of the lesion is related to reflex vasoconstriction in the mucosa and submucosa, shunting of blood away from the mucosa, dilation of mucosal capillaries, and reduction in the rate of flow of blood through the villus. Countercurrent transfer of oxygen from the afferent to efferent vessels in the villus aggravates hypoxemia in the villus by increased shunting of oxygen to the efferent venule. Splanchnic pooling of blood, systemic arterial hypotension, and intestinal vasoconstriction occur in endotoxic shock in dogs, causing similar mucosal lesions. Microthrombosis associated with sluggish flow, DIC, and endotoxemia may contribute to mucosal ischemia by obstructing capillaries in the villi, and mucosal and submucosal venules. Microthrombi in these vessels in association with hemorrhagic mucosal necrosis suggest the possibility of ischemia caused by "slow flow."

Transient or incomplete reduction in perfusion caused by obstruction of the arterial blood supply has a similar effect on the mucosa. The obstruction may be due to *arteriospasm*, perhaps induced by vasoactive mediators such as thromboxane. Mucosa devitalized by hypoxia will become hemorrhagic with continued blood flow. Because the primary problem may not involve a systemic state as complicated as severe shock, the animal may survive long enough to develop an effusive ulcerated or pseudomembranous mucosa, with some prospect of stabilization or repair, if the lesion is not widespread. "Slow flow" caused by reduced arterial perfusion with inadequate collateral flow may be expected to affect the "watershed" areas of a circulatory field preferentially. In the horse this may be the explanation for mucosal lesions at the pelvic flexure and apex of the cecum in which thromboembolism cannot be implicated, but in which mural thrombi in the cranial mesenteric root could have caused significantly reduced perfusion or flushed vasoconstrictive thromboxane into circulation.

Transient or noninfarctive "slow flow" has been proposed as a cause of intermittent colic in horses due to verminous arteritis. It may also play a role in the development of functional obstruction and volvulus in horses with cranial mesenteric arterial lesions.

Ischemia at the periphery of the circulatory field of the caudal mesenteric artery may possibly predispose to rectal perforation in horses. The precarious perfusion of the mucosa at this site may contribute to ischemic ulceration and the development of *rectal stricture in swine*. In many cases, this condition appears to be associated with *Salmonella* infection, and it is discussed further with porcine salmonellosis.

Acute acorn poisoning in the horse may cause severe GI edema and focal hemorrhage, with infarction and ulceration in the cecum and colon. Microscopic lesions in the small and large intestine are consistent with an ischemic pathogenesis, and microthrombi have been associated with mucosal infarcts in the large bowel as well as in other organs.

Non-steroidal anti-inflammatory drugs (NSAIDs) cause ulceration of the cranial small intestine and colon, as well as oral and gastric ulceration, which seem to be related to ischemia, in horses and dogs. In horses, phenylbutazone, even at therapeutic dosages, can result in ischemic damage to the intestinal mucosa. It may be that intercurrent stress or dehydration contributes to the pathogenesis. The right dorsal colon is affected preferentially, resulting in the term *right dorsal colitis;* however, this may be a misnomer as lesions in other parts of the colon and small intestine frequently occur. The NSAID-associated lesions often are marked edema and avascular necrosis, characteristic of ischemia. Lesions may be focal, linear, or extensive and segmental, involving the entire circumference of the bowel (Fig. 1-45A and B). Depending on the duration and severity of the lesion, the mucosa may be congested and edematous, with superficial necrosis and fibrin exudation, or extensively eroded and ulcerated, with fibrinonecrotic exudate. Early in the process, superficial epithelial necrosis and progressive mucosal necrosis and inflammation are evident. *Microvascular injury* with subsequent microthrombosis and ischemic ulceration is considered by some to be the cause of the lesions in the stomach and intestine. This may be the result of direct phenylbutazone toxicity to the microvasculature. The intestinal gross and microscopic lesions of NSAIDs intoxication in horses may be indistinguishable

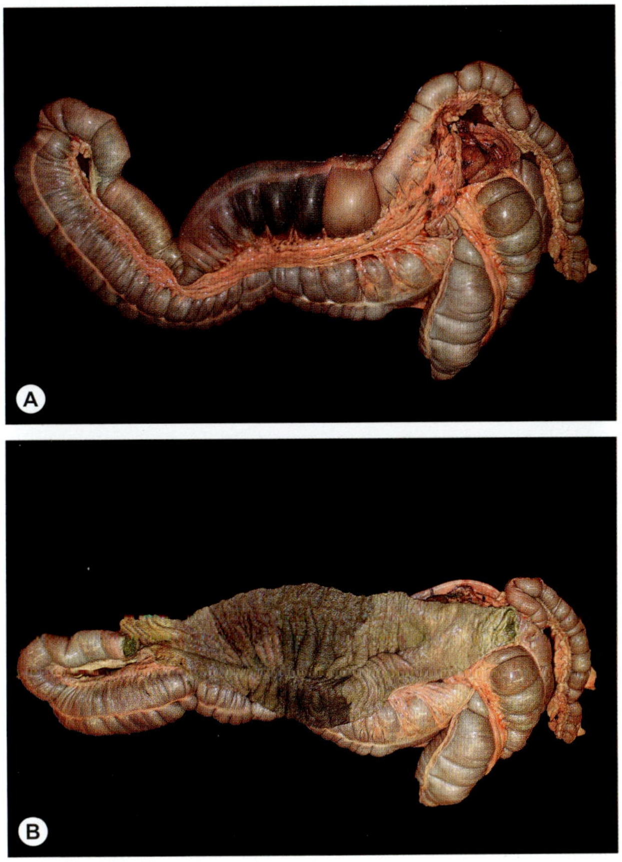

Figure 1-45 Ischemic necrosis and hemorrhage of the right dorsal colon in a horse treated heavily with nonsteroidal anti-inflammatory drugs. **A**. Serosal view. **B**. Mucosal view. (From Mendonça FS, et al. The comparative pathology of enterocolitis caused by *Clostridium perfringens* type C, *Clostridioides difficile, Paraclostridium sordellii, Salmonella enterica* subspecies *enterica* serovar Typhimurium, and nonsteroidal anti-inflammatory drugs in horses. J Vet Diagn Invest 2022;34:412–420.)

from those produced by infectious agents, such as *Salmonella* spp., *C. difficile*, and others. Vasoconstriction or depression of other cytoprotective effects mediated by phenylbutazone inhibition of prostaglandin synthesis could be the cause of the lesions. Animals may develop diarrhea and hypoproteinemia as a result of the extensive mucosal defects.

Minor mucosal lesions may resolve; a sequel to severe colonic damage in horses is colonic stricture. Lesions in the oral cavity associated with NSAID administration are deep crateriform ulcers with a clean granulating base. Concurrent with punched-out ulcers in the glandular mucosa, there may be chronic gastritis and atrophy of the mucosa with loss of differentiation of the cells in the fundus. In the upper small intestine, ulcers may be focal, linear, or segmental and annular. Microscopic lesions that may precede ulceration of the small intestine include mild-to-severe atrophy of villi, epithelial necrosis, mucosal inflammation, and fibrin exudation. Renal papillary necrosis is often concurrent if animals are dehydrated.

Congenital anomalies of the intestine

Segmental anomalies of the intestine are commonly encountered. In early embryonal life, the intestine consists of a simple tube, the lumen of which is lined by epithelial cells of endodermal origin surrounded and supported by an outer layer of connective tissue from the splanchnic ectoderm. As the intestines grow with the developing fetus, they form coiled loops that herniate temporarily through the umbilicus into a peritoneal-lined sac before they are later retracted back into the fetal abdomen. The most plausible cause of segmental defects in intestinal continuity is *ischemia of a segment of gut during early fetal life*, resulting in necrosis of the affected area.

The segmental anomalies of the intestine may vary in degree. **Stenosis** *implies incomplete occlusion or narrowing of the lumen; complete occlusion is referred to as* **atresia**. Atresia is further subdivided into *membrane atresia*, when the obstruction is formed by a simple membrane; *cord atresia*, in which the blind ends of the gut are joined by a cord of connective tissue; and *blind-end atresia*, in which a segment of gut and possibly the corresponding mesentery are missing, leaving two blind ends. All types of segmental anomaly can be produced experimentally by ischemia to a portion of the fetal intestine.

Atresia coli *is the most common segmental anomaly of the intestine in domestic mammals*. It is seen particularly in the spiral colon of Holstein calves, and in the large and small colon of foals; it occurs rarely in cats. Atresia coli may be an autosomal recessive trait in Holsteins. A predisposition for male calves has been described, but this is not consistent among studies. An association has been postulated between pressure on the amniotic vesicle during palpation of the embryo for pregnancy diagnosis before 42 days of gestation, and the development of atresia coli in calves; however, the mechanism of this effect is uncertain. **Atresia intestinalis** is less common. **Atresia ilei** is most prevalent in calves, and rare in foals, lambs, piglets, and pups. These lesions prevent normal movement of gut content and meconium and therefore lead to dilation of the proximal segment and progressive abdominal distension, which may become so extensive in an affected fetus to cause dystocia. The bowel distal to the obstruction is small in diameter, and devoid of content other than mucus and exfoliated cells. Animals fail to pass feces after birth.

Atresia ani (*imperforate anus*) *is the overall most common congenital defect of the lower GI tract*. It may be seen in all species, but is most often encountered in calves and pigs, in which it is considered to be hereditary. The defect may consist only of failure of perforation of the membrane separating the endodermal hindgut from the ectodermal anal membrane, or both anus and rectum may be atretic. Atresia ani may be an isolated abnormality, but is more commonly associated with other malformations, especially of the distal spinal column (spinal dysraphism, sacral or coccygeal vertebral agenesis), genitourinary tract (rectovaginal fistula, renal agenesis, horseshoe kidney, polycystic kidneys, cryptorchidism, duplication of scrotum or penis), and occasionally with intestinal atresia or agenesis of the colon. Vitamin A deficiency during pregnancy has been associated with increased risk of congenital anorectal malformations in several species; this is thought to be related to improper development of the enteric nervous system.

Short colon has been reported in dogs and cats, and is probably the result of abnormal rotation of the midgut and failure to lengthen during fetal life. Clinical signs were subtle and possibly unrelated to the colonic lesion. Affected animals had a shortened colon with the cecum located on the left side of the abdomen. Concurrent anorectal or urogenital abnormalities were observed in some cases. **Anomaly of the colonic mesenteric attachments** has been described and associated with development of colic in a horse because of distortion and convolution of the large colon.

Congenital colonic aganglionosis is somewhat analogous to Hirschsprung disease in humans and occurs in *white foals* that are the offspring of frame overo spotted parents. The disease has not been convincingly demonstrated in other species of domestic animals. Clinically affected foals are predominantly white and develop colic and die generally within 48 hours of birth. Grossly, there is stenosis mainly of the small colon, but the entire colon and rectum may be patent but contracted; the proximal intestine is distended with gas and meconium. Microscopically, *ganglia of the myenteric plexus are absent in the walls of the ileum, cecum, and colon*, although occasional nerve fibers are evident. Except for the few pigmented spots, melanocytes are absent in the skin. Although several gene mutations can cause intestinal aganglionosis, loss of function mutation of the *endothelin receptor type B* gene are observed in horses, rodents, and humans with this condition. The pathogenesis is thought to involve improper migration of cells of the neural crest, from which cutaneous melanoblasts and the myenteric plexus neurons are derived. A similar condition of *megacolon* resulting from segmental colonic aganglionosis has been reported in pigs. Megacolon associated with reduced numbers of myenteric ganglion cells in Clydesdale foals is not clearly congenital and is discussed with intestinal obstruction, as is megacolon in other species.

Intestinal diverticula occur rarely in dogs, cats, and horses. *True diverticula* are congenital lesions involving all layers of the intestinal wall and are distinguished from *pseudodiverticula* resulting from disruption or weakening of the tunica muscularis and not involving all layers of the intestinal wall. They may be incidental but in horses have been associated with idiopathic muscle hypertrophy or other lesions of the small bowel, including neoplasia. Diverticula can cause impaction, obstruction, intussusception, or fistula, and potentially diverticulitis, rupture, and peritonitis.

Persistent Meckel diverticulum is an uncommon embryonic developmental anomaly occurring mostly along the antimesenteric border of the lower small bowel, mainly in swine and horses. It is derived from the omphalomesenteric (vitelline) duct, which is the stalk of the yolk sac. The vitelline membrane can also persist forming a fibrous ligament or *mesodiverticular band* between the distal small jejunum and the diverticulum or umbilicus. **Multiple persistent vitelline duct cysts**, distinct from Meckel diverticulum, have been described on the ileal serosa in a dog.

Hypoplasia of the small intestinal mucosa has been reported in foals with failure of passive transfer, and this may represent defective fetal organogenesis.

Degenerative and inflammatory conditions of the intestine

Acute obstruction typically involves the cranial or middle small intestine; chronic blockage usually involves the ileum and large bowel. Intestinal obstruction may be the sequel to a physical blockage of the lumen resulting from **stenosis** (narrowing, stricture) caused by an intrinsic lesion involving the intestinal wall, **obturation** (occlusion) by an intraluminal mass, or extrinsic compression.

Failure of the intestinal circular smooth muscle to contract blocks the peristaltic wave, causing **functional obstruction**, a clinical syndrome of pseudo-obstruction in which there is no physical occlusion of the lumen of the impacted intestine. **Adynamic ileus**, intestinal obstruction resulting from inhibition of bowel motility, is a common sequel to peritonitis and pain. Circulatory embarrassment of a segment of bowel via embolism or venous infarction also causes functional obstruction without a physical blockage. Many intestinal displacements that produce obstruction such as volvulus, strangulation, or intussusception may cause *ischemia*. The term **strangulation obstruction** refers to an event that simultaneously causes ischemia and physically blocks the intestine. Mucosal hypoxia may be a sequel to venous occlusion caused by physical distension of gut proximal to an obstruction; to local pressure caused by an adjacent mass; or to generalized circulatory failure. The pathogenesis and consequences of intestinal ischemia are dealt with later in this chapter.

Fluid accumulation occurs proximal to an obstruction, derived from ingesta, gastric, biliary, pancreatic, and intrinsic intestinal secretion, and *gas* swallowed or originating from bacterial activity in the gut (Fig. 1-46A and B). Intestinal distension results in luminal sequestration of water and electrolytes and mucosal edema; further fluid secretion into the lumen may be associated with contractile stimuli, and potentially transudation from the peritoneal surface. Upper small-bowel obstruction progresses rapidly to *vomiting* in most species, with dehydration, hypochloremia, hypokalemia, and metabolic alkalosis caused by loss of acid in vomitus and of fluid sequestration in the stomach. If acute complications of ischemia including rupture do not occur, an animal with obstruction succumbs to the *systemic effects of hypovolemia, electrolyte, and acid-base disturbance*.

With obstruction of the lower small intestine or colon, there is usually less pronounced electrolyte and acid-base imbalance because vomition is less severe and absorption of fluid proximal to the obstruction may prevent or delay severe distension and additional fluid secretion. Metabolic acidosis eventually follows, however, with dehydration and catabolism of fat and muscle once food consumption and assimilation ceases. In the horse, obstruction or impaction of the cecum or colon in particular often leads to *local ischemia and rupture* of the colon and, less frequently, of the stomach.

In obstruction, the outstanding gross alteration in the bowel is distension proximal to the point of blockage, caused by ileus

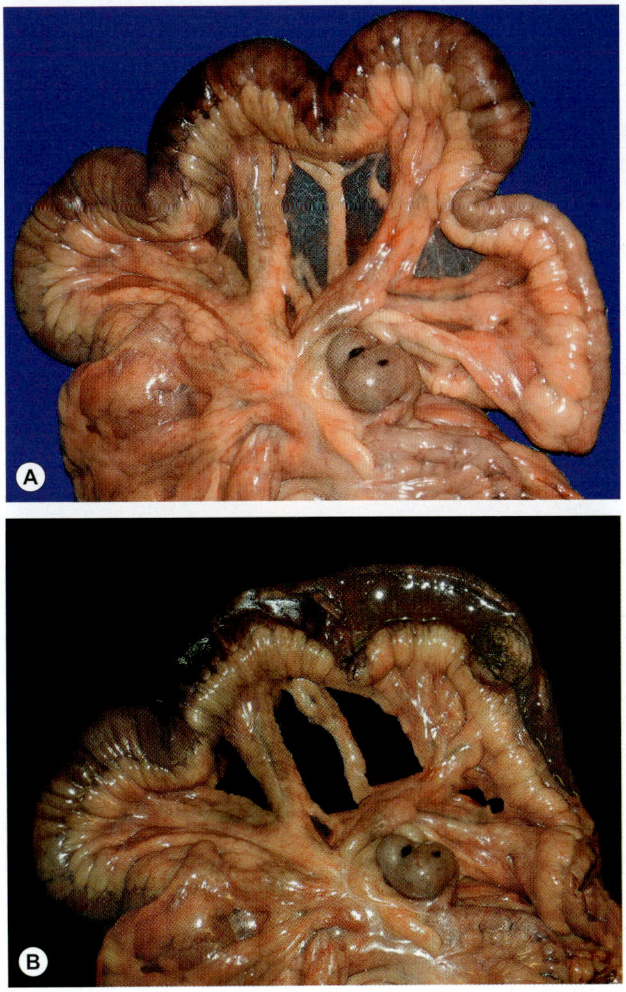

Figure 1-46 Small intestinal obstruction in a dog, caused by a foreign body. Dilation is present proximal to the obstruction, with contraction of the empty intestine distally. **A.** Serosal view. **B.** Mucosal view, small intestine opened. (Courtesy J. Caswell.)

and accumulation of fluid contents and gas. The volume of distension and length of bowel involved is dependent on the location, degree, and duration of obstruction; this may be remarkable with distal lesions such as rectal stricture in pigs, which can cause profound abdominal distension. As distension increases, interference with venous return may develop and the mucosa and submucosa become congested. Devitalization of severely dilated gut or pressure necrosis of the mucosa at the site of lodgment of intraluminal foreign bodies may occur, leading to necrosis, perforation, and peritonitis. Distal to the point of obstruction, the bowel is collapsed and empty.

Physical intrinsic obstruction. Congenital intrinsic obstruction caused by segmental atresia and imperforations is considered under the previous section on congenital anomalies of the intestine. The primary lesions involving the intestinal wall causing **acquired stenosis** include intramural abscesses or hematomas, neoplasms, and fibrosis secondary to ulceration. These lesions can result in partial or complete stenosis and may develop slowly with a course as described for simple chronic obstruction.

Foreign bodies of all kinds are commonly found in the alimentary canal. Small rounded foreign bodies and even some sharp-edged objects may pass through the intestines

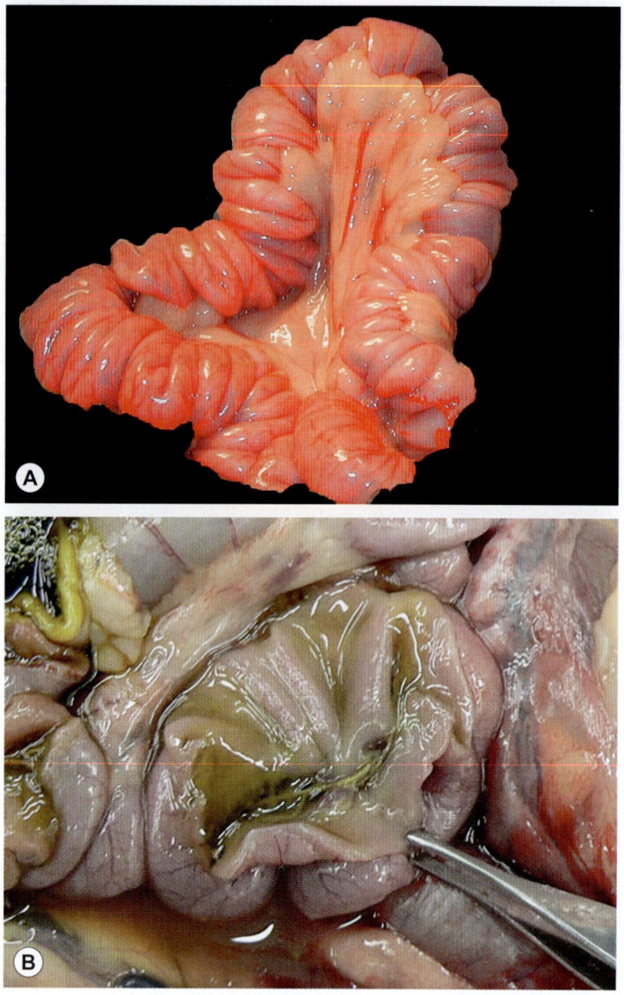

Figure 1-47 A. Pleating of the small intestine of a cat along (B) a **linear foreign body**. (A, Courtesy A. Quain; B, Courtesy A.J. Fales-Williams.)

uneventfully, but for these and many large foreign bodies the course is unpredictable. Some may reside in the intestine for long periods and produce no disturbance until they act as a nidus for the development of an enterolith. Foreign bodies may cause partial or complete intestinal obstruction and compromise the blood supply by luminal distension, which may progress to edema, necrosis, and possibly perforation. Most obstructions occur in the jejunum, although any segment of bowel can be affected. **Linear foreign bodies** such as strips of cloth or string probably occur more commonly in cats compared with dogs, and once ingested may pass through the intestine. However, if they become immobilized, they produce a characteristic lesion. One portion becomes fixed, most commonly around the base of the tongue or by impaction at the pylorus. The free end is then stretched taut distally because of peristalsis, which results in pleating of the distal gut onto the string (Fig. 1-47A). Peristalsis results in progressive mucosal damage (see Fig. 1-47B) along the lesser curvature of intestinal loops that may lead eventually to perforation and peritonitis.

Enteroliths (mineral concretions) are common in the colon of horses and are observed more frequently in some areas, such as California and Florida in the United States. Aged Arabians, Morgans, American Saddlebreds, and donkeys seem to be over-represented. The concretions consist of *magnesium ammonium phosphate*, the source of which is probably

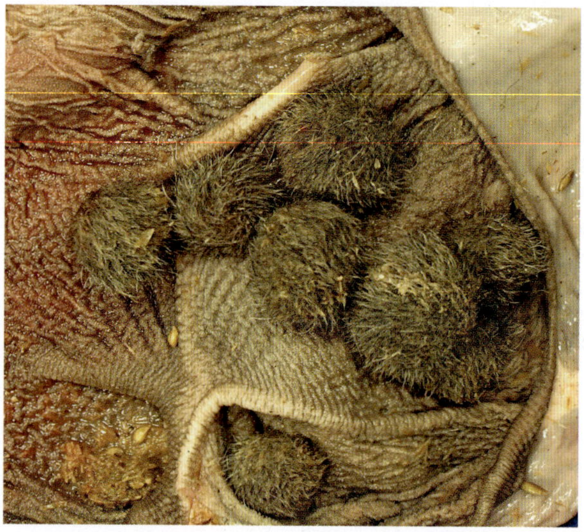

Figure 1-48 Trichobezoars in the rumen of a calf.

grain, bran, alfalfa, or alkaline water. Colonic pH >6.6 seems to contribute to enterolith formation. The mechanism is not completely clear; however, mineral salts are deposited in concentric lamellae around a central *nidus*—a foreign body such as a nail, wire, stone, or particle of feed. They can vary greatly in size, some weighing as much as 10 kg. Enteroliths are usually smooth and spherical (eFig. 1-6) but can be flattened; irregular mineralized masses may also occur, usually centered on a fibrous nidus, such as twine, rope, or netting.

Fiber balls (**phytobezoars** or phytotrichobezoars), which consist largely of plant fibers intermixed with phosphate salts, may be found especially in the colon of horses. They are not as heavy as enteroliths, and are usually round, smooth, and moist with a velvety and occasionally convoluted surface. Response to medical therapy and dissolution of phytobezoars has been reported in horses. Hairballs (**trichobezoars**) sometimes occur in dogs, cats, and ruminants; in ruminants they occur mostly in the forestomachs (Fig. 1-48) and abomasum but can also cause *small intestinal obstruction*. Enteroliths and bezoars in horses are often insignificant; apparently, they are moved about by peristalsis and are passed in the feces. They may obstruct the gut if they become impacted, usually where the colon lumen narrows or changes direction, for example, at the pelvic flexure, and the junction between the right dorsal colon and the small colon. These enterolith impactions cause acute colic and frequently colonic rupture.

Small intestinal obstruction may be caused by parasites that can form ropelike tangled masses in the lumen. This occurs in pigs and foals infested with large numbers of *ascarid nematodes*. It also occurs rarely in sheep heavily infested with *cestodes*. Impaction of the jejunum or ileum is the most common cause of small intestinal nonstrangulating obstruction in horses. Feeding of a high-fiber diet, such as coastal Bermuda grass hay, predisposes to this condition. Gravel and sand have been reported as causes of small intestinal obstruction in cattle and dogs, respectively.

Impaction of the colon is a common cause of simple intestinal obstruction. The impaction cause is often feces in dogs and cats. In horses the cause is digesta, fibrous foreign material, sand, or feces, and can be complicated by intestinal tympany from fermentation if the obstruction is complete. *Obstipation of the colon* in dogs may result from voluntarily suppressed defecation caused by pain from inflammation or neoplasia involving the prostate gland or anal sacs. Impaction with foreign bodies, such as hair or fine bones in the colon or rectum, or the result of stenosis caused by tumors or strictures, is less common. Colonic obstipation also may be associated with trauma to the pelvic area or spinal cord; it is described in Manx cats because of sacral spinal cord anomalies. **Megacolon** ensues if the obstruction persists; however, in small animals megacolon is frequently idiopathic. Examination of the syndrome in cats reveals no histologic abnormalities, and it is suggested that the underlying problem is a disturbance in the activation of smooth muscle myofilaments.

Impaction of the cecum or colon in horses occurs mostly where the lumen narrows at the pelvic flexure and transverse or small colon. Impaction may be precipitated by water deprivation, a dietary change to rough hay or chaff, or poor dentition; recurrent impaction is seen in animals with dental problems. Abnormal motility resulting from altered colonic or cecal peristalsis may explain impaction in the absence of other predisposing causes and is discussed later with pseudo-obstructions of the gut. Ingestion of indigestible *synthetic fibers* has been associated with colonic impaction. In horses grazing poorly covered sandy soils, *sand* may cause chronic colitis and diarrhea, or it may sediment, accumulate, and cause impaction at any level of the large or small colon. *Sand impaction* in horses is often associated with concurrent displacement or torsion. Ingestion of large numbers of *acorns and leaves* may also cause impaction of the intestinal tract in ruminants. Rupture of the bowel may occur if impactions are not treated, and the bowel wall becomes ischemic and devitalized.

Cecal rupture in horses occurs as a complication of impaction, or of parturition in mares. Two distinct forms of cecal rupture are described. In type 1, the cecum is filled with firm dehydrated food; in type 2, the cecum is distended with more normal digesta, often with increased amount of fluid. Type 2 is considered a rare complication of general anesthesia or administration of NSAIDs and is thought to be due to dysfunctional motility.

Physical extrinsic obstructions. Compression of intestine causing obstruction is rather common and is caused by tumors, abscesses, peritonitis, and fibrous adhesions. **Neoplasms** involve the intestine by extension from adjacent viscera, particularly the pancreas. Many abdominal tumors involve the craniodorsal part of the abdominal cavity and thus cause compression of the duodenum. Peritoneal **adhesions** are common, and fibrous bands may stretch from the wall of the bowel to some fixed point, or between two or more points along the bowel or mesentery. In these cases, obstruction develops gradually as fibrous tissue contracts and restricts or adheres the bowel to itself or other abdominal structures. Large firm masses of **abdominal fat necrosis** cause extrinsic obstruction of the small intestine, spiral colon, or descending colon and rectum of cattle. **Pedicles of some tumors**, especially *mesenteric lipomas in older horses*, occasionally entrap loops of the intestine causing obstruction and strangulation. Similarly, the **ovarian suspensory ligaments** may entrap the equine colon if the ovary is enlarged because of neoplasia or inflammation. Incarceration in hernias, discussed with other displacements of the bowel, is also a common cause of extrinsic obstruction of the gut.

Functional obstructions. Adynamic (paralytic) ileus is itself not of specific interest to the pathologist but is a rather common condition. It frequently follows abdominal surgery, especially when the intestines are handled roughly or traumatized. It is also associated with peritoneal irritation of any cause, especially peritonitis. It is the result of neurogenic reflexes that interfere with control of the inhibitory neurons of the myenteric plexus. Continual tonic discharge by these neurons inhibits contraction of circular smooth muscle and prevents peristalsis. Grossly, the intestine is distended with a mixture of gas and fluid, and the wall is flaccid. The defect may be segmental, involving short lengths of the intestinal tract, but many such segments may be involved, especially in diffuse peritonitis. Idiopathic gastric or intestinal ileus may be more common in horses during the postparturient period, and acute colic and gastric rupture may occur in mares as a complication.

Pseudo-obstruction, a clinical syndrome described mostly in dogs, in which there is *no physical occlusion of the lumen* of an impacted intestine, may result from segmental or diffuse neuromuscular dysfunction in the gut. In humans, pseudo-obstruction is classified as failure of nervous or muscular components of the intestine. In dogs, fibrosis and cellular infiltration of the tunica muscularis are the most commonly described lesions leading to pseudo-obstruction. Intestinal leiomyositis was described as the cause of intestinal pseudo-obstruction in several dogs; the consistent microscopic finding was T-lymphocyte infiltration of the muscularis with various stages of degeneration and necrosis of myofibers; the mucosa, submucosa, and neural plexuses were relatively spared. In addition to equine congenital aganglionosis discussed previously, pseudo-obstruction associated with neuronal loss or ganglioneuritis involving autonomic ganglia in the GI tract, systemic dysautonomia, and intrinsic disease of intestinal smooth muscle are recognized among domestic animals. A segment of contracted or thickened bowel may be noted as a cause of obstruction; in neurogenic disease, the affected bowel is often dilated, flaccid, and unable to maintain tone.

Megacolon in Clydesdale foals associated with *hypoganglionosis of the myenteric plexus* has been reported in 4-9-month-old foals from the United States and Australia. The timing of clinical onset of these cases suggests an acquired condition; however, the common breed suggests a genetic basis for the syndrome. The pathogenesis of the condition remains unknown. Some variation in neuron density of the dorsal colonic myenteric plexus has been reported.

Grass sickness in horses, the prototypic **dysautonomia** in domestic animals, occurs chiefly in parts of the United Kingdom, western Europe, and southern South America where it is known as *mal seco*. Anecdotal evidence suggests that cases have occurred in North America. The disease more commonly affects young horses with pasture access during the spring season, and the GI tract is most affected. Grass sickness can occur acutely as colic, tympany, and drooling with rapid progression and is nearly always fatal, usually within 7 days. The condition can also occur as chronic colic of >7 days duration, usually with weight loss or dysphagia. Horses with this form may survive with appropriate management. In acute cases, postmortem findings include gastric and small intestinal distension; often, there is esophageal ulceration caused by reflux. In chronic cases, gross lesions are often not present except for marked emaciation. There also may be impaction of the colon and cecum by dehydrated ingesta in cases of longer duration.

Characteristic *histologic lesions* are present in the intestinal and extraintestinal autonomic ganglia and include chromatolysis, nuclear eccentricity, and karyorrhexis of nerve cell bodies of both peripheral and central neurons. Neuronophagia and smooth round eosinophilic bodies or spheroids within or adjacent to perikarya are also recognized. Significant inflammation is not evident. Lesions in several brainstem nuclei have been described, albeit inconsistently. The severity of lesions has been shown to be correlated with decreased functional cholinergic responses.

Diagnosis can be confirmed in live horses by histologic evaluation of nerve cell bodies of the myenteric or submucosal plexus in surgically obtained ileal samples. Examination of the cranial celiaco-mesenteric ganglia, sympathetic thoracic chain, stellate, and/or superior cervical ganglia provide confirmation of the diagnosis in dead horses. Cytology of the cranial cervical ganglion can be a fast and reliable method for postmortem diagnosis of grass sickness. Immunohistochemical assessment of β-amyloid precursor protein in rectal biopsies may be more sensitive than conventional histologic examination for equine grass sickness diagnosis.

Clostridium botulinum has been suggested to play a role in equine dysautonomia, although this remains unconfirmed and it is not known if the presence of *C. botulinum* type C and/or type C neurotoxin represents secondary bacterial overgrowth or the cause of this syndrome. Significant changes have been described in the GI microbiome of horses with grass sickness, indicating that horses with this disease have a significantly richer, more diverse, and structurally different GI microbiota than healthy control horses. Horses with acute grass sickness have a marked reduction in plasma concentrations of cysteine and methionine, which is thought to be an indication of exposure to a neurotoxic xenobiotic. A possible heritable background has also been suggested but not proved.

Feline dysautonomia, or Key-Gaskell syndrome, is an autonomic dysfunction of unknown etiology, most common in the United Kingdom and continental Europe, with sporadic cases reported elsewhere. A similar syndrome has also been reported in a few dogs, rabbits, hares, sheep, alpacas, and llamas. Cats <3-years-old seem to be preferentially affected. Signs include depression, anorexia, reduced lacrimation and salivation, bradycardia, mydriasis, delayed pupillary light reflex, megaesophagus, constipation, or ileal impaction. Diarrhea is reported in some **dogs** with dysautonomia. The GI signs suggest *disordered motility*, and animals often succumb to the effects of regurgitation, inanition, or aspiration pneumonia, among other problems. Cases tend to occur in clusters, suggesting an environmental toxin or infectious agent. As for horses, exposure to *C. botulinum* and type C neurotoxin has been hypothesized, although no conclusive etiologic associations have been made.

Involvement of functions of both sympathetic and parasympathetic divisions of the autonomic nervous system, and of some functions under voluntary control, is reflected in the distribution of neuronal lesions in autonomic ganglia. Cranial nerve nuclei III, V, VII, and XII, ventral horns of the spinal gray matter, and dorsal root ganglia may be involved. Chromatolysis-like lesions of affected neurons seen by light microscopy have a *distinctive ultrastructural appearance* in dysautonomia: autophagocytic vacuoles, dilated cisternae, and complex stacks of smooth endoplasmic membranes are in the cytoplasm of affected cells. Neuronal lesions including neuronal loss may be transient and difficult to confirm histologically. Although the cause of feline dysautonomia remains unknown, a dietary neurotoxic mycotoxin or xenobiotic may be involved.

Intrinsic disease of intestinal smooth muscle may produce a syndrome of **intestinal sclerosis**, resembling progressive systemic sclerosis or *scleroderma* of humans. In dogs, lesions are restricted to the intestinal tract, where there is diffuse dilation of the small and large bowel. Histologically, mononuclear inflammatory cells infiltrate the smooth muscle of the bowel wall; also, there is atrophy of myofibers and fibrosis. Fibrosis of the small intestinal submucosa has also been reported in horses, and in some cases there is arteriolosclerosis. The cause is unknown, although geographical clustering of cases is described.

Intestinal displacements. Mesenteric volvulus (often referred to as mesenteric torsion) occurs commonly in suckling ruminants, swine, horses, and rarely in cats and dogs. By definition, a volvulus is a twist along the mesenteric axis of the intestine; torsion is a twist along the intestinal axis. The abdomen is distended and, upon opening the cavity, tensely dilated deep red-to-black loops of bowel are usually apparent immediately.

In *swine*, the mesentery of the small intestine and sometimes the large bowel is involved in a volvulus that is usually counterclockwise, when viewed from the ventrocaudal aspect. In volvulus involving the small and large intestines, the apex of the cecum may be pointing cranial in the cranial left quadrant of the abdomen, reflecting the rotation of ~180 degrees. In swine, mesenteric volvulus may be due to gas production from a highly fermentable substrate in the colon, and its subsequent displacement, with progression to mesenteric volvulus. Mesenteric volvulus is a common cause of sporadic sudden death in swine but may occur as a recurrent problem in a herd. Many cases of *intestinal hemorrhage syndrome* in that species are probably misdiagnosed mesenteric volvulus.

Death caused by mesenteric volvulus is common in suckling or artificially reared *calves and lambs*. In these species, vigorous ingestion of large amounts of feed over a short period may predispose to gas formation in the gut, or perhaps hypermotility, which induces volvulus. Usually, only the mucosa of the proximal duodenum and terminal ileum, cecum, and colon is spared from infarction, although occasionally volvulus is restricted to shorter segments of intestine. Similar lesions are occasionally encountered in other species.

In *dogs*, volvulus has been associated with ingestion of large quantities of food, and with exocrine pancreatic insufficiency in German Shepherds. It is occasionally accompanied by gastric volvulus.

Volvulus of various lengths of the small intestine may occur in any species, but is perhaps most prevalent in the horse, where it is a common cause of strangulation obstruction of the bowel.

The large colon of the horse is predisposed to **twisting** by its lack of mesenteric anchorage, and potential mobility. The condition is frequently referred to as large colon torsion because the twist occurs along the colonic axis. However, some authors consider this condition a true volvulus because the twist involves the mesentery between the ventral and dorsal colon at the level of the ceco-colic mesentery. The torsion begins with the right ventral colon rotating medially and dorsally (clockwise as seen from behind); the severity of the rotation can vary between 270 and 720 degrees. If the twist exceeds 360 degrees, there is obstruction of the lumen of the colon with subsequent accumulation of gas, ischemia of most of the dorsal and ventral colon wall, and eventually endotoxemia. Part of the cecum is usually incorporated in the torsion. The equine cecum alone rarely undergoes torsion, and if so, it may be related to hypoplasia of the cecocolic fold. At surgery or autopsy, the usual signs of strangulation obstruction are evident, including dilation and devitalization of the infarcted segment and distension of the cecum if it is not twisted. Postmortem rupture of the diaphragm or abdominal wall may occur because of tympany.

Duodenal sigmoid flexure volvulus is an unusual lesion of adult dairy cattle. The sigmoid flexure of the duodenum is first displaced in a dorsolateral direction, and then rotates about its omental attachment causing obstruction of the proximal small intestine and the common bile duct. The cause is unknown, but this condition has been associated with prior surgical correction of a displaced abomasum.

Intussusception involves the telescoping of one segment of bowel (the intussusceptum) into an outer sheath formed by another, usually distal, segment of gut (the intussuscipiens) (Fig. 1-49A-C). Any level of the gut with sufficient mesenteric mobility may be involved. The naming convention is that the intussusceptum is followed by the intussuscipiens; hence, an ileocolic intussusception is a normograde intussusception in which the ileum has invaginated into the colon. The *cause* is usually not apparent, although linear foreign bodies, heavy parasitism, previous intestinal surgery, enteritis, and intramural lesions such as abscesses and tumors may be associated. It also may be a *terminal, agonal,* or *postmortem event.* The history is that of partial or complete intestinal obstruction, perhaps with bloody feces, and it is most common in young animals.

Intussusception is common in *dogs,* in which most frequently it is ileocolic. It is much less common in cats. Intussusception is also moderately common in lambs, calves, and young horses, where it may involve small intestine, cecum, and colon.

The progressive invagination of the leading edge of the intussusceptum into the distal segment results in the *wall of the intussusception being composed of 3 layers*: 1) the inner entering, 2) middle returning, segment of invaginated bowel, and 3) the outer wall of the receiving segment of gut. It is limited in length by the increasing tension on the mesentery drawn into the lesion, to ~10-12 cm in small animals, and ~20-30 cm in large animals. This tension along one edge of the bowel may cause the mass to become bowed or spiraled.

Tension and compression of mesenteric veins cause the intussusceptum, or a portion of it, to undergo *venous infarction.* It swells with edema and congestion, and the adjacent apposed serosal surfaces become adherent as fibrin and inflammatory cells effuse from the affected bowel. Edema, congestion, inflammation, and adhesion quickly render the intussusception irreducible. Necrosis and gangrene of the invaginated intestine usually develop, but sometimes the intussusceptum sloughs and the remaining viable segments maintain continuity of the gut, or rarely, forms two adjacent blind ends. Intestine cranial to the obstructing intussusception may be dilated and that distal contracted and devoid of content. If obstruction is chronic or partial, there may be hypertrophy of the smooth muscle of proximal bowel. In horses, chronic ileocecal intussusception involves a relatively short (<10 cm) length of bowel. Incidental terminal, agonal, or postmortem intussusception is recognized by the relative absence of congestion, edema, and adhesion of the involuted segment of gut.

Cecal inversion, and cecocolic intussusception in the horse, with inversion of the cecum into itself, or into the right ventral colon (Fig. 1-50), may result in ischemia of the cecum and possibly part of the involved colon; if partial, ischemia usually involves the more distal cecum. Cecocolic intussusception in horses has been associated with typhlocolitis caused by *Salmonella* spp., cyathostomes, or *Anoplocephala perfoliata*.

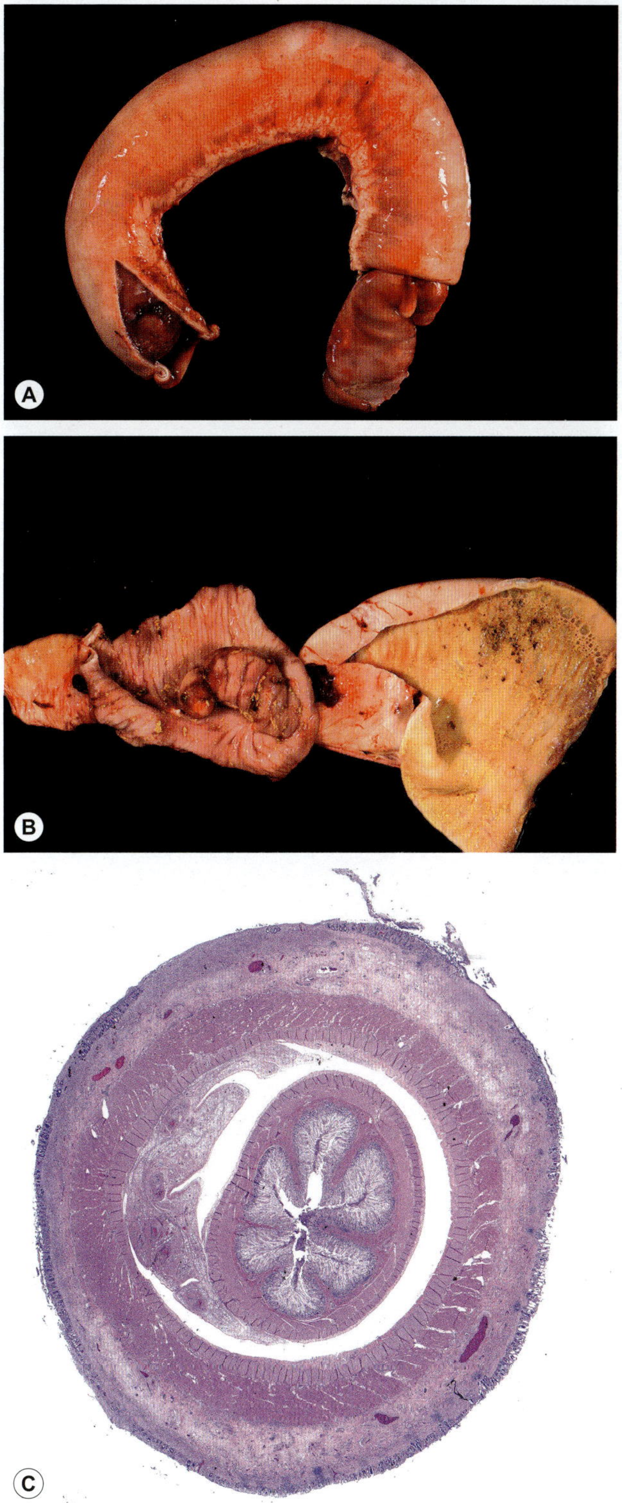

Figure 1-49 A, B. **Intussusception** of the small intestine in 2 dogs. The outer layer of the intussuscipiens has been cut away to expose the inner edematous and congested intussusceptum. (Courtesy T. Walsh.) C. Histologic section showing intussusception with the outer layer (intussuscipiens) removed.

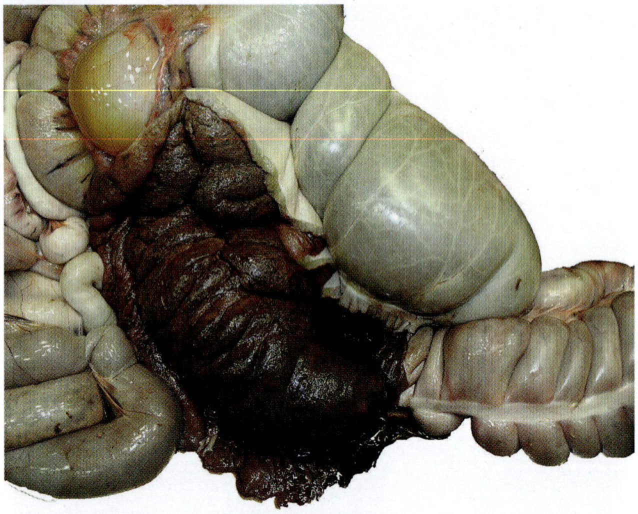

Figure 1-50 **Cecocolic intussusception** in a horse with severe cyathostominosis. The cecum has been completely invaginated into the right ventral colon (open.) The cecal mucosa is completely necrotic. (Courtesy M. Anderson.)

Segmental ischemic necrosis of the small colon may occur in pregnant or postpartum mares, because of mesenteric tension from intussusception and rectal prolapse of the distal large bowel, or perhaps because of laceration of the mesocolon and associated vessels by the feet of the foal during parturition. Colic, and intestinal obstruction, necrosis, rupture, and peritonitis may follow.

Eventration *is displacement of a portion of the gut, usually the small intestine, outside the abdominal cavity*, and it has been described in most domestic animal species. They can be congenital or acquired. Congenital eventrations may be predisposed by a congenital anomaly, as in schistosomus reflexus, patent umbilicus, and congenital diaphragmatic hernia. Acquired eventrations result from trauma and therefore are varied. The displaced intestine protrudes into the abdominal muscle or subcutis, or it may be completely exteriorized. Vaginal eventration may occasionally occur in females following trauma. Diaphragmatic eventration may occur as a consequence of diaphragmatic rupture or malformation.

Cecal and colonic dilation, tympany, torsion, and infarction. In ruminants, cecal dilation and torsion is an uncommon condition. It mainly occurs in animals fed *high-concentrate rations*, but it has been associated with late gestation and ileus from other causes. It usually occurs within 2 months postpartum in cattle. It is rare in other ruminants. About 30% of the carbohydrates in the ration are digested in the cecum of ruminants. Sudden change from a roughage to a grain-based ration results in an increase in the concentration of volatile fatty acids, with only a slight decrease in pH of the cecal contents. An increase in the concentration of dissociated volatile fatty acids, especially butyric acid, causes atony of the cecum, and dilation follows. Cecal dilation occurs more often in cattle that are not receiving mineral supplements, and in one study hypocalcemia was found in 85% of cases of cecal dilation. Although it has been suggested that calcium deficiency may cause cecal dilation, this has not been proved and it is not clear whether hypocalcemia is the cause or a result of cecal dilation. Once the cecum is dilated and distended with watery digesta, various degrees of clockwise or counterclockwise rotation can occur, which may incorporate adjacent terminal ileum or proximal colon. **Cecal infarction** is a rare condition, described in calves, and of undetermined cause. The infarction results in localized peritonitis or less frequently, in cecal perforation with secondary diffuse peritonitis and sepsis. Grossly a clearly demarcated, variably sized, discolored area of necrosis is observed around the midpoint of the cecum, usually on the antimesenteric surface. Microscopically, cecal infarction of calves is seen as transmural ischemic necrosis, with neutrophilic inflammation and thrombosis.

In horses, cecal and colonic tympany has a similar pathogenesis. Readily fermentable carbohydrate, following a sudden change in feed, results in an increase in volatile fatty acid production, which exceeds the buffering and absorptive capacity of the organ. As the pH drops, and fermentation shifts to production of the less well-absorbed butyric and lactic acids, water is drawn into the lumen by osmosis. The large bowel dilates with fluid digesta and gas, and motility is reduced by the effects of the volatile fatty acids. Severe abdominal distension, compression of intra-abdominal organs, reduced cardiac return caused by postcaval compression, and reduced respiratory capacity resulting from compression of the diaphragm may follow, with associated severe pain. Death caused by hypovolemia and acidosis may occur before the large bowel ruptures. In recovered horses, laminitis may occur because of absorption of endotoxin through the cecal mucosa, which becomes eroded and permeable as a result of local acidosis.

Internal herniation is a displacement of the intestine through normal or pathologic foramina within the abdominal cavity without the formation of a hernial sac. It is uncommon. Herniation through a natural foramen occurs mainly in horses. In *incarceration in the epiploic foramen*, a portion of small intestine, usually distal jejunum, may pass down into the omental bursa and become entrapped if the normally short and slit-like epiploic foramen of Winslow is dilated for any reason. In these circumstances, the wall of the omental bursa often ruptures. The cause of epiploic foramen incarceration is not known. Risk factors for the condition include being a Thoroughbred or Thoroughbred-cross, greater height, crib-biting or windsucking behavior, colic episodes in the previous 12 months, and prolonged periods of stall rest within 28 days before the entrapment. Infection by *C. difficile* may be another predisposing factor for this entrapment.

Omental hernia occurs when a loop of intestine passes through a tear in the greater or lesser omentum. **Mesenteric hernia** is the result of passage of intestine through a tear in the mesentery. These are probably traumatic defects and usually involve the mesentery of the small intestine, but occasionally, that of the colon.

Pelvic hernia occurs in young ruminants, and rarely in other species, following castration. During the operation, excessive traction on the spermatic cord may tear the peritoneal fold of the ductus deferens, which fixes the duct to the pelvic wall. A hiatus is formed between the ductus deferens and the lateral abdominal or pelvic walls through which loops of intestine may become incarcerated. Intestine may also become incarcerated by passing through lacerations in the lateral ligament of the bladder, or through entrapment by the remnant of a persistent urachus, by the gastrosplenic ligament, and by mesodiverticular or vitelloumbilical bands in the horse.

External hernia typically consists of a *hernial sac* formed as a pouch of parietal peritoneum; a *covering* of skin and soft tissues; depending on the location of the hernia, a *hernial ring;* and the *hernial contents*. The hernial ring is an opening in the abdominal wall, and this may be acquired, or it may be natural as, for example, the vaginal ring at the inguinal canal. The hernia usually contains a portion of omentum, a freely mobile portion of the intestine, and occasionally, other viscera.

Ventral hernia of the abdominal wall occurs uncommonly in horses, rarely in cattle, and exceptionally in other species, except perhaps following blunt trauma or biting injuries in small animals. These hernias through the abdominal musculature into the subcutaneous tissue may be spontaneous in heavily pregnant females, especially older animals, or be a consequence of blunt trauma, bite wounds, horn injuries, surgical scars, or inflammation, which cause weakening or perforation of the muscle. In pregnant mares, they often occur in the lower flank lateral to the mammae where there is only a single layer of muscle, the transverse abdominal. They may become very large in herbivores because of the weight of the alimentary viscera and pregnant uterus. The lesion must be differentiated from rupture of the prepubic tendon and from postmortem rupture of abdominal muscle in bloated animals.

Umbilical hernia is *common* and is often present as a congenital and perhaps inherited defect. It is most frequent in piglets, foals, calves, and pups, and depends on persistent patency of the umbilical ring. It is the *most common congenital defect in cattle* and has a hereditary component in the Holstein and probably other breeds. In calves, it is also significantly predisposed to by umbilical infection. The hernial sac is formed by the peritoneum and skin; the contents depend on the size of the ring and of the sac. Incarceration of the enclosed intestine is uncommon. Formation of an *enterocutaneous fistula*, a rare complication of umbilical hernia, is seen most frequently in the horse.

Inguinal hernia may evolve to **scrotal hernia** when the herniated viscera pass down the inguinal canal. The internal, or deep, inguinal ring remains patent in intact male animals, but its diameter and the tendency to herniation in the neonate may be inherited. Inguinal hernias are classified as direct or indirect. Inguinal hernias may be direct or indirect.

Direct inguinal hernias are far less common and occur when abdominal contents pass through the internal inguinal ring and come to rest in a subcutaneous position, through a tear in either the peritoneum or the fascia around the deep inguinal ring. This is mostly seen in foals and is thought to result from increased intra-abdominal pressure during passage through the birth canal. These direct inguinal hernias often cause necrosis of overlying skin, can become fixed by adhesions, and strangulate. They are life-threatening.

Indirect inguinal hernias are far more common and *consist of abdominal contents contained within the tunica vaginalis*. These occur as a congenital lesion in the young of many species, and as an acquired problem in older animals. Although size of the inguinal rings may be a factor in neonates, there is usually no apparent cause in acquired cases. The herniated viscus passes through the inguinal and vaginal rings within the vaginal sheath, coming to lie in the scrotum inside the cavity of the tunica vaginalis. If the hernia is scrotal, there may be degeneration of the testes. Routine castration of such animals can lead to eventration through the scrotal incision, and closed castration may cause infarction of the herniated loop of gut.

Congenital inguinal hernia is rare in dogs; West Highland Whites, Pekingese, and Basenjis may be predisposed, and it is more common in males than in females. However, overall, inguinal hernia is much more common in female dogs, which differ from females of other species in having a patent inguinal ring and canal through which the omentum and the uterus may pass. The herniated uterus may become incarcerated when pregnant, or if pyometra develops. In horses, indirect inguinal hernias may rupture through the inguinal canal, coming to rest in a subcutaneous location. These ruptured indirect hernias have a prognosis similar to the direct inguinal hernias described previously.

Femoral hernias develop as an outpouching of peritoneum through the femoral triangle along the course of the femoral artery. They contain omentum and small intestine.

Perineal hernias *occur principally in old male dogs in association with prostatic enlargement and obstipation*. They are precipitated by abdominal straining and are probably predisposed to by weakening of perineal fascia and muscles from some unknown cause, possibly hormonal. They are very unusual in females. Retroperitoneal pelvic fat bulges through a defect between the coccygeus medialis muscle and the cranial border of the anal sphincter. Usually, this is the only tissue to prolapse, and the lesion consists, essentially, of a loss of support on one side of the anal ring. Concomitant with the loss of pelvic support, the rectum deviates, and the prostate and the bladder may move into the pelvis. Further displacement may occur occasionally, and then the latter organs are forced through the ruptured perineal fascia, causing acute urethral obstruction. Perineal hernias are most commonly unilateral, but bilateral hernias may occur.

Diaphragmatic hernias are *common*. The defect in the diaphragm may be congenital, but most often it is acquired, generally as the result of increased abdominal pressure. Although abdominal viscera pass into the thoracic cavity, strangulation of displaced gut is rare. Acquired diaphragmatic hernias are considered more fully in the Traumatic Lesions of the Abdomen and Peritoneum section. **Prepubic hernias** occur in small animals, usually associated with severe trauma to the caudal abdomen that produces rupture of the prepubic tendon.

The **sequelae of herniation** depend largely on location and content, but some generalities apply to all hernias. As long as the hernial contents remain freely movable and reducible, there may be no untoward sequelae. Fixation of the hernial contents (*incarceration*) is a serious development, however, and may result from stenosis or tension of the hernial ring, adhesion between the contents and the sac, or distension of the herniated viscus. This distension may be due mainly to mural congestion and edema in any incarcerated viscus, accumulated gas or ingesta in the intestine, urine in a herniated bladder, and fetuses or pus in a herniated uterus. Incarcerated intestine may become obstructed or undergo ischemic necrosis and perforate, causing peritonitis. Small intestine fixed by incarceration may be predisposed to volvulus.

Displacements of the equine colon. The large colon of the horse is composed of a loop of capacious bowel joined along its length by the short mesocolon, and folded upon itself at the sternal, pelvic, and diaphragmatic flexures. The loop is only fixed at its base, by the cecum, the transverse colon, and mesenteric root. Its volume and lack of attachment make the large

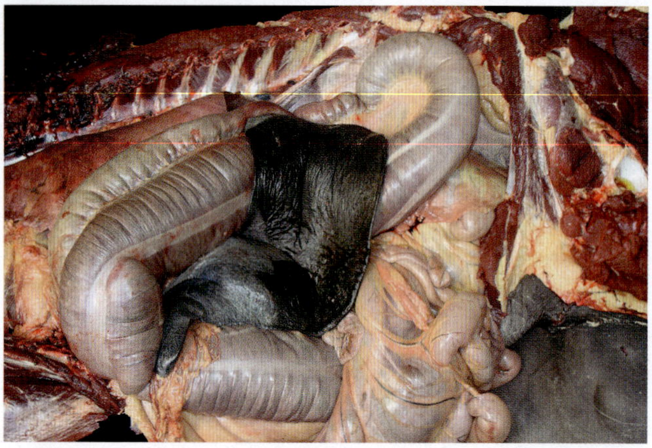

Figure 1-51 Left dorsal displacement (**nephrosplenic entrapment**) of the equine colon. The left segments of the large colon are hanging over the nephrosplenic ligament.

colon prone to displacement or torsion. Equine intestinal displacements are difficult to describe in words. The Glass Horse (see *Further reading* after this section) is an excellent resource providing 3D video animated images to aid understanding of these displacements.

Left dorsal displacement of the colon, variously known as nephrosplenic entrapment, entrapment of the colon by the nephrosplenic, renosplenic, or phrenicosplenic ligament, or by the suspensory ligament of the spleen, is also encountered as a cause of obstruction and colic in horses (Fig. 1-51, eFig. 1-7). The left dorsal and ventral large colon move laterally and dorsally between the spleen and the left body wall and become entrapped above the nephrosplenic ligament, with the spleen to the left and below, the nephrosplenic ligament below, the left kidney on the medial aspect, and the abdominal wall dorsolaterally. As the colon becomes entrapped, it may rotate along its axis with the result that the ventral colon lies dorsally and the dorsal colon lies ventrally. The colon caudal to the entrapment may become curved cranially, with the pelvic flexure rotated through 180 degrees because of tension on the taeniae. If the weight of the displaced colon is supported by the nephrosplenic ligament, compression of the splenic vein will cause splenic congestion. Compression of the colon at the point of entrapment can impair the flow of ingesta, cause local bruising or edema and partial ischemia of the displaced organ, and result in partial or complete impaction. If the gut remains patent, clinical signs are intermittent. The cecum and small intestine may be distended as a result of the colonic obstruction. The cause of left dorsal displacement is unknown but may be related to an anatomic predisposition resulting from a large cleft between the spleen and the left kidney. It is possible that occasionally this entrapment corrects itself during transportation of the carcass after death, which would explain why sometimes a displacement or other gross or microscopic lesions are not seen during autopsy in horses that were euthanized due to recurrent colic.

Right dorsal displacement of the colon involves displacement of the left segments of the large colon to the right of the abdomen. This occurs when the large colon pelvic flexure moves cranially toward the diaphragm (clockwise in the standing animal viewed from above), ending up against the right abdominal wall (eFig. 1-8). This is usually accompanied by a 180-360-degree rotation of the right side of the colon over its longitudinal axis (clockwise in the standing animal viewed from behind). Consequently, when the carcass is opened from the right side of the body, the left colons are visible first. When the carcass is opened from the left of the body, the right side of the colon and the head of the cecum are visible first. It presumably results from displacement and wedging of the large colon because of tympany. This displacement is usually preceded by impaction of the pelvic flexure, which then is bent to the left and migrates cranially in the abdomen toward the diaphragm. This is termed *right dorsal displacement with flexion*. Alternatively, the left colon may move in the opposite direction, caudal and to the right of the base of the cecum, with the pelvic flexure again lying at the sternum. This is termed *right dorsal displacement with medial flexion*. Some degree of torsion may also occur, and obstruction, with mild-to-severe colic, ensues. Surgery is required to correct the displacement, although frequently the condition is lethal.

Colonic torsion (more frequently referred to as **colonic volvulus**) *is one of the most common and grave colic causes in horses*. The loop of large colon, with or without the cecum, may rotate around itself at some point along its length, most frequently on the right dorsal and ventral parts or around the root of the mesentery. The condition is life-threatening because of severe vascular embarrassment and is discussed further under the Intestinal Ischemia and Infarction section. This torsion may be up to 360 degrees and it frequently occurs clockwise with the horse viewed from behind.

Malassimilation and protein-losing syndromes of the intestine. A number of inflammatory and/or idiopathic intestinal syndromes occur in dogs, less commonly in horses, cats, and other species; these occur variably with *chronic nonspecific diarrhea*, *weight loss*, *hypoproteinemia*, and *intestinal malabsorption*. Known collectively as protein-losing enteropathies (PLEs), by which plasma protein is lost through the GI tract lumen, they may include neoplastic or inflammatory conditions with many potential causes including genetic, dietary, idiopathic, immune-mediated, infectious, or noninfectious processes of the intestine and lymphatic system. In each syndrome, protein-rich fluid accumulates in the interstitium and eventually transits into the bowel lumen through mucosal tight junctions, sometimes without epithelial injury or ulceration. In health, lacteals and lymphatics are critical for maintaining intestinal tissue fluid homeostasis, immune cell migration, and transport of lipid-soluble substances from the intestine into the venous circulation via absorption and unidirectional flow of interstitial fluid. The lacteals located in the small intestinal villi are noncontractile blind-ended vessels into which interstitial fluid is first collected prior to its return to the venous supply; thus, drainage of fluid via lacteals is essential for resolving inflammation and fluid accumulation and maintaining homeostasis in the interstitium.

In **dogs**, PLE is mostly caused by chronic enteritis instead of primary intestinal lymphangiectasia (as in humans); PLE in dogs is associated with lymphangiectasia in 50% of cases, and lymphoplasmacytic enteritis in 66% of cases. *Endoscopic or full-thickness intestinal biopsy is usually necessary to establish a definitive diagnosis and prognosis*. These syndromes typically include one or more of several histologic lesions including abnormal lamina proprial inflammation (which may be dominated by eosinophils, lymphocytes, and plasma cells or macrophages), neoplasia (especially lymphoma), proprial amyloid deposition, structural alterations (including crypt hyperplasia and villus atrophy), and lymphatic or lacteal obstruction and dilation (lymphangiectasia) or inflammation (lymphangitis). Several known infectious causes of intestinal surface injury including erosion or ulceration need to be considered but are less common. Fungal (histoplasmosis, cryptococcosis), protozoal (giardiasis, cryptosporidiosis), oomycotic (pythiosis), algal (protothecosis), and even sequelae to severe chronic parvoviral infections may cause such a syndrome, mostly in **dogs** and **cats**. IBD in dogs and cats can be associated with PLE where clear evidence of lymphangiectasis is absent. This may be due to alterations in epithelial permeability secondary to chronic mucosal inflammation. In **horses**, chronic salmonellosis and *Lawsonia* are potential infectious causes of malassimilation and protein loss.

Causes of intestinal protein loss must be differentiated (neoplasia, inflammation, amyloidosis, lymphangiectasia), although the limitations of endoscopic intestinal biopsies should be carefully considered. When inflammatory intestinal disease is recognized histologically, specific associated or complicating agents or causes should be carefully ruled out (although etiologic agents are not always evident), and the clinical history, diet of the animal, and response to previous therapy should be investigated.

***Lymphangiectasia** can be primary or secondary and has been described most commonly in the dog, where it is a relatively rare disease of unknown etiology, and often a diagnosis by exclusion.* It has not been reported in cats, but rare cases are reported in horses. Breed predisposition seems limited to the Soft Coated Wheaten Terrier, Maltese, Shar-Pei, Yorkshire Terrier, and the Norwegian Lundehund, in which lymphangiectasia is part of a syndrome of PLE with IBD and in which gastritis and gastric neoplasia may be concurrent. The disease can occur diffusely, segmentally, or focally within the intestinal tract. **Primary lymphangiectasia** is usually idiopathic with unclear pathophysiology; potential causes include a genetic association due to breed predispositions, lymphatic hypoplasia, or other idiopathic lymphatic anomaly. **Secondary lymphangiectasia** occurs when a primary disease causes obstruction of lymphatic vessels, or when increased venous pressure induces lymphatic hypertension; in dogs, secondary lymphangiectasia is presumed to be more common, although the primary disease or actual cause of lymphatic obstruction is frequently difficult to prove definitively. Experimental obstruction of mesenteric lymphatics produces hypoproteinemia and lymphangiectasia, but not diarrhea and weight loss, suggesting that *the etiology of the clinical syndrome may be more complex than simple lymphatic obstruction.*

Regardless of the cause, lymphangiectasia is seen as dilated lacteals and lymphatics, many of which can be observed grossly, and that often rupture and leak protein-rich fluid into the proprial interstitium and bowel lumen. Malabsorbed lipid may also contribute to diarrhea via the effects of fatty acids on colonic secretion. Ultimately, a syndrome develops that variably involves *chronic diarrhea, wasting, abdominal distension, weakness; typical clinicopathologic anomalies include hypoproteinemia, lymphopenia, hypocalcemia, and hypocholesterolemia.* Mucosal permeability associated with increased proprial hydrostatic pressure likely contributes to significant plasma protein loss. Lymphopenia is thought to be the result of the loss of lymphocyte-rich lymph into the gut. Hypocalcemia is at least in part related to the loss of calcium bound to plasma albumin, altered vitamin D absorption, or formation of soaps with malabsorbed lipid in the gut lumen. Hypocholesterolemia is related to lipid malabsorption and effusion of plasma.

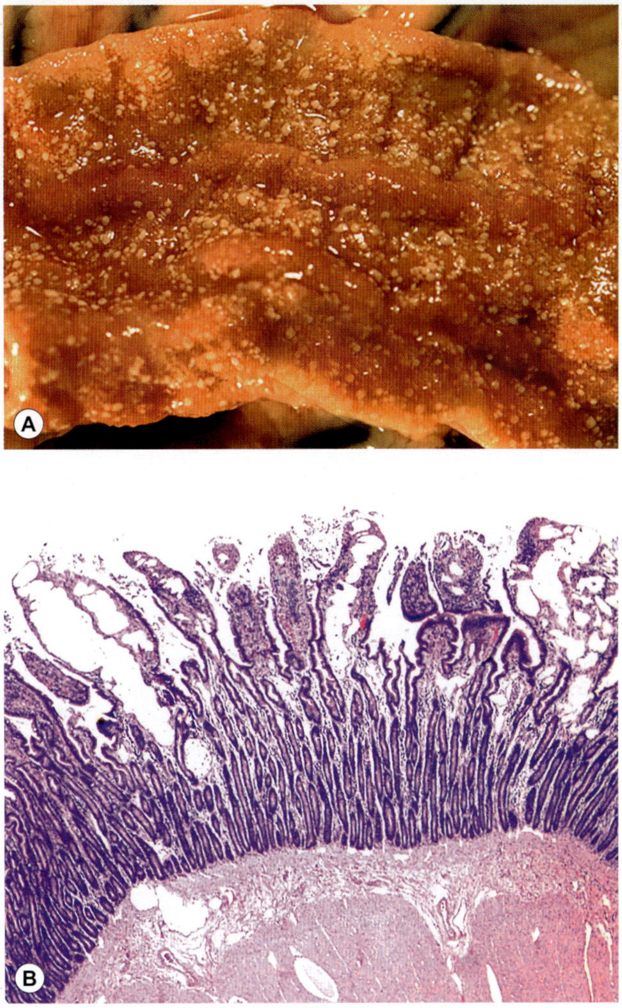

Figure 1-52 **Lymphangiectasia** in the small intestine of a dog. **A.** Mucosa, thickened by edema, is thrown into folds. Many villi contain white chyle-filled lacteals. **B.** Lacteals are dilated, and lymphatics in submucosa and muscularis are open.

The lesion in the small intestine is *dilation of lacteals and often lymphatics* of the submucosa, tunica muscularis, serosa, and mesentery. Villi containing dilated chyle-filled lacteals are often visible grossly as small white foci in a thickened, folded, and edematous mucosa (Fig. 1-52A). Serosal and mesenteric lymphatic vessels may also be prominent, dilated, and white due to accumulation of lymphocyte-rich chyle. In granulomatous lymphangitis, *white, 5-10 mm, nodules are seen grossly. Microscopically, accumulations of macrophages, multinucleate giant cells, lymphocytes, and plasma cells* may be observed on the serosa at the mesenteric border and along lymphatics; rarely, they are found on the liver, diaphragm, other abdominal organs, and pleura.

Villi may be of normal length or there may be evidence of villus atrophy and variable crypt hyperplasia; these changes likely depend on the chronicity of the inflammation. The surface epithelium may appear normal or perhaps slightly attenuated, and lateral interepithelial spaces are often dilated. The lacteals in many villi are distended (mild lacteal dilation is defined at least 50%, moderate dilation at least 75%, and severe 100% of the width of the villus), and lymphatics in deeper portions of the mucosa, submucosa, and muscularis usually are as well (see Fig. 1-52B). Occasional lipid-laden macrophages are present in and around lacteals and lymphatics. Large focal accumulations of lipid-laden macrophages surround lymphatics as a local granulomatous response to leakage of lipid or saponified fat, and along with the ectatic lacteals form the white nodules that may be evident grossly; granulomatous-to-mixed inflammation may also be present in the draining lymph nodes; lipogranulomas along lymphatic drainage tracts are variably consistent features of lymphangiectasia, and probably mostly represent a response to chronic leakage of lipid-laden chyle, rather than a cause of lymphatic obstruction. The lamina propria, submucosa, and possibly the tunica muscularis and serosa are edematous, and the proprial inflammatory cell population may be normal, or with increased lymphocytes, plasma cells, and/or eosinophils (similar to chronic IBD). Dilated crypts filled with cellular debris (so-called crypt abscesses) can be associated with lymphangiectasia; however, this is a nonspecific finding. Some degree of dilation or ectasia of lacteals can be a normal histologic finding, possibly a tissue processing or sampling artifact, so some caution should be exercised before diagnosing lymphangiectasia without evidence of inflammatory response, or of simultaneous lymphatic dilation involving the submucosa or tunica muscularis. Dilation of lymphatics is typically present in the submucosa and muscularis, so various full-thickness intestinal biopsies that include duodenal and ileal samples are much more sensitive than endoscopic biopsies for the definitive diagnosis of lymphangiectasia. A diagnostic challenge is differentiating endothelium lining blood vessels versus lymphatics or lacteals in H&E-stained tissue sections because they are often histomorphologically identical, even if erythrocytes are present in the vascular lumens. Immunohistochemical markers Prox1 and CD31 have been shown to successfully identify and distinguish lymphatic from vascular endothelium, respectively.

Focal intestinal lipogranulomatous lymphangitis is a unique and histologically discrete form of PLE, and likely of intestinal lymphangiectasia in dogs. This is an uncommon variant of chronic canine enteropathy that is thought to be secondary to chronic leakage of lipid-rich fluid from ectatic and ruptured lymphatic vessels. Patients have chronic PLE, usually with chronic diarrhea, anorexia, and weight loss. Gross changes often include thickening or nodules of the intestinal wall (which can mimic neoplasia), the mesenteric border of the small intestine, and along the serosal lymphatics (which can mimic neoplasia). Typical histologic features include variably severe lymphangiectasia, fluid- or debris-filled ectatic spaces that are intact or ruptured lymphatic vessels, along with mural-to-transmural granulomatous or lipogranulomatous lymphangitis and enteritis, often with lipogranulomas expanding the submucosa, muscularis, and serosa, and which can extend along the lymphatics into the adjacent mesenteric adipose tissue. Some chronic cases can also have significant fibroplasia surrounding the inflammatory reaction, which can cause significant luminal narrowing or stenosis. Similar granulomatous or lipogranulomatous inflammation is present in the draining lymph nodes. It is important to differentiate this from other infectious or inflammatory diseases (e.g., fungal, foreign body, other bacteria) and from neoplasia (especially lymphoma); full-thickness intestinal biopsy is generally required to confirm the diagnosis; histochemical stains may be helpful or necessary to rule out infectious causes [PAS, Grocott methenamine silver (GMS), acid fast, etc.].

Amyloidosis occurs when amyloid is deposited in the small intestine and stomach occasionally in animals with systemic amyloidosis, and although this is often an incidental lesion, GI lesions can predominate and contribute significantly to the clinical syndrome. This condition is best described in cats with familial AA amyloid deposition involving various organs and tissues such as the kidney, liver, spleen, and intestine, although the amyloid protein differs in sequence and deposition pattern; renal medullary and liver amyloid deposition in Abyssinian and Siamese cats, respectively, are the most frequent patterns. Significant intestinal amyloidosis causes malabsorption and enteric protein loss, although usually there is no gross evidence of amyloid deposits in the intestine; focal ulceration or hemorrhage may be noted occasionally. Rarely, intestinal amyloid is associated with neoplasia, including intestinal extramedullary plasmacytomas. Microscopically, amyloid is seen beneath the epithelium or expanding the propria in villi, and perhaps around or within vessels in the submucosa (Fig. 1-53). It must not be mistaken for collagen deposition, which is unusual in these locations, although a band of collagenous material is often present at the base of the mucosa in cats. The pathogenic effects of amyloid in the intestine seem to involve either impaired movement of interstitial fluid into lacteals or perhaps increased permeability of capillaries, possibly explaining protein loss into the lumen.

In **granulomatous enteritis**, *chronic inflammatory infiltrates of aggregates of histiocytes, and often multinucleate giant cells, occur in the lamina propria.* With time, the inflammatory reaction typically follows lymphatics transmurally into the submucosa and through the tunica muscularis to the serosa. The submucosa is usually edematous, and mural and serosal lymphatics are prominent. Granulomas may be present in the submucosa and along lymphatics, and affected lymph nodes are hyperplastic, usually with prominent sinus histiocytes, neutrophils, and perhaps eosinophils. Multinucleate giant cells may be present in sinusoids, and granulomas may be evident.

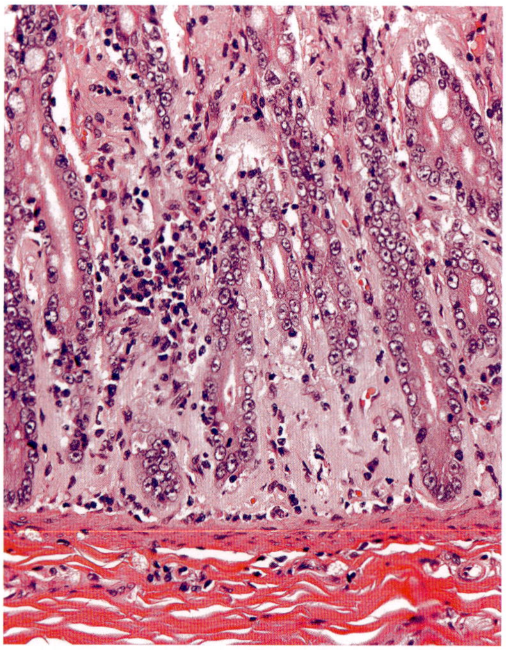

Figure 1-53 Intestine of a cat with deposits of pale amorphous **amyloid** within the deep lamina propria between crypts.

Granulomatous enteritis can potentially occur in *any species*. Paratuberculosis of ruminants, or other intestinal mycobacterioses, *Rhodococcus* sp. in horses, or other intracellular bacterial infections in various species, fungal enteritis (*Histoplasma* sp., *Cryptococcus* sp., or other fungi) in dogs and cats, and oomycotic enteritis (*Pythium* sp., *Lagenidium* sp., *Paralagenidium* sp.) in dogs and horses are several specific examples (see the Infectious and Parasitic Diseases of the Alimentary Tract section). Often the cause is not identified despite attempts to identify etiologic agents by bacterial or fungal culture, PCR assay, or histochemical stains. Advancement in next-generation metagenomic sequencing technology and its associated reduced cost has made this technique more diagnostically possible and useful, and this is likely to lead to more successful identification of specific causative agents.

Transmural granulomatous enteritis is occasionally seen in **dogs** and **cats**. It is generally segmental and perhaps discontinuous in distribution, usually affecting the lower ileum, colon, and draining lymph nodes. There is often marked necrosis at granuloma centers and extensive fibrosis; because of the extent of the attendant fibrosis, these lesions may be stenotic and must therefore be differentiated from invasive and scirrhous carcinoma.

Idiopathic granulomatous enteritis as a cause of wasting and PLE is most commonly seen as a sporadic disease in **horses**. Depending on the duration of the disease, animals may be markedly cachectic, have subcutaneous edema, especially of dependent areas, and there may be hydrothorax, hydropericardium, and ascites. Lesions in the horse usually affect the small intestine; stomach and large bowel are occasionally also involved. Mesenteric lymph nodes are usually enlarged, edematous, with mottled firm gray areas, fibrotic nodules, or, rarely caseous or mineralized foci on the cut surface. Granulomatous pale, caseous, or mineralized foci may be scattered in the liver.

Microscopic granulomatous lesions may be patchy, regional, or diffuse, and they may be mucosal, or transmural, and inflammation often ultimately gains access to draining lymph nodes. In the small intestine, associated villi are mildly to markedly atrophic, and crypts are hyperplastic. Depending on the distribution of the lesions, the epithelium may be normal, or significantly attenuated to low-columnar or cuboidal with an indistinct brush border. Surface ulceration, erosion, or even microerosions may be present through which neutrophils and proteinaceous exudate pass into the lumen. The lamina propria is edematous and contains scattered aggregates of histiocytes and perhaps giant cells, or less commonly, more organized granulomatous foci. Neutrophils and eosinophils are distributed diffusely throughout the lamina propria and may be concentrated in or near granulomatous foci. A heavy population of lymphocytes and plasma cells inhabits the lamina propria, and the infiltrate and edema may separate crypts abnormally from each other.

Miscellaneous conditions of the intestinal tract. Small intestinal bacterial overgrowth (SIBO) is defined as an absolute increase in small intestinal bacterial numbers. SIBO is a recognized entity in humans occurring secondarily to a number of underlying disorders, including hypochlorhydria, exocrine pancreatic insufficiency, hypomotility, partial small-bowel obstruction, radiation injury, or impairment of systemic and local immunity. The existence of genuine bacterial overgrowth in animals remains controversial and is rarely observed or diagnosed by pathologists. Cases of idiopathic SIBO have been described in young, large-breed dogs, and many of these have been responsive to antibiotic therapy, which suggests that the preferred (clinical) diagnosis may be **antibiotic-responsive diarrhea** (ARD). This term is more appropriate in cases that respond clinically to antibiotics and where other (infectious and neoplastic) conditions have been ruled out. Secondary SIBO, however, likely truly exists in dogs, and this term is best used in cases in which a known initiating cause or risk factor is documented. For SIBO and ARD, histologic examination of intestinal biopsies reveals no significant lesions, other than the possible presence of bacterial colonies in mucus on the mucosal surface in some cases.

Intestinal lipofuscinosis (*brown gut*) in dogs is characterized grossly by *tan-brown discoloration of the tunica muscularis* (Fig. 1-54). It may involve any segment of the intestine but is most commonly observed in the lower small intestine; the bladder and mesenteric or peripheral lymph nodes also may be affected. Although the lesion is usually incidental, it is associated with *chronic enteric and/or pancreatic disease*. Lipofuscinosis is reported in Boxer dogs with histiocytic ulcerative colitis (HUC), but a definitive correlation between the 2 conditions has not been established. Increased prevalence of lipofuscinosis has also been reported in dogs consuming high levels of polyunsaturated fats with a *relative deficiency of vitamin E;* the condition is prevented by vitamin E supplementation. Any condition, such as exocrine pancreatic insufficiency, that causes a reduction in the absorption of fats and fat-soluble vitamins, especially in the presence of polyunsaturated fatty acids in the diet, may predispose to lipofuscinosis.

The microscopic lesions of intestinal lipofuscinosis are gray-to-brown granules in the cytoplasm of smooth muscle cells in the tunica muscularis; the reason they tend to accumulate here is unknown. The granules stain positively by PAS and Sudan, are weakly acid-fast with Ziehl-Neelsen, and are

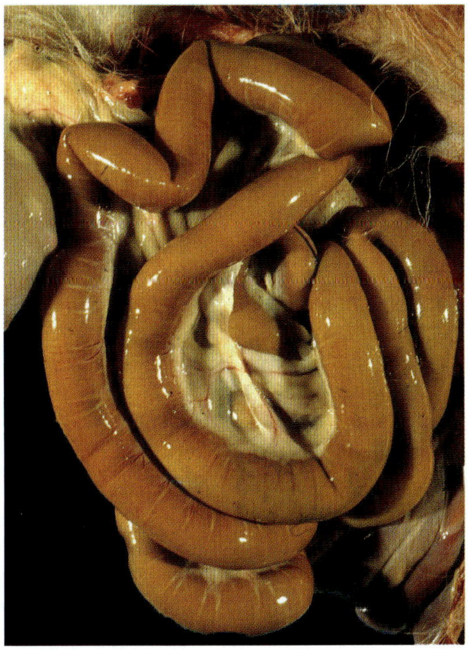

Figure 1-54 Intestinal lipofuscinosis, discoloring the small intestine to a tan hue in a dog.

mildly fluorescent in paraffin section. The granules are termed *leiomyometaplasts*, are oxidized polymerized phospholipids derived from cell membrane lipid peroxidation, and are highly resistant to further endophagocytic degradation. In Cocker Spaniel dogs affected with the inherited storage disease *generalized ceroid-lipofuscinosis*, intestinal lipofuscinosis is also observed and is often accompanied by progressive hindlimb paresis and incoordination.

Muscle hypertrophy of the intestine was historically a common finding in **swine**, but it appears to have diminished in prevalence in most areas. It may be found in apparently healthy swine at slaughter as a uniform thickening of the muscle layers of the *terminal ileum*; the distal 25-50 cm of the small intestine may be involved. The ileum is thickened and turgid; the lumen is small; the tunica muscularis in particular is markedly thickened and the mucosa is folded. This condition must be differentiated from proliferative enteropathy associated with *Lawsonia* infection in swine. *Perforation or rupture* of the intestine may occur following feed impaction in the thickened segment; this may be a secondary to the formation of pseudodiverticula, or as the result of violent peristalsis through the affected and variably obstructed small intestinal segment. Although the underlying basis remains obscure, it is likely that the muscle hypertrophy is secondary to functional obstruction of the ileocecal orifice.

Idiopathic muscle hypertrophy of the distal small intestine also occurs in **horses** (Fig. 1-55A). A similar lesion has been associated with *Anoplocephala* sp. tapeworms at the ileocecal orifice; however, this remains uncertain because many cases also show significant muscle hypertrophy of the *terminal esophagus* (see Fig. 1-55B). The lesions are similar to those described in swine, and the *ileum is the most common site*; however, any segment of the small intestine, and occasionally the large intestine, can be affected. Horses with this condition may have chronic mild colic and anorexia or intermittent diarrhea with progressive loss of weight. Diverticula, and perforation or laceration of the thickened intestinal wall, may also occur.

Idiopathic intestinal smooth muscle hyperplasia has been described in a **goat** and, unlike the condition in horses and swine, only the jejunum was affected.

Pseudodiverticulosis of the small intestine is a rare lesion that is sometimes associated with muscle hypertrophy in pigs and horses. Single or multiple saccular dilations lined by intestinal mucosal epithelium (but not tunica muscularis) are formed secondary to defects in the tunica muscularis and subserosa of the small intestine. Pseudodiverticula (false pulsion diverticula) are distinguished from true diverticula, which are congenital defects involving all layers of the intestinal wall, and they tend to follow the pathway of blood vessels and are mainly located adjacent to the mesenteric attachment.

Intestinal emphysema, or *pneumatosis cystoides intestinalis*, is a rare condition found mainly in weaned *pigs*, in which it is usually an incidental finding in slaughtered animals (Fig. 1-56). Numerous thin-walled gas-filled cystic structures a few millimeters to several centimeters in diameter occur within the intestinal wall and on the serosal surface. These are mainly located in the small intestine, although the large intestine, mesentery, and mesenteric lymph nodes may be involved. Microscopically, the cystic structures appear to be *dilated lymphatics* that are located in the lamina propria,

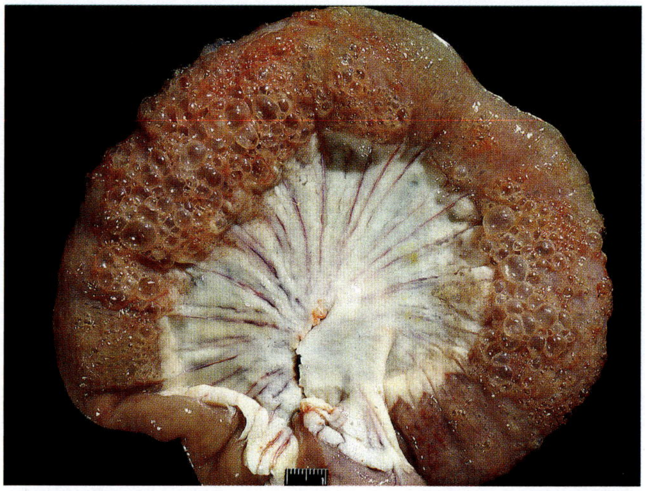

Figure 1-56 Intestinal emphysema in a pig. (Courtesy P. Stromberg.)

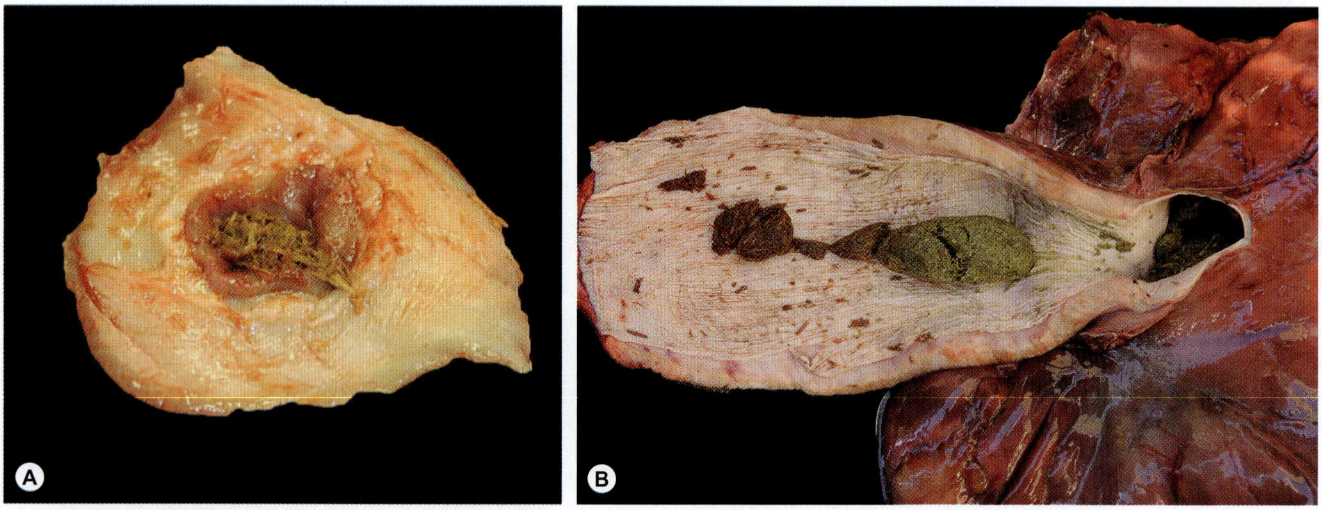

Figure 1-55 A. **Muscle hypertrophy** in the ileum of a horse, cross section. **B.** Idiopathic muscle hypertrophy in the esophagus of a horse, longitudinal section.

submucosa, muscularis, subserosa, mesentery, and mesenteric lymph nodes. A mixed cellular inflammatory reaction may be evident in the walls of the cysts. Although production of gas by bacteria has been implicated, the cause remains obscure.

Jejunal hematoma (hemorrhagic bowel syndrome, intestinal hematoma) has been described mainly in adult lactating *dairy cattle* in North America, with occasional reports from Europe, the Middle East, and South America. The syndrome is usually seen clinically as sudden death, although a few affected animals may have blood in their feces, bloat, and acute abdominal pain for a short time before death. At autopsy, there are one or more short jejunal loops with intramural segmental hemorrhage and luminal clot formation (Fig. 1-57A). The hemorrhage usually distends the intestinal mucosa to the point of complete or partial obstruction of the intestinal lumen (see Fig. 1-57B). Determination of the primary location of the hemorrhage (intramural vs. intraluminal) requires careful dissection, as in the cases of intramural hemorrhage, the compressed and thin intestinal mucosa frequently tears when the intestine is opened, giving the false impression that the blood is intraluminal rather than intramural. *Microscopically*, the interface between the hematoma and nonhematoma portions of the jejunum has an abrupt elevation of the mucosa, and the muscularis mucosa is often split by severe hemorrhage, with one portion adherent to the submucosa and the other to the lamina propria. The elevated mucosa may be completely necrotic or have only necrosis of the surface epithelium (see Fig. 1-57C). Often, the affected mucosa has moderate-to-large numbers of large, gram-positive rods on the luminal surface. Because the percentage of gram-positive rods was found to increase with the degree of autolysis, it has been postulated that this bacterial population is a consequence rather than a cause of the condition. The affected mucosa, but also the more normal-looking adjacent mucosa, has dilated villus lacteals that are either empty or contain abundant erythrocytes and/or pale eosinophilic, hyalinized material. Occasionally, there are small numbers of hemosiderophages in the lamina propria of the affected mucosa. In a few cases, the mucosa may have mild-to-moderate edema, mild neutrophilic infiltration, and small foci of submucosal hemorrhage. Submucosal blood vessels in these areas are usually within normal limits, but a small percentage of cases may have mild-to-moderate vasculopathy with hyaline change of the vessel wall, mild pleocellular perivascular and subintimal inflammatory infiltrates, and plump lining endothelium. Focal neutrophilic peritonitis can rarely be seen in the affected areas of the jejunum. The cause of this entity is not known.

A study of a large number of cases of jejunal hematoma and normal cows did not find a statistically significant relationship between the isolation of *C. perfringens*, *C. perfringens* type A, or the *cpb2* gene and jejunal hematoma, strongly suggesting that *C. perfringens* is not associated with this condition. *Aspergillus fumigatus* has also been hypothesized to play a role due to the fungus in tissue and blood of affected cows; however, this has not been supported by additional studies. No association was found between jejunal hematoma and BVDV, *Salmonella* sp., or copper levels. Dietary factors and high milk yield are associated with jejunal hematoma syndrome, so altered small intestinal microbiome may be a significant predisposing factor. Erosions or lacerations have been suggested as early-stage

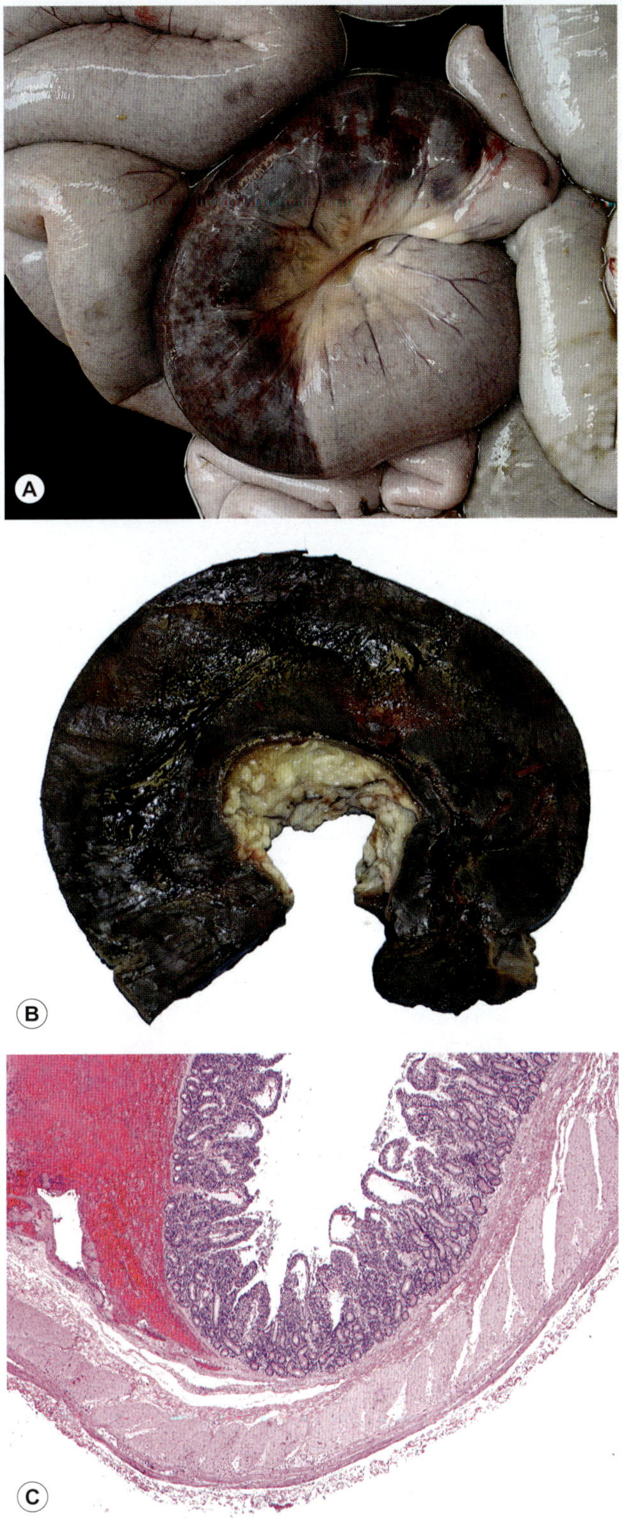

Figure 1-57 Jejunal hematoma (**hemorrhagic bowel syndrome**) in a dairy cow. **A.** Serosal view of hemorrhage in a jejunal loop. **B.** Mucosal view, there is severe intramural hemorrhage with only a narrow remnant of the lumen. **C.** Histologic section with hemorrhage and hematoma splitting the muscularis mucosa. (C from Adaska JM, et al. Jejunal hematoma in cattle: a retrospective case analysis. J Vet Diagn Invest 2014;26:96–103.)

lesions that may progress to mural and luminal hematoma formation. The hematomas seem to occur via propagation of dissecting hemorrhage within the muscularis mucosa; however, the cause of these surface microlesions was not determined; etiologic or infectious agents are unlikely to be primary causes of this disease.

Terminal (regional) ileitis of lambs is a syndrome of unknown etiology, with reduced weight gain, diarrhea, and apparent abdominal pain, usually in 1-4-month-old animals. It is reported from the United Kingdom, continental Europe, and North America. At autopsy, animals are typically in poor body condition, with evidence of diarrhea. There is marked enlargement of the caudal small intestinal mesenteric lymph node. The terminal small intestine is thickened, with transmural edema and a corrugated appearance on the serosal aspect. The mucosa is reddened and thrown into thick transverse nodular folds. There may be superficial erosion and fibrin exudation. The mucosa of the cecum and spiral colon also may be grossly thickened.

Microscopic lesions are always evident in the ileum and consist of moderate-to-severe villus atrophy, crypt hypertrophy, hyperplasia of crypt epithelium, and a heavy mixed inflammatory cell infiltrate in the lamina propria. Microerosions or ulcers may be present, through which neutrophils exude. In the large intestine, the crypt epithelium is hyperplastic, causing thickening of the mucosa, which is infiltrated by a mixed, mainly mononuclear, inflammatory cell population, and is thrown into folds superficially. Peyer patches and submucosal lymphoid aggregates are hypertrophic, with lymphoid hyperplasia.

Intestinal encephalopathy with clinical signs and lesions similar to those traditionally seen in hepatic encephalopathy has been described in horses with colic and/or diarrhea but no hepatic disease. Because those horses had hyperammonemia, it was speculated that this was a consequence of excessive production and absorption of ammonia in the intestine secondary to altered microbial communities associated with intestinal disease. Intestinal overgrowth of ammonia-producing bacteria or reduced populations of ammonia-metabolizing bacteria may be responsible. Hyperammonemic encephalopathy has been described as a rare consequence in horses with intestinal disease due to betacoronaviral infection. An investigation of 13 documented cases of this syndrome did not find any breed, age, sex, or dietary predisposition. As in cases of hyperammonemic encephalopathy related to hepatic or renal disease, the most common microscopic finding in the brain of horses with the disease is the presence of Alzheimer type II astrocytes in the cerebral cortex. In addition to hyperammonemia, laboratory findings often include metabolic acidosis and hyperglycemia.

Several toxic plants are known to cause significant GI lesions, mostly in livestock in various parts the world. ***Baccharis coridifolia*** and ***Baccharis megapotamica*** are found in several South American countries and are some of the most common poisonous plants affecting mostly livestock species and horses in Argentina, Brazil, and Uruguay. ***Baccharis pteronioides*** has been implicated in similar livestock poisoning in the southwestern United States. The numerous toxic principles of these plants include the macrocyclic trichothecene complex of antibiotics. The clinical syndrome produced by both plants is similar and includes dullness, abdominal pain, dehydration, recumbency, dyspnea, and acute death. Gross findings include abundant liquid rumen content, multifocal hemorrhages on serosae of omasum, rumen, lungs, and heart; there are also ulcers on the mucosal surfaces of forestomachs and intestine, as well as myocardial and renal hemorrhage. Major histologic lesions include extensive hemorrhagic necrosis, neutrophilic inflammation, thrombosis, and edema of forestomachs, widespread lymphoid necrosis, and renal tubular necrosis and mineralization.

Chinaberry tree (*Melia azedarach*) is cultivated worldwide as an ornamental plant, which has caused intoxication in pigs, cattle, sheep, goats, and dogs; pigs seem to be most susceptible. The toxic principles (melia toxins A1, A2, B1, B2) are concentrated in the fruit. Neurologic and/or GI clinical signs develop within a few hours of ingestion of the fruits. The former include excitement or depression, convulsions, ataxia, paresis, and coma. GI signs include anorexia, vomiting, constipation, or diarrhea, frequently bloody, and colic. Grossly, the changes observed in different animal species are similar and include intestinal congestion, yellow discoloration of the liver, and brain congestion. *Microscopically*, there is individual cell necrosis randomly distributed throughout the parenchyma or concentrated in the centrilobular zone of the liver, degenerative and necrotic changes in the epithelium of the forestomachs, and lymphoid necrosis.

Oleander toxicosis occurs in several mammalian species, including sheep, goats, cattle, camelids, monkeys, equids, and humans. In addition to the main cardiac lesion produced by intoxication with *Nerium oleander*, intestinal changes are frequently observed in several animal species. In horses and ruminants, it is thought that the changes in the alimentary tract are primarily caused by the highly irritant effect of *oleandrin*, the main glycoside present in oleander. However, it is possible that hypoperfusion caused by cardiac failure contributes to these changes. In a study of 30 equids referred to a veterinary teaching hospital with a diagnosis of oleander intoxication, 85% had GI signs including colic, diarrhea, gastric reflux, intestinal hyper- or hypomotility, and abdominal distension. Gross changes in the alimentary tract of horses and ruminants with oleander intoxication include hemorrhage (Fig. 1-58), edema, and occasionally surface necrosis and pseudomembrane formation in the small intestine. Histologic changes include hyperemia and hemorrhage of the mucosa in the small and/or large intestine, although neutrophilic and/or fibrinonecrotizing enteritis can be seen in more advanced cases.

Astylus atromaculatus is a native beetle of South America that feeds mostly on pollen of crops, but also other plants

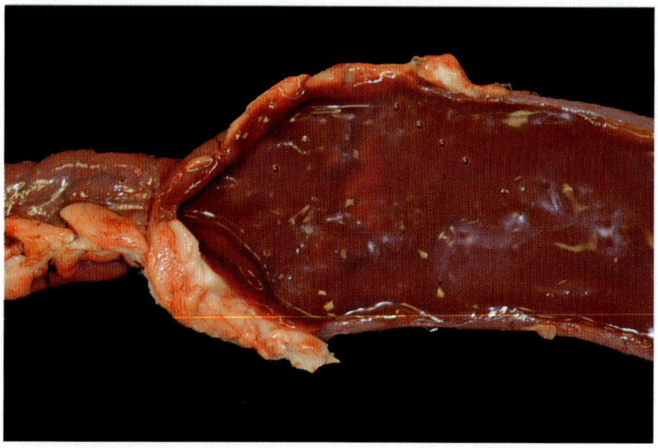

Figure 1-58 Oleander intoxication in a llama. The mucosa of the small intestine is severely hyperemic and hemorrhagic.

(eFig. 1-9A). During a severe drought in the summer of 2022-23 affecting central Argentina and Uruguay, there were several cases of necrotizing enteritis in cattle and sheep associated with ingestion of large numbers of these beetles that were present in the pastures where these animals were grazing. The heavy contamination of the pastures was probably associated with the drought, which reduced significantly the availability of flowers in the crops. The lesions involved mostly the small intestine where multifocal and severe necrotizing enteritis was observed (see eFig. 1-9B and C). Although a toxic substance present in *A. atromaculatus* is suspected to be responsible for the intestinal lesions, a toxic principle of the beetle has not yet been found. Other possible explanations for the mechanism of action of *A. atromaculatus* include initial mechanical injury to the intestinal mucosa by the chitinous exoskeleton of the insects, followed by secondary bacteria invasion, and an allergic reaction to the beetles.

Inflammatory and other syndromes of the large intestine. Various pathologic processes including ischemia, necrosis of the proliferative epithelium by etiologic agents, severe inflammation, and several luminal toxins are responsible for development of focal or diffuse lesions involving the large intestine. Inflammatory infiltrates in the lamina propria are classified based on the inflammatory cell phenotype and may be limited in distribution to the mucosa or be transmural involving all layers of the intestinal wall, and frequently involve the draining lymph nodes. *Typhlitis* and *colitis* may be manifestations of a generalized disease; they may be part of *enterocolitis* involving both small and large intestine, or they may be regional and limited to any specific segment or segments of the intestine. Damaged colonic mucosa provides a potential portal of entry for cross-mucosal translocation of bacteria or toxins. Increased mucosal permeability in the colon permits enteric loss of plasma protein or blood. Colonic flora dysbacteriosis, especially in hindgut fermenters, compromises uptake of volatile fatty acids and water. In any species, damage to the colonic mucosa results in malabsorption of electrolytes and water or altered secretion.

Granulomatous or histiocytic ulcerative colitis. Histiocytic colitis of Boxers and French Bulldogs (HCBF) is a distinctive syndrome described mostly in young Boxers and French Bulldogs. The disease was first described in Boxer dogs (as idiopathic Boxer colitis), then French bulldogs were also observed to be overrepresented; however, isolated cases have been described in various canine breeds. Clinical signs typically include bloody and mucus-rich diarrhea, anemia, hypoalbuminemia, weight loss, and chronic cachexia. The colon of affected dogs with advanced disease is ulcerated, variably thickened, folded, and perhaps dilated and shortened with some segmental or focal areas of scarring and stricture. Mucosal lesions vary from patchy punctate red ulcers to more extensive irregular circular or linear coalescing ulcers, with islands of remnant surface mucosa. The *histologic lesions* are the unique and defining feature of this disease and include severe mucosal ulceration, goblet cell loss, and infiltration of the lamina propria and submucosa by predominantly macrophages or histiocytes (Fig. 1-59A and B) containing abundant cytoplasmic PAS-positive material (see Fig. 1-59C). These cells are also found within and surrounding lymphatics of the tunica muscularis and serosal surface. Their presence in draining lymph nodes, along with lymphoid hyperplasia, explains the localized or generalized lymphadenopathy that often accompanies this syndrome. The cecum can also be involved with similar lesions, although often to a lesser degree.

This condition was long regarded as an idiopathic and possibly immune-mediated disease, although with some reported clinical response to antimicrobials but not corticosteroids, suggesting for decades that bacterial infection was the underlying cause. Intramucosal colonization by selective invasive strains of *Escherichia coli* has been demonstrated; affected dogs have been shown to have impaired killing ability of *E. coli*. The diagnosis is confirmed by visualization of bacteria individually or clustered within phagocytic vacuoles of colonic macrophages via fluorescence in situ hybridization (FISH) in tissue sections (see Fig. 1-59D); traditional chromogenic IHC can also be utilized to confirm the diagnosis. Bacterial strains isolated from affected dogs are able to invade epithelial cells, persist in macrophages, or both. Long-term clinical remission has been demonstrated in cases of HUC of Boxer dogs following eradication of the invasive *E. coli* using appropriate antibacterial therapy, usually fluoroquinolone antibiotics. However, antibiotic resistance, especially to enrofloxacin, has been correlated with invasive *E. coli* isolated from Boxer dogs with nonresponsive or refractory disease. Antimicrobial treatment *guided by susceptibility profiling of E. coli organisms* identified by deep intestinal tissue bacterial culture is strongly associated with a long-term positive outcome in most cases. Severe acute necrotizing colitis and, less commonly, typhlitis or gastritis leading to *ulceration and perforation* has been associated with functional adrenocortical tumors or exogenous glucocorticoid administration, especially following trauma or surgery involving the spinal cord. Perforations can occur anywhere in the colon, but usually occur along the antimesenteric border of the left colonic flexure or proximal descending colon. The pathogenesis of these lesions remains unclear.

Granulomatous or histiocytic colitis of cats is also associated with adherent-invasive *E. coli* (AIEC), which has also been implicated as a cause of malakoplakia of the vagina and urinary bladder in cats. This is probably a rare disease of cats, usually with an elongated history of vomiting, large-bowel diarrhea, hematochezia, mucoid feces, enlarged lymph nodes, and weight loss due to a grossly thickened and ulcerated colonic wall. Histologic lesions are similar to those described in dogs and include ulceration of the colonic mucosa and transmural infiltration of foamy PAS-positive macrophages, along with other mixed leukocytes. Breed predispositions have not been documented yet in cats, although affected breeds have included Oriental Shorthair and Sphynx.

Rectal prolapse occurs most commonly in *swine, sheep*, and *cattle*. It may occur in any animal that has *prolonged episodes of tenesmus or excessive coughing, which increases abdominal pressure*, and is often associated with colitis or lower urinary tract infection or obstruction. In pigs, rectal prolapse occurs more broadly in a herd when the ration contains *zearalenone*, an estrogenic mycotoxin produced by fungi of the genus *Fusarium*. The toxin causes marked swelling and congestion of the vulva and vaginal mucosa, straining, and eventually vaginal and/or rectal prolapse. *Rectal prolapse in sheep* may be the consequence of ingestion of estrogenic pastures and is accompanied by other signs of hyperestrogenism (see Vol. 3, Female Genital System).

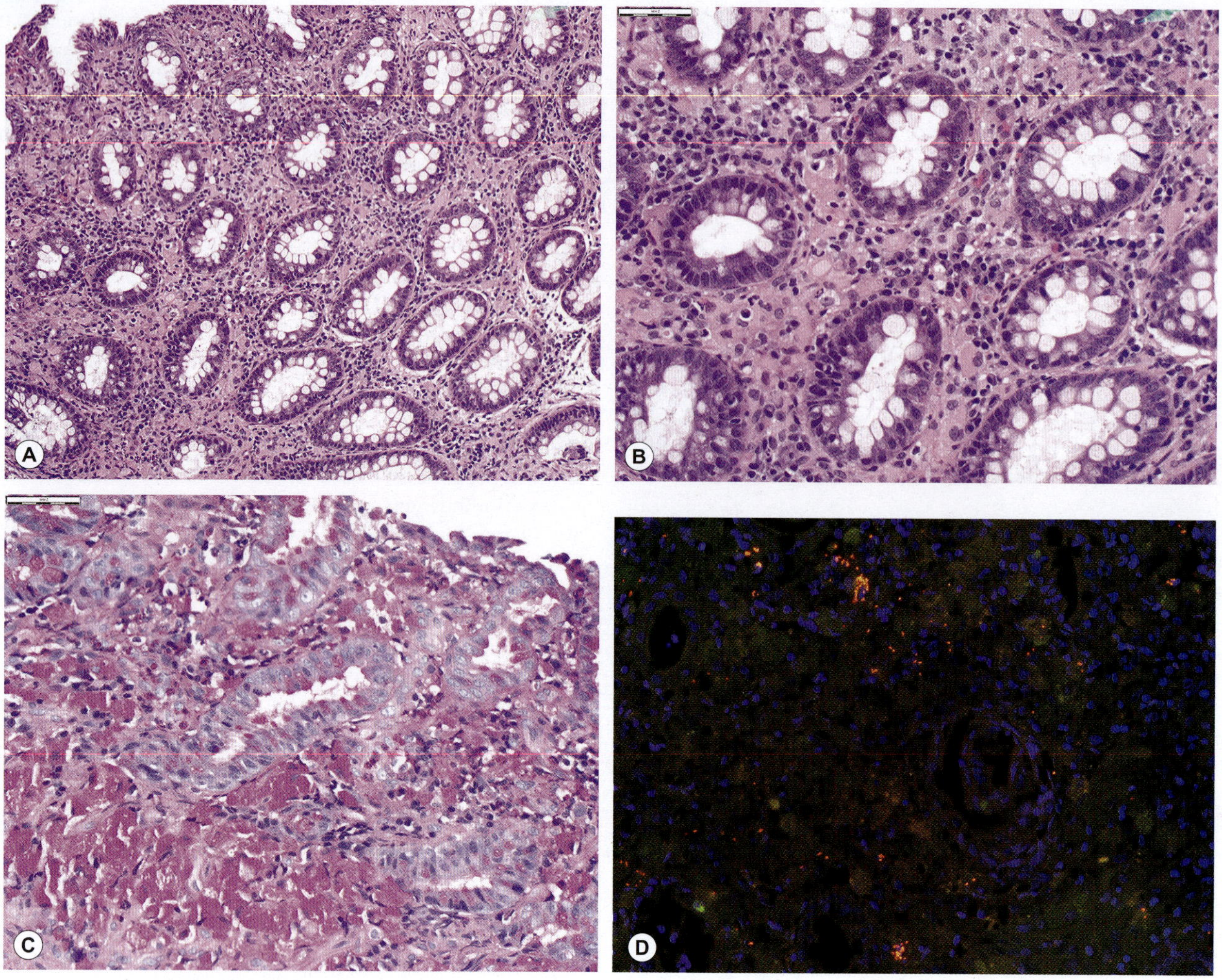

Figure 1-59 **Histiocytic ulcerative colitis** in a Boxer dog. **A, B**. Accumulation of macrophages with abundant cytoplasm throughout mucosa, between base of glands. **C**. Periodic-acid Schiff stain shows positive cytoplasmic staining in proprial macrophages. **D**. Fluorescence in situ hybridization confirms invasive *Escherichia coli* (*E. coli* FISH probe, Cy3 red) within the colon. (D, Courtesy K.W. Simpson.)

The prolapsed rectum is edematous and congested, and there may be necrosis and ulceration of the everted mucosa. These lesions are ischemic in origin owing to interference with venous blood flow from the prolapsed section. The prolapse may involve only the mucosa or all layers of the bowel. In swine surviving slough or amputation of the prolapsed tissue, *rectal stricture* may ensue.

Miscellaneous inflammatory syndromes of the small and large intestine. Mostly dogs and cats, and less commonly cattle and horses, with evidence of malabsorption and/or plasma loss into the GI tract, have microscopic lesions in the mucosa of the small intestine described as *chronic inflammatory bowel disease, lymphocytic-plasmacytic or eosinophilic enteritis, or gastroenteritis*. Eosinophilic gastroenteritis in cats and horses can be a manifestation of systemic eosinophilic syndromes affecting those species. In dogs and cats, IBD continues to be a significantly challenging area for diagnostic pathologists, especially when presented with small endoscopic biopsy samples. In general, for dogs and cats, and probably for other species as well, there is limited correlation between histologic lesions or histologic scores of inflammation in the intestinal tract and clinical signs or clinical activity, and thus patients may have quite variable clinical signs along various scoring systems. This is greatly exacerbated and confused by a general lack of definitive standards for assessing inflammation in the intestinal tract, although several scoring systems have emphasized various histologic features. In the following section, we summarize the current understanding of idiopathic IBD in domestic species (dogs and cats in particular), including several specific disease variants in these species, and discuss various significant challenges and helpful tips for attaining a definitive diagnosis with the tools available to clinicians and pathologists.

Inflammatory bowel disease (IBD) is a clinical syndrome that refers broadly to chronic GI disorders characterized histologically by inflammation. In some cases, a specific cause or etiologic agent is identified, but most cases are idiopathic and presumed to represent GI mucosal immune dysregulation that may be directed to pathogenic or commensal bacteria (or their metabolic byproducts), environmental antigens, or underlying host immune dysfunctions or altered responsiveness. *IBD is one or more of the variants of chronic enteropathy that are distinguished from food- or* *diet-responsive enteropathy, and from antibiotic-associated enteropathy, by their positive clinical response to immunosuppressive therapy but not to dietary or antibiotic therapy alone.* A clinical distinction is often made (at least in dogs) among diet-responsive enteropathy, antibiotic-responsive enteropathy, and IBD, but no studies have demonstrated significant distinguishing histologic GI lesions between them, although intestinal microbiota distinctions have been described. It has proven difficult to develop valid and objective histologic criteria that establish a definitive diagnosis; hence, histologic changes should be interpreted by the clinician in the context of the clinical scenario, response to attempted therapy, and a diagnosis of IBD should be considered only after alternatives such as food intolerance, motility disorders, parasitism, various infectious diseases, and neoplasia (particularly lymphoma) have been ruled out. *IBD is defined as chronic (>3 weeks) history of persistent or recurrent diarrhea or vomiting, weight loss, or altered appetite; histologic evidence of inflammatory cellular infiltrate (although specific criteria have not been universally accepted); lack of evidence for alternative explanations or causes of GI inflammation; lack of response to therapeutic attempts including anthelmintics, antimicrobials, or diet; and a positive clinical response to anti-inflammatory or immunosuppressive therapy.*

The etiopathogenesis of idiopathic IBD is not well understood in any species. It is likely that various factors, including genetics, mucosal immunity, intestinal microbiota, diet, and environment, play a role in pathogenesis. A familial role in dogs has been established for some enteropathies in various breeds, including Boxers, Basenjis, German Shepherds, Rottweilers, and Irish Setters. As molecular techniques to detect intestinal microbes continue to improve, alterations in the intestinal microbial communities in dogs and cats have been described in dogs with intestinal inflammation; in particular, shifts have been noted in major microbial constituents from gram-positive *Firmicutes* species, such as the genus *Faecalibacterium*, to gram-negative proteobacteria in healthy animals compared with those with intestinal inflammation. Although the mechanisms remain unknown, these alterations in the composition of the intestinal microbiome have been termed *dysbiosis*, which seems to be correlated with mucosal inflammation and may drive persistent inflammation. The data have not been universally encouraging, although clinical signs of chronic enteropathy have improved in dogs after fecal microbial transplantation, suggesting a prominent role for dysbiosis in the pathogenesis of IBD. Potential pathogens, such as invasive species of *E. coli* in Boxer dogs and French Bulldogs (and cats) with granulomatous or histiocytic colitis, have been identified. Diet also appears to be important in some cases, and a significant percentage of dogs and cats with chronic enteropathy respond favorably to dietary changes. An immunologic basis for this sensitivity is not always determined, however, so *adverse food reaction* is a more appropriate term than food allergy.

The nature of the inflammatory infiltrate suggests that the loss of tolerance to dietary antigen or antigens produced by the enteric microflora may be implicated, and regulation of innate immune responses may be important during initial loss of mucosal tolerance in dog and cats. Changes in mucosal dendritic cell phenotype and frequency, or in T lymphocyte activity in the mucosa have been detected in dogs with IBD, suggesting altered antigen sampling and subsequent adaptive immune responses; specifically, reduced regulatory T lymphocytes in dogs have been shown to play a role in the loss of tolerance to luminal antigens, increased recruitment of inflammatory cells, and histologic progression of mucosal inflammation.

Lymphocytic-plasmacytic enteritis associated with *familial sensitivity to wheat protein* has been demonstrated in Irish Setters. In Basenjis and in the Norwegian Lundehund, syndromes of hypoalbuminemia, chronic diarrhea, and wasting occur with high prevalence, primarily attributable to lymphocytic-plasmacytic enteritis, with lymphangiectasia in some dogs. Hypergammaglobulinemia commonly occurs in the late stages of the syndrome in Basenjis, and lymphoma develops in a low number of affected animals.

The thoroughness of the clinical and laboratory investigation before the use of endoscopic biopsy for histologic evaluation is influenced by the amount of time and money available to evaluate what are often elusive clinical entities. Endoscopic biopsies are often performed only after empirical dietary or medical therapy has failed to control clinical signs. The microscopic findings commonly associated with IBD lack specificity and reflect chronic mucosal inflammation, which can be the result of several potential causes or etiologies. It is usually not appropriate for a pathologist to issue a definitive diagnosis of IBD without extensive clinical history and in consultation with clinical veterinarians; it is almost always preferred to simply list the histologic findings and to indicate that the changes *could be compatible with a clinical diagnosis of IBD*, which is *a diagnosis by exclusion*. This is a complex diagnostic journey, and clinical veterinarians must play a significant role in ultimately arriving at a diagnosis of IBD.

The **limitations of interpretation of histologic GI samples** should be considered carefully and always kept in mind as we approach the challenge of assessing what are often subtle histologic lesions in these fragile tissues. Ultimately, without an accepted standard of normal, distinguishing true inflammation from normal tissue, and from neoplasia (especially lymphoma) is often difficult and even impossible at times, especially given the great variability in species, breed, specific anatomic localization, age, and other factors. There are significant advantages of endoscopy compared with laparoscopy, including reduced invasiveness and risk to the patient, and increased ability to acquire more individual samples (especially important for IBD, which can be multifocally distributed within the GI tract); however, several additional unique limitations of endoscopy also add confusion to histologic interpretation. These include the type of equipment utilized (limited reach or access to certain anatomic regions of the GI tract; rigid vs. flexible endoscopes; various types of biopsy forceps); expertise of the endoscope operator; surgical tissue artifacts induced during sampling or tissue processing (crush, fragmentation, orientation, etc.); expertise and experience of the pathologist; and even in the best of scenarios, samples obtained are superficial (they typically include only mucosa) and fragile. Some forms of chronic enteropathy are simply impossible to diagnose with endoscopy, including lesions in the mid-jejunum (unreachable by most endoscopes), functional motility disorders, mural or transmural lesions, brush border defects, some secretory diarrheas, adverse food reactions, and antimicrobial-responsive diseases.

With this in mind, histologic evaluation of the GI tract is a significant part of the diagnostic process for chronic enteropathies in small animals in particular. Despite the limitations and the development of novel testing modalities (IHC, and PCR for lymphocyte receptor clonality) that significantly aid the process and improve the confidence in a diagnosis, *morphologic evaluation via histologic assessment remains the gold standard and is the optimal diagnostic tool for achieving a morphologic diagnosis for this disease*. The most effective way to establish confident diagnoses includes an approach in which histologic, immunohistochemical, and clonality data are interpreted *together and in the context* of gross lesions, clinical history, and overall clinical assessment and history of the patient. Because there is considerable evidence that chronic mucosal lymphoplasmacytic inflammation is a precursor to the development of lymphoma in dogs and cats, the two most significant challenges for veterinary pathologists are to distinguish on one hand normal cellularity of the bowel from bona fide lymphoplasmacytic enteritis, and on the other hand to distinguish lymphoplasmacytic enteritis from lymphoma—particularly in the cat, in which small-cell alimentary lymphoma is one of the most common presentations of lymphoma.

Guidelines for interpretation of histomorphologic changes in the stomach, small, and large intestine of companion animals have been defined, although specific features and thresholds continue to be modified as we learn more about the many variations of normal.

The *canine and feline* **stomach** has a variety of *normal anatomic features and common background lesions* that have not been proven to have any functional significance. These include lymphoid nodules within the deep lamina propria, and a substantial amount of fibrous connective tissue within the lamina propria of the pyloric antrum. A dense band of hyalinized fibrous tissue composed of type IV collagen and fibronectin called the *lamina densa, lamina subglandularis,* or *stratum compactum* is unique to the cat and is situated between the muscularis mucosa and the base of the glands. Background lesions of dogs and cats that may or may not be correlated with previous specific stimuli include gastric proprial fibrosis, glandular atrophy, and glandular nesting within the fundic mucosa. Although we often assume that such fibrosis and glandular atrophy are sequelae to previous inflammation or necrosis, such changes have not been correlated with gastric dysfunction or clinical illness. A diagnosis of **gastric mucosal atrophy** in the dog and cat must be made with great care because there is substantial difference in mucosal thickness between various portions of the stomach, and even within the same anatomic region. *Epithelial injury is not usually prominent during gastritis in dogs and cats.* It is uncommon to encounter erosion or ulceration as part of gastritis, and acute ulceration associated with chemical or mechanical injury to the stomach mucosa (such as during ingestion of chemicals or foreign bodies) has little cellular infiltrate; it is therefore often helpful from a pathogenesis viewpoint to distinguish gastric ulceration from gastritis in these species. The cellularity of leukocytes in the GI tract is often assessed, although often skeptically, given the difficulty with interpretation; however, in the stomach there is less overall normal cellularity compared with the small intestine, so assessing cellularity may be more consistently applied in this compartment.

The **small intestine** of dogs and cats is unique; the overall architecture of the small intestine is distinct, with prominent villi covered by well-differentiated epithelial cells with brush borders and supported by highly vascular lamina propria containing variably proliferating crypts oriented at right angles to the muscularis mucosa. Lacteals should be at least subtly evident in the villar propria center, but not too dilated; some dilation of lacteals occurs as an artifact of sample processing, so care should be taken when interpreting lymphangiectasia, especially in superficial-only biopsies. The lamina propria of the small intestine is much more densely cellular and contains less fibrous connective tissue than stomach or colon, and in the normal small intestinal propria there should be a mix of mature lymphocytes and plasma cells, a few eosinophils, and no neutrophils. A unique population of controversial and so-named globule (or globular) leukocytes with distinct large eosinophilic cytoplasmic granules are often observed within the intestinal epithelium of cats; some data indicate that these are CD3 positive (T cells); other data indicate that they are perforin positive, suggesting that they are granular lymphocytes with cytotoxic function. Although frequently observed, they remain poorly understood; they may increase with hypersensitivity reactions, and neoplasia of these cells has been reported.

Historically, various forms of idiopathic inflammation in the **colon** of dogs and cats have been described (idiopathic mucosal colitis, acute mucosal colitis); except for the specific entities discussed in more detail in the following sections, these likely represent variants of idiopathic IBD manifest in the colon of dogs and cats. In the colon of dogs and cats, some unique features should be noted. No villi are present here, the cellularity is notably diminished, and the fibrous connective tissue is notably increased in the colon compared with the small intestine; however, as for the small intestine, the colon should contain a mixture of mature lymphocytes and plasma cells, with a few eosinophils and rare neutrophils. As for the stomach, assessing cellularity consistently may be a credible goal in the colon, simply because it is less cellular normally, and changes can be detected more readily by the astute pathologist. Greater severity of colonic lesions is often reflected in altered surface epithelium, and dense inflammatory infiltrates in the lamina propria; however, the severity of histologic lesions can be surprisingly underwhelming in dogs and cats with severe clinical signs. Chronic inflammation in the colon is often marked by a variably thick and dense layer of fibrous connective tissue in the superficial lamina propria—this can eventually cause separation of seemingly haphazardly oriented glands in the deep propria. Colonic mucosal fibrosis (detection is aided by Masson trichrome staining) is correlated with failure to attain clinical remission and death due to various chronic GI diseases in cats. Unique downgrowth of colonic glands may be seen with chronic colitis, especially in dogs and pigs. Chronic inflammatory lesions of the colon may not be accompanied by prominent hyperplasia or irregularity of colonic glands as in the small intestine, although defective repair in the face of severe or ongoing injury can result in tortuous, basophilic, proliferative crypts and papillary hyperplasia of the epithelial colonic surface. **Colitis cystica profunda** is the presence of dilated mucus-filled colonic glands protruding through the muscularis mucosa into the submucosa or tunica muscularis; this is an uncommon finding in domestic animals that has been described in pigs, dogs, and goats. This is likely a sequel to chronic colitis and local damage to the muscularis mucosa (e.g., from swine dysentery), or it may represent herniation into the space left by involuted submucosal lymphoid tissue.

While seeking to understand normal histologic variation in the GI tract and recognizing that it may be risky to include numbers in this text, the following discussion originates from the consensus statement of Washabau et al. published as the World Small Animal Veterinary Association 2010 guidelines. This should be read and viewed as guidelines only, with eyes open as we continue to learn and hone this important interpretive skill.

Both the gastric body/fundus and the pyloric antrum of the stomach should be evaluated in dogs and cats. The overall **cellularity** in the stomach should be low but is normally higher in the pyloric antrum compared with the fundus. *In the fundus*, 2-4 IELs are considered normal per 500 µm of epithelium. Mixed inflammatory cells are normally observed in the lamina propria, which may include 4-8 lymphocytes, rare eosinophils, and 2-4 plasma cells per 500 µm of epithelium. *In the pyloric antrum*, 8-16 IELs are considered normal; in the lamina propria, 10-20 lymphocytes, 3-5 eosinophils, and 7-14 plasma cells are considered normal. *In the canine duodenum*, villi should be tall and perpendicular to the muscularis mucosa, without villus blunting, atrophy, or fusion, and the normal crypt:villus ratio in adult dogs is ~1:1. There are 3-4 goblet cells per 100 epithelial cells in the villi, and 1 goblet cell per 10 epithelial cells in normal crypts. A single IEL per 5 epithelial cells in *canine* villi, up to 1 IEL per 2 epithelial cells in *feline* villi, and 1 IEL per 20 epithelial cells in small intestinal cryptal epithelium for both dogs and cats are considered normal. In dogs, the small intestinal lamina propria adjacent to crypts normally contains many more leukocytes, including eosinophils, compared with the lamina propria of villi. *In the colon*, villi are not present, but more goblet cells are seen here compared with the small intestine, but with much variation that may change rapidly with manipulation of the colon. IELs are more frequent in the colon compared to the small intestine normally, with 1 IEL per 10 colonocytes in colonic glands; a few mixed leukocytes, including lymphocytes, plasma cells, and eosinophils, are normally present in the intercryptal lamina propria. More than 4 layers of inflammatory cells in the deep intercryptal lamina propria of dogs may be abnormal. *Neutrophils are rare in any portion of the GI tract*, and in general they indicate either loss of surface epithelial integrity or an infectious process.

In addition to cellularity, several **other morphologic features** of the stomach, small intestine, and colon should be assessed, including atrophy and loss of gastric glands, periglandular fibrosis and nesting of gastric glands, altered epithelium (including surface and gastric pits, intestinal villi, intestinal crypts, gastric glands) such as flattening and attenuation of surface epithelium, loss of goblet cells, loss of brush border (small intestine), villus atrophy, and cryptal or glandular dilation or distension and inflammation, lacteal dilation, and lamina propria fibrosis. Although cell numbers in lamina propria are often pondered, assessed, and relied on as a basis for reaching a diagnosis, this is at best highly subjective and should be interpreted cautiously. Severe inflammatory changes can be identified quickly, but it is much more difficult to objectively identify moderate or mild mucosal inflammation. Although subjective assessment of cellularity in the lamina propria is often heavily used in the diagnostic process ("normal" continues to be debated and defined), it is in reality the least sensitive indicator and should be relied on less; *epithelial morphologic changes are the much more sensitive and reliable indicators of injury*; they are also the least prevalent. After the publication of standardized criteria by Washabau et al. in 2010, publications have detailed more simplified systems with fewer and less subjective criteria in an attempt to improve reliability and consistency of assessment. Parameters shown to be most important (and with least divergence among individual pathologists) include gastric parameters (IELs, lamina propria infiltrates, mucosal fibrosis); duodenal parameters (villus atrophy, epithelial injury, IELs, crypt changes, lamina propria infiltrates); and colonic parameters (epithelial injury, crypt dilation, fibrosis, lamina propria infiltrates, goblet cell depletion).

IBD is common in **dogs**, and thus of significant interest to veterinary pathologists. Affected dogs have variable and vague GI signs, including diarrhea, weight loss, vomiting, hypoproteinemia, and anorexia. Two methods of clinical disease activity scoring in dogs are used to assess clinical disease; these include the brief canine IBD activity index (CIBDAI) and the more complex canine chronic enteropathy clinical activity index (CCECAI). Attempts have been made to identify specific risk factors, and results have varied; high clinical activity index, high endoscopic score (which assess gross mucosal lesions), hypocobalaminemia, and hypoalbuminemia (but not histologic score) are usually considered the most significant risk factors for disease.

Evaluation of histologic changes remains a significant challenge because of variation in normal microscopic anatomy as discussed previously, and because inflammatory lesions in the stomach and intestine are often distributed unevenly; most studies have looked to best characterize normal and define lesions in the stomach, duodenum, ileum, and colon, simply because these represent the regions of the GI tract that are reachable by commonly used endoscopes and thus are the most commonly submitted samples as endoscopic biopsies to veterinary pathologists for interpretation.

Most studies have failed to correlate histologic lesions in the GI tract of dogs with clinical disease activity; much of this may arise from understanding the range of normal, and variation among pathologists; a simplified and easily applicable **scoring system** (0 = normal; 1 = mild; 2 = moderate; and 3 = marked) using selected features *in well-oriented endoscopic (or full-thickness) samples* is useful for correlating select histomorphologic changes with clinical activity. *In the canine gastric fundus*, fibrosis is scored from normal (<2 fibrocytes separating glands) to marked (>10 fibrocytes separating glands); IELs are scored from normal (<2 IELs per 50 epithelial cells) to marked (>20 IELs per 50 epithelial cells); lamina propria lymphocytes and plasma cells are scored from normal [<20 cells per 400× field of view (defined as 40× objective, 10× ocular, ocular field number = 22 mm, field of view diameter = 0.55 mm at specimen level; 0.237 mm²)] to marked (>100 cells per 400× field of view); lamina propria eosinophils are scored from normal (<2 cells per 400× field) to marked (>50 cells per 400× field); and lamina propria neutrophils are scored from normal (0 cells per 400× field) to marked (>50 cells per 400× field). In the *canine gastric pyloric antrum*, fibrosis is scored from normal (<10 fibrocytes separating glands) to marked

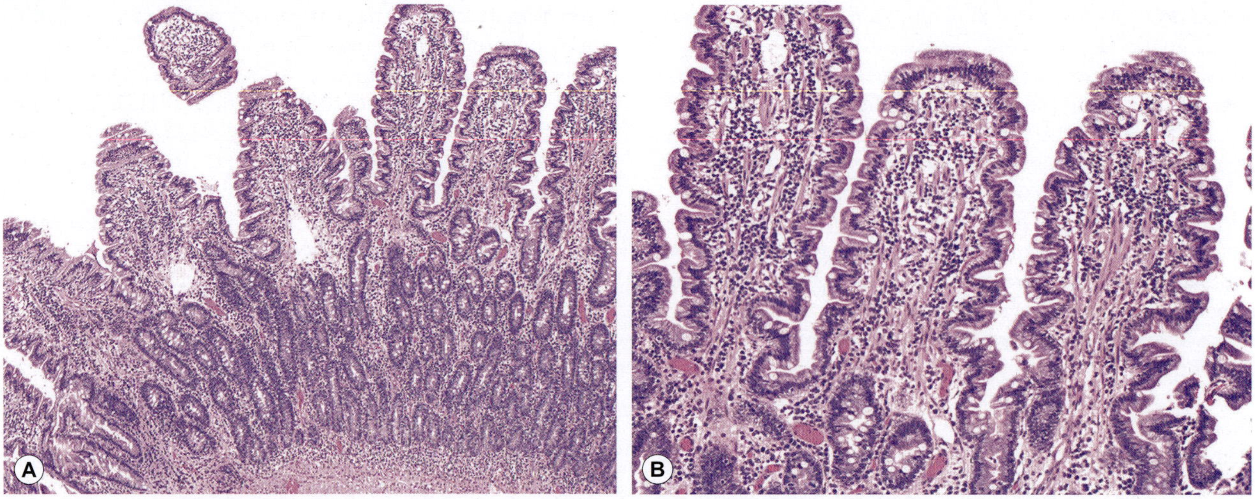

Figure 1-60 **Idiopathic inflammatory bowel disease** affecting the duodenum of a dog. **A.** There is mild villar blunting and surface enterocyte injury, reduced numbers of surface goblet cells, crypt hyperplasia, and diffusely and moderately increased mixed inflammatory cells in the lamina propria. **B.** Moderate increased mixed inflammatory cells including plasma cells, lymphocytes, and neutrophils, as well as scattered eosinophils expand the villar lamina propria.

(>20 fibrocytes separating glands); IELs are scored from normal (<2 cells per 50 epithelial cells) to marked (>10 cells per 50 epithelial cells); lamina propria lymphocytes and plasma cells are scored as per the fundus; lamina propria eosinophils are scored from normal (<2 cells per 400× field) to marked (>50 cells per 400× field); and lamina propria neutrophils are scored as per the fundus. In the canine small intestine (duodenum and ileum), villus stunting is scored from normal (100% normal length) to marked (25% normal length) (Fig. 1-60A); crypt dilation is scored from normal (<2 dilated or distorted crypts containing debris, degenerate neutrophils per 400× field) to marked (>26 dilated or distorted crypts containing debris, degenerate neutrophils per 400× field); lacteal dilation is scored from normal (<25% of villus width) to marked (>75% of villus width); surface epithelial injury is scored from normal (0% erosion or ulceration per section) to marked (>25% erosion or ulceration per section); lamina propria lymphocytes and plasma cells are scored from normal (<25% area of one 400× field) to marked (>75% area of one 400× field); lamina propria eosinophils are scored from normal (<3 cells per 400× field) to marked (>20 cells per 400× field); and lamina propria neutrophils are scored from normal (0 cells per 400× field) to marked (>30 cells per 400× field) (see Fig. 1-60B). Of particular note in regard to crypt dilation, extensive crypt ectasia and inflammation has been termed *cystic mucinous enteropathy* and is likely a severe variant of lymphocytic-plasmacytic enteritis. Rupture of ectatic crypts can eventually occur, and lakes of mucus, reactive histiocytes, and occasional giant cells are present in the lamina propria. *In the canine colon*, crypt dilation is scored from normal (0% dilated crypts per section) to marked (>50% of dilated crypts per section); fibrosis is scored from normal (<2 fibrocytes separating crypts) to marked (>10 fibrocytes separating crypts); goblet cell numbers are scored from normal (0% reduction from normal) to marked (>50% reduction from normal); surface epithelial injury is scored as per the small intestine; lamina propria lymphocytes and plasma cells are scored from normal (<5 cells between crypts) to marked (>20 cells between crypts); lamina propria eosinophils are scored from normal (<2 cells per 400× field) to marked (>20 cells per 400× field); lamina propria neutrophils are scored as per the small intestine; and lamina propria macrophages are scored from normal (<2 cells per 400× field) to marked (>50 cells per 400× field).

Using this simplified system, significant positive correlation was observed between pathologists and between the clinical disease activity scores and the summative histologic score for the small intestine and colon. Significant positive correlation was also noted between clinical disease activity score and individual features, including gastric mucosal fibrosis, duodenal villus atrophy, duodenal lacteal dilation, duodenal lamina proprial lymphocytes and neutrophils, ileal crypt dilation, ileal villus atrophy, colonic fibrosis, and colonic crypt dilation. Therefore, these features likely represent the most objective and descriptive histologic information from the GI tract of dogs, which collectively have repeatable and consistent utility for the very challenging task of interpreting canine GI changes. As previously indicated, establishing a definitive diagnosis of GI inflammation is one hurdle; another is distinguishing inflammatory changes from alimentary lymphoma.

IBD is also very common in **cats**. Affected cats typically have vague clinical signs (like dogs) that include *weight loss*, lethargy, hyporexia, polyphagia, vomiting, and rarely constipation, but cases do not necessarily have persistent diarrhea. As in dogs, establishing a diagnosis is frequently a significant challenge in cats, not only for lack of a definitive standard of normal in the feline GI tract, but because lesions are often unevenly distributed. The distinction between chronic lymphoplasmacytic enteritis and low-grade intestinal T-cell lymphoma in cats is a particular diagnostic challenge, possibly more in cats than in dogs given the high incidence of low-grade intestinal T-cell lymphoma in cats, and that the 2 entities often coexist. In fact, distinction may not be possible in many cases with histology alone. Early reports in cats were vague, had limited discussion of the range of normal histomorphologic features in the feline GI tract, but concluded correctly that features such as mixed small mature lymphocytes and plasma cells within the lamina propria supported a diagnosis of enteritis. The ranges of normal have been defined for various histomorphologic features in the GI tract of cats, including fibrosis, lacteal dilation, crypt distension, proprial cellularity, epithelial damage, and villus atrophy (all discussed above), but most proposed schemes continue to emphasize the subjective characterization of the type and degree of proprial cellular infiltrate, including specific grades for lymphocytic cellularity density within the lamina propria from 1 (mild) to 3 (severe). This emphasis may suggest that anomalies of mucosal architecture (villus atrophy, epithelial cell injury, proprial fibrosis, etc.) are underemphasized, which have been shown to be correlated with gross lesions (endoscopic score) and clinical severity.

A simplified **histologic grading system** for the small intestine has been published for cats (as for dogs), which represents a significant step toward consistency and reliability, again assuming that sufficient numbers of appropriately sampled, processed, and well-oriented samples (especially endoscopic biopsies) are available for evaluation. In the feline small intestine, several significant histomorphologic features were scored as follows: villus atrophy is scored from 0 (no villus atrophy) to 2 (shortened and enlarged villi, crypt:villus ratio <3:1); IEL infiltration is scored as 0 (no epithelial lymphocytic infiltration) or 1 (diffuse epithelial lymphocytic infiltration); the pattern of clusters of IELs are scored as 0 [no IEL nests or plaques (nests are defined as >5 clustered IELs; plaques are defined as >5 epithelial contiguous epithelial cells are obscured by IELs)] or 1 (>1 nest and/or plaque are present); lamina propria lymphocytic cellularity is scored as 1 (mild) to 3 (marked); lamina propria lymphocytic distribution is scored as 0 (apical to basal gradient of small lymphocytes not present) or 1 (apical to basal gradient of small lymphocytes present); lamina propria lymphocyte appearance is scored as 0 (leukocytes present are not monomorphic and are instead of mixed subtype) or 1 (leukocytes present are small and monomorphic lymphocytes); small intestinal crypt hyperplasia is scored from 0 (normal crypts, no crypt hyperplasia) to 3 (marked crypt hyperplasia); lymphocytic inflammation of crypts is scored from 0 (normal crypts) to 3 (marked lymphocytic cryptitis); neutrophilic inflammation of crypts is scored from 0 (normal crypts) to 3 (marked neutrophilic cryptitis); crypt abscesses are scored as 0 (normal crypts) or 1 (<1 dilated crypt filled with fibrin, fluid, degenerate neutrophils, sloughed epithelial cells); crypt epithelial apoptosis is scored as 0 (not present) or 1 (epithelial apoptosis observed); the depth of cellular infiltration is scored as either 0 (absent) or 1 (present) in the submucosa, tunica muscularis, and serosa; and fibrosis is scored both in the lamina propria and in the submucosa as either 0 (not present) or 1 (present). Using this more well-defined scoring system, several histomorphologic features are strongly correlated with a diagnosis of lymphoplasmacytic enteritis (often to the exclusion of lymphoma), including lack of villus atrophy; lack of IELs individually or forming nests or plaques; mixed inflammatory cells instead of monomorphic small lymphocytes; and the lack of submucosal, muscularis, or serosal infiltration. Several other features were less strongly correlated with a diagnosis of enteritis including less prominent cryptal hyperplasia, and more prominent superficial lamina proprial fibrosis. These specific histomorphologic features likely represent the most significant criteria that lead to at least presumptive diagnosis of intestinal inflammation in cats; more confidence in distinction of enteritis from small-cell lymphoma is gained by additional testing including IHC and clonality.

IBD in horses. Several malabsorptive syndromes with similarities to chronic inflammatory enteropathies of dogs and cats have been described in **horses**, and because specific causes are not usually identified, these are often referred to as *idiopathic IBD of horses*. In general, all variants of IBD that have been described (lymphoplasmacytic enteritis, lymphoplasmacytic colitis, eosinophilic enterocolitis, granulomatous enteritis, multisystemic eosinophilic epitheliotropic disease (MEED), and proliferative enteritis) can affect the small and/or large intestine. Affected animals have clinical signs of weight loss, recurrent colic, diarrhea, and lethargy, in order of frequency. Hypoproteinemia and hypoalbuminemia are also common; abnormal intestinal absorption tests, abnormal gross appearance of the intestinal mucosa, and abnormal intestinal mucosal biopsies are common, although histomorphologic data for the range of normal are even more scarce for the equine intestine than for dogs and cats. The etiologies in the horse are unknown, but it is possible that similar mechanisms described earlier are involved. As for other species, definitive confirmation of IBD diagnosis can only be obtained by histologic assessment of intestinal biopsies—which are performed less frequently in the horse due to lack of ability to reach much of the GI tract by endoscopy (limited to the stomach, upper duodenum, and rectum), significant cost, effort, and risk associated with exploratory laparotomy or laparoscopy in horses, and of course a lack of understanding of the range of histomorphologic normal in the equine GI tract.

The approach to equine intestinal biopsies (thorough case workup with history, prior therapeutic attempts, ancillary testing, biopsy collection, tissue preservation and processing, and histologic interpretation) mirrors in principle that of other species discussed previously. The most significant factors to evaluate in the equine stomach include epithelial damage such as attenuation or flattening and loss of terminal differentiation of surface and foveolar epithelial cells, erosions, ulcerations, and isthmus or cryptal mucous cell hyperplasia. In the small intestine, villus atrophy, including blunting, fusion, and altered shape (domed or flattened), is important to assess. Crypts are assessed as for companion animals, and significant changes include irregular branching of cryptal epithelium, crypt dilation and filling of lumens with mucus, eosinophilic fluid, inflammatory cells (so-called crypt abscesses), and crypt loss. Lacteals are often not visible, but lacteal dilation and lymphangiectasia associated with protein-losing enteropathies is reported in horses. It is important to note that in horses (as in other species), dilation of lacteals can be observed secondary to chronic inflammation and obstruction of lymphatic outflow from the mucosa; although specific data are not available for horses, guidelines for dogs are likely appropriate when interpreting this change in horses. Fibrosis is assessed in all segments of the GI tract and may appear as increased collagen and fibroblasts within the mucosa and may also be observed between and separating crypts or gastric glands, and often clustering, nesting, or even replacing glands in the equine stomach. Goblet cell changes are described in rectal biopsies of horses and can include loss of goblet cells, or goblet cell hyperplasia; again, the significance is not always clear but is considered an important indicator of inflammation.

As in other species, the number and pattern of lamina proprial leukocytes including lymphocytes, plasma cells, and eosinophils are often assessed; normal is poorly defined in horses. Changes are usually graded subjectively as mild, moderate, or severe; however, this is typically difficult to interpret, especially for suspected mild or moderate changes. Despite the limitations, cellularity of the propria remains a significant feature to assess because all inflammatory cell types can be increased in the intestine during episodes of inflammation. Expected numbers of leukocytes in different regions of the GI tract of young (<4-years-old) horses without clinical disease have been published; data were reported within an area of interest (defined as 5 nonoverlapping fields of 0.02 mm^2 using a 40× objective). Lymphocytes are the most common, and plasma cells are significantly fewer in all segments of the intestine. Eosinophils are not present in the superficial lamina propria but are present in variable numbers deeper in the lamina propria and are significantly more numerous in the colons compared with the small intestine. Eosinophils are also observed in the submucosa of horses, and more numerous in the colon than in the small intestine. Other publications and our experience indicate that eosinophils are easily recognized throughout the GI tract of horses, and so in a broader population of animals, eosinophils may be under-reported by Rocchigiani et al. because they evaluated young racehorses with strict health management (including parasiticides). Macrophages are uncommon in villus and deep lamina propria and are present as scattered individual cells in all segments of the small and large intestine. Subcryptal leukocytes are 0-3 in most segments of the intestine, and no differences are reported between the small intestine and colon. Paneth cells are present, and often prominent in the small intestinal cryptal epithelium and are significantly fewer in the duodenum than in the jejunum and ileum.

As in other species, the *microscopic changes* in equine intestinal mucosa are often nonspecific, and determination of particular etiologic agents requires further investigation; however, duodenal and rectal microscopic lesions are significantly associated with weight loss in horses, so the use of published equine GI guidelines will surely provide consistency and improve confidence as pathologists work with equine veterinary clinicians to assess and interpret intestinal biopsies (Fig. 1-61). When properly controlled, IHC is used successfully in the equine intestine, but small-cell intestinal epitheliotropic lymphoma is rare, and additional IHC testing is required infrequently. Lymphocyte receptor clonality is used infrequently in horses. The prognosis of horses diagnosed with IBD in most studies is guarded, although the overall prognosis may be fair to moderate if an individual animal responds positively initially to anthelmintic and immunosuppressive corticosteroid therapy.

IBD in ferrets is considered to be a very common disease. The pathogenesis of IBD in ferrets remains unclear; it likely involves (as for other species) a complex interplay of etiologic infectious agents (e.g., helicobacters, ferret enteric coronavirus, *L. intracellularis*, coccidia, and cryptosporidia), diet, genetic factors, and the host immune system, culminating in chronic inflammation in susceptible individuals. Untreated IBD of ferrets can apparently progress to intestinal lymphoma; hence, diagnosis and differentiation of the two require histologic evaluation, and sometimes additional ancillary testing including IHC.

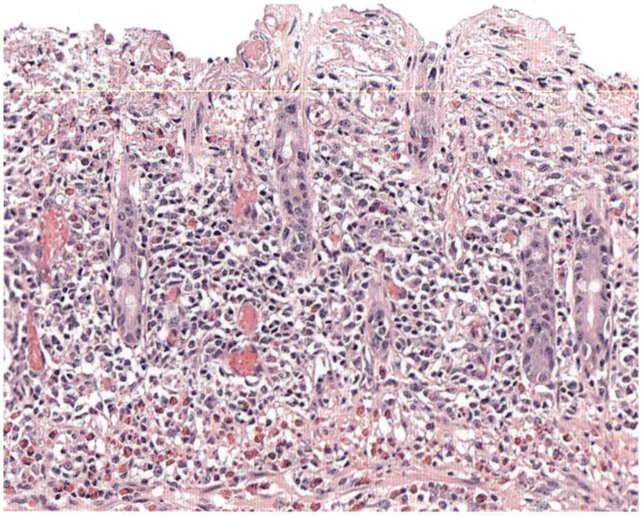

Figure 1-61 Equine inflammatory bowel disease. Infiltration of the lamina propria by many lymphocytes, plasma cells, and a few eosinophils in the colon of a horse.

Diffuse eosinophilic enteritis in cats is likely a unique variant of IBD and is considered distinct from lymphoplasmacytic enteritis with eosinophil infiltrates, which is common in cats and may be associated with hypersensitivity, helminth endoparasitism, toxoplasmosis, food hypersensitivity, and intestinal neoplasia including MCTs and lymphoma. Historically, eosinophilic enteritis in cats was thought to be a manifestation of hypereosinophilic syndrome involving various organs and peripheral eosinophilia in middle-aged or older cats; however, widespread involvement and circulating eosinophilia is not always concurrent and may be limited to cats with eosinophilic syndrome as opposed to diffuse eosinophilic enteritis restricted to the GI tract. Eosinophilic enteritis is morphologically distinguished by the numbers of eosinophils in the intestinal lamina propria (defined as >10 eosinophils per 400× field), and a diagnosis is made when no other inciting cause is identified. Accompanying these changes in severe cases is variably severe muscle hypertrophy, which is correlated with the grossly evident intestinal thickening. The most common clinical signs include vomiting, anorexia, weight loss, diarrhea, and lethargy. Clinical findings include *intestinal thickening*, mesenteric lymphadenomegaly, and possible involvement of other organs, including hepatomegaly and splenomegaly; in general, it seems to be much more severe than eosinophilic gastroenteritis in dogs. Histologic examination reveals *dense focal or segmental infiltrates of well-differentiated eosinophils* in affected tissues; in the small intestine, the eosinophilic infiltrate may be transmural, and as indicated previously is accompanied by grossly visible hyperplasia and hypertrophy of the tunica muscularis, especially in severe cases; the colon may also be involved but is rarely reported. Lymph nodes may have hyperplastic follicles and many mature eosinophils in sinusoids. In addition, eosinophilic lymphadenitis may be variably severe, with fibrosis or even effacement of nodal architecture and replacement by eosinophils in a fibrillar stroma extending through the capsule into surrounding tissue.

A distinct entity with many shared features with eosinophilic enteritis is known as **feline gastrointestinal eosinophilic sclerosing fibroplasia (FGESF)**, which has been reported in domestic cats since 2009; the pathogenesis remains incompletely understood. FGESF is considered an inflammatory disease, although it may appear similar to intestinal neoplasia, and some authors consider this entity to be part of the feline eosinophilic inflammatory disorders (indolent ulcer, eosinophilic plaque, eosinophilic granuloma, and hypereosinophilic syndrome); furthermore, it likely is a variant of, and may develop from, diffuse idiopathic eosinophilic enteritis in cats, and it may share similar initiating factors or causes. Grading of FGESF cases from grade I (low grade, involving a reactive fibroblast layer restricted to the mucosa) to grade III (severe, involving at least 3 intestinal layers) allows differentiation by degree of intestinal fibrosis and may be prognostically helpful. Grade I FGESF is indistinguishable from localized chronic eosinophilic enteritis in cats; true idiopathic eosinophilic enteritis is expected to be restricted to the mucosa; FGESF eventually extends into the submucosa. Most reports are of individual cases in cats, and in-depth pathogenesis studies have not been published. Some have hypothesized a genetic component to FGESF, mostly because long-haired domestic breeds, including the Ragdoll, are over-represented. Other factors that may play a role in development of FGESF include diet, microbiome dysbiosis, intracellular bacterial infection, parasitism, various fungal pathogens, or even hair or plant ingestion. *Eosinophilic inflammation and fibrosis are the key diagnostic features*, and it is likely that prominent fibroblast activation is driven by high levels of proinflammatory mediators such as transforming growth factor–β1. Affected cats have clinical signs of weight loss, anorexia, pale mucous membranes, vomiting, chronic diarrhea, constipation, or intestinal stenosis and obstruction. Gross lesions of FGESF usually include a focal intramural firm mass of the stomach, small intestine, or colon; the mesenteric lymph nodes are often prominent. On rare occasions, involvement of the thoracic lymph nodes is observed, which is likely due to draining of abdominal to thoracic nodes. The histologic features of FGESF are characteristic: there is dense often haphazard deposition of dense collagen trabeculae that can be mistaken for osteoid; trabeculae are separated by proliferative mesenchymal fibroblasts intermixed with inflammatory cells, usually dominated by eosinophils with fewer lymphocytes, plasma cells, and mast cells. The features lead to easy misdiagnosis of this unique lesion as lymphoma, osteosarcoma, or sclerosing intestinal MCT, so care is required to rule out neoplasia in these cases.

Hypereosinophilia syndrome as described in **cats** may be indistinguishable from eosinophilic leukemia and may represent a variant of other eosinophilic diseases in cats. Hypereosinophilia syndrome is a rare systemic disorder of cats with sustained peripheral eosinophilia without a defined or identified cause; many cases progress to involvement of other systems with infiltration of mature eosinophils into various organs, including the GI tract. Cats with hypereosinophilia syndrome (or eosinophilic leukemia) generally have a poor response to therapy and poor overall prognosis, so identification of eosinophilic predominant enteritis in biopsies should prompt the pathologist to further investigate for evidence of peripheral eosinophilia as a precaution and to help distinguish eosinophilic enteritis from the more severe and systemic disease.

Eosinophilic enteritis in horses has been described as part of a distinct *multisystemic eosinophilic epitheliotropic disease (MEED)* and is a rare condition of horses and donkeys in which eosinophils infiltrate various organs, including the GI tract, liver, skin, pancreas, lungs, and lymph nodes. Grossly, the changes are nonspecific, with erosion and possibly ulceration (Fig. 1-62A). Although Standardbreds and Thoroughbreds may be over-represented, several breeds have been affected. The cause remains poorly understood; various hypotheses include hypersensitivity reaction, parasitic insult, eosinophilic myeloproliferative disorder, or a paraneoplastic syndrome associated with lymphoma. Typical clinical signs in affected horses include weight loss, diarrhea, and exfoliative dermatitis; hypoalbuminemia due to enteric loss of protein is often observed. If the lungs, liver, or skin are heavily involved, clinical signs will be attributable to those systems. Peripheral eosinophilia occurs in ~14% of MEED cases, and some reports have described localized or diffuse eosinophilic infiltrates (or eosinophilic granulomas) in the stomach and in the small and large intestine of affected horses; other organs are also affected in some cases.

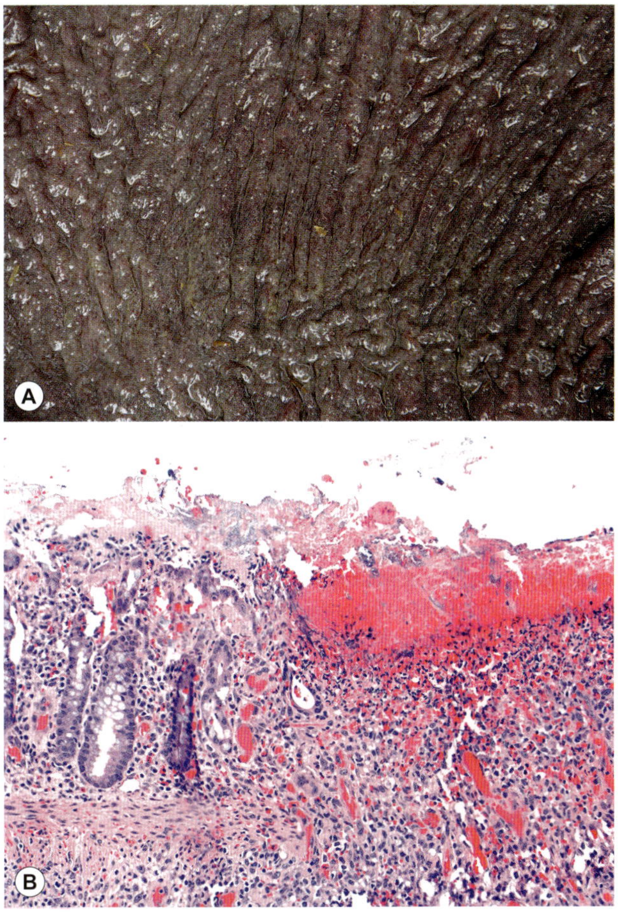

Figure 1-62 Eosinophilic colitis in a horse. **A**. Grossly, there is thickening and edema of the mucosa with multifocal erosions. **B**. The lamina propria, muscularis mucosa, and superficial submucosa are infiltrated by lymphocytes, eosinophils, and plasma cells; the surface is eroded.

Microscopic changes usually include diffuse infiltration of the mucosa, submucosa, and often deeper layers of the enteric wall by eosinophils, mast cells, macrophages, lymphocytes, and plasma cells. Moderate-to-severe villus atrophy and fibroplasia in the lamina propria, as well as hypertrophy of the muscularis mucosa, occur. Eosinophilic granulomas in the mucosa and submucosa consist of central masses of eosinophils, surrounded by macrophages, giant cells, and fibrous connective tissue (see Fig. 1-62B). Eosinophilic interstitial infiltrates and granulomas are also described in the biliary and pancreatic ducts, pancreas, salivary glands, capsule and outer cortex of enlarged firm mesenteric lymph nodes, and near portal tracts in the liver. Epitheliotropism is a common feature, and eosinophils are seen within the intraepithelial spaces of bronchi, bronchioles, gastric, small and large intestine, bile ducts, and epidermis of the skin. Due to frequent eosinophilic inflammation of the GI tract (even if gross evidence of disease is not present), MEED is often considered an uncommon form of idiopathic IBD in horses; at minimum, identification of eosinophilic inflammation in the GI tract of horses should prompt the astute pathologist to consider MEED as a differential diagnosis and prompt further evaluation for evidence of systemic disease (including other explanations for hypereosinophilia, such as parasitism, hypersensitivity, and lymphoma). This can be a difficult task given the wide variety of clinical signs that may be evident. The prognosis of MEED in affected equids is generally poor, even with immunosuppressive therapy.

Eosinophilic gastroenteritis also occurs in horses apart from MEED. In addition to eosinophilic inflammation associated with enteric parasitism, idiopathic focal or multifocal eosinophilic enteritis has been described and termed variably as part of idiopathic IBD, focal or multifocal eosinophilic enteritis, circumferential mural bands, or most consistently idiopathic focal eosinophilic enteritis (IFEE). Focal eosinophilic inflammation in the intestine has been described in association with oomycotic infection (*Pythium* sp.) or encapsulated nematodes; however, a cause of IFEE has not been identified. Affected horses have clinical signs of acute abdominal pain and usually require surgical management; the gross lesions are focal hyperemic circumferential areas of the small intestine or rarely colon, with a locally thickened wall that causes reduced flow of ingesta, and simple intestinal obstruction. Histologically, there is infiltration of eosinophils and macrophages, with fewer lymphocytes, plasma cells, and neutrophils that infiltrate the submucosa and muscularis. As for the other eosinophil-dominant inflammatory conditions, the cause remains unknown and is thought to be an exacerbated inflammatory reaction in the horse intestine; its relation with diffuse eosinophilic enteritis or MEED remain unknown.

Typhlocolitis in dogs is usually associated with frequent small volumes of *diarrhea*, often with mucus or blood, and often accompanied by tenesmus. By far the most common disease of the colon encountered in dogs is **idiopathic lymphoplasmacytic (entero)colitis**, considered earlier in the Inflammatory bowel disease section.

Histiocytic colitis of Boxer and French Bulldogs (HCBF) (discussed earlier) associated with invasive *E. coli* causes characteristic histiocytic inflammation of the colon of these breeds in particular, and regression of clinical signs has been observed after bacterial culture and susceptibility-guided antimicrobial therapy.

Ulcerative colitis with perforation has been reported in dogs with **uremia**, but the mechanism is uncertain. Given the frequency of concurrent vascular lesions including arteritis, fibrinoid necrosis, and mineralization, colonic mucosal damage may be related to mucosal ischemia or a variety of uremic toxins, including increased ammonia formed by bacterial urease in the colon.

Trichuris vulpis, the *canine* whipworm, causes acute or chronic colitis or typhlitis; in heavy infestations there may be significant blood loss because of mucosal damage inflicted by the nematodes. Clinical trichurosis is generally associated with adult trichurid nematodes extending from the cecum and proximal ascending colon into more distal parts of the large intestine. Ulcerative colitis in dogs is also rarely caused by ***Entamoeba histolytica***. Ulcerative granulomatous transmural colitis is common as an enteric manifestation of systemic infection with ***Histoplasma capsulatum*** in cats and dogs; intestinal-only forms can occur in dogs, presumably following the ingestion of the fungus. Other systemic mycoses can affect the GI tract, including ***Cryptococcus*** sp. The oomycete ***Pythium*** or the algal pathogen ***Prototheca*** are uncommon causes of enterocolitis—depending on geographic location, and often but not always part of systemic disease in dogs. **Leishmaniosis** in dogs is often a multisystemic disease, but chronic mixed-cell inflammatory infiltration of the colon along with numerous *L. infantum* amastigotes is usually observed. **Canine parvovirus 2** (CPV2; *Parvoviridae*, *Protoparvovirus carnivoran1*) causes colonic damage, but in virtually all cases, there are more severe lesions in the small intestine. **Canine coronavirus** has also been implicated as a cause of colonic and small intestinal lesions, although most infections are likely clinically and histologically mild. ***Brachyspira*** spp. cause colitis in pigs, chickens, and humans; these organisms colonize the canine colon, although their role in canine diarrhea or colitis remains controversial. ***Campylobacter*** spp. can be isolated from dogs with and without diarrhea but has been implicated as a cause of enterocolitis outbreaks in some dog colonies.

Typhlocolitis in cats is less common than in dogs. *Idiopathic colitis* as a component of idiopathic IBD also occurs in cats, similar to that described in dogs, and is discussed in previous sections on idiopathic inflammatory bowel disease. The protozoal pathogen ***Tritrichomonas foetus*** is associated with persistent large-bowel diarrhea and chronic mucosal colitis in young densely housed cats.

Feline panleukopenia virus (FPLV) causes colonic lesions in about half of clinical cases in cats, and typical lesions are less widespread or severe compared with small intestinal lesions. **Mycotic colitis** has been reported in cats as a hemorrhagic ulcerative colitis with microvascular thrombosis and mucosal invasion by *Candida*, zygomycetes (most of these organisms are now reclassified into the orders *Entomophthorales* or *Mucoromycotina*), or *Aspergillus*; these can be secondary invaders, due to colonic damage and leukopenia associated with FPLV. ***Clostridium piliforme*** is the cause of Tyzzer disease, which is associated with mild-to-severe ulcerative colitis or typhlocolitis (along with myocarditis and hepatitis in some cases) in kittens, as well as foals, and sporadically in puppies, calves, and lambs. This may be a significant cause of morbidity and mortality in young orphaned (and immunocompromised) kittens. Histologic lesions include focal necrosis, dilation of crypts, exfoliation of epithelial cells, and neutrophilic inflammation; in some cases the classic intracytoplasmic basophilic linear stacked bacterial rods are identified, especially with silver-stained tissue sections.

Adherent-invasive *E. coli* (AIEC)-induced colitis has also been described in individual cats, an entity known as **granulomatous or histiocytic colitis of cats**. Similar to HCBF (described above), the disease occurs rarely in cats, usually with an long history of vomiting, large-bowel diarrhea, hematochezia, mucoid feces, enlarged lymph nodes, and weight loss due to grossly thickened and ulcerated colonic wall. Histologic lesions are similar to those described in HCBF of dogs and are ulcers of the colonic mucosa and transmural infiltration of foamy PAS-positive macrophages, along with other mixed leukocytes. Also as in canine cases, regression of clinical signs has been observed after bacterial culture and susceptibility-guided antimicrobial therapy was initiated. Specific breed predispositions have not been noted in cats, although affected breeds have included Oriental shorthair and Sphynx; however, insufficient case numbers have been reported to make breed association conclusions.

Granulomatous or pyogranulomatous inflammation along blood vessels or lymphatics in the wall of the colon or ileocecocolic junction associated with **feline infections peritonitis virus** may grossly mimic a neoplasm.

Necrotizing colitis caused by *Entamoeba histolytica* in cats is seen as severe necrosis of the colon and cecum; a similar condition has been described in older cats, with no apparent etiologic agent and is hypothesized to be secondary to ischemia. Variably severe, often transmural acute ulcerative and fibrinous-to-neutrophilic enterocolitis and intracellular gram-negative bacilli (in neutrophils and macrophages within the lamina propria) are hallmarks of ***Salmonella enterica*** ser. **Enteritidis** and **Typhimurium** infection in cats, and there is usually evidence of septicemic disease as well. ***Anaerobiospirillum*** sp. is also associated with ileocolitis in cats.

Typhlocolitis in horses. The diagnosis of infectious acute colitis or typhlocolitis in horses resolves mainly into the differentiation of salmonellosis, clostridial diseases, and equine neorickettsiosis [Potomac horse fever (PHF), equine monocytic ehrlichiosis]. Although acute colitis can be produced in horses by other agents, they are less common and the role of many of them remains not fully understood. Infectious colitis must also be differentiated from the sequelae of intestinal accidents, NSAID intoxication, intoxication by other agents such as oleander, and thromboembolism involving the large bowel. The pathology of the equine colitis associated with salmonellosis, clostridial disease, PHF, and intoxication by NSAIDs is very similar regardless of the etiology, and an etiologic diagnosis cannot be made based on gross and/or microscopic lesions alone.

Salmonellosis in horses is most frequently associated with ***S. enterica*** subsp. ***enterica*** **serovar Typhimurium**, although other serovars may be associated with sporadic cases of disease. Diarrhea is the main clinical sign of equine salmonellosis.

Equine intestinal clostridial diseases are increasingly well defined. Many of these cases were lumped together in an umbrella category, *colitis X*, a term that was used to refer to severe acute colitis in which all known etiologic agents had been ruled out. This term should no longer be used as it does not describe a specific syndrome but rather a group of diseases for which a final etiology cannot be established. *C. perfringens* type C and *C. difficile* (Fig. 1-63) are the most common clostridial species responsible for equine clostridial

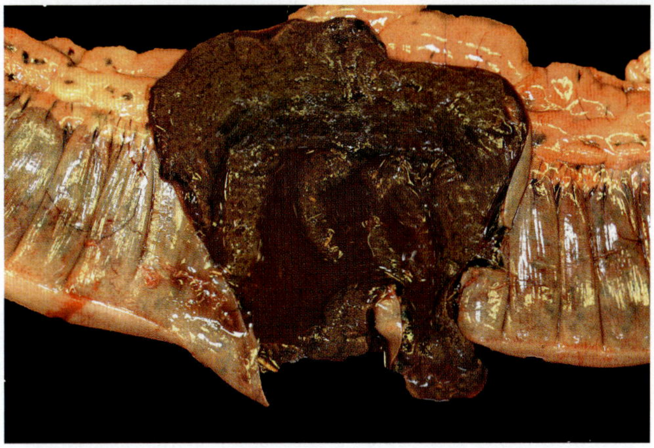

Figure 1-63 **Acute necrohemorrhagic colitis** produced by *Clostridioides difficile* in a horse.

enteric disease. *C. perfringens* type C occurs most commonly in neonates, although disease can be seen occasionally in older horses; diarrhea is a frequent but not consistent clinical sign, with sudden death, the only sign in a few foals. *C. difficile* infection occurs in horses of any age, and it almost invariably produces diarrhea regardless of the age of the affected animal. Coinfection by *C. difficile* and *C. perfringens* type C may occur, mostly in foals. A series of cases of equine enterocolitis associated with *P. sordellii* (formerly *Clostridium sordellii*) has been described.

Equine neorickettsiosis (Potomac horse fever, PHF) is a frequent type of equine colitis, which is restricted to certain geographic areas where the disease is endemic. Traditionally, ***Neorickettsia risticii*** was considered the only etiology of PHF. However, ***Neorickettsia findlayensis*** has been isolated from affected horses and assumed to also be responsible for some cases of PHF. In foals, ***Rhodococcus equi*** causes neutrophilic ulcers involving lymphoid tissue in the cecocolic mucosa, and cecal and colic lymphadenitis. ***C. piliforme*** is an uncommon agent of colitis in horses, the disease being seen mostly as hepatitis. Other bacterial agents, including ***Actinobacillus equuli***, and others, have been associated with acute colitis in horses, but definitive evidence of their role in these infections is lacking.

Histoplasmosis is rare in the horse, and has been reported once in a horse with salmonellosis and ulcerative colitis. Extensive mucosal involvement by **larval cyathostomes** and **strongyles** and, rarely, ulcerative typhlitis resulting from **anoplocephalid tapeworms**, may also cause chronic diarrhea and wasting. Coinfection by *Listeria monocytogenes*, *S. enterica* ser. Typhimurium, and cyathostomes probably led to granulomatous typhlocolitis in a horse.

Ciliate protozoa may be seen over the colonic mucosa and occasionally within the lamina propria of horses at autopsy due to death from a variety of enteric and non-enteric problems; the protozoa are usually not associated with tissue inflammatory changes and are considered normal inhabitants of the intestine with no proven pathogenic role in enteric disease. Intralesional protozoa, however, have been reported in a horse with diffuse eosinophilic colitis; the relation between the protozoa and the colitis was not definitively established.

Chronic diarrhea and possibly cachexia may also result from persistent ulceration of the cecum or colon caused by

ischemic mucosal lesions. These may be the product of arterial thromboembolism and slow flow, or less likely, corrected strangulation with reflow. The use of **NSAIDs** also has been associated with cecal and colonic ulceration and plasma protein loss. *Right dorsal colitis*, in which ulcerative lesions are mostly observed in the right dorsal colon, may be associated with colic, and acute or chronic diarrhea. The specific cause of extensive ulceration may be difficult to determine. A history of administration of NSAIDs, and lesions in the renal papilla and upper alimentary tract, suggests intoxication by those agents.

Typhlocolitis in pigs. The differential diagnosis of typhlocolitis in swine mainly revolves around identifying swine dysentery and other spirochetoses, *Salmonella* enterocolitis, and *L. intracellularis* infection. Other agents may also be involved.

Swine dysentery caused by *Brachyspira hyodysenteriae* involves only the cecum and spiral colon. It is a catarrhal to mildly fibrinohemorrhagic erosive mucosal typhlocolitis. The colonic content is fluid and usually blood tinged. A similar but milder disease, **intestinal spirochetosis**, is associated with *Brachyspira pilosicoli*, which causes distinctive microscopic lesions as it colonizes the apex of surface epithelium. ***Salmonella* enterocolitis**, mainly resulting from *Salmonella* Typhimurium causes a fibrinous, erosive to focally ulcerative condition, mainly of the cecum and colon, but occasionally involving the small intestine, especially the terminal ileum. The intestinal content is fluid but usually not bloody. Mesenteric lymph nodes are prominent. *Rectal stricture* appears to be a product of ischemic proctitis, probably related in many cases to infection with *Salmonella* Typhimurium.

L. intracellularis infection is readily recognized by the consistent involvement of the terminal ileum by adenomatosis, with or without hemorrhage, or by necrotic ileitis.

In **postweaning colibacillosis**, catarrhal to mild fibrinohemorrhagic enterocolitis occurs in piglets after weaning.

C. perfringens* type C** and ***C. difficile are also increasingly important causes of enteritis with occasional typhlocolitis in neonatal piglets. Necrotizing or pseudomembranous inflammation occurs in both, with acute stages of *C. difficile* infection being neutrophilic and marked by mesocolonic edema.

Fibrinohemorrhagic typhlitis is caused by heavy infestations with ***Trichuris suis***, especially in weaned pigs with access to pastures and yards. Under similar circumstances, ***Cystoisospora suis*** infection may also cause ileotyphlocolitis.

Typhlocolitis in ruminants. Diagnostic considerations in cattle >2-3-months-old with acute-to-subacute fibrinohemorrhagic typhlocolitis include salmonellosis, BVD, coccidiosis, adenoviral infection, and winter dysentery (coronavirus). Lesions of the oral cavity and upper alimentary tract may be expected but are not necessarily present in **BVD**. **Bovine coronavirus** (BCoV) causes microscopic lesions in colonic crypts in cattle with winter dysentery similar to those observed in calves with BCoV colitis; fibrinous or hemorrhagic typhlocolitis may be seen grossly. **Salmonellosis** affects all age groups from neonate to adult and may frequently involve both the small and large intestine in catarrhal-to-fibrinohemorrhagic enteritis; mesenteric lymph nodes usually are enlarged. **Coccidiosis** may involve the ileum and large intestine. **Bovine adenovirus** infection may cause severe hemorrhagic enterocolitis, with few lesions elsewhere. **Arsenic**, other **heavy metals**, and **oleander**, **oak** or **acorn poisoning** also may cause hemorrhagic typhlocolitis and dysentery. Rarely, **trichurosis** causes hemorrhagic mucosal typhlitis in calves.

Chronic fibrinous or ulcerative typhlocolitis may occur in **salmonellosis, BVD**, and **coccidiosis**.

Granulomatous typhlocolitis associated with chronic diarrhea and wasting may occur in **paratuberculosis**, concurrently with granulomatous ileitis and mesenteric lymphadenitis. The mucosa of the large bowel in these cases is thickened and rugose. Impressions of affected mucosa or ileocecal lymph node will contain acid-fast bacilli. Paratuberculosis in sheep and goats is usually associated with wasting, but often not diarrhea. The large bowel may be involved in a minority of cases; the ileum is consistently affected.

In **sheep**, hemorrhagic typhlocolitis may be present in animals with **bluetongue** and **peste-des-petits ruminants (PPR)**; it is rarely the only lesion. **Salmonellosis** may cause fibrinohemorrhagic enteritis in lambs and pregnant ewes, and typhlitis caused by **trichurosis** will occur rarely, although small numbers of parasites are common in weaners. **Coccidiosis** may be implicated in hemorrhagic ileotyphlocolitis in lambs and kids, although the small intestine is usually more commonly and severely involved. In goats, enterotoxemia caused by *C. perfringens* type D may cause moderate-to-severe fibrinonecrotic typhlocolitis, which occasionally extends to the terminal small intestine as well. Uremia may cause hemorrhagic lesions associated with vasculitis in the cecum and colon.

Proliferative and neoplastic lesions of the intestine

Neoplasms of the lower GI tract are *infrequent* in domestic animals (see Table 1-1). However, as is the case in the stomach, intestinal proliferative lesions are common among surgical biopsy submissions from dogs and cats, which is in contrast to horses and ruminants. As in the stomach, malignant neoplasms are more common in the intestine than benign neoplasms, and except for lymphomas, *most are carcinomas*. Non-neoplastic epithelial polyps are the most frequently observed, and they occur most commonly in the rectum. Colonic or small intestinal polyp-like lesions in dogs can appear grossly similar but are mostly diagnosed as invasive and metastatic malignant adenocarcinomas. *Lymphoma* is the most common malignant round-cell tumor in most species; it may arise from various regions of the intestine, including the organized intestinal lymphoid tissue; involvement of the GI tract can be part of multicentric disease (see Vol. 3, Hematolymphoid System). *GI stromal tumors* are most common in dogs; these arise either from the interstitial cells of Cajal (GIST) or smooth muscle (smooth muscle tumor).

There appears to be no significant difference in histologic appearance or biological behavior of various neoplasms based on their site of origin in the GI tract (except for terminal rectal inflammatory polyps of dogs, discussed immediately below), but prefixes such as gastric, intestinal, colonic, or rectal are necessary descriptive anatomic terms to improve clarity in communication of lesions and diagnoses.

Non-neoplastic proliferative and reactive lesions of the intestine. Irregular **intestinal epithelial hyperplasia** is a common lesion and can occur as focal polypoid or tubulopapillary proliferation of surface epithelium anywhere in the intestinal tract; the most common site by far is the rectum of middle-aged male **dogs**, and lesions are usually within 10 cm of the anal-rectal margin. The lesion here has been given a variety of names including *inflammatory (colo) rectal polyp, adenomatous hyperplasia, papillotubular or polypoid adenoma, (colo)rectal polypoid carcinoma in situ*, or *simply (colo)rectal polyp;* clear distinction between hyperplastic polyp, adenoma, and carcinoma in situ is not always well defined or articulated and the terms are often used interchangeably. We do not make an argument to distinguish the terms currently based on lack of convincing prognostic or behavioral significance. The term polyp may be best reserved for the non-neoplastic proliferative epithelial lesion occurring mostly in the rectum of dogs, usually a single firm pedunculated or polyp-like mass of 1-cm to several centimeters diameter that is easily managed by adequate surgical excision. Tenesmus, prolapse of the polyp, rectal bleeding following defecation, chronic dyschezia, and diarrhea are the most common signs.

Microscopically, hyperplastic epithelial polyps are comprised of variably well-differentiated proliferative epithelial cells, usually oriented as pedunculated fronds supported by thin fibrous stroma with lamina proprial fibromuscular hyperplasia (Fig. 1-64); some cases are accompanied by significant chronic mixed inflammation. Additional unique features may include surface ulceration, hemorrhage, granulation tissue-like stroma, hyperplastic goblet cells, increased mucus accumulation within dilated crypts or the interstitium, osteoid matrix production, and infiltration of many neutrophils or mixed inflammatory cells. In well-oriented specimens, the tubular pattern is seen as branching crypts lined by generally well-differentiated columnar-to-cuboidal pseudostratified epithelial cells. The papillary type consists of villus-like projections of proprial connective tissue that are covered by a layer of pseudostratified columnar epithelial cells. There may be cellular atypia and dysplasia, cytoplasmic basophilia, loss of nuclear polarity, and prominent nucleoli in the epithelium (changes often attributed to surface trauma due to the polyp location), but in general the proliferative cells of the polyp share histomorphologic features of well-differentiated colonic or rectal epithelium. The number of mitotic figures varies, often within the same polyp. These often appear to originate in the superficial portion of the glands; the deeper portions of the same glands may remain histomorphologically normal, with tubules or slender papillae of hyperchromatic proliferative epithelial cells above them. The stalk of the polyp is often highly vascular and is continuous with the lamina propria or submucosa of the rectum. Hyperplastic polyps are generally well demarcated from the adjacent normal mucosa. The amount of goblet cells and mucin within the epithelium varies considerably, and it is often absent, especially in more dysplastic variants.

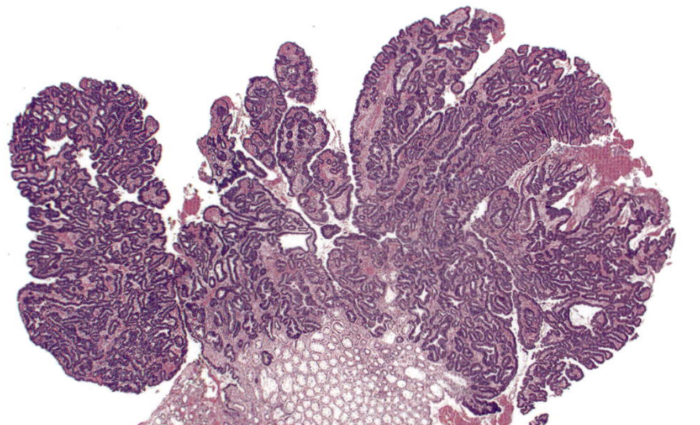

Figure 1-64 Hyperplastic polyp in the rectum of a dog. Arising from the rectal mucosa is a polypoid mass comprising fronds of proliferative epithelial cells.

The vast majority are benign with no evidence of malignant transformation or progresssion; however, in the Miniature Dachshund (in Japan), colorectal *inflammatory polyps* have been shown to progress to adenoma or carcinoma. In general, surgical removal of these lesions in dogs is curative. Given the diagnostic challenge, some are interpreted as adenoma or carcinoma in situ based on histologic or cytologic features; however, due to trauma in this location, mere cellular atypia is insufficient to warrant a diagnosis of adenoma or carcinoma (and probably in situ carcinoma), and so it is important to remember that deep mural or transmural biopsies and/or complete excision of these polyps are essential to rule out local invasion of the basement membrane or infiltration of lymphatics by proliferative epithelial cells. Polyps that are >1 cm in diameter, that are more traumatized, or that are more inflamed tend to have cells with a more pleomorphic appearance. With incomplete surgical excision, local recurrence may be more likely in cases with greater atypia or pleomorphism, multiple masses, or those with greater diffuse colonic involvement.

In other species, polyps are less common. Hyperplastic polyps are reported in the stomach and duodenum of predominantly middle-aged male **cats** with vomition, hematemesis, and possibly anemia. As for dogs, surgical excision is almost always considered curative.

In **cattle**, intestinal polyps are usually an incidental finding, except when they are large enough to cause partial intestinal obstruction. The tumors are raised, often pedunculated, gray-to-brown masses on the mucosal surface. They may occur singly, in grapelike clusters, or they are scattered along the intestinal mucosa. Microscopically, they resemble benign rectal polyps in the dog. Adenomatous polyps are described in **sheep**, although mostly in the context of concurrent intestinal carcinoma. Grossly similar but histologically distinct hyperplastic polyp-like lesions occur in the small intestine of **lambs** and **goats** with chronic proliferative coccidiosis. The proliferative lesions caused by *L. intracellularis* in **horses** and **swine** may impart a polypoid appearance to the intestinal mucosa grossly, and microscopically should not be mistaken for adenomatous neoplasia.

Idiopathic hypertrophy of intestinal smooth muscle occurs commonly in horses and pigs, less frequently in cats, and has been described in rabbits, dogs, and small ruminants. Affected animals are usually nonclinical, and either localized or diffuse segmental thickening of the small intestine (ileum is most common) is observed as an incidental finding at autopsy; however, acute intestinal obstruction can occur in some severe cases. The intestine has a grossly thickened and pale muscular wall, and histologically, there is muscle hypertrophy with myofiber enlargement; necrosis, hemorrhage, inflammation, or fibrosis can be present simultaneously. Cats, horses, and rabbits can develop individual or multiple intestinal diverticula or pseudodiverticula secondary to intestinal smooth muscle hypertrophy.

Intestinal hamartomas are rarely described in dogs and a single horse. These are polypoid lesions identified in the distal large intestine. In dogs, they appear as disorganized or haphazard aggregates of proliferative tubular epithelial cells and possible ganglion cells (*ganglioneuromatosis*) that may extend into the submucosa; they are supported by increased fibrous connective tissue or smooth muscle that is continuous with the muscle layer of the intestine. A single cecal polyp in a horse was composed of irregular but well-differentiated vascular channels and was diagnosed as a vascular hamartoma.

Mural or intramural **intestinal hematomas** are rarely described in the small intestine of dogs and the colon of horses. They are presumed to occur secondary to trauma including foreign body or blunt-force abdominal trauma, associated with inflammation and ulceration, as a consequence of clotting or platelet dysfunction, or they are idiopathic. Affected patients have abdominal pain, vomiting, and even obstruction. Before histologic evaluation, the differential diagnoses should include neoplastic disease, localized inflammation, or abscessation.

Neoplasms of epithelial cells. Intestinal adenomas are distinct from hyperplastic epithelial polyps, although historically the distinction and terminology has not been clear (discussed previously with hyperplastic polyps), and they are often grossly and histologically similar. Adenomas are probably rare in the intestine and colon; they are described most frequently in the rectum of dogs and probably comprise ~50% of all canine rectal tumors (although in many studies they are grouped with rectal polyps). Adenomas arise from intestinal, colonic, or rectal crypts or glands; they form distinct papillary often-pedunculated luminal lesions extending from a stalk and are composed of proliferating hyperchromatic epithelial cells forming branching tubular structures surrounded by variably inflamed lamina propria. Adenoma is defined by greater atypia of the proliferating epithelial cells but with no evidence of invasion; however as discussed previously, traumatized hyperplastic polyps also may have significant cellular atypia and inflammation. The distinction between polyp and adenoma is often impossible to make and likely has minimal prognostic significance. Canine intestinal adenomas have been classified by morphologic subtype (tubular, villous, tubulovillous), but this is not known to be associated with prognosis. Within some adenomas, areas of anaplastic or dysplastic epithelial cells are observed, and some authors have termed such lesions carcinoma in situ or mucosal carcinoma; in either case, the prominently dysplastic epithelial cells do not invade the muscularis mucosa or submucosa. Features that distinguish adenoma from carcinoma in situ are poorly defined, and there is no conclusive evidence of significant biologic behavior or prognostic difference between them. Distinct from humans, and with the exception of inflammatory colorectal polyps of the Miniature Dachshund of Japan (previously discusssed), there is no definitive evidence that canine intestinal adenomas progress to carcinomas regardless of their histologic features or size. Superficial endoscopic samples (especially of inflamed or traumatized polyps or adenomas) can easily be mistaken for carcinoma if only cytologic features are assessed; on the contrary, *intestinal and rectal carcinoma cannot be definitively ruled out without complete excision, or deep mural biopsies*.

The prevalence and distribution of **intestinal carcinomas** vary among species. In dogs, small intestinal and colonic carcinomas are relatively uncommon, especially compared with gastric carcinomas. In contrast, feline small intestinal and colonic adenocarcinomas are relatively common compared with the rare gastric carcinoma. In other species, where they are in general rare, carcinomas involve the small intestine more commonly than the large intestine or stomach.

Intestinal adenocarcinomas in dogs occur most frequently in the proximal small intestine and the large intestine; the mean age of affected dogs is 8-9 years. The etiopathogenesis of intestinal and colonic carcinomas in dogs is uncertain, and there may be progression to malignancy from benign adenomas in a minority of cases. Intestinal adenocarcinoma in the dog has been used as a model of human colon cancer due to some common features in tumorigenesis. Regulation of β-catenin, E-cadherin, and cyclooxygenase-2 are altered in malignant colonic epithelial cells in some cases, as they are in humans. In addition, adenomatous polyposis coli (APC), a protein encoded by the tumor suppressor gene *APC*, is frequently altered in sporadic canine colon adenomas and adenocarcinoma as it is in human colon tumors, and changes in this gene may be an early event in tumor development. Intestinal carcinomas may be more prevalent in males, with a breed predisposition in Boxers, Collies, Poodles, and German Shepherds. Weight loss, persistent vomiting, anorexia, emaciation, and abdominal distension are the most common signs with small intestinal carcinomas; more frequent signs in dogs with distal colonic or rectal carcinomas are large-bowel diarrhea, tenesmus, hematochezia, and dyschezia. Anemia can occur due to chronic persistent hemorrhage of ulcerated neoplasms.

Intestinal carcinomas **grossly** appear as firm, pale, gray-white annular thickening (scirrhous fibrosis) and possible stenosis of the intestinal wall (Fig. 1-65A), or as an intraluminal papillary or polypoid mass protruding from the intestinal wall (see Fig. 1-65B). With either gross presentation, there is often scirrhous fibrosis and stenosis leading to dilation proximally and possibly thickening of the tunica muscularis. Intestinal carcinomas are often highly locally infiltrative (see Fig. 1-65C) and widely metastatic, mainly via the lymphatics (see Fig. 1-65D) to mesenteric lymph nodes, and less commonly to other abdominal nodes, liver, spleen, and lungs. Gross or histologic evidence of metastasis at the time of resection of small intestinal lesions predicts a markedly reduced postsurgical survival time; even dogs without such evidence may still succumb to metastatic disease, albeit with longer survival. Approximately 50% of intestinal adenocarcinomas metastasize to colonic, iliac, and other pelvic and abdominal nodes; ~30% metastasize more widely, to abdominal organs or the lung. For rectal carcinomas the data vary, but newer studies indicate a metastatic rate of 10-30%. Implantation of neoplastic cells on serosal surfaces (see Fig. 1-65A) may result in obstruction of omental and diaphragmatic lymphatics, leading to ascites. In a few cases, malignant cells may spread retrograde in the lymphatics of the abdomen and pelvic limbs, causing edema of the abdominal wall and legs. Dogs with annular colorectal carcinomas have a much shorter survival period than dogs that have a single, pedunculated polypoid tumor in this location.

The **microscopic appearance** is similar, regardless of species or location. A few develop as tubular and papillary proliferations of well-differentiated columnar epithelial cells; these typically project into the intestinal lumen, and this form is

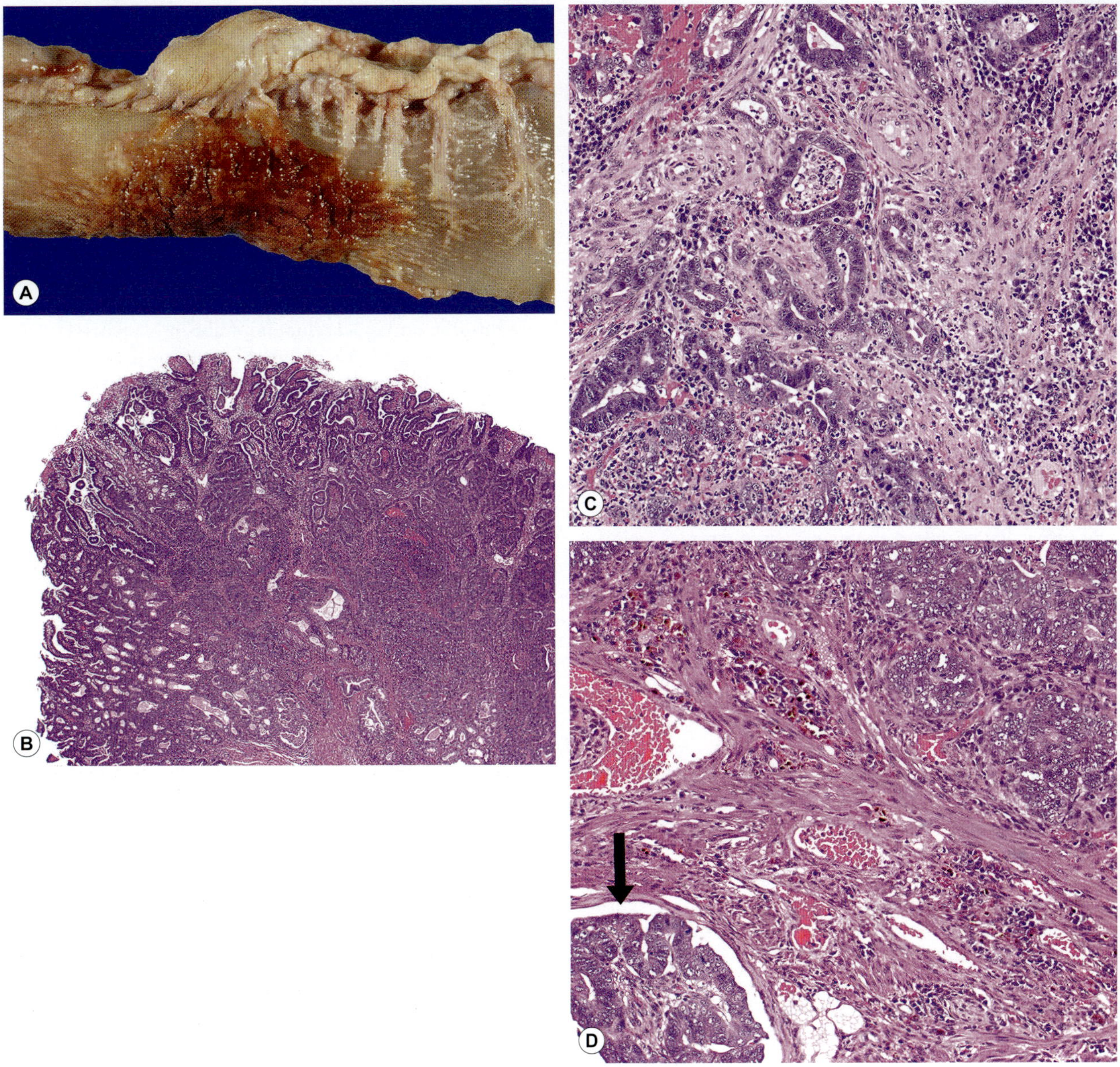

Figure 1-65 Intestinal carcinoma in a dog. **A**. Serosal hemorrhage and plaque-like masses of desmoplastic fibrous tissue and neoplastic cells on the serosa and along serosal lymphatics of the colon. **B**. Colorectal adenocarcinoma composed of a polypoid mass formed by haphazardly oriented immature basophilic neoplastic intestinal epithelial cells. **C**. A key defining feature of carcinoma is infiltrative growth of neoplastic epithelial cells surrounded by fibroplasia and inflammation, extending deep to the muscularis mucosa into the submucosa. **D**. Lymphatic invasion in the submucosa (arrow) is a feature of intestinal carcinoma.

perhaps most commonly seen with colonic carcinomas in cats. Malignant lesions are distinguished from hyperplastic polyps or benign adenomas solely because *they display at least some invasion into the underlying lamina propria, submucosa, or tunica muscularis*, which can be exceedingly difficult or impossible to detect in superficial endoscopic biopsies.

The earliest recognizable histologic lesion of intestinal carcinomas is *local effacement of glandular mucosal architecture* at the site of origin by proliferating polygonal mucus-producing epithelial cells. Neoplastic epithelial cells infiltrate the lamina propria and then invade sequentially through the basement membrane into the submucosa and tunica muscularis, infiltrating lymphatics, and sometimes veins. They are often highly infiltrative and readily penetrate the serosal surface of the intestine where they exfoliate into the peritoneal cavity to establish neoplastic implants on omentum and mesentery, which is termed **carcinomatosis**. The tumor also spreads early via lymphatic and venous routes, so that even if surgical excision can be achieved in the case of early diagnosis, cure is rare because metastasis has likely already occurred.

Histologic features can be quite variable, and usually more than one histologic subtype occurs within the same neoplasm, although there is no established behavioral, prognostic, or therapeutic significance to different histologic patterns. *Most are scirrhous mucus-producing carcinomas* that generate abundant mucus-filled and neoplastic epithelium-lined lakes throughout the intestinal wall, which are further surrounded by prominent and abundant fibrous stromal proliferation (scirrhous or desmoplastic response). The degree of cytologic maturation of the neoplastic epithelial cells may be quite low, with prominent cellular atypia, lack of well-differentiated columnar cells, brush border, or distinct goblet cells; however, the diagnosis of carcinoma is obvious given the transmural invasive behavior accompanied frequently by abundant mucus production. It is not uncommon to find the wall of the intestine markedly expanded by large prominent lakes of mucus or fibroplasia with only rare clusters or individualized or clusters of neoplastic epithelial cells floating in the mucus or aggregated along the margins. The neoplastic cells may also form *signet ring* (epithelial cells with nucleus displaced to the periphery by a single large clear cytoplasmic vacuole), *medullary* (solid nests or trabeculae of cells with a few irregular glands), *adenosquamous* (areas of distinct squamous differentiation), or commonly *adenocarcinoma not otherwise specified* (features of specific subtypes are not evident) patterns with variable scirrhous reaction, so that the diagnosis of intestinal carcinoma may be quite challenging to distinguish from stromal neoplasia or postinflammatory reactive fibrosis. In almost all cases, however, the tumor cells do produce mucus, the visualization of which may be aided by special staining techniques (PAS, Alcian blue). Use of IHC (pan-cytokeratin) may be useful to search for neoplastic cells in lesions with significant fibroplasia.

The histologic diagnosis is best made with a *full-thickness biopsy*, as the submucosal and transmural portions of the neoplasm are often larger and more readily identified as malignancy than the mucosal portion of the lesions, which endoscopic biopsies may not capture. Alternatively, especially when large deep ulcerative lesions are biopsied endoscopically, only the necrosis, inflammation, and fibrosis that accompany neoplastic cells may be captured. An erroneous diagnosis of carcinoma may be easily made when attempting to distinguish early carcinoma from dysplastic repair of recent ulceration (more common in the stomach); full-thickness biopsies are again the more reliable endoscopic sample in such cases.

Intestinal adenocarcinoma in cats is the second most common GI neoplasm (lymphoma is the most common). Carcinomas of the intestine are more prevalent in Siamese cats than in other breeds. As in dogs, a higher prevalence is reported in males than in females. The mean age of cats with intestinal carcinoma is 10-11 years. Disease develops more frequently in the small intestine, although the colon has been reported to be frequently involved; the ileum seems to be a common site, followed by the jejunum. Carcinomas also arise in the large intestine of cats, and when located at the ileocecal junction, both the large and small intestine can be involved. The clinical signs and gross appearance are similar to those described for dogs.

The microscopic appearance of intestinal carcinomas in cats is similar to dogs and other species, and most are well-differentiated mucinous-type adenocarcinomas (or adenocarcinoma not otherwise specified) except that osteochondroid metaplasia of the stroma may be a feature. The rare carcinomas involving the large intestine have tended to be papillary, better differentiated, and less scirrhous than carcinomas involving the small intestine. Wide surgical excision with or without chemotherapy is the treatment of choice; the prognosis is typically poor. Lymphatic or vascular invasion is thought to be less frequently observed in cats compared with dogs, but ~50% of cats in some studies had metastases in mesenteric lymph nodes at the time of diagnosis of intestinal carcinoma. Similar to dogs, feline intestinal carcinomas are highly infiltrative, so even if transection site margins can be achieved surgically, mural margins are often not complete, leading to a high rate of carcinomatosis, usually in close proximity to the primary tumor. No significant histomorphologic features or immunohistochemical markers of feline intestinal carcinoma have been demonstrated, although lower mitotic counts in neoplastic cell populations are correlated with longer progression-free survival (mean mitotic count was 18 per 2.37 mm^2; however, specific thresholds for mitotic counts have not been defined for intestinal carcinomas in cats).

Intestinal adenocarcinoma of sheep is relatively common in New Zealand, the United Kingdom, Scotland, Iceland, Norway, and southeastern Australia; in New Zealand and Australia there is a high prevalence in meat-production breeds, which may be related to exposure to bracken fern or other unidentified carcinogens. Heavy use of certain fertilizers and pastures with the weed *Cynosurus cristatus* have also been linked to an increased incidence of intestinal carcinoma in New Zealand sheep. Tumors occur mainly in animals ≥5-years-old. Clinically affected sheep lose weight and have abdominal distension caused by ascites, but most cases are incidental findings at slaughter.

Neoplasms are usually located in the middle or lower small intestine (Fig. 1-66A and B), and rarely in the colon. They are dense, firm, white, well-demarcated nodules, 0.5 to several centimeters long, and up to 1 cm thick; they may form annular constrictive bands at the affected site. Polyps or plaques may protrude into the lumen or occasionally from the serosal surface; mucosal ulceration is uncommon. The intestine is dilated proximal to the lesion; carcinomatosis on serosal surfaces is common, and these appear as opaque-to-white plaques or diffusely thickened areas, which must be differentiated from mesothelioma. Obstruction of serosal lymphatics by tumor emboli may lead to ascites. Lung and liver metastases are rare.

Microscopically, there are solid sheets or nests of well-differentiated to highly anaplastic polyhedral, cuboidal, or columnar epithelial cells that may form irregular acinar structures. They may be distributed singly, or in small aggregates, and are often difficult to detect in the heavy fibrous desmoplastic response. The neoplastic cells infiltrate the bowel wall along lymphatics, vessels, and nerve trunks, through to the serosal surface, whence they spread to the mesenteric lymph nodes. This is apparently followed by retrograde lymphogenous metastasis back to the intestinal wall proximal to the primary tumor; these are particularly responsible for constriction of the gut lumen. Sclerotic masses with anaplastic epithelial cells, many of which are PAS-positive, are located on the serosal surfaces of the abdominal organs but rarely infiltrate the parenchyma. Argentaffin cells may form part of some intestinal carcinomas, especially in lymph node metastases. Mineralization and osseous metaplasia may develop in the stroma.

Intestinal carcinomas are generally rare in **cattle** (see Fig. 1-66C), **goats, horses**, and **swine**. In horses, intestinal adenocarcinomas represent <1% of equine neoplasms and are found less frequently than intestinal lymphoma. In cattle, intestinal adenocarcinoma is associated with bracken fern, papillomavirus, or carcinoma involving the forestomachs. Most of these tumors in cattle are **adenomas** and 3 types are recognized: 1) sessile plaque; 2) adenomatous polyp; and 3) proliferative adenoma of the ampullae (where the bile and pancreatic ducts open into the duodenum). Intestinal

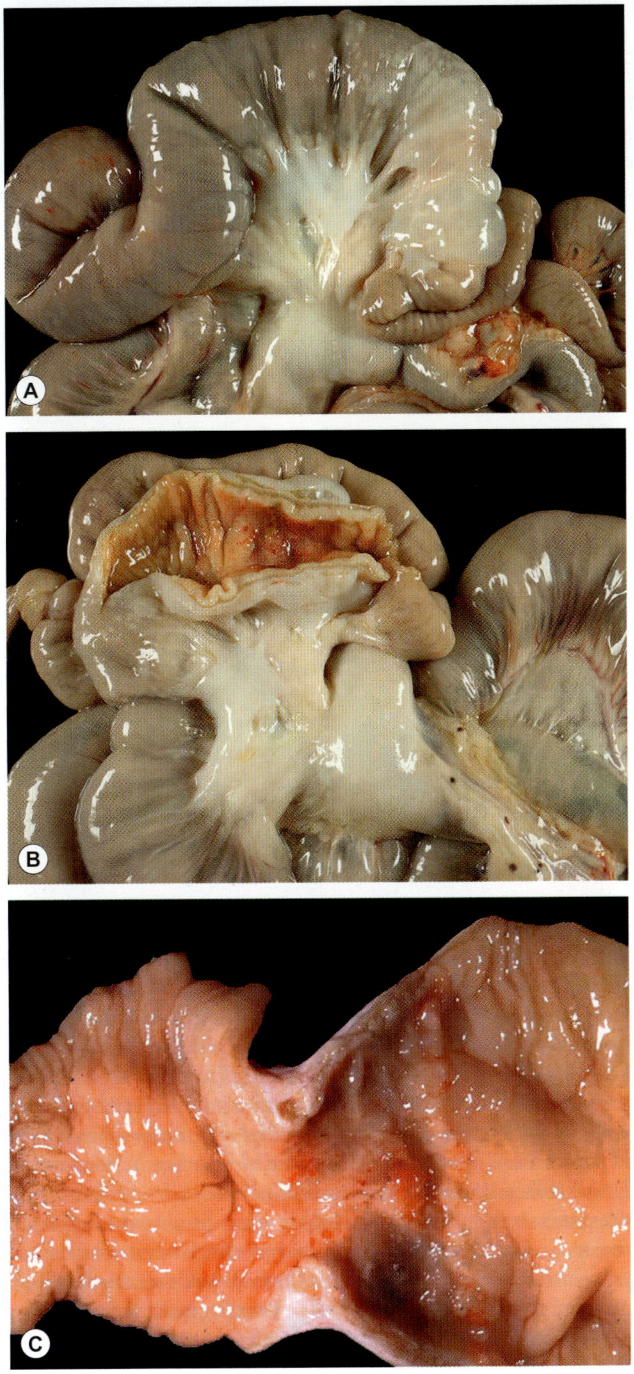

Figure 1-66 Intestinal adenocarcinoma in ruminants. **A**. Thickened and dilated small intestine segments in a sheep. **B**. Opened section of (A.) (A, B courtesy K. Thompson.) **C**. Intestinal carcinoma in a cow with annular thickening. (Courtesy Noah's Arkives.)

carcinomas are usually an incidental finding at meat inspection. The location, morphology, and routes of metastasis are similar to those described for sheep, except that serosal lesions are less obvious. Hematogenous spread to the liver, lung, kidney, uterus, and ovaries may occur in cattle.

Neuroendocrine carcinomas (carcinoids) arise from neuroendocrine cells that are scattered in the mucosa of a wide variety of organs, including the stomach and intestine. These cells secrete low–molecular-weight polypeptide hormones, such as secretin, somatostatin, and cholecystokinin, or they are part of the APUD group, producing compounds such as serotonin (5-hydroxytryptamine). Carcinoid tumors of the GI tract are *rare* in domestic animals. They have been reported mainly in aged dogs and very rarely in the cat, cow, and horse. In **dogs**, most carcinoids are located in the duodenum, colon, and rectum, and only rarely in the stomach and lower small intestine. They may cause intestinal obstruction or anemia resulting from ulceration and hemorrhage. Associated diarrhea in some cases can speculatively be attributed to hypersecretion of functional polypeptide hormones. Rectal carcinoids may protrude from the anus and resemble adenomatous polyps.

Macroscopically, carcinoids are usually lobulated, firm, dark-red to cream-colored masses, a few millimeters to perhaps 2 cm in diameter, that seem to arise deep in the mucosa, often forming submucosal or subserosal nodules, with ulceration of overlying mucosa. They tend to infiltrate locally, transmurally, and into the mesentery.

Carcinoids have a *distinct histomorphologic neuroendocrine appearance*. Round or oval-to-polyhedral cells have abundant finely granular eosinophilic or vacuolated cytoplasm and vesiculate nuclei with prominent nucleoli. They form nests, packets, ribbons, rosettes, or diffuse sheets in the mucosa, submucosa, and/or tunica muscularis of the intestine, supported by finely vascularized fibrous stroma. Amyloid has rarely been described with carcinoids, and megalocytes or multinucleate giant cells are observed occasionally. A *diagnosis* of carcinoid is based on the distinct histomorphologic pattern, cytoplasmic argentaffinic and argyrophilic granularity, immunohistochemical identification of specific secretory products, and the typical ultrastructural appearance. The histochemical reactions may be negative, especially in rectal carcinoids, and they also may be lost during fixation in formalin or by autolysis prior to fixation. These cells are routinely positive with immunohistochemical staining for neuron-specific enolase and chromogranin, as are most neuroendocrine tumors, and with one or more of the specific immune probes related to the peptides being produced. An increased concentration of specific secretory products may be detected in circulation.

When available, electron microscopic ultrastructural examination likely helps to differentiate carcinoids from intestinal MCTs. Carcinoid cells have dense, round-to-oval, membrane-bound, 75-300-nm, secretory granules in the cytoplasm. They have abundant rough endoplasmic reticulum, and the plasma membrane forms interdigitating processes. Carcinoid cells are PAS negative and are not metachromatic with Giemsa stains. Data on biological behavior of intestinal carcinoids in dogs are limited; most reported cases have been malignant. There may be extensive invasion of the gut wall and veins with metastasis, especially to the liver. The few cases that have been described in other species have features similar to those described in dogs.

Goblet cell carcinoids (adenocarcinoids, mucinous carcinoids) are described in the appendix of humans, with features of both carcinoids and adenocarcinomas. A single report of such a tumor in the rectum of a dog describes merged regions of mucinous adenocarcinoma and carcinoid; the carcinoid component was prominent and metastatic.

Neoplasms of mesenchymal cells of the GI tract have been variably defined and now broadly include nonangiogenic and nonlymphogenic intestinal mesenchymal tumors (**NIMTs**), which have been recently more precisely subclassified as intestinal smooth-muscle tumors (leiomyoma and leiomyosarcoma), gastrointestinal stromal tumors (GISTs) which originate from the pacemaker or interstitial cells of Cajal, intestinal neurogenic tumors, and various other uncommon mesenchymal neoplasms.

Intestinal smooth-muscle tumors include only leiomyoma and leiomyosarcoma; historically, other intestinal mesenchymal tumors were incorrectly classified here, but now thanks to immunohistochemical studies, it is well recognized that these are distinct lesions—although they remain difficult to differentiate from other intestinal sarcomas grossly and microscopically. Previous studies that did not utilize IHC to distinguish smooth-muscle tumors from GISTs should thus be read with caution.

Leiomyoma and leiomyosarcoma are the 2 extremes of a morphologic continuum of neoplastic lesions arising from smooth muscle of the GI tract, and they are probably not as uncommon as historically thought. Leiomyosarcomas are ~38% of all abdominal sarcomas, and 22-24% of those arose from the small intestine. The jejunum is the most commonly reported anatomic location for leiomyosarcoma; the most common location of all abdominal sarcomas is the spleen. Smooth-muscle tumors arising from the stomach are mostly benign, but those arising from the intestine are more often malignant. Because these arise from the tunica muscularis (or the muscularis mucosa), they tend to grow into the intestinal lumen and cause obstruction. Clinical signs often include weight loss, lethargy, anorexia, possibly anemia resulting from intestinal hemorrhage, abdominal pain, palpable abdominal masses, diarrhea, vomition, and dehydration or other signs of GI obstruction. Smooth-muscle tumors are often a single focal lesion that can grow quite large, with invasion of variable layers of the intestinal wall and eventually adjacent tissues. Smooth-muscle tumors are solid and often white, firm, fibrous masses on section; larger more aggressive neoplasms often have central necrosis due to local ischemia from rapid growth and expansion.

Histologically, smooth-muscle neoplasms are composed of swirling interwoven bundles of variably uniform fusiform mesenchymal cells, many with abundant eosinophilic cytoplasm and a central nucleus with blunted ends. Other features that can be present include a nuclear palisading and trabecular pattern, although these are apparently less frequent in intestinal smooth-muscle tumors than in those arising from other anatomic locations. Aggressive lesions often resemble benign lesions grossly and sometimes histologically, and the distinction between the 2 can be challenging. The most reliable features of malignancy in canine smooth-muscle tumors include differentiation (similarity to normal tissue), nuclear atypia (abnormal shape, karyomegaly, or prominent nucleoli), proliferative activity [mitotic count >9 per 2.37 mm^2 or increased Ki67 labeling index (although this is poorly defined)], multinucleation, evidence of infiltrative growth, and necrosis (absent, <50%, or >50% of the tumor). Similar to descriptions of tumors in humans, these features are probably best assessed together, and multiple of these features should be present to warrant a diagnosis of leiomyosarcoma. As examples, nuclear atypia and significant tumor necrosis likely indicate leiomyosarcoma; nuclear atypia and mitotic count >9 per 2.37 mm^2 supports a diagnosis of leiomyosarcoma; a neoplasm with an elevated mitotic count but lacking nuclear atypia and necrosis is probably more accurately diagnosed as leiomyoma; mitotic count alone is probably insufficient to warrant a diagnosis of leiomyosarcoma.

IHC can be helpful to definitively diagnose smooth-muscle tumors, and specifically to distinguish them from other mesenchymal tumors of the intestine. Smooth-muscle tumors express αSMA diffusely but not CD117 (c-kit) or discovered on GIST (DOG)-1. Approximately 70% express desmin diffusely or multifocally; estrogen and/or progesterone receptors are expressed in up to 30%, although these have no known prognostic significance for intestinal lesions. Most smooth-muscle tumors are probably benign, although the occurrence of leiomyosarcomas in the intestinal tract is likely higher than historically thought. Metastasis seems to be correlated with increased proliferative activity (mitotic count or increased Ki67 labeling) and tumor necrosis. Tumor-related deaths are correlated with the overall size of the neoplasm, cellular and nuclear atypia, mitotic count, necrosis, differentiation, and lack of desmin expression. The overall reported metastatic rate for leiomyosarcomas is ~15%. Mesenteric invasion and metastasis observed at diagnosis or during surgery in dogs (and thus warranting a diagnosis of leiomyosarcoma) may not actually negatively affect the long-term prognosis, so (as in humans) tumor size and location may still represent the most significant prognostic factors.

Gastrointestinal stromal tumors (GISTs) are distinct from smooth-muscle tumors, although they are common GI sarcomas that have historically been erroneously grouped with smooth-muscle tumors. GISTs arise from the interstitial cells of Cajal, which are pacemaker cells located in myenteric or submucosal plexuses of the GI wall, and have many similarities to smooth-muscle tumors, including both their gross and histologic appearance. The prevalence of GISTs in dogs is difficult to assess because of historical misclassification as smooth-muscle tumors, but GISTs are probably uncommon neoplasms in dogs and less frequent in other species, including cats. They are most common in the intestine, especially the distal intestine and cecum, with only rare gastric GISTs reported; however, the primary site is not known to have prognostic significance. The presentation will be similar to smooth-muscle tumors of the intestine, and clinical signs include anorexia, weight loss, lethargy, anorexia, anemia, abdominal pain, palpable abdominal masses, diarrhea, vomition, and GI obstruction. GISTs (like smooth-muscle tumors) arise from the wall of the intestine, so they are usually single focal lesions that grow by expansion, sometimes forming exophytic or cavitated cystic masses that can be visible from serosal and/or mucosal surfaces, which may be ulcerated. They are mural masses and can be transmural with infiltrative growth into the intestinal wall, or into adjacent tissues (Fig. 1-67A). GISTs are composed of spindle cells arranged as interlacing fascicles, or in a storiform whorling pattern, with oval nuclei, and a somewhat basophilic cytoplasm with indistinct cell borders. Most are of spindle morphology in dogs (see Fig. 1-67B), although other patterns recognized (mostly in humans and less frequently in dogs) include myxoid, fascicular, and epithelioid types. A minority of cases in dogs may have an epithelioid morphology in which pleomorphic polygonal neoplastic cells with increased cytoplasm are arranged in sheets supported by fibrous, myxoid, or fatty vascular stroma. The epithelioid variant, although rare, may reflect some degree of neural differentiation. There may be nuclear pleomorphism, lymphocytic and plasmacytic inflammation, and areas of hemorrhage and necrosis in all patterns of GISTs. The mitotic rate can vary widely but is usually higher in GISTs than in smooth-muscle tumors, with an average of 7-8 per 2.37 mm^2. GISTs may have more

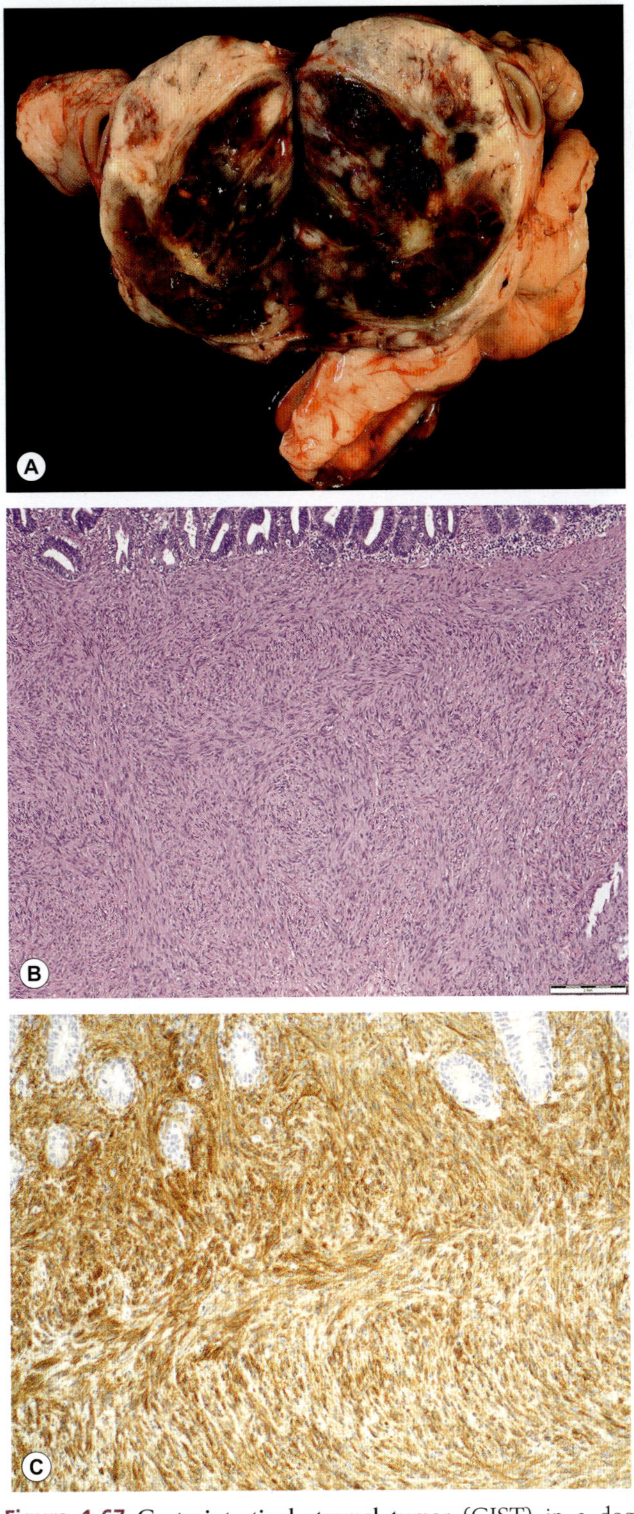

Figure 1-67 Gastrointestinal stromal tumor (GIST) in a dog. **A.** Small intestinal GIST arising from the wall of the small intestine. (Courtesy T. Walsh.) **B.** Neoplastic spindle cells arranged in bundles. **C.** CD117 (c-KIT) IHC demonstrates strong cytoplasmic immunoreactivity in the neoplastic spindle cells.

necrosis, hemorrhage, and inflammation and may be quicker to invade locally and cause intestinal perforation compared with smooth-muscle tumors. Despite these features, GISTs cannot be reliably distinguished from smooth-muscle tumors without the use of IHC.

The defining feature of a GIST is at least some neoplastic cells with positive cytoplasmic immunoreactivity with CD117 (c-KIT, tyrosine kinase receptor) (see Fig. 1-67C) *or DOG1 (discovered on GIST1)*. Some GISTs may also display immunoreactivity to α-SMA; smooth-muscle tumors do not demonstrate immunoreactivity to CD117 or DOG1. The intensity of IHC may also be significant prognostically for GISTs; patients with neoplasms with weak cytoplasmic immunoreactivity for c-KIT had a significantly worse prognosis and shorter survival time than patients with GISTs with moderate or strong cytoplasmic c-KIT staining. Immunoreactivity for S100, desmin, neuron-specific enolase, CD34, and PGP 9.5 has been documented in some cases, but these are inconsistent. Although the prognostic significance of these IHC markers remains unknown, some authors have hypothesized that some GISTs have myogenic or neurogenic differentiation.

When GISTs were initially reported as distinct from other intestinal sarcomas based on retrospective IHC studies, they were thought to be more aggressive clinical lesions with frequent metastasis to the liver and lymph nodes; however, this has not proven to be true. The reported metastatic rate of GISTs is ~30%, which is somewhat higher than malignant smooth-muscle tumors (15%). There have been no significant patient outcome differences in metastatic rate, recurrence rate, progression-free interval, or progression-free survival for dogs with GISTs compared with dogs with leiomyosarcomas. High mitotic count, incomplete surgical margins, and weak cytoplasmic c-KIT staining intensity remain important prognostic factors for GISTs in dogs; however, despite distinctions in cell of origin and anatomic location for GIST and smooth-muscle tumors, the behavior of these neoplasms appears to be similar. Large intestinal tumors may also cause *paraneoplastic hypoglycemia*, owing to the production of insulin-like growth factors. Production of erythropoietin resulting in erythrocytosis also has been documented in dogs.

Intestinal GISTs in horses have been described; most occur in the distal intestine including the colon, cecum, and rectum. IHC confirmation [CD117 (c-kit)] has been demonstrated in horses. Most GISTs are encountered as incidental lesions discovered at autopsy or during surgery, although they (or other intestinal sarcomas) may cause intermittent bouts of colic, hematochezia, or obstruction. They are encapsulated, firm, often multinodular, pale-tan or hemorrhagic masses in the muscularis or subserosa, protruding on the serosal surface, or rarely, as somewhat pedunculated tumors projecting from the serosa or into the lumen. Histologic features are as expected for other species, and neoplastic mesenchymal cells are arranged in interconnected trabeculae or interwoven bundles, and sometimes whorls or palisades supported by mucinous-to-myxoid matrix. Areas of inflammation, hemorrhage, or necrosis can be seen; the mitotic rate is usually low. Malignancy including localized infiltrative growth or metastasis is not described in horses. A GIST has been described in a **goat**, which originated in the rumen. The diagnosis was confirmed by positive immunoreactivity for CD117, although the neoplasm was also immunoreactive for smooth muscle actin (SMA); metastasis was also documented in the liver.

Other sarcomas of the intestine are reported in various species and include neurogenic (**neurofibroma**) or **nerve sheath (schwannoma) tumors**. Nerve sheath or perineural tumors arise from Schwann cells or perineural cells and are similar to those described in other tissues. They probably arise more commonly in the distal intestine (colon, cecum) and are composed of neoplastic spindle cells forming storiform whorls or palisades (Antoni type A pattern is most common, but Antoni type B pattern can also be evident). By definition they lack immunoreactivity for both SMA and c-kit (CD117), although they may also exhibit immunoreactivity for S100, PGP 9.5, GFAP, and vimentin; however, this can be variable. Given the variable IHC results and morphology reported of these uncommon lesions, nonangiogenic and nonlymphogenic intestinal mesenchymal tumors (NIMTs) that also lack immunoreactivity for both SMA and c-kit are most appropriately termed **non-GIST non-smooth muscle NIMTs**.

Proliferative mesenchymal lesions involving the ganglia include ganglioneuromatosis and ganglioneuroma. In **ganglioneuromatosis**, ganglion plexi proliferate in the intestinal wall; these are thought to be hyperplastic lesions that may develop as a congenital lesion that progressively enlarges as the animal ages. Ganglioneuromatosis has been described in young dogs, a calf, and a young horse, mostly as a poorly demarcated nodular lesions that can affect various segments of the intestine. The lesion arises from the submucosal ganglia and consists of proliferative ganglion cells in clusters supported by interlacing nerve fibers and perineural sheaths. In contrast and even more uncommon is the **ganglioneuroma**, which is a neoplasm of ganglion cells that has been described in single case reports to affect the intestine of a dog, cat, and horse. This occurs as a solitary well-demarcated nodule of ganglion cells with a few mitotic figures. Infiltrative or invasive growth behavior is not reported, and the malignant potential is thought to be quite low.

Various **other sarcomas** have been reported in the intestinal tract, including fibrosarcoma, myxosarcoma (dog, horse), extraskeletal osteosarcoma (dogs), hemangiosarcoma (cat, dog); these are all uncommon and have features or immunohistochemical reactivity as expected for these sarcomas in other anatomic locations.

Neoplasms of round cells. Intestinal lymphoma occurs in most species, and variants of lymphoma are especially common in cats and dogs. These neoplasms may be primary to the GI tract or as part of the systemic or multicentric form of the neoplasm (see Vol. 3, Hematolymphoid System). Primary GI lymphoma is defined as malignant lymphocytic infiltrates in the stomach or intestine as the major system involved and to which treatment is directed; there may also be involvement of other abdominal organs, lymph nodes, or bone marrow, although lesions are not present in the thorax or peripheral lymph nodes. In addition, lymphoma can develop at other sites and then spread to the GI tract; this also would not be considered primary intestinal lymphoma.

Lymphoma is the most common GI neoplasm in companion animals, which is unsurprising given the huge number of lymphoid cell populations normally present in the GI tract; the disease is more prevalent and more complex in cats than in dogs. It can be segmental within any portion of the GI tract or diffuse. Although the GI tract may be involved in advanced multicentric lymphoma in dogs, such cases are rarely submitted for biopsy because the diagnosis has already been made based on lesions elsewhere. Most samples submitted for histologic assessment are from cases suspected of having primary GI lymphoma, and in cats, almost all cases examined at biopsy are primary within the stomach or intestine.

In both dogs and cats, tumors may arise from clonal expansion of lymphocytes in MALT, lamina propria, or intraepithelial layers; they can be of T-cell, B-cell, or NK-cell phenotype. Following the pattern set by WHO, neoplastic lymphocytes can be classified by 4 specific and prognostically significant features: neoplastic cell nuclear size (small = 1-1.25× RBC; intermediate = 1.5× RBC; large = >2× RBC); histologic grade (low = 0-5 mitotic figures/0.237 mm^2; intermediate = 6-10 mitotic figures/0.237 mm^2; or high >= 10 mitotic figures/0.237 mm^2); immunophenotype (B, T, or non-B non-T, by immunohistochemistry); and growth pattern (mucosal or transmural, when possible). Additional important information can be gleaned by flow cytometry (more markers are available for use in fresh lymph node aspirates) and receptor clonality by PCR assay (PARR).

Lymphoma of the canine intestine can appear in several situations and syndromes. Large B-cell lymphoma is the most common type of lymphoma in dogs, and intestinal involvement can certainly occur, although lesions are often present in other organs as well. Primary enteric lymphoma is less common than multicentric lymphoma in dogs; prevalence is higher in males. Most occur in the small intestine, although other sites can also be affected. Most patients with intestinal lymphoma have historically had poor long-term survival and prognosis (mean survival time of ~60 days), and many deaths occur due to progression of the disease within weeks to months after the initial diagnosis; lymphoma restricted to the intestine has longer survival (mean 121 days) compared with GI lymphoma with nodal involvement, although few specific prognostic indicators have been identified. Most dogs with primary GI lymphoma were reported historically to be of B-cell phenotype; however, T-cell lymphoma is now more common. The reason for a shift from B-cell to T-cell dominance in dogs and cats is unknown but is likely related to greater understanding of the various subtypes of T-cell lymphoma in the GI tract (although shifting naming convention and acronyms bring frustration and confusion to the area). Recent work has substantially increased understanding and recognition of intestinal low-grade small-cell lymphoma (also called low-grade alimentary lymphoma/LGAL, monomorphic epitheliotropic intestinal T-cell lymphoma/MEITL; formerly *enteropathy-associated T-cell lymphoma*/EATL type 2), an indolent disease in which small neoplastic lymphocytes infiltrate the mucosa and often the epithelium. An important diagnostic task for pathologists is to distinguish lymphoma (especially low-grade small-cell lymphoma) from chronic intestinal inflammation. Compared with the indolent course of intestinal low-grade small-cell lymphoma, high-grade large-cell intestinal lymphoma (also called high-grade alimentary lymphoma/HGAL, or enteropathy-associated T-cell lymphoma (EATL); formerly *EATL type 1*) in dogs has larger neoplastic lymphocytes (eFig. 1-10) in the mucosa that may have cytoplasmic granularity and that often infiltrate transmurally; this is probably the most common primary form of GI lymphoma in the dog.

Several other less frequent subtypes or variants of intestinal lymphoma are described in the literature. Indolent or follicular B-cell lymphoma arising from MALT in the canine colon and rectum is rare. Rare cases of B-cell intestinal lymphoma with Mott cell differentiation have been reported. GI lymphomas in the Miniature Dachshund are apparently mostly intestinal and colorectal, and usually of large B-cell phenotype; they tend to develop in younger dogs, and patients have prolonged survival. Anaplastic large T-cell lymphoma involving the intestine has been described as a unique rare and aggressive transmural disease in dogs.

Eosinophil recruitment occurs and is likely related to the production of IL3 and IL5 by neoplastic lymphocytes in many cases of large-cell lymphoma (HGAL or EATL). In addition, these neoplasms may display cytoplasmic granules (they are best seen by cytology) and may express the IHC marker granzyme B; however, this currently has no known prognostic significance.

The most frequent clinical signs include anorexia, vomiting, diarrhea, weight loss, and lethargy. Hypoproteinemia, probably associated with enteric protein loss, occurs in ~30% of affected dogs. Gross lesions often include nodular soft-to-firm cream-colored masses located in the small intestine, stomach, and colon (in that order of frequency); they are located in the submucosa and often protrude into the intestinal lumen; the overlying mucosa may be ulcerated. The diagnosis of lymphoma in such cases is usually readily evident during autopsy. Some lesions develop as locally extensive or diffuse thickening of the intestine, and several sections of the gut can be affected simultaneously. The mesenteric nodes are often enlarged, and the liver can be involved at the time of presentation. The microscopic lesions of canine intestinal lymphoma when masses are present are straightforward: there is accumulation and often effacement of intestinal parenchyma including mucosa, submucosa, and possibly the tunica muscularis by densely cellular nodules and sheets of monomorphic neoplastic lymphocytes, which appear histomorphologically indistinguishable from multicentric lymphoma in most cases. Neoplastic lymphocytes infiltrate and efface intestinal parenchyma, but usually are not prominently necrotic; this, along with the lack of mixed pleomorphic inflammatory cells, can be helpful to distinguish lymphoma from IBD lesions in some cases. However, many lymphomas in dogs (and cats) do have lymphocytic and variable plasmacytic infiltrates within the lamina propria. The distribution of severe infiltrative disease can be diffuse or multifocal in lymphoma or IBD, and because lymphomas may arise in some cases from a background of chronic inflammation, mixed neoplastic and inflammatory cells are commonly encountered. When distinguishing histomorphologic features of infiltrating cells are not clear, or when mural or transmural infiltration by neoplastic lymphocytes is not observed, several additional features are helpful to distinguish the chronic lymphoplasmacytic inflammation of IBD from intestinal lymphoma.

The most significant histologic features that support a **diagnosis of lymphoma** include intra-epithelial lymphocytes (IELs) and epithelial injury, which is more frequent and more severe in lymphomas than in IBD. Most (but not all) cases of intestinal lymphoma have increased IELs within the surface epithelium, and intraepithelial infiltrates involving both surface and cryptal epithelium are more commonly observed in intestinal lymphoma than in IBD. The pattern of IELs is a significant feature to note: IELs occur as single cells (more common in IBD), nests (>5 clustered IELs, more common in lymphoma), or plaques (>5 epithelial cells obscured by clustered IELs, also more common in lymphoma), and can be observed in a few villi. *Importantly though in dogs (in contrast to cats), a significant number of IBD cases have increased IELs, and in many of these cases, nests and plaques can be observed in both surface and cryptal epithelium; thus, the occurrence of intraepithelial nests and plaques that are a strong indicator of low-grade small-cell epitheliotropic lymphoma (LGAL, formerly EATL type 2) in cats are not predictive of lymphoma in dogs*. Thus, epitheliotropism is a much less significant diagnostic parameter for lymphoma in dogs. Additional histomorphologic features supporting a diagnosis of lymphoma instead of IBD in dogs include a monomorphic population of lymphocytes in lamina propria and transmural infiltration. In challenging and histologically equivocal cases, additional testing including IHC and PARR may be necessary; however, it is important to recall that these should be viewed as ancillary tests and thus should be performed in this order (histology ◂ IHC ◂ PARR). Interpretation of test results is always best performed together in context, which will lead to improved accuracy and confidence in diagnosis in this confusing area.

IHC is an excellent and often essential complementary technique to histologic assessment of intestine and diagnosis of intestinal lymphoma. Common antibodies for IHC in cats and dogs include CD3 for T lymphocytes, and CD79a, CD20, PAX5 (paired box gene 5, a nuclear transcription factor, staining is evident in nuclei), and less commonly B-lymphocyte antigen 36 (BLA.36) for B lymphocytes, ionizing calcium-binding adaptor molecule-1 (IBA1) or macrophage marker antibody 387 (MAC387) for macrophages, granzyme B for natural killer (NK) cells, and the proliferation marker Ki67. IHC (CD3) is especially helpful for distinguishing IBD from lymphoma, although its value lies mostly as an aid in observation and confirmation of the number and pattern of distribution of lymphocytes within the lamina propria, and to confirm the presence of individual or subtle nests and plaques of IELs within surface and cryptal epithelium, which can be more difficult to discern in H&E sections when there is significant concurrent inflammation. Additional IHC such as Ki67 may be helpful because its expression is significantly higher in canine intestinal lymphomas compared with IBD.

Clonality testing is now commonly used especially to identify lymphomas in cases of significant concurrent inflammation in the intestine (and other organs), and although clonality can be assessed by flow cytometry and southern blotting, PCR is by far the most common method utilized because it can be used in formalin-fixed paraffin-embedded tissues. This test is based on the amplification of the complementarity determining region (CDR) 3 of the T-cell receptor and the immunoglobulin heavy-chain genes for B cells; the assumption driving interpretation of this test is that neoplastic lesions are clonal (or oligoclonal) and derived from one or a few cells, whereas reactive inflammatory lesions are polyclonal and derived from a heterogeneous population of lymphocytes. Interpretation of PARR can also be challenging in difficult or equivocal cases, and especially when early or emerging neoplasia is suspected; it is therefore unwise to interpret PARR results in these cases without the specific context of histomorphologic features of the intestinal lesions and IHC. Several studies have shown that PARR results can be misleading for various reasons, including low numbers of neoplastic cells in a strong inflammatory background, poor quality or nonrepresentative samples, PCR assays and primers with insufficient antigen receptor coverage (not all primer sets for multiplex PCR are created or designed equally robust), overall assay sensitivity, presence of pseudoclones (due to low template DNA recovery), presence of oligoclones (reduced natural T-cell repertoire due to age or immune status of an individual), lack of expertise or training in interpreting PCR results, or other technical reasons. In summary, various testing modalities should be utilized for diagnosis of intestinal lymphomas in dogs, *with histomorphology of appropriately sampled and processed endoscopic or surgical biopsy samples of affected intestine as the cornerstone diagnostic modality*, which can then be supplemented or confirmed by IHC and/or clonality PARR testing. Even with a flawless stepwise approach, some cases are diagnostically equivocal, which further reveals the difficulty in detecting subtle changes in normal from development of significant lesions within the GI tract over time.

Lymphoma of the feline intestine is common and can also occur in several scenarios and syndromes. Historically, most feline intestinal lymphomas have been associated with the highly lymphomagenic FeLV infection, but even with reduced incidence of FeLV infection, lymphoma in cats has increased, likely due specifically to GI lymphomas—because mucosal T-cell lymphomas were underdiagnosed before widespread use of IHC and PARR. As for dogs (although the disease is more thoroughly and clearly described in cats), intestinal lymphoma can manifest as nodules of neoplastic lymphocytes that exhibit mucosal effacement and infiltrative growth with transmural invasion (eFig. 1-11). Although this is certainly more straightforward diagnostically for pathologists, it is well recognized that mucosal lymphomas involving the epithelial and/or the lamina proprial compartments of the intestine can be much more histomorphologically subtle and develop long before transmural invasion and progression actually occur. Recognizing that many early lymphomas probably develop as patchy or focal disease coincidentally arising with or from within the GI inflammation of IBD, the differentiation of early mucosal lymphoma from IBD in cats is thus especially challenging and of great interest to pathologists and primary care veterinarians everywhere. Fortunately, much work has been published demonstrating key diagnostic features of feline intestinal lymphoma.

Enteric lymphoma in cats is distinct from mediastinal or multicentric lymphoma and refers to primary GI or alimentary lymphoma, with variable involvement of extraintestinal sites including lymph nodes, liver, and spleen. As in dogs, enteric lymphoma is broadly categorized by pattern and location as transmural or mucosal (lamina proprial and/or intraepithelial), neoplastic lymphocyte nuclear size (small = 1-1.25× RBC; intermediate = 1.5-2× RBC; and large = >2× RBC), histologic grade (low = 0-5 mitotic figures/0.237mm^2; intermediate = 6-10 mitotic figures/0.237mm^2; and high >10 mitotic figures/0.237mm^2), and phenotype (T cell or B cell, by IHC). Overall, most intestinal lymphomas in cats are of T-cell phenotype, although studies have varied as to the actual percentages present. Most transmural lymphomas in cats are high grade, composed of large (or less commonly small) cells, and can be of T- or B-cell phenotype. Transmural intermediate- to large-cell lymphomas are less frequent in cats but are usually composed of LGL (the granules are often easier to observe cytologically); many express the cytotoxic marker granzyme B by IHC (the histochemical stain PTAH may be helpful in some casess to identify subtle cytoplasmic granules), and these are likely a more behaviorally aggressive variant of GI lymphoma in cats.

Most *B-cell lymphomas of the feline GI tract* are large cell, are found in the stomach and the distal small intestine, the cells exhibit no epitheliotropism, they are infiltrative and often transmural, and have shorter mean survival times. The diagnosis of *feline intestinal transmural lymphoma* when masses are present is straightforward, and care should be taken to evaluate other organs for multicentric disease. Neoplastic B lymphocytes are usually large and cause effacement of intestinal parenchyma including mucosa, submucosa, and possibly tunica muscularis by nodules, plaques, or sheets of dense monomorphic neoplastic lymphocytes.

In contrast, most *T-cell lymphomas in the feline intestine* are small cell, are present in the small intestine (specifically the jejunum), are limited to the mucosa (many exhibit epitheliotropism), and have prolonged survival times with an indolent course of disease. This type of lymphoma corresponds closely to human monomorphic epitheliotrpic intestinal T-cell lymphoma (MEITL, formerly known as *EATL type 2*), based on the WHO classification; these are often called small-cell or simply low-grade intestinal or alimentary lymphoma, and are the most common form in cats (estimated to be up to 65-75% of GI lymphoma cases), and can be of particular challenge diagnostically. Small-cell low-grade lymphoma is uncommonly identified in the stomach or colon of cats and is not reported in the literature in these organs without small intestinal involvement.

Low-grade intestinal lymphoma shares many clinical, ultrasonographic, and gross features with IBD in cats and is considered by some to be an appropriate animal model for human small-cell intestinal lymphoma. Affected cats have chronic progressive weight loss, vomiting, anorexia, lethargy, and sometimes diarrhea (although this is less in cats than in dogs); the clinical signs are indistinguishable from chronic IBD. They often have intestinal thickening, and the loss of the normal layered appearance of the intestinal wall noted during radiographic or ultrasound evaluation, which can be focal or diffuse. Mesenteric lymphadenopathy, hepatomegaly, and splenomegaly may also be present. Diagnostic imaging is probably more helpful to evaluate other organ involvement (lymph nodes, liver, etc.), and less helpful for diagnosis of lymphoma. Endoscopic visualization of the intestine is often reported, though again, the changes are nonspecific and unreliable for diagnosis of lymphoma or to distinguish from other chronic enteropathies.

The cause of intestinal lymphoma remains incompletely understood, and though FeLV, dysbiosis, chronic intestinal inflammation, or *H. pylori* infection are all hypothesized to be associated with the development of GI lymphoma in cats, there is insufficient evidence to confirm these associations. Assessments of cobalamin and folate are often performed as part of the clinical workup and are helpful indicators of disease location (folate is absorbed in the proximal small intestine, cobalamin is absorbed in the distal small intestine), and although altered absorption of these B vitamins occurs with various chronic enteropathies, they have not been diagnostic for intestinal lymphoma, or in distinguishing lymphoma from other chronic enteropathies.

The **diagnosis** of *feline intestinal mucosal lymphomas* is complex and potentially confusing, especially because distinction from IBD is expected; but this is a frequent task and expectation for veterinary pathologists. *The gold standard for diagnosis of feline intestinal mucosal lymphoma is histologic examination of appropriately sampled and appropriately oriented intestinal biopsy specimens*. Specimens presented for histologic assessment should be evaluated using the stepwise criteria discussed previously. Specific histomorphologic features strongly correlated with a diagnosis of mucosal lymphoma in cats (often to the exclusion of lymphoplasmacytic enteritis) include: villus atrophy; IELs individually and forming nests or plaques (eFig. 1-12); dense infiltration of the lamina propria or epithelium by monomorphic small or large lymphocytes (Fig. 1-68A and B); a lack of mixed inflammatory cellular infiltration of the lamina propria; and infiltration of submucosa, tunica muscularis, or serosal layers by monomorphic lymphocytes (which is typically not evident in endoscopic samples). Several other features less strongly correlated with a diagnosis of intestinal lymphoma in cats include: an apical-to-basal gradient of small monomorphic lymphocytes; lymphocytic cryptitis; prominent cryptal hyperplasia; less prominent superficial lamina proprial fibrosis; and more prominent deep lamina propria and submucosal fibrosis. Although these specific histomorphologic features likely are the most significant criteria that lead to at least presumptive diagnosis of intestinal lymphoma in cats, *features of inflammation and lymphoma often occur simultaneously in the GI tract* (such as IELs individually or forming inconsistent or subtle nests in a few or a single villus within a mixed cellular proprial infiltrate, or areas of monomorphic dense lymphocytic infiltrates within a mixed cellular proprial infiltrate), leading to ambiguity. Thus, in some cases, histologic evaluation as the sole diagnostic test may be insufficient to confidently establish a diagnosis; in cases of early or emerging lymphoma, distinction from IBD may be impossible. Improved confidence in a diagnosis of lymphoma and differentiation from lymphoplasmacytic enteritis in cats can be gained by additional testing modalities including IHC and PARR.

IHC is an excellent and often essential complementary technique to histologic assessment of intestine (see Fig. 1-68C). As for dogs, the value of IHC in this context is probably not solely for the differentiation of T- versus B-cell phenotype, but rather IHC allows better assessment of monomorphic populations of T or B cells, and it provides better visualization of patterns of infiltration both in the lamina propria and in the epithelium; in particular, individual IELs or subtle nests formed are more readily evident in IHC-stained sections, compared with standard H&E-stained sections. Common antibodies for IHC in cats (as for dogs) include CD3 for T lymphocytes, and CD79a, CD20, PAX5, and BLA.36 for B lymphocytes, MAC387 for macrophages, granzyme B for NK cells, and Ki67 for cellular proliferation. In addition, the phosphorylated signal transducer and activator of transcription (pSTAT) 5 is highly expressed in neoplastic lymphocytes but not in lymphocytes of lymphoplasmacytic enteritis in cats, so this marker may become an increasingly important marker for lymphoma in cats and other species.

Clonality testing is now commonly used in cats, especially for early, equivocal, or suspect cases; it is particularly useful for differentiating lymphoma from enteritis or for identification of early or emerging lymphomas. As indicated for dogs, various testing modalities should be utilized for diagnosis of subtle intestinal lymphomas in cats, *with histomorphology of appropriately sampled and processed endoscopic or surgical biopsy samples of affected intestine as the cornerstone diagnostic modality*, which is then supplemented or confirmed by IHC and/or PARR testing. A report showed that >50% of clinically healthy and apparently normal cats had evidence of histologic lesions and clonal T-cell arrangements in the small intestine consistent with a diagnosis of lymphoma. Thus, *it is imperative that pathologists and clinicians avoid diagnosis or reclassification of cases based on clonality results alone, and results should always be carefully interpreted collectively with clinical and other test data to avoid misdiagnosis*. Regardless, and as is true for dogs,

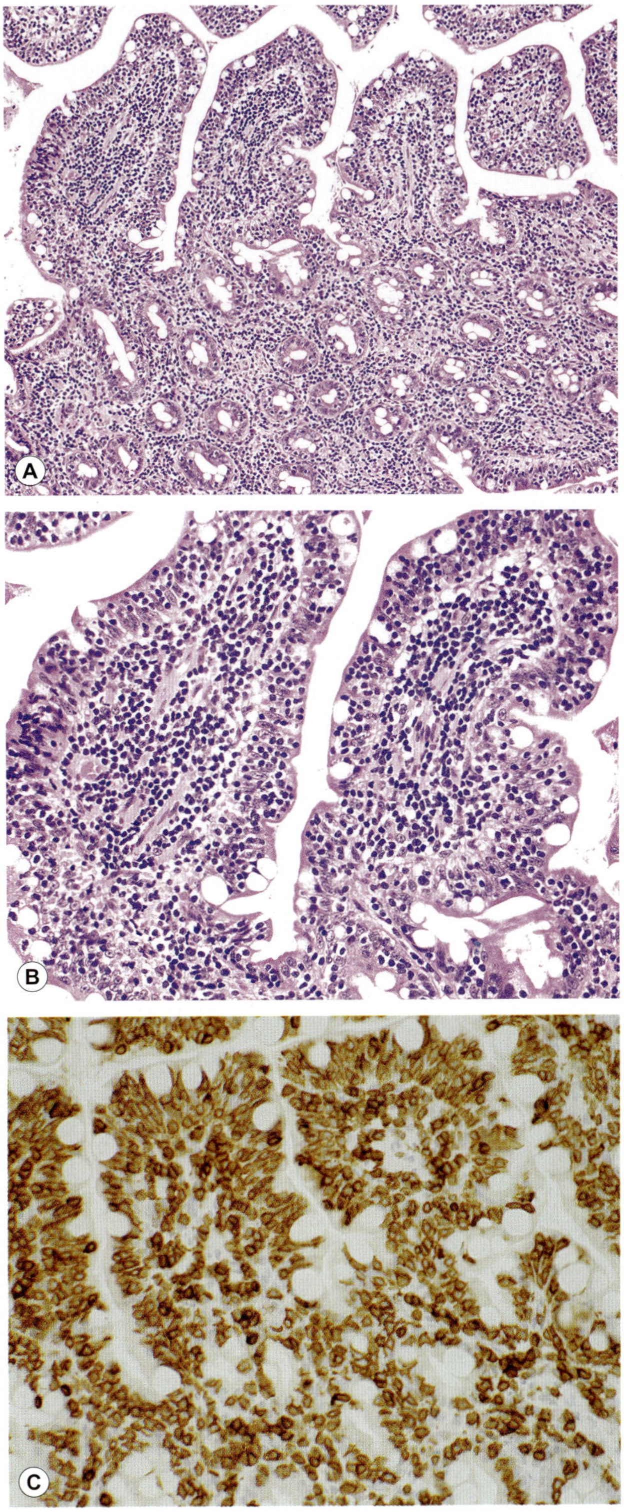

Figure 1-68 Small-cell low-grade epitheliotropic **intestinal lymphoma** (LGAL) in a cat. **A.** There is dense infiltration of the lamina propria by monomorphic small round lymphocytes, which also infiltrate the overlying surface enterocytes of small intestinal crypts and villi. **B.** Monomorphic small lymphocytes are seen individually and forming nests and plaques within the epithelial layer, often making visual distinction of the epithelium and lamina propria difficult. **C.** Diffuse strong cytoplasmic CD3 immunoreactivity of the lamina propria and intraepithelial lymphocytes confirming a diagnosis of T-cell lymphoma (T-cell clonality was also confirmed in this case.)

even with a flawless stepwise approach, some cases of chronic enteropathy in cats remain diagnostically equivocal.

Equine intestinal lymphoma is relatively common and is reported as the most common intestinal neoplasm of the horse. Intestinal lymphoma in horses most frequently involves the small intestine, and less commonly is present in the colon, or both small and large intestinal tract. As for other species, affected horses are usually middle-aged to older, and they have chronic diarrhea, weight loss, anorexia, PLE and malabsorption syndromes, or intestinal obstruction. Gross lesions include intestinal wall thickening that can be localized or diffuse but is most commonly single or numerous mural masses, nodules, or plaques, with lymph node involvement is some cases. As is true for other species, intestinal lymphoma can occur as mucosal disease in which the features are intestinal thickening grossly, and histologically are consistent with small-cell or large-cell T-cell lymphomas, or as focal or multifocal infiltrative neoplastic masses consistent with T-cell–rich large-B-cell lymphoma (TCRLBCL, see later). Mucosal lymphoma in horses is seen either as infiltration of small CD3-positive T cells infiltrating lamina propria, with prominent epitheliotropism occurring as individual cells, nests, or plaques, and rarely extending into the submucosa (similar to small-cell low-grade intestinal lymphoma, formerly *EATL type 2*), or as infiltration of sheets of large lymphocytes in the lamina propria but without epitheliotropism, and usually also extending transmurally into the submucosa and muscle layers of the intestinal wall, some with individual cell epitheliotropism of the villi and cryptal epithelium, and usually with infiltration into the submucosa and muscle layers of the intestinal wall (similar to large-cell high-grade intestinal lymphoma or EATL, formerly *EATL type 1*). Small-cell low-grade intestinal lymphoma should be carefully distinguished from IBD in horses, and *the key diagnostic differentiating feature of nests and plaques of IELs* is highly suggestive, as in other species. Some cases of equine intestinal lymphoma have numerous eosinophils or plasma cells; the significance of these cells is not known, although paraneoplastic eosinophilia has also been associated with intestinal lymphoma in the horse.

T-cell-rich large-B-cell lymphoma (TCRLBCL) is well-described in horses, mostly as transmural infiltration of a mixed population of medium-to-large atypical B lymphocytes (PAX5, CD20, or CD79a positive) with a smaller variable intermixed population of CD3-positive T lymphocytes; epitheliotropism is not a consistent feature of these neoplasms. TCRLBCL cases are thought to be part of, or progress to multicentric lymphoma, so in these cases, care should be taken to evaluate for possible involvement of other organs or lymph nodes at the time of diagnosis. The mitotic count forms the basis for the grading scheme for equine intestinal lymphomas, which is based on lymphoma grading for dogs: grade 1 (low) neoplasms have 0-5 mitoses/0.237 mm^2, grade 2 (intermediate) neoplasms have 6-10 mitoses/0.237 mm^2, and grade 3 (high) neoplasms have >10 mitoses/0.237 mm^2. Ki67 has also been measured in equine intestinal lymphomas, but probably due to few cases and published reports, proliferation has not been specifically correlated with prognosis or survival. IHC can be helpful to further characterize the patterns and presence of epitheliotropism in horses.

The prognosis for horses with intestinal lymphoma is overall relatively poor. Horses with mucosal T-cell lymphomas had shorter median survival times (25-90 days) compared with horses with TCRLBCL (187 days); however, progression and nodal metastasis may be more likely in TCRLBCL cases, and no significant difference in survival was identified by subtype. Equine herpesvirus 5 been linked to colonic lymphoma (TCRLBCL); the significance or prevalence of this more broadly remains unclear.

Intestinal lymphoma of ruminants is generally part of the adult multicentric form of the disease. There is association of multicentric B-cell lymphoma in ruminants with BLV, and intestinal lesions are rare, but are probably part of that syndrome. The lesions resemble intestinal transmural lymphomas described in other species. Most important in cattle is lymphoma of the abomasum, which is one of the most common anatomic sites in adult cattle.

Intestinal lymphoma in swine occurs, but is apparently quite uncommon. A survey of pigs at slaughter showed that lymphoma was the most common reported spontaneous neoplasm of pigs, and diffuse B-cell phenotype was the most common diagnosis. The intestine is usually transmurally thickened by neoplastic lymphocytes, which can invade the mucosa or produce nodules, may ulcerate, or appear simply as diffusely thickened intestine with surface necrosis and fibrinonecrotic membrane. Affected pigs typically have other organ systems involved, including lymph nodes, genitourinary, respiratory, and hepatobiliary systems. Cases of multicentric B-cell lymphoma have been seen in young pigs with gross lesions in the GI tract reminiscent of other common infectious disease of growing pigs [porcine proliferative enteropathy (PPE), circoviral-associated diseases, or intestinal and systemic salmonellosis]. Intestinal lymphomas may be more common than reported in pigs, but are not often thoroughly worked up diagnostically for definitive diagnosis in production systems. There are no known specific causes, and presumably lymphomas arise from the MALT or proprial lymphocytes, although the GI tract is usually not the only system involved, and they tend to be part of multicentric disease involving many other organs.

Intestinal mast cell tumors (MCTs) in dogs are uncommon; affected patients have nonspecific clinical signs such as vomition, diarrhea, and melena. These are invasive round-cell tumors that can resemble carcinoids or lymphomas; *definitive diagnosis requires histochemical* (toluidine blue, Giemsa) *and possibly IHC* (CD117) *confirmation* because GI mast cells usually have minimal metachromatic cytoplasmic granules. Primary MCTs of the GI tract arise from mucosal mast cells, which differ significantly from connective tissue mast cells, such as those found in the skin and from which the much more common cutaneous and subcutaneous MCTs arise. In the GI tract, mast cell neoplasms occur more commonly in the oral cavity; involvement of the stomach or intestine is quite uncommon.

Gross lesions are nonspecific, and composed of tan, firm, thickened, and possibly ulcerated, mural nodules. Histologic features of intestinal MCT include effacement of native tissue architecture by granular round cells accompanied by variable numbers of eosinophils. They generally grow in infiltrative cords, but occasionally form neuroendocrine-like packets surrounded by a delicate fibrovascular stroma. There is a wide range in cytologic appearance. Some tumors are populated by moderately well-differentiated mast cells with abundant cytoplasmic granularity easily demonstrated with toluidine blue. Others are populated by anaplastic and pleomorphic round-or-spindle cells, sometimes with giant nuclei or forming syncytia, in which cytoplasmic granules (even with metachromatic staining) are difficult to observe. Those with abundant metachromatic granules must be differentiated from connective tissue MCTs metastatic to the GI tract, in which case lesions should be sought in the skin and elsewhere. There can be marked variation in the number of eosinophils in the tumor, and they are not definitive because eosinophils are also common in some intestinal lymphomas, and as part of the background cell population in normal lamina propria.

Feline intestinal mast cell tumors (MCTs) are also uncommon, but probably more common than intestinal MCTs in dogs, and may account for 2-15% of feline neoplasms, although most of these are cutaneous or splenic. In the intestinal tract, they occur as focal or multifocal plaques, or as diffuse luminal or mural lesions in the distal small intestine and colon. The clinical signs are similar to other intestinal neoplasms of cats and may include vomiting, inappetence, weight loss, depression, or abdominal distension; palpable abdominal masses may be detected, and lesions that become obstructive may cause acute painful abdomens. Ultrasound or radiographic imaging will detect focal or multifocal intestinal wall thickening or masses. In contrast to most cutaneous MCTs in cats, *intestinal MCTs usually have unique histomorphology*, and are described as well-differentiated, moderately differentiated, or poorly differentiated with considerable histomorphologic variation. The neoplasms can involve the mucosa, submucosa, or tunica muscularis; many are transmural (eFig. 1-13A). Interestingly, although ulceration of the GI mucosa occurs commonly with systemic or cutaneous MCTs in cats and dogs owing to histamine stimulation of acid production by gastric parietal cells, GI ulceration is not typically a feature of mucosal MCTs of intestinal origin, except perhaps in the case of mucosal effacement by the tumor.

In the intestine, neoplastic mast cells are arranged in sheets or possibly packets (resembling carcinoids, see eFig. 1-13B) supported by fine fibrous-to-collagenous stroma. Histochemical stains (toluidine blue, Giemsa) may reveal granules, but even if negative by histochemical stains, mast cell neoplasia cannot be definitively ruled out because intestinal mast cells are frequently poorly granulated (see eFig. 1-13C). The neoplasms may also closely resemble lymphoma, such as large-granular lymphoma, especially when subtle cytoplasmic granularity is evident. *Well-differentiated intestinal MCTs* are composed of uniform round cells with cytoplasmic metachromatic granules; *moderately differentiated intestinal MCTs* are composed of oval-to-spindle neoplastic mast cells with considerable variation in nuclear size and shape and indistinct metachromatic cytoplasmic granules, even with histochemical staining; *poorly differentiated intestinal MCTs* are composed of pleomorphic polygonal-to-spindle cells arranged in bundles and cords, with large often elongated and prominent nucleoli, with indistinct metachromatic cytoplasmic granules. Moderately or poorly differentiated intestinal MCTs in cats can be easily confused with carcinoids, fibrosarcomas, or histiocytic sarcomas; histochemical staining is helpful to confirm mast cells, although the cytoplasmic metachromatic granules may be absent or subtle. The degree or density of cytoplasmic granules is apparently not correlated with tumor differentiation, but poorly differentiated tumors have significantly higher mitotic counts (6/2.37 mm^2) and Ki67 index (15%) compared with well-differentiated tumors (0/2.37 mm^2 and 5%, respectively), and mitotic counts >2 are associated with a shorter survival time. Most stain immunohistochemically positive for mast cell tryptase and c-KIT (CD117), but negatively for CD3 (distinguishing them from T-cell lymphoma), cytokeratin (distinguishing them from carcinoma), and chromogranin and synaptophysin (distinguishing them from carcinoid). No specific c-KIT expression pattern or exon mutation patterns have been associated with prognosis and survival of cats with intestinal MCTs. Immunoreactivity of feline intestinal MCTs may be variable, and some caution should be exercised because GISTs are also expected to be positive for c-KIT; however, the spindle morphologic features and lack of metachromatic granules of stromal tumors should readily allow differentiation.

Metastatic disease is frequent, and usually involves mesenteric lymph nodes and liver. The long-term prognosis of feline intestinal MCTs is quite poor, and significantly worse for poorly differentiated tumors.

Extramedullary plasma cell tumors of the intestine are *uncommon neoplasms in dogs*, and rare in cats and other species. They are encountered most frequently in the submucosa of the distal colon and rectum of dogs, where they are associated with signs of large-bowel diarrhea and bleeding.

Histologically, they resemble plasmacytomas of the skin, oral cavity, or larynx. The tumor is formed by solid packets of pleomorphic round cells with various degrees of plasmacytoid maturation, especially at the periphery of the tumor. There is frequent nuclear hyperchromasia and convolution. The cells are typically arranged in solid endocrine-like packets surrounded by a delicate fibrovascular stroma, and there may be AL-type amyloid deposition among the tumor cells. A few syncytial plasmacytoid or histiocytic cells may be evident. Most of the tumor growth is submucosal, with possible infiltration into the deep half of the lamina propria. Most tumors have a discrete local growth habit amenable to surgical cure. A small proportion are more aggressive, poorly differentiated, and include invasion of the tunica muscularis, and some spread to regional lymph nodes and spleen, perhaps producing a monoclonal gammopathy, although this is not commonly reported.

Differentiation of some extramedullary intestinal plasma cell tumors from lymphoma or carcinoids may be challenging; the use of IHC is usually helpful. *Plasma cell tumors* are positive for MUM1/IRF4 and immunoglobulin light chains; *lymphomas* are expected to be positive for CD20, PAX5 (B cells), or CD3 (T cells); and *carcinoids* are histochemically positive for argentaffinic and argyrophilic granules, or show immunoreactivity by IHC for neuron-specific enolase, chromogranin A, or other antibodies for specific peptides being produced, and have a typical ultrastructural appearance.

INFECTIOUS AND PARASITIC DISEASES OF THE ALIMENTARY TRACT

Viral diseases of the alimentary tract

Foot-and-mouth disease

Foot-and-mouth disease (FMD) is a highly contagious viral infection of all cloven-hoofed animals. **Foot-and-mouth disease virus** (FMDV; *Picornaviridae, Aphthovirus vesiculae*) belongs to the genus *Aphthovirus* (aphtha = ulcer). FMD is a problem of worldwide concern, being enzootic in large areas of Africa, Asia, and parts of Europe and South America. FMDV imposes serious trade restrictions that effectively thwart the development of a healthy agricultural economy. FMD is an acute febrile condition with the formation of vesicles in and around the mouth, on the feet, teats, and mammary glands. The disease is not notable for high mortality, except in sucklings, but morbidity is very high, with a concomitant loss of production efficiency.

FMDV is highly resistant under many circumstances, but is inactivated by direct sunlight, because of drying and increase in temperature, and by moderate acidity (pH <5.0). The acid production that accompanies rigor mortis in carcasses and meat inactivates the virus. However, the alteration in pH is not dependable and the virus survives in viscera, lymph nodes, and bone marrow for an indefinite period under refrigeration. Next to the movement of infected animals, contaminated animal products are likely the most common mechanism of spread. FMDV may survive on hay and other fomites for several weeks.

The persistence of FMDV is of epidemiologic significance, especially where control policies involve slaughter rather than vaccination. The importance of a carrier state in the epidemiology of FMD is uncertain. The carrier state has been observed in cattle, sheep, goats, and African buffalo (*Syncerus caffer*), but not in pigs, although the latter play a significant role in transmission because of the high number of viral particles that they produce. The carrier state may persist for up to 2 years postinfection in cattle, even in animals with a significant level of virus-neutralizing antibody. Sheep and goats are considered to be frequent inapparent sources of dissemination of the virus because disease can be mild and lesions difficult to identify. Infection in wild ruminants is an obstacle to control. African buffalo can carry FMDV for at least 5 years. Field outbreaks have been associated with buffalo-cattle contact in Africa, but these appear to be rare. Although Asian water buffaloes (*Bubalus arnee*) may be affected in FMD outbreaks, it is not known whether they remain carriers.

Of equal importance to the persistence of the virus is its *antigenic heterogeneity and instability*. There are 7 principal antigenic serotypes, namely the classical A, O, and C types, and SAT1, SAT2, SAT3, and Asia-1. These can be distinguished by serologic tests. Six of the 7 serotypes (O, A, C, SAT1, SAT2, SAT3) are known to occur in Africa, 4 (O, A, C, Asia-1) in Asia, and 3 (O, A, C) in Europe and South America, although pandemics blur these geographic distinctions. These serotypes are sufficiently different immunologically that *infection with 1 type does not confer protection to the other* 6. Within these 7 major types there are antigenic subtypes, each different, to various degrees, from the parental virus type. Generally, the subtypes cross-protect to a useful degree, but exceptions do arise and become recognizable, especially when vaccination fails. *Antigenic drift* can be demonstrated experimentally; new subtypes can be produced by passing the virus in immune or partially immune animals, or by growing the virus in vitro in immune serum. There are >70 distinct virus antigenic variants of natural origin.

As virus strains differ in antigenicity, they also differ in virulence, and a given strain is likely to exhibit diverse virulence phenotypes. Certainly, there is considerable variation in the severity of the disease produced in a given host species in different outbreaks. Virulence also varies among species. Although most strains affect a wide range of susceptible animal species, there have been occasional viruses that show a distinct predilection for one species. An example is the porcinophilic strain that originated in China in the late 1990s and spread to Taiwan, destroying the local swine industry.

The main portal of virus entry and primary site of early viral replication is the epithelium of the pharynx and lung. Affected pharyngeal epithelium is often associated with MALT. Subsequent to the first round of replication, there is widespread viremic dissemination to other surface epithelia, with subsequent development of lesions in sites of mechanical or physiologic stress, such as oral, pedal, and/or teat stratified epithelia. The resulting cellular degeneration and lysis result in the formation of **epidermal vesicles**, *which are the hallmarks of the disease*.

Virus is present at high titer in the vesicular fluid and is present in large amounts in expired air from acutely infected animals, which is the main source of interhost virus spread—pigs in particular release large quantities of airborne virus. Virus persists in lesions for 3-8 days after the appearance of significant neutralizing antibody titers in serum, but seldom beyond day 11 from the onset of clinical illness. It is believed that FMDV is localized in epithelial cells of the oropharynx during persistent infection of ruminants, and virus can be detected in esophagopharyngeal fluid for a considerable period.

Within a week of development of neutralizing antibodies, virus titer in circulation declines. Ordinarily, serum antibody titers decline progressively and fairly rapidly. The duration of persistence of antibody is correlated with the initial titer. In general, animals are resistant to reinfection with homologous strains by natural exposure for ~2-4 years; susceptibility increases as the antibody titer declines.

The characteristic **lesions** of FMD are only seen in those animals that are examined at the height of disease. As the infection progresses, lesions heal or are obscured by secondary bacterial infection. Lesions develop mainly in areas subject to trauma: the *oral mucosa*, especially the *tongue*; the *interdigital cleft*; and the *teats* in lactating animals. In cattle, there is appreciable loss of weight and the buccal cavity may contain much saliva. In the living animal, there is diffuse buccal hyperemia and mild catarrhal stomatitis, but the hyperemia disappears at death. Vesicles form on the inner aspects of the lips and cheeks, the gums, hard palate, dental pad, and especially on the sides and rostral portion of the dorsum of the tongue. Sometimes they form on the muzzle and exterior nares. The primary vesicles are small but coalesce to produce *bullae* that may be 5-6 cm across; these bullae rupture in 12-14 hours, leaving an intensely red, raw, and moist base to which shreds of epithelium may still adhere (Fig. 1-69). The eroded-to-ulcerated area may be replaced by regenerated epithelium in <2 weeks. Secondary infection may complicate this course.

Foot lesions occur in most cases. There is inflammatory swelling with blanching of the skin of the interdigital space in ruminants, coronet in swine, and heels in all species a day or so before vesicles form. The swellings persist until the vesicles rupture and the resultant erosions heal; healing may be considerably delayed on the feet. Vesicles may also occur in the other sites, but much less frequently.

A *more severe form of the disease*, without vesiculation, does occur in young animals and occasionally in adults. In these, death is common, as a result of *myocarditis*. Poorly defined pale foci of variable size are seen anywhere within the ventricular muscle. Although historically referred to as "tiger-heart," these gross lesions are no different from those generated in any other syndrome of severe, acute myocardial damage, but necrosis of fibers may be striking. Viral replication in young ruminants also occurs in skeletal muscle cells. Animals that survive the acute phase of FMDV infection (or are not slaughtered during depopulation) can progress to develop a set of chronic lesions. Chronic lesions include myocardial necrosis and scarring, heat intolerance, pancreatitis with acinar

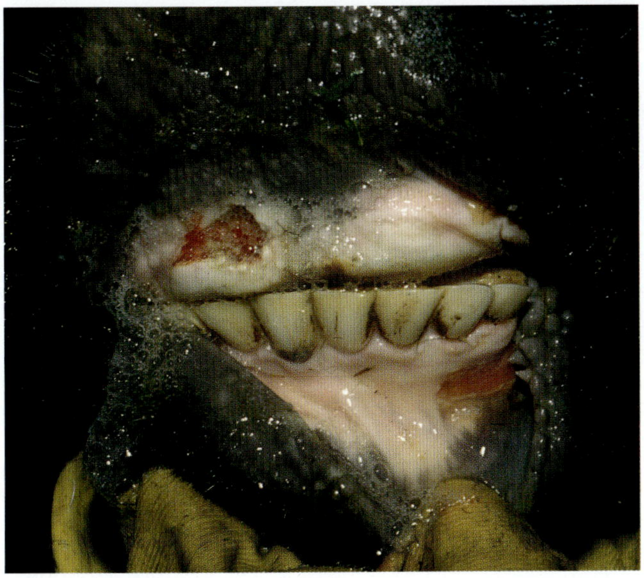

Figure 1-69 Foot-and-mouth disease. Ruptured vesicle on the gingiva of a cow.

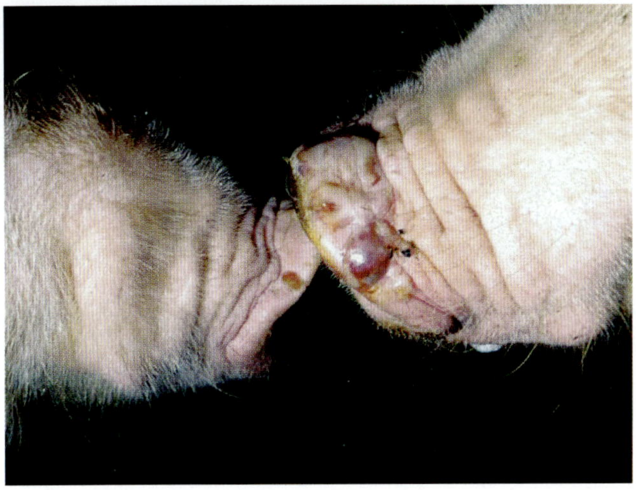

Figure 1-70 Foot-and-mouth disease. Vesicles on the snouts of 2 pigs. (Courtesy Noah's Arkives.)

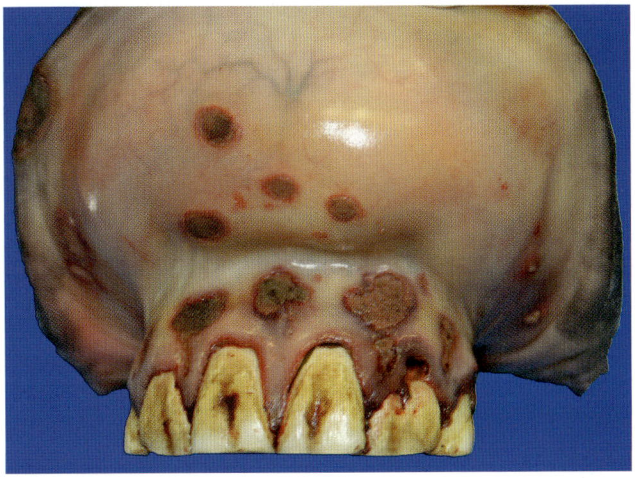

Figure 1-71 Vesicular stomatitis. Ulceration of vesicular lesions in the oral mucosa of a horse.

necrosis, and regeneration. Diabetes mellitus occurs in experimental cases, as does hypophysitis, leading to a constellation of endocrinopathies because of a range of expressions of pituitary dysfunction.

In **sheep**, the infection runs a milder course, although there may be exceptions. Lesions may be subtle or not develop. When lesions do develop, the *dental pad* is the preferred site in the oral cavity. Lingual lesions tend to occur on the caudal dorsal portion as under-running necrotic erosions rather than vesicles. These are small and easily missed, and they heal within a few days. *Lameness* may be prominent in acute outbreaks. Typical vesicles develop in the interdigital cleft, on the coronet, and the bulb of the heel. Occasionally, they may involve the entire coronet and lead to eventual shedding of the hoof. Vesicles also occasionally occur on the teats, vulva, prepuce, and on the pillars of the rumen. The peracute form with myocardial necrosis may occur in lambs. The disease in **goats** is similar to that described for sheep. Both species may be inapparent carriers, and many outbreaks worldwide have been due to transport of inapparently infected small ruminants.

In **pigs**, lesions occur in the usual sites, although more commonly on the feet than in the mouth. Sloughing of the hooves leads to severe lameness. Lesions also may be present on the snout and behind its rim (Fig. 1-70), and on the teats of lactating sows. Abortion and stillbirth of infected piglets are recorded. The peracute form, with high mortality caused by myocarditis, occurs in sucklings, often before vesicle formation is noticed in sows.

FMD must be differentiated from other viral diseases that cause vesicular lesions in the oral cavity, teats, and feet, and sudden death among cloven-footed animals, especially the young, including vesicular stomatitis, vesicular exanthema, senecavirus A infection, and swine vesicular disease in susceptible species, and in the later stages, from diseases producing erosive or ulcerative lesions of the oral cavity. *Gross lesions alone cannot differentiate these entities*. Definitive **diagnosis** requires virus isolation and characterization, demonstration of viral antigen by ELISA, or detection of viral genome by PCR in lesional material. The regulatory status of FMD dictates that this must be carried out in accredited laboratories. In areas where vaccination is performed, vaccinated animals need to be differentiated from infected animals.

Vesicular stomatitis

Vesicular stomatitis (VS) affects horses, cattle, and pigs and may also affect wildlife species such as white-tailed deer, raccoons, feral swine, and some rodents. Experimentally, various rodent species are susceptible and persistence has been demonstrated in hamsters. Also, persistence of viral RNA has been shown in both experimentally and naturally infected cattle, but the reservoir of the virus is unknown. *The disease is important because it causes a loss in production, especially in dairy herds, and it must be differentiated from FMD in cattle and pigs*. VS is the only vesicular disease occurring naturally in horses (Fig. 1-71). Sheep and goats do not appear to be susceptible to the disease, but a severe, although nonfatal, influenza-like syndrome may occur in infected humans.

Vesicular stomatitis virus (VSV; *Rhabdoviridae*, genus *Vesiculovirus*; type species: *vesicular stomatitis Indiana virus*, VSIV). VSV particles are ~80 × 120 nm, bullet shaped, and enveloped, with a helical nucleocapsid containing a negative-sense single-stranded RNA genome. There are several serologically and immunologically distinct types of VSV based on epitopes of the surface glycoproteins, including New Jersey, Indiana, Piry, Isfahan, and Chandipura. The 2 most common serotypes of VSV infecting domestic animals in the Americas are New Jersey and Indiana.

VS is enzootic in Central and South America and occurs sporadically elsewhere in the rest of the Americas. It has a seasonal occurrence; outbreaks occur in the warmer seasons and usually cease with the onset of cold weather. The seasonal nature of the disease suggests that it is transmitted by *insects*; however, insect transmission is not essential and *contact transmission* has been proved experimentally. VSV has been isolated from both biting and nonbiting insects, and black flies have transmitted the virus to pigs. Biting insects most likely become infected from feeding on lesions rather than blood, because viremia is transient, if present. Nonbiting insects act as mechanical carriers of the virus. It is not known how the virus spreads from one geographic area to another. There is some indication that VSVs adapt to specific regions, developing distinct genotypes based on specific vectors or reservoirs in an ecologic area. The intact mucosa is resistant to infection, but abrasions in a susceptible site readily result in infection when contaminated with saliva or exudate from a lesion. Environmental factors that increase the chance of causing abrasions to the skin, teats, or oral mucosa may predispose to infection.

Morbidity in lactating dairy cows may be as high as 100%, although only ~60% of the affected animals drool or froth around the mouth. The lesions of VS occur mainly on the *oral mucosa*; occasionally, they do occur elsewhere, including on the *feet*, and in swine and horses, foot lesions are common. This is by no means a dependable feature, and outbreaks of the disease in cattle have been described in which the lesions were predominantly on the *teats*.

The incubation period following exposure by abrasion is 24-72 hours. Experimentally, VS New Jersey virus inoculation in cattle led to viral replication at the inoculation site from 24-48 hours and in the draining lymph nodes within the first 24 hours. In horses, experimental inoculation in the oral cavity and lips also led to local viral infection of the inoculation site, tonsil, and retropharyngeal lymph nodes. The viremic phase seems to be short-lived because the virus cannot be cultured from blood. Secondary lesions are rare. In cattle, intramuscular injections will not initiate the disease, a distinguishing feature from FMD. After experimental infection of swine, infectious viral particles can be recovered from a wide variety of tissues within 6 hours postinfection, including salivary gland, tonsils, snout, skin, and lymph nodes. However, infective virus, viral antigens, and nucleic acids cannot be demonstrated 6 days postinfection.

Specific virus-neutralizing antibodies persist for months in swine, and years in cattle. There is no evidence that animals with persistent antibodies may act as a source of infection to herdmates. Animals are immune against homologous but not heterologous strains of the virus.

The lesions of VS are indistinguishable from those of FMD. Initially, in cattle, there is a raised flattened pale-pink to blanched papule a few millimeters in diameter in or near the mouth. These papules rapidly become inflamed and hyperemic. In the course of a day or so they develop into vesicles 2-3 cm in diameter, and by coalescence may involve large areas. The shallow erosions that follow rupture of vesicles heal within 1-2 weeks unless secondary infections occur; in the mouth, the latter are common. Oral lesions heal rapidly in swine, but coronary band lesions often become secondarily infected to the point where the claw may separate and slough. Serous rhinitis, with the development of tags of necrotic mucosa, has been described in experimentally infected swine.

The first microscopic changes are seen in the deeper layers of the spinous layer, where the virus replicates. Increasing prominence of the intercellular spaces and stretching of the desmosomes are accompanied by a reduction in volume of the cell cytoplasm. This dissociation of cells proceeds to distinct intercellular edema (*spongiosis*) followed by further cytoplasmic retraction until the affected epithelial cells float freely in enlarging vacuoles, which in turn are loculated by strands of cytoplasmic debris. There is no hydropic degeneration of the epithelial cells and the nuclei until now remain normal. *There are no inclusion bodies*. With the onset of epithelial cell necrosis, there is a pleocellular inflammatory reaction in the mucosa and underlying lamina propria. Electron microscopic examination of epithelial cells adjacent to the vesicles confirms the intercellular edema and keratinocyte necrosis seen under the light microscope. The microscopic appearance of the lesions is not diagnostic. In light of the similarity of VS to FMD, *laboratory confirmation of VS is essential*. Vesicular fluid and mucosa from the tongue are good sources of the virus. *Diagnosis* is accomplished mainly through tissue culture, complement fixation, ELISA, and PCR.

Vesicular exanthema of swine

Vesicular exanthema of swine virus (VESV; *Caliciviridae, Vesivirus exanthema*) is the type species of the genus *Vesivirus*. Virions consist of nonenveloped, 30-40-nm, icosahedral capsids, with typical cup-shaped surface structures (calyces). The viral genome is positive-sense single-stranded RNA and encodes for only one major polypeptide. There are 13 immunologically distinct serotypes, which vary in virulence.

In 1973, a virus that is biophysically and morphologically similar to VESV was recovered from sea lions (*Zalophus californianus*) with vesicles on their flippers, off the coast of California near San Miguel Island. Several strains of this virus, called **San Miguel sea lion virus** (SMSV; *Caliciviridae*), produce milder but otherwise identical lesions to those of vesicular exanthema (VE) when inoculated into swine, and SMSV is classified as a serotype of VESV. The host range of SMSV is very broad and includes cetaceans, cattle, horses, and reptiles. One serotype, SMSV7, has been isolated from opaleye fish (*Girella nigricans*), and it produces lesions identical to VE when inoculated into swine, with horizontal transmission to contact swine. Evidence of SMSV infection continues to be identified in fish and marine mammals. It is thought that VE of swine arose through the feeding of ocean fish to swine, with some adaptation of the virus allowing for very efficient spread through swine.

Most outbreaks of VE were associated with feeding of raw garbage containing pork waste, indicating that the disease was transmitted by direct contact and fomites. VESV now exists only as viral stocks archived in freezers and should be considered a *disease of historical significance only*. The possibility of a recurrence remains, however, if swine are fed uncooked tissues from ocean-origin fish or marine mammals.

Swine vesicular disease

Swine vesicular disease (SVD) is a highly contagious viral disease of pigs; vesicles form around the coronary bands and heels of the feet, and, to a lesser extent, on the mouth, lips, tongue, and teats. *Clinically, the disease is indistinguishable from the other vesicular diseases of swine*, including FMD, VS, and vesicular exanthema of swine. The disease was first recognized in Italy in 1966, and it has since been reported from Hong Kong, the United Kingdom, continental Europe, and Asia. The economic importance of SVD is related less to the rather limited losses in production and more to the fact that it is difficult to differentiate from other vesicular diseases and hence restricts trade.

Swine vesicular disease virus (SVDV; *Picornaviridae*, variant of genus *Enterovirus B*, coxsackievirus B5), a small RNA virus, is a porcine variant of human coxsackievirus B5, which is a serotype of human *Enterovirus B*. SVDV is highly resistant to environmental factors. Unlike FMDV, it is not inactivated at the low pH in muscle commonly associated with rigor mortis.

Many outbreaks of SVD appear to originate by feeding raw garbage containing pork products. Transmission within and among affected herds is by direct contact, especially during the early stages of the disease, or by exposure to the virus in the environment, where it is very persistent. The portal of entry is most likely oral or by exposure of excoriated skin. Following contact with infected pigs, vesicles develop within 2 days and consistent virus isolation from tonsil is possible for 1-7 days. Viremia lasts for 2-3 days. SVDV has a strong affinity for the epithelial cells of the coronary band, tongue, snout, lips, lymphoid follicles of the tonsils, myocardial cells, and brain. Virus titers in tissue decrease with the appearance of circulating antibodies, which peak after 2-3 weeks and apparently persist for years. Secretions and excretions have high viral titers for 12-14 days. Feces may contain virus for up to 3 months. Pigs may become carriers, with stress reactivating viral shedding several months postinfection.

Clinically, *vesicles are most common on the feet*. Oral lesions occur in only ~10% of affected pigs. The foot lesions appear first at the junction between the heel and the coronary band. Initially, there is a 5-mm-wide, pale, swollen area that encircles the digit. In later stages, a 1-cm-wide band of necrotic skin is located along the coronet. Vesicles on the mouth, lips, and tongue occur in clusters, and they are small, ~2 mm in diameter, white, and opaque. They coalesce and rupture within 36 hours and may be covered by a pseudodiphtheritic membrane resulting from secondary bacterial infections. Affected pigs usually recover in 2-3 weeks.

The development of vesicles tends to follow a similar course as that reported for FMD. The virus infects individual epithelial cells in the spinous layer, which leads to focal areas of keratinocyte degeneration and vesicle formation. There is an intense leukocytic reaction in the necrotic areas, which is mainly neutrophilic. As with the other vesicular diseases, after 1 week there are indications of epithelial regeneration.

Nervous signs and lesions of *mononuclear meningoencephalomyelitis* have been reported in field outbreaks and reproduced experimentally in SVD. Lesions involve most areas in the brain and sometimes the spinal cord and are centered on ganglia and spinal nerve roots. Clinically, the severe lameness tends to overshadow any nervous signs that might be present.

Laboratory diagnosis depends on demonstration of the agent by virus isolation, antigen ELISA, or PCR, in accredited laboratories, on account of its regulatory status.

Senecavirus A1 infection

Senecavirus A1 (SVV; Seneca Valley virus, *Picornaviridae, Senecavirus valles*), discovered in 2002, is only the second member of the genus *Senecavirus*. SVV has a 25-30-nm, nonenveloped capsid with icosahedral symmetry and a linear single-stranded RNA genome of positive polarity and ~7.3 kb. SVV causes a mild infection in pigs with clinical signs and lesions indistinguishable from other vesicular diseases that is therefore an important differential diagnosis for FMD. Lesions are found most frequently on the snout, lips, tongue, and feet and consist of vesicles that eventually rupture to create ulcers. In piglets born to infected sows, sudden death, diarrhea, dehydration, and lethargy were described. The only lesion described in those piglets was mesocolonic edema.

Bovine viral diarrhea

Bovine viral diarrhea virus (BVDV; *Flaviviridae*, genus *Pestivirus*) is an RNA virus that includes 4 species of veterinary importance, **BVDV1** and **BVDV2** (previously referred to as genotypes 1 and 2, and currently designated *Pestivirus bovis* and *Pestivirus tauri*, respectively), **classical swine fever virus** (CSFV, Hog cholera virus; *Flaviviridae, Pestivirus suis*), and **border disease virus** (BDV; *Flaviviridae, Pestivirus ovis*). BVDV is widespread in cattle populations, and this or closely related viruses can infect most even-toed ungulates, including swine. Although evidence for BVDV infection has been found in farmed and free-ranging wildlife in North America, the risk of transmission of the disease from wildlife to cattle remains unknown. As an RNA virus, BVDV is highly mutable because of the error-prone nature of the RNA polymerases responsible for replication of viral RNA. As a result, "swarms" of viral mutants or "quasispecies" circulate within an infected individual and among individuals in a population. Although most viral variants lack a selective advantage, or suffer deleterious point mutations, preventing them from becoming dominant, the ability to generate mutants enables BVDV to evade host responses, and to establish chronic or persistent infections in some circumstances. Although low virulence would seem to promote prolonged viral shedding, high virulence may be advantageous as it favors the emergence of quasispecies capable of causing severe disease and high virus shedding.

Viral genotype may be linked to specific manifestations of BVDV infection; noncytopathic (NCP) BVDV2 has been associated with thrombocytopenia, for instance. However, there is a range of virulence among both BVDV1 and BVDV2 isolates, ranging from subclinical infections or mild clinical disease to fatal syndromes.

RNA recombination between homologous viruses (BVDV) or between BVDV and heterologous viral or host RNAs, usually involving the region encoding the nonstructural protein NS2-3 of NCP virus, results in a shift in biotype of either genotype of virus, from the more common **NCP biotype**, in which inapparent persistent infection is produced in cultured cells, to a **cytopathic (CP) biotype**, capable of inducing cytoplasmic vacuolation and apoptotic death of cells in tissue culture. Recombination splits NS2-3, resulting in a small NS3 protein, which induces apoptosis, and is a marker for CP BVD viruses. Reversion of CP viruses to an NCP biotype also occurs, less commonly. *Cytopathogenicity in vitro is not directly related to virulence in vivo*.

HoBi-like pestivirus (HoBiPeV; *Flaviviridae, Pestivirus brazilense*), also known as **BVDV3**, or atypical pestivirus, was identified in fetal bovine serum imported from Brazil into Europe. These viruses are genetically and antigenically related to BVDV and cause disease similar to that traditionally associated with BVDV infection. HoBiPeV may not be detected by conventional BVDV detection techniques. Current BVDV vaccines confer limited cross-protection against HoBiPeV. These viruses have been identified in Brazil, Southeast Asia, and Europe.

BVDV gains access to the oropharyngeal mucosa by ingestion or inhalation, and primarily replicates in oropharyngeal lymphoid tissues, including tonsils. The outcome of the ensuing viremia is the product of the genotype and virulence of the virus, and the immune and pregnancy status of the host. Infection of immunocompetent, seronegative, nonpregnant animals usually results in subclinical infection or mild clinical disease. Affected animals develop slight fever, leukopenia, and specific neutralizing antibodies, the outcome in 70-90% of BVDV infections. In a few situations, animals, mainly those >6-months-old, develop a more obvious clinical syndrome, with high morbidity and low mortality—classical **BVD**. The infecting agent is usually an NCP BVDV. After an incubation period of 5-7 days, the affected animals develop fever, leukopenia, and viremia that may persist up to 15 days. The virus is present in leukocytes (buffy coat), especially lymphocytes and monocytes, and in plasma. There is a transient decrease in the number of B and T lymphocytes and a decline in responsiveness of lymphocytes to mitogen stimulation. Clinically, lethargy, anorexia, mild oculonasal discharge, and occasional mild oral erosions and shallow ulcers are found. Diarrhea may occur. In dairy herds, there is a transient drop in milk production. Affected animals develop neutralizing antibodies that peak in 10-12 weeks, and probably are immune for life.

A syndrome of **severe acute BVD**, with high morbidity and mortality in all age groups of susceptible animals, has been recognized since the early 1990s. Sometimes termed BVD type 2, because it is caused mainly, although not exclusively, by primary infections with BVDV2, this syndrome usually has a peracute-to-acute course, with fever, diarrhea, or pneumonia, and sudden death. Not all BVDV2 isolates are highly virulent. In some cases, a **thrombocytopenic syndrome**, seen clinically as epistaxis, hyphema, mucosal hemorrhages, bleeding at injection sites, and bloody diarrhea, is superimposed on the alimentary syndrome caused by BVDV2, or occurs independently. The pathogenesis of BVD type 2 is most frequently linked to increased strain virulence. However, production of inflammatory cytokines, in response to widespread infection of mononuclear phagocytes, has also been postulated as a cause for the severe disease seen clinically. The mechanism of thrombocytopenia is not completely defined, although infected megakaryocytes in the bone marrow undergo necrosis.

Fetal infections may occur in pregnant, immunocompetent, seronegative, acutely infected females, and in persistently infected (PI) counterparts. The outcome of fetal infection depends on the stage of gestation. The most serious consequences occur if an NCP BVDV crosses the placental barrier during the first 4 months of gestation. It may result in fetal resorption, mummification, abortion, congenital anomalies, or, if the calf survives, a **PI** calf. PI calves remain viremic for life and are immunotolerant to homologous NCP BVD viruses because of failure of the immature fetal immune system to recognize the infecting viral antigens as foreign.

PI calves may be clinically normal, weak, or undersized at birth. They may appear normal, but are often unthrifty, and may have a rough or curly hair coat. The prevalence of these calves in a herd is usually <2%, but may be as high as 25-30% in herds in which a large number of naive cows, early in pregnancy, have been exposed to NCP BVDV. *Most PI calves succumb to mucosal disease* (see later), usually between the ages of 6 months and 2 years. The offspring of the few animals that reach sexual maturity and become pregnant are also PI, which can result in families of animals PI with BVDV. PI animals are viremic and lack antibody to the infecting virus (are antigen positive but seronegative), which they shed constantly, acting as the *most important source of infection in the population*.

In PI animals, virus is present in a wide variety of tissues, and antigen can be demonstrated by IHC in skin biopsies—in follicular and interfollicular keratinocytes, matrix cells of the hair bulb, and dermal papillae. The use of skin biopsies for diagnosis of persistent infections by IHC or ELISA has been exploited diagnostically, but it should be recognized that acutely infected animals may have virus in skin biopsies as well, and detection of BVDV antigen in skin is therefore not specific for PI animals. Lesions in PI animals are minimal and subclinical, despite the widespread infection of virtually all tissues.

Mucosal disease is a clinicopathologic syndrome occurring in PI animals that subsequently become infected with a closely related CP strain, or probably more commonly, when the virus causing persistent congenital infection spontaneously undergoes recombination involving NS3 sequences. The result is an overwhelming infection that destroys cells, and to which the animal is incapable of responding. A condition of *low morbidity but very high mortality*, mucosal disease occurs most commonly in cattle that are 6 months to 2 years of age. Although deaths may occur within a few days of illness, and almost always within 2 weeks, some cases may survive for months. The incubation period after experimental infection with a CP strain in an animal PI with an NCP BVDV is usually 7-14 days but may be considerably longer. Mucosal disease occurred in yearling steers shortly after vaccination with a multivalent vaccine containing modified-live BVDV. Genetic studies of the BVDV isolate obtained from the affected animals, combined with epidemiologic evidence, were considered as strong evidence that the BVDV vaccine was the cause of mucosal disease.

Basically, there are *2 forms of clinically severe BVDV infection:* mucosal disease in PI animals, and the severe acute form of BVD caused by primary infections with very virulent strains of virus. At autopsy, one cannot confidently differentiate spontaneous cases of severe acute BVD caused by BVDV1 or BVDV2 from each other, or from cases of mucosal disease, other than by the more hemorrhagic character of some cases of severe acute BVD caused by BVDV2 isolates. Tentative differentiation of mucosal disease from severe acute BVD rests on the epidemiologic picture; antigenic or molecular characterization of the involved viruses is required for definitive diagnosis of the various syndromes.

Fulminant severe acute BVD or mucosal disease closely resemble rinderpest clinically and grossly. At the onset the animal is febrile, with serous-to-mucoid nasal discharge. Discrete oral lesions are preceded by acute stomatitis and pharyngitis, the mucosae being hyperemic and pink and covered by a thin gray film of catarrhal exudate. There is severe diarrhea and tenesmus with feces containing little or no blood or mucus. Affected animals become lethargic, anorexic, and dehydrated; they drool, are polypneic and tachycardic, and may die quickly.

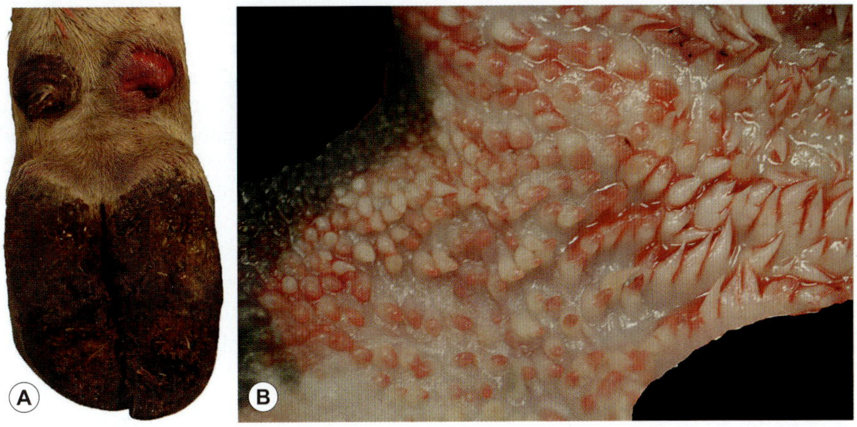

Figure 1-72 Bovine viral diarrhea (BVD). **A.** Erosive-ulcerative dermatitis of pastern in BVD. (Courtesy D. O'Toole.) **B.** Blunting and hemorrhage of buccal papillae due to BVDV–induced necrosis. A few remaining normal papillae are long with sharp points. (Courtesy R. Moeller.)

In more chronic cases, the development of the oral lesions is like that found in acute cases; however, by the time they die there is usually some evidence of healing. The watery diarrhea of the early phase gradually gives way to feces that are passed frequently, are scant in volume, and contain a large proportion of mucus flecked with blood. Late in the clinical course, there is lethargy, emaciation, ruminal stasis, and frequent attempts at defecation accompanied by severe tenesmus. Interdigital dermatitis, dermatitis of pasterns (Fig. 1-72A), coronitis, and laminitis affecting all 4 feet may be present in chronically affected animals, resulting in lameness. In these too, the skin is dry and scurfy, especially over the neck, withers, back, perineal and preputial areas, and vulva, whereas that on the medial aspect of the thighs and forelegs becomes moist and dirty yellow.

At autopsy, the **gross lesions** vary considerably, especially in acute cases, in which either upper alimentary or intestinal lesions rarely may be absent, and less so in the chronic disease, in which a broader pathologic picture often is present, perhaps partially obscured by healing or evolution of lesions.

Crusts, erosions, and shallow ulcers are present on the muzzle and nares of many affected cattle. There is loss of epithelium from much of the oral cavity. The most conspicuous oral erosions are on the palate, the tips of the buccal papillae (see Fig. 1-72B), and the gingiva. Many, especially on the papillae, the hard palate, and in the pharynx, are sharp punched-out ulcers, and expose a denuded, intensely hyperemic lamina propria. In more chronic cases, ulcers may have a margin of thickened proliferative epithelium. The tongue is not always affected; when present, lesions may be evident on all surfaces (Fig. 1-73A).

Esophageal lesions are usually present, most commonly in the upper third. In some acute cases, the lesions are shallow erosions, rather than ulcers. The erosions are more-or-less linear but otherwise irregular, have a dirty brown base, and little or no hyperemia, and may be covered by shreds of necrotic epithelium in animals that have not been swallowing (see Fig. 1-73B). In more advanced cases, discrete ulcerations occur. In many chronically affected animals, the ulcers are beginning to heal and have yellow-white slightly elevated plaques of proliferative epithelium at the periphery of the mucosal defect.

Lesions are found in the *reticulorumen and omasum,* but usually not in the esophageal groove. The ruminal content in chronically affected animals with prolonged anorexia is usually scant and dry. In most acute cases, the ruminal content is unusually liquid and putrid. The lesions on the wall of the rumen resemble those present elsewhere in the upper alimentary tract and, although they occur anywhere, they are best seen on the pillars and other smooth or nonvillus portions of the mucosa. The omasal lesions are most numerous along the edges of the leaves, sometimes causing a scalloped margin or perforation.

The morphogenesis of the lesions in the squamous mucosa of the upper alimentary tract begins with necrosis of the

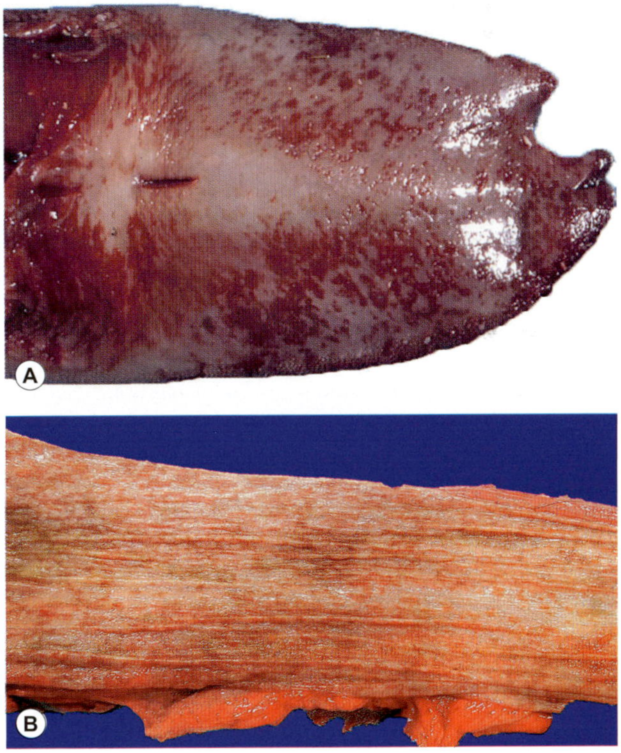

Figure 1-73 Bovine viral diarrhea. **A.** Confluent ulcers on the ventral surface of the tongue. **B.** Longitudinal erosions and ulcers in the esophageal mucosa. (Courtesy R. Moeller.)

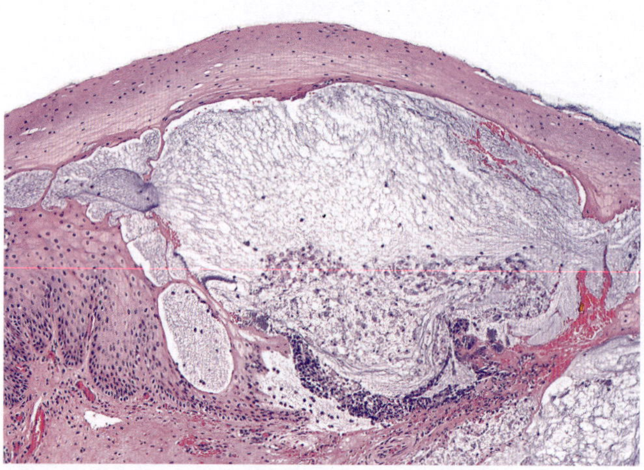

Figure 1-74 Bovine viral diarrhea. Histologic appearance of acute esophageal vesicle due to bovine viral diarrhea virus. (Courtesy J.P. Garcia.)

epithelium (Fig. 1-74). Individual cells and groups of cells deep in the epithelium are eosinophilic and swollen, with pyknotic nuclei. These foci enlarge progressively and form areas of necrosis that extend to, and may involve, the basal layer. In the early stages, there is little or no inflammation of the lamina propria, but leukocytes infiltrate the necrotic epithelium. These necrotic foci enlarge progressively tending to coalesce and may form small cleavage vesicles along the proprial-epithelial junction, leading to erosions or ulcers as necrotic epithelium is abraded away. The ulcerations of the squamous epithelium of the upper alimentary tract are accompanied by inflammation in the lamina propria, especially where this forms papillae.

Changes are regularly present in the *abomasum*. The sides of the rugae bear ulcers that may be punctate to 1 cm or more in diameter. The histologic changes in the glandular epithelium of the abomasum are epithelial necrosis, mainly in the depths of the glands, and accompanying interstitial inflammation.

The mucosa of the *small intestine* often appears normal over much of its length. However, in some cases the mucosa of the small intestine may have patchy or diffuse congestion. In rare cases, fibrin casts may be in the lumen of the small bowel.

In acute cases, it is usual to find dark *coagulated blood and fibrin overlying and outlining Peyer patches*, the covering of which is eroded. This, when present, is a very distinctive lesion that was only paralleled in the now-eradicated rinderpest. Severely affected Peyer patches are often obvious through the serosa as red-black oval areas up to 10-12 cm long on the antimesenteric border of the gut (Fig. 1-75A). Less acutely affected Peyer patches may be overlain by a diphtheritic membrane, whereas in milder or more chronic cases, the patches may be depressed and covered by tenacious mucus. Mesenteric lymph nodes may or may not be enlarged.

Lesions in the *large bowel* are highly variable. The mucosa may be congested, often in a "tiger-stripe" pattern following the colonic folds, a reflection of tenesmus. In acute cases, there may be fibrinohemorrhagic typhlocolitis. In more chronic cases, fibrinous or fibrinonecrotic lesions and focal or extensive ulceration may be present at any level of the large bowel, but particularly in the cecum and rectum.

The characteristic **microscopic lesion** in the intestinal mucosa is *destruction of the epithelial lining of the intestinal crypts*. In the duodenum, only a few crypts are affected, but more crypts are affected more severely in the lower reaches of the small intestine and in the cecum and colon. Affected crypts are dilated and filled with mucus, epithelial debris, and leukocytes. Remaining crypt-lining cells are attenuated in an attempt to cover the basement membrane. Reparative hyperplasia of crypt lining is rarely encountered. Crypt dropout may be evident microscopically. In the cecum and colon, extensive damage to crypts and associated collapse of the lamina propria are the probable cause of ulceration seen grossly. Congestion of mucosal capillaries, and in acute or ulcerated cases, effusion of fibrin and neutrophils from the mucosal surface may be evident.

The microscopic lesions of Peyer patches are distinctive, although not specific, in BVD. In the acute phase of the disease, severe acute inflammation in the mucosa over Peyer patches accompanies almost complete destruction of the underlying glands, collapse of the lamina propria, and lysis of the follicular lymphoid tissues. Later in the course of the disease, dilated crypts, lined at least in part by cuboidal epithelium and filled with necrotic epithelial cells, mucus, and inflammatory cells, appear to *herniate* into the submucosal space previously occupied by involuted lymphoid follicles (see Fig. 1-75B). Crypt herniation, although characteristic of BVD, is not specific as it can be seen in a few other diseases. Peyer patches should be sought assiduously at autopsy because their gross and microscopic appearance may provide useful evidence for diagnosis.

Microscopically, the mesenteric and sometimes other lymph nodes have a diminished population of lymphocytes and necrosis of germinal centers. By IHC, there is a marked decrease in most lymphocyte subpopulations.

An important microscopic lesion is *hyaline degeneration and fibrinoid necrosis of submucosal and mesenteric arterioles* (see Fig. 1-75C). A mild-to-moderate mononuclear inflammatory cell reaction is frequently present in the walls of the vessels and in perivascular areas. The vascular lesions also may be present in a variety of other organs, such as the heart, brain, and adrenal cortices, which may make it difficult to differentiate the disease from MCF. The vascular lesions in acute mucosal disease are less consistently present and are usually milder, and there is *involution of lymphoid tissue in BVD*, in contrast with the lymphoproliferation characteristic of MCF.

Coronitis may extend completely around the coronary band, with some separation of the skin-horn junction causing disturbance and overgrowth of the horn. Dermatitis may extend from the coronet up the back of the pastern. Milder dermatitis is generalized, with scurfiness, especially from the ears to the withers. In sections of the skin of animals with chronic mucosal disease, there is hyperkeratosis and parakeratosis with focal accumulations of necrotic epithelium with intense hyperemia of the adjacent superficial dermis. The epithelial lesions are basically similar to those in the squamous mucosa of the upper alimentary tract. Necrosis often extends deeply to or through the basal layers; it results in minute erosions or ulcerations. There is massive infiltration of macrophages and some lymphocytes in the underlying dermis. These deeper lesions occur in the inner aspects of the legs and the perineum, and there is exudation of serum in these areas. The overlying degenerate epithelium becomes disorderly and eventually is lifted off.

Some animals with chronic disease develop *mycotic infections* secondary to lesions in the forestomachs, abomasum, and Peyer patches. The lesions are areas of hemorrhagic necrosis

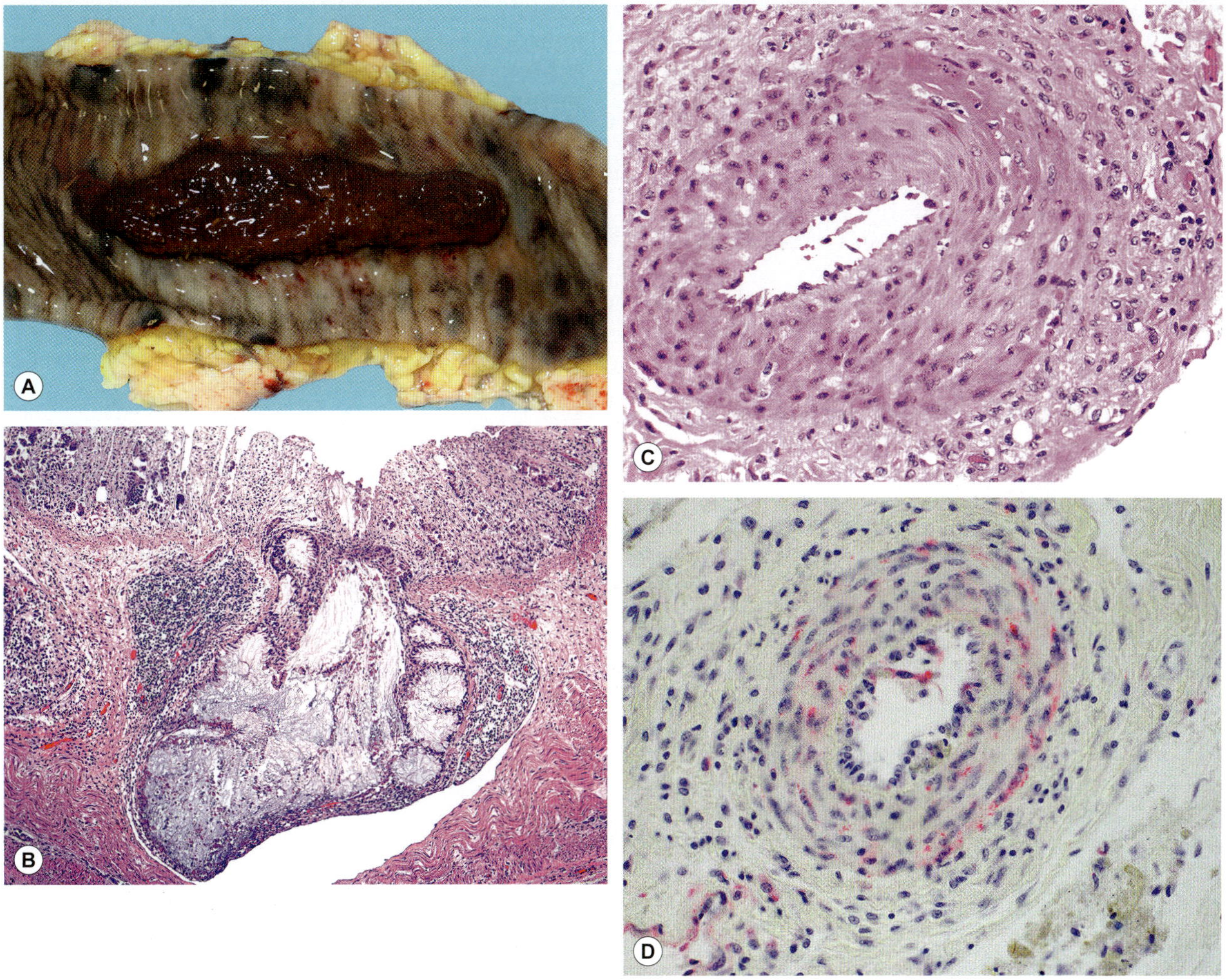

Figure 1-75 Bovine viral diarrhea. **A**. Fibrinohemorrhagic exudate over ileal Peyer patch. (Courtesy R. Moeller.) **B**. Herniation of intestinal crypts into the submucosa replacing necrotic lymphoid follicles in Peyer patch. Mucus and inflammatory exudate are in the cystic glands. **C**. Hyaline degeneration and fibrinoid necrosis of mesenteric arteriole in a calf with bovine viral diarrhea virus (BVDV)–associated mucosal disease. **D**. Positive immunoreactivity in smooth muscle wall of the mesenteric arteriole shown in (C). IHC for BVDV antigen.

involving the mucosa, submucosa, and sometimes deeper layers of the wall. Fungal hyphae are found invading the stroma and causing thrombosis in venules.

Infection of oocytes and cumulus cells in the ovaries has been well documented, causing speculation concerning ovarian dysfunction and reduced fertility in animals surviving BVDV infection.

After *experimental inoculation with virulent BVDV2*, animals are febrile by 7 days postinfection. Prominent clinical signs are anorexia, depression, and episodes of profuse watery and bloody diarrhea that persist until the animal is moribund at 13-14 days postinfection. Pregnant animals may abort. Leukopenia and thrombocytopenia are often marked. In cases with severe thrombocytopenia, hemorrhage may be evident clinically.

Lesions are found in the digestive and respiratory systems. There is mild tracheitis, bronchitis, and bronchiolitis, which can progress to secondary bacterial pneumonia. Strains may vary in their ability to infect the pulmonary tree and result in disease. Intestinal lesions strongly resemble those seen in mucosal disease, with severe lymphoid depletion and necrosis of epithelial cells. However, with these BVDV2 infections, there is often also a significant amount of hemorrhage evident externally, as described previously, and there may be extensive subserosal hemorrhages in the thoracic and abdominal cavities. Similarly, edema may be more noteworthy in this form than in mucosal disease. Severe necrotizing vasculitis, especially arteritis, is noted in various organs but is most readily identifiable in lymphoid tissue. Meningoencephalitis associated with neuronal infection by BVDV2 has been reported.

By IHC, there is widespread viral antigen within epithelial cells (including oral and esophageal epithelium), smooth muscle cells (see Fig. 1-75D), and mononuclear phagocytes in various organs, although lesions often do not correspond to the sites of antigen staining.

BVDV and secondary infections. BVDV infection suppresses interferon production and impairs lymphocyte function, monocyte proliferation and chemotaxis, humoral antibody production, neutrophil function, and bacterial clearance. These changes are fairly persistent in chronically infected animals and in those with mucosal disease. The failure of immunogenic response may be associated with immunotolerance, or destruction of immunocompetent cells, which is reflected in lymphopenia. In addition to a lack of humoral antibody response, there is also depression of cell-mediated immunity, as indicated by a poor response of cultured peripheral lymphocytes to various mitogens. The impairment of neutrophil function in cattle infected with BVDV may explain in part the apparent susceptibility of such cattle to *secondary bacterial infections*.

Fetal infection with BVDV. In addition to the early embryonic death and abortions that can be ascribed to BVDV, infections of seronegative immunocompetent dams, usually between 90 and 120 days of gestation, may result in a wide spectrum of *teratogenic lesions*, including microencephaly, hypomyelinogenesis, cerebellar hypoplasia and dysgenesis, hydranencephaly, hydrocephalus, and defective myelination of the spinal cord. Ocular lesions, such as microphthalmia, cataracts, retinal degeneration, atrophy and dysplasia, and optic neuritis, have all been associated with fetal infections by BVDV (see Vol. 1, Nervous System; Vol. 1, Special Senses Vol. 3, Female Genital System). Infections of the immunocompetent fetus, usually after 135 days of gestation, result in antibody production that is detectable in precolostral serum samples of the newborn calf.

Fetal infection later in gestation may produce lesions unrelated to teratogenesis in the fetus, including alimentary tract lesions. Punctate hemorrhages with 1-3 mm ulcers may be profuse in the oral cavity, excepting the dorsum of the tongue, and in the esophagus, larynx, trachea, conjunctiva, and abomasum. The fetal lesions of squamous epithelium evolve in somewhat the same manner as those described earlier, with focal hemorrhages in the lamina propria and epithelial necrosis beginning in the basal layer.

BVDV infection in pigs. The prevalence of naturally occurring antibodies to BVDV in swine has increased dramatically with seroconversion in different countries from 2% to 43%. Antibodies to BVDV may complicate the diagnosis of classical swine fever, especially in those countries considered to be free of this disease. Cattle and modified live virus vaccines containing contaminated fetal bovine serum are considered to be common sources of infection for swine. Infection of pigs with BVDV usually occurs without clinical signs, allowing an opportunity for the virus to spread without detection. There are sporadic reports of disease in pigs associated with BVDV infection, including stillbirth, and poorly viable piglets, some showing tremors. A few 2-4-week-old pigs in infected herds are anemic, have a rough hair coat, growth retardation, wasting, and diarrhea. Affected pigs fail to develop neutralizing antibodies to the infecting homologous BVDV. Littermates that remain normal develop neutralizing antibodies. The suggestion is that the infections are congenital. In pigs infected postnatally with BVDV; usually no lesions, or very mild lesions, are observed. Experimental in utero BVDV infection of sows may result in prenatal and perinatal deaths, PI immunotolerant or normal pigs. Many of these conditions resemble the effects of in utero infection with NCP BVDV in cattle.

Border disease

Border disease is a congenital infection of sheep and goats, usually with one of several NCP genotypes of **border disease virus** (BDV; *Flaviviridae, Pestivirus ovis*), a pestivirus antigenically related to BVDV and CSFV, but apparently also with some BVDV2 strains. The disease was first reported in lambs from border areas between England and Wales; embryonic and fetal death, abortion, mummification, and birth of weak lambs or kids occur. The affected animals have an abnormal body conformation, long hairy fleece, clonic rhythmic tremors ("hairy shakers"), unthriftiness, and poor viability (see Vol. 1, Nervous System; Vol. 1, Integumentary System; Vol. 3, Female Genital System).

A syndrome resembling mucosal disease has been reported in lambs that survived the initial border disease; they were PI with an NCP BVDV. Immunohistochemical examination of tissues from PI sheep reveals viral antigen in smooth muscle cells of hollow organs and blood vessels, epithelial cells in the GI tract, lymphocytes, neurons, and glial cells. When CP BDV is superimposed on persistent infection, affected sheep develop chronic diarrhea, wasting, nasal discharge, and polypnea. Macroscopic lesions are particularly present in the cecum and colon and in a few sheep, also the terminal ileum. There is marked thickening of the gut wall caused by subserosal and mucosal edema and diffuse polypoid hyperplasia of the mucosa, which is hemorrhagic and focally ulcerated.

The *microscopic lesions* in the gut are similar to those described for mucosal disease in cattle. Lymphoid cell reactions are evident in the choroid plexus, portal triads of the liver, kidney, myocardium, thyroids, lungs, spleen, and lymph nodes. In addition, some lambs have marked hypertrophy and edema of the muscularis of the terminal ileum. The lesions in the latter resemble "terminal ileitis," and that is the reason why BVDV should be considered a possible cause of that syndrome of yet undetermined etiology.

The pathogenesis of fetal infections, resultant border disease, and related enteric lesions in sheep appear to be similar to the multitude of conditions associated with NCP BVDV prenatal infections in cattle. Seronegative ewes infected before 80 days of gestation may produce PI, immunotolerant, chronically viremic lambs.

Rinderpest

Otherwise known as "cattle plague," rinderpest was an *acute or subacute highly contagious disease of cattle, domestic buffalo, and some other species of even-toed ungulates, including buffaloes, large antelope, deer, giraffes, wildebeests, and warthogs, with erosive or hemorrhagic lesions of all mucous membranes*. After a global eradication campaign, including limitations on animal movement and the use of a highly efficacious vaccine, *the disease was eradicated from the planet*, with the virus last detected in 2001 in wild buffaloes in Meru National Park in Kenya, located on the edge of the Somali ecosystem, the last known remaining reservoir. For several years after that, studies in the region detected antibodies to the rinderpest virus (RPV) in cattle, but it is thought that they came from old vaccinations. More recent surveillance confirmed the absence of the virus in the region. Vaccination against rinderpest is no longer used anywhere in the world. Before eradication, pandemics of rinderpest occurred in the Middle East and sub-Saharan and equatorial Africa. The infection impacted heavily on wildlife populations in close contact with cattle, and wildlife was important in virus spread.

Rinderpest virus (RPV; *Paramyxoviridae, Morbillivirus pecoris*) is a highly pleomorphic single-stranded RNA virus with a core diameter of 120-300 nm and a spiked envelope. The virus is highly fragile under ordinary environmental conditions; it is incapable of surviving more than a few hours outside the animal body under normal circumstances.

Fever and its attendant signs usher in the **clinical syndrome**, with early leukopenia. Fever reaches its peak in ~3 days and falls with the onset of diarrhea, which may be bloody. There is severe abdominal pain, anorexia, ocular and nasal discharge, tachypnea, fetid breath, occasional cough, lethargy, severe dehydration and emaciation, and prostration. Death occurs in 5-8 days. Explosive outbreaks with high morbidity and mortality were more likely to occur in naive populations. Vaccinated or recovered animals usually had lifelong immunity. Secondary bacterial, viral, protozoal, and rickettsial infections were common.

The **gross changes** in rinderpest are characteristic but not pathognomonic. They are similar to BVD and mucosal disease (Fig. 1-76A), and they also bear some similarities with MCF. The lesions in the upper alimentary tract are *necrotizing and erosive or ulcerative*.

The **histologic lesions** of stratified squamous epithelium originate in the spinous layer. Entrance into the epithelium may be via infected Langerhans cells that then pass virus along to adjacent cells. Irregularly shaped rafts of acanthocytes are infected with virus as evidenced by IHC. These same cells then undergo degeneration and necrosis. Multinucleate syncytia form in the epithelium (see Fig. 1-76B) and these may have *cytoplasmic and nuclear inclusions*. Abrasion causes the necrotic tissue to lift off and produce shallow erosions or ulcers. This occurs so readily that they are usually the first lesions observed. Their margins are sharp, and the bases are reddened by the underlying congested capillaries. The initial minute erosions enlarge and coalesce to form extensive defects.

Lesions in the intestine are severe and severity is correlated with the amount of lymphoid tissue in subjacent areas. Consequently, the greatest mucosal damage is seen in the ileum and the proximal colonic patch. Peyer patches are almost universally involved. These areas become hemorrhagic and necrotic (see Fig. 1-76C) and are associated with necrosis of the overlying mucosa, leaving deep ulcers.

There is replication of virus at all levels of intestine, with both crypt and villus epithelium involved. Replication is associated with the formation of inclusion bodies, both nuclear and cytoplasmic, degeneration, necrosis, denuding of epithelium, formation of crypt abscesses, and, if prolonged enough, villus atrophy. The formation of syncytia within gut epithelium is a rare event, in contrast with the oral cavity lesions, where it is seen with some regularity.

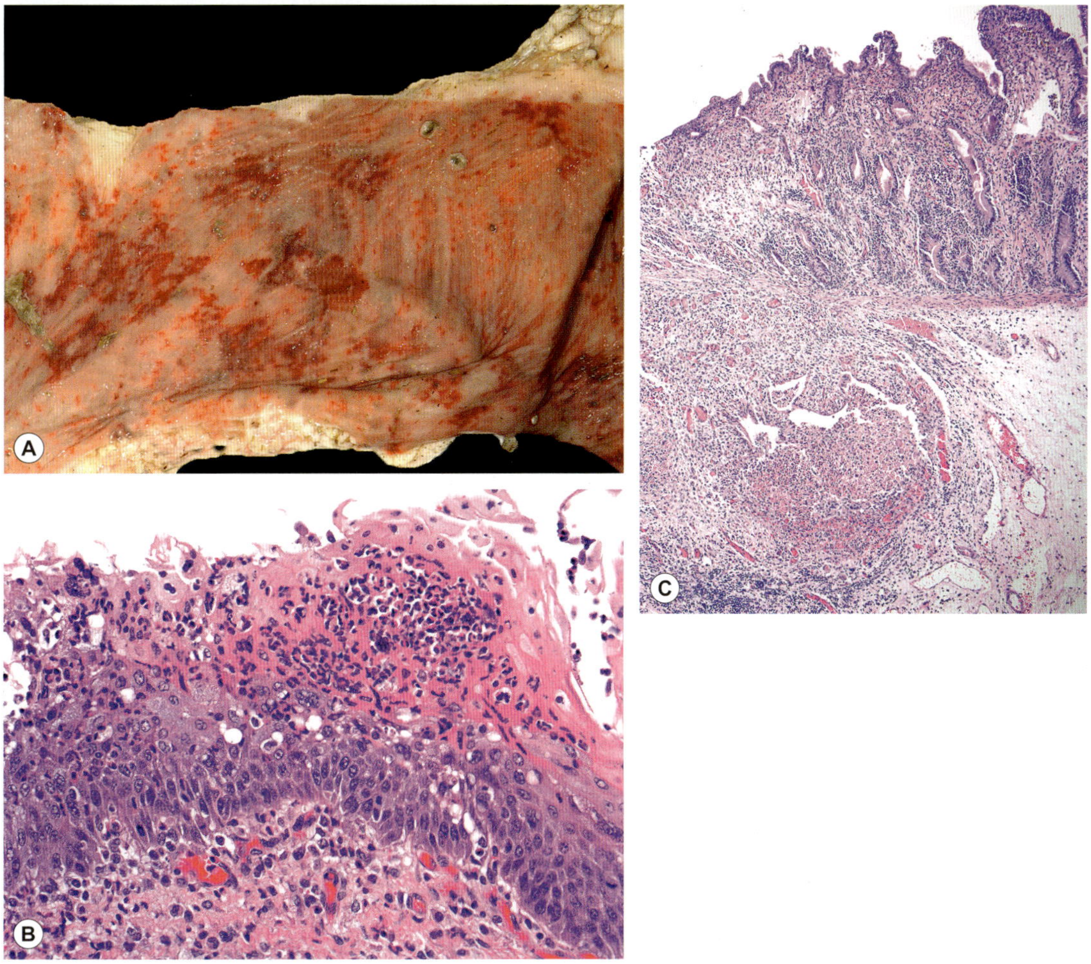

Figure 1-76 Rinderpest. A. Multifocal-to-coalescing fibrinohemorrhagic colitis in a cow. (Courtesy Elizabeth Clark, U.S. Department of Agriculture, Animal and Plant Health Inspection Service, Plum Island, NY.) **B.** Necrosis and disorganization of superficial epithelium with the formation of syncytial cells in the tongue of a cow. **C.** Peyer patch necrosis in ileum of a cow.

Receptor affinity dictates that *RPV is trophic for lymphoid tissues*. Infection and replication have been documented in both lymphocytes and macrophages. Necrosis of follicular lymphocytes is extreme, and gross inspection, which reveals little abnormality of nodes, is misleading.

Although the gross lesions of rinderpest resemble those of severe acute BVD, mucosal disease, and MCF, *rinderpest is distinguished microscopically most readily by the presence of syncytia and inclusion bodies*.

Peste des petits ruminants

PPR is an acute viral disease of sheep and goats that closely resembles rinderpest and is also known as kata, *stomatitis-pneumoenteritis complex*, goat plague, ovine rinderpest, and pseudo-rinderpest. The disease was first recognized in West Africa and is now distributed in north and sub-Saharan Africa, the Arabian Peninsula, Anatolia, the Indian subcontinent, including Pakistan, Nepal, and Bangladesh, and China. **Peste-des-petits-ruminants virus** (PPRV; *Paramyxoviridae, Morbillivirus caprinae; Small ruminant morbillivirus*) is closely related to RPV, with which it shares common antigenic determinants. The virus cross-reacts with RPV in immunodiffusion and complement fixation tests. It may be differentiated from RPV using monoclonal antibody techniques and cDNA probes. In April 2015, the Food and Agriculture Organization of the United Nations and the World Organization for Animal Health launched the PPR global control and eradication strategy with the goal of global eradication by 2030.

The clinical signs, pathogenesis, and lesions of PPR in sheep and goats in general are similar to those of rinderpest (Fig. 1-77A and B), except that PPR is more acute in onset, especially in goats, and follows a more rapid course. Goats have been reported to be more susceptible than sheep in some outbreaks. West African goats appear to be more susceptible than European varieties, and, among the former, the dwarf varieties are most susceptible. Another difference is the marked involvement of the respiratory tract; affected animals have dyspnea, hyperpnea, and cough. There is also marked serous-to-mucopurulent nasal and ocular discharge. Erosion/ulceration of the oral and pharyngeal epithelium may be diffuse, and pseudomembranes are characteristically observed in the oral cavity (see Fig. 1-77A and B). The erosions can spread into the pharynx.

The pulmonary lesions of PPR are similar to pneumonia caused by CDV in dogs and measles virus infections in humans. The gross respiratory tract lesions include fibrinonecrotic tracheitis, and consolidation, atelectasis, and dark-red discoloration of the cranioventral lung lobes. Some animals have fibrinous pleuritis (see Vol. 2, Respiratory System). Hemorrhagic colitis is almost always present (Fig. 1-78A). Microscopically, there is mild-to-severe tracheitis, bronchitis and necrotizing bronchiolitis, and diffuse proliferative *interstitial pneumonia*, with formation of alveolar syncytial cells. Other microscopic lesions include diffuse colitis (see Fig. 1-78B and C), multifocal hepatic necrosis, and severe lymphocytolysis in lymphoid tissues. Syncytial cells are conspicuous, particularly in the oral mucosa, pulmonary alveoli, liver, and lymphoid tissues.

Eosinophilic cytoplasmic and nuclear inclusions are present in the epithelial cells of the colonic crypts (see Fig. 1-78C) and renal pelvis, abomasal mucosa, air passages, type II pneumocytes, and syncytial cells. Viral antigen may be demonstrated in the same cells and in the brain, rumen, abomasum, heart, and myocytes of the tongue with appropriate immunohistochemical techniques. The primary viral lesions often are complicated by secondary bacterial infections.

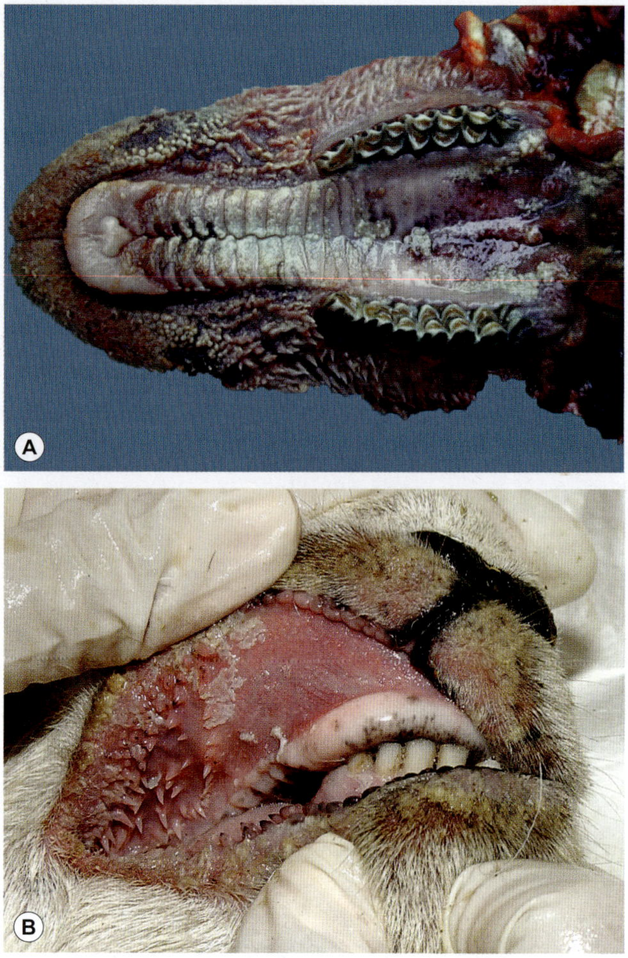

Figure 1-77 Peste des petits ruminants. **A.** Oral ulceration and fibrinonecrotic inflammation in a sheep. (Courtesy S. Perl.) **B.** Ulceration and fibrinonecrotic pseudomembrane on the oral mucosa of a sheep. (Courtesy Plum Island Animal Disease Center.)

Concurrent infection with PPRV and pestivirus was diagnosed in stillborn twin lambs that grossly showed several anomalies typical of border disease, including scoliosis, brachygnathism, prognathism, arthrogryposis, hydranencephaly, cerebellar hypoplasia, and hairy fleece. Microscopically, these lambs had epidermal syncytial cells and necrotizing bronchitis/bronchiolitis with PPRV detected by IHC in the skin, lungs, kidneys, rumen, and thymus.

Experimental inoculation of PPRV into cattle or pigs does not produce clinical disease, but these animals will resist subsequent challenge with RPV. These species are considered to be dead-end hosts because they do not seem to spread the infection to other species. Natural infection or vaccination of sheep and goats with RPV protects them against PPRV.

A zoo outbreak of PPR that involved several species of wild ungulates has been reported, and Indian buffalo are also susceptible. The distribution of the virus in free-ranging wild ungulates has not been investigated.

Malignant catarrhal fever

Malignant catarrhal fever (MCF) is an infectious disease primarily of ungulate species in the order *Artiodactyla*, principally in the families *Bovidae, Cervidae*, and *Giraffidae*. MCF is also known as malignant head catarrh, and snotsiekte. Lesions

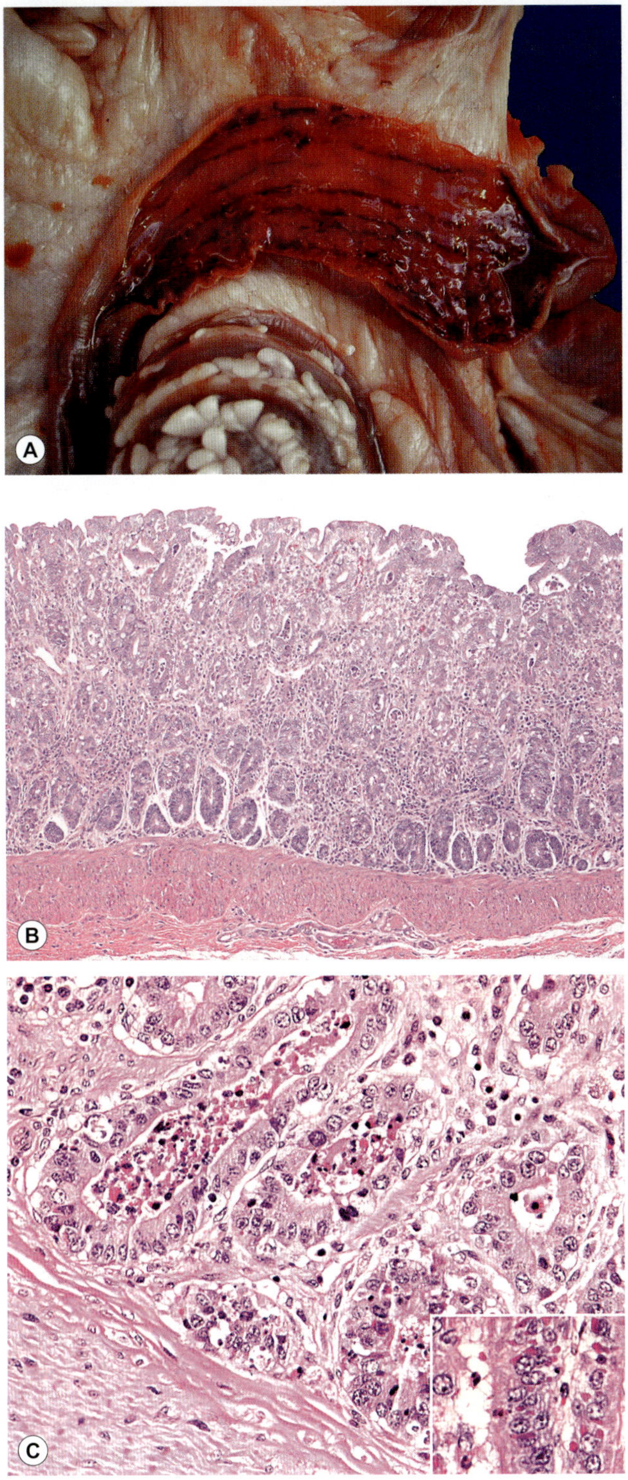

Figure 1-78 **Peste des petits ruminants**; hemorrhagic colitis in a goat. A. Colon with diffuse hemorrhage. (Courtesy S. Perl.) B. Necrohemorrhagic colitis with severe lymphoid depletion. C. Dilated and necrotic glands; numerous acidophilic, intracytoplasmic inclusion bodies are present in gland epithelial cells (inset).

include *lymphoproliferation, vasculitis, and mucocutaneous erosions and ulcers*.

MCF is distributed worldwide. It is generally sporadic, although severe herd outbreaks have been reported in feedlot, dairy, and range cattle, in farmed bison and deer, and in zoos. Among cervids, all species except fallow deer are probably susceptible. Other susceptible species of ruminants include banteng, Cape buffalo, and greater kudu. *Lethality in susceptible species approaches 100%*, although there are rare recorded cases of chronic infection and recovery from MCF, especially in infected cattle, goats, bison, and pigs. Although the agent is transmissible, the disease is apparently not contagious among cattle or bison by direct contact.

MCF is caused by cross-species infections with members of the MCF virus group of ruminant gammaherpesviruses (family *Orthoherpesviridae*, subfamily *Gammaherpesvirinae*, genus *Macavirus*). Of the 10 members of the MCF virus group that have been identified, at least 6 are associated with clinical MCF under natural conditions: 1) **alcelaphine gammaherpesvirus 1**, wildebeest-associated malignant catarrhal fever virus (AlGHV1, MCFV; *Macavirus alcelaphinegamma1*), carried by wildebeest (*Connochaetes* spp. and others); 2) **ovine gammaherpesvirus 2**, sheep-associated malignant catarrhal fever virus (OvGHV2; *Macavirus ovinegamma2*), endemic in domestic sheep; 3) **caprine gammaherpesvirus 2** (CpGHV2; *Macavirus caprinegamma2*), endemic in domestic goats; 4) **caprine gammaherpesvirus 3** (CpGHV3) causing MCF in white-tailed deer and red brocket deer; 5) **alcelaphine gammaherpesvirus 2**, hartebeest-associated malignant catarrhal fever virus (AlGHV2; *Macavirus alcelaphinegamma2*), carried by hartebeest (*Alcelaphus* sp.) and topi (*Damaliscus* sp.) and causing MCF in Barbary red deer and bison; and 6) **ibex MCF virus** (Ibex-MCFV), carried by the Nubian ibex and producing MCF in bongo and anoa.

Related gammaherpesviruses, as yet unassociated with MCF, have been detected in a number of bovids. Gammaherpesviruses of ruminants are highly cell-associated lymphotropic herpesviruses, difficult or impossible to isolate, which are typically transmitted from adults to offspring within the first 2-3 months of life, probably via free virus shed in nasal secretions. In the natural host, infection is latent or inapparent, with intermittent virus shedding, although disease has been incited in sheep by experimental aerosol inoculation of a large dose of OvGHV2.

Most natural outbreaks of MCF are due to 2 agents originally incriminated in MCF outbreaks: AlGHV1and OvGHV2. **AlGHV1** is responsible for the "African" or **wildebeest-associated (WA-MCF)** form. **OvGHV2** causes **sheep-associated (SA-MCF)**. Each member of the MCFV group has a subclinical reservoir host species and, for those known to be pathogenic, one or more clinically susceptible host species that develop clinical disease. The division is not absolute and lesions and/or disease can be induced in some reservoir species when the challenge dose is sufficiently high. Nevertheless, as a general rule, reservoir species are well adapted to subclinical infection and efficiently shed cell-free virus; MCF-susceptible species are poorly adapted and shed little, or more commonly no, cell-free virus. This absence of viral shedding accounts for end-stage hosts.

The **classical form** of MCF resulting from AlGHV1 and OvGHV2 is identical in clinical and pathologic terms. However, the epidemiology of the 2 agents has important differences. The most important wildebeest species, the blue or brindled wildebeest (*Connochaetes taurinus*) carries AlGHV1. Wildebeest calves become infected during the first 2-3 months of life when they are also viremic and shed cell-free AlGHV1 in nasal and ocular secretions. Most wildebeest >7-months-old are serologically positive for AlGHV1. In utero infections have also been reported. Wildebeest are infected for life and transmit AlGHV1 to their calves without showing clinical signs.

Wildebeest calves are considered to be the main source of infection for cattle in East Africa. They may shed virus in nasal and ocular secretions until they are 3-4 months of age. Transmission to cattle may occur even without intimate contact, suggesting aerosol spread.

Viremia apparently ceases with the development of active neutralizing antibodies in animals >6-months-old. It may be reactivated during late pregnancy or periods of stress, such as transportation. Although AlGHV1 produces MCF in many captive exotic species of ruminants, apparently most species that are exposed in their native habitat do not develop disease. AlGHV1 has been transmitted and adapted to domestic rabbits, as well as to hamsters, rats, and guinea pigs, in which it produces MCF-like lesions.

The etiologic agent of **SA-MCF** has never been isolated from sheep; however, PCR probes have permitted its differentiation. *Most sheep have PCR-detectable specific OvGHV2 sequences in cells*, and identical sequences are detectable in spontaneous cases of SA-MCF. Experimental transmission of OvGHV2 between sheep has been accomplished using an aerosol of virus-infected nasal secretions, and natural transmission from adults to offspring probably involves this route, producing very high rates of infection in the sheep population, where it can be considered ubiquitous. The other gammaherpesviruses associated with MCF have also been suspected histologically and implicated by molecular techniques.

MCF has been reproduced by infecting bison via intranasal nebulization with sheep nasal secretions containing OvGHV2. MCF caused by OvGHV2 occurs spontaneously and experimentally in pigs, and the relative rarity of the disease in swine may be due to lack of exposure to ruminant gammaherpesviruses under most conditions of husbandry. Most sheep are presumed to be carriers of OvGHV2, and for a long time, it was thought that spontaneous MCF did not occur in this species, although clinical signs and lesions resembling MCF were produced in sheep experimentally exposed to a high dose of aerosolized OvGHV2. However, sporadic, MCF-like vascular disease in sheep is likely due to OvGHV2.

SA-MCF occurs where bovids and deer come in contact with sheep. There is considerable variation in the susceptibility of various ruminant species to SA-MCF. Domestic cattle (*Bos taurus* and *Bos indicus*) appear to require high levels of exposure to induce disease. Bali cattle or banteng (*Bos javanicus*), the domestic water buffalo (*Bubalus bubalis*), American bison (*Bison bison*), and most species of deer, with the exception of fallow deer (*Dama dama*), seem to be highly susceptible. MCF has been one of the most serious diseases of farmed deer in New Zealand, Australia, and the United Kingdom. Numerous case outbreaks have also been reported in captive North American cervids.

The *mucosa of the upper respiratory tract and/or the tonsil* is the most likely natural route of entry for the agents of MCF. Both WA-MCF and SA-MCF can be transmitted to susceptible hosts with large volumes of whole blood or lymphoid tissues administered intravenously, but not by cell-free filtrates, indicating that the agents are cell associated, probably with lymphocytes. The incubation period of MCF is usually 2-10 weeks, but may on occasion be much longer.

Antibodies against the gammaherpesvirus involved can be detected in animals with MCF, and often in herdmates, implying subclinical infection. Development of antibodies does not prevent a fatal outcome.

The **pathogenesis**, clinical signs, and lesions are similar, whichever agent induces MCF. Viremia in WA-MCF usually starts ~7 days before the onset of fever and persists throughout the course of the disease; *marked T-lymphocyte hyperplasia occurs*. A population of LGL appears to be latently infected and transformed by gammaherpesviral infection, and OvGHV2 genome has been detected in CD8+ T cells, the predominant cell infiltrating around vessels in the brains studied. These cells are probably cytotoxic T lymphocytes or T-suppressor cells, but the mechanism by which they mediate the lesions of MCF is unclear. Dysfunction of this cell population may result in derepression of T-lymphocyte replication, permitting lymphoproliferation. Deranged cytotoxic T-cell activity may then create the epithelial and vascular lesions, through a type of graft-versus-host response, attacking epithelium of the respiratory and GI systems, as well as medium-sized arteries throughout the body. This is a unifying, but unproved, hypothesis explaining the lymphadenopathy, mucosal epithelial lesions, and vasculitis characteristic of MCF. Vascular lesions may mediate infarction of some affected tissues.

There is wide variation in the presenting **clinical syndromes**, which are potentially pansystemic. The *head-and-eye form* is the most common presentation in domestic cattle. Quite consistently, affected animals have enlarged lymph nodes, although this may be less the case in bison, and there is usually some degree of ocular and oral disease, and exudative dermatitis. There is edema of the eyelids and palpebral conjunctivae and congestion of the nasal and buccal mucosae. Photophobia is accompanied by copious lacrimation. There is conjunctivitis and an increasing circumferential rim of bilateral corneal opacity, starting at the limbus and progressing centripetally. Corneal ulceration occurs in some cases, but in those that die quickly, the infiltration of the filtration angle may be all that is seen, and this is easily overlooked. Hypopyon may be seen. In some cases, there are nervous signs, such as hyperesthesia, head pressing, trembling, nystagmus, incoordination, and behavioral changes. Other animals may have gastroenteritis with diarrhea, which may be bloody in acute cases. This is most commonly seen in deer. The disease may take an acute course of ~1-3 days, particularly in animals with hemorrhagic enteritis. Those with less severe gastroenteritis, central nervous signs, or generalized disease may linger for as long as 9-10 days. Mortality in MCF has been considered to approach 100% of clinical cases, but recovery may occur, although chronic ocular lesions and vasculitis persist. Clinical signs in bison are more subtle than those in cattle, with a high percentage of animals dying without clinical signs being observed or with animals dying very soon after the onset of clinical disease.

Gross changes involve various organs and are the consequence of 3 basic microscopic lesions: widespread *arteritis-phlebitis* of medium caliber vessels, *lymphoid proliferation* and production of atypical lymphoblastoid cells, and *mucosal ulceration* in digestive, urinary, and respiratory tracts. Gross changes may not be present in occasional animals that die of peracute MCF, and in these the diagnosis must rest on the detection of the characteristic histologic changes, and demonstration of the genome of an implicated gammaherpesvirus in tissue. The carcass is dehydrated and may be emaciated if the course has been prolonged. Conjunctivitis may be evident. The muzzle and nares are heavily encrusted and, if wiped, often reveal irregular eroded or ulcerated surfaces; in some cases, there may be only a slight serous discharge. Cutaneous lesions, especially in SA-MCF, are common, but often overlooked. The affected areas include the thorax, abdomen, inguinal regions, perineum, udder, and occasionally the head. There may be, acutely, more-or-less generalized exanthema with sufficient exudation to wet and mat the hair, and to form detachable crusts; in unpigmented skin there is obvious hyperemia. The crusts may become several millimeters thick, and there is patchy loss of hair. Sometimes these cutaneous changes begin locally about the base of the hooves and horns, the loin, and perineum; they may remain localized or become generalized. In severe cases, the horns and hooves may slough. Caprine gammaherpesvirus 2 has been associated with syndromes in deer that include dermatitis and alopecia, alone, or in combination with GI or neurologic disease.

The respiratory system may have minor or severe lesions. When the course is short, the nasal mucosa may only have congestion and slight serous exudation. Later, there is a copious discharge. Lesions are most severe in the rostral third of the nasal cavity, corresponding to the zone of stratified squamous epithelium. In some cases, fibrinous tracheobronchitis may occur.

The lower alimentary mucosae may have no significant lesions in the peracute disease, although *oral lesions are present in most cases of* MCF (Fig. 1-79). Minor erosions are first observed on the lips adjacent to the mucocutaneous junction. Sometimes apparently normal epithelium on the surface of the tongue peels off in sheets. Later, erosive and ulcerative lesions may involve a large area of oral mucosa, frequently occurring on all surfaces of the tongue, the dental pad, the tips of the buccal papillae, gingivae, hard and soft palate, and the cheeks. In some areas, the cheesy or tattered necrotic epithelium may not be sloughed at the time of inspection. Esophageal erosions or ulcers, similar to those that occur in the other diseases causing ulcerative stomatitis, occur in MCF, and are most consistent in the cranial portion. Lesions of the same sort may be present in the forestomachs. Focal ulceration or generalized hyperemia may be evident in the abomasal mucosa. In deer especially, hemorrhagic or fibrinohemorrhagic typhlocolitis may be a prominent finding.

The *liver* may be slightly enlarged. Close inspection will reveal, in some cases, diffuse mottling with white foci, which are periportal accumulations of mononuclear cells. There may be numerous petechiae and a few erosions of the mucous membrane of the gallbladder.

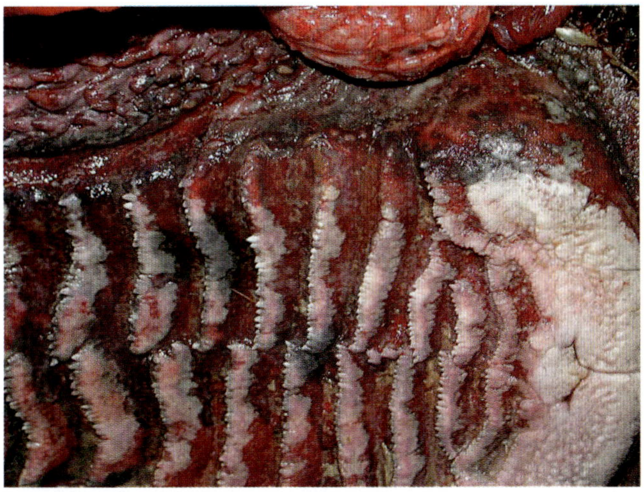

Figure 1-79 Malignant catarrhal fever. Ulcerative lesions in the hard palate of a bison.

Characteristic lesions may occur in the *urinary system*. Renal changes are not always present. They are infarcts or 2-4 mm foci of mononuclear interstitial nephritis (Fig. 1-80A). They may be numerous enough to produce a mottled appearance and may form slight rounded projections from the capsular surfaces. The pelvic and ureteral mucosa frequently has petechial and ecchymotic hemorrhages. Similar lesions are present on the mucosa of the urinary bladder, or there may be more severe hemorrhage associated with erosion and ulceration of the epithelium, and hematuria. Superficial lesions may occur in the vagina and vulva, similar to those of the oral cavity and skin.

Enlargement of lymph nodes is a characteristic lesion of MCF in most species, perhaps except in bison, where lymphadenopathy was found in one large study in only 62% of cases. This lesion is almost invariably present in cattle. All nodes may be involved, or some may appear grossly normal. Affected nodes may be many times the normal size, and some, including hemolymph nodes, which are usually too small to recognize, may become quite obvious. There is edema of the affected nodes and the pericapsular connective tissue. On microscopic examination, it is apparent that the increase in size is due to *lymphocytic hyperplasia*. Some of the nodes are congested or hemorrhagic. The spleen is slightly enlarged, and the lymphoid follicles are prominent.

Most animals may have *meningoencephalitis* as a result of *vasculitis* that may be accompanied by meningeal edema and is one of the most consistent histologic lesions of the disease.

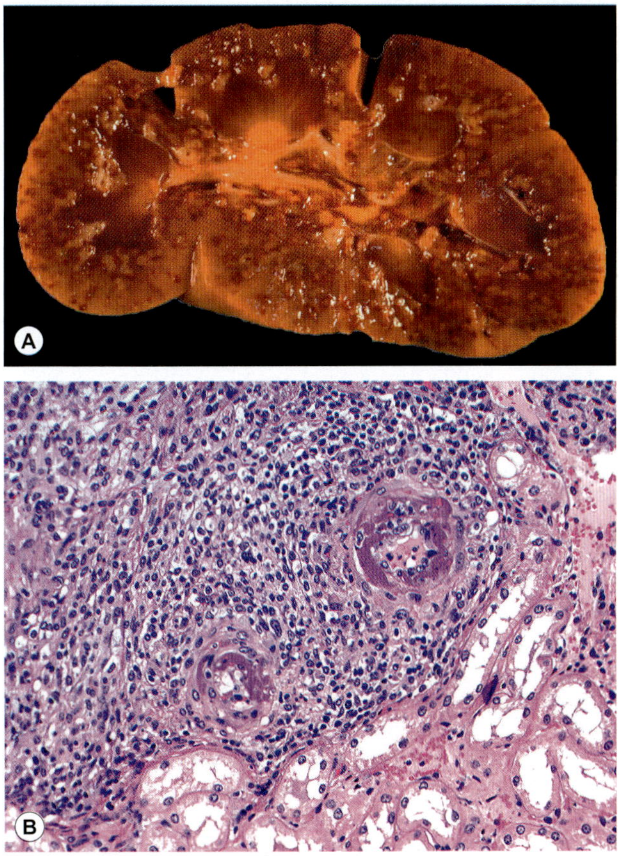

Figure 1-80 Malignant catarrhal fever. A. Multifocal mononuclear interstitial nephritis. **B.** Perivascular mononuclear cells and fibrinoid necrosis in the wall of small arterioles in the kidney. (Courtesy D. O'Toole.)

The **histologic changes** usually must be relied on for the diagnosis of MCF, and its differentiation from similar diseases, although access to molecular detection of specific gammaherpesviral infections is increasing. The characteristic histologic changes found in lymphoid tissues and in the adventitia and walls of medium-sized vessels, especially arteries in any organ, are perivascular accumulations of mainly mononuclear cells, and fibrinoid necrotizing vasculitis (see Fig. 1-80B). These changes may be focal or segmental and may involve the full thickness of the wall, or be confined more or less to one of the layers. When the intima is involved, there is often endothelial swelling. Thrombi are difficult to demonstrate in damaged vessels. The media may be selectively affected, or occasionally, the adventitia alone. Severely affected segments of vessel are replaced by a coagulum of homogeneous, eosinophilic material, in which fragmented nuclear remnants are seen. The perivascular accumulation of cells is particularly characteristic. They are mainly lymphoid cells with large open nuclei and prominent nucleoli; small lymphocytes and plasma cells may be present occasionally. The vascular lesions may be more subtle in other species (especially bison, deer, and elk) than in cattle, and in bison this lesion tends to be less widely disseminated than in cattle.

Cattle that recover from SA-MCF also have distinctive vascular lesions 90 days after clinical onset. Concentric fibrointimal plaques, disrupted inner elastic lamina, focally atrophic tunica media, and vasculitis of variable severity are evident in many organ systems.

In *lymph nodes*, there is active proliferation of lymphoblasts, which form extensive homogeneous populations of cells in the T-cell–dependent areas of the interfollicular cortical and paracortical zones. In bison, lymphoid hyperplasia is either absent or subtle in paracortical areas of lymph nodes. Focal areas of hemorrhage and necrosis associated with arteritis may be seen in all areas of the nodes. The lymphoid reaction in the spleen varies from marked lymphoid cell hyperplasia in the periarteriolar sheaths, to atrophy and depletion of lymphocytes. In addition, there is marked proliferation and infiltration of lymphocytic and lymphoblastic cells, mainly perivascular in distribution, in various organs. The lymphoreticular proliferation may become so severe in some organs that it is difficult to determine whether it is hyperplastic or neoplastic.

Microscopic arteritis similar to that present in other organs occurs in the nervous system of many cases. Necrotizing arteritis, plasma exudation into the meninges or perivascular space, and the predominantly adventitial lymphocytic response are, in the brain of cattle, *unique to MCF* and allow it to be differentiated from other mononuclear encephalitides. Degenerative changes in nervous parenchyma can be explained on the basis of the vascular changes.

The lesions in the *skin and squamous mucosae* of the alimentary tract consist of a lichenoid infiltrate, as the altered and proliferating lymphoid population moves into the upper dermis and then the epidermis. Often typical arteritis, involving small and medium-sized vessels, is present in underlying tissue. Groups of epithelial cells become necrotic, with swollen, strongly acidophilic cytoplasm; ultimately the full thickness of epithelium in affected areas undergoes necrosis and ulcerates. Granulomatous mural folliculitis (GMF) was the prominent microscopic finding in alopecic sika deer infected with CpGHV2; OvGHV2 has been detected in infected follicular keratinocytes within areas of GMF in goats.

The mucosa of the abomasum may be infiltrated by lymphocytes and undergo mucous metaplasia or focal ulceration. The mucosa of the lower alimentary tract, especially the cecum and colon in deer, may similarly be heavily infiltrated by lymphocytes, often with fibrin and blood exuding into the lumen where surface and glandular epithelium has undergone necrosis and collapsed, sometimes over wide areas. Submucosal arterioles in the affected areas of the abomasum and intestine are affected by the characteristic arteritis.

The *mottling of liver and the focal nephritis* seen grossly are due to the perivascular accumulation of mononuclear cells in the hepatic portal triads and in the renal cortices. In the liver, these cuffs may be very large and invest the branches of the hepatic artery, which may undergo fibrinoid necrosis. Microscopic lesions are frequently present in the kidneys, even though gross lesions are not; they consist of vasculitis involving the smaller arteries and afferent arterioles. Extensive diffuse lymphocytic infiltrates disrupt the normal renal cortical architecture, and in some cases, infarcts appear to be associated with vasculitis involving arcuate arteries.

Ophthalmitis often occurs, and its presence is a useful differential criterion from other ulcerative diseases of the alimentary tract. Corneal edema, secondary to vasculitis, is responsible initially for the opacity (Fig. 1-81). Later, there may be lymphocytic infiltration of various structures within the globe. There is retinal vasculitis and, in some cases, hemorrhagic or inflammatory detachment of the retina in focal areas. Lymphocytic optic neuritis and meningitis may be seen.

Differentiation of acute severe BVD and mucosal disease from MCF is sometimes difficult, but MCF usually affects one or more organ systems or tissues (liver, kidney, bladder, eye, brain, tracheobronchial tree) not involved in mucosal disease, and MCF typically produces lymphoid hyperplasia in cattle; lymphoid tissue in BVDV infections is expected to be atrophic. Arteritis may be seen in some cases of BVDV infection, mainly in the submucosa in the lower alimentary tract. Fortunately, *arteritis is present in more than one tissue in all cases of MCF*, whether peracute, acute, or mild with recovery, although it may be necessary to examine many sections to find it. The best organs to examine for vascular lesions are the brain and leptomeninges, carotid rete, kidney (renal arcuate vessels and rete mirabile), liver, adrenal capsule and medulla, salivary gland, and any area of the skin or alimentary tract with gross

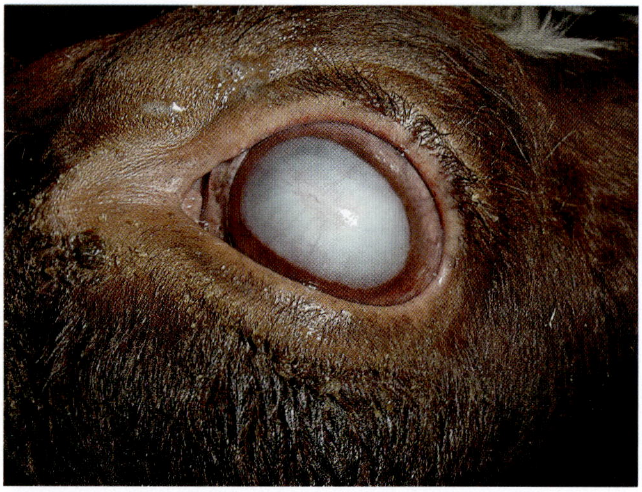

Figure 1-81 Malignant catarrhal fever. Corneal edema in a cow. (Courtesy A.P. Loretti.)

lesions. In bison, no single tissue can be relied on to establish a morphologic diagnosis of MCF, and a range of tissues should be examined to confirm or rule out the disease. A combination of arteritis, lymphoid hyperplasia, and lymphocytic infiltrates into affected epithelia is very characteristic of MCF.

Bali cattle as well as other species of cattle and buffalo are affected with a disease that closely resembles MCF, and both diseases occur geographically together in Indonesia. **Jembrana disease** is caused by a *lentivirus* (JDV; *Retroviridae, Lentivirus bovjem*) distinct from but genetically related to bovine immunodeficiency virus. JDV was initially described in Bali, where it is endemic, and has now spread to other islands in Indonesia, including Kalimantan, West Sumatra, and Java. JDV causes a severe lymphoproliferative response. Gross changes include lymphadenopathy, splenomegaly, and hemorrhages associated with vascular damage. Microscopically, lymphoid tissues of all organs have proliferating lymphoblastic cells. This is particularly marked in the enlarged peripheral lymph nodes and spleen, where proliferating lymphoblastic cells are present throughout the parafollicular T-cell areas; and B-cell follicles are atrophied. Proliferation of T lymphocytes and atrophy of follicles in lymph nodes and spleen, with lymphoid infiltrates in various organs in Jembrana disease, appear similar to lesions of MCF.

Bluetongue and related diseases

Bluetongue (BT) is caused by a reovirus: **Bluetongue virus** (BTV; *Sedoreoviridae, Orbivirus caerulinguae*). There are at least 26 recognized serotypes of BTV, distinguished initially by virus neutralization tests and more recently by RT-PCR amplification of the serotype-specific genome segment 2. Immunity to one serotype does not confer resistance against another and may cause sensitization, with a more severe syndrome following infection by a second type. Apparently not all serotypes are pathogenic.

Epizootic hemorrhagic disease (EHD) of deer and other ruminants, including cattle, is caused by epizootic hemorrhagic disease virus (EHDV; *Sedoreoviridae, Orbivirus ruminantium*), which is a virus in another serogroup of genus *Orbivirus*. **Ibaraki disease**, recognized in cattle in Japan, is caused by EHDV2, a variant of EHDV; seropositive animals also have been found in Taiwan and Indonesia, and an identical virus has been isolated in Australia.

BTV, EHDV, and related viruses are spread by vector-competent *Culicoides* spp., also known as midges or gnats. The virus multiplies by a factor of 10^3-10^4 in the *Culicoides* within a week of the infected blood meal being ingested, and transmission can occur after infection of the salivary glands, 10-15 days after the initial blood meal. Transovarial transmission of virus in *Culicoides* does not occur.

BTV circulates in a broad belt across the tropics and warm temperate areas, from about latitude 49° N to 35° S, with incursions or recrudescence during the *Culicoides* season, annually, or at irregular longer intervals in cooler temperate areas. The condition is enzootic or seasonally epizootic in most of Africa, the Middle East, the eastern Mediterranean basin, the Indian subcontinent, the Caribbean, northern Australia, and the United States. It appears sporadically in the Okanagan valley of western Canada. It also has made persistent incursions into the Iberian peninsula, Corsica and Sardinia, Italy, the Balkans, and northern Europe, including the United Kingdom, perhaps associated with climate change. Seasonality of infection toward the periphery of its distribution probably reflects the unavailability of vectors because the virus may be able to overwinter in latently infected cells in the skin of sheep, which express virus once vector feeding occurs again.

Sheep, goats, and cattle are the primary susceptible domestic species. Severe disease has been described in numerous species of wild and domestic ruminants. South American camelids traditionally have been considered resistant to BT, but serosurveys have identified apparently subclinical infection of alpacas, and lethal cases of BT have been reported in llamas and alpacas. Sheep are the domestic species most highly susceptible to BT, but there is considerable variation in expression of the disease, depending on the breed, age, and immune status of the sheep, the environmental circumstances under which they are held, and the strain of virus. Typically, indigenous breeds seem more resistant to clinical disease than do exotics. Goats, although susceptible to infection, rarely have clinical signs; however, disease has occurred in goats in the Middle East and India. Infection in cattle usually produces only inapparent infection or mild clinical disease. In Africa, a wide variety of nondomestic ungulates and some small mammals may be infected inapparently; mortality has occurred in naturally or experimentally infected topi, Cape buffalo, and kudu. In North America, wildlife species, particularly white-tailed deer, black-tailed or mule deer, elk, bighorn sheep, bison, and pronghorn antelope are also infected. BT is responsible for significant mortality in all these species except elk, which usually develop mild or inapparent infection, and bison, which are infrequently demonstrated to be seropositive. Clinical cases of BT have been described only in individual South American camelids. Vaccine inadvertently contaminated with BTV and administered to dogs caused significant mortality, but BTV is not normally considered a pathogen in dogs.

EHD occurs in North America, Europe, Africa, and Asia. In North America, the white-tailed deer is extremely susceptible, and widespread epizootics have occurred among this species in the United States. The rate of survival is much higher among black-tailed deer and pronghorn antelope; elk are only very mildly affected.

Although sheep are not considered to develop disease when infected with EHDV, occasional mild clinical signs and lesions resembling BT have been reported in sheep inoculated with some Australian isolates. In Japan, the Ibaraki virus strain of EHDV produces a clinical syndrome resembling BT in cattle, but not in sheep.

BTV and EHDV circulate together in North America. Both viruses may be involved simultaneously in outbreaks of hemorrhagic disease in wild ruminants, and both have been isolated from *Culicoides* in a single locality at the same time. The role of cattle as reservoirs of BTV is uncertain. Cattle may act as reservoirs in that the virus will be associated with erythrocytes for the lifespan of that cell. Detectable viremia in cattle is thought to be <9 weeks.

The **pathogenesis** of BT, EHD, and Ibaraki disease is fundamentally similar in all species in which disease is seen. Primary viral replication following insect bite occurs in regional lymph nodes and spleen. Viremia ~4-6 days after inoculation results in secondary infection of endothelium in arterioles, capillaries, and venules throughout the body, but especially in lung microvascular endothelium. Microscopic lesions, fever, and lymphopenia begin a day or so later, about a week after inoculation. BTV in the blood appears to be closely associated with, or in, both leukocytes and erythrocytes, and it may co-circulate with antibody.

Endothelial damage caused by viral infection initiates local *microvascular thrombosis and permeability*. This is reflected microscopically by swollen endothelium, and fibrin and platelet thrombi in small vessels, with edema and hemorrhage in surrounding tissue. These lesions in turn mediate the full spectrum of gross findings. These are fundamentally *ischemic necrosis* of many tissues; *edema* caused by vascular permeability; and *hemorrhage* resulting from vascular damage compounded (Fig. 1-82A and B), in severe cases, by consumption coagulopathy, with thrombocytopenia and depletion of soluble clotting factors. Differences in the expression and activity of vasoactive and procoagulant and anticoagulant mediators by infected pulmonary endothelium may explain the greater propensity of sheep to have clinical signs, compared with cattle.

BT in sheep is highly variable; it may cause inapparent infection or acute fulminant disease. Typically, leukopenia and pyrexia occur, even in mild infections, coincident with viremia. The degree and duration of fever are not correlated with the severity of the syndrome otherwise.

In the early phase, there is hyperemia of the oral and nasal mucosa, drooling, and nasal discharge a day or two after the onset of fever. Hyperemia and edema of the eyelids and conjunctiva may occur, and edema of lips, ears, and the intermandibular area becomes apparent. Hyperemia may extend over the muzzle and the skin of much of the body, including the axillary and inguinal areas. Focal hemorrhage may be present on the lips and gums, and *the tongue may become edematous and congested or cyanotic*, giving the disease its name. Infarcted epithelium thickens and becomes excoriated; erosions and ulcerations develop along the margins of the tongue opposite the molars, and the mucosa of much of the tongue may slough.

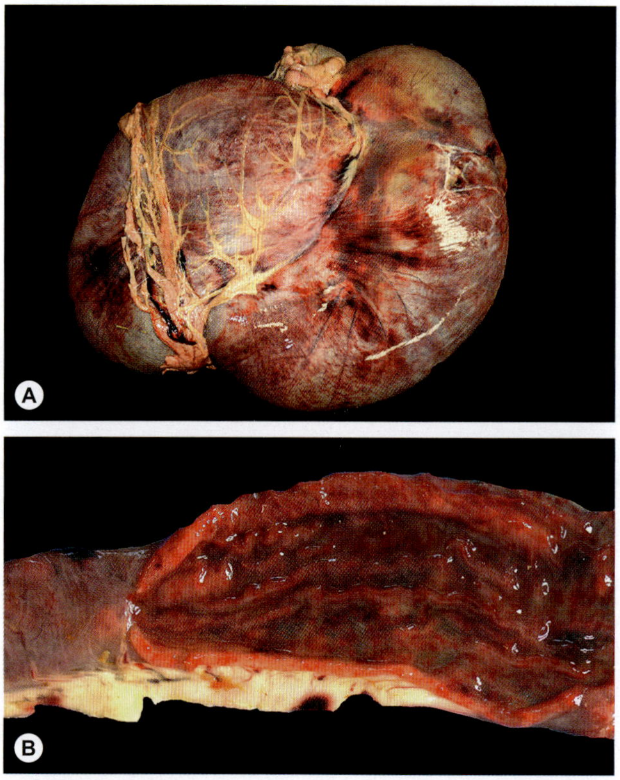

Figure 1-82 Epizootic hemorrhagic disease in a pronghorn antelope. **A.** Subserosal hemorrhage of the reticulorumen. **B.** Hemorrhage in the small intestine.

Excoriation and ulceration also occur on the buccal mucosa, the hard palate, and dental pad (eFig. 1-14A). The affected areas of the skin also may become encrusted and excoriated with time, and a break in the wool can result in parts or much of the fleece being tender or cast. The coronet, bulbs, and interdigital areas of the foot may become hyperemic. Coronary swelling and streaky hemorrhages in the periople may be evident as a result of lesions in the underlying sensitive laminae. These hemorrhages may persist in the hoof as brown lines that move down the hoof as it grows. A defect parallel to the coronet also may be evident in the growing hoof in recovered cases.

Internally, in acute cases there is *subcutaneous and intermuscular edema*, which may be serous or suffused with blood. Superficial lymph nodes are enlarged and edematous. Bruise-like gelatinous hemorrhages and contusions, which may be small and easily overlooked if not numerous, often are present in the subcutis and intermuscular fascial planes. Focal or multifocal pallid areas of streaky myodegeneration may be present throughout the carcass, sometimes partly obscured by petechiae or ecchymoses. Resolving muscle lesions may be mineralized or fibrous. Stiffness, reluctance to move, and recumbency seen clinically are due to these muscle lesions.

Necrosis may be present deep in the papillary muscle of the left ventricle, and elsewhere in the myocardium. The lesion that is perhaps most consistent and closest to pathognomonic for BT is *focal hemorrhage*, petechial or up to 1 cm wide × 2-3 cm long, in the tunica media and adventitia at the *base of the pulmonary* artery (see eFig. 1-14B). These hemorrhages are visible from both the internal and adventitial surfaces and may be present in clinically mild cases with few other lesions. Petechiae may also be present at the base of the aorta and in subendocardial and subepicardial locations over the heart.

There also may be edema and petechiae or ecchymoses in the pharyngeal and laryngeal area. In severe cases, the lungs may assume a purple hue, with marked edematous separation of lobules, and froth in the tracheobronchial tree, probably because of pulmonary microvascular damage and heart failure (see eFig. 1-14C). Animals with pharyngeal or esophageal myodegeneration suffer from dysphagia, or regurgitate, and may succumb to aspiration pneumonia.

Hyperemia, occasionally marked hemorrhage, or in advanced cases, ulceration of the mucosa may occur on rumen papillae, the pillars of the rumen (see eFig. 1-14D), and the reticular plicae. In convalescent animals, stellate healing ulcers or scars on the wall of the forestomachs may be apparent.

Microscopically, acute lesions consist of microvascular thrombosis, and edema and hemorrhage in the affected sites recognized at autopsy. In squamous mucosa and skin, capillaries of the proprial and dermal papillae are involved, resulting in vacuolation and necrosis of overlying epithelium. In acute lesions, there is a mild, local neutrophilic infiltrate, and a similarly mild mononuclear reaction in the dermis or propria in uncomplicated chronic lesions, which may granulate if widely or deeply ulcerated. Similar microvascular lesions are associated with necrosis and fragmentation of infarcted skeletal and cardiac muscle. Muscle during the reparative phase follows the usual course of regeneration of fibers or fibrous replacement, depending on whether or not the sarcolemma retains its integrity.

In **cattle**, *clinical BT is rarely apparent;* in endemic areas it may never be evident. Mortality is low and it is often attributed to secondary infection. Clinical disease may be a function of hypersensitivity in previously exposed animals, and disease in experimentally infected animals is poorly defined. Fever, loss of appetite, and leukopenia are usually seen after an incubation period of 6-8 days, and there may be a drop in milk production in dairy cattle. There is reddening of the epithelium of the mucous membranes, and of thin exposed skin, especially notable on the udder and teats. Edema of the lips and conjunctiva may be present. Drooling may become profuse, and as the disease progresses over the next several days, hyperemia and congestion of the mucosae become more intense. Ulcerations of the gingival, lingual, or buccal mucosa occur, most consistently on the dental pad. There may be necrosis of epithelium on the muzzle. Muscle stiffness is a feature of the disease in some animals. Laminitis, with hyperemia and edema of the sensitive laminae at the coronet, may be apparent, and in some cases, hooves on affected feet may eventually slough. Sloughing or cracking of crusts of necrotic epithelium may also occur on the affected parts of the skin, but the ulcerative or erosive defects heal readily. Viral antigen and thrombosis are present in small vessels in affected tissues during the acute phase.

Although traditionally **South American camelids** have been considered to be resistant to BTV, individual cases of the disease have been described in alpacas and llamas with lesions, including hydrothorax, hydropericardium, pulmonary edema, myocardial hemorrhage, and pericarditis, but no alimentary tract lesions. Experimental inoculation of llamas and alpacas with BTV serotype 8 produced seroconversion, but minimal and mild clinical signs and no significant gross or microscopic lesions.

EHDV can also induce disease in cattle. Clinically and pathologically, EHD in cattle is similar to BT.

Ibaraki disease has been described in Japan; the signs and lesions of Ibaraki disease are similar to those of BT and EHD in cattle, although more severe in some cases. There may also be difficulty in swallowing in 20-30% of clinically affected animals, and the swollen tongue may protrude from the mouth. At autopsy, in addition to the lesions observable externally, there may be congestion, erosion, or ulceration of the mucosa of the abomasum, and less commonly, the esophagus and forestomachs. Ischemic necrosis and hemorrhage of the striated muscle in the tongue, pharynx, larynx, and esophagus cause the difficulty in swallowing seen clinically, and similar changes are seen in other skeletal muscles. Necrotizing aspiration pneumonia is a sequel to dysphagia in some animals.

The **hemorrhagic diseases** in bighorn sheep, pronghorn antelope, and white-tailed and black-tailed or mule deer in North America resemble BT in sheep. White-tailed deer and pronghorn may develop a particularly severe and fulminant hemorrhagic disease, with high mortality. There may be necrosis of velvet antler, and hooves may slough in survivors. BT in goats, although usually inapparent, can resemble BT in sheep.

BT in sheep must be differentiated from FMD, PPR, BVD, EHD, contagious ecthyma, and photosensitization. In cattle, BT must be differentiated from FMD, VS, EHD, BVD, MCF, and photosensitization. In Japan, Ibaraki disease of cattle in addition must be differentiated clinically from ephemeral fever virus infection. A diagnosis of BT is confirmed by PCR or virus isolation. Serology is of little value as many clinically normal animals are seropositive to BTV.

In addition to the systemic disease described, *abortion*, perhaps unobserved, and birth of progeny with various *congenital defects* may follow BTV infection of pregnant sheep and cattle. In sheep, BTV infection of ewes early in gestation may result in hydranencephaly. Anomalous calves produced by BTV-infected cattle have excessive gingiva, an enlarged tongue, anomalous maxillae, dwarflike build, and rotations and contractures of the distal extremities. Porencephaly, hydranencephaly, and arthrogryposis are also reported in calves infected in utero with BTV. Antibody may be sought in neonates that have not sucked, and attempts should be made to isolate virus, because some prenatally infected animals may have immune tolerance, and persistent infection. Anomalies of the brain are considered further in Vol. 1, Nervous System.

Parapoxviral infections

Bovine papular stomatitis occurs worldwide. *It is generally not a clinically significant infection*, but needs to be differentiated from other more serious diseases affecting the oral cavity and skin. Bovine papular stomatitis is usually an indicator of immunity problems associated in many cases with poor colostrum administration. It is caused by bovine papular stomatitis virus (BPSV; *Poxviridae, Parapoxvirus bovinestomatitis*), genus *Parapoxvirus*, which is closely related to pseudocowpox virus that causes pseudocowpox in cattle and milker's nodules in humans. The disease in humans is usually very mild. BPSV is morphologically similar to, and shares antigens with, orf virus of sheep and goats (see Vol. 1, Integumentary System). However, analysis of the genome indicates that these viruses are distinct.

BPSV is relatively host specific. As with many of the poxviruses, neutralizing antibody is not readily demonstrated. Infection does not confer significant immunity, and successive episodes of lesions and relapses can occur. The disease is more common in calves than in older animals, although the susceptibility of, or recrudescence in, the latter may be increased by intercurrent debility, disease such as BVD, infectious bovine rhinotracheitis, or other stressors.

The *papular lesions* of this disease occur on the muzzle and in the rostral nares, on the gums, the buccal papillae, the dental pad, the inner aspect of the lips, the hard palate (Fig. 1-83A), the floor of the oral cavity behind the incisors, the ventral and lateral (not dorsal) surfaces of the tongue, and occasionally in the esophagus (see Fig. 1-83B) and forestomachs.

The initial lesions, which are likely to be detected on the muzzle or lips, are erythematous roughly round macules, ~2 mm-2 cm in diameter. Shortly, the central portion becomes elevated as a low papule, although the elevation is not easy to see, and by the second day a gray central zone of epithelial hyperplasia has developed on which there is superficial scaliness and necrosis. A central necrotic area may slough to form a shallow craterous defect surrounded by a slightly raised red margin. Lesions may coalesce. The course of individual lesions is about a week.

Histologically, there is focal but intense hyperemia and edema in the papillae of the lamina propria, with accumulation of a few mononuclear leukocytes. The epithelium is thickened, sometimes to twice its normal depth, by hyperplasia and ballooning degeneration in the deeper layers. The cytoplasm of affected cells is clear, and the nucleus may be shrunken. *Dense eosinophilic inclusion bodies lie in the vacuolated cytoplasm*, especially in cells at the active margin of the lesion (see Fig. 1-83C). These inclusion bodies are present during the initial period of the infection but are difficult to see in the more advanced lesions. In the central, more advanced part of

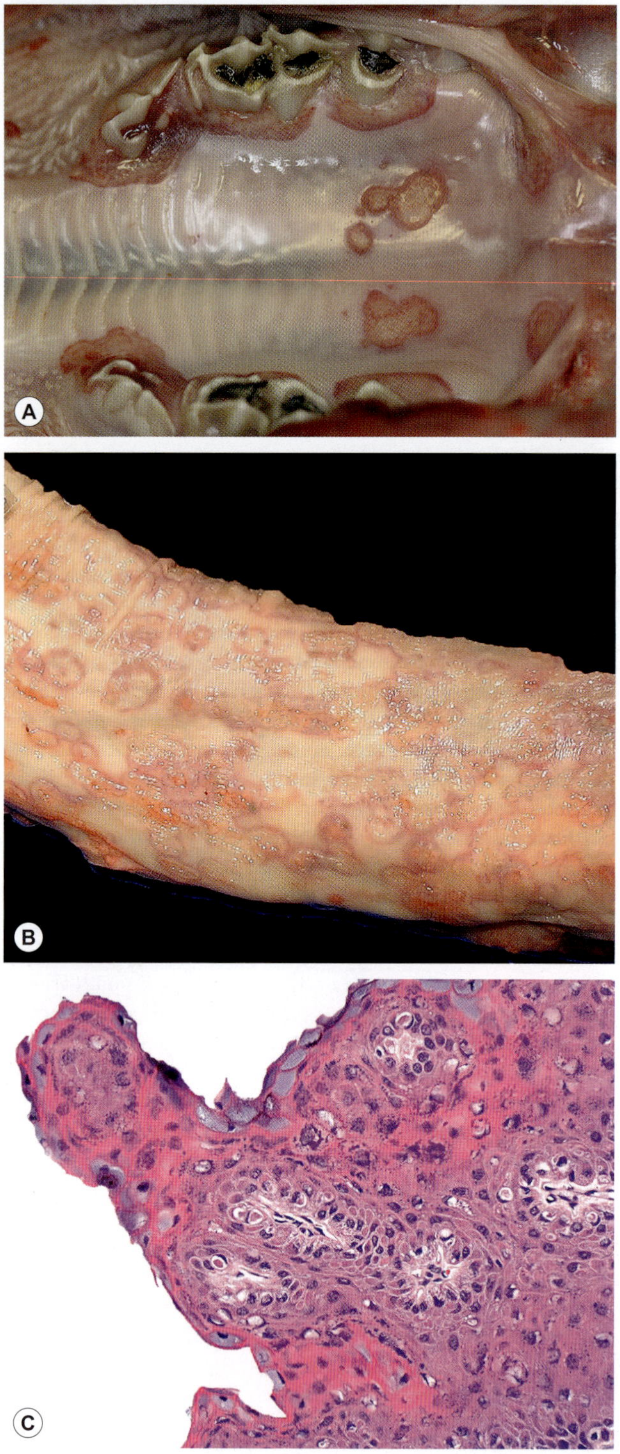

Figure 1-83 Bovine papular stomatitis. A. Lesions in the palate of a cow. **B**. Lesions in the esophagus of a bull. (Reprinted with permission from Jeckel S, et al. Severe oesophagitis in an adult bull caused by bovine papular stomatitis virus. Vet Rec 2011;169:317.) **C**. Proliferative stomatitis in a calf with intracytoplasmic inclusion bodies.

the lesion, a mainly neutrophilic infiltrate into the superficial propria and epithelium is associated with erosion of the upper layers of necrotic cells. The basal layer survives and may be very flattened in eroded areas. Vesicles do not form.

A *chronic form* has been reported, with necrotic and proliferative stomatitis, seen histologically as extensive parakeratotic

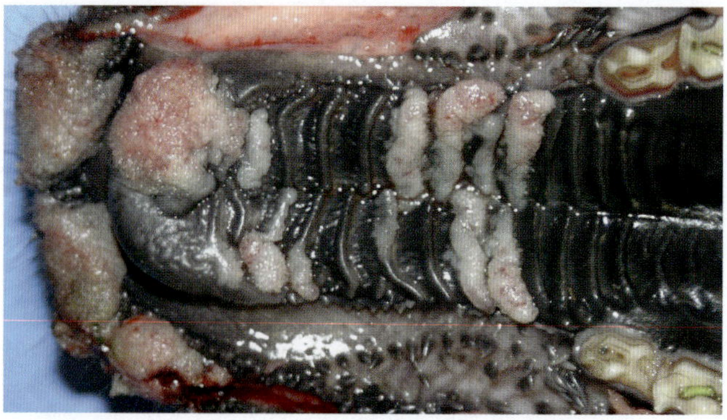

Figure 1-84 Contagious ecthyma. Multifocal proliferative stomatitis in the lips, dental pad, and hard palate of a lamb.

hyperkeratosis, pseudoepitheliomatous hyperplasia, and occasional intracytoplasmic inclusion bodies.

Papular stomatitis is probably more common and widespread than reports indicate. Variation in the extent and gross appearance of the lesions is to be expected, depending on the usual host-parasite factors and the nature of superimposed infections. They may predispose to the development of necrotic stomatitis and must be differentiated from the lesions of BVD, FMD, alimentary infectious bovine rhinotracheitis, and other causes of ulcers and erosions in the upper alimentary tract. The infection can be transmitted to humans to produce small papules that may persist for several weeks on the skin, usually of the fingers or forearms.

Coinfection with vaccinia virus and a parapoxvirus with 85-86% homology with BPSV was described in dairy cattle in Brazil. Affected cows had gross and histologic lesions similar to those of bovine papular stomatitis on the teats and udder.

Rapid diagnosis is readily accomplished by demonstration of characteristic parapoxvirus particles in negatively stained material from lesions examined under the electron microscope, or by PCR. Histology is highly suggestive when the characteristic inclusion bodies are present, but challenging in more chronic lesions when no inclusion bodies are seen.

Contagious ecthyma, also called **contagious pustular dermatitis** or **orf**, is a parapoxviral disease (ORFV; *Poxviridae, Parapoxvirus orf*) of sheep and goats seen mainly as *proliferative scabby lesions on the lips, face, udder, and feet* (see Vol. 1, Integumentary System). The disease also has been reported in camels and a gazelle. Lesions may extend into the oral cavity, involving the tongue, gingiva, dental pad, and palate (Fig. 1-84). Involvement of the esophagus and forestomachs occurs but is very unusual. In general, the evolution of the alimentary lesions is similar to papular stomatitis of cattle, although they are more exudative and usually much more proliferative. *Intracytoplasmic inclusion bodies* similar to those observed in bovine papular stomatitis also can be observed in the initial stages of the infection. Morbidity may be high, and death can occur in suckling animals. In the upper alimentary tract, lesions may consist of focal red, raised areas, which coalesce to form papules followed by pustules. The latter rupture, and on the muzzle and in the mouth they may become covered by a gray-to-brown scab, although scab formation may not occur in the mucosa of the upper alimentary tract. As with bovine papular stomatitis, rapid diagnosis is readily accomplished by demonstration of characteristic parapoxvirus particles in negatively stained material from lesions examined under the electron microscope, or by PCR. Histology is highly suggestive when the characteristic inclusion bodies are present. Because the inclusion bodies are transient, their absence does not preclude a diagnosis of contagious ecthyma.

Herpesviral infections

Bovine alphaherpesvirus 1, infectious bovine rhinotracheitis virus (BoAHV1; *Orthoherpesviridae, Varicellovirus bovinealpha1*) has been associated with a wide range of clinicopathologic syndromes in cattle. These include necrotizing rhinotracheitis, conjunctivitis, infectious pustular vulvovaginitis and balanoposthitis, vesicular lesions of the udder, abortions, and systemic infections in neonates. Like all herpesviruses, BoAHV1 establishes subclinical latent infections. The clinical significance of BoAHV1 infections in other animal species for which serologic evidence of exposure has been shown, such as the bison, remains unknown.

A *systemic form* of the disease, which usually involves the alimentary tract, may occur spontaneously in neonatal calves (in which it may be congenital, or acquired shortly after birth) and in feedlot cattle. It has been reproduced experimentally in young calves.

The pathogenesis of systemic infection with BoAHV1 is poorly understood. Colostrum-deprived calves are especially susceptible, and the disease can be prevented by feeding colostrum from actively immunized dams. The virus probably spreads from the mucosa of the upper respiratory tract to other tissues by circulating leukocytes. Peripheral blood mononuclear leukocytes may exhibit apoptosis in response to BoAHV1, but the significance of this is unknown.

Experimental infection of calves with NCP BVDV followed by BoAHV1 inoculation results in dissemination of the latter to a variety of tissues. BVDV impairs cell-mediated immunity, and this may allow BoAHV1 to escape from the respiratory tract and lead to a systemic infection. Dual infections of BVDV and BoAHV1 occur under field conditions, but coinfection of these 2 viruses is not a prerequisite for the disease to develop.

Clinically affected animals have hyperemic oral and nasal mucosae, and focal areas of necrosis, erosion, and ulceration on the nares, dental pad, gums, buccal mucosa, palate, and the caudal, ventral, and dorsal surfaces of the tongue. Characteristically, the lesions tend to be punctate with a slightly raised margin; the necrotic areas are covered by a gray-white layer of fibrinonecrotic exudate, which leaves a raw red base when removed.

The **lesions** may be present in the oral cavity and extend into the esophagus, usually only the upper third, the forestomachs, and rarely the abomasum. In the oral cavity and esophagus, the erosions and ulcers may be irregular, circular, or linear, and often they have a punched-out appearance and a hyperemic border (Fig. 1-85). The ruminal lesions, which are most commonly located in the dorsal and cranioventral sacs, vary considerably. The earliest lesions consist of foci of necrosis and hemorrhage, a few millimeters in diameter. In some cases, the necrosis may involve almost the entire surface of the ruminal mucosa, which becomes covered by a thick, dirty gray layer of exudate, resembling curdled milk, which adheres tightly to the wall (Fig. 1-86). Similar lesions may be evident in the reticulum and abomasum. Focal areas of necrosis result in the formation of holes, as large as 1.5 cm in diameter, in the leaves of the omasum. In addition, these calves may have focal areas of necrosis covered by a fibrinous pseudomembrane in

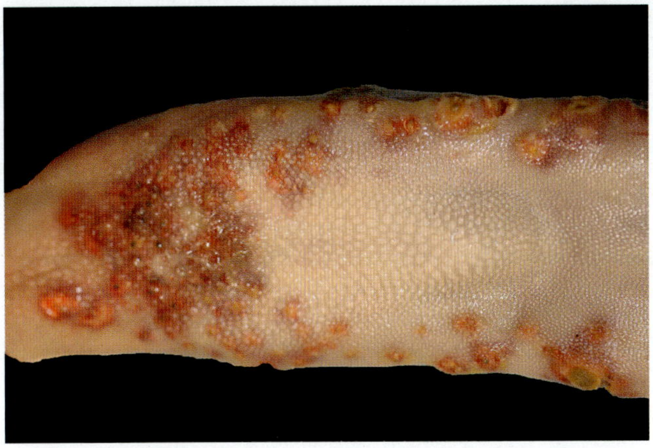

Figure 1-85 Infectious bovine rhinotracheitis. Mucosal necrosis of the tongue in a neonatal calf. (Courtesy R. Moeller.)

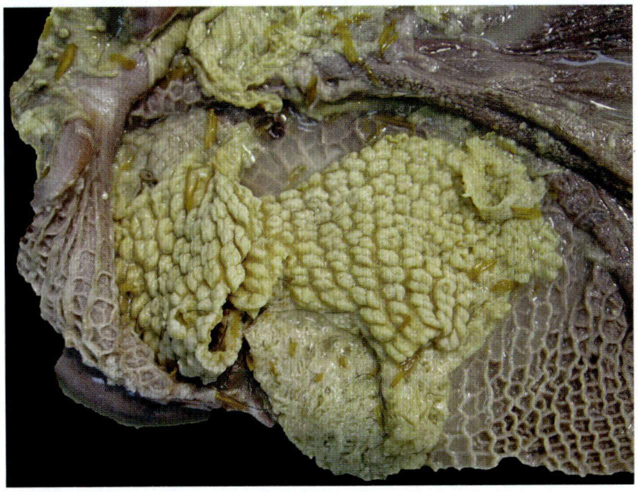

Figure 1-86 Infectious bovine rhinotracheitis. Fibrinonecrotic inflammation in rumen and reticulum in a neonatal calf. (Courtesy V. Psychas.)

the abomasal mucosal folds, which may coalesce to form 2-3 cm areas of necrosis. The intestines are red and dilated, and the serosal surface may be covered by a thin layer of fibrinous exudate.

The enteric lesions may be accompanied by changes in the upper respiratory tract. When present, the respiratory lesions are similar to those described for older cattle, although they are milder and generally limited to the nasal mucosa, larynx, and upper third of the trachea (see Vol. 2, Respiratory System). Gray-to-yellow, 2-5-mm necrotic foci may be evident macroscopically on the capsular and cut surfaces of the liver, the adrenal cortices, the spleen, and in Peyer patches.

Microscopically, the lesions in the squamous mucosa of the upper alimentary tract and forestomachs are *focal areas of necrosis, erosion, and ulceration. Severe* necrosis may involve the entire papilla or the mucosa more diffusely. *Nuclear inclusions* may be present in epithelial cells in the periphery of the lesion, although these are an inconsistent finding. They are more likely to be found if tissues are collected in the early stages of the disease and fixed in Bouin fluid. The abomasal lesions consist of necrosis of glandular epithelial cells. Affected glands are dilated and filled with necrotic debris. Focal necrotic lesions involving crypts and lamina propria may be present in

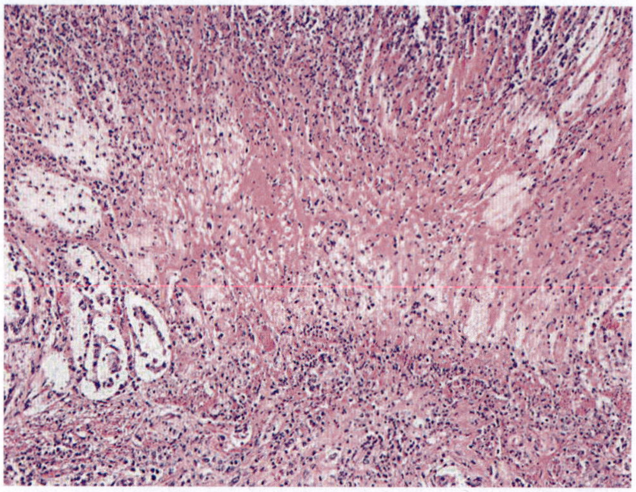

Figure 1-87 Infectious bovine rhinotracheitis. Necrosis of epithelium in intestinal crypts in the small intestine of a neonatal calf. (Courtesy R. Moeller.)

both the small intestine and large bowel (Fig. 1-87). Abomasal and intestinal lesions may predispose to the development of *secondary mycosis*, which is a common complication.

Foci of coagulative necrosis may occur in the liver, lymph nodes, thymus, Peyer patches, spleen, and adrenal cortices. Typically, there is little inflammation associated with the necrosis. Herpesviral inclusions are inconsistently seen in cells at the periphery of the necrotic foci. In a study of systemic BoAHV1 infection in neonatal calves in California, a large proportion of affected calves had histologic lesions compatible with BoAHV1 only in the adrenal gland. Although most of those animals had enteritis and/or colitis, these lesions were considered to be due to other enteric pathogens (coronavirus, cryptosporidia, rotavirus, and attaching-and-effacing *E. coli*).

The lesions in the upper alimentary tract of cattle associated with BoAHV1 infection must be differentiated from those of calf diphtheria, bovine papular stomatitis, and BVD. The ruminal lesions must be differentiated from those of bovine adenoviral infection and nonspecific rumenitis. The liver lesions may be confused with focal necrosis associated with septicemias, for example, listeriosis or salmonellosis (see Vol. 2, Liver and Biliary System).

Caprine alphaherpesvirus 1, goat herpesvirus (CpAHV1; *Orthoherpesviridae, Varicellovirus caprinealpha1*) has been isolated from neonatal goat kids in various parts of the world. CpAHV1 is different from, but shows genomic similarity to, other viruses of this group, such as BoAHV1, bovine alphaherpesvirus 5 (BoAHV5; *Orthoherpesviridae, Varicellovirus bovinealpha5*), suid alphaherpesvirus 1 (SuAHV1, PRV), cervid alphaherpesvirus 1 (CvAHV1; *Orthoherpesviridae, Varicellovirus cervidalpha1*), and rangiferine herpesvirus 1. CpAHV1 is associated with 2 different syndromes in goats depending on the age of the animals at the time of infection. In neonatal kids, CpAHV1 causes an often severe and generalized disease *affecting the digestive tract where it produces erosions and ulcerations*. Infection in adult goats remains inapparent (adult goats may be latent carriers) or may cause respiratory distress, abortion, vulvovaginitis, or balanoposthitis (see Vol. 3, Female Genital System). CpAHV1 is able to establish latent infection in trigeminal ganglia and to cause immunosuppression. Although capable of infecting sheep, cattle, and goats, severe disease caused by CpAHV1 is restricted to goats.

The disease in neonatal kids is seen clinically as fever, conjunctivitis, ocular and nasal discharges, dyspnea, anorexia, abdominal pain, weakness, and death, usually within 1-4 days after the onset of clinical signs. Affected kids have leukopenia and hypoproteinemia.

Macroscopic lesions are most obvious throughout the entire alimentary tract. Round or longitudinal erosions, which have a hyperemic border, are evident in the oral mucosa. These are particularly prominent on the gums around the incisor teeth and to a lesser extent in the pharynx and esophagus. Focal red areas of necrosis, which may be slightly elevated above the surrounding mucosa, occur in the rumen. In the abomasum, numerous longitudinal, red erosions are located in the mucosa. The most severe lesions occur in the *cecum and spiral colon*, which are dilated, with a thickened wall, and contain focal to large areas of mucosal necrosis and ulceration, frequently covered by a diphtheritic membrane. The contents are yellow and mucoid. Hemorrhagic foci may be visible in the bladder mucosa.

Microscopically, the lesions in the upper alimentary tract are typical areas of necrosis and erosion of squamous epithelial cells. The epithelial cells at the periphery of necrotic areas are swollen and vacuolated, and these may contain typical *intranuclear herpesviral inclusions*. There is marked inflammatory reaction in the underlying lamina propria. The abomasal lesions consist of acute foci of mucosal necrosis. Inclusions are particularly evident in this area. Lesions in the cecum and colon are more extensive and consist of large areas of mucosal ulceration and necrosis, which may involve the entire thickness of the wall. The submucosa is edematous and markedly infiltrated by inflammatory cells. The mesenteric nodes are edematous and germinal centers are depleted of lymphoid cells. Focal areas of necrosis with a mild inflammatory cell reaction also may be present in the liver, urinary bladder, and kidney.

Canid alphaherpesvirus 1 (canine herpesvirus, CaAHV1, CHV; *Orthoherpesviridae, Varicellovirus canidalpha1*) causes systemic disease of neonatal puppies with foci of necrosis and hemorrhage in a wide variety of organs, especially the lungs and renal cortices (see Vol. 3, Female Genital System). Focal areas of necrosis may occur in the intestine as part of the systemic syndrome. A similar syndrome also has been described in an adult dog. As with most other herpesviruses, the trigeminal ganglion is an important latency site for CaAHV1. However, latency of CaAHV1 also occurs in the lumbosacral ganglia and retropharyngeal lymph nodes. Latently infected dogs may or may not shed virus, and shedding may occur continuously or intermittently.

Felid alphaherpesvirus 1, feline viral rhinotracheitis virus (FeAHV1; *Orthoherpesviridae*; *Varicellovirus felidalpha1*), causes oral lesions. Primary infection by FeAHV1 may be followed by viremia with the virus distributed to several distant organs. Viruses antigenically related to FeAHV1 have been isolated from dogs with diarrhea, but descriptions of lesions are not available.

Natural infections with **suid alphaherpesvirus 1** (pseudorabies virus, Aujeszky disease virus, SuAHV1, PRV; *Orthoherpesviridae, Varicellovirus suidalpha1*) often result in necrotizing tonsillitis. Experimental infection of pigs with SuAHV1 may cause necrotizing enteritis of the distal small intestine. The enteric lesions are focal areas of necrosis of the cryptal mucosa, muscularis mucosa, and tunica muscularis.

Immunohistochemically, antigen is documented in the dome area, the lymphoid follicles of Peyer patches, and ganglion cells of submucosal and myenteric plexuses.

Necrotizing enterocolitis in adult horses caused by **equid alphaherpesvirus 1** (equine herpesvirus, equine abortion virus, EqAHV1; *Orthoherpesviridae, Varicellovirus equidalpha1*) has been reported rarely. A single case with similar intestinal lesions was reported in a yearling filly. At autopsy there were areas of hemorrhage, necrosis, and ulceration, some several centimeters in diameter, of the mucosa in both the small and large intestines. Microscopically, these lesions consisted of erosions and ulcerations of the mucosa, and necrosis of cryptal epithelial cells in adjacent areas. Cryptal epithelial cells and some proprial mononuclear cells may have acidophilic and amphophilic nuclear inclusions.

Adenoviral infections

The adenoviruses that have been associated with enteric infections in humans, cattle, swine, horses, sheep, cervids, camelids, and dogs belong to the family *Adenoviridae*, genera *Mastadenovirus*, and *Atadenovirus* (*Barthadenovirus* as of 2024). Serosurveys show that widely divergent serotypes occur both within and between host species, and their distribution is worldwide. All serotypes are morphologically similar; the virus consists of a nonenveloped icosahedral capsid, 70-80 nm in diameter, which has 252 capsomeres. Virus neutralization tests and molecular methods are used to distinguish serotypes. Adenoviral infection of cells causes *intranuclear inclusions*. Adenoviruses are relatively heat resistant and can survive for several days at room temperature. Most adenoviruses are transmitted by feces, aerosols, or possibly fomites, to susceptible, usually suckling or recently weaned, animals. Infected animals may remain carriers for weeks.

Adenoviruses are highly host specific. Infections in both humans and animals appear, in general, to be subclinical, and disease seems to occur more commonly in immunologically compromised individuals. Most infections are systemic; certain strains have a tropism for the respiratory tract, and others for the alimentary tract, vascular endothelial cells, or hepatocytes. Their enteric manifestations are considered here.

Bovine adenoviruses. Serotypes of bovine adenovirus (BAdV) are in the genera ***Mastadenovirus*** and ***Atadenovirus***, and have been renamed, such as bovine adenovirus 1 (BAdV1; *Adenoviridae*) becomes taxon species *Bovine mastadenovirus A*. Infection has been mainly associated with keratoconjunctivitis and respiratory disease. Many strains have been isolated from normal cattle. Serotypes 3, 4, 7, and 10 have been associated with enteric disease. It appears that after an initial viremic stage, the virus localizes in the *endothelial cells* of vessels in a variety of organs, resulting in thrombosis with subsequent focal areas of ischemic necrosis.

Clinically, enteric infections with BAdV occur sporadically in 1-8-week-old calves and in feedlot animals. Affected animals have fever and diarrhea that may contain blood, and some animals will die peracutely from dysentery. They are dehydrated and the mucous membranes of the muzzle and mouth are congested. Dry, encrusted exudate may cover the muzzle, and there may be serous-to-mucopurulent ocular and nasal discharges.

Macroscopic lesions may be present in the forestomachs, abomasum, and intestine. Those in the forestomachs are irregular, raised, 2-4 mm, red-to-gray necrotic areas, on the mucosa of both the dorsal and ventral sacs of the rumen. In some cases, the areas of necrosis coalesce to give rise to diffuse necrotizing rumenitis. Ulcers up to 1.5 cm in diameter may be located on the ruminal pillars, and these may be visible through the serosa. Similar lesions may be evident in the omasum. The abomasal mucosal folds are edematous and congested, with focal necrosis and ulceration in the mucosa that, like those in the forestomachs, may be visible on the serosal surface.

The intestinal lesions vary from slight dilation and distension with excessive fluid to severe multifocal or diffuse necrosis, which may be covered by a pseudodiphtheritic membrane. In young calves, the lesions are most severe in the jejunum and ileum, especially over the Peyer patches. In feedlot cattle, the lesions may be most prominent in the colon. The mucosa is dark-red, and there is marked edema of the mesocolon. The mesenteric lymph nodes are enlarged and edematous.

Microscopically, foci of ischemic necrosis are evident in the intestinal mucosa, and in more advanced lesions, the necrosis extends across the muscularis mucosa. Fibrinocellular exudate often covers the mucosal surface. Intestinal crypts are dilated, lined by flat epithelial cells, and usually contain necrotic debris (Fig. 1-88A). There is usually marked submucosal edema, congestion, and fibrinous exudation. Foci of necrosis are evident in the lymphoid follicles of the Peyer patches, which are also depleted of lymphocytes. *Large basophilic-to-amphophilic inclusions* completely or partially fill the endothelial cell nuclei in the vessels of the lamina propria and submucosa of affected areas of the rumen, abomasum, intestine (see Fig. 1-88B), and kidney. The endothelial cells are swollen and necrotic, and some veins and lymphatics contain thrombi. Similar inclusion bodies may occasionally be seen in nuclei of enterocytes. Typical inclusions also may be found in endothelial cells of vessels and sinusoids of the adrenal glands, mesenteric lymph nodes, liver, spleen, glomeruli and interstitial capillaries in the kidney, and in the mucosa of the urinary bladder.

Confirmation of enteric BAdV infection depends on the demonstration of the virus in tissue through electron microscopy, in situ hybridization, PCR, or virus isolation in cell culture. The latter is often difficult because different serotypes and strains of the virus require specific cell cultures, and several blind passages may be required before CP changes are evident.

Porcine adenovirus. According to serosurveys, the 5 serotypes of porcine adenovirus (PAdV; *Adenoviridae*), genus *Mastadenovirus*, are all common. Serotype 4 appears to be the most widely distributed strain of the virus in Europe and North America. Subclinical infections are most common in swine, and PAdV may be isolated from feces of normal pigs; PAdVs are actually of more interest as viral vaccine vectors than as pathogens.

The importance of adenoviruses as a cause of enteric disease in the field remains controversial. When disease occurs, the **macroscopic** lesions in the intestine consist of excessive yellow watery-to-pasty contents and moderate enlargement of the mesenteric lymph nodes, which cannot be differentiated from other causes of diarrhea in neonatal pigs.

Microscopically, and in contrast to the situation in calves, in which inclusions are located mainly in the nuclei of endothelial cells, *inclusions in pigs are in enterocytes* in the distal jejunum and ileum, where primary viral replication likely occurs. The infected nuclei are enlarged, round, and displaced to the apical portion of the cell. The villi may be short and blunt. There may be a moderate mononuclear cell reaction in the lamina propria. Inclusions are also found in the squamous

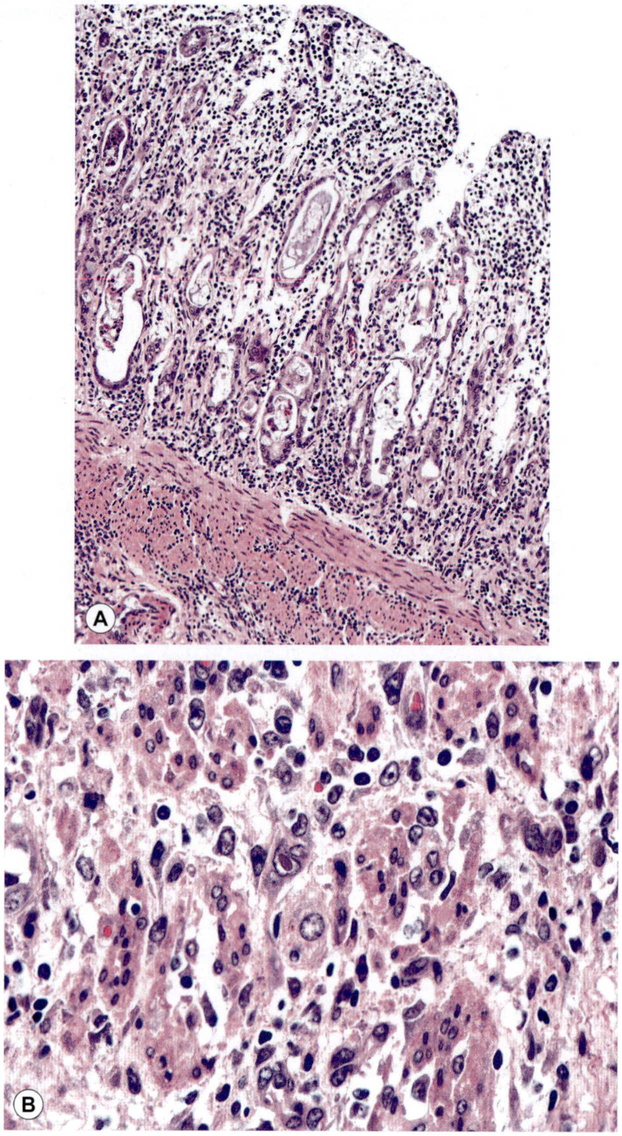

Figure 1-88 Bovine adenoviral infection. **A**. Colonic necrosis with dilated glands. **B**. Large basophilic-to-amphophilic inclusion bodies in the nuclei of endothelium in the vessels of the intestinal lamina propria. (Courtesy C. Buergelt.)

epithelial cells of the tonsils and in endothelial cells of capillary and small blood vessels throughout the body.

The significance of adenoviral inclusions in enterocytes must be interpreted with caution. A survey in Canada revealed that 4.4% of 5-day to 24-week-old pigs had adenoviral inclusions in enterocytes, mainly in the ileum. More than 50% of the pigs had diarrhea; however, other enteropathogens were also found in most of these animals.

Equine adenovirus. Two serotypes of equine adenovirus (EAdV), genus *Mastadenovirus*, designated **EAdV1** and **EAdV2**, have been isolated to date. EAdV1 has a worldwide distribution, and it is mainly responsible for upper respiratory tract infections in foals <3-months-old; EAdV2 has been isolated mainly from horses with GI tract infections.

EAdV2 has been isolated in Australia from foals with diarrhea. Rotavirus also was identified in the feces of these foals. A serologic survey showed that 77% of adult horses in the area had neutralizing antibodies to this particular serotype.

An unidentified alimentary tract adenoviral infection has been reported in an Arabian foal that did not have lesions of combined immunodeficiency. The foal had diarrhea and progressive weight loss over a 2-month period. The macroscopic lesions consisted of ulcers in the distal esophagus and nonglandular mucosa of the stomach. The intestine contained soft-to-semifluid ingesta. Histologically, there was necrosis and ulceration of the esophageal and gastric squamous mucosa. Typical adenoviral inclusions were found at all levels of the small intestine. These were most commonly located in the villus epithelial cells, less often in the crypts, and only occasionally in the submucosal glands. There was focal-to-diffuse villus atrophy through the small intestine.

Adenoviruses in other species. The family *Adenoviridae* is classified into 5 genera. Members of genera *Mastadenovirus* and *Aviadenovirus* infect exclusively mammals and birds, respectively. Seven serotypes of **ovine adenovirus** (OAdV) have been isolated from **sheep**. Serotypes 1-6 belong to the genus ***Mastadenovirus***. However, serotype 7 is phylogenetically different from mastadenoviruses and was renamed as *Ovine adenovirus D*, and subsequently *Ovine atadenovirus D*, the type species in genus ***Atadenovirus***. Serotypes 1, 2, and 3 have been recovered from feces of normal sheep, and lambs with enteritis and pneumoenteritis. Experimental inoculation of specific-pathogen-free lambs with OAdV4 did not cause disease, but the virus was reisolated from feces and nasal secretions for several days postinfection. However, occasionally, there are reports of enteritis associated with abundant adenoviral inclusions in lambs and kids. In the former, inclusions were found predominantly in the lamina propria; in the latter they were mostly epithelial.

Goat adenovirus (GAdV) serotypes 1 and 2 can cause enteritis and diarrhea in goat kids; GAdV1 is a serotype of *Ovine atadenovirus D*, which also includes serotype 7 and isolate 287.

Two distinct but serologically related adenoviruses have been isolated from **dogs**. **Canine adenovirus 1** (CAdV1) infection is usually subclinical, but it may cause infectious hepatitis, and diarrhea may be present in these cases. The virus has a particular tropism for hepatocytes and endothelial cells. The serosal hemorrhages in the GI tract and possibly the diarrhea may be related to vascular damage in the serosa and mucosa, respectively (see Vol. 2, Liver and Biliary System). **CAdV2** is usually associated with upper respiratory infections in dogs (see Vol. 2, Respiratory System). Viruses serologically similar to CAdV2 have been isolated from feces of diarrheic dogs. DNA fingerprinting of two of these isolates indicated that they are distinct from CAdV2. It may be that the fecal isolates are due to swallowing of virus originating from upper respiratory tract infections.

Deer atadenovirus A (OdAdV1; *Odocoileus adenovirus 1*, now *Barthadenovirus cervi*) is the cause of hemorrhagic disease that caused high mortality in **mule deer** species in California in the 1990s and that has since been diagnosed as a frequent cause of herd mortality in other deer species in other states of the United States and Canada. Experimentally, OdAdV1 has been demonstrated to be noninfectious to cattle and sheep.

There are 2 manifestations of the disease in deer: systemic and localized. Both forms were experimentally reproduced in black- and white-tailed deer. The disease mimics the orbivirus

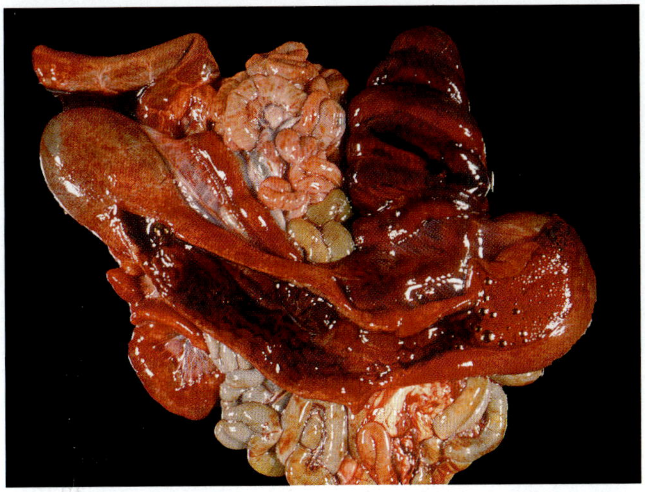

Figure 1-89 Adenoviral hemorrhagic disease. Disseminated hemorrhages throughout the gastrointestinal tract of a deer. (Courtesy L. Woods.)

hemorrhagic diseases in that it triggers DIC through endothelial cell necrosis; however, OdAdV1 targets first endothelial cells of medium and large vessels; BT and EHD viruses target primarily the microvasculature. With *systemic infection*, gross findings include pulmonary edema and/or GI hemorrhage (Fig. 1-89).

Microscopically, there is widespread vasculitis with endothelial cell hypertrophy and necrosis, disruption of the tunica intima, leukocytic margination, fibrinoid necrosis, and leukocytic infiltration of the tunica intima and sometimes media. Intranuclear inclusion bodies are seen primarily in the endothelium of large vessels in the lungs and serosa and submucosa of the intestine and less often in endothelium of interalveolar septal capillaries in the lungs and lamina propria of the intestines. *Localized infection* is seen grossly as necrosis and ulceration of the upper alimentary tract. Microscopically, there is necrosis of various tissues in areas of gross lesions, but vasculitis with intranuclear inclusions is frequently not present.

Coronaviral infections

Coronaviruses cause disease affecting a number of organ systems in a variety of species. Among domestic mammals they mainly cause enteric infections, although coronaviruses are implicated in pneumonia in swine and cattle, and in feline infectious peritonitis (FIP).

Coronaviruses have a single-stranded RNA genome. They are pleomorphic or roughly spherical and vary in size from ~70 to 200 nm in diameter, averaging 100-130 nm. They have a phospholipid-bearing envelope, probably derived in part from host cell membrane. They gain their name from the characteristic "corona" of petal- or droplet-shaped radial surface projections ("peplomers") visible under the electron microscope in negatively stained preparations.

The coronaviruses infecting each species of host appear to be distinctive; some species are infected by more than one type of coronavirus. There are antigenic relationships among viruses from various hosts, and experimental cross-infection will occur between some host species, usually without pathologic consequences. Persistent infections can occur.

Coronaviruses are classified in the family *Coronaviridae*, subfamily *Orthocoronavirinae*, as genera *Alphacoronavirus*, *Betacoronavirus*, and *Deltacoronavirus*. Species of domestic mammalian veterinary significance include:

- Genus *Alphacoronavirus*
  - Subgenus *Tegacovirus*
    - Species *Alphacoronavirus 1*—canine coronavirus (CCoV), feline coronavirus (FCoV), porcine respiratory coronavirus (PRCoV), transmissible gastroenteritis virus (TGEV; *Alphacoronavirus suis*)
  - Subgenus *Pedacovirus*
    - Species *Alphacoronavirus porci* (porcine epidemic diarrhea virus, PEDV)
- Genus *Betacoronavirus*
  - Subgenus *Embecovirus*
    - Species *Betacoronavirus 1*—bovine coronavirus (BCoV), canine respiratory coronavirus (CRCoV), equine coronavirus (EqCoV), porcine hemagglutinating encephalomyelitis virus (HEV)
- Genus *Deltacoronavirus*
  - Subgenus *Buldecovirus*
    - Species *Deltacoronavirus suis* (porcine deltacoronavirus, PDCoV, PoCoV_HKU15)

Viral replication in the intestinal epithelium by coronaviruses is similar in all of the species studied. Coronavirus infects and replicates in the apical cytoplasm of absorptive enterocytes on the tips and sides of intestinal villi. Virions are probably taken up by the apical border of the cell, by fusion with the plasmalemma. Replication and maturation appear to involve budding of virions from the cytosol through the membrane and into the lumen of vacuoles or cisternae in the smooth endoplasmic reticulum, where they accumulate. Virions are found in tubules of the Golgi apparatus. They may exit via that route from infected cells, by exocytosis at the apical cell membrane, or on the lateral cell surface, because viral particles are often seen lined up between microvilli or in the basolateral intercellular space between infected cells. Virus also may be released by lysis of infected cells. Coronaviruses also infect some mesenchymal cells in villi and probably mesenteric lymph node.

Changes in the infected cell occur by ~12-24 hours after infection. Mitochondria in virus-infected cells swell, cisternae of smooth and rough endoplasmic reticulum dilate, the cytoplasm of infected cells loses its electron density, and cells lose their columnar profile. The terminal web is fragmented; microvilli swell and become irregular, perhaps in association with blebbing of the apical membrane. Damaged epithelium may lyse in situ, releasing virus retained in cytoplasmic vacuoles, or it may exfoliate into the lumen. Profuse diarrhea usually begins about the time that early cytologic changes are becoming apparent, but before there is extensive epithelial exfoliation.

Exfoliation of damaged epithelium may be massive over a relatively short period, leading to the development of *villus atrophy*, the severity of which largely reflects the degree of initial viral damage. Villi may appear fused along their sides or tips, and during the exfoliative phase some villi with denuded tips may be present. The enterocytes present on villi shortly after the initial exfoliative episode are mainly poorly differentiated low columnar, cuboidal, or squamous cells, with stubby irregular microvilli. Within 2-3 days, villi begin to regenerate and the epithelium becomes progressively more columnar, although still lacking a well-developed brush border and its complement of enzymes. Defective fat absorption is reflected in the accumulation of lipid droplets in the cytoplasm of enterocytes on villi. This is particularly marked over the period of ~2-5 days after experimental inoculation.

With progressive epithelial regeneration from the crypts, the *villus fusion*, which may be the result of adhesion of temporarily denuded lamina propria of adjacent villi, regresses. Separation begins along the basal margins of the adhesions and progresses toward the tips of the villi. There may be focal acute inflammation in the lamina propria of temporarily denuded villi, and a mild mononuclear infiltrate in the stroma of collapsed villi. Although several cycles of viral replication may occur, poorly differentiated enterocytes appear relatively refractory to infection, and the virus titer falls, presumably as local immune mechanisms also come into play. Hyperplasia of epithelium in crypts usually results in eventual resolution of the villus atrophy, restoring normal function.

The diarrhea that occurs is a result of electrolyte and nutrient malabsorption, with some contribution by secretion by crypt cells, and probably by poorly differentiated surface epithelium in the reparative phase. Mechanisms of diarrhea in villus atrophy are discussed in the Pathophysiology of Enteric Disease section. Remission of signs occurs within ~4-6 days as regeneration of villi occurs, providing that the animal survives the dehydration, electrolyte depletion, and acidosis brought about by diarrhea.

Diagnosis is achieved by detection of viral particles by negative-staining electron microscopy or detection of the virus by fluorescent antibodies, IHC, PCR, and/or virus isolation.

Swine coronaviruses. Four coronaviruses cause GI signs in swine: in genus *Alphacoronavirus*, porcine epidemic diarrhea virus (PEDV, *Alphacoronavirus porci*), transmissible gastroenteritis virus (TGEV, *Alphacoronavirus suis*); in genus *Betacoronavirus*, porcine hemagglutinating encephalomyelitis virus (PHEV, *Betacoronavirus 1*); and in genus *Deltacoronavirus*, porcine deltacoronavirus (PDCoV; *Deltacoronavirus suis*). PEDV, TGEV, and PDCoV produce vomiting and diarrhea in suckling piglets, with high morbidity and mortality caused by severe enteritis. PHEV also causes vomiting and wasting disease in suckling piglets, but mainly mediated by infection of the central and peripheral nervous system (see Vol. 1, Nervous System).

Transmissible gastroenteritis (TGE) may affect swine of any age, causing vomiting, severe diarrhea, and, in piglets, high mortality. The disease is recognized throughout most of the world. The epidemiology of TGE depends on the overall immune status of the herd and of the various age groups within the herd. Introduction of TGEV into a naive herd results in rapid spread of disease with high morbidity affecting all age groups. Sows and older pigs have transient inappetence, and possibly diarrhea and vomiting. Signs may be more severe in sows exposed to high virus challenge from infected baby pigs. Agalactia may occur in recently farrowed sows, perhaps related to TGEV infection of the mammary gland. *Suckling piglets develop severe diarrhea*, and mortality may approach 100% in piglets <10-14-days-old. Older pigs usually develop less severe signs and have lower mortality. In herds with enzootic infection, high piglet mortality may occur in the offspring of recently introduced naive sows, and diarrhea with lower mortality may occur in piglets greater than ~2-3-weeks-old as milk intake and concomitant lactogenic immunity wane. Infected pigs in the late suckling or weanling age group may runt. TGE is more prevalent in the winter, perhaps because the virus is not resistant to summer environmental conditions of warmth and sunlight. Baby pigs that are chilled also seem less able to survive the effects of infection.

The severity of disease in baby pigs is partly related to their inability to withstand dehydration because of their small size, and to their susceptibility to hypoglycemia. Probably as significant is the differentiation, and low rate of turnover, of small intestinal epithelium in the neonate. The surface epithelium is mature and has an extensive vesicular network in the apical cytoplasm associated with the uptake of macromolecules and colostrum during the first day or two after birth. Crypts are short and relatively inactive. Therefore, the population of epithelium susceptible to infection on each villus is large, and the capacity to regenerate new enterocytes is small. By ~3 weeks of age, epithelium is actively proliferative. Virus production by infected enterocytes in older pigs seems less efficient, and replacement of cells lost to infection is more rapid, contributing to the relative resistance seen in swine greater than ~3-weeks-old.

Piglets with TGE have the nonspecific gross appearance at autopsy of undifferentiated neonatal diarrhea. The stomach may contain a milk curd or bile-stained fluid. The small bowel is flaccid and contains yellow frothy fluid with flecks of mucus; chyle is not usually evident in mesenteric lymphatics because there is fat malabsorption.

The microscopic lesions are those of villus atrophy resulting from exfoliation of surface enterocytes (Fig. 1-90A and B), the severity of which is a function of the age of the pig and the stage of the disease. In young piglets, the lesions are most severe about the time of the onset of diarrhea. In later phases or in older pigs there may be subtotal to moderate atrophy, and the mucosa may be lined by cuboidal to low-columnar epithelium, with irregular nuclear polarity and an indistinct brush border. Severe atrophy is readily recognized at autopsy of neonatal piglets by examination of the mucosa under a dissecting microscope. Lesions are most common in the middle and lower small intestine, and villi in the duodenum are usually tall and cylindrical. Lesions may be patchy, and several areas of the lower small intestine must be examined before atrophy is considered not to be present. In animals beyond the neonatal age group, atrophy may not be so severe and readily recognized under the dissecting microscope, and the contrast with the normally shorter villi in the duodenum of older pigs is not as marked. Histologic assessment of the gut is essential.

Porcine respiratory coronavirus (PRCoV) is genetically and antigenically extremely close to TGEV. It cross-reacts serologically, and vaccinated sows successfully induce passive immunity against TGEV enteric infections. PRCoV is spread by inhalation and infects lining cells of the upper respiratory tract. Mild bronchointerstitial pneumonia results from experimental infection, and the agent has been associated with outbreaks of respiratory disease.

Porcine epidemic diarrhea virus (PEDV), an *Alphacoronavirus* antigenically distinct from TGEV, has been reported for many years from Europe and Asia. In 2013 a diagnosis of this condition was made in Iowa, from where it spread quickly to several other states of the United States and Canada. Traditionally, the disease was considered to be essentially similar to TGE in epidemiology, pathogenesis, and lesions, but milder. However, the US epidemic occurred as explosive epidemics of diarrhea and vomiting affecting all ages, with 90-95% mortality in suckling pigs. Clinically, grossly, and histologically, disease produced by PEDV cannot be differentiated from TGE. Differences in virulence have been

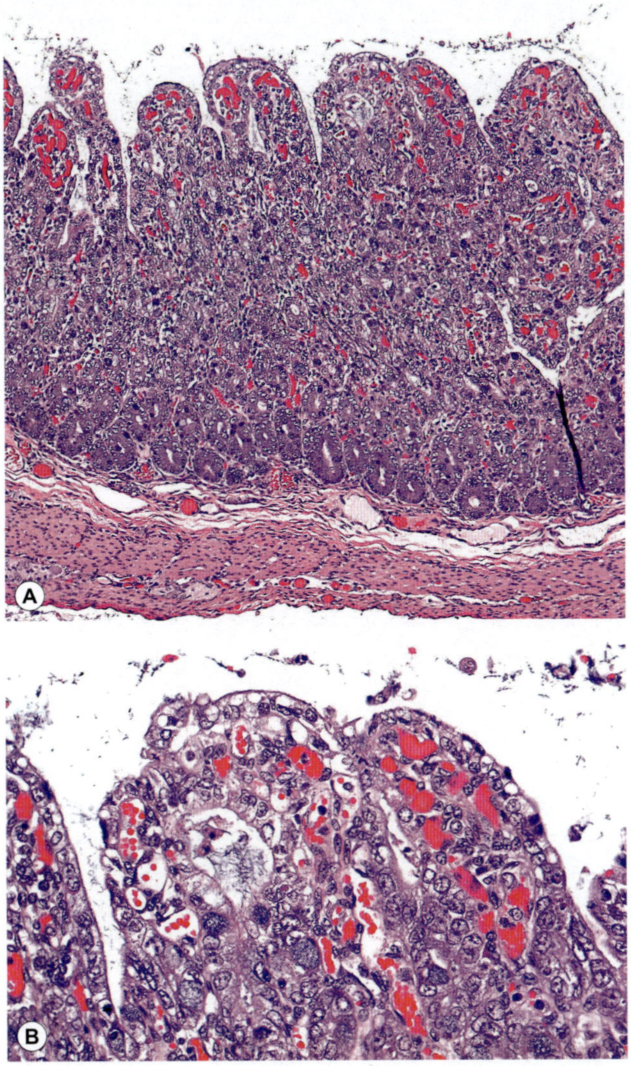

Figure 1-90 Transmissible gastroenteritis in a pig. **A.** Atrophy of villi in the small intestine. **B.** Severely attenuated enterocytes on surface of atrophic villi.

observed between various strains of this virus. It was suggested that coinfection with *C. perfringens* type A enhances disease in weaned pigs with PEDV infection. The diagnosis should be confirmed by PCR or IHC. Although PEDV is related to TGEV, tests for TGEV will not detect PEDV.

Porcine deltacoronavirus (PDCoV), a *Deltacoronavirus* first detected in Hong Kong in 2012 and now present in North America, causes infection that is clinically similar to, but distinct from, PED and TGE. It causes diarrhea and vomiting in all age groups and mortality in nursing pigs. Mortality rates appear to be lower than in cases of PED. However, the prevalence of PDCoV in mainland China has increased, and there have been human cases of PDCoV infection.

Bovine coronavirus. In **neonatal calves**, bovine coronavirus (BCoV) infection is a common cause of diarrhea, either alone or in combination with other agents, particularly rotavirus and *Cryptosporidium*. The disease may be severe in combination with BVDV infection. BCoV is capable of infecting absorptive epithelium in the full length of the small intestine, and in the large bowel. Viral antigen is also found in macrophages in the lamina propria of villi and in mesenteric lymph nodes. In field infections, microscopic lesions are found most consistently in the lower small intestine and colon. Calves with BCoV infection usually develop mild depression but continue to drink milk despite developing profuse diarrhea. With progressive dehydration, acidosis, and hyperkalemia, the animals become weak and lethargic; death can ensue as a result of hypovolemia, hypoglycemia, and potassium cardiotoxicosis. Diarrhea in survivors resolves in 5-6 days.

At **autopsy**, affected animals have the gross nonspecific lesions of undifferentiated neonatal calf diarrhea. Rarely, mild fibrinonecrotic typhlocolitis is recognized in calves with coronaviral infection. Mesenteric lymph nodes may be somewhat enlarged and wet.

Virus replication is cytocidal and initially occurs throughout the length of the villi in all levels of the small intestine, eventually spreading throughout the large intestine up to the end of the large colon and rectum, causing malabsorptive diarrhea. Large concentrations of BCoV can be typically found in the spiral colon. Infected epithelial cells die, slough off, and are replaced by immature cells. The **microscopic** lesions of coronaviral infection in calves vary with the severity and duration of the infection; *villus atrophy and fusion in combination with mild colitis is typical* (Fig. 1-91A). In the calf *small intestine*, villus atrophy is rarely as severe as that seen in neonatal swine with TGE. Rather, villi are moderately shortened, or have subtotal atrophy with stumpy, club-shaped, or pointed tips, and villus fusion may be common. In the early phase of the clinical disease, villi are often pointed and covered by cuboidal-to-squamous epithelium. Exfoliation of epithelium and microerosion may be evident. Later, the epithelium is cuboidal to low-columnar, basophilic, with irregular nuclear polarity and an indistinct brush border. Cryptal epithelium is hyperplastic. The lamina propria may contain a moderate infiltrate of mainly mononuclear inflammatory cells, some of which may have pyknotic or karyorrhectic nuclei. In the early stages of infection, necrosis of cells in mesenteric lymph nodes is associated with viral replication. Peyer patches in animals examined after 4-5 days of clinical illness often appear involuted and are dominated by histiocytic cells. Whether this is the result of viral activity or the effect of endogenous glucocorticoids is unclear.

In the *colon* during the early phase of infection, surface epithelium may be exfoliating, flattened, and squamous or eroded in patchy areas. Some colonic glands may be dilated, lined by flattened epithelium, and contain exfoliated cells and necrotic debris (see Fig. 1-91B). A moderate mixed inflammatory reaction is present in the lamina propria, and neutrophils may be in damaged glands or effusing into the lumen through superficial microerosions. Later in infection, some dilated debris-filled colonic glands will remain, but other glands will be lined by hyperplastic epithelium, and the surface epithelium will be restored to a cuboidal or low-columnar cell type. Goblet cells are usually relatively uncommon. Colonic lesions may be recognizable in tissues from animals submitted dead, even though postmortem change has obscured changes in the small intestine.

Live calves in the early stages of clinical disease are the best subjects for confirmation of an etiologic diagnosis. In calves becoming ill at <7 days of age, enterotoxigenic *E. coli* (ETEC) is the main alternative diagnosis. Rotavirus, *Cryptosporidium*, attaching-effacing *E. coli* (AEEC), and combined infections must be considered in calves 5-15-days-old. Infectious bovine rhinotracheitis, salmonellosis, and BVD must also be considered. Both salmonellosis and BVD may be associated with

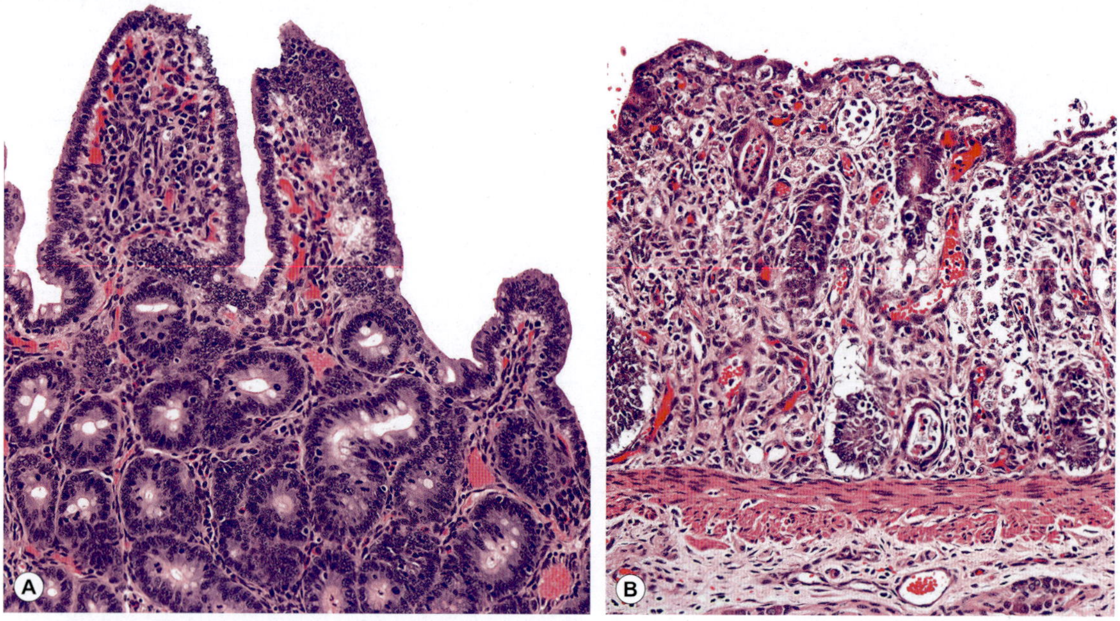

Figure 1-91 Bovine coronaviral infection. A. Blunted and fused villi with cuboidal surface epithelium in the small intestine. **B.** Attenuation of surface epithelium and necrosis of gland epithelium in the colon.

depletion of Peyer patches and colitis that can be confused with that of coronaviral infection; neither is common in the strictly neonatal age group (<7-14 days of age).

Respiratory tract infection may also occur, albeit infrequently, in calves and feeders infected with BCoV. The virus replicates in the epithelium of the nasal turbinates and tracheobronchial tree, and *respiratory infection may precede, be concurrent with, or follow enteric infection.* Calf pneumonia caused by BRCoV can be observed in calves 6-9-months-old. Affected animals may develop fever, serous-to-mucopurulent nasal discharge, coughing, tachypnea, and dyspnea. Respiratory infections may play a role in maintaining the virus within a herd, and significant, but poorly characterized, pneumonia has been reported in some experimentally infected calves. In addition, coronaviral infection may predispose to subsequent respiratory bacterial infections or contribute to more severe respiratory disease as part of the shipping fever syndrome. Virus may be identified in tissue or nasal secretions by immunofluorescence or IHC.

Winter dysentery is a syndrome in adult cattle that has been associated with BCoV in a number of areas around the world. Animals develop usually self-limiting blood-tinged diarrhea, nasolacrimal discharge or cough, anorexia, and drop in milk production. The morbidity rate is high (50-100%), but the mortality rate is usually low, typically <2%. Winter dysentery outbreaks are predominantly seen in young postpartum dairy cows, which then experience a 25-95% drop in milk production. Occasional cases are also observed in adult dairy and beef cattle. Despite its name, cases of winter dysentery can be observed throughout the year. The pathophysiologic characteristics of winter dysentery are mostly attributed to lesions of the colonic mucosa. *Grossly,* the colon of affected animals has linear congestion and hemorrhage along the crests of mucosal folds, and there may be a large amount of blood mixed with colonic contents (Fig. 1-92). The *histologic lesions* are similar to those seen in calves with classical BCoV diarrhea, although

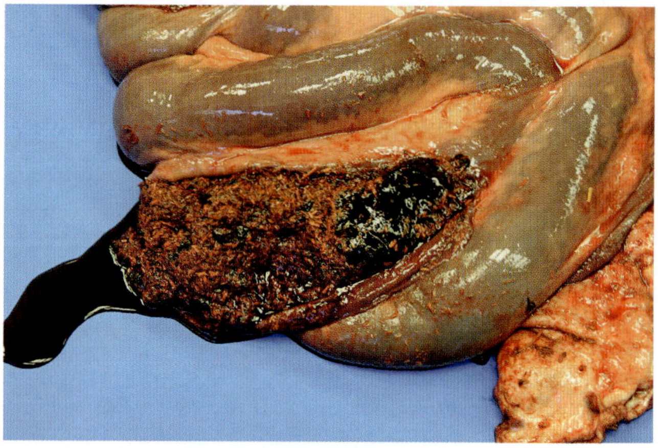

Figure 1-92 Winter dysentery. A large amount of blood mixed with intestinal content is present in the lumen of the spiral colon of a cow.

they are mostly restricted to the colon with only occasional lesions seen in the terminal small intestine. Large amount of BCoV can be detected in colonic epithelium by IHC. Coronaviruses are commonly demonstrated in the feces of cattle with winter dysentery; seroconversions occur, and seroprevalence increases in affected herds. Coronavirus antigen is found in the colonic glands of affected animals, in which there is necrosis and exfoliation of epithelial cells. Certain management practices, notably housing animals in stanchions and use of equipment that handles both manure and feed, have been associated with the development of winter dysentery.

Canine coronavirus. Canine coronavirus (CCoV) is widely prevalent in the dog population. Although dogs of all ages appear to be susceptible to infection by CCoV, the condition is an *uncommon, transient, generally nonfatal diarrhea in puppies.* Fatal infections have been reported in pups previously infected with parvovirus. Infection with a pantropic canine coronavirus has caused a deadly acute systemic disease; concurrent in most cases with canine parvovirus 2c infection. However, there are some more virulent strains of CCoV, capable of causing significant enteric disease in the absence of coinfection. Some of these strains may also cause fatal systemic disease involving lethargy, inappetence, vomiting, hemorrhagic diarrhea, ataxia, and seizures.

Viral replication occurs in the enterocytes of the small intestine, and in experimental infections in neonatal puppies, the lesion resembles the *villus atrophy* associated with coronaviral infection in other species. Diarrhea begins as early as 1 day after inoculation and in most animals by 4 days. Onset of signs coincides with the development of moderate villus atrophy and fusion. Enterocytes on villi become cuboidal, contain lipid vacuoles, and have an indistinct brush border. Lesions are most consistent and severe in the ileum. Resolution of villus atrophy within 7-10 days is associated with remission of signs.

Colonic infection by CCoV was not demonstrated by immunofluorescence in experimental animals, although mild colonic lesions were described, including loss of sulfomucins from goblet cells and some epithelial shedding. However, in a report of lesions caused by spontaneous CCoV infection, colonic infection and lesions were demonstrated. There was watery content in the lumen of the small and large intestine, and fibrin mixed with blood was evident in the cecum and colon. Mesenteric lymph nodes were enlarged and edematous. Villus atrophy in the jejunum was inconsistent, but there was necrotic debris in many glands in the cecum and colon. Virus-infected cells were exfoliating into the lumen.

In the infections with pantropic coronavirus, gross lesions were mostly confined to the small intestine and included pink-to-red intestinal mucosa that occasionally had a slightly dry and rough surface with rare petechiae. Regional mesenteric lymph nodes and spleen were enlarged and congested. Microscopic lesions included villus atrophy and fusion together with dilated crypts containing degenerate and necrotic cells.

Feline and other enteric coronaviruses. Our understanding of the enteric implications of coronaviral infections of **cats** is still incomplete. It appears that feline enteric coronavirus (FECV) can establish persistent infection in the intestine, which in rare cases may be clinically apparent. Infection is very common. When it occurs, diarrhea is usually mild or moderate, perhaps with some blood, and kittens are most susceptible. Viral antigen is in cells on the tips of villi, and mild villus atrophy has been observed. Approximately 13% of all infected cats are not able to clear the virus, which persists for long periods of time in the colonic epithelium. During replication, mutations may occur in the viral genome giving rise to feline infectious peritonitis virus (FIPV), which causes the highly lethal FIP, a disease of far greater clinical significance.

Coronaviruses have been recovered from the feces of **sheep** with transient diarrhea, and they have been associated with severe villus atrophy in several spontaneous outbreaks of diarrhea. No experimental confirmation of the pathogenicity of coronavirus in sheep is available. Cases of colitis similar to those described in cattle with bovine coronaviral infection have been described in sheep and thought to be caused by ovine coronavirus; this has, however, not been confirmed.

Equine coronavirus (ECoV) is a betacoronavirus that has been recognized as an emerging virus from adult horses with fever and enteric signs in Japan, the United States, Europe, Saudi Arabia, and Oman. The disease occurs predominantly in adult horses, and there is an apparent seasonality to ECoV qPCR-positive cases in the United States, with a higher detection rate during the colder months of the year. Both outbreaks and individual cases of ECoV infection occur, and they have been described in racing, pleasure, and show horses, but less frequently in breeding stock. Morbidity of 10-83% occurs in ECoV infection in adult horses. Lethality is low; fatal cases have been associated with necrotizing enteritis leading to disruption of the intestinal mucosa, and septicemia, endotoxemia, and hyperammonemia-associated encephalopathy. Clinically, ECoV infection of adult horses causes anorexia, lethargy, and fever. Diarrhea and/or colic are not consistently observed, but horses with ECoV infection can sometimes develop acute neurologic signs. The neurologic signs may be caused by hyperammonemia, secondary to disruption of the intestinal barrier.

Gross changes are compatible with nonspecific enteritis, including congestion of the mucosa and liquid intestinal contents. *Microscopic findings* include necrotizing enteritis with marked villus blunting, epithelial cell necrosis that is most marked at the tips of the villi, neutrophilic and fibrin infiltration of the lamina propria, crypt necrosis, microthrombosis, and hemorrhage. Occasionally, crypt enterocytes contain single, round intracytoplasmic eosinophilic inclusion bodies. In cases with hyperammonemic encephalopathy, Alzheimer type II astrocytosis is present throughout the cerebral cortex.

Rotaviral infections

Members of the genus ***Rotavirus*** in the family *Sedoreoviridae* infect the GI tract of most mammals and birds. Based on the capsid protein VP6, rotaviruses are classified into 9 species or groups, A through J. *Group A rotaviruses (RVA) are the most diverse and common*, infecting all species of domestic animals, as well as humans, laboratory animals, and wildlife. Additional viral antigens subdivide groups into subgroups and serotypes. Based on VP7 and VP4 external capsid proteins, RVA can be subdivided into G and P serotypes, respectively; there are 14 G serotypes and 20 P serotypes. The serotypes isolated most commonly from piglets with diarrhea are P[7],G5, P[6],G4, P[7],G3, and P[7],G11. Individual rotavirus serotypes have a surprisingly broad host range. Non–group A rotaviruses infect pigs and ruminants, among domestic animals.

The ability to infect cells, and the serotype specificity of rotaviruses, are conferred by elements of the outer capsid. The viruses are probably host specific, with little significant zoonotic potential. However, if epidemiologic circumstances are favorable, cross-species transmission may occur.

Rotaviruses infect the absorptive enterocytes and occasionally goblet cells covering the tips and sides of the villus distal half (ruminants) or the entire villus (pigs), mainly in the jejunum and ileum. Virus production and the pathogenesis of infection are similar in all species studied. Rotaviruses adhere to cell receptors (e.g., integrins, sialic acid), and inner capsid components are internalized into the cell. Granular "viroplasm" containing incomplete virions is seen in the apical cytoplasm of infected cells, and virions acquire their complete capsid after budding into dilated cisternae of endoplasmic reticulum, where they accumulate. Elongate tubular structures are found in the nuclei and rough endoplasmic reticulum of some infected cells.

Enterocytes with CP effect and viral antigen are most prevalent 18-24 hours after experimental infection, and they tend to diminish in number rapidly, so that by 3-4 days after infection few cells containing viral antigen are present. Ultrastructurally, infected enterocytes lose cytoplasmic electron density, and mitochondria swell, as does the cell generally. Swollen rarified cells and syncytia may occur in the enterocytes at the villus tip. These cells are shed readily, particularly if autolysis intervenes. Syncytial cell formation has been recognized in porcine, bovine, and laboratory animal infections. Microvilli become irregular and somewhat stunted, and there may be some blebbing of membranes. Infected cells exfoliate into the intestinal lumen, and virus is released by lysis of damaged epithelium before or after exfoliation.

The *pathogenesis of diarrhea with rotavirus* involves 3 mechanisms. First, malabsorption occurs secondary to destruction of enterocytes. Second, a vasoactive agent is released from infected epithelial cells and causes villus ischemia and activation of the enteric nervous system. Third, rotaviruses encode a nonstructural protein, NSP4, which acts as a *secretory enterotoxin*. This is the first viral pathogen known to produce a toxin.

Exfoliation of infected epithelium over a relatively short period results in villus atrophy. The mucosal surface is covered by cuboidal, poorly differentiated epithelium that has an ill-defined microvillus border and may contain lipid droplets in the cytoplasm. Diarrhea is probably mediated by electrolyte and nutrient malabsorption, perhaps exacerbated by the effect of cryptal secretion. It begins about the time of early viral cytopathology 20-24 hours after infection and may persist from a few hours to a week or more. Regeneration of the mucosa by new epithelium emerging from crypts, and differentiating on reformed villi, is associated with remission of signs in animals surviving the effects of diarrhea.

Rotaviruses are widespread, if not ubiquitous, among populations of most species, and they are relatively resistant to the external environment. Protection against infection in neonates is apparently largely conferred by *lactogenic immunity*. Many individuals in a population probably undergo inapparent infection. Disease is seen in the various species when viral contamination of the environment is heavy, perhaps as a result of intensive husbandry practices, and lactogenic immunity is waning or absent. Although rotaviral infection is usually associated with young animals, and viral receptors on cells diminish with age in some species, naive older animals may become infected and, eventually, diarrheic.

Bovine rotaviral infection. Rotaviral infection is mainly implicated in *diarrhea of neonatal beef and dairy calves*, both suckled and artificially reared, although there are reports of its association with diarrhea in adult cattle. Combinations of agents, including rotavirus, are frequently involved in outbreaks of diarrhea in neonatal calves. Diarrhea may be produced in calves by rotaviral infection alone, but the condition is usually considered to be relatively mild or transient compared with that induced by ETEC or BCoV. Rotavirus may be implicated in animals developing signs at any time up to ~2-3 weeks of age, and it is more commonly encountered in animals >4-5-days-old. Rotaviral diarrhea is most severe in calves that have slower enterocyte regeneration times. Rotavirus has a prepatent period of 1-3 days, and diarrhea lasts 2-5 days if uncomplicated.

The *gross lesions* of rotaviral infection are the nonspecific findings of undifferentiated neonatal diarrhea in calves. *Microscopic lesions in the small intestine cannot be differentiated from those of coronaviral infection*. They may vary somewhat depending on the severity of the initial viral damage and the stage of evolution of the sequelae. Blunt club-shaped villi, mild-or-moderate villus atrophy, and perhaps villus fusion may be present (Fig. 1-93). Villi are covered by low-columnar, cuboidal, or flattened surface epithelium with a poorly defined brush border. There is usually a moderate proprial infiltrate of mononuclear cells and eosinophils or neutrophils, and hypertrophic crypts may be evident. The distribution of lesions may vary between animals and perhaps with time after infection within an individual animal because the onset of maximal viral damage may not occur synchronously throughout the full length of the intestine. Lesions and viral antigen always should be sought in the distal small intestine, and preferably at several sites along its length. Rotavirus does not cause gross or microscopic lesions in the colon, in contrast to coronavirus.

Swine rotaviral infection. Rotaviral infection is widespread and enzootic in most swine herds, and subclinical infection of piglets is common. Rotaviruses A and C are the most common species of the *Rotavirus* genus reported in swine. Although rotavirus A has been traditionally considered the most prevalent and pathogenic in swine, rotavirus C has emerged as a significant cause of enteritis in newborn piglets. Swine rotaviral infection assumes particular importance as a cause of diarrhea in pigs with reduced lactogenic immunity, either as a result of early weaning or after normal weaning. High environmental levels of virus may result in disease in piglets suckling the sow, but in these circumstances the signs are usually relatively mild. Rotavirus may be a cause of "3-week," "white," or postweaning scours in piglets 2-8-weeks-old.

The signs may resemble those of TGE, although rotaviral infection is considered to be less severe. Vomition is less commonly encountered than with TGE, but depression, diarrhea, and dehydration are usual. The character of the feces varies with the diet. Steatorrhea occurs in white scours of suckling piglets. Rotaviral infection in swine is frequently associated with other causes of diarrhea, including *E. coli*, coccidia, adenoviral infection, and *Strongyloides*.

The *gross and microscopic lesions* and pathogenesis of rotavirus infection in pigs resemble those of TGE (Fig. 1-94). As in TGE, the severity of lesions seems inversely related to age.

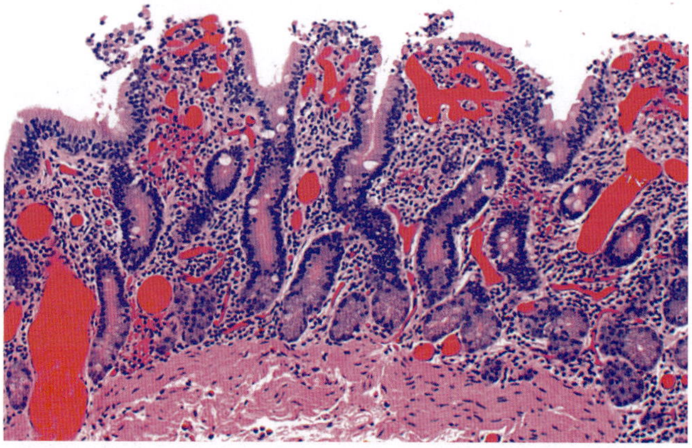

Figure 1-93 Bovine rotaviral infection. Blunted villi with severely attenuated surface epithelium. (Courtesy J. Edwards.)

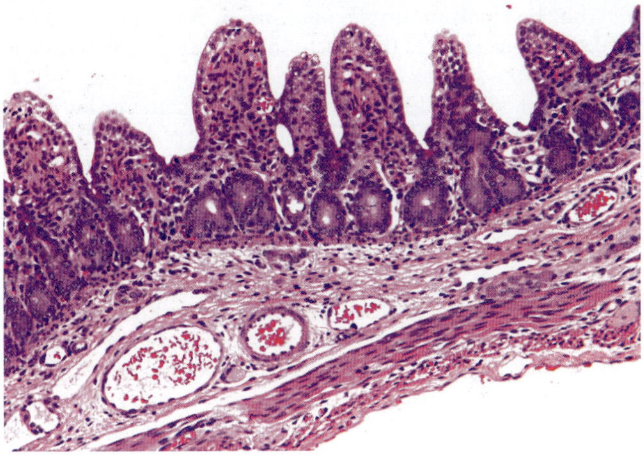

Figure 1-94 Rotaviral infection. Villus atrophy and fusion in the small intestine of a piglet.

Rotaviral infection in other species. Neonatal lambs have proved a useful model for the demonstration of the importance of lactogenic immunity in preventing disease caused by rotavirus. Rotavirus may cause diarrhea in neonatal lambs alone or in combination with ETEC and/or *Cryptosporidium* spp. In older, weaned lambs, an outbreak of diarrhea with 17% mortality was reported, produced by a novel ovine rotavirus group A G8 P strain and no other intestinal pathogens associated. The pathogenesis and lesions of rotaviral infection in lambs are like those caused in other species, with the exception that viral infection of the colon may occur.

Equine rotavirus is endemic to many horse populations. In **foals** <3-4-months-old, rotaviral infection is considered a major cause of diarrhea, although mortality is rare. Outbreaks have been reported in many areas of the world. Equine rotaviruses are ubiquitous in horse populations and dual infections with more than one strain of rotavirus have been reported. Only group A rotaviruses had been detected in horses, but in 2021, a rotavirus group B of ruminant origin causing severe watery-to-hemorrhagic diarrhea in foals 2-7-days-old was found in central Kentucky. Coinfections with other pathogens, including *Salmonella* spp., *Cryptosporidium* spp., and equine coronavirus, have also been observed. The natural and experimental disease resembles that seen in other species, with significant viral infection limited to enterocytes in the small intestine, where villus atrophy occurs. Because rotavirus-associated lethality is rare, very little information is available about gross and microscopic lesions of foals infected with this pathogen.

In young **puppies**, especially those <1-2-weeks-old, diarrhea, occasionally fatal, may be caused by rotaviral infection. In experimentally infected pups, green fluid content filled the lower small bowel and colon, and moderate villus atrophy was induced by exfoliation of epithelium from the distal half of villi.

Rotavirus has also been associated with diarrhea in **kittens**, although rotavirus also can be isolated from subclinically infected kittens.

Rotaviral infection should be sought in cases of diarrhea in young animals of any species, and it should be particularly suspected in animals with villus atrophy in the small intestine. Rotavirus is part of the syndrome of undifferentiated neonatal diarrhea in any species.

Toroviral and astroviral infections

Bovine torovirus (formerly Breda virus; *Tobaniviridae, Torovirus banli*) has been documented as the sole pathogen from diarrheic calves, usually in calves <3-weeks-old. However, the virus has been found with similar frequency in diarrheic and nondiarrheic calves, which questions the belief that this virus causes enteric disease. Lesions in bovine torovirus–infected calves are similar to those of coronaviral infections.

Astroviral infections occur in calves but are mostly subclinical. Less frequently, this virus has been found in diarrheic calves. The disease has, however, not been reproduced experimentally, and the role of astrovirus in diarrhea of calves and other animals remains undetermined. Astrovirus also produces encephalitis and inflammation in other organs in cattle.

Parvoviral infections

Viruses in the family *Parvoviridae* are small, nonenveloped ~18-26 nm particles, with icosahedral symmetry and a short single-stranded DNA genome. They replicate and produce inclusion bodies in the nucleus of infected cells. Members of the genus *Protoparvovirus* infect many species of domestic and laboratory animals and include within the species *Protoparvovirus carnivoran1*, the unranked **canine parvovirus 2** (CPV2), **feline panleukopenia virus** (FPLV), and **mink enteritis virus** (MEV). Among syndromes associated with parvoviral infection are diseases in cats (FPLV), dogs (CPV2), and mink (MEV; distinct from Aleutian mink disease virus) dominated clinically by enteritis, diarrhea in neonatal calves, and reproductive wastage in swine (**porcine parvovirus**; species: *Protoparvovirus ungulate1*).

The occurrence and severity of enteric signs are determined by the degree and extent of damage to epithelium in intestinal crypts. This seems to be a function of 2 main factors. The first is the availability of virus, which is influenced by the rate of proliferation of lymphocytes, and therefore their susceptibility to virus replication and lysis. The second factor is the rate of proliferation in the progenitor compartment in intestinal crypts. If many cells are entering mitosis, large numbers will support virus replication and subsequently lyse. Destruction of cells in the intestinal crypts, if severe enough, ultimately results in focal or widespread villus atrophy and perhaps mucosal erosion or ulceration.

Maximal infection of cryptal epithelium occurs during the period ~5-9 days after infection. Regeneration of cryptal epithelium and partial or complete restoration of mucosal architecture will occur if undamaged stem cells persist in most affected crypts and the animal survives the acute phase of clinical illness. In some survivors, focal villus atrophy is associated with persistent dilated crypts containing cellular debris, and with local "dropout" of crypts completely destroyed by infection. In rare animals that have recovered from acute disease, chronic malabsorption and PLE are associated with persistent areas of ulceration caused by more extensive loss of crypts and collapse of the mucosa.

The low rate of replication of intestinal epithelium in germ-free cats explains failure to produce significant intestinal lesions and clinical panleukopenia in experimentally infected animals. In spontaneous cases, the lower prevalence of parvoviral lesions in the colon and stomach, compared with the small intestine, reflects the relatively lower rate of epithelial proliferation in those tissues. The consistency of epithelial lesions in the mucosa over Peyer patches probably results from high local concentrations of virus derived from infected lymphocytes in the dome and follicle. This may be coupled with local stimulation of epithelial turnover by cytokines released by T lymphocytes in the vicinity. Variations in the rate of epithelial proliferation related to age, starvation, and refeeding, or concomitant parasitic, bacterial, or viral infections, may also influence the susceptibility of crypt epithelium to infection, and therefore affect the extent and severity of intestinal lesions and signs.

Diarrhea in parvoviral infections is mainly the result of reduced functional absorptive surface in the small intestine. Effusion of tissue fluids and blood from a mucosa at least focally denuded of epithelium probably also contributes to diarrhea. Dehydration and electrolyte depletion are the result of reduced fluid intake, enteric malabsorption, effusion of tissue fluid, and, in some animals, vomition. Hypoproteinemia is common, and anemia may occur because of enteric blood loss; both are exacerbated by rehydration. Anemia reflects hemorrhage into the gut.

Proliferating cells in the *bone marrow* also are infected during viremia. Lysis of many infected cells is reflected in hypocellularity of the marrow caused by depletion of myeloid and erythroid elements, particularly the former. Megakaryocytes also may be lost but seem the least sensitive cell population in the marrow. The number of neutrophils in circulation drops quickly in severely affected animals. This is due to failure of recruitment from the damaged marrow, and peripheral consumption, especially in the intestine. Transient neutropenia, of ~2-3 days' duration, occurs consistently in cats, and less commonly in dogs. In surviving animals, regeneration of depleted myeloid elements from remaining stem cells restores the circulating population of granulocytes within a few days. Neutrophilia with left shift may occur during recovery.

Lymphopenia, relative or absolute, results from *viral lymphocytolysis* in all infected lymphoid tissue. Relative lymphopenia is more consistently observed in dogs than neutropenia. When lymphopenia and neutropenia occur together, *the combined leukopenia may be profound in both dogs and cats*. In dogs surviving the lymphopenic phase, circulating lymphocytes return to normal numbers within 2-5 days, as regenerative hyperplasia occurs in lymphoid tissue throughout the body. Lymphocyte numbers increase rapidly, sometimes producing lymphocytosis in recovering dogs. However, there may be transient immunosuppression in gnotobiotic pups subclinically infected with CPV2. Transient depression of T-cell response to mitogens occurs in cats a week after experimental infection with FPLV. But immunosuppression by these agents appears to be of little clinical significance.

Most infected cats and dogs do not develop clinical disease. When it occurs, signs usually begin during the late viremic phase, ~5-7 days after infection. Severe enteric damage is the major cause of mortality. Shedding of infective virus in feces begins ~3-5 days after infection when Peyer patches and cryptal epithelium first become infected. Virus shedding persists until coproantibody appears to neutralize virus entering the gut, ~6-9 days after infection. Virus-infected cells may still be detected in crypts and Peyer patches at this time, and virus complexed with antibody may be found in feces or intestinal content by direct electron microscopy. However, attempts to demonstrate virus in tissues or feces after several days of clinical disease, or at death, are often thwarted by the fact that virus is neutralized by antibody present in tissue fluids. Persistent or sporadic shedding of virus by recovered animals may be the result of virus replication in cells entering mitosis days or weeks after they were infected during the viremic phase.

Infection of the fetus during late prenatal life by FPLV causes *anomalies of the CNS*, mainly hypoplasia of the cerebellum; anomalies of the CNS have not been reported in puppies with CPV2, although there is evidence from PCR studies that CNS lesions in puppies can be induced by fetal CPV2 infections. Infection of proliferating cardiac myocytes in young puppies with CPV2 results in mononuclear myocarditis and sequelae of acute or chronic heart failure (see Vol. 3, Cardiovascular System), but this is rarely seen in populations with a high prevalence of maternal immunity. A tentative association has been made between infection of kittens with FPLV and myocarditis, as well as subsequent cardiomyopathy.

Feline panleukopenia is caused by strains of species *Protoparvovirus carnivoran1*, including feline parvovirus (FPLV), which is responsible for 90-95% of cases, and canine parvovirus, responsible for <10% of the cases. FPLV infects all members of the *Felidae*, as well as mink, raccoons, and some other members of the *Procyonidae*. FPLV is ubiquitous in environments frequented by cats, and infection is common, although generally subclinical. The disease panleukopenia (infectious feline enteritis, feline distemper) usually occurs in young animals exposed after decay of passively acquired maternal antibody, but it may occur in naive cats of any age. Clinical signs of several days' duration, including pyrexia, depression, inappetence, vomiting, diarrhea, dehydration, and perhaps anemia, may be evident in the history. However, many cases, particularly poorly observed animals or those prone to wander, may be presented as "sudden death." Lesions of the CNS in kittens are considered in Vol. 1, Nervous System.

At **autopsy**, external evidence of diarrhea may be present, the eyes may be sunken, and the skin is usually inelastic, with a tacky subcutis reflecting dehydration. Rehydrated animals may have edema, hydrothorax, and ascites resulting from hypoproteinemia. There is pallor of mucous membranes and internal tissues in anemic animals. Gross lesions of internal organs most consistently involve the thymus and the intestine. The thymus is markedly involuted and reduced in mass in young kittens. Enteric lesions may be subtle and easily overlooked. Hence, it is mandatory that the intestine be examined microscopically despite the apparent absence of gross change.

The intestinal serosa may appear dry and nonreflective, with an opaque ground-glass appearance. Uncommonly in cats, there may be petechiae or more extensive hemorrhage in the subserosa, muscularis, or submucosa of the intestinal wall. The small bowel may be segmentally dilated and can acquire a hose-like turgidity in places, perhaps because of submucosal edema (Fig. 1-95A). However, turgidity is difficult to assess in the intestine of the cat. The content is usually foul smelling, scant, and watery, and yellow-gray at all levels of the intestine. The mucosa may be glistening gray or pink, with petechiae, perhaps covered by fine strands of fibrin. Patchy diphtheritic lesions may be present, especially over Peyer patches in the ileum. Flecks of fibrin and sometimes casts may be in the content in the lumen. Formed feces are not evident in the colon. Lymph nodes may be prominent at the root of the mesentery. Gross lesions elsewhere in the carcass are usually restricted to pulmonary congestion and edema in some animals, and pale gelatinous marrow in normally active hematopoietic sites.

Microscopic lesions are consistently found in the intestinal tract in fatal cases and are usual in lymphoid organs and bone

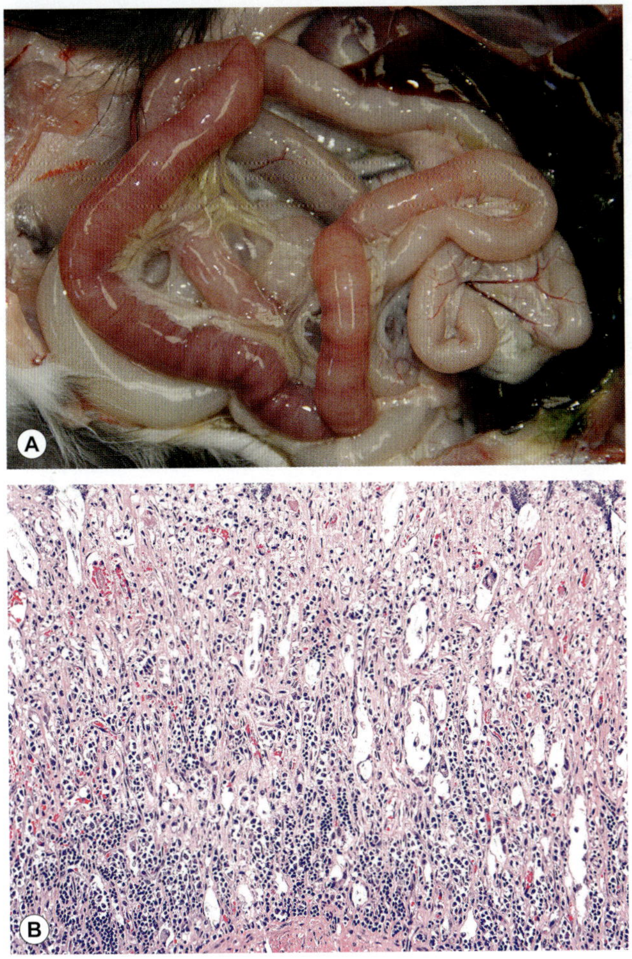

Figure 1-95 **Feline panleukopenia virus** infection. **A.** Dilated and hemorrhagic small intestine in a young cat. **B.** Necrosis and dilation of intestinal crypts in a cat.

marrow. The *intestinal lesions* vary with the severity and duration of the disease. Lesions may be patchy, and several levels of gut should be examined, preferably including the ileum and, if possible, Peyer patches. During the late incubation period and early phase of clinical disease, crypt-lining epithelium is infected. Intranuclear inclusions may be found, and damaged epithelium containing inclusions exfoliates into the lumen of crypts. Crypts are dilated and lined by cuboidal or more severely attenuated cells. The lamina propria between crypts contains numerous neutrophils and eosinophils at this time, and some emigrate into the lumen of crypts, where they join the epithelial debris.

Subsequently, severely damaged crypts may be lined by extremely flattened cells, and by scattered large, bizarre cells with swollen nuclei and prominent nucleoli (see Fig. 1-95B). Enterocytes covering villi are not affected. But as they progress off the villus, they are replaced by a few cuboidal, squamous, or bizarre epithelial cells, so that villi in affected areas undergo progressive atrophy. If cryptal damage is severe and widespread, the mucosa becomes thin and eroded or ulcerated, with effusion of tissue fluids, fibrin, and erythrocytes. Inflammatory cells are usually sparse in the gut of such animals, and superficial masses of bacteria may be present, occasionally accompanied by locally invasive fungal hyphae. In less severely affected animals with disease of longer duration, corresponding to ~8-10 days after infection, scattered focal dropout of crypts, or focal mucosal collapse and erosion or ulceration, may be evident. In these animals, remaining crypts recovering from milder viral damage show regenerative epithelial hyperplasia. Mucosal lesions are often most marked in the vicinity of Peyer patches.

Lesions in the *colon* generally resemble those found in the small bowel, although they are often less severe or more patchy in distribution. Colonic lesions are present in about half of fatal cases of panleukopenia. Gastric lesions resulting from damage to mitotic epithelium are relatively uncommon in cats. They are recognized by flattening of basophilic cells lining the narrowed isthmus of gastric fundic glands, with some reduction in number of parietal cells in the upper portion of the neck of glands.

Lesions of *lymphoid organs* during the early phase of the disease consist of lymphocytolysis in follicles and paracortical tissue in lymph nodes, thymic cortex and splenic white pulp, and gut-associated lymphoid tissue. Lymphoid necrosis has been associated with induced apoptosis of virus-infected lymphocytes. Lymphocytes are markedly depleted in affected tissue and large histiocytes are prominent, often containing the fragmented remnants of nuclear debris. Follicular hyalinosis (amorphous eosinophilic material in the center of depleted follicles) may be seen. Erythrophagocytosis by sinus histiocytes may occur in lymph nodes, especially those draining the gut. Severely depleted Peyer patches may be difficult to recognize microscopically. Later in the course of clinical disease, corresponding to the period beyond ~7-8 days after infection, prominent regenerative lymphoid hyperplasia may be found.

In severely affected animals at the nadir of the leukopenia, virtually all proliferating elements in the *bone marrow* may be depleted. The extremely hypocellular, moderately congested marrow is only populated by scattered stem cells. Milder lesions mainly affect the neutrophil series, generally sparing megakaryocytes and the committed erythroid elements. During the later phases of the disease, marked hyperplasia of stem cells, and eventually of amplifier populations in the various cell lines, is evident.

In the *liver*, dissociation and rounding up of hepatocytes, and perhaps some periacinar atrophy and congestion, may be evident. This is probably associated with dehydration and anemia. Pancreatic acinar atrophy also is common, reflecting inappetence. The lungs may be congested and edematous. In leukopenic animals, few leukocytes are seen in circulation in any organ.

A **diagnosis** of feline panleukopenia may be made on the basis of the characteristic microscopic intestinal lesions, in association with evidence of involution or regenerative hyperplasia of lymphoid and hematopoietic tissues. *Inclusion bodies* may be sought in these tissues, but are usually present in significant numbers only during the late incubation and early clinical period. Cryptal necrosis is also reported in the intestines of some cats with FeLV infection, which must be differentiated from feline panleukopenia. Application of immunohistochemical techniques may identify viral antigen in tissue as late as 8-10 days after infection. Viral antigen also may be identified in intestinal content or feces by ELISA or PCR testing.

Infection with CPV2 with clinical signs and lesions indistinguishable from those caused by FPLV have been described, albeit rarely, in cats. Coinfection of CPV2 and FPLV have also been described in cats with clinical disease.

Canine parvovirus 2 (CPV2) resulted from mutation of a closely related virus, likely an FPLV-like virus from wild carnivores, such as foxes. It appeared spontaneously and virtually simultaneously in populations of dogs on several continents in 1978, and rapidly spread worldwide. Retrospective serologic studies suggest that it was circulating unnoticed in western Europe by 1976. In addition to domestic dogs, several species of wild canids, including coyotes, gray wolves, and raccoon dogs, are susceptible to infection.

Enteric disease caused by this virus was epizootic for several years in naive populations of dogs, affecting animals of all ages. As the prevalence of antibody caused by natural infection and vaccination increased, the problem subsided to one of an enzootic disease. It now affects those animals with reduced levels of passively acquired maternal immunity or scattered naive individuals. A complication of CPV2 enteritis is severe dysbiosis.

During the epizootic period, mononuclear viral myocarditis caused by CPV2 was prevalent in the offspring of naive dams unable to protect pups with maternal antibody during the first 15 days of life, when replicating myocardial cells are susceptible to parvoviral damage. Myocardial disease in pups caused by CPV2 is now fairly uncommon, as most dams have antibody. Enteric and myocardial diseases rarely occur together in the same individual or cohort of animals. Occasional cases of generalized parvoviral infection have been reported in susceptible neonates. Necrosis and inclusion bodies are found in organs such as the kidney, liver, lung, heart, gut, and vascular endothelium. They are presumably related to mitotic activity during organogenesis.

Dogs with typical disease caused by CPV2 become anorectic and lethargic and may vomit and develop diarrhea, perhaps in association with transient moderate pyrexia. Relative or absolute lymphopenia or leukopenia of 1-2 days' duration may occur. Diarrhea may be mucoid or liquid, sometimes bloody, and is malodorous. After a period of 2-3 days, dogs succumb to the effects of dehydration, hypoproteinemia, and anemia, or begin to recover.

Gross findings at autopsy of fatal cases are those of dehydration, accompanied by enteric lesions characteristic of the disease. There is often segmental or widespread subserosal intestinal hemorrhage, which may extend into the muscularis and submucosa (Fig. 1-96A). The serosa frequently appears hemorrhagic and finely granular because of superficial fibrinous effusion (see Fig. 1-96B). Peyer patches may be evident from the serosal and mucosal aspects as deep-red oval areas several centimeters long. The intestinal contents may be mucoid or fluid and are frequently hemorrhagic. The mucosa is usually deeply congested and glistening or covered by patchy fibrinous exudate. Severe mucosal lesions may be widespread or segmental, and their distribution is irregular; thus, tissues from several levels of the small intestine should be selected for microscopic examination. Gross changes in the colon are similar but less common. The stomach may have a congested mucosa and contain scant bloody or bile-stained fluid. Mesenteric lymph nodes may be enlarged, congested, and wet, or be reduced in size. Thymic atrophy is consistently present in young animals, and the organ may be so reduced in size as to be difficult to find. The lungs often appear congested and have a rubbery texture.

The **microscopic lesions** in the stomach, small intestine (see Fig. 1-96C), colon, lymphoid tissue, and bone marrow caused by CPV2 infection do not differ significantly from those described earlier in cats with panleukopenia. Gastric lesions are perhaps more frequently encountered in dogs with parvoviral infection. Small intestinal lesions are invariably severe in fatal cases. The colon is involved in a minority of animals. Increased immunoreactivity to caspase 3 has been described in enterocytes and intestinal inflammatory cells of dogs infected with CPV2, indicating that apoptosis is an important form of cell death in dogs with parvoviral enteritis. Pulmonary lesions such as alveolar septal thickening by mononuclear cells, congestion, and effusion of edema fluid and fibrin into the lumina of alveoli may be related to terminal gram-negative sepsis and endotoxemia, which is common in fatal cases. Periacinar atrophy and congestion in the liver are attributable to anemia, hypovolemia, and shock, and prominent Kupffer cells probably reflect endotoxemia. Some studies have shown that viral inclusions may occur in tongue epithelium cells as well. Although these inclusions are nuclear, they often appear to be in the cytoplasm (pseudocytoplasmic). A case of erythema multiforme as a result of CPV2 infection of keratinocytes has been described in a dog with concurrent parvoviral enteritis; viral inclusions were present in oral and skin epithelial cells.

The diagnosis of parvoviral enteritis in dogs follows the principles described for that of panleukopenia in cats. PCR, IHC (see Fig. 1-96D, inset), or antigen ELISA are confirmatory. The disease must be differentiated from canine coronavirus infection, which is very rarely fatal, and from canine intestinal hemorrhage syndrome, shock gut, intoxication with heavy metals or warfarin, infectious canine hepatitis, and other causes of hemorrhagic diathesis. Involution of gut-associated lymphoid tissue and cryptal necrosis caused by parvovirus must be differentiated from similar lesions seen occasionally in canine distemper.

Canine bocaparvovirus 1, canine minute virus (CnMV; *Parvoviridae, Bocaparvovirus carnivoran1*) has been mainly described associated with enteritis in young dogs. The virus is most closely related to bovine parvovirus 1 and is genetically and antigenically unrelated to CPV2. Serologic studies demonstrate that this virus is widespread in dogs, although most infections are very mild or subclinical. However, in some cases CnMV causes diarrhea or sudden death in neonatal puppies. Although some cases are associated with primary infection by CnMV, coinfections with other pathogens seem to be common. CnMV is capable of transplacental transmission to the fetus, and exposure of pregnant dams was associated with fetal resorption, or birth of dead or weak pups. CnMV causes enteric or respiratory signs in puppies <3-weeks-old. Enterocyte hyperplasia in the duodenum and jejunum with large intranuclear viral inclusion bodies is evident, but the crypt necrosis characteristic of infection by CPV2 does not occur. Interstitial pneumonia and myocarditis are variably present in naturally infected puppies, with death occurring sporadically.

Another parvovirus, carnivore chaphamaparvovirus-1 (CaChPV1; *Chaphamaparvovirus carnivoran1*) localizes in canine villar endothelial cells, has been associated with diarrhea in puppies, and may be an enteric pathogen.

Bovine parvoviral infection. Bovine parvovirus 1 (BPV1; *Parvoviridae, Bocaparvovirus ungulate1*, formerly *Bovine parvovirus*) has 3 significant subspecies: **BPV1, 2, and 3**. BPV has

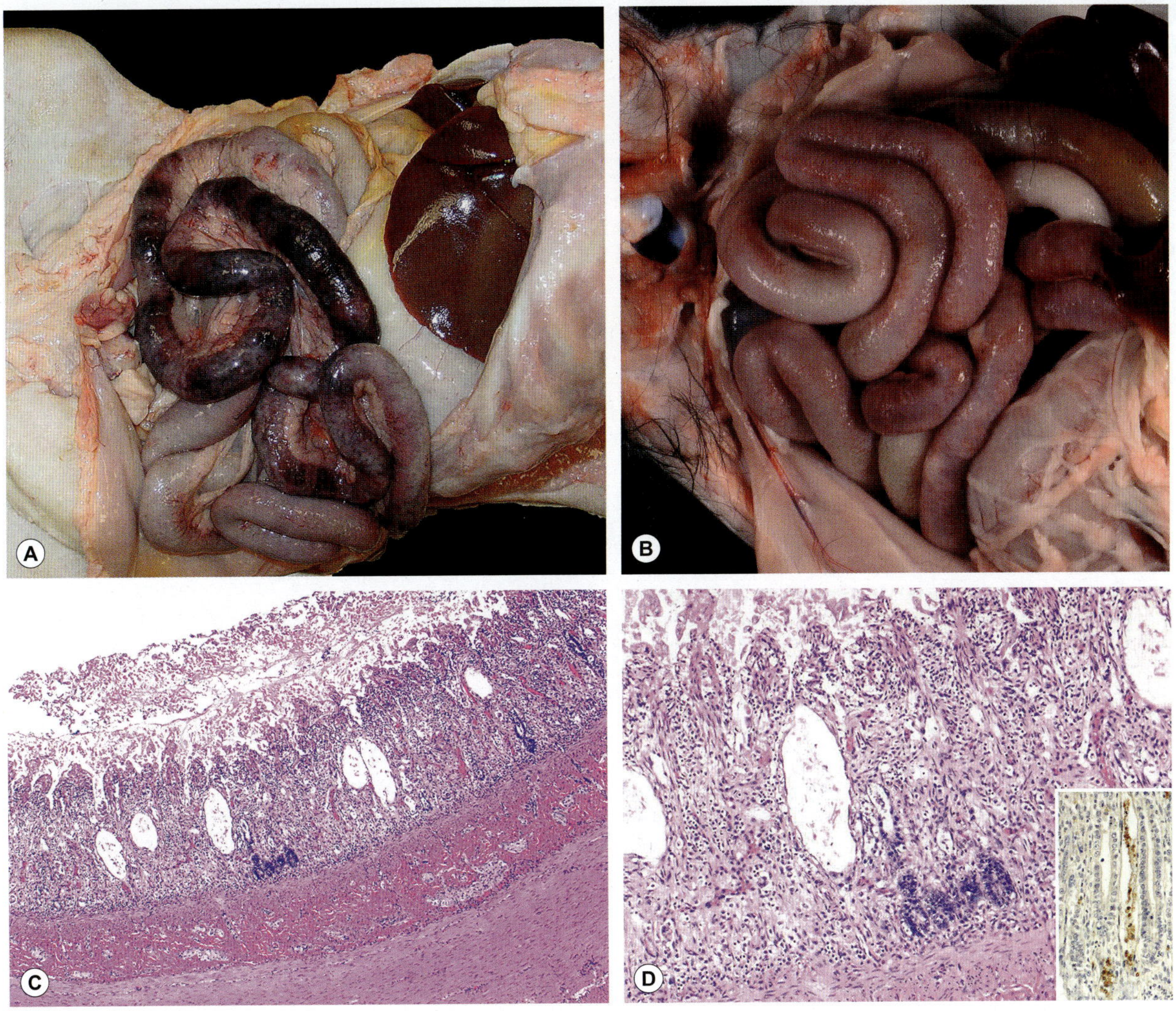

Figure 1-96 Canine parvoviral infection. **A**. Segmental subserosal hemorrhage and mild fibrinous exudation on intestinal serosa in canine parvovirus 2 (CPV2) infection. (Courtesy J. Ortega-Porcel.) **B**. The serosal surface is hemorrhagic and finely granular. **C**. Segmental loss and dilation of intestinal crypts and collapse of proprial stroma in the small intestine. **D**. Remnants of hyperplastic cryptal epithelium persist deep in lamina propria. Inset: strong cytoplasmic immunoreactivity in remnant cryptal epithelial cells. IHC for CPV2.

been recognized for many years and occurs widely in cattle populations on all continents. It has been isolated from the feces of normal and recently diarrheic calves as well as from conjunctiva and aborted fetuses. *The status of BPV1 as an enteric pathogen is unclear*, although it is believed to cause diarrhea in neonatal calves and respiratory and reproductive disease in adult cattle. Virus shedding is not always associated with diarrhea, and it may be part of a mixed infection in diarrheic animals. Serologic prevalence of antibodies to BPV is high, with 83% of cattle and 100% of herds being positive over 2 years of testing in one study. However, in recent studies of calf diarrhea, BPV was associated with diarrhea in only 5.5% of cases. It is rarely diagnosed as a cause of death, and unless sought specifically by culture, direct electron microscopy, or molecular probe, it would be missed in cases of diarrhea. Its significance may be greatest in neonatal calves and animals exposed while passive maternal antibody levels are waning, or in animals in the postweaning period.

The pathogenesis of infection with BPV1 resembles that in carnivores. Initial viral replication following oral inoculation is in tonsils and gut, with spread to systemic lymphoid tissues, resulting in transient lymphopenia. Viral antigen has been identified in the nuclei of epithelium in intestinal crypts and in cells in the thymus, lymph nodes, adrenal glands, and heart muscle. Transient lymphocytolysis in infected tissues, and exfoliation of epithelium in crypts of the small and large intestine, with moderate villus atrophy, depletion of colonic goblets, and mixed inflammatory cell infiltration of the mucosa, have been seen experimentally. Intranuclear inclusions are present when lesions are prevalent. Gross lesions other than abnormally fluid content in the gut are subtle or absent. Intravenous inoculation of BPV into young calves causes severe watery diarrhea and prostration. Milder diarrhea occurs in calves infected orally. The severity of the disease may be potentiated by concurrent infection with other enteric pathogens, or other factors that may increase intestinal epithelial proliferation.

Bacterial diseases of the alimentary tract

Virulence of bacterial pathogens

Evolutionary processes for bacterial survival, persistence, and proliferation are controlled by virulence genes and are subject to complex mechanisms of regulation of expression. Similarly, evolutionary processes for resisting the effects of bacteria on the host are determined by genetic factors and equally complex regulatory processes in the host. *Bacterial virulence can be resolved into 5 components:* 1) attachment; 2) colonization or entry into the host; 3) evasion of host defense; 4) multiplication and/or spread within the host, and damage to the host, by direct virulence attributes, or by stimulation of an immunoinflammatory response; and 5) transmission to other susceptible animals. The interplay between host and pathogen has been extensively studied for a number of important enteric bacterial pathogens, including *Salmonella* spp., *E. coli*, and several clostridial species.

Genes encoding a range of virulence characteristics in pathogenic bacteria, including adhesion factors, toxins, proteolytic enzymes, and other agents that promote tissue invasion, are often clustered in discrete regions of the genome known as *pathogenicity islands* or *plasmids*. These appear to be sites of relative instability and are thought to facilitate the horizontal transfer of virulence factors between bacteria, and their continued evolution. Similarities in the regulatory mechanisms for pathogenicity islands of important enteric pathogens, including *Salmonella*, *Shigella*, *Vibrio*, *Yersinia*, *E. coli*, and *Clostridium*, are providing new insights into the reasons why strains of many genera of bacteria vary greatly in their host range and ability to cause disease. Among the factors in the mucosal barrier that resist pathogen virulence, there is growing interest in the role of the luminal microbiota and their metabolites. Disruption of the intestinal microbiota may facilitate virulence factors of invading pathogens listed earlier.

Colibacillosis

Escherichia coli has several virulence attributes that result in disease in animals. Principally, these promote *colonization or adhesion* to the mucosa; they cause *metabolic dysfunction or death of enterocytes*; they affect the *local or systemic vasculature*; or they promote *invasion and septicemia*. Disease syndromes caused by *E. coli* in domestic animals can be related to the combinations of virulence attributes expressed. Many terms have been applied to the mechanisms of action of *E. coli*, with some becoming obsolete and others applying mainly to *E. coli* infections of laboratory animals and humans, rather than to domestic animals.

"Enterotoxigenic" *E. coli* (ETEC) cause secretory small-bowel diarrhea stimulated by enterotoxins produced by *E. coli* colonizing the mucosa of the small intestine. This condition is an important, common cause of diarrhea in neonatal animals of many species, and in postweaning pigs. The enterocytes of animals affected with ETEC remain morphologically normal.

"Enteropathogenic" *E. coli* (EPEC) in humans and animals may colonize the mucosa of the intestine by a mechanism involving adhesion-effacement (**"enteroadherent" *E. coli*** or AEEC). Some do not produce recognized toxins, but are associated with villus atrophy and erosions of enterocytes. Other strains of *E. coli*, many of which are attaching-effacing, in addition secrete *cytotoxins* (Shiga toxins = verotoxins) that have an effect locally or systemically. Depending on the manifestation of this effect, such *E. coli* have been categorized as **"Shiga toxin–producing"** (STEC) = **"verotoxin-producing"** (VTEC), or **"enterohemorrhagic"** (EHEC). EHEC are a serious cause of foodborne illness in humans and have been incriminated as a cause of hemorrhagic enterocolitis in calves <1-month-old. The reservoir for EHEC that cause human disease is thought to be ruminants.

Shigatoxigenic infections in swine that are not attaching-effacing are associated with some outbreaks of postweaning *E. coli* enteritis and also cause edema disease of weaned pigs, which is a systemic toxemia.

"Enteroinvasive" *E. coli* (EIEC) can be internalized by surface enterocytes and subsequently disseminate through the body to become septicemic. Although EIEC are poorly documented in domestic animals, **septicemic colibacillosis** is a common manifestation of *E. coli* infection caused by strains adapted to avoid specific or innate systemic defense mechanisms, often in compromised hosts. The intestine is not necessarily the portal of entry and there may not be alimentary disease. The signs of *E. coli* septicemia are mainly referable to bacteremia, endotoxemia, and the effect of bacterial localization in a variety of tissue spaces throughout the body.

Enterotoxigenic colibacillosis caused by ETEC is one of the major forms of diarrhea in neonatal pigs, calves, and lambs, as well as in humans.

Two major attributes confer virulence on these strains of *E. coli*. These are the ability to colonize the intestine, and the capacity to produce toxins that stimulate the secretion of electrolytes and water by the intestinal mucosa. *Colonization and enterotoxin production must occur together for disease to ensue.* The diarrhea produced by ETEC is of the secretory type and accompanied by relatively minor microscopic evidence of inflammation, and by little or no architectural change in the mucosa. As a result, overt enteritis is usually not evident at autopsy, and the disease is part of the syndrome of undifferentiated diarrhea of neonatal animals.

Intestinal colonization results from the adhesion of *E. coli* to the surface of enterocytes on villi in the small intestine, and proliferation there (Fig. 1-97A). By adhering to the mucosa, bacteria are able to resist the normal peristaltic clearance mechanisms. Large numbers of organisms, of the order of $>10^7$ per gram of mucosa, or 20-30 per enterocyte, cover the surface of villi. The ability to attach to enterocytes is conferred on ETEC by pili and may be enhanced by the presence of a capsule.

Fimbriae or **pili** [also known as *colonization factor antigens* (*CFA*), with specific names in transition to a system of "F" numbers] are rodlike or filamentous projections from the cell wall of *E. coli* that attach to specific glycoconjugate receptors on the surface of enterocytes (see Fig. 1-97B). They are distinct from type 1 fimbriae, which do not promote colonization of the gut. Fimbriae are polymers of protein (pilin) subunits, which are coded by plasmid [F4 (K88), F5 (K99), F18; some F6 (987P)] or chromosomal [F6 (987P), F17, F41] DNA. They are antigenically distinct, permitting recognition by specific antibody.

Fimbrial adhesins include **F5** (K99) and **F41** in strains affecting calves, lambs, and pigs; **F42, F165, F17, F18** in calves and pigs; and **F4** (K88), **F6** (987P), **F18** in pigs. Combinations of adhesins may be expressed by the same strain of ETEC;

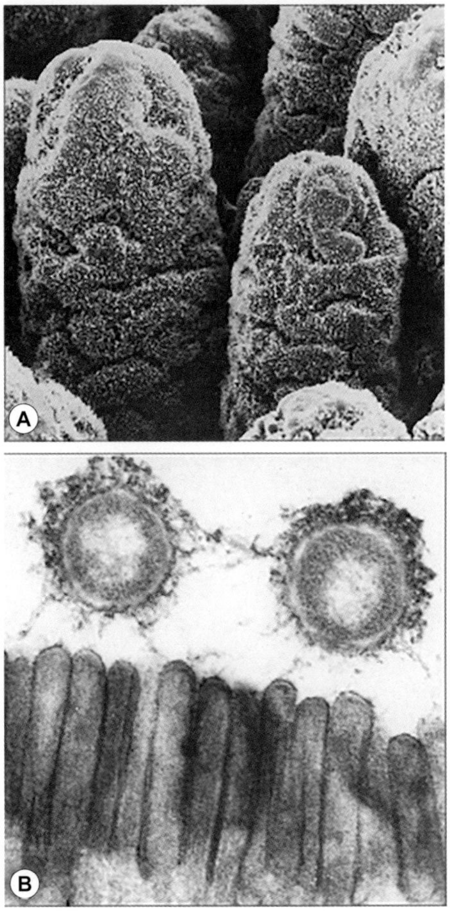

Figure 1-97 Enterotoxigenic colibacillosis. A. Scanning electron micrograph of *E. coli* adherent to the surface of villi in a calf. **B.** Transmission electron micrograph of fimbriate *E. coli* adherent to microvilli in the small intestine of a calf. (Courtesy J.J. Hadad and C.L. Gyles.)

typically, F41 is expressed by strains also expressing F5 and seems to be of minor importance. Bacteria possessing F4 colonize the entire small bowel; those with F5, F6, and F41 mainly adhere in the jejunum and ileum.

Susceptibility to bacterial fimbrial adhesins, especially F5 and F6, appears to be somewhat age related; the ability of fimbria-bearing *E. coli* to colonize the small intestine is greatest in animals only a few days of age. F5 receptors on enterocytes decline in availability with age; F6 receptors are shed into the lumen in older pigs, facilitating clearance of bacteria from the mucosa, and interfering with colonization. F18 receptors are not found in neonatal pigs, but are produced with increasing age to weaning. Stimulation of maternal immunity to fimbrial antigens causes secretion of lactogenic antibody, which combines with adhesins in the gut lumen, preventing colonization of the gut of suckling animals.

A nonfimbrial plasmid-encoded *adhesin involved in diffuse adherence* of *E. coli* to enterocytes in humans also occurs in strains from pigs associated with edema disease and postweaning diarrhea, often in combination with F18.

Enterotoxigenic strains of *E. coli* produce 2 classes of plasmid-encoded proteins—heat-labile toxin (LT) and heat-stable toxin (ST)—which act locally in the intestine to alter secretion and absorption of electrolytes and water by enterocytes. However, these toxins usually do not alter enterocyte morphology.

Heat-labile toxin is a large immunogenic plasmid-encoded molecule, with 2 subgroups (LTI and LTII) and composed of a small A subunit with two fragments (A1 and A2), which links A1 to a large pentamer of 5 B subunits. LTI is antigenically similar to cholera toxin; LTII toxins have B subunits that differ from LTI. The B subunits bind to ganglioside receptors (GM1 gangliosides) on the enterocyte surface; the toxin complex then dissociates, and the A1 subunit is internalized into the cell. It operates via an adenylate cyclase pathway to cause chloride secretion by enterocytes, sodium, and water following osmotically from the mucosa. Cotransport of sodium chloride by enterocytes, and associated water uptake, is probably also shut down at the same time. LT may also promote mucosal secretion by stimulation of local prostaglandin production, the enteric nervous system, and cytokine activation. LT has been shown to decrease host defenses through interference with antimicrobial peptide production by human enterocytes. LT has a latent period before the development of secretion, but the effects on the cell are irreversible.

Heat-stable toxin is classified as STa and STb based on biological properties and is plasmid encoded. STa causes an increase in cyclic guanosine monophosphate, which inhibits Na/Cl cotransport and therefore water absorption by surface enterocytes; in crypt epithelium, it promotes Cl^- and water secretion. STb acts through a different mechanism than STa and is mainly produced by ETEC associated with pigs. STb causes increased intracellular calcium, chloride secretion, and may cause secretion by stimulation of prostaglandin E2 and 5-hydroxytryptamine production. In pigs, STb can cause exfoliation of surface enterocytes, resulting in mild atrophy of villi.

Enteroaggregative *E. coli* heat-stabile toxin (EAST1) has also been reported in ETEC isolated from pigs and cattle. This toxin has been associated with *E. coli*–induced diarrhea in children. However, the role of EAST1 in *E. coli* disease in pigs and cattle is not certain.

Enterotoxigenic colibacillosis is among the most common causes of diarrhea in **neonatal pigs**, from a few hours to ~1 week of age. ETEC are present in the environment and are ingested. Commonly, serogroups O8, O45, O138, O141, O147, O149, and O157, expressing F4, are involved in enterotoxigenic colibacillosis in piglets, although the prevalence of F4-bearing strains may be declining because of vaccination of sows. Less commonly, F5, F6, and F41 pilus adhesins are involved. STb is the most common toxin produced by porcine ETEC; when LT is found, it is in association with STb, which may be encoded on the same plasmid. STa also occurs in strains of ETEC in swine, alone or in combination with other enterotoxins.

At autopsy, enterotoxigenic colibacillosis cannot be readily separated from the other common causes of undifferentiated neonatal diarrhea without laboratory assistance. Generally, there is dehydration, usually with evidence of diarrhea, or a history of its occurrence in the herd. Lipopolysaccharide (LPS) from the bacterial cell membrane may promote inflammatory cascades and contribute to shock. Other than the characteristic fluid content in the flaccid small and large bowel, usually with clotted milk still in the stomach, the internal findings are unremarkable.

In contrast to the viruses and *Cystoisospora*, *ETEC usually does not cause significant villus atrophy* or other morphologic changes in the intestine. Small clumps, or a continuous layer of gram-negative coccobacilli may be found on the surface of enterocytes on villi in mucosal tissue sections, most consistently in the terminal jejunum and ileum. Some neutrophils may be present in the proprial core of villi, and transmigrating the epithelium into the lumen.

The involvement of ETEC expressing F4 in postweaning diarrhea of pigs >3-weeks-old, and distinct from postweaning colibacillosis caused by VTEC, discussed later, may be related to colonization of the intestine in weaned pigs in which rotavirus infection, changes in diet, or villus atrophy associated with hypersensitivity to dietary protein constituents provide adhesin-bearing *E. coli* with a competitive advantage. It causes diarrhea for up to a week or so, with ill-thrift, but is uncommonly fatal, although a syndrome probably caused by endotoxic shock, similar to that associated with shigatoxigenic stains associated with postweaning colibacillosis, described later, may occur.

In **calves**, many cases of undifferentiated neonatal diarrhea are accounted for by enterotoxigenic colibacillosis, usually involving strains of serogroups O8, O9, O20, O64, O101 with fimbrial adhesins F5 and F41, and producing STa. Infection is typically restricted to the first 4-5 days of life, probably because of the loss of receptors for F5 in older calves.

ETEC must be differentiated from the other major causes of undifferentiated diarrhea in neonatal calves—BCoV, rotavirus, and *Cryptosporidium*—which typically dominate in calves older than a few days of age. However, ETEC is commonly found in combination with BCoV or rotaviral infection.

The **gross findings** in calves with enterotoxigenic colibacillosis are the nonspecific appearance of diarrhea and dehydration. The infection is differentiated in tissue sections from the other infectious causes of this syndrome by the *absence of severe villus atrophy* (Fig. 1-98A) and by gram-negative *bacteria on the surfaces of villi* in the distal small intestine (see Fig. 1-98B). As in piglets, application of a variety of presumptive or specific tests for ETEC in the intestine confirms the diagnosis.

Enterotoxigenic colibacillosis is a significant problem in **lambs** in some areas. The serotypes involved, pathogenesis, and diagnosis of the condition are similar to those in calves. Synergism with rotaviral infection may occur.

There are several reports of ETEC isolated from **foals** with diarrhea. The organisms have pili, probably F41, and secrete LT or STa. However, their capacity to produce disease in foals is unproved. Diarrhea has not ensued in foals inoculated with F4-bearing *E. coli*, despite the presence of F4 receptors on enterocytes, and it seems that ETEC has little significance in this species.

Strains of *E. coli* have been associated with diarrhea in neonates of **other species** of animals, especially young dogs, where they mainly produce STa. Generally, the enterotoxigenicity and other attributes of virulence have not been well described in strains from other species.

Enteropathogenic *E. coli* (EPEC) are those that cause direct damage to the mucosa, through a *characteristic mechanism of attachment to, and effacement of, epithelium. These* **AEEC** are more common in humans than in animals, where they are most important in pigs, cattle, dogs, and rabbits, although they also have been isolated from cats. Control of attaching-effacing activity resides in the *locus for enterocyte effacement* (LEE), a chromosomal pathogenicity island. EPEC have a complicated and sequential relationship with host cells. Long polar fimbriae may mediate initial bacterial interaction with the enterocyte. Secretion of bacterial proteins ensues, including *intimin*, which is an adhesin. A second protein, the *translocated intimin receptor*, is transported via a type III secretion system into the enterocyte cytoplasm, emerging on the cell membrane as the intimin receptor. In response to translocated EPEC proteins, the cell's cytoskeleton is reorganized, resulting in formation of cupped *pedestal-like structures* beneath the attached bacteria, and the subsequent loss of microvilli (Figs. 1-99A and B, and 1-100). Paracellular permeability increases as tight junctions between enterocytes loosen, and neutrophils migrate between cells into the lumen.

In animals and humans, some strains of AEEC are pathogenic despite failure to secrete enterotoxins or cytotoxins. A heavy layer of plump coccobacilli may be found over the

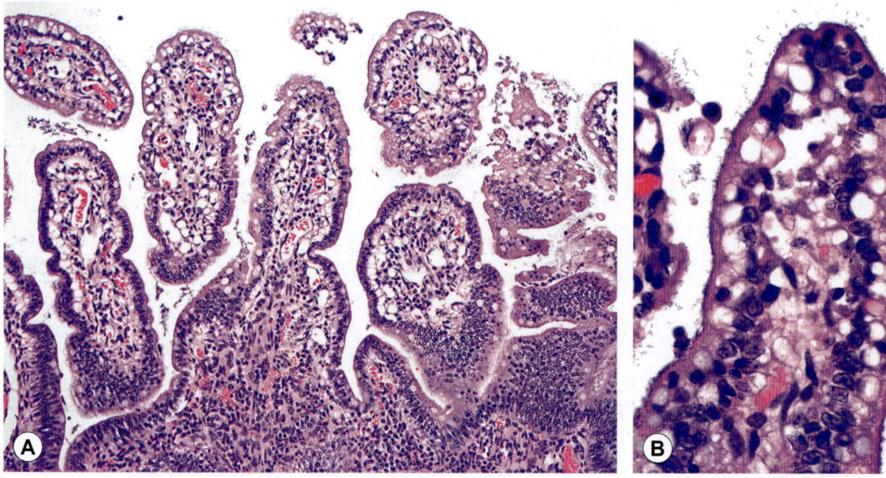

Figure 1-98 Enterotoxigenic colibacillosis in a calf. **A.** Atrophy of villi is not evident and surface epithelium is normal. **B.** Higher magnification of (A); numerous bacteria are attached to the epithelial surface.

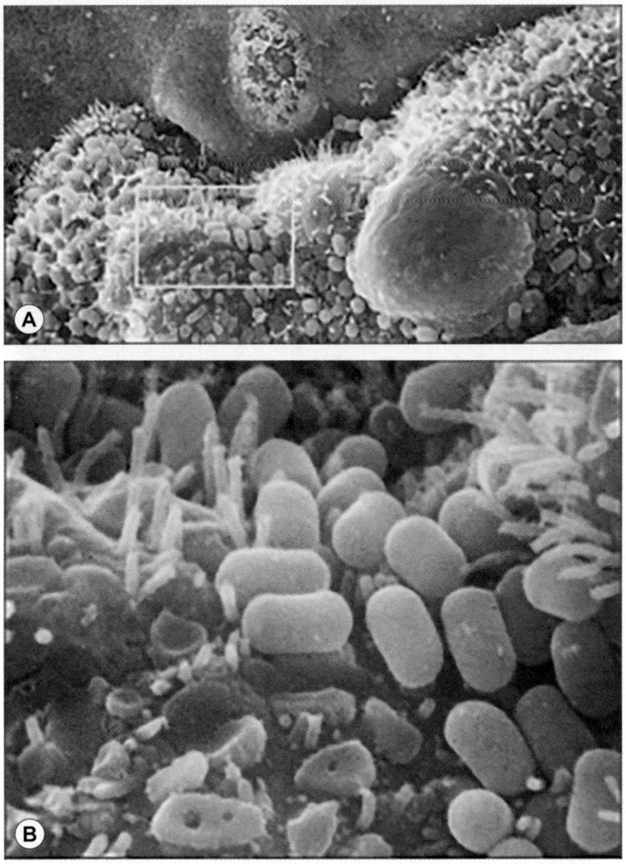

Figure 1-99 Attaching-and-effacing *Escherichia coli* infection. **A, B**. Scanning electron micrograph of the colon of a calf. Cells infected by attaching-effacing *E. coli* have irregular microvilli, in comparison to uninfected background cells. **B**. Area outlined is shown at higher magnification; adherent bacteria can be seen on pedestals projecting from the surface of enterocytes. (Courtesy M. Schoonderwoerd and R. Clarke.)

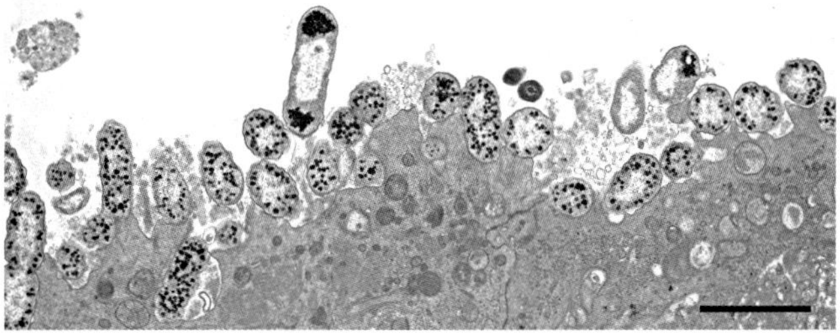

Figure 1-100 Attaching-and-effacing *Escherichia coli* infection. Transmission electron micrograph of intestinal enterocytes with *E. coli* on pedestals projecting from surface of infected cells. (Courtesy A. Armien.)

luminal aspect of enterocytes on villi throughout the small intestine, and on the surface of the large intestine. *The degree of diarrhea seems related to the extent of bacterial colonization, which is most consistent in lower small intestine and large bowel.*

Enterocytes to which bacteria are adherent are initially attenuated and lose the apical part of the cytoplasm. At low magnification, this gives a ragged, irregular, scalloped appearance to the mucosal surface. These cells round-up or contract and exfoliate from the mucosa singly or in clumps, resulting in mild-to-severe atrophy of villi in the small bowel, and attenuation of surface cells, or microerosions in the large intestine. Fusion of villi may occur in the small intestine, and goblet cell numbers are depleted in both large and small bowel. There is moderate mucosal congestion and local infiltration by neutrophils.

Diarrhea is presumably related to maldigestion and malabsorption of nutrients and electrolytes in the small intestine, perhaps with the additive effect of increased mucosal permeability, overloading the colon, the absorptive ability of which is also compromised by damage to surface cells. *Microscopic diagnosis is based on recognition of bacteria on the mucosal surface associated with changes in the enteric mucosa. Very fresh tissues are required for this purpose.*

In **pigs**, EPEC belonging to serogroups O45 and O103, infecting the small and large intestine, are responsible for some cases of postweaning diarrhea. In young **dogs**, and occasionally in cats, EPEC have been associated with diarrhea, often as a component of co-infections with viral or protozoal agents. Microscopic lesions characteristic of AEEC are typically found in the jejunum and ileum, less commonly in the colon, and in dogs, sometimes in the stomach.

A distinct subset of EPEC is the STEC, also known as **EHEC**. In addition to their ability to attach and efface, these strains produce cytotoxic Shiga toxins (Stx1 and its homologue Stx2 with its variants, c, d, e, f). Shiga toxin 1 is structurally identical to the Shiga toxin produced by *Shigella dysenteriae*, which has a profound CP effect. Because of their effect on Vero cells in culture, these *E. coli* are also referred to as **VTEC**. Shiga toxins, encoded in the genome of bacteriophages, are composed of an A subunit that has enzymatic activity and a B subunit that binds the toxin to the glycolipid receptor globotriaosylceramide (Gb3) on the cell surface. Once endocytosed and transferred via the Golgi apparatus to the rough endoplasmic reticulum, the toxin inhibits protein synthesis, which may be lethal to the target cell, and via separate mechanisms may induce apoptosis. The presence or absence of Gb3 on cell surfaces is a major determinant of the distribution of tissue susceptibility to Shiga toxins, which mainly affect intestinal epithelium and vascular endothelium. Some EHEC also produce hemolysins, which may assist survival in the gut by increasing iron availability. Acid tolerance may also promote colonization efficiency by enhancing survival in the stomach.

The EHEC strains produce disease predominantly in humans, although involvement of domestic animals has been highlighted in the public health arena because of the tendency for cattle and some other species to carry the organism subclinically, adherent to epithelium over lymphoid follicles in the rectal mucosa. Different variants of the Stx encoded by phage have been associated with clinical disease and carrier states in cattle. The most widely recognized EHEC serotype is **O157:H7**, a major pathogen in humans, although >200 other STEC serotypes have been identified. In addition to Shiga toxin production, virulence is attributable to attaching-and-effacing capability, encoded on the LEE.

In **calves <4-weeks-old** (generally >3-days-old, and most commonly in the second week of life), strains of EHEC (O5:NM, O8:H9, O26:H11, O103:H2, O111:NM, O111:H8, and O111:H11) have been associated with a syndrome of *erosive fibrinohemorrhagic enterocolitis*, with the development of dysentery. Fever is not characteristic, and animals may remain bright until the effects of dehydration and blood loss

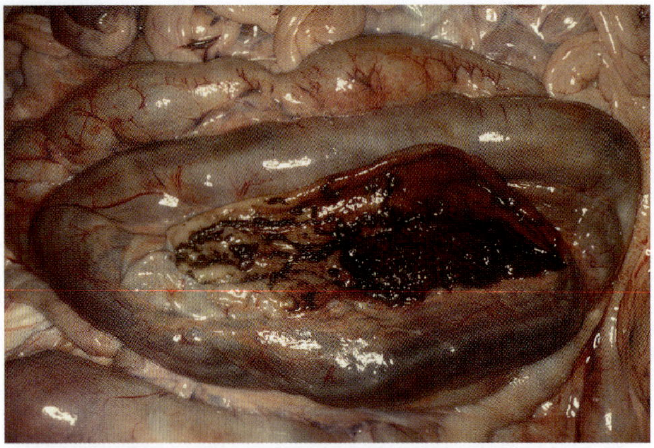

Figure 1-101 Attaching-and-effacing ***Escherichia coli*** infection. Fibrinohemorrhagic enteritis in the ileum of a calf.

supervene. Death may occur within several days of onset of illness, but some cases will recover in 7-10 days.

At autopsy, **gross lesions** are usually confined to the spiral colon and rectum, although the ileum and cecum are occasionally involved with mild fibrinous or fibrinohemorrhagic enteritis/typhlitis. In the colon, changes vary from mild patchy congestion of the mucosa to marked mucosal reddening, with adherent mucus, necrotic debris, and blood; colonic contents are fluid and frequently blood tinged (Fig. 1-101). There may be congestion of the margins of mucosal folds in the rectum, or overt fibrinohemorrhagic proctitis. Mesenteric lymph nodes are often enlarged, especially along the ileum, and occasionally there are lesions (arthritis, serositis) suggesting septicemia.

Microscopically, in affected small intestine the profile of villi is ragged or markedly scalloped, and they are blunted, moderately atrophic, or fused. Epithelial cells on villi in small bowel and on the colonic surface where lesions are most severe are short, rounded up, and in some cases exfoliating singly or in small clumps, causing focal microerosions. Cells in some areas may be markedly attenuated. The microvillus border is indistinct and covered by a heavy layer of prominent gram-negative coccobacilli (Fig. 1-102). Lesions in the large bowel may extend down into glands, which may be dilated, lined by flattened epithelium, and filled with sloughed epithelium and leukocytes. In the small intestine, foci of bacterial adhesion may be patchy, on the sides of the upper third of villi, with extensive surrounding areas of normal epithelium. Crypts in areas of atrophic small intestine may be elongate, with numerous mitotic figures. In severely affected bowel, the mucosa and submucosa are congested, edematous, and occasional microvascular thrombi may be present. Sloughed enterocytes, erythrocytes, neutrophils, fibrin, and bacteria are in the lumen.

In **dogs**, STEC have been associated with dysentery, and in some dogs, hemolytic uremic syndrome and cutaneous edema and ulceration. In Greyhounds, the syndrome involving this triad has been termed *cutaneous and renal glomerular vasculopathy* and has been attributed to consumption of beef contaminated with O157:H7 *E. coli*, and other STEC. Renal and cutaneous lesions are attributable to vascular damage caused by Shiga toxin (see Vol. 2, Urinary System; Vol. 1, Integumentary System).

Edema disease is a distinct syndrome in pigs, seen as sudden death, or the development of nervous signs associated

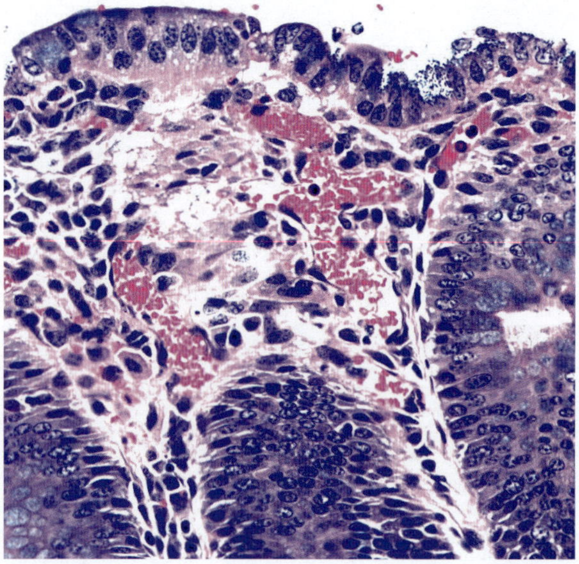

Figure 1-102 Attaching-and-effacing ***Escherichia coli*** infection. Adherent bacteria on the surface of necrotic enterocytes in the colon of a calf.

with enteric colonization by STEC, especially serotypes O138, O139, and O141. The disease occurs most commonly in pigs within a few weeks after weaning, or after other change in feeding or management. Colonization may be related to transient enterocyte malabsorption soon after weaning, which allows for increased dietary protein accumulation in the gut lumen. It often occurs in association with outbreaks of postweaning *E. coli* enteritis. Rare reports exist of edema disease in suckling and mature animals. The disease may be sporadic or occur as an outbreak, usually affecting the best animals in a group, and mortality often approaches 100% of affected animals. Edema disease and postweaning *E. coli* enteritis have apparently declined in prevalence in parts of North America, perhaps with the use of concentrate rations based largely on soybeans and corn, rather than other grains.

Bacterial colonization of the gut is mediated by *F18ab fimbriae*. Susceptibility of pigs is genetic and related to the presence of receptors for the fimbriae. A *Shiga toxin (Stx2e)* producing vascular injury and edema has been incriminated in the pathogenesis of edema disease, and vaccination with Stx2e toxoid almost entirely prevents edema disease.

Some strains of *E. coli* that cause edema disease also produce secretory enterotoxin. Diarrhea is not a usual concomitant of edema disease in individual animals. Significant gross or microscopic lesions in the intestinal mucosa do not occur in edema disease, which appears to be a *classical enterotoxemia*, the active principle being absorbed from the gut and acting at a distant site. However, the means by which the toxin enters the circulation is unknown. Stx2e can bind to erythrocytes, which may promote its dissemination from the intestine.

Experimentally, the target of Stx2e, like other Shiga toxins, is *vascular endothelium*, particularly of small arteries and arterioles. Preferentially affected organs include the spinal cord, cerebellum, eyelid, and colon. However, a study to determine preferential binding sites for Stx2e found receptors in a variety of tissues, not just the aforementioned. Stx2e causes *angiopathy*, which, in its early stages in experimental intoxication, is recognized by swelling of endothelial cells and mild intramural and perivascular hemorrhage. Pyknosis and karyorrhexis of smooth muscle nuclei, often accompanied by fibrinoid degeneration or hyaline change in the tunica media, may be seen in subacute spontaneous cases. Proliferative mesenchymal elements are found in the tunica media and tunica adventitia in more advanced cases. However, inflammation is not at any stage a prominent component of the angiopathy, nor of the associated edema in most sites, and thrombosis of vessels is rarely encountered. Edema is probably caused by vessel damage during the early stages of the angiopathy. The lesions are distinct from those expected with endotoxemia.

Swine with edema disease may die without premonitory signs. Others may have anorexia, or, more characteristically, show nervous signs, usually of <1 day's duration. An unsteady staggering gait, knuckling, ataxia, prostration and tremors, convulsions, and paddling occur. A hoarse squeal, the hoarseness attributed to laryngeal edema and dyspnea, also may be noted clinically.

At autopsy, **gross lesions** in acute deaths may be subtle or absent. Typically, *edema is variably present in one or more sites*. However, it may be mild and must be carefully sought, especially by "slipping" the suspected area over subjacent tissue. Subcutaneous edema may be present in the frontal area and over the snout, in the eyelids, and in the submandibular, ventral abdominal, and inguinal areas. Internally, there may be some hydropericardium, and serous pleural and peritoneal effusion, perhaps accompanied by mild or moderate pulmonary edema. More commonly, the serous surfaces merely appear glistening and wet. Edema of the mesocolon, of the submucosa of the cardiac glandular area of the stomach over the greater curvature, and of mesenteric lymph nodes is most consistently found. The gastric submucosal edema should be sought by carefully cutting through the muscularis to the submucosa; the lesion is best appreciated by making several slices through the serosa and external muscle to the submucosa on the greater curvature over the body of the stomach. The edema fluid is clear and slightly gelatinous (Fig. 1-103). It is rarely blood tinged, and overt hemorrhage is usually not present in uncomplicated edema disease. The stomach is often full of feed, but the small intestine is relatively empty and the mucosa is grossly normal. The colon may contain somewhat inspissated feces.

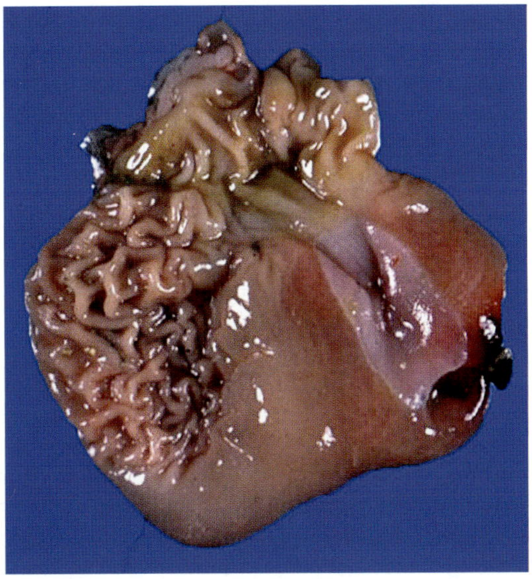

Figure 1-103 Edema disease. Edema of stomach wall in a pig. (Courtesy Noah's Arkives and A. Doster.)

In swine dying after a more prolonged clinical course, gross edema is often not present, although enlargement of mesenteric lymph nodes is present in a large proportion of cases. A few pigs may show foci of yellow malacia, usually bilaterally symmetrical, in the brainstem at various levels from basal ganglia to medulla.

Microscopically, edema in the sites of predilection mentioned earlier is the main lesion in swine dying acutely. It is generally devoid of much protein and contains a few erythrocytes and inflammatory cells. A proportion of animals also will have meningeal edema and distended perivascular spaces in the brain. Vascular lesions may not be well developed in pigs dying suddenly. When present, they usually consist of edema, hemorrhage, myocyte necrosis, and hyaline degeneration in the tunica media. Angiopathy is more consistently found in cases of longer standing. Affected vessels may be found in any tissue in the carcass, but most commonly in the brain and intestinal tract (submucosa of stomach, intestine, and mesentery). Brain edema and focal encephalomalacia in the brainstem are associated with lesions in cerebral vessels; necrosis may be a sequel to edema and ischemia. *Cerebrospinal angiopathy of swine* is probably a manifestation of edema disease.

A **diagnosis** of edema disease is based on nervous signs or sudden death in growing pigs, in association with typical gross and microscopic lesions, when they are present. In acute cases, heavy growth of hemolytic *E. coli* of one of the serotypes known to produce Stx2e is essential.

Edema disease must be differentiated from enteritis and endotoxemia resulting from *E. coli* in postweaning pigs; from mulberry heart disease in animals dying suddenly; and from salt poisoning, *Salmonella* meningoencephalitis, and other infectious encephalitides, in animals with nervous signs.

Postweaning *E. coli* enteritis (coliform enteritis of weaned pigs) typically occurs during the first week or two following weaning, or after some other change in feed or management. Postweaning diarrhea may be caused by classical enterotoxigenic F4 (K88) *E. coli*, but it is often associated with hemolytic *E. coli* of the same serotypes primarily implicated in edema disease, as well as serotype O149. The 2 diseases often occur in the same population of pigs, although usually affecting different animals. However, several other pathogens have been found in feces of pigs with postweaning E. coli enteritis, suggesting that at least some of these agents may be also associated with the condition. Agents detected included *B. pilosicoli*, *C. perfringens*, *Cryptosporidium* spp., *Cystoisospora suis*, ETEC, *L. intracellularis*, PCV2 and PCV3, rotavirus A, B, C, and H, *S. enterica* spp. *enterica*, and *Trichuri suis*. Typically, postweaning colibacillosis is a disease of high morbidity and variable mortality, with loss of condition in pigs suffering prolonged illness. Diarrhea is usually yellow and fluid and stains the perineum. Deaths that occur may or may not follow a prior episode of diarrhea and often appear to be related to endotoxemia.

In fatal cases, there may be blue-red discoloration of the skin and evidence of dehydration. **Grossly**, deep-red *gastric venous infarcts* are present in some cases (Fig. 1-104). The small intestine is flaccid. The mucosa may be normal in color and the content creamy. In other animals, the mucosa of the distal small intestine is congested and the contents watery and perhaps blood tinged or brown with flecks of yellow mucus or

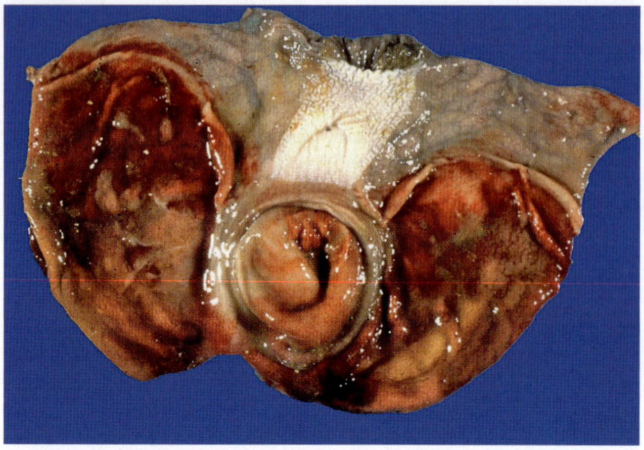

Figure 1-104 Gastric infarction. Deep-red areas of venous infarction in the gastric mucosa associated with postweaning colibacillosis in a pig.

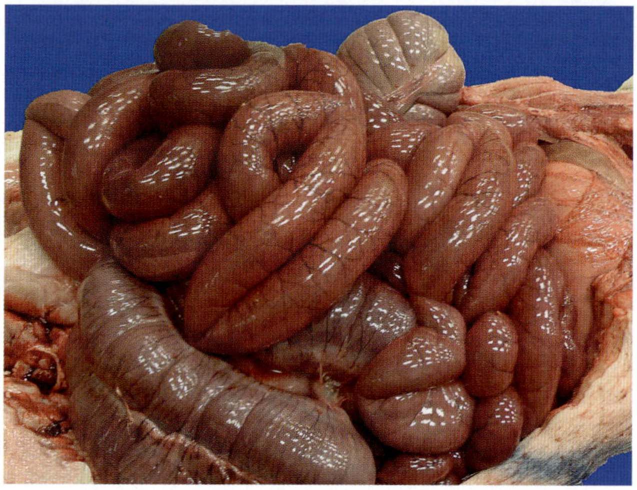

Figure 1-105 Postweaning colibacillosis. Acute enteritis, with congested, flaccid small intestine in a pig. (Courtesy Iowa State University Veterinary Diagnostic Laboratory.)

fibrin (Fig. 1-105). Cecal and colonic lesions are usually mild, but there may be some congestion and fibrinous exudate in the proximal large bowel. Mesenteric lymph nodes may be somewhat enlarged, congested, and juicy. Other organs are usually unremarkable grossly.

The **pathogenesis** of postweaning *E. coli* enteritis caused by non-F4 *E. coli* is poorly understood, and the microscopic histopathology is not well described. In swine with diarrhea, *E. coli* may be attached to the surface of villi by F18ac fimbriae (Fig. 1-106). Experimentally, stress and decreased mucosal immune functions associated with early weaning have been associated with ETEC and postweaning diarrhea. Like edema disease, high protein levels in the intestinal lumen at weaning may play a role in colonization and disease development. Atrophy of villi does not seem to be evident, and diarrhea is presumed to be mediated by enterotoxins. Mortality may be ascribed to dehydration in animals with prolonged diarrhea and few gross intestinal or extraintestinal lesions. In animals dying of more acute disease, there is local microvascular thrombosis in sections of congested mucosa, and the gross and

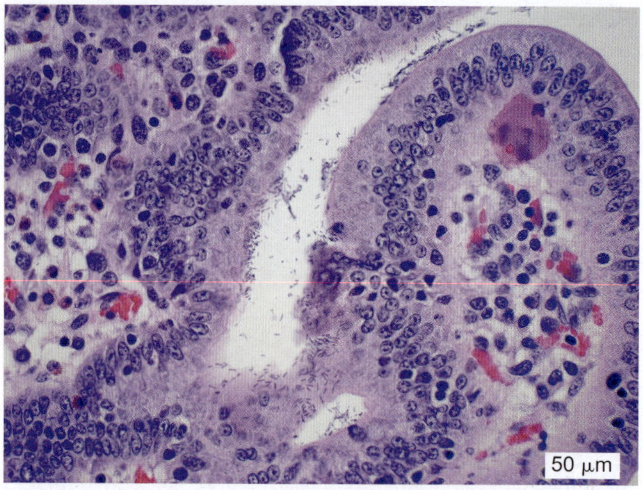

Figure 1-106 Postweaning colibacillosis. *Escherichia coli* attached to the epithelial surface of the villus in postweaning colibacillosis in a pig. (Courtesy Iowa State University Veterinary Diagnostic Laboratory.)

microscopic lesions in other organs, especially those related to gastric mucosal and submucosal thrombosis and venous infarction, are suggestive of endotoxemia. Hemolytic *E. coli* of the implicated strains are consistently isolated in virtually pure culture from the lower small intestine and colon. However, they are present in the spleen and liver in only a few cases, suggesting terminal bacteremia.

The factors predisposing to the massive colonization of hemolytic *E. coli* are unclear. Loss of lactogenic immunity, a favorable environment for proliferation of bacterial strains with specific nutrient requirements, and promotion of epithelial colonization by the effects of antecedent rotaviral infection have been variously implicated.

A **diagnosis** of postweaning colibacillosis is suggested by the gross lesions in animals dying acutely or subacutely, and it is confirmed by culture and serotyping of associated strains of *E. coli*. Reduced rectal temperature, alkaline feces, and reduced skin elasticity, possibly indicating dehydration, have been described in pigs with postweaning *E. coli* enteritis, and these findings may help with the diagnosis. The fatal disease must be differentiated from edema disease, proliferative hemorrhagic enteropathy, salmonellosis, and swine dysentery. Postweaning diarrhea caused by uncomplicated rotaviral infection, TGEV, or associated with attaching-effacing O45:K "E65" *E. coli* is usually nonfatal.

Enteroinvasive *E. coli*. Strains of *E. coli* infecting humans and certain other species are recognized that have the capacity to invade or to be internalized by surface enterocytes of the small and large intestine, in which they multiply. In this sense, they resemble *Shigella* in primates, and *Salmonella* in several species. The enteroinvasiveness of *Shigella* and some strains of *E. coli* appears to be correlated with a high–molecular-weight plasmid coding for outer membrane proteins involved in invasion. Multiplication of the organism within epithelial cells results in *local erosion and ulceration*, associated with acute inflammation in the mucosa.

Among domestic animals, *enteroinvasive colibacillosis has only been confirmed experimentally in neonatal swine*, using a strain of O101 *E. coli*. Spontaneous enteritis that appears to be due to EIEC is rarely encountered in piglets up to weaning and in calves <2-weeks-old. Diarrhea in experimentally infected piglets is described as gray-yellow, watery, and containing small clots. The gross findings may not be remarkable, or the intestine may appear congested compared with that in most diarrheic piglets. In spontaneous cases suspected of being due to EIEC, the gastric fundus also may be congested, and this is correlated with the venous infarction visible microscopically. Experimental enteroinvasive colibacillosis in piglets causes villus atrophy that is comparable in severity to that induced by the common viruses of neonates. Enterocytes appear cuboidal or flattened and some are seen lysing. The lamina propria is edematous; capillaries are congested and infiltrated by neutrophils and other inflammatory cells. In spontaneous cases, thrombi may be evident in proprial capillaries and submucosal lymphatics. Neutrophils and tissue fluid effuse into the lumen between villi through epithelial discontinuities. Similar microthrombosis, proprial inflammation, enterocyte destruction, and effusion may be found in the cecum and colon. Intracellular organisms of O serogroup 101 were demonstrated by immunoperoxidase staining in the experimental study, but are not generally recognized in spontaneous cases suspected to be due to EIEC. Edema and neutrophil accumulation in sinusoids of mesenteric lymph nodes are present. Experimental enteroinvasive colibacillosis in piglets has been associated with malabsorption and protein loss into the gut, presumably a result of villus atrophy and effusive enteritis, respectively.

There is convincing evidence that select invasive *E. coli* are involved in the histiocytic and ulcerative colitis of Boxers, French Bulldogs, and possibly other breeds. In these dogs, *E. coli* are noted within lamina proprial macrophages and mesenteric lymph nodes. A role for this agent in disease development is supported by improvement of clinical signs and mucosal inflammation after its removal from the mucosa by antimicrobial therapy. Evidence indicates that a genetic predisposition to this invasive *E. coli* exists in these breeds. There are similarities between this *E. coli* and AIEC described as playing a role in human IBD.

Septicemic colibacillosis. Generalized systemic infection with *E. coli* occurs commonly in *calves*, and less commonly or sporadically, especially among young animals of the other domestic species. Predisposition to infection is a prerequisite for *E. coli* septicemia. This usually results from reduced transfer or absorption of maternal colostral immunoglobulin, or from intercurrent disease or debilitation. But certain strains of *E. coli*, especially O8, O9, O15, O26, O35, O45, O78, O86, O101, O117, and O137 in calves and lambs, and O115 in pigs and calves, are particularly associated with septicemia and may possess characteristics that enhance their ability to invade and proliferate systemically in compromised animals.

Among factors conferring virulence upon these strains are plasmids coding for colicin V (Col V). Col V plasmids carry genes coding for aerobactin, a bacterial hydroxamate siderophore permitting survival in low-iron extracellular environments; outer membrane proteins resisting bactericidal effects of serum, such as complement activation; and hydrophobic properties that impede phagocytosis, conferred by a capsule. Some produce cytolethal distending toxin, or fimbriae that impede phagocytosis. Endotoxin released by dying bacteria causes the vascular damage and shock associated with *E. coli* septicemia.

The portal of entry of *E. coli* causing septicemia probably varies somewhat. The navel in the neonate, the upper respiratory tract and possibly the tonsil, and the intestine in neonates and older animals are likely sites. In calves, adhesins such as P, F17, AfaE-VIII, and CS31A may promote enteric colonization and invasion. Enteritis is not a necessary, or even common, concomitant of colisepticemia in animals.

Colisepticemia is most commonly a disease of neonates and may vary from peracute septicemia and endotoxemia resulting in sudden death, to subacute or chronic disease in which signs are related to sites of bacterial localization, especially in the meninges, joints, and eyes.

The lesions associated with colisepticemia in young animals of any species, especially calves, lambs, and foals, may vary from subtle to obvious. Mortality in hypogammaglobulinemic neonates may occur acutely with little in the way of abnormal gross findings. These may be limited to mildly congested or blue-red, slightly rubbery lungs, and a firm spleen, perhaps with evidence of omphalitis. *Microscopic changes* in the lungs include thickening of alveolar septa by mononuclear cells and neutrophils, and effusion of lightly fibrinous exudate and a few neutrophils into alveoli. There may be a corona of neutrophils around white pulp in the spleen, and neutrophils may be present in abnormal numbers in circulation in many organs, including lung and hepatic sinusoids. Kupffer cells also may be prominent in sinusoids in the liver. Fibrin thrombi may be evident in pulmonary capillaries, glomeruli, and hepatic sinusoids. Some calves develop acute interstitial nephritis with foci of neutrophil accumulation, which with time evolve into the so-called "white-spotted kidney" in surviving animals.

Grossly, *more severe acute cases* show evidence of serosal hemorrhage, with perhaps some serosanguineous pericardial fluid. The lungs may be deep red-blue, rubbery, and fail to collapse. Interlobular septa may be slightly separated by edema, and froth or fluid may be present in the major airways. Meningeal vessels may be congested, and the meninges wet. The abomasum or stomach may have focal superficial ulcers, or more extensive deep-red areas of venous infarction. There may be evidence of diarrhea and dehydration, with congestion of the small intestine. *Microscopic lesions* resemble those previously described, with more severe congestion, thrombosis, and edema in the lungs, and perhaps other tissues. In cases not examined for some time after death, clumps of small bacilli may be seen in vessels throughout the body. The vascular permeability, thrombosis, and hemorrhage reflect endotoxemia and its sequelae.

Subacute cases may develop localized infection on serous surfaces, in the joints and meninges. Fibrinous peritonitis, pleuritis, and pericarditis, fibrinopurulent arthritis and meningitis, and hypopyon are commonly found, alone or in various combinations. Affected animals may have a history of lameness ascribable to arthritis, nervous signs caused by meningitis, or general debilitation. Microscopic examination reveals the lesions already described in animals with active systemic disease, with the addition of extensive congestion and edema of inflamed serous surfaces, associated with an acute fibrinous inflammatory exudate.

In *lambs*, congestion and edema of the mucosa of turbinates and sinuses, perhaps with mucopurulent-to-hemorrhagic sinusitis, have been described. Fibrinous polyserositis and arthritis are sporadic manifestations of *E. coli* septicemia in growing or adult swine and must be differentiated from the more significant *Haemophilus*, *Mycoplasma*, and streptococcal infections causing these lesions. Colisepticemia is a sporadic cause of mortality in litters of young puppies.

Diagnosis of colisepticemia is based on the isolation of *E. coli* in large numbers from more than one parenchymatous organ or other internal site, other than mesenteric lymph node (preferably the liver, spleen, lung, or kidney), or from a site of serosal localization, in conjunction with compatible gross and/or microscopic lesions.

"Watery mouth," a syndrome of drooling, depression, loss of appetite, and abomasal and abdominal distension, is associated with *E. coli* infection/bacteremia in lambs <3-days-old in the United Kingdom. At **autopsy**, affected lambs are in poor condition. They may have unclotted milk and mucinous fluid in the distended abomasum; there is gas in the abomasum and intestine, and meconium retention is common. It is hypothesized that *E. coli* colonize the bowel, and in some manner cause loss of motility and functional obstruction. Fluid and gas accumulate in the abomasum. Bacteremia/septicemia is terminal.

Salmonellosis

The **taxonomy of *Salmonella*** is based on molecular genetic analysis. The genus *Salmonella* is considered to be composed of 2 species, ***Salmonella bongori*** and ***S. enterica***. There are 6 subspecies of *S. enterica* [*enterica* (I), *salamae* (II), *arizonae* (IIIa), *diarizonae* (IIIb), *indica* (VI), and *houtenae* (IV)] and many (>2,500) antigenically distinct serovars. About 60% of *Salmonella* serotypes belong to *S. enterica* subsp. *enterica* and occur in birds and mammals. Members of *S. e. enterica* are the predominant cause of salmonellosis in humans and domestic animals, but <50 of these serovars have been isolated from mammals or birds with some frequency worldwide. The remainder of *S. enterica* and *S. bongori* serovars are found in ectothermic animals or the environment. In conventional terminology, the serovars have been treated as species, but in the new terminology the names of serovars are capitalized, but not italicized (e.g., *S. enterica* subsp. *enterica* serovar Typhimurium when first used, followed later by *Salmonella* Typhimurium). They are usually named on the basis of the locality in which the serovar was first isolated or identified, or on their host association and the clinical syndrome they may produce. Characterization of isolates at the subserotype level, by phage typing, plasmid profile analysis, or other molecular techniques, is desirable when there is evidence of zoonotic transmission, or when epidemiologic tracing is necessary.

The **clinical and pathologic syndromes of salmonellosis** typically vary from localized enterocolitis to septicemia; abortion may also occur, with or without obvious systemic disease. Although some serotypes are strongly host adapted, others have a very wide host range. Highly host-adapted serotypes, such as *Salmonella* Typhi (humans), *Salmonella* Dublin (cattle), and *Salmonella* Choleraesuis (swine), tend to produce severe systemic disease in adult, as well as juvenile animals; serotypes with a broad host range, for example, *Salmonella* Typhimurium, tend to affect predominantly young animals in most species, and mainly cause enterocolitis, although septicemia may occur. There may be overlap between the 2 forms of disease, and if the animal survives, a carrier state of variable duration usually follows.

Subclinical carriage of *Salmonella* may be common, depending on the species, and transmission can occur directly, or indirectly, by contamination of feed, water, or the environment, from which the organism is ingested or inhaled. Stressors that compromise immune competence or disrupt the enteric bacterial ecosystem are often implicated in salmonellosis, and disease is usually more common and severe in young animals. The more common *stressors* associated with salmonellosis in domestic animals include transportation, starvation, changes in the ration, overcrowding, pregnancy, parturition, exertion, anesthesia, surgery, intercurrent disease, immunosuppressive drugs, and oral treatment with antibiotics and anthelmintics. Consequent changes in the anaerobic bacterial ecosystem that alter the volatile fatty acid composition of the enteric environment are permissive of *Salmonella* colonization.

There are many examples of enhanced susceptibility to salmonellosis associated with intercurrent disease. The best known is that between the *CSFV* and *Salmonella* Choleraesuis in pigs, an association so close as to have caused early pathologists to disregard the bacterium as a significant pathogen. The disease in adult cattle is usually sporadic, and often there are predisposing conditions, such as parturient paresis, ketosis, mastitis, and parasitic infestations. The stress of anesthesia and surgery may account in part for the serious outbreaks of salmonellosis that occur in hospitalized animals, especially horses, at veterinary schools.

The **pathogenesis of salmonellosis** may be divided into several stages: *access* of the intestinal tract of the host by the bacteria and attainment of the primary site of infection, usually the enterocyte; attachment to the surface (*colonization*); and *invasion* of enterocytes.

For infection to take place, *Salmonella* must be present in sufficient numbers; generally, a minimal infective oral dose of 10^7-10^9 organisms is needed for experimental infection of large domestic animals. However, the minimal infective dose varies with different serotypes and animal species. After ingestion, the *Salmonella* must overcome nonspecific resistance factors, including the bactericidal effects of salivary enzymes, and the acid pH of the gastric environment. Mucus and lysozymes in the glycocalyx, peristalsis, commensal luminal microbial population, and constant sloughing of enterocytes may interfere with attachment. Those organisms that survive the nonspecific resistance factors may colonize and invade enterocytes.

Invading *Salmonella* in some species enter the mucosa through M cells in the Peyer patches, and host specificity of some *Salmonella* serotypes may be associated in part with specific receptor sites on these cells. *Salmonella* have been demonstrated in the Peyer patches as early as 6 hours postinoculation by the oral route. However, in some experimental models, the bacterium can be detected in Peyer patches even earlier than that. Although *Salmonella* has specific tropism for M cells, which are the first cells that the microorganism adheres to, smaller numbers of *Salmonella* may enter through enterocytes in other areas of the small intestine.

In salmonellosis characterized primarily by enterocolitis, the organisms do not usually disseminate beyond the mucosa and the mesenteric lymph nodes, and the ensuing inflammation remains confined to the intestine. In those cases in which bacteremia ensues, the organisms must be able to survive and replicate in macrophages and disseminate to other systemic sites, such as the liver, lung, joints, meninges, or placenta and fetus. In *Salmonella* Dublin infection, the bacteria are present within macrophages in the intestinal mucosa but are free in lymph in the draining lymphatics, and dissemination is likely via lymphatics.

The ability to attach, invade, and penetrate intestinal epithelial cells (including goblet cells) *is crucial to virulence*, and is the first step in the development of salmonellosis. A number of known virulence factors contribute to the pathogenesis of salmonellosis, including motility, pili, or fimbriae, effector proteins modifying the metabolism or causing death of host cells, and LPSs. The information for such virulence attributes is often encoded in chromosomes in clusters of genes known as *Salmonella* pathogenicity islands (SPI).

Invasion of enterocytes, especially those in the ileum, occurs within 12 hours of oral infection. Ability to invade cells is dependent on a type III secretion system encoded in SPI1. Effector proteins are translocated into host cells, where they facilitate bacterial invasion by causing changes in the cytoskeleton and ruffling of the cell membrane at the apical surface of the cell, favoring *Salmonella* invasion. Outer membrane vesicles are secreted from the surface of the bacterium and are internalized by the host cells. These vesicles also carry bacterial proteins into the cell that are important for internalization.

Motility, associated with the presence of flagella, is characteristic of many *Salmonella* serovars. Bacterial motility is generally not considered to be an important virulence determinant. However, it may enhance the movement of bacteria through the glycocalyx and facilitate attachment to specific receptor sites on enterocytes.

Fimbriae (pilus adhesins) encoded in chromosomes and on virulence plasmids are present on salmonellae, and they may play a role in colonization of the gut. Adherence of *Salmonella* to intestinal epithelial cells takes place in 2 stages. The first step is reversible because the organisms can be easily washed off. Weak ionic and nonionic interactions between bacterial and host cell membrane surfaces are thought to be the binding forces responsible for this attachment. The second stage, referred to as *receptor-mediated endocytosis*, is irreversible. It occurs after a few-minutes lag period, with degeneration of the microvilli on epithelial cells, "ruffling" of the cell membrane, and macropinocytosis, resulting in internalization into membrane-bound vacuoles (endosomes) containing *Salmonella*.

The ultrastructural changes of *Salmonella* infection in the intestine were first described in experimental infections of guinea pigs. Large numbers of organisms are present in the lumen, on the surface of the brush border, and in enterocytes. There is an increase in the number of neutrophils in the gut lumen and within intercellular spaces, and some of these contain bacteria. Degeneration of microvilli, with loss of filamentous cores, is associated with close adherence of bacteria. Other changes consist of elongation, swelling, budding and fusion of microvilli, and loss of the terminal web.

The organisms usually invade the cells through the brush border; however, they may also enter the mucosa through the intercellular junctional complex. In the cytoplasm, the bacteria are located within membrane-bound vacuoles, which may also contain remnants of microvilli and cytoplasmic debris. Most organisms remain intact and multiply during their transcellular migration in endosomes. Often, many bacteria are present in a single enterocyte during the early stages of infection, but cellular damage is mild and transient. The *Salmonella*-receptor complex dissociates as a result of the acidification of the endosomal content, allowing the receptor site to return to the apical plasma membrane and repeat the processes of endocytosis. After 24 hours, most bacteria are located within membrane-bound vacuoles in macrophages in the lamina propria. The intracellular survival is mediated by a type III secretion system.

The **lipopolysaccharide (LPS)** moiety of *Salmonella* with smooth cell walls consists of an *O-specific side chain, a core portion, and a lipid A portion*. Most *Salmonella* isolated from animals have smooth cell walls, which influences virulence in several ways. These strains are more invasive and are more successful at avoiding phagocytosis, and lysis in phagolysosomes after invasion, than are "rough" counterparts with incomplete LPS. LPSs reduce the susceptibility of the organisms to the host's cationic proteins; they stimulate local prostaglandin synthesis; and they prevent the activation and deposition of complement on the bacterial surface.

The main function of LPS may be to facilitate survival in the intestinal mucosa and eventual entry into deeper tissues. The involvement of LPS in invasion apparently varies among *Salmonella* serotypes because some strains of *Salmonella* Typhimurium do not require intact LPS to invade epithelial cells in vitro. On the contrary, more host-specific *Salmonella* serotypes, such as *Salmonella* Typhi and *Salmonella* Choleraesuis, require intact LPS or O-side chains. The lipid A portion of LPS is responsible for the endotoxin-mediated effects of *Salmonella* infection that are seen in systemic disease. Septicemia (endotoxemia) typically causes fever, leukopenia, hemoconcentration, lactic acidosis, coagulopathies, hypotension, and death.

Diarrhea in salmonellosis is not mediated by enterotoxins such as those involved in cholera and *E. coli* infections. Rather, *effector proteins* associated with SPI1 induce secretory diarrhea by blocking chloride channel closure; others attract neutrophils and induce apoptosis of enterocytes. Proteins encoded in SPI5 also promote neutrophil recruitment and electrolyte secretion. Mucosal inflammation leads to the accumulation of a number of mediators, including prostaglandin E2, capable of causing hypersecretion of chloride by enterocytes, and consequent passive osmotic movement of water into the lumen. Loss of enterocytes, dying as a sequel to *Salmonella* invasion and neutrophil-induced tissue injury, results in a reduction in absorptive surface area and causes defects in mucosal integrity, through which the protein- and neutrophil-rich exudate leaking from permeable vessels effuses.

Thus diarrhea is an outcome of active secretion of electrolyte, malabsorption resulting from reduced mucosal surface area and enterocyte competence, and inflammatory exudation, which may contain sufficient fibrinogen to form a pseudomembrane over the affected surface. The volume of fluid originating in lesions in the small intestine may overwhelm the capacity of the colon to compensate; as often as not in salmonellosis, the large intestinal mucosa is also involved, further compounding the compromise to electrolyte and water homeostasis in the gut.

Thrombosis of mucosal venules is common in *Salmonella* enteritis and may contribute to loss of mucosal viability. Such lesions may be due in part to the large amounts of **endotoxin** absorbed through the damaged mucosa or released locally.

Salmonella is a strong proinflammatory stimulus, but this pathogen also evolved to take advantage of the inflamed intestinal environment to overcome the microbiota through various mechanisms, for example, resistance to lipocalin, tetrathionate respiration, and others.

Enteritis in salmonellosis is thus seen as *fibrinous or fibrinohemorrhagic exudates over denuded small and large intestinal mucosae*, directly mediated by the apoptosis, necrosis, and/or pyroptosis induced by invading bacteria, and by the necrotizing effects of local neutrophil activity and microvascular thrombosis.

The **systemic outcome of an infection with *Salmonella*** is determined by the genetic virulence determinants of the invading organism and the ensuing innate, humoral, and cell-mediated immune response of the host. Salmonellae are considered to be *facultative intracellular pathogens*, and invading strains must have the ability to survive and replicate within macrophages to cause bacteremia or septicemia. This capacity is conferred by components coded in SPI2, perhaps largely through inhibition of NADPH oxidase-mediated oxidative killing of *Salmonella* in cytoplasmic vacuoles, and in some species by factors encoded in SPI2 and SPI3. The virulence of several serotypes commonly associated with systemic infections in animals, including *Salmonella* Typhimurium, *Salmonella* Dublin, and *Salmonella* Choleraesuis, is enhanced by intracellular survival in macrophages mediated by attributes encoded on virulence plasmids.

Salmonella taken up by resident macrophages elicit a *major immune response* in the host. Initiation of the innate immune response commences with pattern recognition receptors, such as TLR, which recognize conserved bacterial motifs. Ligation of these receptors promotes proinflammatory cytokine production and recruitment of neutrophils. There is considerable controversy about the roles played by cell-mediated and humoral immunity in the pathogenesis of salmonellosis, but *Salmonella* infection results in the release of cytokines by specifically stimulated T lymphocytes. They activate macrophages that phagocytose the organisms, and in such a circumstance, cell-mediated immunity is of paramount importance.

Once salmonellae cross the intestinal epithelium, they may enter the bloodstream via the lymphatics, perhaps carried in macrophages, and cause septicemia or transient bacteremia. Or they may remain indefinitely in the gut-associated lymphoid tissues and mesenteric lymph nodes. Increased susceptibility to salmonellosis in animals with intercurrent disease, or subjected to stress, may be related to relaxation of cell-mediated immunity to the organism. Septicemia may be of variable duration and severity but, as a rule, it is rapidly fatal in young animals. If, however, there is transient bacteremia, the organisms are removed by fixed macrophages, especially those of the spleen, liver, and bone marrow. They may continue to proliferate in such extravascular locations and subsequently may cause another bacteremic phase that may result in fatal septicemia or secondary localization in other tissues.

The carrier state is important in the epidemiology of the disease. Whether *Salmonella* can maintain themselves in the intestinal lumen is not clear; to some extent fecal shedding is likely to depend on intermittent seeding from the bile, or from macrophages in the lamina propria and gut-associated lymphoid tissue. The duration of the carrier state may be prolonged, or animals may rid themselves of the infection, probably by means of cell-mediated immunity. The carrier state is an unstable one, for it appears that if the carrier is subjected to some stress or debilitating disease, it may succumb to disease; this often seems to occur in adult cattle. The carrier animal is a potential threat to any other animal that it contacts, either directly or through the medium of its excreta, or by-products such as bone or meat meal.

Salmonellosis in swine. Many serotypes of *Salmonella* have been isolated from swine, and with poultry and cattle they form an *important reservoir of the organism*. The bacteria are carried in the lamina propria of the intestine, but also in the regional lymph nodes or tonsils of the alimentary tract, and therefore carrier animals may not excrete the organism in the feces.

Historically, several distinct syndromes have been associated with *Salmonella* infections in swine: 1) **septicemic salmonellosis** is usually associated with the host-adapted *Salmonella* Choleraesuis var. Kunzendorf, although enteric lesions may also be present with this serovar. Although important historically worldwide, this serotype is now infrequently identified in North American swine. Sporadic infections and septicemia associated with *Salmonella* Dublin have also been described in nursing pigs. 2) *Salmonella* Typhimurium is now probably the most commonly isolated serotype and causes **acute or chronic enterocolitis**, including necrotizing proctitis, which may rarely lead to rectal stricture. 3) *Salmonella* Typhisuis infection has been associated with infrequent localized outbreaks of **ulcerative enterocolitis** in pigs, as well as caseous tonsillitis and lymphadenitis.

Several other serotypes can also cause sporadic disease in swine, but these are usually transient and occur secondary to other factors, such as immunocompromise, debilitation, or exposure to large bacterial doses. Most outbreaks occur in weaned pigs, and although disease is generally infrequent, infection is quite common. Ongoing concerns about public health and foodborne illnesses related to *Salmonella* contamination of pork products and development or persistence of antimicrobial resistance are beyond the scope of this text, but it drives continued research and expansion of our knowledge of the epidemiology and pathogenesis of *Salmonella*-associated infection and disease.

***Salmonella* Choleraesuis** was once thought to be the cause of classical swine fever because gross lesions of septicemic salmonellosis and acute classical swine fever are similar; *Salmonella* Choleraesuis is recovered from a significant percentage of pigs with classical swine fever. Although rarely identified in modern diagnostic laboratories, *Salmonella* Cholerasuis is isolated almost exclusively from diseased pigs (usually with septicemia). The major clinical manifestations of *Salmonella* Choleraesuis infection are *septicemia and enteritis*, which occur mostly in weaned pigs <5-6-months-old and only rarely in other ages. Clinical signs are first associated with sepsis and include lethargy, pyrexia, and cyanosis of extremities (Fig. 1-107); as the disease progresses, signs may become attributable to localized or system-specific inflammation, such

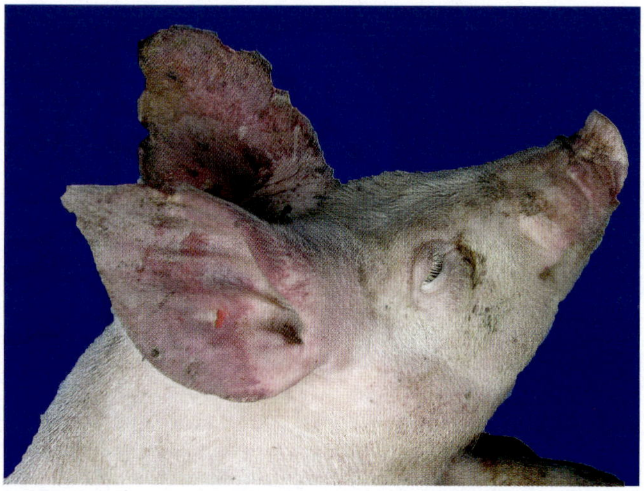

Figure 1-107 Septicemic salmonellosis. Congestion of skin of ears and snout due to microvascular thrombosis caused by endotoxemia in a pig. (Courtesy D. Driemeier.)

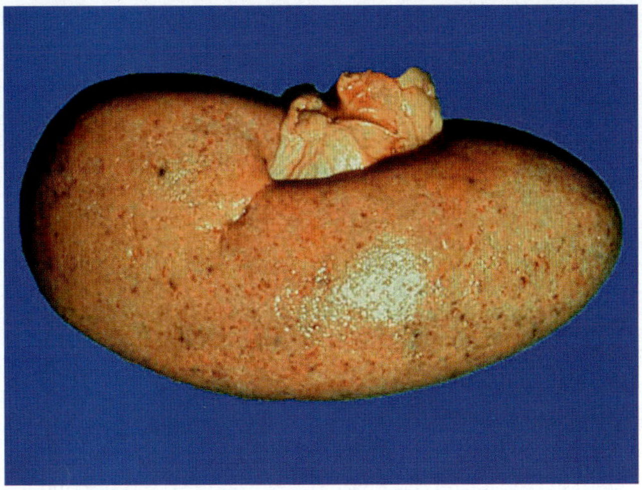

Figure 1-108 Septicemic salmonellosis. Petechiae in the kidney of a pig. (Courtesy Joint Pathology Center.)

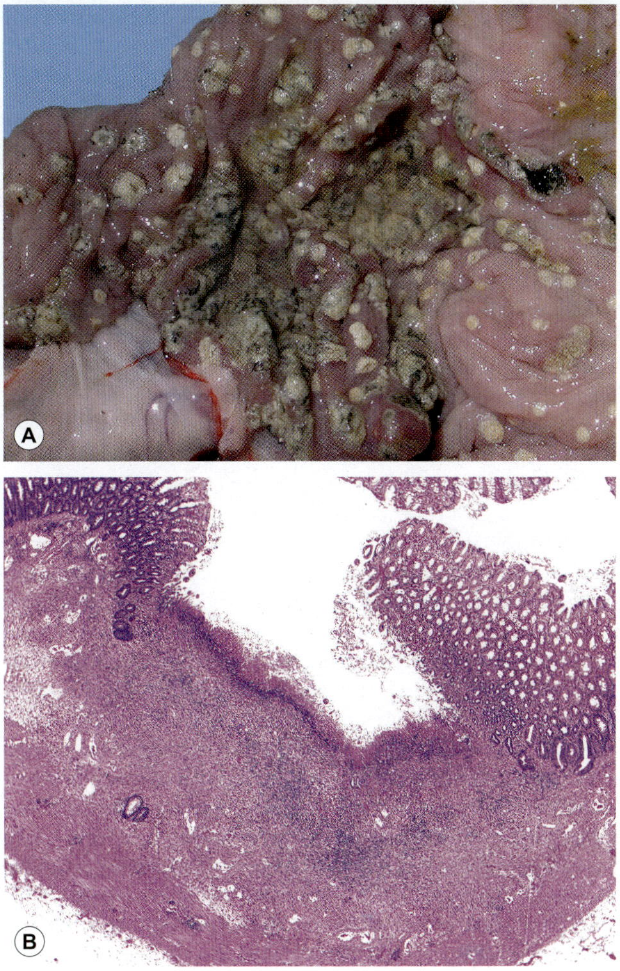

Figure 1-109 Porcine salmonellosis. **A.** Button ulcers in colon. (Courtesy D. Driemeier.) **B.** Deep colonic ulceration with elevated margins.

as diarrhea (enterocolitis), neurologic signs (encephalitis or meningitis), or respiratory distress or dyspnea (fibrinous pneumonia). Cases of *Salmonella*-associated septicemia may be acutely fatal. Sows may abort during the septicemic phase of infection. Pigs that have recovered from this phase may have dry gangrene of the ears and tail, paraplegia, blindness, and diphtheritic fibrinous enteritis. Although not classically associated with enterocolitis, a *chronic or enteric form* may occasionally develop following acute sepsis, with loose yellow feces containing flakes of fibrin, progressive emaciation and debility, and eventual death. Some pigs recover but fail to thrive, often partly owing to chronic bronchopneumonia.

At **autopsy**, the lesions of *Salmonella* Choleraesuis are attributable to sepsis and endotoxemia. There is blue or purple discoloration and ischemic necrosis of the *skin*, especially of the extremities, head, and ears. Petechiae are observed in many organs and tissues, including the skin, spleen, liver, kidney (Fig. 1-108), lung, heart, brain, synovial membranes of joints, GI tract, and lymph nodes. The GI lymph nodes are often prominently enlarged, congested, and hemorrhagic; other nodes throughout the body can also be affected but are usually less prominent. The *lungs* fail to collapse due to acute fibrinous interstitial pneumonia, which is seen grossly as firm and often hemorrhagic lung parenchyma with prominent interstitial and interlobular edema. Bronchopneumonia may also develop and be evident as consolidation of cranioventral lungs with exudate present in the airways on section. The spleen is often enlarged, congested, and firm with sharp edges. The *liver* is also enlarged, often congested, and has focal capsular petechiae or ecchymoses. In many cases, there will also be random yellow-tan areas of necrosis, secondary to embolic dissemination of bacteria; these are referred to as *paratyphoid nodules*.

The *stomach* has intense red-black discoloration due to severe congestion and possibly venous infarction that is observed with endotoxemia in pigs. In animals that survive the acute septicemia and endotoxemia, fibrinous-to-hemorrhagic enterocolitis may develop, which may include the appearance of well-demarcated deep ulcers with elevated irregular surfaces (so-called *button ulcers*, Fig. 1-109A and B), although often there are no lesions in the *intestinal tract*. There may also be polysynovitis and polyarthritis, with increased fluid and synovial hyperplasia.

The **histologic changes** that occur in internal organs in acute disease are mainly associated with *endothelial damage resulting from endotoxin*, and *wide dissemination of bacteria*. The most diagnostically helpful lesions are probably located in the liver, where there are randomly distributed foci of hepatocellular coagulative necrosis, and, depending on the duration and chronicity, these are often infiltrated with variable numbers of neutrophils and macrophages (*parathyroid nodules*). Paratyphoid nodules are also observed in the spleen, lymph nodes, or within other filter organs, such as the lung or kidney. In the spleen, there can also be diffuse histiocytosis and increased parenchymal neutrophils, as well as hemorrhage and scattered clusters of gram-negative bacteria. In small arterioles and capillaries of various organs (especially the gastric mucosa, skin, renal glomeruli, and lung), there is fibrinoid necrosis, leukocytoclastic vasculitis, endothelial hyperplasia, perivascular mixed inflammation, and frequently fibrin thrombosis; gram-negative bacteria are usually evident in large colonies. In the lung (in addition to vascular lesions), there is also diffuse histiocytic-to-fibrinous interstitial pneumonia and prominent edema and recruited alveolar macrophages.

Meningoencephalomyelitis occurs in a small proportion of cases of septicemic salmonellosis, and lesions include vasculitis, petechiation, and increased meningeal and perivascular neutrophils and mononuclear inflammatory cells. Intestinal inflammation can also occur in a subset of cases, and the lesions are indistinguishable from those caused by *Salmonella* Typhimurium.

***Salmonella* Typhimurium** and some other variants are not host adapted, have worldwide distribution, and are now the most common serotypes isolated from pigs. *Salmonella* Typhimurium produces a clinical syndrome of fever, inanition, and often intermittent yellow watery diarrhea that may contain blood and mucus, especially in the later stages. There is often high morbidity with outbreaks occurring within groups of pigs within a few days, but there is usually low mortality. Most pigs recover but may remain *carriers* for variable periods of time; a few may develop rectal stricture. The organism may persist in tonsils, lower intestinal tract, and submandibular and ileocolic lymph nodes.

The **gross lesions** of *Salmonella* Typhimurium are focused mostly in the intestine, where there is enterotyphlocolitis involving the ileum, cecum, and spiral colon (with less frequent involvement of the descending colon and rectum). Of note, the gross lesions of enteric salmonellosis often closely resemble the gross lesions of the necrotizing form of proliferative enteropathy and possibly swine dysentery; however, salmonellosis tends to occur most severely in the spiral colon with less frequent involvement of the small intestine. In addition, pigs with salmonellosis almost universally have mesenteric lymphadenomegaly, which may be less prominent in cases of proliferative enteropathy or swine dysentery. There is prominent thickening of the intestinal wall due to edema, and acute or chronic inflammation and surface erosion or ulceration, with fibrinonecrotic membrane formation (Fig. 1-110). With chronicity, button ulcers can also be observed; mesenteric lymph nodes are usually prominent and enlarged and congested. Systemic dissemination and septicemia (as described previously for *Salmonella* Choleraesuis infection) is uncommonly associated with *Salmonella* Typhimurium.

The **histologic lesions** are most consistently observed in the ascending colon and cecum, where there is localized or more widespread necrosis of intestinal surface and cryptal epithelium with intense infiltration by neutrophils and fibrin with fewer macrophages or lymphocytes. Small-to-medium submucosal arterioles and capillaries are occluded by fibrin thrombi due to leukocytoclastic and fibrinoid vasculitis; as a result, regional ischemic infarction and ulceration develop. Submucosal lymphoid tissue is often necrotic early, but becomes hyperplastic with prominent lymphoid follicles in pigs that survive the acute disease. There is typically abundant luminal and mural fibrinonecrotic debris as well as myriad gram-negative bacterial organisms throughout the tissue.

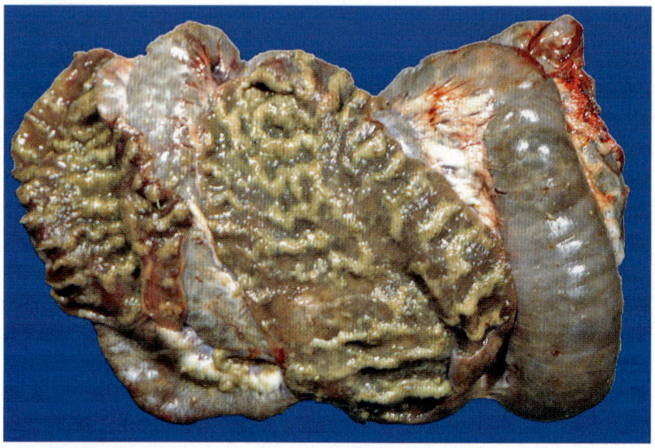

Figure 1-110 Porcine salmonellosis. Fibrinous colitis in a pig.

Rectal stricture is thought to be the *sequel in some cases to ulcerative proctitis of ischemic origin* caused by *Salmonella* Typhimurium. It is characterized clinically by marked progressive distension of the abdomen, loss of appetite, and emaciation. At autopsy, there is marked obstipation, distension, and dilation of the proximal sections of the descending colon caused by narrowing and stricture with fibrosis of the rectum, 1-10 cm cranial to the anus (Fig. 1-111). The stricture is located in an area of the rectum that has an inherently poor blood supply, namely the junction of the circulatory fields of the caudal mesenteric and pudendal arteries. Ulcerative proctitis is consistently found in swine with typhlocolitis caused by *Salmonella* Typhimurium infection, and localized granulation and fibrosis of these lesions are thought to progress in some pigs to stricture.

***Salmonella* Typhisuis** infection is an *uncommon* condition in pigs and is usually described as localized outbreaks. Often referred to as *paratyphoid* in Europe, the disease is known to cause disease in pigs in Americas and Asia. It is a progressive disease of 2-4-month-old pigs with intermittent diarrhea, emaciation, and frequently, massive enlargement of the neck due to caseous necrotizing palatine tonsillitis, cervical lymphadenitis, and parotid sialoadenitis. There is also circular or button-like to confluent mucosal caseous necrosis and ulceration of the ileum, cecum, colon, and rectum. Other less frequent findings are caseous lymphadenitis of the mesenteric lymph nodes, interstitial pneumonia, hepatitis, and pericarditis.

Salmonellosis in horses. The most common serovar in horses in most areas is ***Salmonella* Typhimurium**, and its prevalence is increasing, especially that of multidrug-resistant definitive phage type 104 (**DT104**). Other serovars are usually associated with sporadic cases of disease. *Many horses are* Salmonella *carriers, and when they are stressed, diarrhea follows*. Abortion of pregnant mares has been associated with *Salmonella* Abortusequi. *Salmonella* Infantum has been associated with disseminated infection localizing in a variety of tissues, including muscle, in a horse. Disease occurs more frequently in foals and young horses. GI surgery, hospitalization,

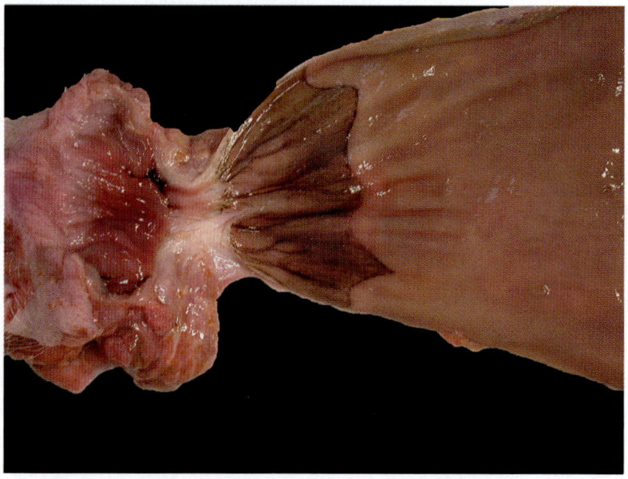

Figure 1-111 Rectal stricture in a pig. A sequel of ulcerative proctitis due to salmonellosis. (Courtesy G. Andrews, Kansas State University Diagnostic Laboratory.)

transportation, overcrowding, and treatment with antibiotics, especially orally, increase the risk of salmonellosis. Resistance to certain antibiotics is associated with *resistance (R) plasmids* that may be transferred to other bacteria, of the same or different species, by conjugation or transduction. Antibiotic-resistant *Salmonella* may not respond to treatment, and antimicrobial therapy may increase the potential for infection and disease because of suppression of the normal intestinal microbiota. Antibiotic-resistant strains have been associated with outbreaks of salmonellosis at veterinary teaching hospitals.

Salmonellosis in horses may be manifested clinically as *peracute* (usually septicemic), *acute*, and *chronic* forms, and as a *subclinical carrier state*.

The **septicemic** form occurs most commonly in foals 1-6-months-old. These animals are usually with their dams at pasture, and predisposing factors are unclear. The infection in foals tends to be fatal. Affected animals are lethargic and develop severe diarrhea, often with characteristic green color, which may contain casts and blood. They are febrile and waste rapidly, to die in 2-3 days. Some survive for a week or more, and these may develop signs of pneumonia, osteitis, polyarthritis, and meningoencephalitis.

The primarily **enteric forms** of the disease are more likely to occur in older horses. Most of the predisposing factors mentioned earlier apply to horses. *Salmonellosis is an occupational hazard of horses*, since many are exposed to long periods of transport, to exertion owing to overwork or excessive training, and to antimicrobial treatment.

Clinically, in the acute disease, diarrhea and fever occur for 1-2 weeks, followed by recovery or death. The chronic form persists for weeks or months. Affected horses pass soft, unformed manure that resembles cow feces. They lose their appetite, with subsequent progressive loss of weight and condition. In later stages, they become dehydrated and emaciated.

The gross lesions are those of enterocolitis and/or septicemia; the former are most consistently found at autopsy. As a rule, the longer the course, the lower in the intestine does one find the most severe lesions.

Grossly, acute septicemic cases have small hemorrhages on the serous or mucosal membranes. The visceral lymph nodes are always enlarged, edematous, and often hemorrhagic. Marked pulmonary congestion and edema, and renal cortical pallor and medullary congestion may occur. The main lesions are in the stomach and intestines. In peracute or septicemic cases, there is intense hyperemia of the gastric mucosa, probably venous infarction, with some edema and scattered hemorrhage. The small intestine may be congested with a mucoid or hemorrhagic exudate. In acute cases, there is diffuse and intense fibrinohemorrhagic inflammation of the cecum and colon overshadowing any lesions in the upper intestine and leading rapidly to superficial necrosis of the mucosa and gray-red pseudomembranes (Fig. 1-112A). In chronic salmonellosis, enteric lesions may be few or subtle. Some animals have extensive or patchy fibrinous or ulcerative lesions of the cecum and colon. In others, raised circumscribed lesions ~2-3 cm in diameter may be evident, with a gelatinous submucosa and ulcerated mucosa. Some such lesions are more fibrinous and resemble button ulcers (see Fig. 1-112B).

Histologic alterations of significance are usually limited to the intestine. However, in septicemic animals, lesions typical of endotoxemia are present in the lung, liver, kidney, spleen, and adrenal. There may be acute ileocecocolic lymphadenitis,

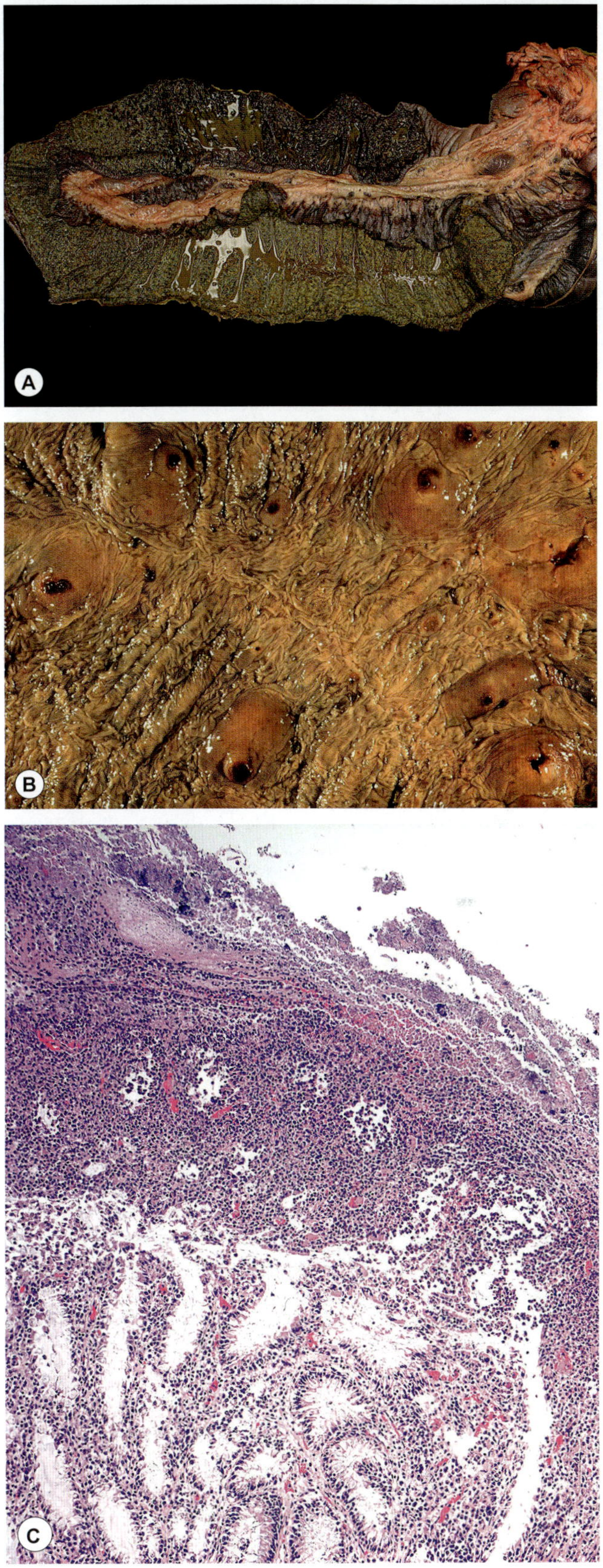

Figure 1-112 Colonic salmonellosis. A. Fibrinonecrotic membrane covering the mucosal surface of the colon of a foal. **B**. Nodular ulcerative lesions in the colon of a horse. **C**. Full-thickness necrosis and effusion from colonic mucosa; several vessels in the lamina propria are thrombosed.

and inflammation in sites of localization, such as growth plates in long bones and meninges. Depending on the duration of the enteric disease, hemorrhage, necrosis, and/or diphtheresis may predominate, but the infiltrating leukocytes are largely mononuclear. The superficial coagulative necrosis of the mucosa may extend over large areas. A layer of fibrinocellular exudate may cover the necrotic mucosa. Fibrin thrombi are frequently present in the capillaries or venules of the lamina propria (see Fig. 1-112C). There is usually marked congestion of submucosal vessels, which is accompanied by considerable edema. These lesions may be indistinguishable from those produced by *C. difficile*, *P. sordellii*, and, in neonatal foals, *C. perfringens* type C. Lesions produced by NSAIDs may sometimes resemble those of salmonellosis.

Salmonellosis in cattle. The serotypes most frequently incriminated are ***Salmonella*** **Typhimurium** and ***Salmonella*** **Dublin**, although several other serotypes can cause salmonellosis in cattle. Both *Salmonella* Typhimurium and *Salmonella* Dublin are distributed worldwide. Wherever *Salmonella* Dublin is found, it tends to be adapted to cattle and to occur in epizootics; other serotypes usually cause more sporadic disease. ***Salmonella*** **Newport** is an emerging pathogen in cattle.

It is unusual to find enteric salmonellosis in **calves** <1-week-old, in contrast to septicemic colibacillosis, which usually affects very young animals. *In calves, salmonellosis is a febrile disease typified by dejection, dehydration, and usually diarrhea*. Diarrhea is not always present, but when it is, the feces are yellow or gray, and have a very unpleasant odor. In older calves, there may be blood, mucus, and/or fibrin in the feces. In less acute cases, there may be delayed evidence of localization in the lung and synovial structures. Morbidity and mortality may be considerable, especially in calves that are confined, such as in vealer operations. Experimental infections in calves indicate that survival is inversely related to the numbers of *Salmonella* in the inoculum, and directly to the age of the calves.

At **autopsy** of a calf with enteric salmonellosis, there is *enlargement of mesenteric lymph nodes and enteric lesions*. There is moderately severe GI inflammation, acute swelling, and hemorrhage of the visceral lymph nodes, and some petechiation of serous membranes. The enteritis is usually fibrinonecrotizing (Fig. 1-113A), although occasionally it may be catarrhal or hemorrhagic. The mucosa overlying the lymphoid tissues may become necrotic and slough. In animals with fibrinous enteritis, the bowel wall is somewhat turgid and the serosa may have a ground-glass appearance. There is often diffuse but usually mild fibrinous peritonitis.

The intestinal lesions are usually most severe in the terminal jejunum and ileum, especially during the early stages of the disease. With time, the proximal jejunum and colon become involved, but the duodenum remains relatively normal. The regional distribution of the lesions may, in part, be related to differences in the level of bacterial colonization of the mucosa. Twelve hours after oral infection of calves with *Salmonella* Typhimurium, the numbers of bacteria are generally lower in the abomasum and duodenum than in the lower intestinal tract; they are relatively constant from the jejunum through to the rectum.

The early **microscopic lesions** in the small intestine consist of a thin layer of fibrinocellular exudate on the surface of short and blunt villi. This is followed by extensive necrosis and ulceration of the mucosa, with fibrin and neutrophils exuding from the ulcerated areas into the lumen. The lamina propria

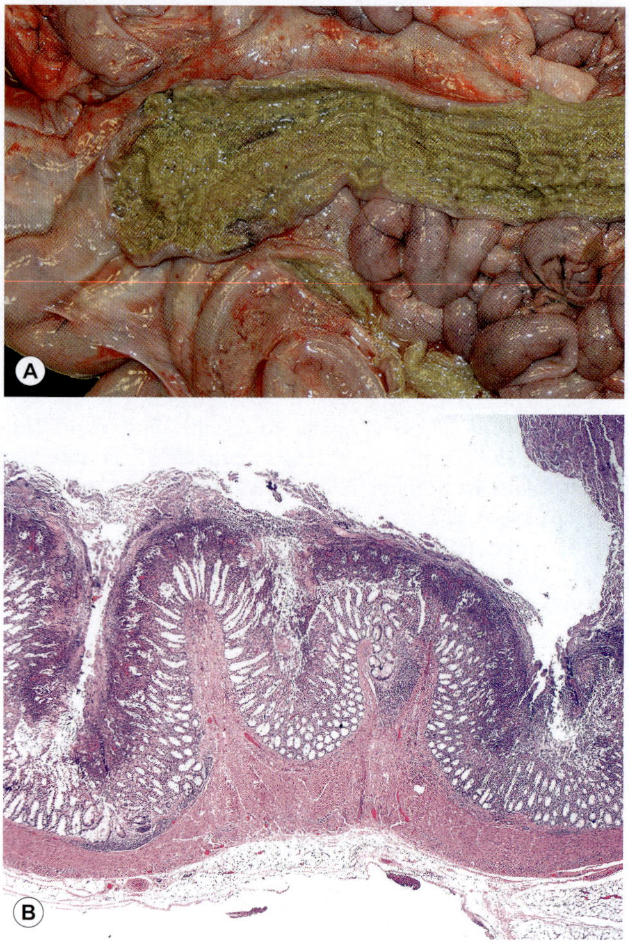

Figure 1-113 Intestinal salmonellosis in a calf due to *Salmonella* Dublin. **A**. Diphtheritic enteritis. **B**. Necrosis of lamina propria, effusion of neutrophils and fibrin, and pseudomembrane formation in the colon.

may be moderately infiltrated by mononuclear inflammatory cells. Fibrin thrombi are often evident in proprial capillaries and venules. There is also marked submucosal edema and the centers of lymphoid follicles in the Peyer patches are completely involuted. Similar erosion, ulceration, and fibrinous effusion occur in the proximal large bowel (see Fig. 1-113B). Scanning electron microscopy of the small intestine reveals large numbers of bacteria on a tattered epithelial surface, with clusters of enterocytes sloughing from short villi and strands of fibrin emerging from the epithelial defects to cover the damaged surface.

Characteristic changes usually occur in the *liver and spleen* but may be absent in peracute septicemic cases. There is often fibrinous cholecystitis. The latter, together with icterus, is characteristic and highly suggestive of infection by *Salmonella* Dublin. In acute cases, the spleen is enlarged and pulpy as a result of congestion, but this is soon replaced by acute splenitis, present as miliary, tiny foci of necrosis, or as reactive nodules. The liver is often pale with many minute *paratyphoid nodules* consisting of areas of lytic necrosis infiltrated by neutrophils. In the spleen, macrophage reaction is sometimes diffuse. Paratyphoid nodules also may be found microscopically in the kidney, lymph nodes, and bone marrow. These probably represent a cell-mediated immune response to embolic bacteria. In those animals that survive the acute phase of the disease, the inflammatory changes in lymphoid tissues progress to an immunologic response, a diffuse reaction of medium and large lymphocytes in the follicles, and plasma cells in the sinusoids. There may be marked cortical atrophy of the thymus. In calves with acute septicemia, pulmonary congestion and edema are visible at autopsy, with interstitial thickening of pulmonary alveolar septa by mononuclear cells in tissue section. There may be thrombosis of septal capillaries, and some effusion of edema fluid and macrophages into alveolar spaces.

In subacute salmonellosis of calves, there may be cranioventral bronchopneumonia, usually with adhesions and abscessation. Purulent exudate is in synovial cavities, and the organism is recoverable in pure culture from such affected joints and tendon sheaths. It may be mixed with *T. pyogenes* and *Pasteurella* spp. in the lungs.

Salmonellosis in **adult cattle** may occur in *outbreaks* as it does in calves, but more often it is sporadic, and it may cause *chronic diarrhea and loss of condition*. The source of infection is usually the carrier animal. Other sources, such as feed containing protein of animal origin, or bone meal, should be considered when the disease is caused by an uncommon serovar. *Abortions* are most common with *Salmonella* Dublin but may occur with any serovar. In some herds, this may be the only clinical evidence of infection, although other animals often excrete the offending serovar in the feces. The *carrier state* of *Salmonella* Dublin infection in adult cattle may persist for years, sometimes for life, in contrast to infections with other serovars, which rarely persist >18 months. Dairy cows may persistently shed *Salmonella*, especially *Salmonella* Dublin, in milk and cause infections in humans who drink raw milk. In cattle admitted to a teaching hospital, a higher risk for shedding was identified in those that were admitted to the hospital in the fall, suggesting a seasonality to shedding. The morbid changes in adult cattle correspond to those in calves except that there is more pleural hemorrhage, and the enteritis may be more hemorrhagic and fibrinous. The histologic changes in the liver and other organs are the same as those seen in calves.

The multidrug-resistant strain *Salmonella* Typhimurium definitive phage type 104 (DT104), first seen in the United Kingdom in the late 1980s, has now spread worldwide and in some parts of the United States is the leading cause of bovine salmonellosis. The potential for this strain to emerge as a major foodborne pathogen has caused great consternation among both agricultural and public health communities. Multidrug-resistant strains of *Salmonella* Newport have also been identified.

Salmonellosis in sheep. As well as abortion caused by ***Salmonella* Abortusovis**, abortion and neonatal death may follow infection of pregnant ewes by any species of *Salmonella*. Although the prevalence of *Salmonella* Abortusovis in the United Kingdom seems to be waning, *Salmonella* Montevideo, however, has been associated with abortions in several flocks in the British Isles. *Salmonella* Brandenburg has been reported in sheep in New Zealand.

Salmonellosis is not a common disease in sheep, but outbreaks are always severe and may cause very heavy losses. Predisposing influences are necessary, and these are usually provided by circumstances that enforce congregation. Deprivation of food and water for 2-3 days may be sufficient and coupled with fatigue is the usual predisposing factor when sheep are transported or confined in holding yards. Deaths usually continue for 7-10 days after debilitating circumstances have been remedied.

The serovars usually found in sheep are ***Salmonella* Typhimurium**, ***Salmonella* Arizonae**, and ***Salmonella* Enteritidis**. *Salmonella* Dublin is increasingly prevalent in the United Kingdom and the midwestern states of the United States. Experimental inoculation of sheep with *Salmonella* Arizonae produces infection but rarely disease. Under natural conditions, this host-adapted organism is frequently considered to be an infection secondary to some other disease, or an incidental finding in apparently healthy animals. Most serovars produce the same sort of disease, which closely resembles that seen in cattle both clinically and at autopsy. The major findings are *fibrinohemorrhagic enteritis and septicemia*.

Salmonellosis in carnivores. *Salmonella* spp. *can often be recovered from apparently healthy dogs and cats*, and carnivores shedding *Salmonella* spp. have been identified as the source of bacteria causing significant disease in humans. However, primary disease in carnivores rarely occurs. *Salmonella* has been recovered in high frequency from normal sled dogs lacking clinical disease, probably because raw meat fed to dogs is often contaminated with *Salmonella*. In dogs and cats, nosocomial systemic infections have also been associated with hospitalization and antibiotic therapy. In **dogs**, salmonellosis can cause bronchopneumonia, acute hemorrhagic gastroenteritis, splenomegaly and lymphadenomegaly, serosal hemorrhages, and hepatic necrosis; however, mostly infection is secondary to other systemic infection or immunocompromise. Septicemia in puppies has been associated with *Salmonella* Dublin infection. Salmonellosis has been identified as a cause of abortion in dogs with bacteremia and has been reported in dogs with lymphoma, possibly associated with immunosuppression and chemotherapy.

Various serovars, including *Salmonella* Enteritidis and *Salmonella* Typhimurium, have been isolated from **cats** with systemic salmonellosis. Most infections appear to be subclinical and associated with immunosuppression or other diseases such as FeLV or FIV infection, or other systemic debilitating or immunosuppressive diseases. Transmission is thought to occur through the fecal-oral route, or via ingestion of contaminated food (including raw meat, wildlife prey, or water). A report documented systemic disease in cats with vomiting, diarrhea, and fever; gross lesions varied somewhat, but included necrotizing-to-hemorrhagic hepatitis, icterus, and lymphadenomegaly. Histology confirmed embolic coagulative necrosis affecting the liver, spleen, and lymph nodes. Fibrinonecrotizing enteritis or colitis was also commonly observed, and myriad gram-negative bacteria were observed in numerous organs. Conjunctivitis and abortions have also been associated with *Salmonella* infection in cats.

Because of their close association with humans, especially children and the aged, dogs and cats that are carriers are considered potential sources of zoonotic infection.

Yersiniosis

Yersinia enterocolitica and ***Y. pseudotuberculosis*** are gram-negative organisms that, in domestic animals, cause *enterocolitis, mesenteric lymphadenitis, septicemia* and, less commonly, conjunctivitis, hepatitis, abortion, neonatal death, epididymitis-orchitis, mastitis, and pneumonia. *Y. pestis*, the cause of plague in animals and humans, is not considered here.

The *epidemiology* of yersiniosis is complex and poorly understood. These organisms may be shed in the feces by subclinical animals in the herd or flock, and by other species, such as rodents and birds, in the environment. The organisms can survive and grow in the environment at low temperatures, and in cool weather environmental contamination by *Yersinia* spp. may be considerable, resulting in significant oral challenge. Disease may in part be due to compromise of cell-mediated immunity, permitting establishment of invading organisms, or recrudescence of latent infection. Often, outbreaks occur under stressful circumstances, such as poor weather, flooding, after transport, during the breeding season, or in animals on a poor plane of nutrition.

Subsequent to ingestion, *the organisms invade through the intestinal epithelium or M cells* overlying Peyer patches and reach the lamina propria or submucosal lymphoid follicles. Enormous recruitment of neutrophils and ensuing destruction of cytoarchitecture of the Peyer patch and overlying epithelium result in the formation of neutrophilic foci in place of follicles in Peyer patches, and microabscesses in the lamina propria of the small or large intestine if invasion occurs elsewhere. *Yersinia* spp. disseminate via lymphatics and hepatic portal venous drainage to mesenteric lymph nodes or to the liver and the systemic circulation.

Pathogenicity in the main *Yersinia* species is associated primarily with the 70-kb virulence plasmid pYV, and with other proteins that are chromosomally encoded. After bacteria are ingested and reach the terminal ileum, they present on their surface the outer membrane protein invasin, which is expressed in stationary growth phase at low temperatures. Invasin facilitates translocation of the bacteria across the intestinal epithelium, after which invasin binds to β1 integrins in the host tissue, which induces the production of chemokines such as IL8. In the Peyer patches, bacteria replicate and express the adhesin YadA, which downregulates the expression of invasin and protects bacteria against phagocytosis. YadA and the protein Ail protect bacteria against the host immune system enabling bacterial propagation to mesenteric lymph nodes and, occasionally, other tissues.

Although *Yersinia* reside extracellularly as microcolonies in neutrophilic foci in the lamina propria of the intestine and lymph nodes, at least some appear to reside intracellularly, since a T-cell–mediated immune response is required to clear infection. Giant cells wall off foci of infection in subacute-to-chronic lesions, hence the specific name *Y. pseudotuberculosis* for the name of the etiologic agent of the disease.

Disease may be gradual in onset, subtle, and chronic, producing a syndrome of diarrhea and ill-thrift in cattle, sheep, and goats. Mild diarrhea and enteritis with low mortality have been reported in Australia in weaned pigs with *Y. pseudotuberculosis*. More fulminant disease, with severe, sometimes hemorrhagic, diarrhea, systemic infection, and prostration, may occur in cattle, some species of deer, especially chital and red deer, water buffalo, and exotic ungulates. Yersiniosis is apparently an uncommon cause of diarrhea, and occasionally fatal enterocolitis, mesenteric lymphadenitis, and systemic infection in carnivores. *Yersinia* also causes sporadic pneumonia and septicemia in foals.

Yersiniosis has been described worldwide, as a cause of disease in sheep, cattle, goats, deer, and pigs. The lesions of *Y. pseudotuberculosis* and *Y. enterocolitica* cannot be differentiated reliably grossly or microscopically. In all species, **gross lesions** in clinically subacute-to-chronic yersiniosis may be mild. They are usually limited to abnormally fluid intestinal content, with congestion, edema, roughening, and perhaps small foci of pallor, focal hemorrhages, erosion, or mild ulceration and fibrin effusion. Raised nodules up to 5 mm in diameter, with depressed centers, or ulcers may be evident in affected large bowel (Fig. 1-114A). Mesenteric lymph nodes are enlarged, congested, and edematous, perhaps with foci of necrosis. There may be mild fibrinous cholecystitis, and pale foci of necrosis scattered in the liver.

The infection is characterized **histologically** by *masses of gram-negative coccobacilli forming microcolonies*, in the lamina propria of villi and around the necks of crypts in the distal half of the small intestine, in Peyer patches, and in the superficial mucosa of the large intestine. Intense local infiltrates of inflammatory cells, predominantly neutrophils, accumulate to form *microabscesses* up to ~300 µm in diameter around the bacteria, and effuse into the lumen through microerosions on the mucosal surface or in crypts. Small foci of inflammation may be present in the crypts. In the small intestine, there may be moderate atrophy of villi and hyperplasia of crypts, associated with increased infiltrates of chronic inflammatory cells. Pyogranulomas surrounded by macrophages or giant cells, and sometimes containing bacterial microcolonies, may be present

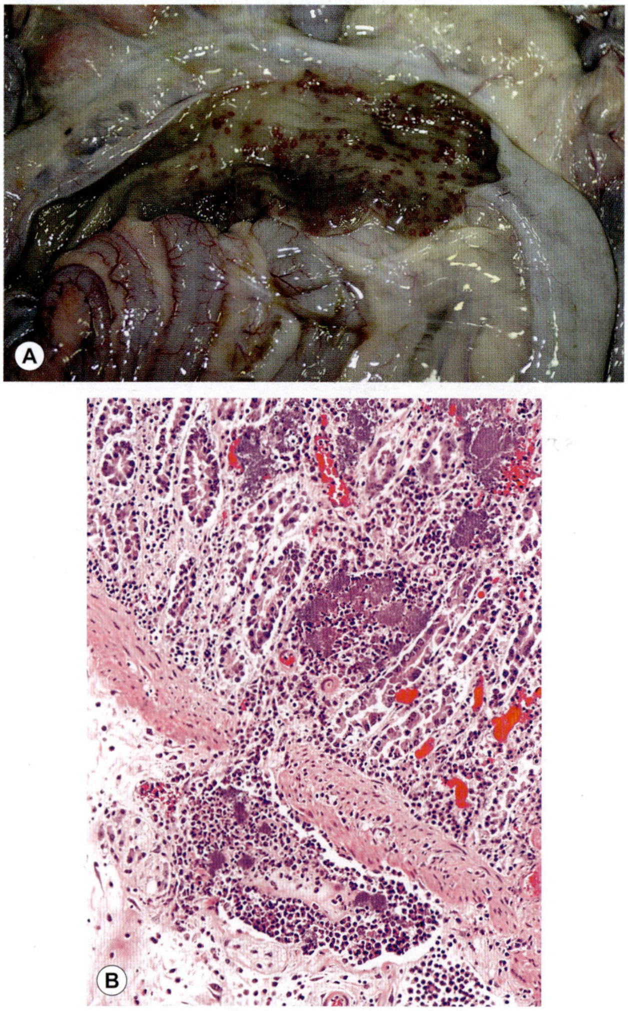

Figure 1-114 ***Yersinia pseudotuberculosis*** **infection** in a goat. A. Ulcerative colitis. (Reprinted with permission from Giannitti F, et al. *Yersinia pseudotuberculosis* infections in goats and other animals diagnosed at the California Animal Health and Food Safety Laboratory System: 1990-2012. J Vet Diagn Invest 2014;26:1–8.) B. Mucosal and submucosal colonies of coccobacilli.

in the subcapsular and medullary sinuses of mesenteric lymph nodes.

In fulminant *Yersinia* infection in all species, there is *fibrinous or fibrinohemorrhagic enterocolitis*, with heavy local mucosal colonization by masses of coccobacilli, and marked neutrophil infiltration (see Fig. 1-114B). Peyer patches may be particularly involved, with grossly visible foci or confluent masses of caseous necrotic debris, as may be found in draining mesenteric lymph nodes, which are enlarged. There may be serosal hemorrhages on the gut, fibrinous peritonitis and pleuritis, and foci of necrosis also may be present in the liver, lungs, and occasionally other parenchymatous organs; the characteristic microcolonies of coccobacilli are usually evident in them. *Caseous mesenteric lymphadenitis*, with mature pyogranulomas containing microcolonies of bacteria, surrounded by neutrophils and giant cells, may occasionally be found as an incidental lesion, or in animals with *Yersinia* abscesses in other organs.

Yersiniosis is **diagnosed** in tissue section by finding characteristic microcolonies of coccobacilli in pyogranulomas or neutrophilic foci (see Fig. 1-114B) and is confirmed by bacterial isolation; IHC is also available for confirmation of the diagnosis. Microscopic lesions may not be detected in the intestinal mucosa of some clinically affected animals from which isolates are made, perhaps because lesions are patchy. Because *Yersinia* spp. are psychrophiles, cold enrichment and culture at temperatures <37° C are used in their isolation.

Lawsonia intracellularis *infections*

Lawsonia intracellularis has been documented in many species, including wildlife, but is a well-recognized cause of proliferative enteritis in a variety of species, including swine, horses, donkeys, deer, rodents, rabbits, guinea pigs, foxes, dogs, ferrets, ratites, poultry, and nonhuman primates. It causes a *characteristic proliferative lesion of cryptal epithelium in the distal small intestine and less frequently in the large intestine* that is usually associated with clinical diarrhea, weight loss, and ill-thrift. Exposure is via the fecal-oral route; the role of feral swine, rodents, or other species as potential sources of *L. intracellularis* in domestic swine has been hypothesized and debated, but specific details and mechanisms remain unclear. Generally, this is a prevalent and important disease in swine globally and is broadly considered an endemic disease associated with significant economic losses in swine production systems worldwide. How and when the disease manifests within any given commercial herd probably depends significantly on exposure and management within a herd; usually, *L. intracellularis* infections occur in the grower/finisher population, and only rarely in breeding stock. Vaccination has been a helpful management tool for many herds.

Formerly referred to as *intestinal adenomatosis complex*, the acute and chronic conditions in swine now known to be caused by *L. intracellularis* including *porcine intestinal adenomatosis, necrotic enteritis*, and *proliferative hemorrhagic enteropathy* are collectively known as **porcine proliferative enteropathy (PPE)**. The intracellular bacterium was initially thought to be *Campylobacter* spp., then putatively identified as *ileal symbiont intracellularis*, until the taxonomy was formalized as *L. intracellularis* in 1995. *L. intracellularis* is a microaerophilic, nonflagellated, gram-negative, curved or S-shaped rod bacterium. Because it is an obligate intracellular organism, successful cultivation of the agent by bacterial culture is difficult and thus uncommonly performed, and instead other methods, including silver-based cytochemical staining, IHC, in situ hybridization, or PCR, are utilized.

The syndrome occurs mostly in postweaned pigs; however, pigs from 3-weeks-old to adults may be affected. The severity of clinical effects varies from mild subclinical disease with reduced growth rate to persistent diarrhea and severe weight loss. Once infected, pigs may shed the organism for weeks. Death may follow a period of diarrhea and progressive cachexia, or it may occasionally occur after perforation of necrotic enteritis, or from peracute hemorrhage. Mortality may be very high. Development of disease is dependent on undefined interactions with other bacteria in the gut because gnotobiotic pigs inoculated with *L. intracellularis* fail to develop disease; conventional pigs are quite susceptible. Experimental studies and mild spontaneous cases suggest that infection occurs first in glandular epithelial cells near lymphoid aggregates of the ileocecocolic region; the cecal and colonic cryptal epithelial cells are infected later in the course of disease.

The **pathogenesis of PPE** is related to active uptake of *L. intracellularis* by epithelial cells, including mature enterocytes and immature crypt cells, although specific receptors for adhesion and cellular entry remain unknown. Once endocytosed by the host cell and established in poorly differentiated crypt cells, the entry vacuole breaks down and the bacteria persist and replicate freely within the apical cytoplasm, causing hyperplasia and propagation of the bacteria throughout the epithelium. Cell division is required for bacterial replication, which may explain its tissue tropism. Bacteria are passed on to daughter epithelial cells and exit via extrusion from the cytoplasm of enterocytes on villi or between crypt openings; possibly there is also transfer of bacteria from crypt to crypt via macrophages through the lamina propria. Disruption of intestinal cell differentiation by the pathogen is theorized to be a central event; however, specific virulence factors of *L. intracellularis* and molecular details of the host cell-pathogen interaction remain undescribed.

The *L. intracellularis*–infected epithelium is thus transformed into a population of mitotically active and poorly differentiated cells. Glands are lined by dysplastic immature pseudostratified columnar epithelial cells with basophilic cytoplasm; goblet cells often are reduced in number. Mucosal glands are elongated, dilated, and branched, resulting in a grossly and histologically thickened mucosal layer (Fig. 1-115A). Hyperplastic glands may protrude multifocally into the underlying submucosal lymphoid tissue or epithelial cells may form elevated plaques above the mucosal surface, leading to the use of the term *adenomatosis* to describe such lesions. Occasionally, microscopic foci of proliferative epithelium may be found in submucosal lymphatics or the regional lymph node. Small intestinal villi in infected animals undergo progressive atrophy and are partially to completely absent in well-established lesions. The proliferative lesion in the crypts is considered a primary lesion, and not a secondary hyperplastic response to increased epithelial exfoliation. *L. intracellularis* organisms are readily recognized as *curved rods* within the *apical cytoplasm of glandular epithelial cells* in silver-stained tissue sections (see Fig. 1-115B) or by IHC (see Fig. 1-115C); these microaerophilic bacteria are difficult to cultivate readily and are rarely isolated by routine bacterial culture techniques. *L. intracellularis* also have been identified ultrastructurally in degenerate cells and macrophages in the lamina propria. Inflammation in areas of uncomplicated adenomatosis is usually not a prominent feature.

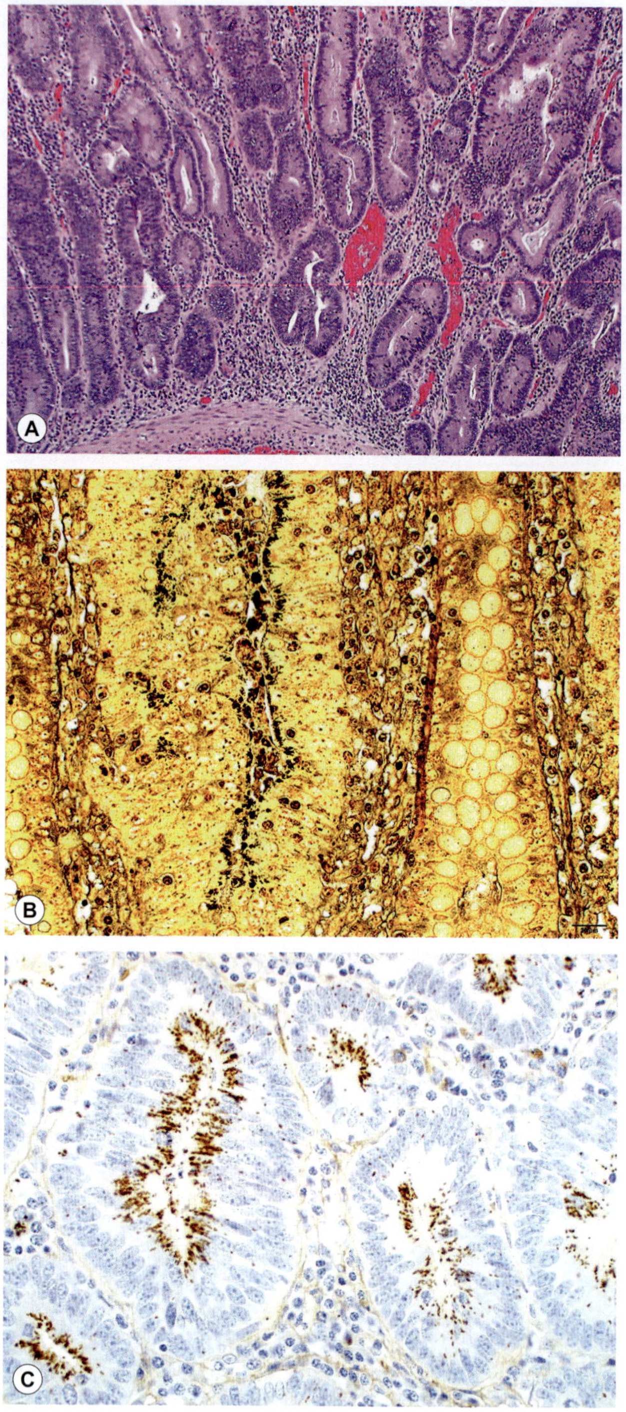

Figure 1-115 Porcine proliferative enteropathy. A. Adenomatous change in glands in the lamina propria. **B.** Masses of silver-stained *Lawsonia intracellularis* organisms in the apical cytoplasm of hyperplastic epithelium lining intestinal glands. **C.** *L. intracellularis* organisms in the apical cytoplasm of hyperplastic epithelium lining intestinal glands by IHC. (Courtesy E.R. Burrough.)

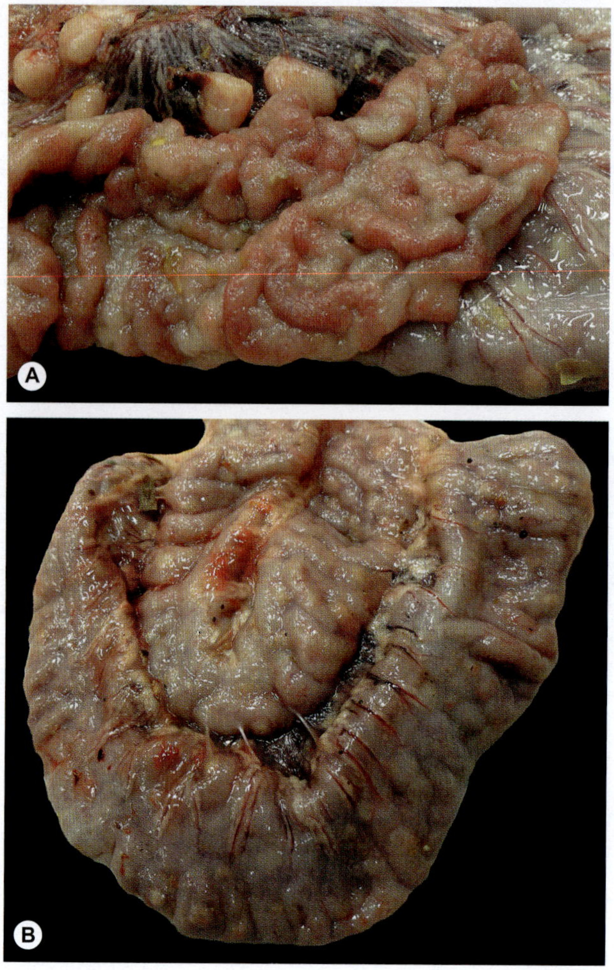

Figure 1-116 Porcine proliferative enteropathy. A. Raised nodular or ridgelike areas of thickened mucosa in the colon, resulting from hyperplasia of glands. **B.** Exaggerated reticular pattern of folds on serosal aspect of the proximal colon. (Courtesy E.R. Burrough.)

In the least complicated forms of the disease, lesions *are always found in the terminal portion of the ileum*, extending proximally for a variable distance, usually <1 m. In a significant proportion of cases, lesions occur in the cecum and proximal spiral colon primarily, or in addition to, the ileum. In mild cases, only a few ridges or plaque-like thickened areas project above the normal mucosa; however, there are typically more widespread lesions with thickened mucosa and irregular longitudinal or transverse folds or ridges (Fig. 1-116A). The mucosal surface in proliferative lesions of the small or large intestine may be intact, but small foci of necrosis or fibrin exudation may be evident. In the affected small or large intestine, hyperplastic mucosal epithelium and some degree of submucosal edema are reflected in the *cerebriform pattern of projections and depressions on the serosal aspect of the intestine, which is often visible from the serosal surface, and is virtually pathognomonic for this condition* (see Fig. 1-116B). Care must be taken with interpretation of early proliferative lesions that lack hemorrhage or necrosis, because other changes including mucosal or submucosal edema, or contraction of the intestine due to postmortem peristalsis can result in subjective thickening of the intestine that closely resembles mild forms of PPE. The ileocolic lymph nodes are enlarged and hyperplastic.

Coagulative necrosis of the proliferative and thickened mucosa commonly occurs and, when extensive areas are affected, this form of the disease is referred to as **necrotic enteritis**. It may be exacerbated by pathogenic anaerobes of the large bowel flora colonizing the affected terminal ileum and large intestine. Necrotic epithelial cells, neutrophils, and fibrin exudation from superficial lesions contribute to the

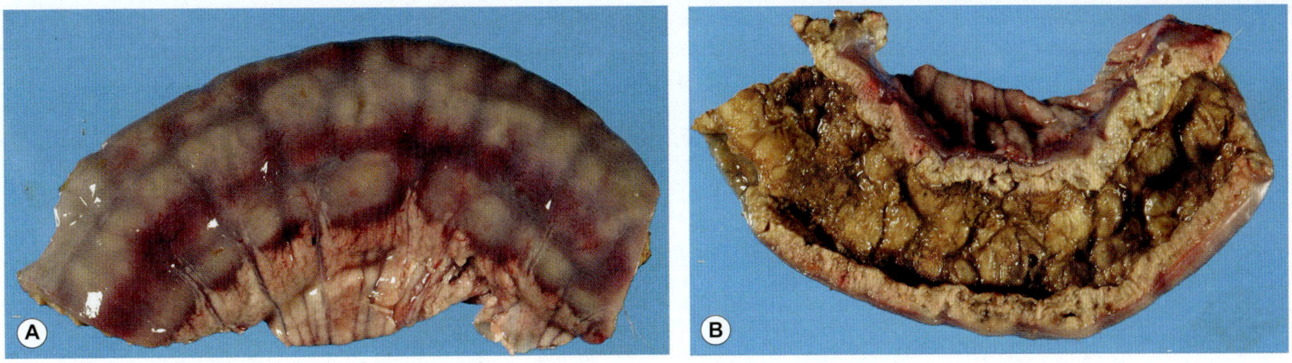

Figure 1-117 **Necrotic enteritis form** of porcine proliferative enteropathy. **A.** The ileal wall is markedly thickened and irregular to rugose. **B.** The mucosal surface is necrotic with accumulation of fibrin and debris.

formation of diphtheritic membranes or luminal fibrin casts, which can be found in the small or large intestine (Fig. 1-117A and B). The cerebriform pattern of serosal folding is usually still evident in necrotic enteritis; the lesions may appear grossly similar to other causes of necrotizing enterocolitis including salmonellosis. Although necrotic enteritis may be associated with other enterocolitides in swine, *PPE caused by* L. intracellularis *infection is the most common primary lesion.*

Acute or subacute intestinal hemorrhage and anemia can also occur as a distinct syndrome referred to as **proliferative hemorrhagic enteropathy**. Some animals exsanguinate and die quickly without hematochezia; others have melena or hematochezia for several days. This syndrome is more common in young adults than in growing pigs. It is usually sporadic and of relatively low morbidity, but up to half of clinically recognized cases may die. Animals that die of *massive intestinal hemorrhage* are pale, and the perianal area may be smeared with blood. The typical cerebriform pattern is often still evident on the serosal surface of the distal ileum, the ileum may contain variable combinations of free blood, fibrin, or clotted blood, and the cecum and colon may contain dark bloody digesta (Fig. 1-118). The ileal mucosa usually resembles that in uncomplicated PPE. Overt regions of hemorrhage or ulceration are rarely discernible grossly, and there appears to be widespread mucosal diapedesis.

Microscopically, the characteristic lesion in all forms of PPE is proliferation of immature cryptal intestinal epithelial cells, often several layers thick and lining the branching and tortuous hyperplastic and dysplastic crypts extending from the muscularis mucosa toward the surface. Coagulative necrosis of the mucosal epithelium may be focal and superficial but can involve the full thickness of the mucosa or even extend into the submucosa. A few islands of viable hyperplastic crypts or glands may remain, and masses of bacteria, presumably fecal anaerobes, are observed among the necrotic debris. With time, granulation tissue develops in ulcerated areas. Even in cases with extensive necrosis, the proximal ileum along the margin of the zone of mucosal necrosis should be carefully examined for hyperplastic epithelium because remnants of mucosa usually can be found. Repeated bouts of epithelial proliferation, necrosis, ulceration, and granulation may result in progressive stricture of the lumen that may be accompanied by hypertrophy of the external muscle layer. This should be differentiated from idiopathic ileal muscular hypertrophy of swine, which is known to occur independent of antecedent PPE. In cases of proliferative hemorrhagic enteropathy, there is still extensive

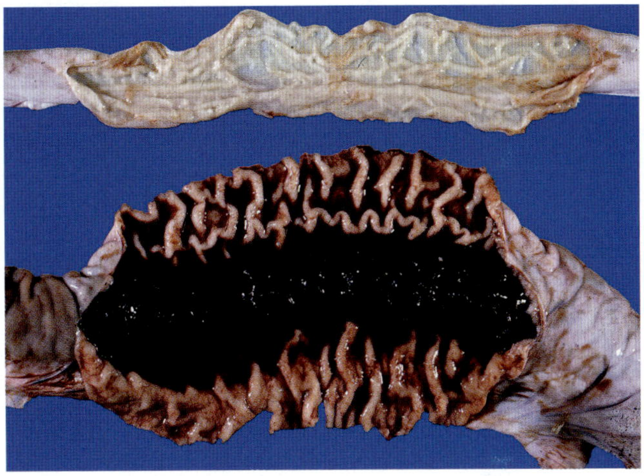

Figure 1-118 **Hemorrhagic form** of porcine proliferative enteropathy. Hemorrhage in the lumen of the terminal small intestine. Normal terminal small intestine (top).

proliferation, erosion, and necrosis of superficial epithelium. An acute inflammatory infiltrate is also often present in the superficial lamina propria. Small mucosal blood vessels are frequently thrombosed, and there is effusion of neutrophils, fibrin, and extensive hemorrhage into intestinal glands, onto the mucosal surface, and into the intestinal lumen.

In **horses**, the lesions and pathogenesis of **equine proliferative enteritis (EPE)** are similar to those of PPE. This disease affects mostly weanling foals and causes fever, anorexia, lethargy, diarrhea (although many affected foals are reported to have normal feces), hypoproteinemia, edema, and weight loss; in North America, most cases occur in fall and winter months. The agent is acquired via the fecal-oral route; however, specific details or the most common sources of infection for horses remain unclear. Rodents and rabbits have been proposed as reservoir hosts, and pigs have been suggested as a potential source of infection for horses, but in most confirmed equine cases there has been no documentation of exposure to pig feces.

Thickening of the mucosa due to epithelial hyperplasia is most commonly observed in the distal small intestine near the ileal-cecal junction; however, gross lesions are not always evident or they are subtle and can be easily overlooked, especially from the serosal surface. In severe or long-standing cases, there can be marked irregular hyperplasia and thickening of the epithelium and the entire mucosa with fibrinonecrotic membrane and variable edema of the submucosa. The microscopic features are similar to pigs and other species, and there is marked irregular hyperplasia of immature cryptal epithelial cells, which line dysplastic and hyperplastic branching glands within the mucosa. As for PPE, EPE is definitively diagnosed by documenting adenomatous proliferation of epithelial cells in the crypts of the small intestine and by demonstrating the intracellular curved bacteria in the apical cytoplasm of enterocytes using silver stains or by IHC.

In all species, including swine, diarrhea is probably related to loss of functional mucosal surface area in the affected distal small intestine and large bowel, whereas ill-thrift or wasting syndromes are attributable to PLE. A presumptive **diagnosis** of proliferative enteritis in any species can be based on typical gross and histologic lesions and supported by Warthin-Starry silver staining to visualize the intracellular apical cytoplasmic bacteria. Confirmation is achieved by IHC using a specific antibody for *L. intracellularis* or by PCR assay.

Campylobacter *infections*

Campylobacter spp. are common causes of GI disease in humans, and some species also may be capable of causing enteritis in animals. ***Campylobacter jejuni*** and ***Campylobacter coli*** are the most studied, but other fastidious *Campylobacter* species are implicated as pathogens in humans and animals. Pathogenic strains penetrate the surface mucus layer, then adhere to and invade the epithelial cells where they avoid delivery to lysosomal compartments and thus prolong their intracellular survival. Central to the pathogenesis of *Campylobacter*-associated disease are type IV and VI secretion systems and the production of toxins, most notably the cytolethal distending toxin. Many human infections are acquired by ingestion of contaminated milk products, water, meat, or other animal products, making this an important potential zoonosis. *Chickens* are common subclinical shedders of *C. jejuni*, and *C. coli* can be frequently isolated from the feces of diarrheic or subclinical swine.

C. jejuni has been associated with diarrhea with blood and mucus in some dogs despite the fact that it can often be isolated from subclinical animals. It has also been isolated from dogs with parvoviral enteritis or other viral infections; preexisting infections may predispose to the development of pathologic effects of *C. jejuni*. The latter has been implicated as the primary pathogen in some canine cases of mild-to-moderate lymphoplasmacytic enterocolitis by associating large numbers of the organism with the lesions and by ruling out other known etiologies. In experimentally infected gnotobiotic and conventional dogs, lesions are limited to mild mucosal colitis. Mild-to-moderate inflammatory lesions limited to the colon have been documented in some pigs in which *Campylobacter* sp. was the only potential pathogen isolated. Young cats are probably subclinical carriers of *C. jejuni*. Several *Campylobacter* spp., including *C. jejuni*, *C. coli*, and *C. fetus* subsp. *fetus*, rarely have been associated with diarrhea and enterocolitis in young foals; the pathogenesis is not clear and infection may be more common in immunocompromised individuals.

Weaner colitis of sheep is described in Australia as a diarrheal syndrome of high morbidity and low mortality and is associated with an unidentified *Campylobacter* sp., not *C. jejuni*. Affected sheep have watery colonic content; chronically affected animals may have edema and loss of body condition suggestive of enteric protein loss. Histologically, there is mild erosive-to-ulcerative typhlocolitis with a layer of bacteria adherent to surface epithelial cells and in crypts. The disease has been reproduced by inoculation of the thermophilic catalase-negative *Campylobacter*-like organism previously isolated from spontaneous cases.

Brachyspira *infections*

Swine dysentery caused by ***Brachyspira*** (formerly *Serpulina, Treponema*) ***hyodysenteriae*** (also by ***B. hampsonii*** and ***B. suanatina***), family *Spirochaetaceae*, is a historically well recognized and now a re-emergent production-limiting disease of swine worldwide, with moderate-to-severe *mucohemorrhagic-to-fibrinous colitis*. **Porcine spirochetal colitis** refers to a less severe nonhemorrhagic colitis caused by ***B. pilosicoli***. Additional *Brachyspira* species, such as ***B. murdochii***, ***B. intermedia***, and ***B. innocens***, have been associated with variably severe disease, but are not considered causative agents of swine dysentery. These latter strains are now frequently identified in herds without evidence of disease, although they are indistinguishable by morphologic and phenotypic features, including biochemical properties and strength of beta-hemolysis. The diagnosis of swine dysentery in pigs thus relies on identification of beta-hemolytic *Brachyspira* sp. from the colon of pigs with appropriate clinical signs, and lesions typical of swine dysentery.

Since 1921, **classical swine dysentery** has been recognized as a highly infectious disease, mainly of weaned pigs. The cause was only identified to be *B. hyodysenteriae* 50 years later as a gram-negative, anaerobic, oxygen-tolerant, strongly beta-hemolytic *spirochete*. The loosely coiled motile organism has periplasmic flagella that facilitate motility and penetration of intestinal content for access to the colonic epithelium. Although the bacterial genus *Brachyspira* includes several species capable of colonizing a wide spectrum of hosts, *B. hyodysenteriae*, *B. hampsonii*, and *B. suanatina* are predominantly pathogens of pigs. Experimental reproduction of swine dysentery in gnotobiotic pigs requires anaerobic bacteria indigenous to the normal colon, along with *B. hyodysenteriae*; there is apparently a *synergistic action between B. hyodysenteriae and the intestinal microbiota*, mainly *Bacteroides* spp. and *Fusobacterium* spp. Several studies have implicated dietary factors, and elevated protein:carbohydrate ratio, altered fermentation activity, and altered hindgut microbiota are considered likely predisposing factors for enhanced pathogenicity of *B. hyodysenteriae* in pigs, although the mechanisms remain poorly understood. Coinfections with other significant swine intestinal pathogens such as *L. intracellularis* can significantly enhance clinical severity, as well as both gross and histologic lesions.

The **pathogenesis** of swine dysentery is still incompletely understood, but gene studies have identified virulence traits for *Brachyspira* that include hemolysins, cytotoxins, outer membrane proteins, motility factors such as flagella, and NADH oxidase, which is thought to be required for the bacterium to successfully colonize the colonic epithelium. *B. hyodysenteriae* first colonizes mucus on the luminal surface of the large bowel before invading the cytoplasm of colonocytes and goblet cells; spirochetes can be observed in silver-stained histologic sections and by electron microscopy or in situ hybridization. This process is likely mediated by flagella and outer membrane proteins that enable the pathogen to successfully colonize the host. Following invasion of enterocytes by the pathogen, there is enhanced and altered mucin secretion, degeneration, and necrosis of epithelial cells, and hemorrhage, which are thought to be mediated by cytotoxins and endotoxin. Exfoliation of surface epithelial cells has been associated with large numbers of spirochetes and other anaerobic bacteria on the mucosa. *Brachyspira* do not usually invade beyond the epithelial cells, and the result is *mucosal colitis*, with superficial erosion with hyperplasia of cells in colonic glands, hypersecretion of mucus, and a mixed inflammatory infiltrate in the lamina propria. Thrombosis of capillaries and venules in the superficial areas of the colonic mucosa is probably due to absorption of endotoxin through the damaged mucosal epithelium. Diarrhea is due to altered ion transportation leading to *malabsorption of fluids and electrolytes in the colon;* this presumably results from damage to the superficial epithelium of the colon, which in the pig normally has tremendous absorptive capacity. Active fluid secretion by the colon, associated with bacterial enterotoxins, probably does not play a major role in swine dysentery.

Transmission by ingestion of feces, or introduction of *subclinical carrier* pigs into a herd, usually precedes an outbreak; vectors including rodents or fomites are also considered risk factors. Once established in a herd, the infection tends to remain *enzootic*, and although treatment can effect rapid clinical amelioration, relapses often occur cyclically in individuals or groups. The morbidity and mortality may reach 90% and 30%, respectively. Immunity is variable following bouts of dysentery, and recovered pigs are apparently protected against subsequent challenge for several months, although some animals remain susceptible.

The disease occurs in pigs 2- or 3-weeks-old, but particularly between 8-14 weeks of age. Once initiated, it spreads rapidly by pen contact. The disease is initially febrile, and the initial diarrheic feces are thin, semisolid, and lack blood or mucus. After 1-2 days, blood and copious mucus appear in the feces and this progresses to watery feces with blood, mucus, and fibrin. Some pigs die peracutely without showing diarrhea, but most pigs recover slowly, although their rate of growth is reduced. Experimentally, the severity of disease depends on overall stress on the animals, diet, body weight, group size, and the quantity and growth phase of the inoculum.

Early intestinal lesions can be subtle and include hyperemia and edema of the colonic walls and mesentery with mucosal exudate containing small amounts of fibrin or blood (Fig. 1-119A). Mucosal lesions become more severe as the disease progresses, and there is increased mucus, fibrin, hemorrhage, and perhaps a fibrinonecrotic membrane forming on the mucosal surfaces of the large intestine and cecum. Lesions

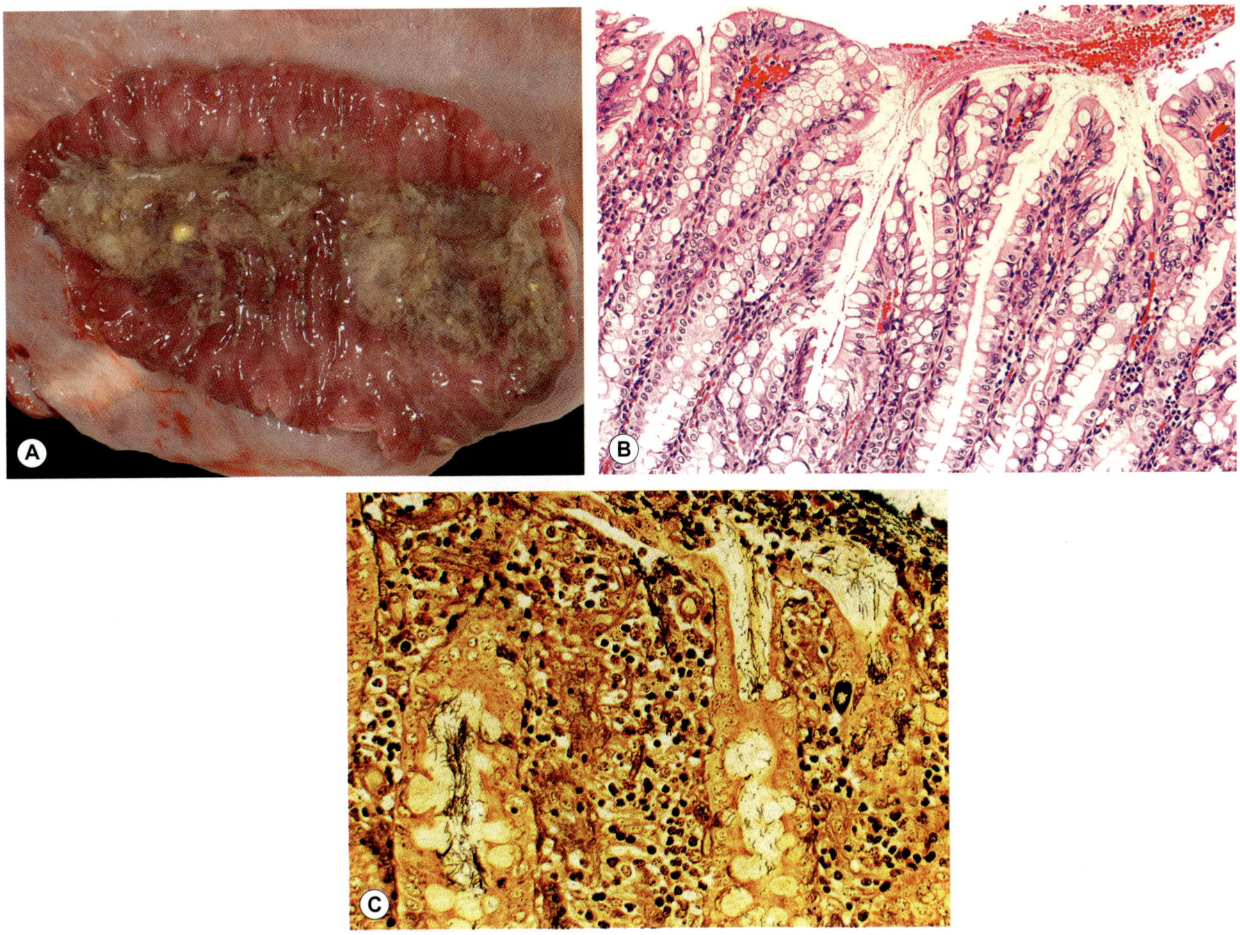

Figure 1-119 Swine dysentery. A. Fibrinocatarrhal exudate on the hemorrhagic colonic mucosa. B. Mucus, fibrin, and hemorrhage covering the mucosa of the colon. There is also goblet cell hyperplasia, increased mucus in the crypts, and lymphoplasmacytic infiltration of the lamina propria. C. Warthin-Starry stain of colonic mucosa with numerous delicate spirochetes. (Courtesy E.R. Burrough.)

can be multifocal, patchy, or involve the entire large intestine. The colonic content in these cases is usually scant, and thick gray to red-brown and greasy in appearance. The most severe lesions can appear similar to those of salmonellosis in extent and severity. The production of mucus in swine dysentery becomes copious in many chronic cases because of *remarkable goblet cell hyperplasia*.

The earliest **microscopic lesions**, which are epithelial erosions and necrosis of the superficial mucosa, are limited to the colon, cecum, and rectum. Thin layers of exudate composed of mucus, fibrin, neutrophils, and erythrocytes cover the areas of damaged epithelium (see Fig. 1-119B). In more advanced cases, these areas become more diffuse and exudation is more copious; however, deep ulceration is not common. There may be minor bleeding or small fibrin thrombi in the superficial vessels of the lamina propria underlying eroded mucosa. There is usually some edema of the lamina propria, submucosa, and serosa, especially in more chronic infections, although thickening of the mucosa and submucosa also occurs due to congestion, fibrin accumulation, and infiltration of leukocytes. In concert with the increased turnover of epithelial cells associated with the superficial erosion, there is hyperplasia of goblet cells as well as epithelial cells deeper in the glands. The crypts become elongated and lined by proliferative basophilic immature epithelial cells with large hyperchromatic nuclei, and few differentiated goblet cells. Crypts often subsequently become dilated and contain necrotic debris; some have marked goblet cell hyperplasia, and copious mucus production. Large delicate spirochetes can be observed within dilated crypts and goblet cells using Warthin-Starry silver staining (see Fig. 1-119C).

Porcine intestinal spirochetosis is caused by one of several weakly beta-hemolytic strains of *Brachyspira* spp., of which ***B. pilosicoli*** (formerly *Anguillina coli*), is by far the most common, and is the type strain. These differ from *B. hyodysenteriae, B. hampsonii, and B. suanatina* in that they are weakly beta-hemolytic. *B. pilosicoli* has a wide host range and has been isolated from a number of other animal species with lesions of intestinal spirochetosis; it may be zoonotic.

Porcine intestinal spirochetosis has been seen in most major swine-producing areas of the world. *Generally, transient watery-to-mucoid diarrhea, without blood, occurs*. Reduced weight gain is a significant clinical finding. As for *B. hyodysenteriae*, gross lesions are limited to the colon and cecum; they may be subtle. Mesocolonic edema, swollen lymph nodes, variable mucosal erosion, and abundant watery large intestinal contents are early gross lesions. Later, the mucosa becomes thickened and in severe cases there is exudation of fibrin, which intermixes with necrotic debris and hemorrhage on the mucosal surface forming a diphtheritic membrane.

Virulence factors of *B. pilosicoli* are also still poorly defined, but motility and chemotaxis for mucus are likely important. The organism is capable of polar attachment by one end of the bacterium to the apical membrane of colonic or rectal epithelial cells, resulting in a palisade of upright bacteria perpendicular to the epithelial cells and displacement or effacement of microvilli. Thus, spirochetes can often be observed histologically as a *false brush border* on the luminal surface early in infection; visualization of the bacteria is enhanced by Warthin-Starry silver stains or fluorescence in situ hybridization. Although the molecular receptors for attachment have not been identified, the organism can invade paracellularly, especially at the extrusion zone between colonic crypt units. *B. pilosicoli* can be observed within colonic crypts, goblet cells, or invading tight junctions into the lamina propria, but is not disseminated systemically in pigs. In chronic infections, there are large numbers of inflammatory cells in the lamina propria, including lymphocytes, plasma cells, and monocytes. There is also goblet cell hyperplasia and crypt hyperplasia so that crypts are lined by immature basophilic mitotically active cells. The diarrhea and ill-thrift characteristic of infection may be related to loss of absorptive function, secondary to disruption of the brush border of enterocytes, and increased exfoliation of poorly differentiated cells and perhaps enteric loss of plasma protein. Given the existence of long-term colonization by *B. pilosicoli* in pigs, it is unlikely that protective immunity develops after infection; however, the immune responses against this organism are poorly understood. Definitive diagnosis of this disease requires identification of the agent by culture, PCR, or FISH, along with either evidence of appropriate clinical disease and/or expected large intestinal lesions in affected animals.

Mild chronic colitis or diarrhea caused by other weakly hemolytic *Brachyspira* sp. (such as *B. intermedia* and *B. murdochii*) are described, but their pathogenicity remains incompletely understood. They are probably mildly pathogenic; however, their presence is not uncommon in domestic pigs and their greatest significance may be that they cause considerable confusion with diagnosis of either swine dysentery or porcine intestinal spirochetosis, both of which are much more economically important diseases.

In **dogs, colonic spirochetosis** with mucosal colitis has also been described, in association with *B. pilosicoli, B. canis*, and perhaps with other *Brachyspira* spp., but a causal relationship has not been definitively established.

Clostridial infections

Most of the important enteric clostridial diseases that occur in herbivores and pigs are caused by 1 of the 7 toxigenic types of ***Clostridium perfringens*** or by ***Clostridioides difficile*** (formerly *Clostridium difficile*). Enteritis in dogs may be associated with NetF-positive strains of *Clostridium perfringens* type A or *C. difficile*, although conclusive evidence of the role of these microorganisms in canine enteric disease is lacking. ***Clostridium piliforme*** causes Tyzzer disease, characterized by multifocal necrotic hepatitis and occasionally enteritis, colitis, and/or myocarditis, in many animal species. ***C. chauvoei*** may affect the tongue causing blackleg-like glossitis (see Vol. 1, Muscle and Tendon). Enteritis produced by *C. chauvoei* has also been rarely described in cattle. ***C. septicum*** causes clostridial abomasitis (braxy) in sheep and possibly calves, discussed earlier in the Stomach and Abomasum section. ***C. botulinum*** causes botulism in horses, cattle, and several other species by ingestion of preformed toxins. ***C. tetani*** is responsible for tetanus in a variety of mammals (see Vol. 1, Nervous System). ***C. spiroforme*** (now reclassified as *Thomasclavelia spiroformis*) is a helically coiled, gram-positive, anaerobic, spore-forming bacillus responsible for *C. spiroforme*–associated enteric disease in rabbits.

The virulence of *C. perfringens* is mostly attributable to its capacity to produce >20 toxins, including 6 so-called major (typing) toxins (i.e., alpha, beta, epsilon, iota, enterotoxin, and necrotic enteritis B-like toxin [NetB]), which are used to classify this microorganism into 7 toxinotypes, designated A-G (Table 1-2). However, no single strain produces this entire toxin set. Besides producing 1 or more of the 6 typing toxins (see Table 1-2), some *C. perfringens* strains produce additional toxins, such as kappa, lambda, beta2, TpeL, and

Table • 1-2

Classification of* Clostridium perfringens *into 7 toxinotypes based on the genes for 6 major exotoxins (alpha, beta, epsilon, iota, enterotoxin, and necrotic enteritis B–like toxin)

	TOXIN GENE					
C. perfringens toxinotype	Alpha	Beta	Epsilon	Iota	Enterotoxin	Necrotic enteritis B–like toxin
A	+	–	–	–	–	–
B	+	+	+	–	–/+	–
C	+	+	–	–	–/+	–
D	+	–	+	–	–/+	–
E	+	–	–	+	–/+	–
F	+	–	–	–	+	–
G	+	–	–	–	–/+	+

+ = toxin gene present; – = toxin gene not present.

NetF, some of which contribute to the virulence of some strains and others may be critical virulence factors of other strains. Some strains may lose their ability to produce one or more of their toxins when stored or cultured, and this complicates the identification of isolates and the assessment of their significance in disease outbreaks. Additionally, plasmid conjugation occurs both in vitro and in vivo, and it is now thought that some previously avirulent strains may become virulent by acquiring toxin genes in vivo.

With the exception of enterotoxin, which is a subproduct of sporulation, the other 5 major typing toxins are produced during active growth. The **alpha toxin** is a lecithinase that acts on cell membranes, producing hemolysis and necrosis of cells. The role of alpha toxin in intestinal disease of mammals is controversial, although most evidence indicates that this toxin on its own does not produce significant intestinal damage.

The **beta toxin** is a pore-forming toxin that induces intestinal necrosis and occasionally a variety of neurologic effects through a yet unknown mechanism. This toxin is exquisitely sensitive to the action of trypsin, which inactivates it in a few minutes; this property is very important for the pathogenesis of beta toxin–related diseases.

The **epsilon toxin** is produced as a relatively inactive prototoxin that is activated by enzymatic digestion. Intestinal trypsin, chymotrypsin, other intestinal proteases, and **lambda toxin** produced by some strains of *C. perfringens* are the main enzymes responsible for activation of epsilon prototoxin. Epsilon toxin is also a pore-forming toxin that induces mainly neurologic, respiratory, and cardiac effects, which are mostly the result of increased vascular permeability, although this toxin can also produce a direct effect on neurons and oligodendroglia in the brain.

Iota toxin is a binary toxin with 2 components, iota a and iota b, which is also elaborated as a prototoxin and activated by proteolytic enzymes.

Beta2 toxin, which despite its name is not related to beta toxin, has been associated with enteric disease in swine and horses caused by *C. perfringens* type A, although conclusive evidence of its pathogenicity is lacking.

C. perfringens type F strains produce **enterotoxin**, which is a specific toxin; the name enterotoxin should therefore not be used to refer to all *C. perfringens* toxins produced in the intestine. Enterotoxin is only elaborated during sporulation and is released upon lysis of vegetative cells. It may also be produced by some other types of *C. perfringens*, but most cases of disease are associated with enterotoxin-producing *C. perfringens* type F, which has been among the most important causes of human food poisoning in the United States over the past few decades. Enterotoxigenic type F strains are also associated with antibiotic treatment–related diarrhea in humans. The significance of enterotoxin in animal disease is limited. It is also a pore-forming toxin.

Most clostridial diseases originating in the intestine are often called **enterotoxemias**, which by definition are diseases produced by toxins generated in the intestine that are absorbed into the circulation and that act on distant organs such as the brain and lungs. However, although several clostridial diseases of the intestine are true enterotoxemias, some of them are not. For instance, disease produced in sheep by *C. perfringens* type D, whose epsilon exotoxin is elaborated in the intestine but in this species exerts its important effects on distant organs such as the brain and lungs, is a true enterotoxemia. The same toxinotype can produce an enterocolitis in goats with, in the chronic cases, no systemic absorption of epsilon toxin, in which case, no enterotoxemia occurs.

The **pathogenesis** of enteric infection with *C. perfringens* and *C. difficile* requires: 1) these microorganisms to be in the intestine (sometimes they can be normal inhabitants of the gut), and 2) a change in the enteric microenvironment favorable to massive expansion of luminal populations of clostridia and/or production of their toxins. Such changes may include a change in feed, abnormally nutrient-rich digesta, antimicrobial therapy, altered pancreatic exocrine function or trypsin inhibitors, reduced motility, and/or primary infections with agents such as coccidia. Intoxication by ingestion of preformed toxin by these microorganisms has not been documented.

Exotoxins are required for *C. perfringens* to induce disease, as has been demonstrated in several animal experiments using so-called reverse genetics, in which bacterial strains genetically engineered to remove one or more toxin genes were inoculated into animals. The absence of a particular toxin gene eliminated the virulence, which was restored when that gene was reintroduced into the genome.

Clostridioides difficile produces 3 main exotoxins: toxin A, which is an enterotoxin, toxin B, which is a cytotoxin but also an enterotoxin, and *C. difficile* transferase (CDT) which is an ADP-ribosyltransferase. Tissue damage is probably due to the effects of one or of both toxins, which glycosylate and inactivate Ras GTPases, disabling signaling pathways in the cell. As well, they glycosylate Rho and interfere with its ability to regulate cytoskeletal actin. Under the influence of these toxins, the cytoskeleton condenses, tight junctions open, cells round up, and undergo apoptosis. They also cause release of proinflammatory mediators, attracting neutrophils, and activate secretion stimulated by the enteric nervous system. Hence, intestinal content is fluid, and there is focal or diffuse small intestinal or colonic epithelial necrosis, through which neutrophils may exude into the lumen, producing a so-called "volcano" lesion. Thirty-four toxinotypes of *C. difficile* have been described based on sequence variations in the genes for the A and B toxin molecules. Some of these isolates produce also CDT, and there are also rare strains that are negative for toxins A and B but positive for CDT and can cause disease. Toxinotypes have diverse toxin production patterns: A+B+CDT−, A−B+CDT+, A+B+CDT+, A−B−CDT+. There are also nontoxigenic strains, which are not included in the toxinotyping scheme.

Clostridium piliforme, the cause of Tyzzer disease and the only gram-negative pathogenic clostridia, is an obligate intracellular pathogen that in the alimentary tract infects small intestinal or colonic epithelial cells causing necrosis and inflammation. The pathogenesis of Tyzzer disease is not clearly dependent on toxin production, although some strains do produce cytotoxic proteins.

Diagnosis of disease by the toxin-producing clostridia is mostly dependent on demonstration of toxin in gut content or feces of affected animals, by the most specific test available. Although large numbers of a particular type of *C. perfringens* in the intestine suggest causation of the disease, some types of this organism are commonly present in the gut in a variety of circumstances, and their mere presence can therefore not be considered diagnostic. *C. perfringens* type A is by far the most ubiquitous toxinotype in the intestine of animals, and isolation of this type alone is the least significant from a diagnostic standpoint. However, other types (e.g., types B and C) are less frequently found in the intestine of healthy animals, which makes isolation of these types more diagnostically significant.

***Clostridium perfringens* type A. *C. perfringens* type A** is the toxinotype most commonly found in the environment and in the intestine of clinically healthy animals. Its major toxin is the alpha toxin; and some strains may also produce a variable number of other so-called minor toxins. This is one of several clostridia that produce gas gangrene in humans and animals. The production of gas gangrene in wound and puerperal infections is mostly mediated by alpha toxin with assistance by perfringolysin O. *C. perfringens* type A has been associated with several alimentary syndromes in mammals, including enteritis in foals, enterocolitis in adult horses and neonatal piglets, enterotoxemia and hemorrhagic enteritis in lambs and neonatal calves and older cattle, and diarrhea and hemorrhagic enteritis in dogs. However, absolute proof of involvement of *C. perfringens* type A in these alimentary syndromes of mammals is lacking.

Many strains of *C. perfringens* type A produce beta2 toxin, and although initially it was thought that this toxin had a role in porcine clostridial enteritis, similar percentages of diarrheic and nondiarrheic pigs carry the beta2 toxin gene, which questions the possible involvement of this toxin in enteric disease of pigs. Involvement of beta2 toxin–producing *C. perfringens* in enterocolitis of horses also has been suggested, but never proved.

A very rare disease of lambs with acute intravascular hemolysis, known as **yellow lamb disease**, has also been associated with type A infections and, on at least one occasion, with type D infection. Affected animals may be found dead or moribund, and jaundice and hemoglobinuria may be evident clinically. At autopsy, icterus, anemia, hemoglobinuric nephrosis, and other changes of severe, acute, intravascular hemolysis are prominent. Microscopically, the most prominent changes are centrilobular hepatic necrosis and hemoglobinuric nephrosis, both presumably associated with acute intravascular hemolysis and anemia. This hemolytic disease must be distinguished from other causes of acute intravascular hemolysis such as leptospirosis, necrotic hepatitis, and bacillary hemoglobinuria caused by *C. novyi* type B and D, respectively, and copper poisoning. Presumably, the hemolytic effect of alpha toxin is responsible for the intravascular hemolysis. Given that type A strains and alpha toxin are commonly found in the intestines of ruminants, diagnosis of this condition cannot be confirmed by detection of either of these and it has to be established presumptively based on clinical, gross, and microscopic findings coupled with ruling out other possible causes of intravascular hemolysis. It has been suggested that the disease is associated with unusually high alpha toxin–producing type A strains, although this has not been confirmed.

Some strains of *C. perfringens* type A and some type F have been associated with diarrhea, sometimes bloody, in dogs. **Hemorrhagic canine gastroenteritis** (canine GI hemorrhage syndrome) is a sporadic, peracute, hemorrhagic gastroenteritis. Epidemiologic evidence suggests that NetF-positive type A strains may be responsible for the disease. This, however, has not been definitely confirmed, and Koch postulates have not been fulfilled. Dogs with the peracute hemorrhagic disease are often found dead lying in a pool of bloody excreta; sometimes hemorrhagic diarrhea is noted before death. Autopsy reveals hemorrhagic enteritis and colitis, and sometimes hemorrhagic gastritis is present. Colonic lesions tend to be more severe. Microscopically, there is hemorrhagic necrosis of the GI mucosa, which extends from the luminal surface into the mucosa. Numerous rods may cover the necrotic intestinal mucosa or be distributed through the detritus, but they do not invade the intact tissue.

***Clostridium perfringens* type B. Infection by *C. perfringens* type B** has been reported from Europe, South Africa, the Middle East, and most recently from New Zealand, but not from the Americas. It causes "lamb dysentery," usually in lambs up to 10-14-days-old, dysentery in calves of approximately the same age, and perhaps dysentery in foals within the first few days of life.

In lambs, death may occur without premonitory signs, but there is usually abdominal pain, especially when animals are forced to rise, and passage of semifluid dark feces mixed or coated with blood. The abdomen is often bloated. In a more chronic form in older lambs, which is known as "pine" in England, there is unthriftiness and depression, reluctance to suckle, and a peculiar stretching when the animal rises; such cases are reputed to respond well to specific antiserum.

Typical **gross lesions** are usually present, although in exceptional peracute cases they may be absent. The characteristic lesion is *extensive necrohemorrhagic enteritis*. The peritoneal cavity often contains a small amount of serous or blood-stained fluid. In cases with more severe and deeply penetrating mucosal ulcerations, there may be overlying peritonitis with red fibrin strands on the local mesentery, and intestinal adhesions. On the mucosal surface, the ulcers are irregular but well defined by a sharp margin and rim of intense hyperemia, and they may be covered by a yellow fibrinonecrotic pseudomembrane; they may coalesce to form extensive areas of necrosis. There may be transmural emphysema. Usually, the intestinal contents are blood stained and may appear to be composed of pure blood, but in lambs that live for 3-4 days, there may be little or no hemorrhage evident. **Histologically**, the wall of the intestine is hemorrhagic, and the areas of necrosis extend deeply into the mucous membrane, in some cases penetrating to the external muscle layers and serosa. There are large numbers of typical bacilli in the necrotic tissue, but few inflammatory cells.

The lesions present in other organs are those of severe toxemia. The liver is usually pale and friable but may be congested. The spleen is normal or slightly enlarged and pulpy. The kidneys may be enlarged, edematous, pale, and soft. The pericardial sac contains abundant clear gelatinous fluid with or without fibrin strands, the myocardium is pale and soft, and epicardial and endocardial hemorrhages are almost constant. The lungs are often congested and very edematous. Occasionally, foci of symmetrical encephalomalacia similar to those observed in cases of type D enterotoxemia may be observed in subacute and chronic cases.

The disease in **calves** caused by type B *C. perfringens* closely resembles that in lambs, usually affecting sucklings <10-days-old, with a course of 2-4 days, prostration, and dysentery. Older calves up to 10-weeks-old are sometimes affected. It appears that calves are more likely to recover, albeit slowly, than are lambs. The intestinal lesion is *acute hemorrhagic enteritis* with extensive mucosal necrosis and patchy diphtheritic membrane formations, especially in the distal jejunum and ileum. Information on the disease in **foals** is very scant as only a few cases in this species have been reported.

***Clostridium perfringens* type C. *C. perfringens* type C** is present worldwide and causes disease mostly in neonatal individuals, particularly in lambs, calves, foals, and piglets. Occasionally, type C disease occurs in adult individuals of several species. The main virulence factor of *C. perfringens* type C is beta toxin as demonstrated in animal experiments using toxin mutants of this microorganism in rabbits, mice, and goats. Synergistic action by *C. perfringens* enterotoxin has been demonstrated experimentally, and it is possible that such synergism also occurs in spontaneous disease. *Beta toxin is trypsin-labile*, and circumstances such as low trypsin levels in neonatal animals, trypsin inhibitors in the diet, and/or very high levels of toxin are critical in the pathogenesis of type C disease. The high susceptibility of neonatal animals to type C disease is considered to be a consequence of the trypsin inhibitor effect of colostrum, a mechanism apparently aimed to protect immunoglobulins present in the colostrum. "Pig-bel," also known as "enteritis necroticans," is a necrotizing enteritis of humans caused by *C. perfringens* type C, which was the most important cause of human deaths in the 1960s in Papua New Guinea and still occurs sporadically in that island and other countries of the region. The disease has been associated with consumption of trypsin inhibitors in sweet potatoes, a significant component of the diet in Papua New Guinea. This, coupled with the low level of protein in the diet, results in low trypsin in the intestine, which allows persistence of beta toxin in the intestinal lumen. Intraduodenal inoculation of *C. perfringens* type C in combination with trypsin inhibitor produces acute necrohemorrhagic enteritis and/or enterotoxemia in guinea pigs, rabbits, lambs, and goats.

The diseases caused by type C in **lambs, calves, piglets, goat kids**, and **foals** are very similar. Affected animals are usually neonates, which contract the disease within the first few days of life, often within the first few hours. Sick lambs may shiver, have abdominal pain and distension, diarrhea, and prostration, and die within 12 hours or less. Frequently, lambs with type C disease are found dead without clinical signs having been observed. In lambs, the **gross** intestinal changes are acute necrohemorrhagic enteritis that may be segmental and can sometimes be confused with intestinal strangulation. The most prominent changes occur in the jejunum and ileum, the lumens of which may contain free blood, which forms a clotted cast in fresh cadavers. Sometimes there is merely acute hyperemia of a segment of jejunum with edema of the wall, scant creamy intestinal content, and a few small ulcerations of the mucosa. A fibrinous pseudomembrane may be observed over the mucosa of the small intestine. The peritoneal cavity contains a small quantity of blood-stained serous fluid, and the local mesentery and peritoneum are often mildly to severely hyperemic and bear red strands of fibrin. The mesenteric nodes are enlarged, edematous, and congested. There is usually excess pericardial fluid and pulmonary interstitial edema. Ecchymoses on the serous membranes are nearly constant, and in a few cadavers, all tissues, but especially the meninges and brain, are liberally sprinkled with small hemorrhages. There might be terminal bacteremia by *C. perfringens* with bacterial embolism in various organs.

Histopathologic changes in lambs with type C disease are not specific but can be highly suggestive of this infection. The changes consist of acute necrosis that involves mostly the intestinal mucosa, although it can progress to be transmural in severe cases. In most cases this is coagulative necrosis, but in animals that survive longer, the mucosa is completely replaced by a fibrinous pseudomembrane. Thrombosis of mucosal and submucosal vessels is a common finding. Inflammatory infiltrate is usually not a striking feature, although a band of viable and degenerate neutrophils separating the necrotic superficial mucosa from the more normal looking deeper mucosa may be observed in subacute cases. Diffuse or multifocal distribution of gram-positive bacilli free in the intestinal lumen is common. Although they may be in close contact with the mucosa and attachment has been suggested, no definitive evidence of attachment has been demonstrated in *C. perfringens* infections of ruminants.

In **adult sheep**, *C. perfringens* type C causes **"struck,"** a disease of pastured animals that has a mortality rate of 5-15% in some areas. Death usually occurs suddenly with terminal convulsive episodes, but less acute cases may adopt a straining position that probably indicates acute abdominal pain. In adult sheep, diarrhea or convulsions rarely occur. Gross and microscopic lesions are similar to those described in lambs except that small intestinal ulceration may be prominent and the mucosal necrosis is deeper, with a peripheral leukocytic rim separating the more-or-less normal deeper layers of the intestine.

Calves with type C disease have abdominal pain, some have diarrhea of sudden onset, and death may be preceded by spasmodic convulsions. Occasionally, sudden death occurs without premonitory clinical signs. The **gross and microscopic lesions** in calves are similar to those described in lambs.

C. perfringens type C also causes necrohemorrhagic enteritis, mostly in neonatal **piglets**. Rarely, epizootics occur in 2-4-week-old and weaned pigs. The disease occurs as epizootics in affected herds and regions and may then remain enzootic. Poor hygienic conditions, overcrowding, and antibiotic treatment are thought to be predisposing factors in some outbreaks. Clinical disease can be peracute, acute, or chronic, with signs of the acute and peracute condition including intense abdominal pain, depression, and bloody diarrhea, which begins 8-22 hours after exposure to *C. perfringens* type C. Sow feces contain small numbers of type C organisms, and these multiply rapidly in the small intestine of piglets, outcompeting other bacteria and becoming the dominant organisms in the population. The course of the disease is usually 24 hours or less in 1-2-day-old piglets, but chronic disease (usually in older animals) can persist for 1 or 2 weeks; diarrhea without blood and dehydration is persistent. Marked anal hyperemia can be observed just before death in both acute and chronic forms.

The receptor for beta toxin has been identified as CD31. Beta toxin binds to small intestinal mucosal endothelial cells of piglets with type C infection. Beta toxin–induced endothelial cell damage may play an important role in the early lesion development of *C. perfringens* type C enteritis in pigs. However, the initial action of beta toxin may be on the superficial enterocytes. It is possible that a combined action of the toxins on the enterocytes and endothelial cells occurs. The predominant lesions occur in the small intestine, especially the jejunum, but the cecum and spiral colon are often involved, and occasionally lesions are confined to the large intestine.

Gross lesions are similar in all areas of the intestine, and in acute cases consist of intestinal and mesenteric hyperemia, extensive necrosis of the intestinal mucosa, which may be covered by a pseudomembrane (Fig. 1-120A), and blood staining of the contents. There may be emphysema of the intestinal wall, which becomes fragile. Mesenteric lymph nodes are red, and sanguineous peritoneal and pleural fluid is present. Fibrinous intestinal adhesions may develop.

Histologically, the hallmark of acute disease in young piglets is *segmental hemorrhagic necrosis* of the intestinal wall, which starts in the mucosa but usually progresses to affect all layers of the intestine. Lesions are morphologically similar in all segments of intestine; the luminal surface is covered by a pseudomembrane composed of degenerate and necrotic desquamated epithelial cells, cell debris, inflammatory cells including neutrophils, lymphocytes, plasma cells, and macrophages, fibrin (see Fig. 1-120B), and a variable number of large, thick bacilli with square ends and occasional subterminal spores. These bacteria occur singly or in clusters, free in the lumen, or covering the margin of the denuded mucosal surface. Although the bacterial population is usually greater in the central intestinal lumen, a few bacilli also can be seen in crypts and glands and invading necrotic lamina propria. Superficial epithelium and superficial layers of lamina propria are necrotic, with a homogeneous acidophilic appearance, scattered pyknotic or karyorrhectic nuclei, and an inflammatory cell infiltrate of neutrophils and mononuclear cells. Fibrin thrombi occluding superficial arteries and veins of the lamina propria and submucosa are characteristic of this condition. Fibrin also can be seen in mucosal and submucosal lymphatics and in the interstitium. Diffuse edema with variable amounts of protein and inflammatory cell exudate can be seen throughout all intestinal layers, including serosa. The mucosa is severely thickened by edema and inflammatory exudate. As the infection progresses, necrosis goes deeper, including epithelium of crypts and glands and, later, all intestinal layers. Severe congestion of subserosal vessels is observed throughout the course of the infection. Lesions are usually diffuse, although they can be multifocal. Mucosal necrosis without hemorrhage may be observed in older pigs with chronic disease.

The disease caused by *C. perfringens* type C in **foals** has been reported from the United States, Canada, Australia, and several European countries. It usually occurs in foals <4-days-old, although occasional cases may also occur in older foals and adult horses. Typical clinical signs include weakness, yellow-to-brown watery diarrhea, colic, and dehydration. Affected foals usually die in <24 hours. Sudden death without clinical signs being observed, as well as neurologic signs, may also occasionally occur. The reason for the neurologic signs

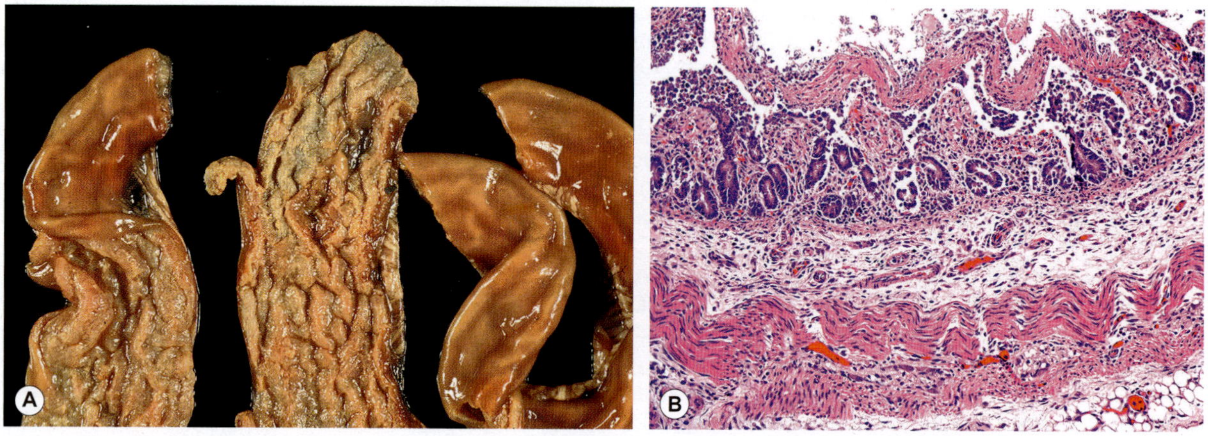

Figure 1-120 Necrotizing enteritis in a piglet, caused by ***Clostridium perfringens* type C.** **A.** Fibrinonecrotic membrane covers the mucosal surface. (Courtesy P. Blanchard.) **B.** Necrosis of the superficial mucosa, which is covered by a pseudomembrane.

has not been elucidated as no gross or microscopic changes have been described in the nervous system of foals with *C. perfringens* type C disease. **Gross lesions** are those of *acute hemorrhagic necrotizing enteritis*, usually in the distal two-thirds of the small intestine (Fig. 1-121A and B), although in some cases most of the small and large intestine may be affected. The **microscopic lesions** are similar to those for *C. perfringens* type C infection in other species (see Fig. 1-121C) and in foals, histologically, the lesions are very similar to those caused by *C. difficile* and *Salmonella* spp. In a series of cases of combined infection with *C. perfringens* type C and *C. difficile* in foals, both the gross and microscopic histopathology were indistinguishable from those in foals infected with either of these 2 microorganisms individually.

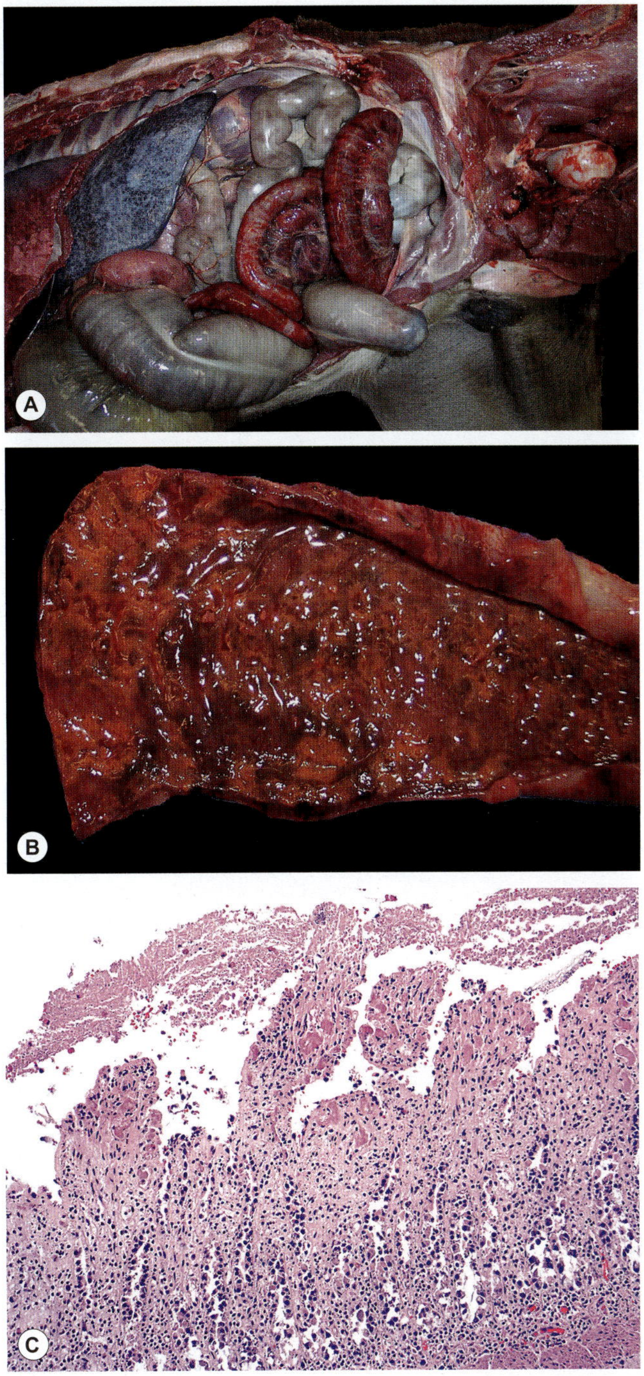

Figure 1-121 Hemorrhagic and necrotizing enteritis caused by ***Clostridium perfringens* type C** in a newborn foal. **A.** Serosal view. **B.** Mucosal view. **C.** A fibrinous pseudomembrane covers the mucosa, and numerous fibrin thrombi occlude mucosal vessels. (Reprinted with permission from Diab SS, et al. Pathology of *Clostridium perfringens* type C enterotoxemia in horses. Vet Pathol 2012:49:255–263.)

A disease clinically and pathologically identical to that described in sheep has been experimentally produced in **goats** inoculated intraduodenally with *C. perfringens* type C. A presumptive diagnosis of type C disease can be established based on clinical and pathologic findings, but confirmation of the disease relies on detection of beta toxin in intestinal contents and/or feces. However, because this toxin is so sensitive to trypsin, failure to detect this toxin in intestinal content does not preclude a diagnosis of *C. perfringens* type C infection. Because this microorganism is infrequently found in the intestine of normal animals, isolation is considered to have some diagnostic significance.

***Clostridium perfringens* type D.** Enterotoxemia ("overeating disease" and formerly known as "*pulpy kidney disease*") caused by *C. perfringens* type D is an important disease of sheep and goats with a worldwide distribution. It occurs occasionally in cattle and poorly documented cases have been described in a few horses. The rarely observed subacute and chronic forms of the disease in sheep have been called *focal symmetrical encephalomalacia* (FSE), because for many years they were thought to be a different disease, but FSE is only one of the pathologic manifestations of the subacute and chronic forms of type D enterotoxemia. By definition, type D isolates must produce both alpha and epsilon toxins, although some type D isolates can express several other toxins. However, it has been demonstrated by the use of reverse genetic experiments in animal models that ***epsilon toxin** is required and sufficient to cause all the clinical signs and lesions of type D enterotoxemia in sheep and goats*; alpha toxin does not seem to have a role in the pathogenesis of the disease. Epsilon toxin is the third most potent clostridial toxin (after botulinum and tetanus toxins) and, for a few years (2002–12) it was considered a class B select agent by the USDA and CDC in the United States. Activated epsilon toxin apparently facilitates its own absorption through the intestinal mucosa, and it is then transported to several target organs, including the brain, heart, lungs, and kidneys. In the brain and possibly also in other organs, epsilon toxin affects endothelial cells, producing the lesions described later. Epsilon toxin also acts directly on neurons and oligodendrocytes within the brain.

Sheep and goats suddenly fed large amounts of grain or concentrate are highly susceptible; thus, the synonym *overeating disease*. The manner in which overeating leads to clostridial enterotoxemia is complex and not fully understood. Cultures of *C. perfringens* type D given orally are largely destroyed in the rumen and abomasum. However, when the intestinal environment is favorable, the few organisms that reach the intestine proliferate rapidly and produce toxin. It was accepted traditionally that the critical factor for type D enterotoxemia to occur is undigested starch in the small intestine, providing a suitable substrate for these saccharolytic bacteria, which allows them to proliferate to immense numbers—perhaps $>10^9$ organisms per gram of intestinal contents—and produce correspondingly large amounts of toxin. However, it has been demonstrated in vitro that the absence of glucose in a culture medium stimulates epsilon toxin production. Therefore, it is possible that starch in the intestine stimulates the growth of C. *perfringens* type D; the absence of glucose stimulates epsilon toxin production. When the animal is suddenly provided with excessive quantities of food, particularly starch-rich food, there is a delay before the ruminal flora can adapt. In this period, undigested or partially digested starch may escape into the intestine, and C. *perfringens* type D is likely to take advantage of it. The lack of digestion of starch also would be responsible for the absence of glucose in the small intestine. The epsilon prototoxin is a relatively inactive prototoxin; it is fully activated by digestive enzymes, especially trypsin and chymotrypsin, but also by some proteases produced by some strains of C. *perfringens* (e.g., lambda toxin). This is the reason why most cases of type D disease occur in animals 2-weeks-old or older, when trypsin activity in the intestine has been restored after the trypsin-inhibitory effect of colostrum has ceased.

Epsilon toxin facilitates its own absorption from the intestine, probably in part by increasing the permeability of the mucosa. No damage to the intestinal mucosa, except for occasional congestion and mild hemorrhage, is observed in sheep, as opposed to goats, in which severe necrotizing colitis and/or enterocolitis are frequently observed. The acute disease in goats likely has a similar pathogenesis as in sheep, but the chronic disease, with lesions confined to the intestine, appears to be caused by local effects of epsilon, and perhaps other, C. *perfringens* type D toxins. Although very little information is available in cattle, probably the disease develops in the same way as in sheep.

Traditionally, it was thought that type D enterotoxemia occurred in lambs and goat kids >2-weeks-old or adult sheep and goats. However, a few cases of type D disease in neonatal lambs and goat kids have been reported; lambda toxin produced by some strains of C. *perfringens* was thought to be responsible for the activation of epsilon toxin in the absence of trypsin. In most lambs with type D enterotoxemia, the course is acute and the animal is found dead without clinical signs being observed or after a short period of acute neurologic and respiratory signs, including convulsions and tachypnea, and often bawling as from severe pain. Animals that survive longer may have drooling, tachypnea, hyperesthesia, wide stance, blindness, opisthotonos, and terminal coma or convulsions. In older sheep or younger but vaccinated sheep, subacute or chronic cases are most frequently seen. Neurologic clinical signs are characteristic of the subacute and chronic forms of type D disease and include blindness, ataxia, head pressing, and paraparesis. Diarrhea occasionally may be observed, although this is not a common clinical sign in sheep type D disease.

Grossly, in sheep dead of acute enterotoxemia, the carcass is usually well nourished. In those with a course of 1-2 days, there may be occasional evidence of scours about the rump, although diarrhea is rarely observed. Often there is excessive straw-colored pericardial, thoracic, and abdominal fluid with strands of fibrin (Fig. 1-122) that clots on exposure to air, congestion and edema of the lungs that may be severe enough to produce froth in all the respiratory passages, and hemorrhage beneath the endocardium of the left and occasionally right ventricle of the heart. Hemorrhages may be seen beneath other serous membranes, such as the epicardium, as well as blotchy hemorrhages beneath the parietal peritoneum. Sometimes the liver is congested and the spleen enlarged and pulpy. There is no GI inflammation visible at autopsy, although the content of the small and large intestine may be moderately fluid, and short lengths of the small intestine occasionally may be distended with gas and be hyperemic.

The so-called "pulpy kidney" (softening of the renal parenchyma) has been suggested to be associated with accelerated autolysis, although no conclusive evidence that this is the case exists. This is not a diagnostic feature of type D enterotoxemia, and the expression "pulpy kidney" should not be used to refer to this disease. *Glucosuria* is present in a relatively small percentage of animals with type D enterotoxemia, and it is a useful, although infrequent and nonspecific, diagnostic indicator when detected. The absence of glucosuria does not preclude a diagnosis of type D enterotoxemia.

In **adult sheep**, the **gross lesions** are the same as those in lambs but are more consistent and more advanced. Brain gross lesions may occur in lambs and older sheep with subacute or chronic enterotoxemia, and these are sufficiently unique to be of diagnostic significance. They include herniation of the cerebellar vermis (Fig. 1-123) and/or FSE (Fig. 1-124). The most common distribution of FSE involves the corpus striatum, thalamus, and cerebellar peduncles; there are some minor variations of the pattern, but the lesions are always of the

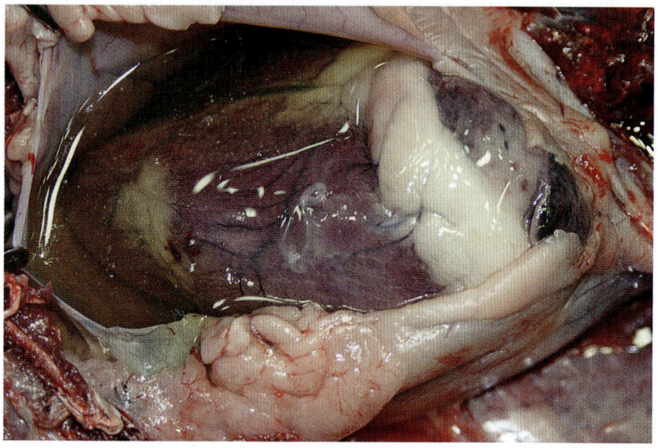

Figure 1-122 ***Clostridium perfringens*** **type D enterotoxemia.** Hydropericardium with fibrin strands in a sheep.

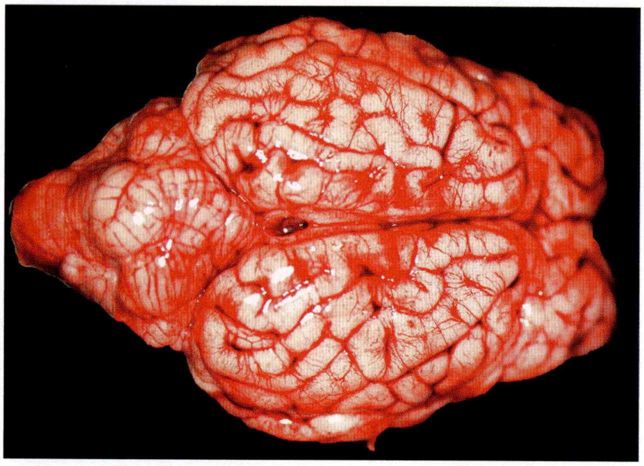

Figure 1-123 ***Clostridium perfringens*** **type D enterotoxemia.** Coning of the cerebellum in a lamb. (Courtesy B. Barr.)

same type. Less frequently, FSE can be seen also in the substantia nigra, white matter of the frontal gyri, rostral cerebral peduncles, and other areas. The white matter is preferentially affected in all these areas. *FSE is pathognomonic* and therefore diagnostic of *C. perfringens* type D enterotoxemia.

The **histologic changes** in the brain of sheep with type D enterotoxemia are unique and pathognomonic, and although they are present in most cases, occasionally, they may be absent. The most consistent change, observed in ~90% of acute and subacute cases, is intramural and probably also perivascular, proteinaceous edema, also known as *microangiopathy*, which is seen mostly as homogeneous acidophilic accumulations of protein within and/or around the wall of small- and medium-sized arteries and veins (Fig. 1-125A). Although it was always believed that the edema was only perivascular, it was recently demonstrated that fluid also accumulates within the vascular wall (see Fig. 1-125B).

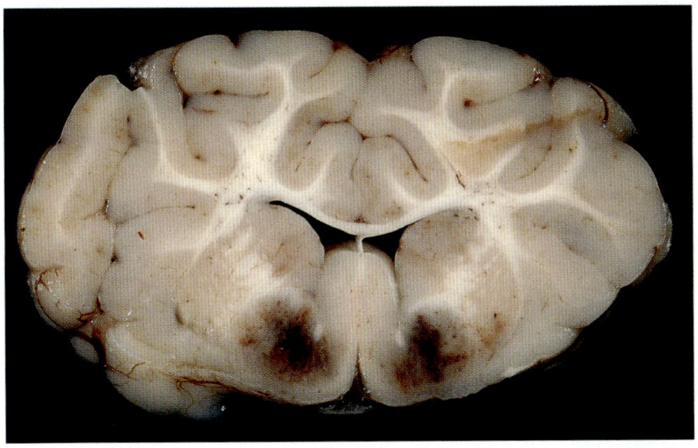

Figure 1-124 ***Clostridium perfringens*** **type D enterotoxemia.** Focal symmetric encephalomalacia in a sheep. Hemorrhage and softening in internal capsules. (Courtesy University of California-Davis Anatomic Pathology.)

Occasionally, accumulation of *hyaline protein droplets* around (and probably also within the wall of) small vessels is also seen. These lesions are first evident a few hours after the onset of clinical signs. Apparently, no other conditions of sheep produce this highly proteinaceous intramural or perivascular edema in the brain, and this change therefore should be considered *diagnostic* for type D enterotoxemia in this species. In subacute and chronic disease, FSE can be observed. This lesion is usually multifocal degeneration of white matter, hemorrhage, astrocyte and axonal swelling, and dilated myelin sheaths. Intramural and perivascular edema, and FSE in the brain, are always bilateral and roughly symmetrical, and they have been described most frequently in corpus striatum, thalamus, midbrain, cerebellar peduncles, and cerebellar white matter. These areas are not exclusively affected, and lesions sometimes can be seen in other parts of the brain, such as cortex and hippocampus. Usually, no significant histologic changes are found in the intestine of sheep dying from enterotoxemia. Specific histologic changes were not observed in kidneys of experimentally inoculated lambs autopsied immediately after death, supporting suggestions that renal changes previously described in cases of type D enterotoxemia are due to postmortem autolysis. Thus, microscopic changes in kidneys should not be considered a diagnostic indicator of ovine enterotoxemia.

Ultrastructurally, severe damage to vascular endothelium is apparent, and there is swelling of protoplasmic astrocytes. The foot processes around blood vessels and the processes around neurons are most severely swollen. Neurons and oligodendrocytes are also affected. IHC has revealed that Alzheimer precursor protein 1 (APP1) is very early upregulated in axons surrounding areas of vasculopathy, suggesting that neuronal stress is an early event in ovine enterotoxemia.

Type D enterotoxemia may be seen in both **adult goats and kids**. As in sheep, the disease occurs mostly in animals 2-weeks-old or older, but cases in neonatal goat kids have also been observed associated with lambda-positive *C. perfringens* type D strains. As in sheep, 3 forms of the disease are recognized in goats: acute, subacute, and chronic. The *acute disease*

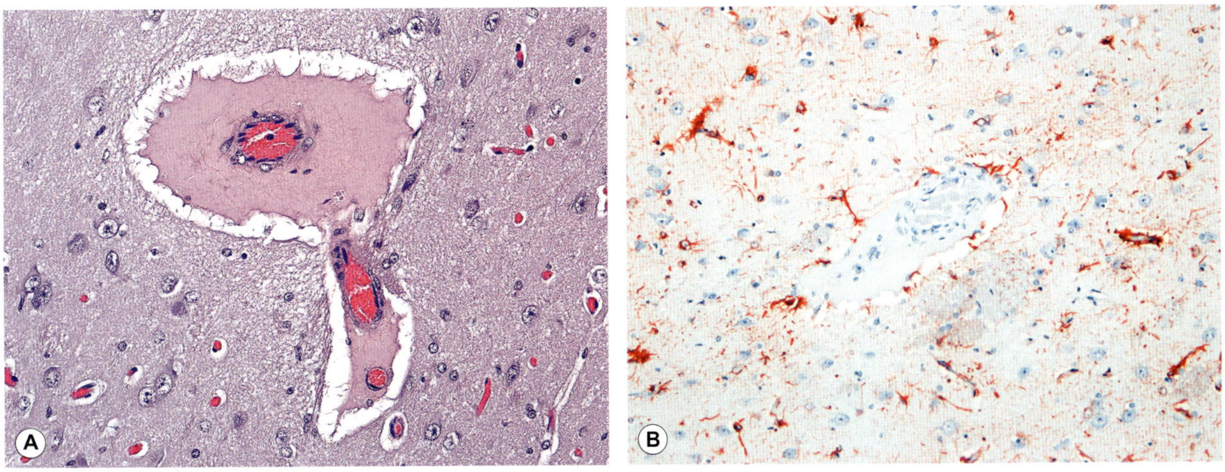

Figure 1-125 ***Clostridium perfringens*** **type D enterotoxemia. A.** Perivascular proteinaceous edema in the corpus striatum of a sheep. (Courtesy J.P. García.) **B.** Terminal ends of astrocyte feet pushed outward due to fluid accumulation within the vascular wall. IHC (glial fibrillary acid protein.) (Reprinted with permission from Garcia JP, et al. Comparative neuropathology of ovine enterotoxemia produced by *Clostridium perfringens* type D wild-type strain CN1020 and its genetically modified derivatives. Vet Pathol 2015;52:465–475.)

is similar to that seen in lambs, and usually manifests as sudden death. In the *subacute form*, diarrhea and severe abdominal discomfort, with or without neurologic signs, occur. Affected animals usually die within 1-2 days of the onset of clinical signs. The *chronic form* of the disease may last for a few days or weeks. Weight loss and diarrhea are its main clinical features. The principal gross lesions in the acute form of the disease are similar to those seen in sheep, except that gross brain lesions are absent. In the subacute and chronic disease, there is mild-to-severe mesocolonic edema, hyperemia, and ulceration of the mucosa (Fig. 1-126A), especially of the distal small intestine, cecum, and spiral colon. The affected areas may be covered by a layer of fibrin that reveals multifocal-to-diffuse ulceration when peeled off. The intestinal contents are olive-green to red and mucoid and frequently contain strands of fibrin. The mesenteric lymph nodes are enlarged and edematous. Hydropericardium, ascites, and pulmonary edema can be seen in the subacute form but not in the chronic form of the disease. FSE similar to that described in sheep has been described in one case of subacute enterotoxemia in goats.

Microscopic changes are usually absent in acute cases, but intramural vascular and probably perivascular edema similar to that described in sheep may be observed in <20% of the cases. The main microscopic lesions in subacute and chronic forms are seen in the colon and, occasionally in the caudal segments of the small intestine. These lesions vary from a mild pleocellular leukocytic reaction in the lamina propria to neutrophilic and fibrinonecrotizing enteritis, colitis, and/or enterocolitis (see Fig. 1-126B). Changes in the lungs may be similar to, but are less consistent than, those seen in lambs. Only rarely has FSE been described in subacute type D enterotoxemia of goats. The reasons for the different manifestations of enterotoxemia in sheep and goats are unknown.

Information on type D enterotoxemia in **cattle** is sparse, and the disease seems to occur very rarely in this species. A spontaneous disease with gross brain lesions similar to those observed in FSE of sheep is occasionally seen in cattle. However, a causal relationship between the lesions and *C. perfringens* type D or its epsilon toxin has not been established in any of these cases, and the etiology of these lesions in cattle remains undetermined.

Experimental results indicate that **cattle** are susceptible to *C. perfringens* type D infection and its epsilon toxin. However, natural type D disease in this species seems to be a rare occurrence. Microangiopathy similar to that described in sheep and goat enterotoxemia was described in the brain of two 1-day-old calves and in a heifer, in which epsilon toxin was detected in the intestinal content.

A **diagnosis** of type D disease in sheep can be established based on FSE and/or intramural vascular or perivascular edema in the brain. The same applies for goats in the rare cases in which these lesions are present. The absence of these lesions in either species does not preclude a diagnosis of enterotoxemia. Although it has been suggested that epsilon toxin may be produced in the intestine after death, this has never been proved, and *demonstration of epsilon toxin in intestinal content is therefore considered diagnostic for the disease in both animal species*. It is likely that the same diagnostic criteria apply for enterotoxemia in cattle, although much less information is available about the disease in this species and diagnostic criteria have not been established in cattle.

***Clostridium perfringens* type E.** ***C. perfringens* type E** has been blamed for enterotoxemia of lambs, calves, and rabbits.

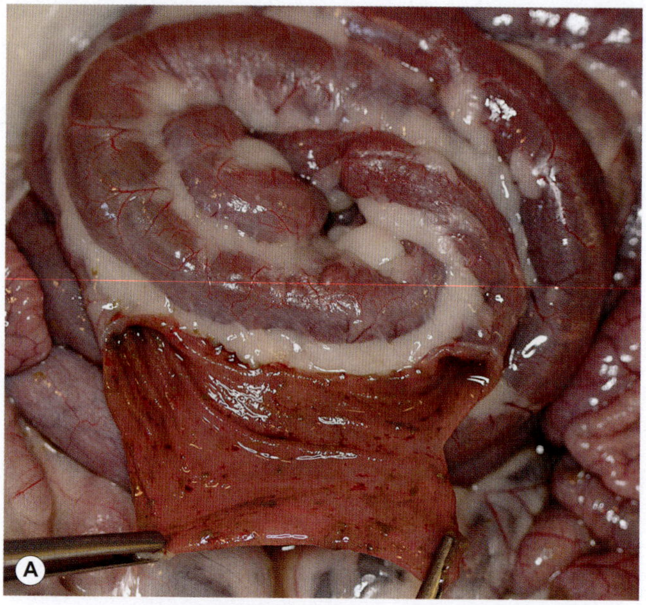

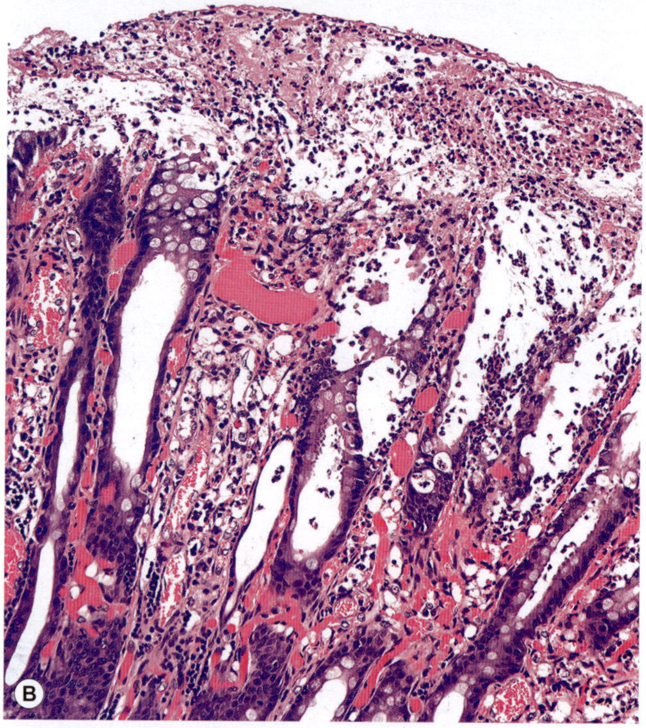

Figure 1-126 ***Clostridium perfringens* type D enterotoxemia** lesions in the colon of a goat. **A.** Mucosal hemorrhage and ulceration. **B.** Mucosal necrosis, neutrophil exudation, and incipient pseudomembrane formation.

Pathogenesis of type E infections is not very well understood, although it is assumed that iota toxin plays an important role.

In the few reported cases of this condition in calves, the animals died acutely and had a congested ulcerated abomasum and hemorrhagic enteritis that occurred segmentally along the small intestine. Mesenteric nodes were enlarged and red, and pericardial effusion and serosal hemorrhages were present. No comprehensive descriptions of clinical disease, gross and microscopic lesions of type E enterotoxemia in other ruminants are available.

The few diagnoses of type E enteritis in calves that have been reported were based on isolation of *C. perfringens* type E from the intestinal content of sick animals. This procedure, however, is not universally accepted as a diagnostic criterion for *C. perfringens* intestinal diseases because this organism is present in many healthy animals.

Although *C. perfringens* type E also has been suspected as a cause of enterotoxemia in rabbits, cross-reactivity of the iota toxin with the toxins of *Clostridium spiroforme* (now reclassified as *Thomasclavelia spiroformis*), a known agent of enterocolitis in rabbits, has created doubt regarding the role of *C. perfringens* type E in disease in rabbits.

***Clostridium perfringens* types F and G. *C. perfringens* type F** by definition encodes alpha toxin and enterotoxin, and is responsible for a highly prevalent food poisoning and antibiotic-associated diarrhea in humans. The pathogenesis of the disease is almost exclusively dependent on the action of the enterotoxin, with the effect of alpha toxin being negligible. However, although it was formerly believed that enterotoxin-secreting type A strains (now reclassified as type F) cause recurrent diarrhea, sometimes bloody in dogs and horses, recent evidence suggests that this is not the case, and the role of *C. perfringens* type F in enteric disease of animals remains undetermined.

***C. perfringens* type G** is responsible for necrotic enteritis in chickens, which is thought to be mediated exclusively by its main virulence factor, necrotic enteritis-like B toxin. To date, no type G strains have been found to be responsible for enteric or other disease in mammalian species.

***Clostridioides difficile*.** Formerly *Clostridium difficile*, is a gram-positive rod that may be found in the soil and gut of many animal species. *C. difficile* is the most commonly identified cause of antibiotic-associated and nosocomial diarrhea in humans, but, for several years, it has also been associated with cases of colitis and diarrhea in people who have not been treated with antibiotics or exposed to hospital environments (community-associated *C. difficile* infections).

C. difficile disease occurs spontaneously in several animal species, including mainly horses, rabbits, pigs, nonhuman primates, ostriches, and black-tailed prairie dogs. *C. difficile* has been isolated from cattle with enteritis but also infected by other pathogens, and although it is very likely that this microorganism plays a role in enteritis of cattle, final evidence to support this assertion is lacking. The role of *C. difficile* in enteric diseases of several other animal species, including dogs and cats, has not been fully determined. It is possible that *C. difficile* causes disease in dogs and cats ranging from mild diarrhea to severe colitis; however, infection and diarrhea do not appear to be associated with antibiotic administration in contrast to people. However, *C. difficile* can be isolated from a small percentage (1-5%) of healthy dogs and cats that carry *C. difficile* in their intestinal tract, and higher percentages are found in young animals, animals in veterinary hospitals, and animals that visit human hospitals as part of therapy programs. Importantly, most dogs and cats carrying *C. difficile* do not get sick. Therefore, isolation of *C. difficile* or detection of its toxins from intestinal content of dogs with diarrhea does not necessarily indicate causality. The microorganism has also been isolated from sheep and goats but its role in enteric disease of these species is not known.

C. difficile disease has been reproduced experimentally in several animal species that are used as models for human disease, including Syrian hamsters, guinea pigs, mice, rats, and rabbits. Lesions in most nonhuman mammals are similar to those in humans but vary extensively in severity and distribution within the GI tract. Differences in distribution of lesions within the GI tract also exist between different age groups of the same animal species. Highly virulent ribotypes responsible for severe human outbreaks (i.e., 027 and 078) have been associated with disease in several animal species, prompting speculation that animal-to-human transmission and/or vice versa occurs. Final evidence of this is, however, lacking.

Pathogenesis of *C. difficile* disease in domestic animals is likely mediated by toxins A (an enterotoxin) and B (a cytotoxin and also an enterotoxin). Much controversy exists about the relative importance of each of these toxins in the pathogenesis of *C. difficile* infection. However, animal experiments using toxin mutant strains of *C. difficile* (i.e., strains that do not produce toxin A or B or both) have shown that both toxins are able to cause lesions and disease. Other *C. difficile* toxins such as CDT are thought to have a synergistic role in the pathogenesis of infection by this microorganism.

The major predisposing factors for *C. difficile* disease in most species are antibiotic therapy and, at least for humans and horses, hospitalization. Cases occur, however, in animals not known to have been subjected to either of these predisposing factors. Although clindamycin and vancomycin therapy pose a higher risk than other antibiotics for many animal species, disturbance of normal flora with development of *C. difficile* disease can occur after administration of almost any antibiotic, including those that are effective against *C. difficile* itself. However, in horses, the disease has been associated most frequently with the administration of β-lactam antibiotics, probably because of the prevalence of their use.

Confirmation of a **diagnosis** of *C. difficile* disease should be based on identification of toxins A, B, or both in gut content or feces by tests with high sensitivity and specificity, mostly ELISAs. However, because of the low carrier rate of this microorganism in some animal species (e.g., horses), isolation of toxigenic strains of this microorganism from intestinal content and/or feces is considered diagnostically significant for *C. difficile* infection by some authors. Typing of isolates is necessary because nontoxic strains can occur and isolation of those is of no diagnostic significance.

In **horses**, *C. difficile* causes enteritis, enterocolitis, and/or colitis. Diarrhea and colic have been reproduced in foals using inocula of *C. difficile* spores and vegetative cells. Horses of any age can be affected, and although there are exceptions, it is generally accepted that the distribution of lesions throughout the intestinal tract seems to be dependent on the age of the horse. In foals <1-month-old, the small intestine is invariably affected; the colon and cecum may or may not have lesions. In older foals and adult horses, the disease has a more caudal distribution, affecting the colon and sometimes the cecum, and generally sparing the small intestine. Although this age-related distribution of lesions within the GI tract is seen in most cases, exceptions do occur and lesion distribution should not be used to confirm/rule out *C. difficile* infection in horses.

The **clinical signs** of *C. difficile* disease in horses are highly variable, nonspecific and may occur with highly variable severity. The main clinical sign is diarrhea, which may be accompanied by hyperemic mucous membranes, prolonged capillary refill time, pyrexia, tachycardia, tachypnea, dehydration, abdominal distension, and colic. The mortality rate in foals and adults is 0-42%. A syndrome known as *duodenitis-proximal* *jejunitis*, characterized clinically by large volumes of enterogastric reflux, has been known since the early 1980s. Although an association has been suggested between *C. difficile* and duodenitis-proximal jejunitis, a conclusive relationship has been neither proved nor ruled out.

C. difficile gross and microscopic lesions may be characteristic but are not pathognomonic, as other infectious (*C. perfringens* type C, *Salmonella* spp., and *Neorickettsia* spp.) and noninfectious (NSAIDs) causes of intestinal disease can produce very similar lesions. **Grossly**, the serosa of the small and large intestine is multifocally red or blue as the result of intense hyperemia and/or hemorrhage (Fig. 1-127). The wall of the small intestine can be slightly thickened; the mucosa is often diffusely reddened and may have an overlying, multifocal, tan-to-orange pseudomembrane. The wall of the colon and cecum is typically diffusely and severely thickened by clear-to-hemorrhagic, gelatinous submucosal and mucosal edema; the mucosa is multifocally or diffusely dull-green or red and may be multifocally covered by a tan or light-green pseudomembrane (Fig. 1-128). The intestinal content in young foals is often hemorrhagic but may be yellow and pasty or green-brown and watery. In older foals and adult horses, the colon and cecum are characteristically filled with large amounts of green or light-brown watery contents, and occasionally dark-brown or red, hemorrhagic watery contents (Fig. 1-129). Bloody content may be present caudally to the small colon and rectum. When present, gross lesions outside the GI tract are those of endotoxic shock and/or DIC, including serous or serosanguineous pericardial effusion, pulmonary congestion and edema, and multifocal subendocardial and subserosal petechiae and ecchymoses.

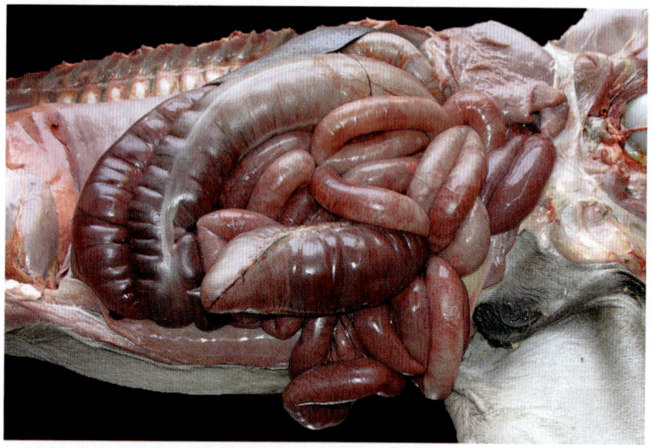

Figure 1-127 ***Clostridioides difficile***–associated enterocolitis in a foal. Marked congestion and hemorrhage of the small and large intestine serosal surfaces. (Reprinted with permission from Diab SS, et al. *Clostridium difficile* infection in horses: a review. Vet Microbiol 2013;167:42–49.)

Microscopic lesions in horses are mostly restricted to the GI tract, and they can be present in the small and/or large intestine. They are almost identical to those seen in horses with *C. perfringens* type C infection and consist mainly of multifocal-to-diffuse, often hemorrhagic, coagulative necrosis of the mucosa, which may be covered by a pseudomembrane, frequently accompanied by submucosal edema and congestion. Thrombosis of small-to-mid-size blood vessels in the mucosa and/or submucosa is a very frequent, although not constant, finding, and it is especially useful in those cases in which autolysis has partially masked the mucosal necrosis. Mild-to-moderate mucosal and submucosal fibrinoneutrophilic infiltration with fewer plasma cells, lymphocytes, and macrophages is frequently observed. The so-called "volcano" lesions, as described in the human disease, are patchy focal erosions on the small intestinal or colonic mucosa through which fibrin and neutrophils exude, are not very frequently seen in horses; a possible reason is that, at the time of autopsy and sample collection, the lesions are usually too advanced to show the delicate volcano-like lesions. Few-to-numerous clusters of short and thick, gram-positive rods can be observed in the intestinal lumen and/or on the surface or within the necrotic mucosa.

Coinfection of foals with *C. difficile* and *C. perfringens* type C can also occur. The clinical signs, gross and microscopic lesions are almost identical to those produced by either of these microorganisms alone.

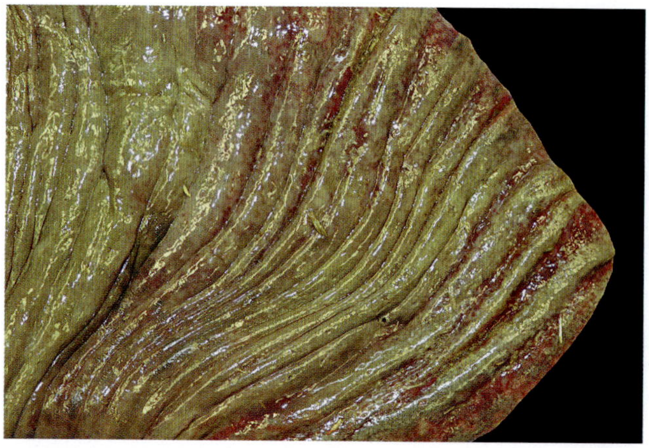

Figure 1-128 ***Clostridioides difficile***–associated disease in a horse. Fibrinonecrotizing colitis and mucosal edema. (Reprinted with permission from Diab SS, et al. *Clostridium difficile* infection in horses: a review. Vet Microbiol 2013;167:42–49.)

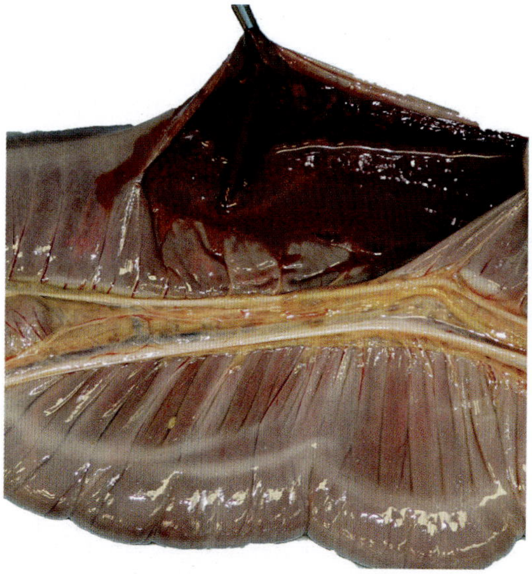

Figure 1-129 ***Clostridioides difficile***–associated enterocolitis in a horse. Dark-red content in the large colon.

C. difficile is recognized as a cause of diarrhea resulting from fibrinous colitis in **neonatal pigs** under about a week of age, and the disease has been reproduced experimentally using pure cultures of the organism. Piglets have diarrhea, dyspnea, scrotal edema, and mild abdominal distension. Affected litters experience lost productivity (mainly shown as decreased weaning weight). **Grossly**, hydrothorax and characteristic, although not pathognomonic, edema of the mesocolon (Fig. 1-130) are evident grossly, usually in association with patchy-to-extensive fibrinous typhlocolitis (Fig. 1-131A), with yellow pasty-to-fluid content and feces.

Microscopically, fibrinous colitis similar to that described in horses is a common lesion, with colonic serosal and mesenteric edema and infiltration of mononuclear inflammatory cells and neutrophils in the lamina propria. Segmental erosion and ulceration of colonic mucosal epithelium are common, and volcano lesions may be seen in acute cases of the disease (see Fig. 1-131B). Occasionally, deeper necrosis of the mucosa and colonic wall may occur.

Information on *C. difficile* infection in domestic **dogs** and **cats** is scant, and the role of this microorganism in canine and feline enteric disease is currently unclear. Although a possible association between the detection of *C. difficile* toxins in feces of dogs and disease has been reported in various studies, diagnostic criteria for *C. difficile* infection in these species have not been defined. This is complicated by the fact that the prevalence of *C. difficile* in normal dogs and cats may be up to 50%, and *C. difficile* toxins also have been detected in a small percentage of subclinical dogs. Descriptions of lesions of *C. difficile* infections in dogs or cats are not available.

A role for *C. difficile* in enteric disease of **cattle** has been proposed in several studies, but no conclusive evidence has been provided to confirm or rule out this possibility. This microorganism, including the highly virulent ribotypes 027 and 078, and its toxins, has been detected in the intestine of healthy and diarrheic calves. Ribotype 078 is the predominant strain in cattle in North America. The fact that several of the highly virulent ribotypes of *C. difficile* for humans have been found in cattle suggests that zoonotic transmission (and/or vice versa) may occur. There is growing concern that some *C. difficile* infections may be acquired from ingestion of *C. difficile* spores in contaminated foods of animal origin. Although a correlation between fecal *C. difficile* and its toxins and calf diarrhea was found, frequently, this microorganism is detected in diarrheic calves together with other enteropathogens (e.g., BCoV, bovine rotavirus, *Cryptosporidium* spp.), and ascribing the enteropathogenic effects to one of these pathogens alone is difficult. One study failed in the attempt to provoke diarrhea in calves by oral administration of virulent *C. difficile* strains. The role of *C. difficile* in enteric diseases of sheep and goats is unknown.

In **duodenitis-proximal jejunitis**, also known as *proximal enteritis* or *ulcerative duodenitis*, signs of upper small intestinal ileus occur, including depression and nasogastric reflux. Although the etiology is not known, there is mounting evidence that the disease is caused by *C. difficile*. At surgery or **autopsy**, there is fibrinous enteritis or ulceration involving the duodenum, and a variable amount of more distal small bowel. The lesions may be segmental and circumferential, only a few centimeters long, or more diffuse, involving much

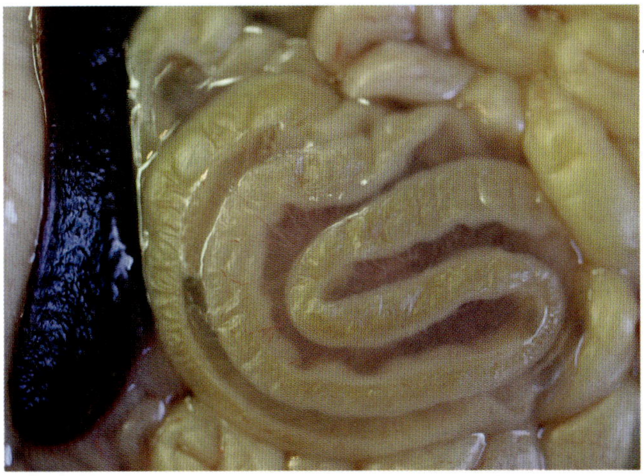

Figure 1-130 ***Clostridioides difficile***–associated enterocolitis. Marked edema of the mesocolon in a neonatal piglet.

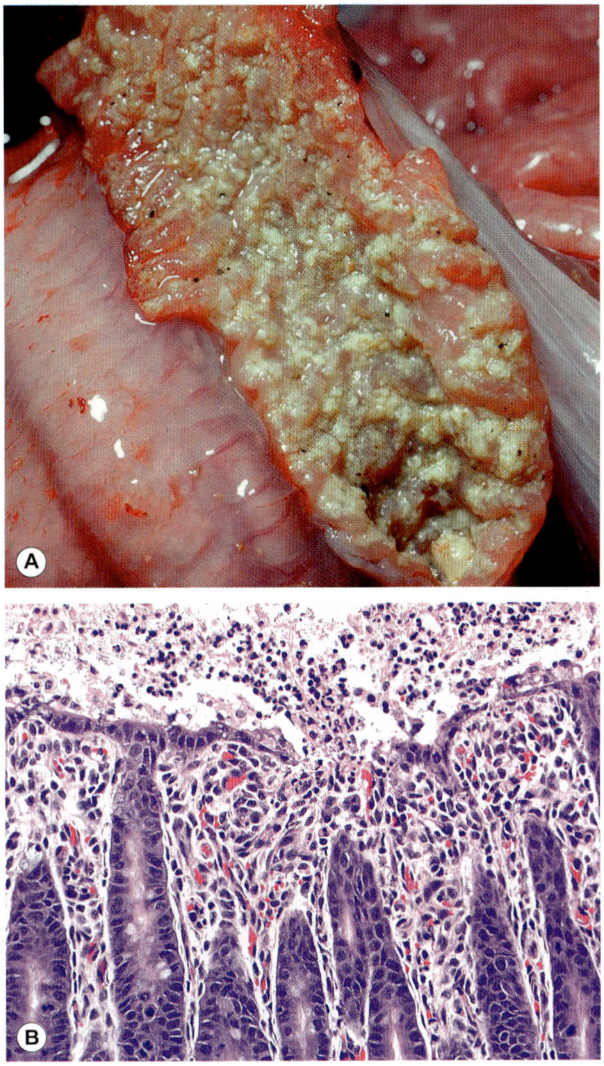

Figure 1-131 ***Clostridioides difficile***–associated disease in a neonatal piglet. **A.** Fibrinonecrotic colitis. The colonic mucosa is covered by a pseudomembrane. (Courtesy W.R. Kelly.) **B.** Effusion of neutrophils through the superficial epithelium (**volcano lesion**).

of the small intestine, but sparing the ileum. The affected segment of bowel may be thickened, congested, or hemorrhagic on the serosal aspect, and there may be fibrinous peritonitis with adhesions, and pancreatitis. Perforation may occur. If the lesion is of some standing, there may be significant stricture at the site. Affected animals often have a distended stomach, with abnormal fluid content, and gastric ulcers, particularly of the pars esophagea. Perforation or rupture of the stomach may occur. Duodenal lesions always should be sought in foals with gastroesophageal ulceration. **Microscopically**, there is edema and congestion, with progressive necrosis from the tips of villi in early lesions, advancing to mucosal or transmural acute fibrinonecrotic enteritis, grading to the development of granulation tissue and fibrosis in the bed of more chronic ulcers.

Clostridium piliforme. Tyzzer disease is caused by the obligate intracellular bacterium *C. piliforme*, the only gram-negative organism among the pathogenic clostridia. It is a disease of many species of mammals, among them horses, cats, dogs, rabbits, hamsters, and cattle, although there seem to be bacterial strain differences that determine host susceptibility. Affected animals are often very young or appear to be immunocompromised in some way. Cases in horses tend to occur every year in the same ranches.

The *classical triad of lesions* in most animal species include changes in the heart, intestinal tract, and liver. However, this triad of lesions does not occur in all animal species. In horses, for instance, lesions are always observed in the liver, and much less frequently in the intestine and the heart. The *liver* is the organ affected most frequently in most animal species. Animals become infected initially through the epithelium of the ileum, cecum, and colon, where, when present, inflammation may vary from subtle catarrhal to fibrinohemorrhagic. Bacilli can be observed faintly in H&E preparations but are better demonstrated using silver stains, often forming characteristic "pick-up-sticks" arrays, in the cytoplasm of enterocytes.

Ultimately, in most cases the bacilli disseminate elsewhere in the body, especially to the liver and myocardium, where they cause acute-to-subacute necrotic lesions. *C. piliforme* cannot be cultured in conventional media, and **diagnosis** is usually based on histologic examination by demonstration of the classical intracellular bacilli. PCR demonstration of *C. piliforme* in tissues of affected animals is diagnostic. The disease is discussed more fully in Vol. 2, Liver and Biliary System.

Paraclostridium sordellii (formerly *Clostridium sordellii* and *Paeniclostridium sordellii*) has been associated with necrohemorrhagic enterocolitis of adult **horses**. Grossly and microscopically, the lesions are very similar to those seen in cases of salmonellosis and enterocolitis caused by *C. difficile*, *C. perfringens type* C, or NSAIDs. The disease was diagnosed based on gross and microscopic changes associated with detection of *P. sordellii* in intestinal tissue and/or contents by culture, PCR, and/or IHC, and ruling out other known causes of enterocolitis. Conventional and molecular Koch postulates have, however, not been fulfilled, and definitive evidence of the role of *P. sordellii* and its toxins in enteric disease of horses is lacking.

Paratuberculosis (Johne disease)

Paratuberculosis is caused by ***Mycobacterium avium* subsp. *paratuberculosis*** (MAP) infection. MAP is classified as a subspecies within the *M. avium* complex based on DNA hybridization studies and other genotypic and phenotypic tests. MAP in culture is slow growing, and its dependence on the iron chelator mycobactin classically has been its key distinguishing phenotypic characteristic. Genetically, the **IS900** insertion sequence element seems unique to MAP and has been used broadly as a detection tool in animals and humans. Highly homologous but not identical IS900-like sequences have been detected in other mycobacteria. At least 2 distinct MAP strains are known to cause paratuberculosis in various hosts, and these are generally referred to as *type I, or S strain* first isolated from sheep, and *type II, or C strain* first isolated from cattle. Type I strains have been isolated mostly from sheep, particularly in Australia; there are rare reports of cattle infected with type I strains. Type II strains, however, are the most common; they have a broad host range and have been isolated from domestic and wildlife species as well as nonruminants. The strains have distinct phenotypic, genotypic, host preference, virulence, and pathogenic traits that continue to be clarified.

Paratuberculosis is most common in *domestic ruminants*, but spontaneous disease also occurs rarely in a number of free-ranging and captive nondomestic ruminants, camelids and rabbits, equids, swine, and captive primates. Wild mammals, including lagomorphs, rodents, and carnivores, and several species of wild birds are naturally infected with MAP, but do not necessarily develop disease. MAP has been recovered from tissue and blood samples of human patients inflicted with *Crohn disease*, a chronic granulomatous enteritis of importance in humans that shares several pathologic and immunologic features with paratuberculosis. These findings are suggestive of a causal relationship; however, this has not been confirmed and it seems more likely that MAP is coincidental or plays a potentially opportunistic role in these cases.

The **epidemiology and pathogenesis** of paratuberculosis are best understood in cattle and are assumed to be similar in other species. MAP is transmitted predominantly by the fecal-oral route, either directly by ingestion in feces or indirectly via MAP-contaminated milk, colostrum, or water. Organisms may be present in semen or urine and may cross the placenta, particularly during advanced disease. A distinct age-dependent susceptibility to MAP infection is observed; the infectious dose for adults is considerable higher than for neonates. The basis for this is unknown, and control programs aimed at blocking transmission are almost exclusively focused on neonates. Paratuberculosis is often categorized into 3 (or 4) stages: *silent infection, subclinical infection, clinical disease (and advanced clinical disease)*, based on severity of clinical signs, potential for shedding of MAP organisms into the environment, and ease of diagnosis. Of particular importance is the subclinical period, which can last 2-5 years before infected animals develop clinical signs. Because shedding of MAP into the environment by subclinical cows is variable and progressive, this period represents a significant risk for spread of the infection to susceptible herdmates. This long and unpredictable incubation period has given rise to the concept of *the iceberg effect* because in any infected herd, although only a few animals may have clinical signs of paratuberculosis, a much greater number of animals are likely MAP infected. Sheep, goats, and cervids are considered to be more susceptible to MAP infection than cattle, and have a shorter incubation period before development of clinical signs. Survivability of MAP in the environment is proposed to have a significant effect on the epidemiology of MAP infection in animals; however, the biologic relevance of these factors for transmission of infection is still unclear.

MAP gains access to the small intestinal mucosa and subepithelial dome via microfold (M cells) or epithelial cells overlying submucosal Peyer patches. Macrophages are the preferred host cell for MAP, and the ability of pathogenic mycobacteria including MAP to inhibit phagosome-lysosome fusion is fundamental to its survival and persistence within the host. Experimental in vitro and in vivo work indicates that MAP-infected cattle develop a proinflammatory immune response early after intestinal infection, which is probably driven by innate intestinal T lymphocytes including gamma-delta T cells and NK cells. However, in animals that fail to clear the infection, the early proinflammatory response eventually gives way to an apparently ineffective but robust MAP-specific antibody response. This transition is correlated with the progression from subclinical to clinical disease in affected adults, but the mechanisms for this remain largely unknown. The rate of disease progression and the length of the subclinical period of paratuberculosis are irregular and can be protracted; clinical cows are rarely <2-years-old. The reasons for this remain unclear, although there is likely a complex interplay of factors, including age of initial exposure, dose, re-exposure over time, environment, nutrition, production stage, and genetics. As an animal progresses toward clinical disease, the population of MAP within the intestinal mucosa increases and live MAP are shed in the feces more frequently and in greater numbers. Appetite often remains normal, and intermittent-to-progressive diarrhea may persist for weeks before eventual development of hypoproteinemia, cachexia, emaciation, and death.

The major lesions of paratuberculosis are usually confined to the distal jejunum, ileum, large intestine, and draining lymph nodes; however, the infection is generalized and the organism is widely distributed in lymph nodes, and can be cultured from a variety of parenchymatous organs or even blood in fulminant infections. Diarrhea during paratuberculosis is related to the *granulomatous inflammatory response in the lamina propria of the small intestine*, and the associated villus atrophy that develops. Malabsorption and filtration secretion caused by the inflamed small intestinal mucosa overload the capacity of the colon to resorb electrolytes and fluid. The function of the colon itself may be compromised by MAP infection, especially in severe or advanced cases. There is malabsorption of amino acids, enteric loss of plasma protein, and hypoproteinemia causing reduced productive efficiency, and when negative nitrogen balance occurs, a decline in body condition, and ultimate emaciation.

The **gross lesions** of paratuberculosis include small intestinal mucosal lesions that may be segmental or continuous and can be distributed from the duodenum to the rectum. Lesions are usually best developed in the *caudal jejunum, ileum, and upper large intestine*. The ileocecal valve is considered by some to be the site that is affected earliest and most consistently; however, lesions in the ileocecal valve can be variable. The classic intestinal change is *diffuse thickening of the mucosa*, which is folded into transverse rugae, the crests of which may be congested (Fig. 1-132A). Mucosal thickening is due to accumulation of predominantly macrophages, as well as edema fluid, in the mucosa and submucosa. The mucosa and/or serosa may have a slightly granular appearance because of increased cellularity and edema (see Fig. 1-132B). *The ileocecal and mesenteric lymph nodes are enlarged, pale, and edematous. Lymphangitis is common*, and the lymphatic vessels can often be traced as thickened cords from the intestinal serosa through the mesentery to the mesenteric nodes (Fig. 1-133). In some cases, mucosal lesions are subtle and lymphangitis is the only readily recognizable gross lesion, which is specific enough to justify a presumptive diagnosis of paratuberculosis at gross postmortem examination. Additionally, there is marked loss of muscle mass and serous atrophy of fat depots, intermandibular edema, and fluid effusion in various body cavities. Plaques of intimal fibrosis and mineralization may be evident in the thoracic aorta.

When gross lesions are well developed, the characteristic **microscopic lesions** of *transmural granulomatous enteritis* (Fig. 1-134A and B) *and lymphangitis* are obvious (Fig. 1-135), although in cattle with minimal gross lesions, microscopic abnormalities can be more subtle. Depending on the severity and stage of the infection, villi are moderately to markedly atrophic; macrophages are increased in number and are focally or diffusely distributed in the lamina propria, submucosa, muscle layers, or the serosa of the intestine. Epithelioid

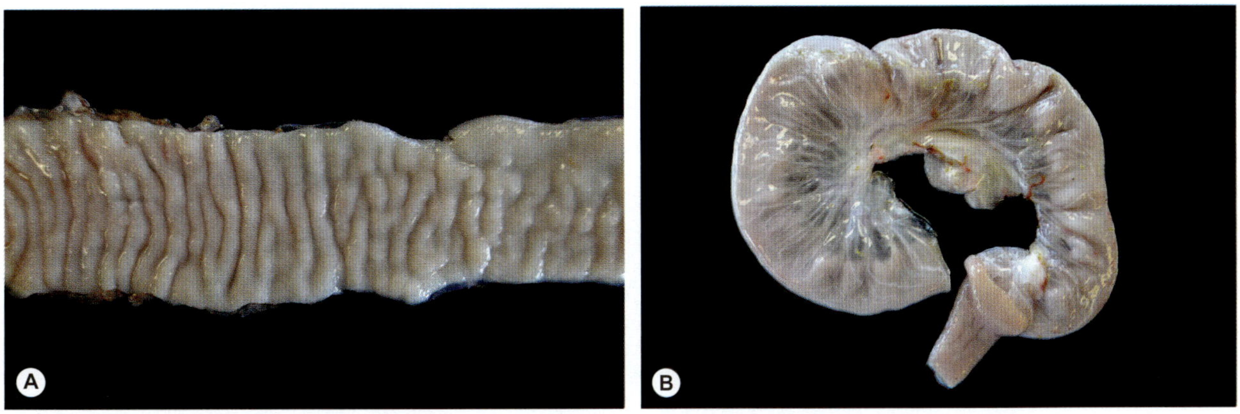

Figure 1-132 Paratuberculosis in a sheep. **A**. Mucosal surface is diffusely and markedly thickened with prominent mucosal folds, due to granulomatous enteritis. **B**. The small intestine is thickened with prominent dilated and thickened serosal lymphatics. (Both courtesy J. Asin.)

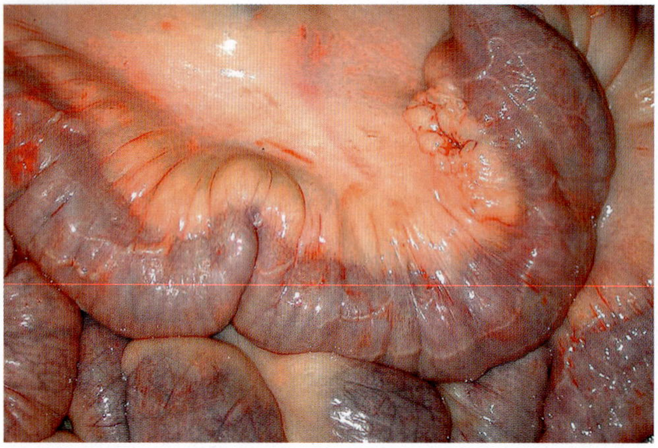

Figure 1-133 Paratuberculosis. Serosal edema and lymphangitis in a goat. (Courtesy J. Caswell.)

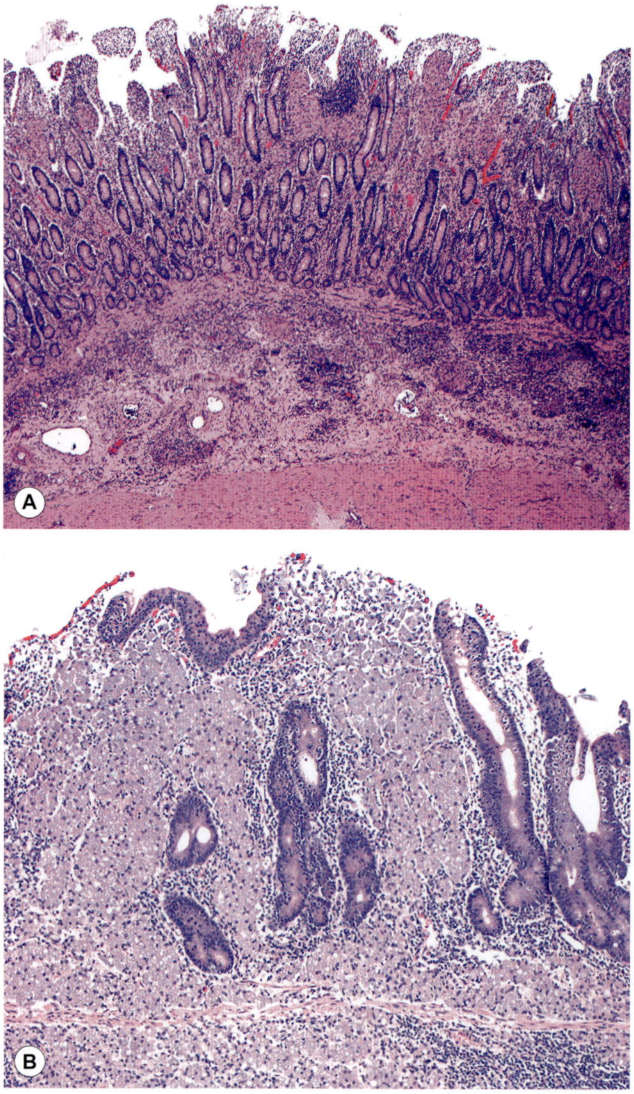

Figure 1-134 Paratuberculosis. A. Blunt atrophic ileal villi, and hyperplastic crypts. Note heavy inflammatory infiltrate in lamina propria and submucosa. **B.** Aggregate of macrophages in hypercellular lamina propria.

macrophages and Langhans-type multinucleate giant cells are often present in aggregates or diffuse sheets. The inflammatory infiltrate may abnormally separate and displace crypts, which are elongate and lined by hyperplastic epithelial cells. Crypts may be distended with mucus and exfoliated cells, probably because of compression and obstruction of their mouths by inflammatory cells and edema. Foci of necrosis may occur within these aggregates of macrophages, but in cattle, formation of classic tuberculoid granulomas with caseation and mineralization is extremely rare.

Granulomatous lymphangitis is one of the most consistent changes, and inflammatory cells can be observed along the lacteals of villi, or in the submucosa (see Fig. 1-135). Initially, the lymphatics are surrounded by lymphocytes and plasma cells, and many contain plugs of epithelioid cells in the lumen. Granulomas may form in the wall and project into the lumen. These nodules may undergo some central necrosis. *Granulomatous lymphadenitis* occurs in ileocecal or mesenteric lymph nodes in advanced cases. In the early stages, there are increased numbers of macrophages within the subcapsular sinuses; with time, these progress to nodular or diffuse infiltrates of epithelioid macrophages and giant cells that replace much of the lymph node cortex and infiltrate the medullary sinusoids.

Of the other organs and tissues from which MAP can be isolated in cattle, *focal granulomas* attributable to MAP have only been described in the liver, hepatic lymph nodes, and very rarely, the kidney and lungs. Granulomas are most common in the liver and are found in portal triads or scattered throughout the hepatic parenchyma. *Acid-fast bacilli* are usually demonstrable in these lesions.

In **sheep and goats**, paratuberculosis mainly occurs in adults as *chronic wasting*; there may be breaks in the wool in sheep, and submandibular edema resulting from hypoproteinemia. Feces are often normal and may be soft and unpelleted, but overt diarrhea is unusual except intermittently in the terminal stages of disease. The reason for this is unknown but may be related to the innately greater efficiency of electrolyte and fluid absorption in the colon of these species. In farmed deer, paratuberculosis is clinically similar, but there are reports of disease in animals well under a year old.

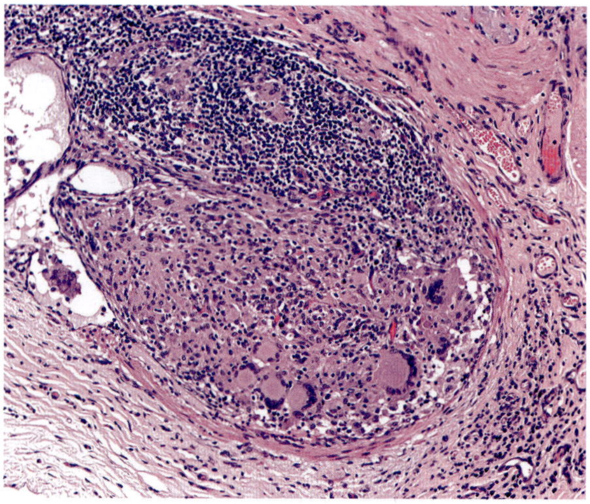

Figure 1-135 Paratuberculosis. Subserosal granulomatous lymphangitis with prominent giant cells in a cow.

In sheep, goats, and deer, a distinct age and dose susceptibility pattern has been described such that animals exposed to higher doses of MAP at earlier ages probably progress faster and develop more severe disease. Goats are thought to be more susceptible to MAP infection than are sheep or cattle. Enteric **gross lesions** in sheep and goats tend to be more sporadic and subtle than in cattle. Lesions appear to occur most commonly in the distal jejunum and ileum, and can range from focal or multifocal subtle lesions that are easily missed at postmortem examination, to diffuse and severe intestinal thickening with prominent transverse ridges and mesenteric adhesions. There may be lymphadenomegaly and lymphangitis as seen in cattle. **Microscopically**, there can be focal or multifocal accumulations of epithelioid cells and lymphocytes, with relatively few organisms; this is the *paucibacillary form*. Others may have a dense transmural intestinal inflammatory infiltrate with abundant organisms; this is the *multibacillary form*. Microscopic lesions also tend to be most severe in the distal jejunum and/or the ileocecal valve. Goats and sometimes sheep develop foci of tubercle-like caseous necrosis, often with mineralization and fibrosis in the mucosa, submucosa, serosa, and lymphatics of the intestine or in the lymph nodes. These nodules may be grossly visible as white 1-4 mm foci. Scattered lymph nodes elsewhere in the body, and liver, lung, spleen, and other organs, may contain granulomas in sheep and goats. Pigmented strains of MAP have been described in sheep, and in these cases the mucosa and lymph nodes may be discolored orange.

The organism is usually readily demonstrable by acid-fast staining within macrophages and giant cells in the lesions, especially in diffuse multibacillary forms of the disease (Fig. 1-136). However, some clinical cases may have multifocal paucibacillary lesions in sheep, so an extensive search must be made for individual macrophages or giant cells bearing low numbers of acid-fast bacilli. Antibodies with well-defined specificity for MAP have allowed the development of IHC tests, but these are typically not helpful when there are very few organisms. PCR techniques are useful for confirming the diagnosis in individual cases. Culture can be reliable to detect MAP in goats because they tend to be infected with the cattle strain; however, culture of MAP from sheep is difficult because of its fastidious growth requirements.

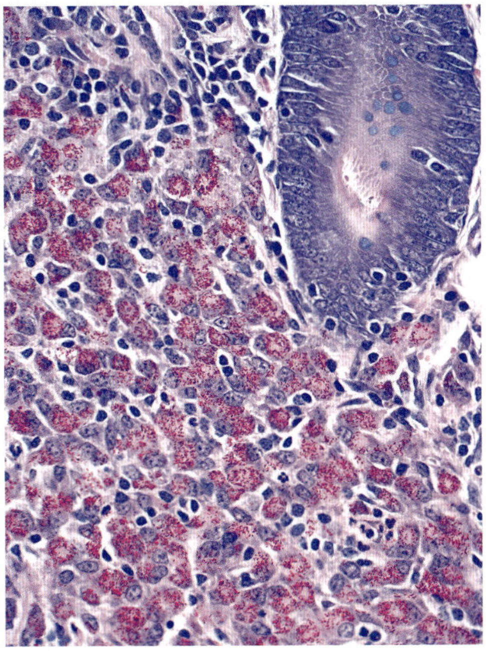

Figure 1-136 Paratuberculosis. Large number of acid-fast bacteria (modified Ziehl-Neelsen stain) in the cytoplasm of macrophages and giant cells in the small intestine of a cow.

Paratuberculosis can also occur in South American **camelids**. Gross and microscopic changes are similar to those described in cattle and small ruminants, but disseminated infection with acid-fast organisms in the lung, liver, and spleen has also been observed.

Rhodococcus *infections*

Rhodococcus equi is an intracellular pathogen found in soil and as part of the normal intestinal flora of horses and other animals. This microorganism is a major pathogen of horses, and it also causes disease in pigs, cattle, and camelids. *R. equi* pneumonia also occurs in HIV-infected or otherwise immunocompromised humans.

R. equi isolated from foals and many recovered from humans carry an ~81-kb plasmid named pVAPA1037. This plasmid is essential for disease in horses; removal of this plasmid results in loss of the capacity of *R. equi* to replicate in macrophages. The genes on the virulence plasmid are divided into 4 groups, but only the genes within 1 of those groups, the PAI region, have been evaluated and reported to play significant roles in virulence. In particular, the PAI-encoded, virulence-associated protein A (*vapA*) and its positive regulators (*virR* and *ORF8*) are critical for resistance to macrophage attack and for bacterial multiplication in vivo. A *R. equi vapA* knockout mutant is incapable of intracellular replication and unable to establish a persistent infection in severe combined-immunodeficient mice. There are both virulent and avirulent strains in nature, and on farms where disease caused by *R. equi* is endemic, there is a much higher proportion of virulent forms. Virulence factors may not be necessary for production of disease in an immunocompromised host. *R. equi* is usually associated with *neutrophilic bronchopneumonia of foals*. Abdominal lesions are identified in ~50% of foals with *R. equi* pneumonia that are presented for autopsy and include any of the following, alone or in combination(s): pyogranulomatous enterotyphlocolitis, pyogranulomatous lymphadenitis of the mesenteric or colonic lymph nodes, large intra-abdominal abscesses, and peritonitis. The development of intestinal lesions appears to be dose related, in that experimental reproduction of the disease requires repeated oral infection. In natural disease, continual exposure to bacteria in swallowed respiratory exudate is probably an important source of infection in those animals with pneumonia.

Gross lesions may occur throughout the small and large intestines but are usually most severe over Peyer patches in small intestine, and in the cecum, large colon (Fig. 1-137A), and related lymph nodes. Mucosal lesions are multifocal irregular, elevated, and crateriform with central ulcers up to 1-2 cm in diameter, often covered by purulent or necrotic debris (see Fig. 1-137B and C). Edema of the wall of the gut may be severe. Mesenteric or colonic lymph nodes often are massively enlarged by edema and caseous or purulent foci that may obliterate the structure of the node. Occasionally,

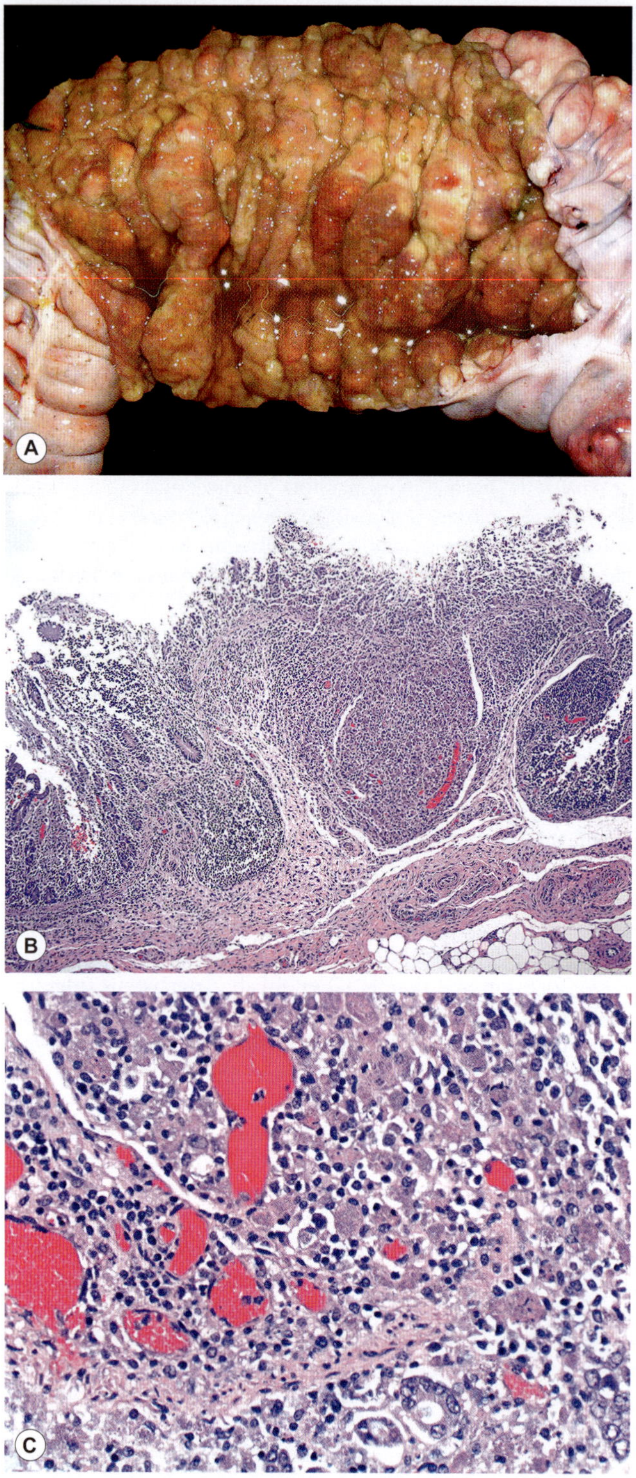

Figure 1-137 ***Rhodococcus equi*** infection in a foal. **A.** Craterous ulcerated lesions on colonic mucosa. (Courtesy L. Minatel.) **B.** Pyogranulomatous enteritis with surface ulceration in the colon of a foal. **C.** Closeup view of macrophages containing myriad intracellular *R. equi* bacterial organisms.

massively enlarged abscessed lymph nodes (Fig. 1-138) are found without evidence of concurrent enteritis or colitis.

Microscopically, the infection seems to occur by penetration of the specialized epithelium over Peyer patches or intestinal lymphoid follicles. An initial neutrophilic response

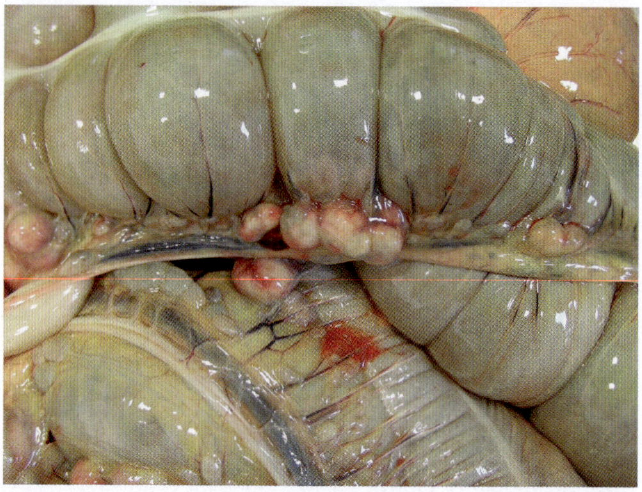

Figure 1-138 ***Rhodococcus equi*** infection. Enlarged cecal and colic lymph nodes. (Courtesy L. Minatel.)

occurs, and erosions of the epithelium develop subsequently. Macrophages and neutrophils accumulate in the lamina propria. The macrophages contain intracytoplasmic aggregates of *R. equi* but do not destroy them (see Fig. 1-137B and C). Later necrosis of lymphoid follicles occurs, and deep ulcers develop that contain masses of neutrophils, macrophages, and multinucleate giant cells. Pyogranulomatous lymphangitis and mesenteric lymphadenitis characterize the chronic enteric disease. Gross and microscopic lesions are highly suggestive of *R. equi* infection, and final confirmation of the diagnosis should be based on detection of the microorganism by culture and/or PCR assay.

Enterococcus *infections*

Enterococcus **spp**. are gram-positive cocci that are common inhabitants of the environment and GI tract of clinically healthy humans and several animal species. However, some enterococci, mainly ***Enterococcus hirae*** and ***E. durans***, may colonize extensively the mucosal surface of the small intestine in piglets, puppies, foals, calves, and suckling rats, in a manner similar to that of EPEC, and produce diarrhea. These bacteria adhere to the microvillus surface of enterocytes by fine filamentous pili. In tissue section, they form a layer of small cocci crowded on the entire surface of epithelial cells, from the tips to the base of villi. There may be mild-to-moderate villus atrophy and some desquamating enterocytes.

The organisms from rats have been described, on genetic grounds, as *E. ratti*; those from piglets have been described as *E. villorum* or *E. porcinus*, which may be synonyms. *E. faecalis* that had numerous virulence traits and was resistant to various antimicrobials was isolated from young kittens with enteritis, diarrhea, and up to 15% mortality. These kittens had been given probiotics that contained enterococci.

Malabsorption associated with reduced brush border enzyme activity may explain diarrhea in all animal species. Although in spontaneous cases in piglets, *Enterococcus* is frequently associated with other pathogens, the organism isolated from foals produced diarrhea when inoculated alone into gnotobiotic pigs. Because several species of *Enterococcus* are commonly found in the intestine of healthy animals, the definitive diagnosis is challenging and should be based on gross and microscopic changes, coupled by detection of *Enterococcus* spp. and ruling out other causes of enteric disease.

Bacteroides fragilis *infections*

Bacteroides fragilis is a nonspore-forming obligate anaerobe that is part of the normal enteric flora. Some enterotoxin-secreting strains have been associated with diarrhea in piglets, calves, lambs, foals, and humans. This enterotoxin is a *protease*, and probably damages the zonula adherens at the tight junction between enterocytes. Enterotoxigenic strains or cell-free culture filtrates cause secretion in ligated lamb or calf intestinal loops, and bacterial inocula cause diarrhea when administered orally to gnotobiotic piglets.

Bacteria do not adhere to the surface. Enterocytes round up and exfoliate, with villus attenuation and crypt elongation and hyperplasia. Infiltration of neutrophils is common. Damage may be seen in both the small and large intestines. Ultrastructurally, affected cells lose their intercellular interdigitations, microvilli are shortened or absent, and the terminal web is disrupted. The diagnosis can be challenging to confirm because *B. fragilis* can be found in the intestine of normal animals of most species.

Anaerobiospirillum *infections*

The genus *Anaerobiospirillum*, small spiral gram-negative bacteria, comprises 2 species, *Anaerobiospirillum succiniciproducens* and *A. thomasii*, which have been isolated from dogs and cats, although only a few studies have related them to diarrhea. In **cats**, ileocolitis has been associated with *Anaerobiospirillum*, although confirmation of its role in enteric disease is lacking. Cats may be subclinical, lethargic, and anorexic, or have vomiting and diarrhea. Microscopically, exfoliated epithelial cells and neutrophils are in dilated crypts in the ileum and colon, and bacteria stained with silver can be found in the lumen of crypts, in goblet cells, and sometimes in the lamina propria. Septicemia may occur, and renal failure has been associated.

Chlamydial infections

Members of the family *Chlamydiaceae* are *obligate intracellular parasites*. While members of the family have undergone various reclassifications, whole-genome sequencing data have led to the designation of 2 different genera in the family, *Chlamydia* and *Chlamydiifrater*. The species of known clinical significance all belong to the genus *Chlamydia*, which includes *C. abortus*, *C. pecorum*, *C. psittaci*, *C. pneumoniae*, *C. felis*, *C. caviae*, *C. trachomatis*, *C. suis*, and *C. muridarum*. In addition to the 9 species with known clinical significance, the *Chlamydia* genus includes 11 additional species of unknown significance. Species belonging to *Chlamydiifrater* are found in birds and their significance is not known.

Among all the *Chlamydiaceae* species, only ***C. pecorum*** and ***C. suis*** are associated with enteritis, in cattle and pigs, respectively. Other syndromes associated with *Chlamydiaceae* in domestic animals include respiratory disease, polyarthritis, orchitis, hepatitis, conjunctivitis, abortion, and encephalomyelitis.

The intestinal tract is the natural habitat for ***Chlamydia pecorum***. Most infections are probably inapparent, but the intestine may be an important portal of entry in the development of systemic infections leading to hepatitis, arthritis, encephalitis, and pneumonia in ruminants. Enteritis may accompany or presage these diseases, and occasionally, *C. pecorum* causes severe enteric disease in calves. Also, subclinical calves with *C. pecorum* intestinal infections may suffer up to 48% reduction in growth rates. This is associated with conjunctival reddening, increased serum globulin, and decreased plasma albumin and insulin-like growth factor–1. Based on these results, it was suggested that suppression of chlamydial subclinical infections may be a major contributor to the growth promoting effect of feed-additive antibiotics.

Following oral infection, *C. pecorum* infects mainly the enterocytes on the tips of ileal villi. These cells are in the G1 phase of the cell cycle, which is required by *Chlamydia* for multiplication. *C. pecorum* also infects other cells, including goblet cells, enterochromaffin cells, and macrophages, and the latter cells may transport the organisms systemically before being destroyed by them.

C. pecorum adsorbs to the brush border of enterocytes and enters the cell by pinocytosis. Following multiplication of organisms in the supranuclear region, the cells degenerate. *C. pecorum* is released into the gut lumen and the lamina propria, where it infects endothelial cells of lacteals, whence they are released and become systemic.

GI disease caused by *C. pecorum* is usually a problem of **calves** <10-days-old, but it may affect older calves and can produce recurrent diarrhea. Watery diarrhea, dehydration, and death are often accompanied by lesions, although not necessarily signs, of hepatitis, interstitial pneumonia, and arthritis. *Gross lesions* may occur in the abomasum and throughout the intestinal tract but are most consistent and severe in the *terminal jejunum and ileum*. Mucosal edema, congestion, and petechiae, sometimes with ulceration, are usually observed. Serosal hemorrhages and focal peritonitis may occur. *Histologically*, chlamydial inclusions may be demonstrable with Giemsa, Jimenez, Macchiavello, or IHC staining. Central lacteals and capillaries are dilated, and neutrophils and monocytes infiltrate the lamina propria. Occasionally, granulomatous inflammation occurs in the intestinal submucosa and extends into the mesentery and to the serosa, producing the peritonitis observed grossly. Crypts in the small and large intestine may be dilated, lined by flattened epithelium, and contain inflammatory exudate. The centers of lymphoid follicles in Peyer patches are necrotic.

Chlamydia suis in **swine** has been associated with conjunctivitis, rhinitis, pneumonia, enteritis, reproductive disorders, and subclinical infections. *C. suis* has been recognized in the intestinal mucosa of swine, with approximately equal frequency in diarrheic and nondiarrheic animals. Enteric chlamydial infections of pigs with *C. suis* are frequent and often subclinical. After experimental inoculation of *C. suis* into gnotobiotic piglets, there was moderate diarrhea, anorexia, weakness, and body weight loss. Microscopic changes consisted of necrosis and exfoliation of enterocytes on the apical half of villi, resulting in mild-to-severe villus atrophy in the distal jejunum and ileum. Lymphangitis and perilymphangitis were also evident in affected gut. Chlamydial replication was particularly marked at 2-4 days postinoculation and primarily located in the small intestinal villus enterocytes. Further sites of replication included large intestinal enterocytes, lamina propria, submucosa, and the mesenteric lymph nodes. In weanling pigs, similar lesions, but no diarrhea, were induced.

Neorickettsia infections (equine neorickettsiosis)

Equine neorickettsiosis is a condition also described as *equine monocytic ehrlichiosis*, *equine ehrlichial colitis*, and *Potomac horse fever* (*PHF*), which was first defined clinically in 1979, with signs of fever, leukopenia, depression, loss of appetite, colic, diarrhea, and lameness. Until very recently, the etiologic agent of equine neorickettsiosis was considered to be only ***Neorickettsia ristici*** (formerly *Ehrlichia risticii*). However, a newly identified *Neorickettsia*, ***N. findlayensis***, was detected in horses with equine neorickettsiosis in Canada. Experimental inoculation of 2 naive ponies with *N. findlayensis* produced neorickettsiosis, and the bacteria were reisolated from both of them, fulfilling Koch postulates. Antibody titers against *N. findlayensis* were higher than those against *N. risticii*.

Neorickettsia spp. are members of the order *Rickettsiales*, which are *obligate intracellular bacterial pathogens*. Equine neoricketisiosis typically occurs in the summer. It was first described in the Potomac River valley of Maryland, Virginia, and Pennsylvania, but it is now found in most areas of the United States and Canada, with cases also reported in Brazil and Uruguay, where it has been known for many years as *churrido*. Considering the current distribution of the disease, the name *PHF* is no longer appropriate, and the term equine neorickettsiosis is preferred.

Neorickettsia spp. replicate within the phagosome in the host cell and use trematodes as hosts. The life cycle of the fluke includes freshwater snails from which it goes back into water, where it is ingested by the larval stages of several aquatic insects, including caddis flies and mayflies. The main mode of infection is most likely by accidental ingestion of infected adult insects in water containers. Insectivorous birds and bats are definitive hosts, and themselves become infected with *Neorickettsia* spp. Experimental infection has been produced with oral administration of infected insects and subcutaneous inoculation of *N. risticii*. All attempts to transmit the disease using ticks have so far failed.

The disease may be highly variable. Many infected horses seem not to get sick. Others develop severe colic, subcutaneous edema, laminitis, and shock; mortality can be up to 30% in untreated cases. Abortions of pregnant mares have been attributed to *N. risticii* infection.

The incubation period in experimental infections is ~9-14 days, and diarrhea begins 1-3 days after the onset of fever. Not all experimentally infected animals develop disease.

At **autopsy** of spontaneous cases, small vesicles are reported in the oral cavity, and epicardial hemorrhages and pulmonary congestion and hemorrhage, compatible with endotoxemia, are described. These are not reported in experimental cases, nor is laminitis. The lesions in the GI tract are the most significant, in both spontaneous and experimental cases. In some animals there may be focal or more extensive erosions in the gastric mucosa, sometimes with overlying fibrinous exudate. Lesions in the small intestine are generally limited to segmental areas of mucosal congestion or hyperemia, with occasional focal ulcers or hemorrhage, and are much less consistent and severe than those in the *cecum and colon*. The content of the large bowel is abnormally fluid and may have a brown or red-brown color, and foul odor. In the cecum and colon, there may be 5-10-cm patches of hyperemia, aggregates of small ulcers a few millimeters in diameter, and petechial hemorrhages. Sometimes the mucosa of the entire cecum is widely hyperemic. Ulcers and petechial hemorrhage are more severe and consistent in the right dorsal colon. The small colon is usually unaffected grossly.

Microscopic lesions are most consistent in the large intestine, although similar changes may be occasionally evident in the small bowel. In areas of gross hyperemia, there is marked congestion and superficial hemorrhage in the mucosa. Associated with these lesions are superficial epithelial necrosis, erosion, and fibrin effusion. The mucosal surface is denuded, or perhaps covered by fibrinocellular exudate, and the epithelium in the upper half of crypts is attenuated. Deeper parts of crypts are dilated and may contain necrotic epithelium and inflammatory cells. An abnormally intense mixed inflammatory cell population is in the lamina propria, and sometimes the submucosa. Lymphoid tissue in the gut, mesenteric lymph nodes, and spleen is moderately involuted, compatible with the effects of the stress of systemic illness.

Organisms are not evident in H&E-stained tissue. They are visible in the large colon, and less consistently, in the cecum, small colon, and small intestine, with *modified Steiner silver stain*. They appear as small clusters of 10-15 fine brown dots, <1 µm in diameter, in the apical cytoplasm of epithelial cells deep in crypts, or as more numerous, smaller black structures in the cytoplasm of macrophages in the periglandular lamina propria, or in a few glandular epithelial cells. Ultrastructurally, small dense elementary bodies may be found, alone or in small clusters in vacuoles in the cytoplasm of macrophages, mast cells, and crypt epithelium, or as morulae-aggregates of larger, more open organisms, in the same locations. *N. risticii* can be identified in feces or peripheral blood buffy coat by PCR, providing a more sensitive and specific means of detection.

Mycotic, oomycotic, and algal diseases of the alimentary tract

Mycotic infections

The GI mucosa is a significant portal of entry for various fungal agents, and because *fungal invasion is a common sequel to many mucosal diseases and lesions*, it may be the precursor to systemic infection. Many of the most common mycotic infectious are particularly or uniquely common in immunocompromised patients (e.g., *Candida* and *Aspergillus*), and heavy fungal challenge, disruption of the normal flora or the physical GI barrier by a primary lesion, and/or lowered host resistance are probably required for establishment of mycotic disease in the GI tract. However, other pathogens are probably capable of causing disease without immunocompromise (e.g., the oomycetes). Recent technologic advances, morphologic, and molecular phylogenetic analyses have resulted in reclassification, regrouping, and renaming of various organisms, which causes significant confusion in veterinary and human medicine.

Mucormycosis is the preferred name for infections caused by several of the most common organisms associated with alimentary tract mycoses, including the group of organisms formerly known as zygomycetes, which is now considered an obsolete term. Reclassification has abolished the order *zygomycetes*, and placed the order ***Mucorales*** in the subphylum *Mucoromycotina*, so infection is now known as *mucormycosis instead of zygomycosis*. The *Mucorales* include several families that are apparently capable of causing rhinocerebral, pulmonary, GI, cutaneous, renal, or disseminated disease in humans and animals; specific families (and genera) reported mostly in animals include *Mortierellaceae* (*Mortierella*), *Mucoraceae* (***Mucor***, ***Rhizomucor***, ***Rhizopus***), and *Lichtheimiaceae* [***Lichtheimia*** (formerly *Absidia*)]. Other organisms formerly classified more broadly as zygomycetes include the family *Entomophthoraceae* (*Basidiobolus* and *Conidiobolus*) and are considered separately later in this chapter.

Mucoralean fungi are mostly saprophytic organisms found in a variety of organic substrates. Transmission likely occurs when spores are inhaled or through contamination of food material that is ingested by the patient; epithelial injury is thought to play a significant role in the ability of these organisms to gain access to various tissues in the respiratory or GI tracts. Fungi may produce localized granulomatous inflammation in Peyer patches or be carried to regional mesenteric lymph nodes. Fungal hyphae in mesenteric lymph node granulomas of clinically normal feedlot cattle are recognized and indicate that *invasion by these agents across the intestinal mucosa does not lead invariably to systemic disease*. Once in tissues though, the spores of *Mucorales* can germinate and undergo filamentous growth; in some animals, angioinvasion leads to vascular thrombosis and tissue necrosis in the host. Lesions can occur anywhere in the GI tract, including the forestomachs of ruminants, and in the mesenteric lymph nodes, and are typically necrosis and hemorrhage, or variably severe granulomatous inflammation causing thickening or mass-like lesions in affected tissue. Microscopically, there is necrosis, thrombosis, and vasculitis, or variably severe granulomatous to pyogranulomatous inflammation, often with prominent multinucleate giant cells, asteroid bodies, and/or the Splendore-Hoeppli phenomenon in affected tissues.

Mucorales in their invasive mycelial form are broad (6-25 µm), coarse, irregular hyphae with infrequent septation, and random branching, sometimes surrounded by an eosinophilic sleeve in tissue sections; angioinvasion is often observed. Cytochemical staining is usually helpful, including PAS or GMS to identify and evaluate morphologic features of the invading fungi.

Cases of mucormycosis in cattle are mostly seen following rumen acidosis caused by grain overload, mastitis, downer cow syndrome, parturition, or subsequent to immunosuppression or prolonged antimicrobial usage. Fungi have been reported in cattle secondary to erosive viral diseases, including infectious bovine rhinotracheitis and BVD, and can cause mycotic abomasitis in calves with bacterial septicemia. These fungi can be found at any level of the GI tract; however, the rumen and omasum are the most common sites. These organisms have a propensity to invade mucosal and submucosal blood vessels, producing *thrombosis and venous infarction*. Characteristic gross lesions are focal or multifocal areas of edema and red-black discoloration caused by venous stasis and hemorrhage. Histologic lesions include mucosal-to-transmural necrosis of the GI wall, and there may be a relatively mild inflammatory response to the fungi. Dissemination to the liver and more distant organs via the portal and systemic circulations is not uncommon. Mucormycosis has been described historically as various zygomycoses in horses, pigs, dogs, cats; all are sporadic, and usually involve the integumentary, respiratory, or GI tract, and may progress to disseminated disease.

Entomophthoromycosis is the preferred name for infections caused by organisms of the orders *Basidiobolales* and *Entomophthorales*, which are genera ***Basidiobolus*** and ***Conidiobolus***, respectively. These are both environmental saprophytic organisms, and both were formerly classified broadly as *zygomycetes*. The most identified species causing basidiobolomycosis in animals is *Basidiobolus ranarum*, and conidiobolomycosis described in animals is most often caused by species *Conidiobolus lamprauges* and *C. incongruus*. Entomophthoromycosis involving the GI tract is far less common and sporadic than mucormycosis, probably because transmission is thought to occur mostly via inhalation (especially for *Conidiobolus* sp.); however, infections have been rarely reported in dogs. *B. ranarum* has been associated with subcutaneous, respiratory, or intestinal infections involving the stomach, small intestine, and distal colon in dogs; *Conidiobolus* sp. has been more commonly associated with cutaneous or rhinofacial and nasopharyngeal lesions in humans, horses, dogs, and sheep. Transmission is likely via inhalation, ingestion, or by percutaneous inoculation of spores. Affected patients have nonspecific clinical signs that are dependent on the anatomic location and severity of the lesions. Grossly, there can be localized severe granulomatous-to-pyogranulomatous inflammation, with intra-lesional thin-walled and poorly septate hyphal organisms. Family *Entomophthoraceae* hyphae are 5-25 µm in diameter, with thin irregularly parallel walls, infrequent septa, and rare random branching. They are characteristically surrounded by a wide sheath or sleeve of eosinophilic material in tissue section; the Splendore-Hoeppli phenomenon is described. Although hyphae of *B. ranarum* are usually larger and stain more strongly by PAS than do hyphae of *Pythium insidiosum* (5-25 µm vs. 4-10 µm, respectively), GI basidiobolomycosis shares several histomorphologic features with GI oomycosis (discussed later in this chapter) and can be difficult to distinguish based only on histomorphology, so additional testing such as culture or molecular analysis is often warranted to definitively determine the causative agent. Much less is known about conidiobolomycosis in animals, which is reported rarely in dogs, sheep, and deer. Most appear as upper respiratory disease due to rhinocerebral, nasopharyngeal, and rarely disseminated disease. Confirmation of the specific pathogen involved has been by culture or molecular techniques.

Aspergillosis in animals occurs as localized infections or as widely disseminated disease and is caused by organisms in the genus *Aspergillus*, which are saprophytic filamentous fungi commonly found in soil or decaying organic matter in the environment. Most cases of aspergillosis in animals involve the respiratory system, with less frequent infection of other systems; all are much more common in immunocompromised patients. Transmission presumably occurs via inhalation, although tissue predilection is described in some species. Affected animals have signs attributable to the anatomic location most affected; in the GI tract there can be thickening of the bowel wall, or hemorrhagic and fibrinonecrotic exudate.

Aspergillus has relatively uniform, narrow (3-6 µm), septate hyphae, typically with acute-angled dichotomous branching. In **ruminants**, *Aspergillus* spp. are known to cause mycotic pneumonia, placentitis, and gastroenteritis; the abomasum is affected most commonly. *Mycotic ileitis and colitis* in **cats** caused by *Aspergillus* spp. has been described and may be associated with feline parvoviral infection or antibiotic therapy. Intestinal lesions can be subtle, particularly in the face of concurrent intestinal pathogens, but are described as hemorrhagic and necrotizing; dissemination to other organs can also occur and the lung appears to be the favored site in cats. Mycotic enteritis in **dogs** with widespread fungal dissemination is a rare sequel to parvoviral (CPV2) enteritis.

Definitive **diagnosis** of mycotic-induced inflammatory lesions requires culture, which may be difficult, and molecular genetic identification of the isolate. A presumptive diagnosis may be based on morphologic characteristics of organisms in tissue sections; histochemical or immunohistochemical staining may add confidence to the likely agent. Major etiologic differential diagnoses include mycobacteria, actinomycotic, or nocardial agents.

Candidiasis refers to diseases caused by various ***Candida*** spp., which are commensal inhabitants of the alimentary and biliary tract of animals, existing as *budding yeasts* in association with mucosal surfaces. With alterations affecting the mucosal surface (especially squamous epithelial mucosal surfaces) or of the mucosal flora, these yeasts become opportunistic pathogens and invade the underlying tissue as *branching, filamentous pseudohyphae and hyphae that replace the yeast forms. Candida* spp. are occasional opportunistic invaders of nonsquamous epithelium of the alimentary tract, but other opportunistic fungi are more likely to be associated with nonsquamous epithelial surfaces, particularly in older animals. *Candidiasis is mainly a disease of keratinized squamous epithelium in young animals, especially pigs, calves, and foals.*

Only a few of the almost 200 *Candida* species are known to cause candidiasis; in animals the most important are ***Candida albicans*** and ***C. tropicalis***. Changes in the mucosal flora usually result from systemic antimicrobial therapy that reduces the numbers of anaerobic bacteria and allows proliferation of *Candida* spp. Immunosuppression, environmental and social stress, and treatment with chemotherapeutic, anticancer, or anti-inflammatory agents may also predispose to candidiasis. An important factor in the virulence of *Candida* spp., especially *C. albicans*, is the ability to adhere to, colonize, and invade the epithelium. Adherence to the epithelium is mediated by a family of *adhesins* produced by the yeast. Biofilm formation, especially in immunocompromised patients, is a major virulence factor during candidiasis.

Candida is a *polymorphic fungus* that can grow as an ovoid 3-6 μm yeast (with budding), as elongated ellipsoid pseudohyphae (chains of tubular yeast), or as true hyphae; binding of the yeast to the epithelium induces the well-known yeast-to-hypha switch. Epithelial damage may be induced by yeast-produced enzymes, including proteinases and catalases, or by host cell–produced enzymes such as neutrophil myeloperoxidase. These enzymes contribute to local damage, which permits deeper penetration into squamous epithelium and perhaps promotes systemic dissemination. Accumulation of keratin caused by anorexia may also contribute to the severity and distribution of lesions in all species by increasing the substrate available to the fungus.

In **pigs**, *Candida* spp. often invade the parakeratotic material that accumulates on the *gastric squamous mucosa;* apparently, these infections are mostly relatively insignificant. *Thrush* is the term for candidiasis of the oral cavity, which is seen occasionally in young pigs, especially those with concurrent disease. Lesions may be confined to the tongue, hard palate, or pharynx, but often involve the esophagus and gastric squamous mucosa as well. Grossly, the lesions are yellow-white, smooth, or wrinkled plaques loosely adherent to the mucosa. Histologically, there is vacuolar degeneration of the epithelium, which contains many yeasts, pseudohyphae, hyphae, and aggregates of neutrophils and bacteria within and beneath the stratum corneum. Vascular congestion, mild inflammation, and erosion and ulceration of the epithelium may all be present.

In **calves**, candidiasis occurs following prolonged antimicrobial therapy and in association with rumen putrefaction. Lesions are most often seen in the *ventral sac of the rumen*, but may involve the omasum, reticulum, and occasionally the abomasum. Grossly, the lesions resemble those of *thrush* in pigs, but the keratin layer tends to be thicker, less diffuse, and light gray. Omasal leaves may be adhered together by fungus-laden keratin layers. *Nakaseomyces glabratus (*formerly *Candida glabrata)* in the abomasum has been implicated as a cause of diarrhea in calves, especially during winter months. Disseminated candidiasis occurs more often in calves than in pigs, probably because of the relatively prolonged survival of calves with alimentary lesions. Epithelial ulcers in cases of candidiasis in calves should prompt a search for alimentary herpesviral infection.

Gastroesophageal candidiasis in **foals** also involves the squamous epithelium, and lesions are typically *adjacent to the margo plicatus*. Colic and anorexia can be observed and are probably related to development of ulcers, which may perforate and cause peritonitis.

In **dogs**, *Candida* spp. have been described as the cause of mycotic stomatitis (thrush), peritonitis, and rarely systemic disease or sepsis; these cases have occurred mostly in immunocompromised patients. In tissues, identification of appropriate lesions composed of foci of necrosis, neutrophilic inflammation, and one or more of the yeast's polymorphic forms permits a provisional identification of *Candida* spp. Silver or PAS stains enhance the organisms in section.

Cryptococcosis is a mycosis caused by the environmental saprophytic yeasts of the genus ***Cryptococcus;*** most cases occur in subtropical or temperate climates. Cryptococcosis is usually caused by various organisms from the *Cryptococcus neoformans* and *C. gattii* complexes, which are associated with bird feces and decayed wood, respectively; other *Cryptococcus* species have been identified sporadically. *C. neoformans* has long been thought to primarily affect immunocompromised patients; *C. gattii* may affect patients with intact immune systems. *C. neoformans* infections have been reported in many animal species, and most are of respiratory, cutaneous, or disseminated infections in domestic cats, and respiratory or CNS disease in dogs. Cryptococcosis involving the GI tract of animals is uncommon, although the incidence may be higher than previously thought, and so may represent a significant emerging disease (or it is more commonly recognized). Several cases of abdominal cryptococcosis in dogs and cats have been reported in Australia; most had mesenteric and intestinal lesions. Infections are described mostly in young dogs, and no breed or sex predispositions are known.

Infection probably occurs following inhalation, or less frequently after ingestion of spores or yeasts, with localized invasion (from the sinonasal cavity into the CNS through the cribriform plate of the ethmoid bone), or systemic dissemination into abdominal or thoracic cavities. Clinical signs are related to the site of infection (respiratory, intestinal, neurologic, ocular), but most cases are disseminated infections, so signs are nonspecific and include lethargy, weight loss, inappetence, and possibly abdominal or thoracic effusion. Imaging may reveal lymphadenomegaly, mass lesions or GI thickening, or involvement of other organs; destruction of bones has been described with sinonasal cryptococcosis. Diagnosis can be aided by serology, and cytologic examination of aspirates, impression smears, or body fluids may reveal organisms; however, as for other mycoses, fungal culture or molecular techniques are required to confirm the diagnosis.

Gross lesions are attributable to the major organ system affected. In the GI tract, there is thickening of the intestinal wall or discrete mass formation that can be obstructive. Histologic findings are multifocal coalescing, mural-to-transmural pyogranulomatous inflammation, often with significant fibroplasia. Inflammation is centered on blastoconidia with narrow-necked budding and a prominent, thick, H&E nonstaining, polysaccharide capsule; the mucicarmine stain is helpful to identify the capsule. Most cases with a documented cause were *C. neoformans* or *C. gattii*, although we have seen a case of *C. albidus* (renamed as *Naganishia albida*) causing lymphadenitis and small intestinal tumorlike masses resulting in intussusception and small intestinal obstruction in a midwestern US dog. Clinical treatment can be successful if the intestinal masses can be excised; if disseminated disease is identified, long-term antifungal therapy is required. There is potential zoonotic risk for humans, particularly those who are immunocompromised.

In **cats**, cryptococcosis is mostly associated with *C. gattii* and is a disease of the respiratory tract, or disseminated disease; GI involvement is rare.

Histoplasmosis is caused by ***Histoplasma capsulatum***, a *dimorphic soilborne fungus* that exists in the environment as a mycelial form within organic matter and within the host as a yeast. Although the fungus has worldwide distribution in subtropical and temperate regions, histoplasmosis is endemic in the midwestern and southern United States, including the Mississippi, Ohio, and Missouri river valleys. In Canada, it is thought to be limited to south-central Canada, along the Ottawa and St. Lawrence River valleys with only sporadic cases reported elsewhere. It is an important disease of humans, cats, and dogs, and occasionally occurs in other species. Infection generally occurs via *inhalation of spores*, and possibly *by ingestion* of microconidia or macroconidia in the mycelial phase that exhibit thermal dimorphism and transition to yeast forms within host macrophages where they replicate, resist host defense mechanisms, and are eventually disseminated via lymphatics to various organs, including the liver, spleen, and GI tract. Disease is only rarely reported in immunocompetent individuals, where most are self-limiting upper or lower respiratory tract infections, but animals that are immunocompromised or receive large doses of organism have greater risk of developing disease. In dogs, the young or sporting/working breeds are reported to have increased risk.

Given the major route of exposure, infection in **dogs** is usually confined to the lungs, but dissemination is common to the GI tract, and less commonly to the skin, bone, liver, spleen, or brain. Rare cases of histoplasmosis confined to the GI tract suggest exposure by ingestion, potentially of infected sputum. The terminal ileum and colon appear to be the most frequent site in the GI tract, this may be due to the increased lymphoid tissue present in this location. *Disseminated histoplasmosis* is predominantly a disease of young dogs that usually have nonspecific signs, including weight loss, generalized lymphadenopathy, hemorrhagic diarrhea, anorexia, lethargy, and possibly tenesmus, especially if the colon is involved. **Cats** are more commonly affected than dogs, and disseminated disease is most often observed, involving the lungs, lymph nodes, liver, spleen, kidney, adrenal glands, bone marrow, eyes, and GI tract; primary *intestinal histoplasmosis* is probably rare in cats.

Horses appear to be relatively resistant to histoplasmosis, although sporadic cases have been reported in a variety of organs, including the intestine. ***Epizootic lymphangitis*** is an endemic chronic contagious disease of working horses in developing countries that is caused by several variants of *H. capsulatum*, and generally is a disseminated infection involving the skin and lymph nodes with only rare involvement of ocular or respiratory tract.

Gross intestinal lesions may be absent, or there may be hemorrhagic enterocolitis, or the lesions may mimic neoplasia as they cause granulomatous nodular thickening of the intestinal wall with mucosal ulceration. Mesenteric lymph nodes are often markedly enlarged, and peritoneal effusion may be present. Characteristic histologic lesions are *multifocal and coalescing transmural granulomatous inflammation* of the stomach, or small and/or large intestine (Fig. 1-139A). Nonulcerated areas of the mucosa and draining lymph nodes contain multifocal-to-diffuse infiltrates of macrophages laden with *H. capsulatum* organisms within cytoplasmic vacuoles. Oval-to-round, 2-5 µm yeasts with a characteristic central spherical basophilic body surrounded by a clear halo (see Fig. 1-139B) usually can be readily observed with H&E stain; however, PAS or GMS stains highlight the organisms in tissues (see Fig. 1-139C). Fungal culture is mentioned frequently in the literature but is probably used infrequently. Antigen detection testing is commonly used for clinical diagnosis, but identification of organisms in tissue by biopsy or by cytopathology (needle aspirates of the lymph nodes, liver, or spleen; rectal or colonic scraping) is needed for confirmation of the definitive diagnosis. Microscopic diagnosis of GI histoplasmosis is not difficult, but grossly the disease must be distinguished from intestinal lymphoma and from colitis of other types.

Oomycotic infections

Oomycosis is infection by aquatic oomycetes (water molds), which are unique organisms more closely related to algae than fungi, although the disease they cause usually closely resembles various mycoses. In domestic species, these are primarily associated with ***Pythium insidiosum***, and less frequently ***Lagenidium giganteum***, or ***Paralagenidium*** sp. These organisms have long been associated mostly with tropical and subtropical climates but can also occur in more temperate regions. *P. insidiosum* zoospores display chemotaxis toward animal hair, intestinal mucosa, and wounds, including those caused by insect bites. Therefore, the lesions commonly involve systems with direct contact with water containing infectious zoospores. Immunocompetent individuals are frequently affected, implying that immunosuppression is less significant for oomycosis, and pathogen exposure and load plays a significant role. Infection is probably acquired through direct contact with water containing zoospores; in animals with cutaneous wounds, the most common manifestation is cutaneous disease with extension to local lymph nodes and dissemination via lymphatics, although GI disease is also frequently observed in dogs.

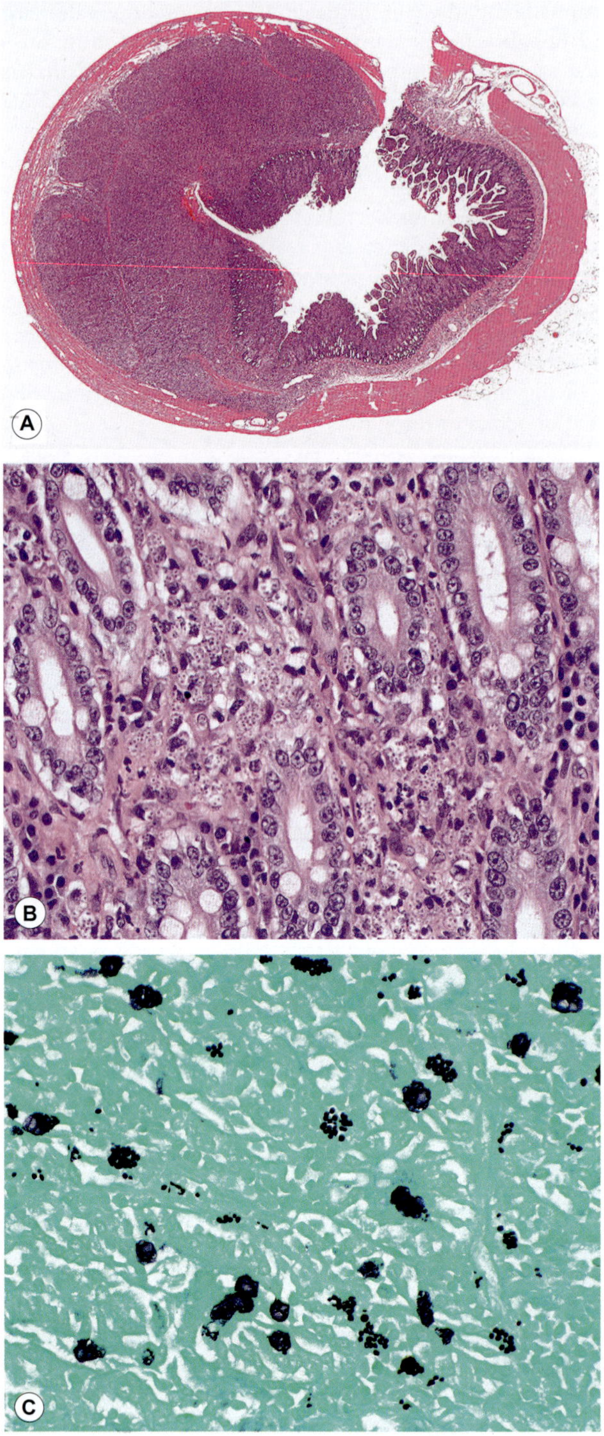

Figure 1-139 Histoplasmosis. A. Marked expansion of the mucosa and submucosa by macrophages containing *Histoplasma capsulatum* organisms. (Courtesy J. Caswell.) **B.** Histologic view of the intestine with numerous 2-5 µm *H. capsulatum* organisms within macrophages. (Courtesy J. Caswell.) **C.** Grocott methenamine silver staining reveals 2-5 µm *H. capsulatum* organisms within macrophages.

Pythium insidiosum is the causative agent of **pythiosis**, a severe, progressive, and potentially fatal disease mostly affecting dogs. Best recognized as a cause of *cutaneous lesions in horses* (see Vol. 1, Integumentary System), *P. insidiosum* can cause distinct disease forms including vascular, ocular, GI, and rarely systemic disease, mostly in dogs and horses but sporadically in calves and sheep. In contrast to horses, the GI form is the most common in dogs. Concurrent cutaneous and GI lesions are rare in the same animal. Affected patients have nonspecific clinical signs, including lethargy, inappetence, or more specific GI signs such as vomiting, diarrhea, or even intestinal obstruction. **Gross lesions** include distinct nodule formation, or thickening of the gastric, small intestinal, or colonic wall that can extend into the adjacent omentum and mesentery. The gastric outflow region, the distal small intestine, and the colon are the locations reported most commonly. Lymphadenomegaly is frequently observed, and the gross lesions are usually detected by diagnostic imaging such as radiography and ultrasound. In some cases, small, firm, white-or-yellow necrotic coagula, known as *leeches* or *kunkers*, may be embedded in the inflamed nodules.

Histologic lesions are multifocal coalescing mural-to-transmural pyogranulomatous inflammation (Fig. 1-140A), lymphangitis, lymphadenitis, and sometimes peritonitis with extensive omental adhesions. Granulomatous-to-pyogranulomatous inflammation, *often with increased and prominent numbers of eosinophils*, are observed in many cases (see Fig. 1-140B). While not pathognomonic, *this eosinophilic infiltration should raise concern for pythiosis*. In contrast to many fungal agents, the characteristic hyphal organisms are often difficult to detect by light microscopy within H&E-stained sections, and typically appear as subtle negative-staining fungal hyphal elements within the inflamed tissue. *P. insidiosum* hyphae are 3-8 µm wide (average 5 µm) with nondichotomous acute-to-right-angle branching, and rarely septate filaments, best observed in the areas of necrosis or centers of granulomas using special cytochemical staining, especially the GMS or other silver stains (see Fig. 1-140C), because these organisms are typically only weakly positive by PAS stains and can be readily overlooked with PAS staining only. Similar lesions are reported in horses, sheep, and cats. A diagnosis of pythiosis should be confirmed by identifying the agent using culture, serology, or PCR. Successful treatment has been described in dogs.

Other oomycotic infections of the GI tract are much less common in dogs, and rare in cats. *L. giganteum* has been identified as a cause of progressive cutaneous, subcutaneous, and disseminated disease that can resemble pythiosis. *L. giganteum* in dogs (and rarely in cats) mostly causes cutaneous ulcerative dermatitis with regional lymphadenopathy but rarely involves the GI tract in any species. The gross and histologic lesions of disseminated disease, however, are indistinguishable from pythiosis; eosinophils are also a prominent histologic feature. *Paralagenidium karlingii* shares morphologic features with *L. giganteum*, but seems to be limited to cutaneous and subcutaneous disease in dogs. While the histomorphologic features of *P. karlingii* organisms are similar to *P. insidiosum*, *L. giganteum* are distinct and typically much larger, 10-20-µm (average 13 µm) hyphae with infrequently septate irregular nonparallel walls; they also are difficult to detect in H&E-stained sections and are best visualized by GMS or other silver staining techniques. Although cytology from aspirates or impression smears, serologic detection of antibodies, and histologic examination are all highly beneficial, the morphologic variability in tissues of many of these agents causing mycoses and oomycoses in animals necessitates culture or molecular techniques (PCR, sequencing) to achieve a definitive diagnosis.

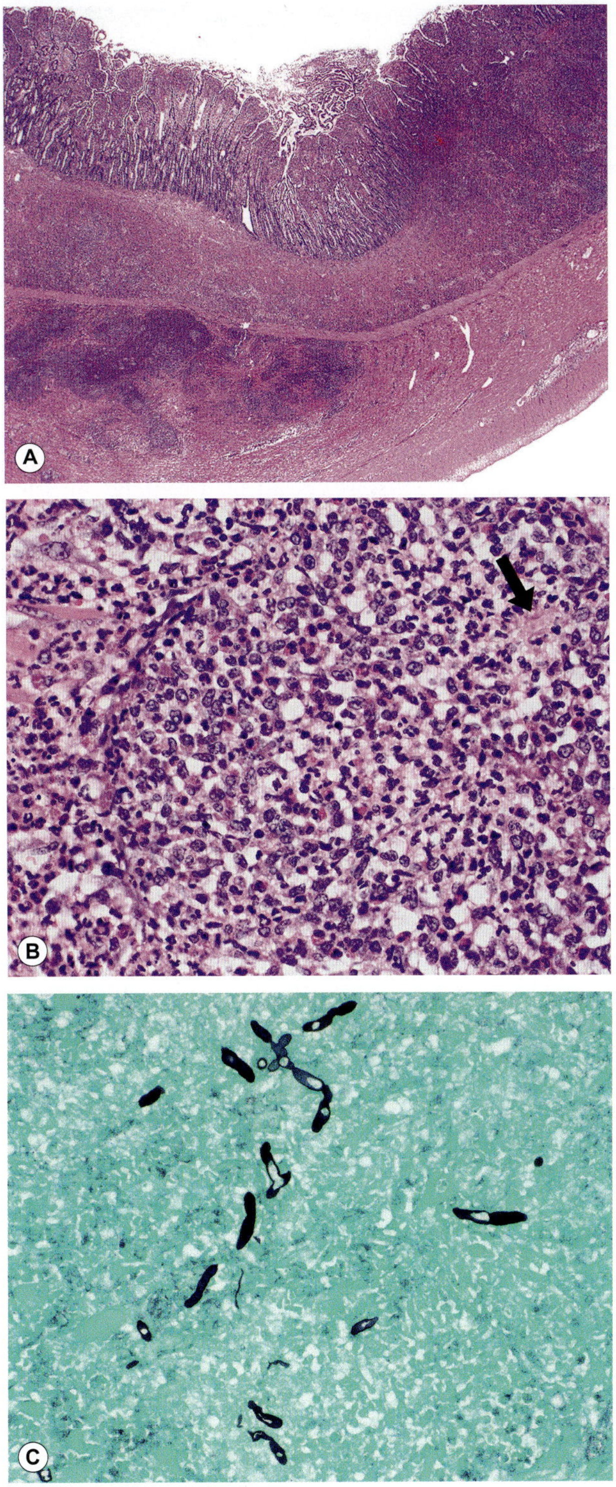

Figure 1-140 **Pythiosis** in a dog. **A**. Marked nodular mural expansion (mucosal, submucosal, and muscle layers) of the small intestine due to severe mixed inflammation. **B**. Macrophages, eosinophils, and neutrophils surround central necrotic regions that contain indistinct oomycotic hyphae that are difficult to visualize in H&E-stained sections (arrow). Eosinophils are often prominent and should raise suspicion of pythiosis. **C**. Grocott methenamine silver highlights numerous 3-8-μm-wide hyphal structures with nondichotomous branching and occasional septa, consistent with the oomycete *Pythium insidiosum*.

Algal infections

Protothecosis is infection caused by ***Prototheca*** spp., which are *opportunistic achlorophyllic unicellular algae* that in some scenarios can be pathogenic for humans and animals. They are ubiquitous in some environmental niches, including raw and treated sewage, water, feces, plant sap, and tree slime; they also can be contaminants of various substrates including cow's milk. Seven species are described, but are grouped into 2 main lineage clusters, of which the major organisms important for domestic animals are ***Prototheca zopfii*** and ***P. wickerhamii***. These 2 are the major causes of disease in animals, with both occurring occasionally in the same animal.

Lesions caused by *Prototheca* spp. are predominantly *cutaneous* infections of cats and humans, *mastitis* in cows and goats, upper respiratory infection in goats and horses, and as *GI* or *disseminated* infections in dogs. The **pathogenesis** of protothecosis is not completely understood. Traumatic inoculation is thought to lead to cutaneous infection in humans and cats. An environmental pathogen in dairy cows, *P. zopfii* probably gains access to the mammary gland by invasion of the teat canal. In dogs, the colon has been proposed as a primary site of infection, with dissemination to other organs, including the eyes, brain, liver, kidneys, bone marrow, and skin. The prognosis following dissemination in dogs is usually considered poor. Factors predisposing to the development of intestinal protothecosis in dogs are poorly understood. Immunosuppression may account for the sporadic occurrence of disease in dogs; Collies and Boxer dogs have been over-represented in some reports, suggesting breed-related susceptibility. Perhaps *Prototheca* spp. are opportunistic invaders of existing mucosal lesions. Cattle, horses, and wild pigs can shed *Prototheca* spp. in feces without apparent clinical disease.

Clinical signs in dogs with intestinal protothecosis often include chronic, episodic, and intractable, hemorrhagic large-bowel diarrhea, with progressive weight loss. *Hemorrhagic and ulcerative colitis* is the first and most consistent enteric lesion. In dogs with disseminated disease, signs may be vague and intestinal lesions may be subtle; dissemination via the hematogenous or lymphatic routes most commonly involves the eyes, CNS, kidneys, and heart. Mesenteric lymph nodes may be enlarged. **Histologically**, the cellular host inflammatory response to infection can vary; granulomatous-to-pyogranulomatous and ulcerative colitis is typical. Intracellular and extracellular algal organisms are observed in variable numbers, depending on the severity of disease in affected tissue. In cases of disseminated disease, granulomas containing organisms can be found in various organs.

Prototheca in tissue sections stained with H&E can be difficult to visualize, so cytochemical stains such as PAS or GMS are helpful. The algae are unicellular, nonbudding, round-to-oval spherules with a refractile capsule, 5-12 μm (*P. wickerhamii*) to 10-25 μm (*P. zopfii*) diameter. Wedge-shaped endospores are within a single sporangium in *Prototheca* spp. Other potentially pathogenic algal organisms that also undergo endosporulation, such as *Chlorella*, contain PAS-positive cytoplasmic starch granules that are PAS negative after diastase digestion; this test can be helpful for differentiation of these organisms. Culture, cytology, and fluorescent antibody tests can be helpful ancillary detection techniques, although, as for other similar diseases, culture, PCR, or sequencing are best to achieve definitive diagnosis.

Parasitic diseases of the alimentary tract

Gastrointestinal helminthosis

Helminths are parasitic organisms that cause a wide variety of diseases in animals. They can be classified into nematodes (roundworms), trematodes (flukes), and cestodes (tapeworms). The diagnosis of disease resulting from GI helminths must be made with knowledge of their pathogenic potential and the mechanisms by which it is expressed. *Parasites are much more common than the diseases they cause*, and thus **helminthiasis**, *the state of infection*, must be clearly distinguished from **helminthosis**, *the state of disease*.

According to their action on the host and pathogenesis of disease, GI helminths can be grouped into 5 distinct categories:

1. The first group, including some nematodes and cestodes, **resides free in the lumen of the intestine**, where they compete with the host for nutrients in the intestinal lumen. They are generally of low pathogenicity, except for rare massive infections, and are not likely to be lethal, except if they cause intestinal luminal obstruction. If present in sufficient numbers, some cause subclinical disease such as inefficient growth, or clinical disease in the form of ill-thrift; others are essentially nonpathogenic. Ascarids including adult small strongyles (cyathostomes) of horses, tapeworms such as *Moniezia* and *Taenia* spp., and *Physaloptera* in the stomach of carnivores fall into this group.
2. A second group of helminths, all nematodes, primarily cause **blood loss**. These worms feed on the mucosa causing surface damage and bleeding, or they actively feed on blood. Anemia and hypoproteinemia result in production loss, clinical disease, and death. *Haemonchus* in the abomasum, hookworms in the intestine of carnivores and ruminants, large strongyles of horses, and *Oesophagostomum radiatum* in cattle are the main examples.
3. The third group, composed of nematodes and some trematodes, mainly causes **protein-losing gastroenteropathy**, usually associated with inappetence and diarrhea. In the abomasum, *Ostertagia* and *T. axei* cause mucous metaplasia and hyperplasia of gastric glands, achlorhydria, and diarrhea. In the small intestine, *Cooperia*, *Nematodirus*, *Strongyloides*, *Trichostrongylus*, and larval paramphistomes in sheep and cattle cause villus atrophy. This may cause malabsorption of nutrients, electrolytes, and water; an additional significant effect is the loss of endogenous protein into the GI lumen, which occurs secondary to chronic mucosal inflammation. Heavy infestations of *Trichuris* spp. cause erosion, which results in loss of absorptive function, effusion of fluid, or in severe cases, hemorrhagic exudate.
4. The fourth group, composed of nematodes and trematodes, causes **physical trauma to the intestinal wall** by burrowing into or inciting inflammation within the mucosa or submucosa. In the stomach, various species of spirurids embed in the mucosa or establish in cystic spaces in the submucosa. In the intestine, acanthocephala cause local ulceration by their thorny holdfast organ; larval stages of equine cyathostomes and *Oesophagostomum* spp. become encapsulated in the mucosa or submucosa. Protein loss may occur from ulcerated areas, or when larvae emerge from the mucosa or submucosa. Some are silent, but there is potential for gastrointestinal perforation or for development of sepsis related to the trauma-induced inflammation caused by these parasites. Adhesion of inflamed serosal surfaces associated with nodules or perforations may impair intestinal motility.
5. Finally, some intestinal helminths have **effects at sites distant from the gut**. This is usually the result of migrating larval stages of the worm, either in definitive or intermediate hosts. Larval *Habronema*, ascarids, hookworms, and equine strongyles may cause lesions in a variety of extraintestinal sites in the definitive host. Larval ascarids and taeniid metacestodes may cause lesions or signs because of migration in nonenteric locations in accidental or intermediate hosts.

A **diagnosis of helminthosis** should be reserved for cases in which 3 criteria are met: 1) the helminth is present in numbers consistent with disease; 2) the lesions typically caused by the agent are evident; and 3) there is a syndrome compatible with the pathogenic mechanisms known to be associated with the worm.

Helminthic diseases of the abomasum and stomach

Ostertagiosis is the disease caused by a complex of related genera and species of trichostrongylid nematodes, including *Ostertagia*, that predominantly parasitize the *abomasum of ruminants*. The nomenclature of these worms is in a state of flux; for the sake of simplicity, the disease that they cause will be termed ostertagiosis. *Ostertagiosis is probably the most important parasitism in grazing sheep and cattle in temperate climate zones throughout the world*. It causes subclinical production losses, and clinical disease of diarrhea, wasting, and in many cases, death. ***Ostertagia ostertagi*** and the associated *O. lyrata* infect cattle. Sheep and goats are infected by ***Teladorsagia circumcincta*** (formerly *O. circumcincta*). Cross-infection by these genera occurs between sheep and cattle but is of minor significance. Other species of *Ostertagia* and related genera, including *Marshallagia*, *Spiculopteragia*, and *Camelostrongylus*, infect wild ruminants, including farmed deer; some may also parasitize the abomasum of cattle, sheep, and goats. Their behavior in general resembles that of *Ostertagia* and *Teladorsagia*.

The life cycle is direct. Third-stage larvae exsheath in the rumen and enter glands in the abomasum where they undergo 2 molts and then emerge as early fifth-stage larvae to mature on the mucosal surface, beginning 8-12 days after infection in *T. circumcincta* infections in sheep, and ~17-21 days after *O. ostertagi* infection in cattle. However, a proportion of larvae ingested may persist in glands in a hypobiotic state at the early fourth stage, only to resume development and emerge at a future time, perhaps many months hence. The prepatent period is ~3 weeks.

When infection is not heavy, proliferative immature mucous cells surrounding encysted larvae form raised pale nodules in the mucosa. Confluence of these lesions in heavily infected animals leads to the development of *coalescing areas of irregularly thickened mucosa with a convoluted surface pattern*, likened to *Morocco leather* (Figs. 1-141A-C). During larval development, the normal architecture of the gastric mucosa is altered by *interstitial inflammation* and *mucous metaplasia and hyperplasia of the epithelium lining glands* (Fig. 1-142A and B). In sheep infected with *T. circumcincta*, mucous metaplasia and hyperplasia occur in infected and surrounding glands early during infection, reaching a peak about the time of larval emergence onto the mucosal surface. In cattle with *O. ostertagi*, only glands infected with larvae undergo significant mucous change until about the time larvae emerge from the glands (see Fig. 1-142B), when the mucosal proliferative change becomes more widespread and involves adjacent uninfected glands. Metaplasia and hyperplasia of mucous neck cells

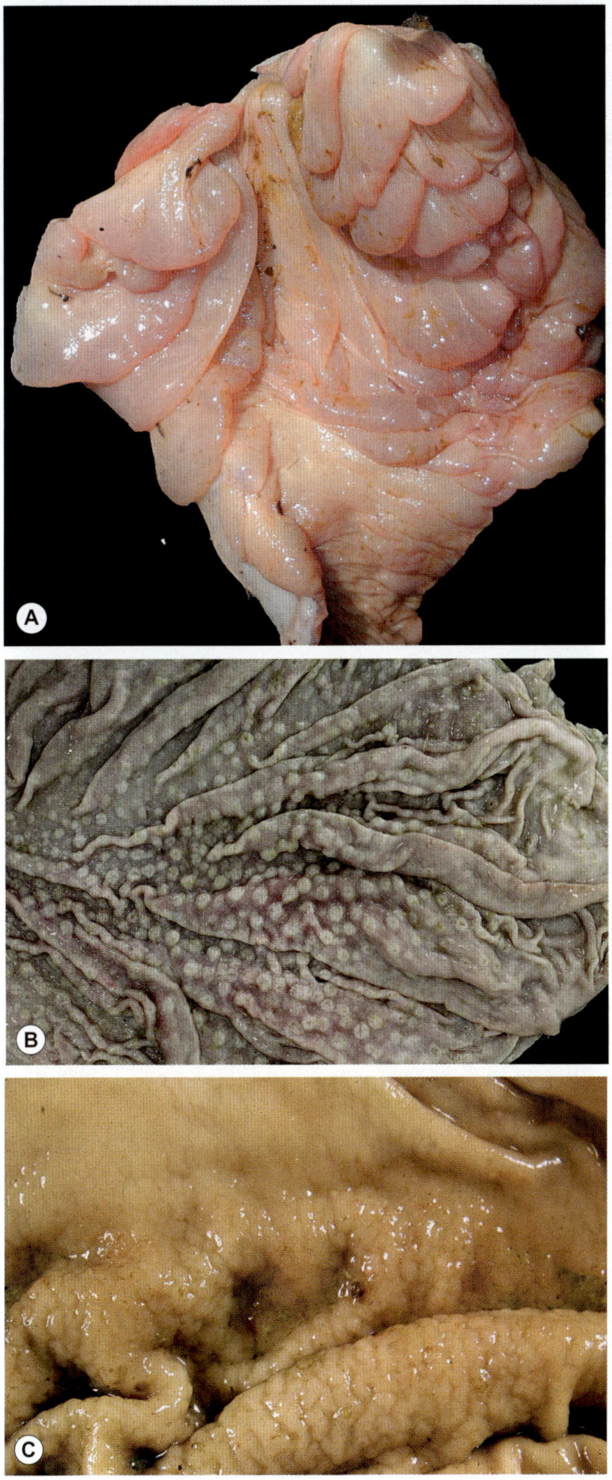

Figure 1-141 Ostertagiosis in ruminants. **A.** Acute edematous abomasitis in a cow. (Courtesy E. Odiozola.) **B.** Multifocal-to-coalescent nodules in a sheep. (Courtesy J. Corpa-Arenas.) **C.** Confluent thickening of hyperplastic glandular mucosa in a sheep.

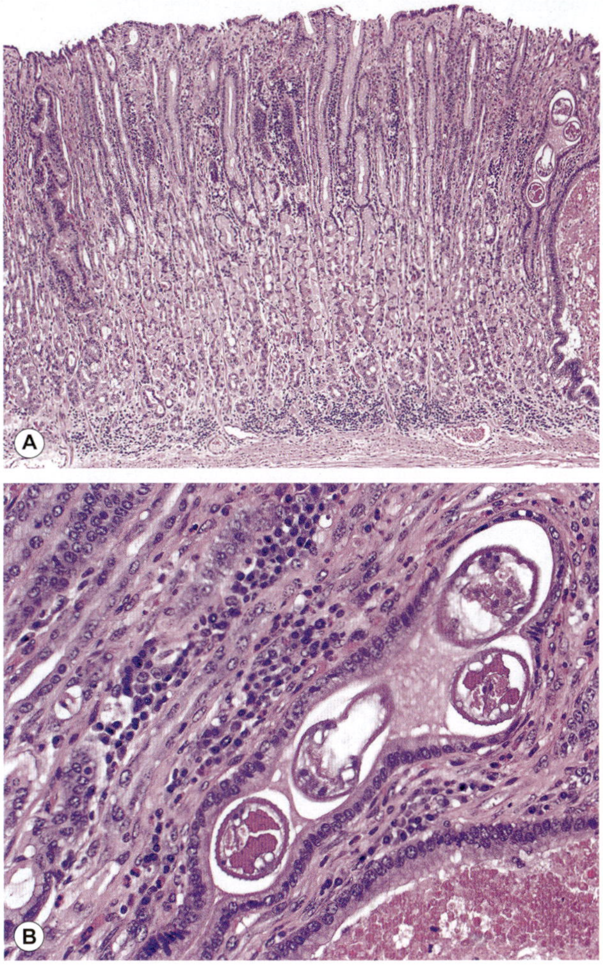

Figure 1-142 Ostertagiosis in the bovine abomasum. **A.** Interstitial lymphocytic, plasmacytic, and eosinophilic abomasitis, with extensive mucous metaplasia and hyperplasia of fundic mucosal epithelium. **B.** Larval and immature adult *Ostertagia ostertagi* within ectatic abomasal glands in a cow.

are accompanied by a mixed population of inflammatory cells in the lamina propria, including lymphocytes, plasma cells, eosinophils, and possibly a few neutrophils; globule leukocytes are commonly observed in glandular epithelium. There may be edema of the lamina propria associated with permeability of proprial vessels.

Widespread replacement of parietal cells by mucous neck cells results in progressive and massive decline in hydrogen ion secretion, with severe cases having a pH of up to 7 or more. This increased abomasal pH results in elevated levels of gastrin in the circulation. Mucosal lesions also lead to achlorhydria, elevation of plasma pepsinogen levels, and local vascular permeability with the loss of plasma protein. The permeability of the mucosa is also increased, which is reflected in back-diffusion of pepsinogen from the lumen of glands to the propria, and ultimately to the circulation. Intercellular junctions between poorly differentiated mucous neck cells are also permeable to plasma protein in tissue fluids, emanating from the leaky small vessels in the inflamed lamina propria. Significant loss of protein occurs into the lumen of the abomasum.

The cardinal signs of ostertagiosis in sheep and cattle are *loss of appetite, diarrhea, and wasting.* Plasma protein loss into the gastrointestinal tract, in combination with reduced feed intake, seems largely responsible for the weight loss and hypoproteinemia that occur in clinical ostertagiosis, and for loss in productive efficiency that occurs in subclinical disease.

Clinical ostertagiosis occurs under 2 sets of circumstances. The first is known as **type I disease** and is seen in lambs or calves at pasture during or shortly after a period of high availability of *infective larvae*. It is due to the direct development, from ingested larvae, of large numbers of adult worms, over a relatively short period and causing chronic gastritis. In contrast, acute gastritis occurs in **type II disease** due to the synchronous maturation and emergence of large numbers of *hypobiotic larvae* from the mucosa, and this form occurs when intake of larvae is likely low or nonexistent. It may occur in yearlings during the winter in the northern hemisphere, or during the dry summer period in Mediterranean climates. Coincident environmental stress likely exacerbates disease.

The **diagnosis** of ostertagiosis is indicated at autopsy by an *abnormally elevated abomasal pH* (>4.5) in association with *typical gross lesions* of the mucosa. The adult worms are brown and threadlike, up to 1.5 cm long, but very difficult to see on the mucosal surface with the unaided eye. *Abomasal contents and washings* should be quantitatively examined for emergent or adult *Ostertagia* and other nematodes. A *portion of the mucosa should be digested* to permit recovery and quantitation of pre-emergent stages. Significant worm burdens in sheep are in the range of 10,000-50,000 or more. In cattle >40,000-50,000 adult worms may be present, and in outbreaks of type II disease, hundreds of thousands of hypobiotic larvae are often detected in the abomasal mucosa. In addition to widespread mucous metaplasia and hyperplasia in dilated glands observed histologically in the abomasum, *Ostertagia* are recognized by the prominent longitudinal cuticular ridges (synlophe) that project from the surface of worms cut transversely. If the parasites have been lost through attrition or recent treatment, the diagnosis must be presumptive, based on the characteristic mucosal lesions.

A positive association between *O. ostertagi* antibodies and abomasal lesions was found in cattle, and measurement of *O. ostertagi* serum antibodies is a useful indicator of parasite-associated abomasal lesions. Abomasal ostertagiosis is accompanied by increased levels of plasma gastrin and pepsinogen, both of which are occasionally used as diagnostic tools for ostertagiosis.

Hemonchosis is a common and severe disease in some parts of the world. *Haemonchus* species require a period of minimum warmth and moisture for larval development to occur on pasture. As a result, they tend to be *most important in tropical or temperate climates with hot wet summers*. ***Haemonchus contortus*** infects mainly sheep, goats, and camelids; ***H. placei*** occurs mainly in cattle. Although *H. contortus* and *H. placei* will infect the heterologous host, the host-parasite relationship appears to be less well adapted, and the species do appear to be genetically distinct. Other species of *Haemonchus* can infect several ruminant species, but they are of less clinical significance. ***Mecistocirrus digitatus*** causes disease very similar to hemonchosis in cattle, buffalo, and sheep in Southeast Asia and Central America.

By exploitation of hypobiosis or retardation of larvae, populations of *H. contortus* are able to persist in the abomasum of the host through periods of climatic adversity, such as excessive cold or dryness. Disease is common in animals experiencing the synchronous "*spring rise*" or periparturient development and maturation of previously hypobiotic larvae, and in young animals heavily stocked at pasture during periods of optimal larval development and availability.

Haemonchus is ~2 cm long and is commonly called the *large stomach worm, or barber pole worm*; the white ovaries and uterus of female adults are prominently viewed coiled within their deep-red bodies. The male is shorter and uniformly deep-red. These worms are equipped with a buccal tooth or lancet, and *fourth-stage and adult worms ingest blood*. Third-stage larvae are ingested and enter abomasal glands, where they molt to the fourth stage and persist as hypobiotic larvae, or emerge as late fourth-stage larvae to continue development in the lumen. The prepatent period for *H. contortus* in sheep is ~15 days; for *H. placei* in cattle ~26-28 days; and for *M. digitatus* ~61-79 days.

Hemonchosis may occur as *peracute or acute disease*, resulting from the maturation or intake of large numbers of larvae. It may cause more insidious *chronic disease* if worm burdens are lower. The pathogenicity of *Haemonchus* infection is the result of their voracious blood-sucking activity, which causes anemia and hypoproteinemia.

Individual *Haemonchus* worms in sheep cause the loss of up to ~0.05 mL of blood per day, which in heavily infected lambs can amount to as much as one-tenth to one-fourth of the blood volume lost per day; plasma loss is concomitant and may be several hundreds of milliliters. *Profound anemia and hypoproteinemia* occur rapidly in heavily infected animals, and affected animals succumb quickly, some even before complete maturation of the worm burden. Less heavily infected animals may be able to withstand the anemia and hypoproteinemia for a period, and they compensate by expanding erythropoiesis and increasing hepatic synthesis of plasma protein. However, they are unable to compensate adequately for the enteric iron loss, despite intestinal reabsorption, and they ultimately succumb some weeks later to *iron-deficiency anemia* when iron reserves are depleted. Low-level infections may contribute to subclinical loss of production or ill-thrift through chronic enteric protein and iron loss. Poor diet and especially low-protein rations compound the effect.

The clinical syndrome may vary somewhat. Some animals are found dead, without previously observed illness. Others lack exercise tolerance, fall when driven, or are reluctant to stand or move, all due to profound anemia. Edema of dependent portions, especially the submandibular area or head in grazing animals, is often observed (Fig. 1-143A). In primary hemonchosis, there is no diarrhea; diarrhea may occur if intercurrent infection with large numbers of other GI helminths occurs.

The **postmortem** appearance of animals with hemonchosis is dominated by the extreme pallor of anemia, apparent on the conjunctiva and throughout the internal tissues. The liver is often pale and friable, and there is usually edema of subcutaneous tissues and mesenteries, with hydrothorax, hydropericardium, and ascites reflecting the severe hypoproteinemia. The abomasal content is usually fluid, and dark red-brown due to variably well-digested blood. The abomasal rugae may be edematous because of hypoproteinemia, and petechiae or ecchymoses may be evident on the surface. In freshly dead animals, the worms will be visible to the observant by the naked eye (see Fig. 1-143B); with more advanced autolysis and dead worms, they are much less obvious and free in the lumen.

Microscopically, there is abomasitis with increased numbers of mucosal and submucosal lymphocytes, eosinophils, and mast cells. Leukocyte levels in the abomasal mucosa peak 5 days after infection, and then may decrease; however, mast cell numbers remain high. Sheep that are resistant to *H. contortus* may have more numerous mucosal mast cells. Centrilobular hepatic necrosis due to anemia can be present.

In clinically affected sheep and goats, usually 1,000-12,000 worms are found. The severity of the disease is a function of the number of worms and to some extent, the size of the

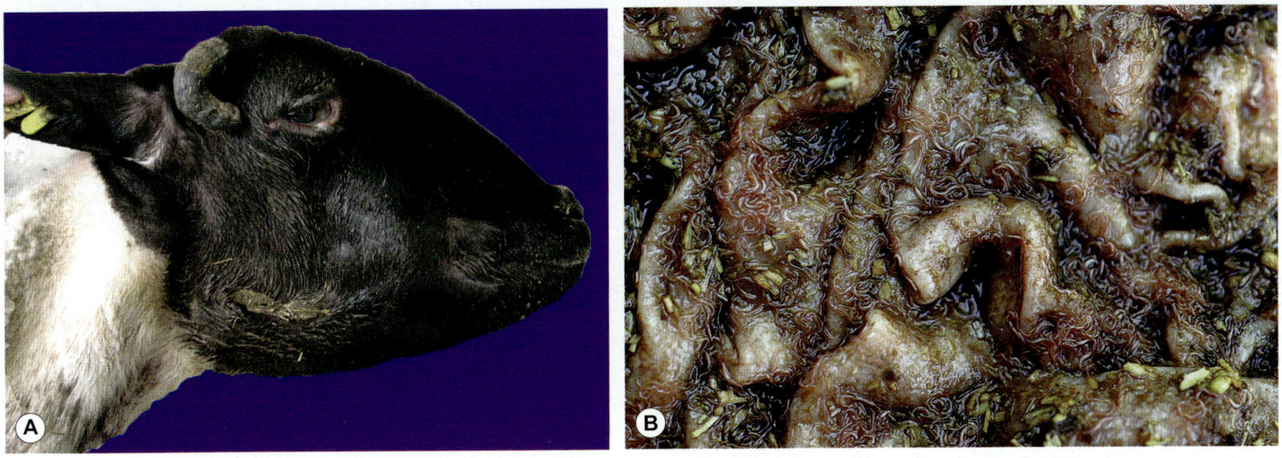

Figure 1-143 **Hemonchosis.** A. Severe submandibular edema (bottle-jaw) in a sheep. B. *Haemonchus contortus* organisms in abomasal content in a sheep. (Both courtesy V. Psychas.)

animal. In lambs, 2,000-3,000 worms are considered a heavy burden, whereas in adult sheep and goats, 8,000-10,000 are associated with fatal infection. A high egg count is usually found on fecal flotation because *Haemonchus* is a prolific egg-layer. However, in peracute prepatent infections, no eggs will be present in feces. In recently treated animals, no worms may be present, and the diagnosis may have to be presumptive. On the contrary, treated animals returned to contaminated pasture may succumb to reinfection within 2-3 weeks. A serologic test targeting a somatic antigen has been developed.

Trichostrongylus axei infects the *abomasum of cattle, sheep, and goats*, and the *stomach of horses*. It has a direct life cycle. Third-stage infective larvae enter tunnels in the epithelium of the foveolae and neck of gastric glands in both fundic and pyloric areas. The worms live throughout their life *partly embedded in intraepithelial tunnels* at about this level of the mucosa. They molt to the fourth stage about a week after being ingested and to the fifth stage by ~2 weeks after infection. The prepatent period is ~3 weeks in calves and sheep, and ~25 days in horses.

Infections with *T. axei* are usually part of a *mixed GI helminthosis*, mostly with *Ostertagia* spp. in ruminants. However, in all hosts this species alone is capable of inducing disease if present in sufficient numbers. In light infestations, there may be no changes visible in the abomasum other than congestion of the mucosa. The gross lesions present in heavy *T. axei* infections reflect the hypertrophy of glands, and superficial erosion. *Circular or irregularly raised white plaques or nodules of thickened infected mucosa* are present, often with a thick layer of mucus.

After a period of several weeks, *mucous metaplasia and hyperplasia are seen histologically in mucosal glands*. In severely affected animals, erosion of the mucosa develops accompanied by effusion of neutrophils, eosinophils, and tissue fluid. Fibroplasia may occur in the superficial propria in eroded areas.

Infection in horses is uncommon and is usually related to sharing pasture with sheep or cattle. In chronically infected horses, white raised plaques or nodules are present in the mucosa, covered by tenacious mucus and surrounded by a zone of congestion (Fig. 1-144). Mucosal lesions may be confluent in heavily infected animals, and erosions and superficial ulceration may be encountered. Infection may extend into the proximal duodenum, where polypoid masses of hypertrophic glandular mucosa are occasionally observed.

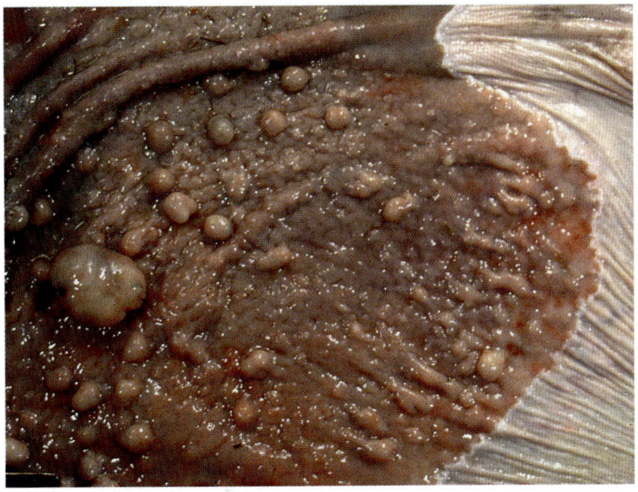

Figure 1-144 **Trichostrongylosis.** Hypertrophic gastritis in the glandular mucosa of a horse. (Courtesy P. Stromberg.)

Achlorhydria develops in heavily infected sheep and cattle associated with *diarrhea*, particularly in cattle. Dehydration may prove severe in scouring calves. Plasma pepsinogen and gastrin levels increase, and hypoproteinemia and *wasting* occur due likely to increased permeability and plasma protein loss into the GI tract.

Although *T. axei* is not commonly seen as a primary cause of disease in any species, it should be sought at autopsy of animals with signs of wasting and perhaps diarrhea. The typical gross lesions in the stomach are distinctive in horses. In ruminants, they must be differentiated from those caused by *Ostertagia*, with which animals may be infected intercurrently. The worms are very fine, and gastric washes or digestion are required to recover them quantitatively. The *distinctive intraepithelial location of T. axei* in section differentiates it from other nematodes inhabiting the abomasum of ruminants and the stomach of horses.

Gastric parasitism in horses. The most common parasites of the equine stomach are *larvae of botflies* of the genus ***Gasterophilus***, which are not helminths, but most convenient to consider here. There are 6 species of the genus, the most common ones being ***Gasterophilus intestinalis, G. nasalis***, and ***G. haemorrhoidalis***, and the uncommon ones being *G. pecorum*, *G. nigricornis*, and *G. inermis*. Flies deposit ova on hairs of the face, intermandibular region, or lower body and legs. The eggs hatch spontaneously or when stimulated by licking, then first-stage larvae penetrate the oral mucosa, molt, emerge, and migrate down the alimentary canal.

Gasterophilus intestinalis is the most common species, and in the stomach, it attaches to the squamous epithelium of the cardia to complete subsequent molts. ***G. nasalis*** are found frequently in the pyloric and duodenal epithelium; *G. pecorum* tends to congregate in the pharynx. Larvae leave the stomach and pass in the feces to pupate. Those of *G. pecorum* and *G. haemorrhoidalis* may attach themselves for a short while to the wall of the rectum. It is generally assumed that the larvae of *Gasterophilus* have little effect on their host, although they fasten themselves to the epithelium by chitinous oral hooks, bore into the mucosa (Fig. 1-145), and produce focal erosions and ulcerations that often exceed the number of larvae, suggesting that they move about on the mucosa. Lesions may also be found in the glandular and pyloric regions of the stomach. With time, ulcers extending into the submucosa may cause chronic inflammation, and the margins of ulcers in the squamous epithelium become hyperplastic.

The **spirurid nematodes *Draschia megastoma, Habronema majus***, and ***H. muscae*** are also parasitic in the stomach of horses. The adult worms are 1-2 cm long. *D. megastoma* burrows into the submucosa to produce large tumorlike nodules (Fig. 1-146); the latter 2 species are probably insignificant, although they may cause mild erosive gastritis. *Stomoxys calcitrans* is the intermediate host of *H. majus*; various muscid flies, including the common fly *Musca domestica*, are the intermediate hosts for *D. megastoma* and *H. muscae*. The *Habronema* larvae in the equid feces are swallowed by their intermediate host larvae and persist through pupation and maturation of the fly. They leave the host fly via the proboscis when it seeks moisture near mucous membranes. Larvae deposited on or in cutaneous wounds, or in the eye, invade the skin or conjunctiva and provoke an intense local reaction, which becomes granulomatous and densely infiltrated with eosinophils (see Vol. 1, Integumentary System). Occasionally, *Draschia* and *Habronema* larvae may be found in the brain or in the lungs where they may become encapsulated and mineralized.

In contrast, *D. megastoma* burrows into the submucosa of the gastric fundus, usually near the margo plicatus where they provoke granulomatous and eosinophilic nodular inflammatory reactions that may be up to ~5 cm in diameter, often with a small fistulous opening to the lumen (see Fig. 1-146). The nodules generally produce no clinical disturbance, although they may lead rarely to abscessation, adhesions of the stomach to the spleen, or gastric perforation if they become secondarily infected.

Gastric parasitism in swine is not of great clinical or pathologic importance and is rare in pigs reared in modern total confinement systems. *Ascaris suum* normally inhabits the small intestine but may migrate or reflux and be found in the stomach after death. *Hyostrongylus rubidus* is probably the most significant parasite of the stomach of swine; this and the various spirurids are more common in pigs allowed to forage. *Ollulanus tricuspis* is reported in pigs. It is more commonly encountered in cats and is discussed with gastric parasitism in dogs and cats.

H. rubidus is a trichostrongylid nematode with a typical life cycle. Third-stage larvae are thought to enter fundic glands in the stomach, where they develop and molt twice before emerging to the gastric surface ~18-20 days after ingestion as preadult and adult worms. The lesions produced by *Hyostrongylus* resemble those caused by *Ostertagia* in ruminants. There is ectasia, *mucous metaplasia, and hyperplasia of the epithelial lining of infected and neighboring glands*. The lamina propria is edematous and infiltrated by lymphocytes, plasma cells, and eosinophils, which transmigrate the epithelium into dilated glands. Lymphoid follicles develop deeper in the propria, and surface epithelial erosions may become prominent. In heavy infections, these proliferative epithelial and glandular nodules may become confluent and result in irregularly thickened convoluted mucosa, most notable in the fundus and along the lesser curvature of the stomach. Adult worms are red and threadlike and are difficult to see in the gastric mucus with the naked eye. Most infections do not result

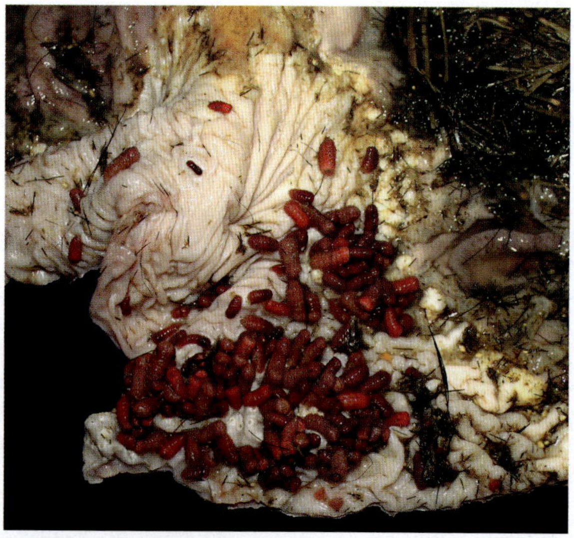

Figure 1-145 ***Gasterophilus* larvae** on the gastric mucosa of a horse. (Courtesy A. Barragán.)

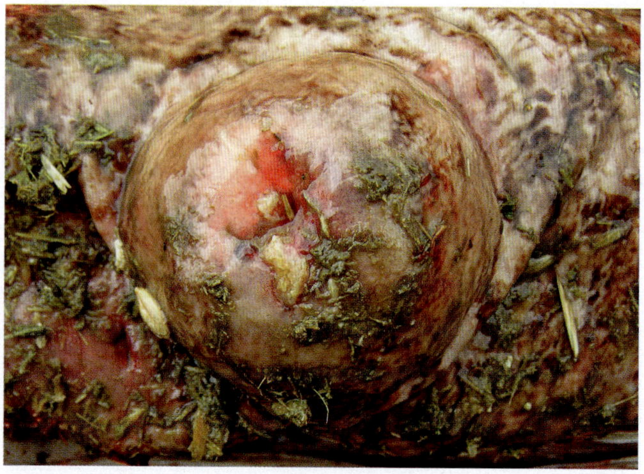

Figure 1-146 ***Draschia megastoma*–induced nodules** in the glandular region near margo plicatus of the stomach in a horse. (Courtesy L. Minatel.)

in clinical signs or loss of production, although loss of plasma protein, inappetence, diarrhea, and reduced weight gain and feed efficiency (so-called thin sow syndrome) has been documented in heavy *Hyostrongylus* infections.

Spirurid nematodes parasitizing the porcine stomach include *Physocephalus sexalatus, Ascarops strongylina, A. dentate,* and *Simondsia paradoxa. Physocephalus* and *Ascarops* use dung beetles as intermediate hosts. ***Ascarops*** and ***Physocephalus*** are common in many parts of the world in swine with access to grazing. Large numbers of parasites are required to cause ill-thrift. Nematodes in affected pigs may be free in the lumen or partly embedded in the mucosa, which may be congested and edematous, or eroded and ulcerated with fibrinous exudate on the surface. There may be chronic interstitial inflammation and fibrosis in the mucosa. ***Simondsia*** is found in swine in Europe, Asia, and Australia. The caudal portion of the female worm is globular and is embedded in palpable nodules up to 6-8 mm in diameter in the gastric mucosa. ***Gnathostoma doloresi*** causes gastric ulcers and granulomas in pigs in eastern Asia. *G. hispidum* may cause lesions in the liver, and submucosal nodules in the gastric wall of pigs, similar to those produced by *G. spinigerum* in carnivores.

Gastric parasitism in dogs and cats. Gastric parasites are uncommonly encountered in the stomach of dogs and cats at autopsy, and most are incidental findings, or postmortem migrants from the intestine.

***Gnathostoma spinigerum**, G. binucleatum, and G. procyonis* occur in the stomach of dogs and cats, and of a variety of nondomestic carnivores. It is more common in areas with warm climates. The life cycle of this spirurid nematode involves copepods as an aquatic invertebrate intermediate host, and a variety of fish, amphibian, or reptiles as second intermediate or paratenic hosts. Ingested third-stage larvae may migrate in the liver leaving tracks of necrotic debris and eventually fibrosis. In heavy infections, lesions associated with larval migration may be found elsewhere in the abdominal and pleural cavities, and in the skin. Adults are found in inflamed and fibrotic nodules up to ~5 cm in diameter that open into the gastric lumen through a pore that may also contain protruding nematodes. Infection with *Gnathostoma* is usually subclinical; however, illness and death may be associated with disturbance of motility, chronic vomition, and occasional rupture of verminous nodules on to the gastric serosa, leading to peritonitis.

Several ***Physaloptera***, spp., including *P. praeputialis* (cat), *P. rara* (dogs and wild canids and felids), and *P. canis* (dog), are found in the stomach of dogs and cats. These spirurid nematodes use arthropod intermediate hosts (grasshoppers, beetles, cockroaches) and probably some vertebrate transport hosts. The adult worms can be 1-6 cm long in dogs and 1-3 cm in cats (dependent on species) and may be mistaken for small ascarids. They are found free in the gastric lumen or more commonly attached as individuals or in small clusters to the gastric mucosa, which may result in the formation of small erosions and ulcers. These nematodes are not highly pathogenic, although even light worm burdens may cause chronic intermittent vomiting; higher worm burdens (>10 adults) have greater potential to cause vomiting, as well as delayed gastric emptying, and significant gastric mucosal damage.

Cylicospirura felineus and members of the genus **Cyathospirura** may be found in the stomachs of domestic and wild felids. *Cylicospirura* are usually found in the submucosal nodules, like those formed by *Gnathostoma; Cyathospirura* are usually found free in the lumen, or sometimes associated with *Cylicospirura* in gastric nodules. The life cycle is unknown; the pathogenicity of these species is poorly defined but is likely low.

Ollulanus tricuspis is a small trichostrongyle, ~1 mm long, which inhabits the stomach of cats and swine. It is viviparous, and third-stage larvae developing in the uterus of the female are transmitted in vomitus. As a result, infection is usually not detected by fecal examination, and infection with this species may go unnoticed. In some parts of the world, it is common, particularly in cat colonies and cats that roam. Clinical signs and gross lesions caused by *O. tricuspis* are uncommon. *Vomition, anorexia,* and *weight loss* are the signs most frequently associated with infection. The worms lie beneath the mucus on the surface of the stomach, or partly in gastric glands. Infection is associated with increased numbers of lymphoid follicles deep in the gastric mucosa, increased interstitial connective tissue in the mucosa, and numerous globule leukocytes in the gastric epithelium. Heavy infection results in mucous metaplasia and hyperplasia of gastric glands, causing the surface of the stomach to be thrown into thickened convoluted folds, grossly resembling idiopathic hypertrophic gastritis of dogs. Gastric glands are often separated by the heavy reactive fibrous stroma in the mucosa. In gastric biopsies, this suite of microscopic changes in the mucosa should be recognized as characteristic of *Ollulanus* infection, even if worms are not present. *Ollulanus* are characterized in section by the numerous longitudinal cuticular ridges (synlophe) recognized as projections on the surface of sectioned worms.

Helminthic diseases of the intestine

Strongyloides spp. (threadworms) parasitize all species of domestic animals considered here. Ruminants are infected by *S. papillosus*; horses by *S. westeri*; swine mainly by *S. ransomi*; dogs by *S. stercoralis*; and cats by *S. felis, S. planiceps* (= *S. catti*), and *S. stercoralis* in the small intestine, and by *S. tumefaciens* in the colon.

The parasitic worms are parthenogenetic females, which produce larvae capable of direct infection of the host, or of uniquely developing into a facultative free-living generation of males and females. Infection by free-living filariform third-stage larvae takes place by skin penetration, or to a lesser extent by ingestion and subsequent penetration of the GI mucosa. Larval migration occurs primarily through the nasofrontal region and the lungs, during which larvae are carried up the mucociliary escalator and swallowed before establishing as parasitic adults in the small intestine.

Strongyloides spp. larvae establish and persist within tunnels in the epithelium (but not beneath the basal lamina) at the base of villi or in upper crypts (Fig. 1-147) mostly in the proximal small intestine. Adult worms are 2-6 mm long, which varies by species. If present in sufficient numbers, they cause villus atrophy, crypt epithelium hyperplasia and immaturity, or erosion of the surface epithelium, and mixed eosinophilic-to-lymphocytic inflammation.

Strongyloides ransomi causes diarrhea in suckling piglets in some parts of the world. Heavy infestations result in moderate-to-severe clinical disease in young piglets; adult nematodes are evident in mucosal scrapings at autopsy, although specific gross lesions are usually absent. Larvae migrating through the lungs may cause minor hemorrhage, alveolar septal damage,

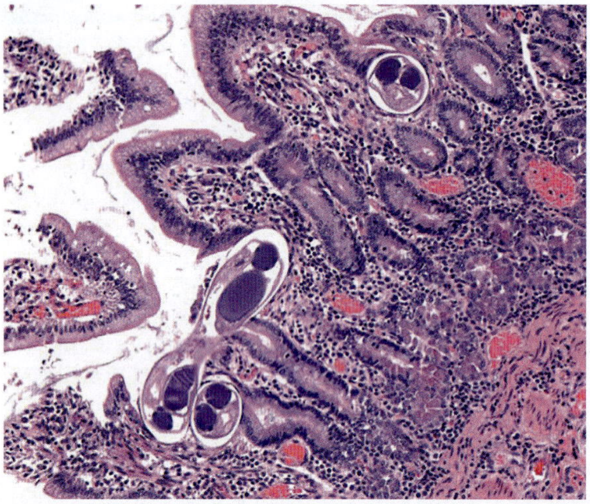

Figure 1-147 ***Strongyloides westeri*** in tunnels at the base of moderately atrophic villi in the intestine of a foal with diarrhea.

and scattered aggregates of lymphocytes and plasma cells. Duodenal villus atrophy results in malabsorption, luminal protein loss, diarrhea, and eventually debilitation of affected piglets.

Strongyloides westeri infects foals and is associated with diarrhea that can be fatal in heavily infected individuals. It has been hypothesized that skin penetration by third-stage larvae permits simultaneous entry of *Rhodococcus equi*, an important bacterial pathogen of foals; however, this remains unproven, and millions of larvae are necessary to cause fatal infections experimentally.

Strongyloides papillosus may cause diarrhea and occasionally death of suckling ruminants, although only if there is heavy parasitic burden. A syndrome of sudden death caused by cardiac failure associated with heavy infections of *S. papillosus* has been described; however, the pathogenesis remains unclear.

Strongyloides stercoralis primarily infects dogs, and autoinfection can result in development of several parasitic generations in the same host, which can result in rapid expansion of parasitic populations. Multiorgan involvement is described, but this probably only occurs with high parasite burdens in the face of severe immunosuppression. Infection is most commonly fatal in puppies up to 2-3-months-old from kennel environments. Affected dogs are dehydrated and emaciated with blood-tinged diarrhea, but the intestine may be grossly unremarkable. Histologically, there is villus atrophy and mononuclear interstitial infiltration in the duodenum of affected dogs. Adult nematodes are embedded within the superficial mucosa, and larvae may be observed in granulomas in the intestinal lamina propria and submucosa. Multifocal interstitial pneumonia may be due to pulmonary migration of larvae. *S. stercoralis* also infects humans, and there are rare reports of natural zoonotic transfer from dogs to humans; immunocompromised humans appear to be more susceptible.

Strongyloides felis may cause mild focal granulomatous or eosinophilic interstitial pneumonia in cats because of larval migration through the lung. There may be crypt hyperplasia due to worms in the small intestine, but diarrhea is uncommon. ***S. tumefaciens*** in cats has rarely been associated with chronic diarrhea. It differs from the other species discussed previously because it causes proliferation of colonic submucosal glands and results in parasitic nodules.

Intestinal trichostrongylosis is caused by various members of the genus ***Trichostrongylus*** that parasitize the proximal small intestine of ruminants worldwide. They cause significant subclinical inefficiency in production, or diarrhea, ill-thrift, and in some cases, death. The most important species infecting sheep and goats are ***Trichostrongylus colubriformis, T. vitrinus***, and ***T. rugatus***; others include *T. longispicularis, T. falculatus, T. capricola, and T. probolurus. T. colubriformis and T. longispicularis* also parasitize cattle. Although some *T. axei* may be found in the duodenum of cattle and sheep, this species is primarily parasitic in the abomasum. The lesions and pathogenesis of disease caused by *Trichostrongylus* spp. are probably similar, although some evidence suggests that *T. vitrinus* is more pathogenic than *T. colubriformis* and *T. rugatus*.

Trichostrongylosis is most important in zones with a cool climate at some time of the year, but without extreme winters; it is a significant problem in sheep-grazing areas of New Zealand, Australia, South Africa, South America, and the United Kingdom. The life cycle is direct; ingested third-stage larvae exsheath in the acidic abomasal environment and establish preferentially in the proximal small intestine of sheep. A small proportion of the population colonizes the abomasal antral mucosa near the pylorus. The larvae enter tunnels in the superficial intestinal mucosa above the basal lamina at the base of villi, and they persist throughout their life at least partially embedded in the epithelium. Larvae develop over 2 weeks into adults with a prepatent period of 16-18 days.

The disease is marked clinically by variable depression, inappetence, diarrhea, and wasting; wool and muscle growth can be hindered, and secondary osteoporosis has been described. *Gross lesions* observed in animals with severe infections are nonspecific and may include cachexia, dehydration, dark-green diarrhea, serous atrophy of internal fat depots, and atrophy of skeletal muscle. Hypoproteinemia results in mesenteric edema and serous effusion into body cavities. Mesenteric lymph nodes are enlarged, intestines are flaccid and contain thin watery green foul-smelling feces. The proximal third of the small intestine usually contains the parasites, and a worm count in the small bowel may reveal 15,000-80,000 adults in severe clinical infections; subclinical or mild disease is associated with fewer worms.

The severity of *histologic lesions* within an individual animal is correlated with the local density of worms: changes include villus atrophy, crypt hyperplasia, goblet cell hyperplasia, and proprial inflammation with variable infiltration of lymphocytes, plasma cells, eosinophils, and globule leukocytes. The diagnosis is based on recovery of substantial populations of *Trichostrongylus* spp. in association with the clinicopathologic syndrome. Mixed infections with other parasitic genera are common.

Nematodirus spp. infect the proximal third of the small intestine of ruminants. The most important species are *N. helvetianus*, which infects cattle; *N. spathiger, N. filicollis*, and *N. abnormalis*, which infect sheep, goats, and cattle; and *N. battus*, a parasite mainly of sheep, which also causes disease in calves.

The life cycle is direct, although infective larvae within eggs of *N. battus* and *N. filicollis* require a period of conditioning by cold (overwintering) before hatching. The epidemiologic pattern is thus one of infection of susceptible lambs by larvae produced by the previous year's lambs, which has led to devastating outbreaks of spring disease in mostly temperate areas of the world. Larvae of *N. spathiger* and *N. helvetianus* are not delayed in hatching, and their epidemiologic pattern resembles that of *Trichostrongylus* spp. in grazing animals. *Nematodirus* spp. often form part of a mixed population of worms in parasitic gastroenteritis of grazing lambs and calves, although the disease may also occur in confined nonpastured calves. Ingested infective third-stage larvae enter the deeper layers of the mucosa and intestinal crypts, then emerge at the fourth or fifth stage to reside coiled among the villi with their caudal ends protruding toward the lumen; they do not normally penetrate the epithelium.

Lambs and calves with nematodirosis develop severe dark-green diarrhea, dehydration, anorexia, wasting, and cachexia that may persist for several weeks before recovering, or they may die acutely. Disease is presumably related to malabsorption and loss of appetite. Gross lesions at autopsy are nonspecific and limited to watery mucoid intestinal contents. Clinical disease is associated with populations of 10,000-50,000 or more *Nematodirus* adults.

Histologic lesions of villus atrophy, crypt hyperplasia, and mixed inflammation in the intestine are observed in heavy infections but are usually mild compared with those induced by *Strongyloides* or *Trichostrongylus*.

***Cooperia* spp.** infect the upper small intestine of ruminants. The important species include *C. curticei*, mainly in sheep and goats, and *C. pectinata*, *C. punctata*, and *C. oncophora*, mainly in cattle. The latter is regarded as the least pathogenic of the three. Although both sheep and cattle may host mixed burdens of helminths containing or dominated by populations of *Cooperia* spp., this parasite seems to be more significant in cattle, especially in cool temperate regions.

Cooperia spp. have a typical trichostrongylid life cycle, but larvae have the capacity to undergo hypobiosis to carry the population through periods of climatic adversity. The normal prepatent period is 16-20 days. Like *Nematodirus* spp., *Cooperia* spp. do not tunnel beneath the epithelium, but rather brace or coil themselves at the base of villi to maintain their place in the intestine. In light infections, the worms are concentrated in the proximal third of the small intestine, although in heavier infections parasites are more evenly distributed along the intestine.

Heavy burdens of *Cooperia* spp. in calves of >70,000-80,000 nematodes may be associated with inappetence, reduced weight gain, or weight loss and diarrhea, with PLE. Villus atrophy and inflammation are variable, and the diagnosis is confirmed by finding large numbers of the coiled *Cooperia* spp. adults among small intestinal villi.

Hookworm infections are caused by members of the family *Ancylostomatidae*, which infect **dogs, cats, ruminants**, and **swine**. Hookworms of the genus *Globocephalus* appear to be of little significance in swine. In dogs, ***Ancylostoma caninum***, ***A. braziliense***, and ***A. ceylanicum*** occur. The former is most common in tropical, subtropical, and warm temperate zones of Africa, Australia, Asia, and North America, where adequate humidity for larval development occurs. *A. braziliense* occurs in dogs and cats in the tropics and subtropics; *A. ceylanicum* is found in both species in Sri Lanka and Southeast Asia. ***Uncinaria stenocephala*** occurs in dogs in cool temperate regions of Europe and North America. ***A. tubaeforme*** only occurs in the cat.

Ancylostoma spp. are capable of infecting the host by 4 routes: 1) orally, with direct development to adult worms in the intestine; 2) by skin penetration, resulting in movement through the bloodstream to the lungs and then by tracheal migration to the pharynx and the intestine; 3) by the lactogenic transmission of third-stage larvae mobilized from dormancy in the skeletal muscle of parturient female dogs; and 4) occasionally by prenatal transplacental transmission of mobilized larvae. The latter route of transmission does not apparently occur in *A. braziliense* infection. Some larvae of *A. caninum* may become arrested at the third stage in the intestine, to resume development at a later time.

Ancylostomosis is the result of *persistent blood loss, anemia, and hypoproteinemia* in affected individuals. *Ancylostoma* spp. usually inhabit the small intestine, where they move about the surface and intermittently attach several times a day to feed. They penetrate deeply into the mucosa, sometimes to the muscularis mucosa, as they take a plug of host tissue into their large buccal capsule. Host tissue is lacerated by large teeth, and parasite-produced anticoagulant is released locally, which permits persistent blood flow. Blood loss is maximal while worms are attaining maturity 12-16 days after infection, and then again during the peak period of egg production after 3-4 weeks of infection. The prepatent period for *A. caninum* is ~15 days.

There is considerable variation in the blood-sucking activity, and therefore the pathogenicity, of members of the genus. *A. caninum* consumes 0.01-0.2 mL of blood per worm per day, which in young puppies and kittens can represent a significant percentage of their blood volume. Anemia in ancylostomosis is at first normochromic and normocytic; however, suckling pups with ancylostomosis are susceptible to rapid development of microcytic hypochromic anemia because of their poor iron reserves and the low iron levels in the dam's milk.

Acute fatal ancylostomosis occurs most commonly in 2-3-week-old pups infected via the lactogenic route. Heavy infections acquired by this route may result in death from acute anemia and hypoproteinemia before eggs are present in the feces. Chronic anemia may also lead to mortality of pups after a longer course. Percutaneous infection occurs in older dogs housed in suboptimal conditions in which moisture and temperature are conducive to larval development. Dermatitis caused by larval penetration may be observed between the toes or on ventral contact surfaces of the body. Ancylostomosis in older dogs usually causes anemia, exercise intolerance, weakness, and emaciation. Watery feces may contain mucus or blood; however, the major effect of ancylostomosis is due to increased loss of erythrocytes, iron, and plasma protein.

Animals that succumb to ancylostomosis are extremely pale, and often have edema of subcutaneous tissue and mesentery, as well as serous effusion into body cavities attributable to hypoproteinemia. If recent exposure to heavy percutaneous infection has occurred, there may be dermatitis, and multifocal hemorrhages throughout the pulmonary parenchyma because of larval migration. The intestinal mucosa is often diffusely red or has pinpoint red foci where adults have fed. Adults are 1-1.5 cm long, translucent, and gray or red depending on when they last consumed blood and dispersed over the mucosa of the small intestine and less commonly into the large intestine. In a young pup, as few as 50-100 worms may cause fatal infection, and they may be easily overlooked.

Uncinaria stenocephala mainly infects by the oral route, and percutaneous infection is inefficient, although dermatitis may occur; prenatal and lactogenic transmission appear not to occur. This species sucks little blood and is less pathogenic than *A. caninum*; however, heavy infections with this species (burdens of >1,000 adults) may cause clinical disease and occasional mortality in pups due to protein loss and malabsorption. Nonspecific signs of infection include lethargy, inappetence, and ill-thrift and perhaps diarrhea; hypoproteinemia may be observed, but anemia does not occur. The lesions are similar to those of ancylostomosis. The intestinal mucosa may appear grossly thickened with hemorrhage at sites of attachment. Histologic lesions may include moderate villus atrophy, crypt hyperplasia, irregularity and immaturity of surface epithelial cells, and mild aggregates of inflammatory cells secondary to the damage induced by deep attachment of adult worms.

All of these hookworms are zoonotic. In humans, *A. braziliense* is most commonly associated with cutaneous larva migrans; other hookworm species larvae less commonly cause eosinophilic pneumonitis, myositis, or ocular lesions. *A. caninum* has been shown to mature to adulthood and cause eosinophilic enteritis in humans.

The hookworms of **ruminants** include the following: in cattle, *Bunostomum phlebotomum*, and in India and Indonesia, *Agriostomum vryburgi*; in sheep, *B. trigonocephalum*, and in India and Southeast Asia, Africa, and South America, *Gaigeria pachyscelis*. The life cycle of these nematodes is typical of hookworms. *Bunostomum* spp. third-stage larvae infect by the oral or percutaneous routes; *Gaigeria* spp. only infect by the percutaneous route. Eggs and larval stages on the ground are extremely susceptible to desiccation, so hookworm disease in ruminants is most common in tropical or subtropical areas during wet seasons. Stabled animals in cooler temperate areas may be affected by larvae invading the skin from contaminated bedding. The prepatent periods are 7-8 weeks and 10 weeks for *Bunostomum* spp. and *Gaigeria* spp., respectively.

Both *Bunostomum* spp. and *Gaigeria* spp. cause *anemia and hypoproteinemia*, especially in animals <1-year-old. These species often occur with mixed GI helminth burdens, and their effects are at least additive to those of the other worms. As few as 20-30 *Gaigeria* spp. will cause anemia and hypoproteinemia in lambs and kids, although several times that the number are necessary to cause severe disease and death. The size of the animal, iron reserves, plane of nutrition, especially the level of protein, all influence the pathogenicity of these species.

Gross lesions are nonspecific, secondary to anemia and hypoproteinemia. *Bunostomum* spp. are often found in the distal half of the small intestine; *Gaigeria* spp. tend to be concentrated in the duodenum. Hemorrhage at attachment sites may be evident on the epithelial surface in the infected areas of intestine. Given that relatively low numbers of worms can cause disease, and their unique distribution, careful and thorough evaluation is needed in suspect cases.

Oesophagostomum and *Chabertia* infection

Oesophagostomum **infection** occurs in **sheep**, **cattle**, and **swine** and is caused by members of the genus *Oesophagostomum*. Two species in sheep, ***O. columbianum*** and ***O. venulosum***, are most significant; the former is considerably more pathogenic and is particularly important in warm temperate-to-tropical areas. After ingestion, infective third-stage larvae penetrate the intestinal wall and encyst deep in the mucosa, inciting the formation of inflammatory nodules in the wall of the intestine. After ~1 week, they molt, emerge, and mature into adults in the colon, and a proportion of fourth-stage larvae encyst within nodules in the colonic submucosa. Adult worms in the colon may be pathogenic for lambs, and burdens of only a few hundred *O. columbianum* are associated with anorexia, mucoid feces or diarrhea, and ill-thrift.

Gross lesions associated with clinical oesophagostomosis are nonspecific and include emaciation, enlarged mesenteric lymph nodes, and thickened and congested colonic mucosa in which adult worms may be observed within the mucus layer. Histologic changes include hyperplasia of goblet cells, and variable mixed inflammation of the lamina propria, with many eosinophils and prominent intraepithelial globule leukocytes. Colonic nodules housing fourth-stage larva are the reason for the common name (pimply gut) and are composed of a central necrotic or mineralized core and remnants or fragments of the larva surrounded by eosinophils, giant cells, macrophages, and fibrous connective tissue. Similar nodules may be found in the liver, lungs, mesentery, and mesenteric lymph nodes. They may cause adhesion to adjacent abdominal viscera, intussusception, or peritonitis; however, most nodules are incidental. *O. venulosum* is a much less significant parasite and may cause small nodules in the cecum and colon.

Two species occur in **cattle**, ***Oesophagostomum radiatum*** and ***O. venulosum***, and the former is the most significant. The life cycle is similar to that of *O. columbianum*. Clinical disease caused by *O. radiatum* includes loss of appetite, reduced productive efficiency, anemia, hypoproteinemia, and possibly diarrhea; these occur mostly due to hemorrhage at sites of mucosal damage from either larval emergence or adult worms. The range of 1,000-10,000 adult *O. radiatum* is probably required to cause disease in calves. Nonspecific gross lesions include pallor, edema, and cachexia attributable to anemia and hypoproteinemia. Colonic lymph nodes are enlarged, and the colonic mucosa is grossly thickened and folded because of edema and mixed inflammation in the lamina propria; repeated exposure to infective larvae may result in the accumulation of large numbers of fourth-stage larvae within inflammatory nodules in the colon, but this has little pathogenic significance in cattle.

In **swine**, several species occur in the large intestine; however, *Oesophagostomum dentatum* and *O. quadrispinulatum* are most widespread. Oesophagostomosis in swine is usually a mild subclinical disease with occasional diarrhea, reduced weight gain, and inefficiency of feed conversion, especially during the period of emergence of larvae and maturation of adult parasites in the lumen of the large intestine. Adult nematodes are 1-2 cm long, white, and are present in mucus along the intestinal surface. The life cycle, gross and histologic lesions are typical of the genus. Lesions resolve following the emergence of larvae.

Chabertia ovina is a robust 1-2 cm long worm that inhabits the colon of sheep, goats, and cattle. It is mainly a problem for sheep in cooler climatic zones. Phylogenetic analysis based on ribosomal DNA sequence data indicates that *C. ovina* is clustered within the subfamily *Oesophagostominae*. The life cycle of *Chabertia* spp. resembles that of *Oesophagostomum* spp.; third-stage larvae encyst in the wall of the small intestine, then emerge to mature in the cecum and colon. Adults penetrate deeply to the muscularis mucosa, so hemorrhage is related to physical trauma to the mucosa, and hemorrhage and significant loss of plasma protein occur at numerous attachment sites. Disease in sheep is associated with mature adults in the colon, and nonspecific clinical signs include ill-thrift and soft feces with mucus and blood. Grossly, the lesions include edema of all layers of the colonic wall, enlargement of colonic lymph nodes, and hemorrhagic foci at attachment sites of adult nematodes in the proximal spiral colon. Pathogenic burdens may be as few as 150 adults. Histologic changes are nonspecific and consist of widespread mononuclear infiltration in the mucosa and submucosa and hyperplasia of goblet cells.

Equine strongylosis is caused by members of the family *Strongylidae*, which are common nematode parasites of the cecum and colon in horses, and are usually present as mixed infections. The subfamily *Strongylinae*, or **large strongyles**, includes the important genus ***Strongylus*** and the less significant genera *Triodontophorus*, *Oesophagodontus*, and *Craterostomum*. Members of this group are plug feeders or blood suckers, and *Strongylus* spp. undergo extensive extraintestinal migrations. In sufficient numbers, adult large strongyles may cause ill-thrift and anemia as the result of active erythrophagia and blood loss from sites of recent feeding activity. The subfamily *Cyathostominae*, or **small strongyles**, includes 8 genera of nematodes. Adults of this group feed mainly on intestinal contents and are of little pathogenic significance; however, simultaneous emergence of large numbers of larvae from the gut wall may cause disease.

Strongylus vulgaris is the best-known large strongyle and is relatively common; it is widely considered to be the most significant nematode parasite in horses; however, infection levels have considerably decreased with the advent and widespread use of highly efficacious anthelmintics. Larval forms cause endoarteritis in the mesenteric circulation, resulting in arterial infarction of the large bowel and colic; the adults cause anemia and ill-thrift. Infective third-stage larvae are ingested from pasture and exsheath in the small intestine to penetrate the intestinal mucosa and molt to the fourth stage. They enter small arterioles, where they migrate along the endothelium to reach the cranial mesenteric artery within 3 weeks. Following a 3-4-month maturation period, immature adults or fifth-stage larvae return to the wall of the cecum or colon via the arterial lumen, where they encapsulate in the subserosa forming 5-8 mm nodules. The nodules eventually rupture into the lumen of the large bowel, especially the cecum and right ventral colon, where the parasites mature in another 1-2 months, ~6-7 months after initial infection. Some larvae may become aberrantly trapped and encapsulated in mesenteric arterioles prior to reaching the large intestine and remain there to die eventually.

Syndromes associated with aberrant migration include cerebrospinal nematodiasis and aortic-iliac thrombosis. Lesions of the cranial mesenteric, cecal, and colic arteries may lead to colic due to reduced perfusion and thromboembolism, or perhaps owing to impingement upon autonomic ganglia in the vicinity of the arterial root at the aorta. Although many older horses are infected with adult worms or have arterial lesions, the complications of colic and infarction caused by this parasite are most common in young horses. An acute syndrome of pyrexia, anorexia, depression and weight loss, diarrhea or constipation, colic, and infarction of intestine occurs in foals infected with large numbers of larvae; this is not often observed in animals previously exposed to infection.

Strongylus edentatus now rarely causes infection. Its life cycle includes extensive larval migration. Third-stage larvae enter the intestinal wall and pass in the portal system to the liver, where they incite inflammatory foci. Here they molt to the fourth stage and, ~30 days after infection, begin migrating through the hepatic parenchyma. Inflammatory reaction in the liver consists of necrotic debris, eosinophils, neutrophils, and mononuclear cells with variable amounts of fibrous connective tissue and hemorrhage. By 8-10 weeks after infection, larvae migrate from the liver via the hepatic ligaments. Parenchymal scars and tags of fibrous tissue on the hepatic capsule, especially the diaphragmatic surface, are commonly found during postmortem examination of horses, and are thought to be a legacy of migrating *S. edentatus*; however, the prevalence of these lesions has not decreased along with the reduction in incidence of infection, and definitive association of these lesions with migrating large strongyles has not been established. Larvae may be encountered in the retroperitoneal tissue, often associated with local hemorrhage, or they can be observed in aberrant locations, including the omentum, hepatic ligaments, and diaphragm, where they induce the formation of eosinophilic granulomas. Omental adhesions also may be a sequel to aberrant larval migration. In the flank, larvae persist for several months, molting to the fifth stage before returning from the right flank via the cecal ligament to the cecum and colon. Here they form nodules and edematous or hemorrhagic plaques in the intestinal wall, eventually perforate to the lumen, where they mature and begin to lay eggs ~10-12 months after infection. Lesions associated with the larval migration of *S. edentatus* are usually incidental findings at autopsy.

Strongylus equinus is very rare today. Exsheathed third-stage larvae penetrate to the deeper layers of the wall of the ileum, cecum, and colon, molt to the fourth stage, and produce hemorrhagic subserosal nodules, before moving to the liver through the peritoneal cavity. They migrate in the hepatic parenchyma for 6-7 weeks, then leave the liver, probably via the hepatic ligaments, to the pancreas and peritoneal cavity, where they molt to the fifth stage ~4 months after infection. They regain the lumen of the cecum and right ventral colon by an unknown route, probably by direct penetration from the peritoneal cavity or pancreas. Pancreatic damage is usually mild and is mainly manifested by slight periductal infiltration of eosinophils.

Hemomelasma ilei is the term applied to slightly elevated subserosal hemorrhagic plaques, up to 1-2 × 3-4 cm, usually found along the antimesenteric border of the distal small intestine, or rarely on the large bowel (Fig. 1-148). The lesion is considered incidental and has long been associated with trauma by migrating larvae of *S. edentatus* in particular, but may be caused by larvae of any of the *Strongylus* spp. As with

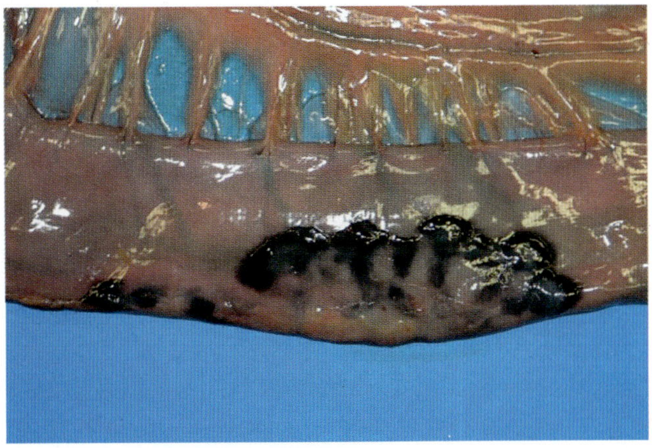

Figure 1-148 Hemomelasma ilei. Large subserosal plaques of resolving hemorrhage on the small intestine of a horse.

the hepatic lesions historically associated with migration of large strongyles, the incidence of hemomelasma ilei has not apparently declined with the reduction in incidence of large strongyle infections over the last 25 years. Histologic changes are edema, hemorrhage, a mixed population of leukocytes and variably mature fibrous tissue; depending on the stage of the lesions, erythrophagocytosis by macrophages can be prominent.

Triodontophorus spp. are also large strongyles found in horses and appear to be less pathogenic than *Strongylus* spp. The most important species is *Triodontophorus tenuicollis*, which can be associated with significant blood loss; these parasites attach to the mucosa of the colon in clusters, causing local congestion and ulceration.

The **small strongyles**, or **cyathostomins (cyathostomes)**, are a group of >50 distinct species; these parasites are highly prevalent worldwide. They are essentially nonpathogenic as adults despite the fact that tens or many hundreds of thousands may be in the content of the large bowel. Cyathostominosis is a disease mostly of horses >1-year-old, and little resistance is apparent to repeated infection.

The clinical syndrome *larval cyathostominosis* occurs because of simultaneous emergence of inhibited third-stage larvae from the intestinal mucosa and is a significant cause of morbidity and mortality in horses. The cyathostomins have a direct life cycle, and infective third-stage larval cyathostomins are ingested, migrate into the deep mucosa or submucosa of the cecum and large colon to encyst and molt before emerging to the lumen to molt again and mature into adults. Encysted third- or fourth-stage larvae may undergo hypobiosis or developmental inhibition to persist in nodules in the colonic wall for as long as 2 years. The timing during which inhibition occurs is dependent on the climate: inhibition occurs during cooler months of the year in temperate climates, and during the hot summer in tropical climates. The most devastating damage occurs when large numbers of encysted inhibited larvae emerge en masse to continue their development in the intestinal lumen. This occurs in the late winter, spring, and early summer in northern temperate climates. Development of widespread anthelmintic resistance by cyathostomins, particularly encysted larval stages, is well documented.

Affected horses may be of any age; clinical signs are nonspecific and include diarrhea, edema, anorexia, and weight loss. Mucosal nodules formed by encysted larvae are evident grossly, and usually only a few millimeters in diameter, slightly raised red or black (Fig. 1-149A); visualization of the nodules and the accompanying encysted larvae is enhanced by transillumination of the intestine. With severe infections, there will be edema and congestion of the mucosa and submucosa. Histologic lesions include variable mixed inflammation centered on still-encysted larvae in the submucosa or more diffusely throughout the lamina propria (see Fig. 1-149B).

Ascarid infections are caused by various members of the family *Ascarididae* and are common; ascarids are important parasites of swine, horses, dogs, cats, water buffalo, and to a lesser extent, cattle. They do not normally occur in sheep and goats. Their importance is related to incidental and sometimes significant lesions caused by larval migration in the tissues of definitive and accidental hosts, and to the effects of adult worms in the small intestine of the definitive host.

Ascaris suum is a large parasite usually found in the upper half of the small intestine of swine; females are up to 40 cm long. The life cycle is direct, with a prepatent period of ~8 weeks. Following ingestion, eggs hatch and release third-stage larvae in the intestine. The larvae penetrate the cecal or colonic mucosa to be carried in the portal blood to the liver, then pass to the lungs, where they break out of capillaries into alveoli, as early as 3-5 days after infection. Larvae move up the respiratory tree to the pharynx, where they are swallowed, and arrive in the intestine to mature. After returning to the intestine, most larvae gradually move to the distal small intestine and are expelled 14-21 days postinfection, a phenomenon likely mediated by parasite-specific immunoglobulin A–producing plasma cells, eosinophils, and intraepithelial T lymphocytes. The pathogenicity of adult ascarids in the intestine is poorly defined. Heavy infections may be evident within the intestinal lumen and can potentially result in obstruction or rare perforation (Fig. 1-150). In young swine, ~80-100 worms may depress feed intake and the efficiency of feed conversion; however, most pigs harboring patent infections are clinically normal. *Ascaris lumbricoides* in humans interferes with carbohydrate, fat, and protein absorption, and *A. suum* probably has a similar influence.

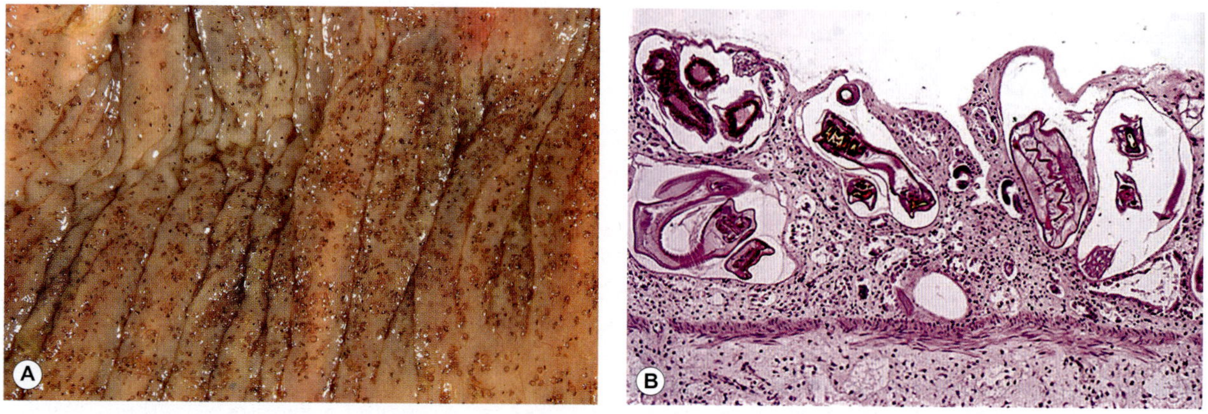

Figure 1-149 Equine cyathostominosis. **A.** Colonic mucosa studded with 2-5 mm nodules formed by larval cyathostomins. (Courtesy R. Foster.) **B.** Encysted larvae in the lamina propria surrounded by mixed inflammatory infiltrate. (Courtesy A. Peregrine.)

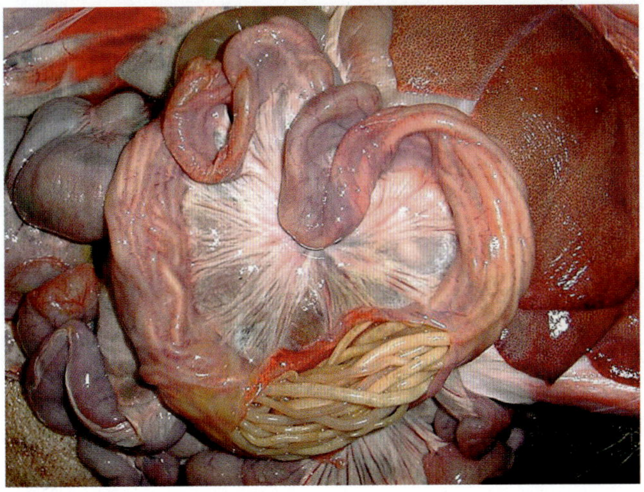

Figure 1-150 **Ascarid** infection. A heavy burden of *Ascaris suum* impacted in and obstructing the small intestine in a pig. (Courtesy A. Peregrine.)

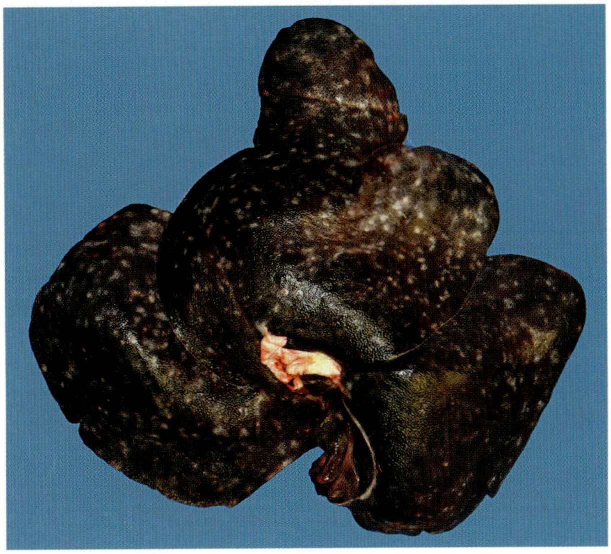

Figure 1-151 **Ascarid** infection. Effects of migrating *Ascaris suum* larvae in a pig include multifocal hepatitis and scarring in the liver (milk-spot liver.)

Larval migration induces lesions in the liver and lungs (Fig. 1-151); dyspnea (commonly referred to as thumps) may occur in piglets if large numbers of larvae migrate through the lungs. Gross lesions in pigs associated with pulmonary migration of ascarids are largely limited to numerous focal hemorrhages scattered over and through the pulmonary parenchyma. Migrating *A. suum* in the liver do not cause clinical disease but can result in considerable economic loss from liver condemnation at slaughter inspection. The lesions are related to mechanical damage caused by migrating nematodes, subsequent repair, and hypersensitivity reactions to excretory and secretory products of the larvae. Hemorrhagic tracks are initially present near portal areas and throughout lobules and are visible through pinpoint slightly depressed red to pale areas, that progress to fibrosis and scarring of portal tracts.

Microscopically in the lung there is eosinophilic bronchiolitis, with bronchiolar epithelial hyperplasia and dysplasia, and possibly eosinophilic or histiocytic vasculitis. Larvae or their remnants are usually present in the lung, and may be present in alveoli, alveolar ducts, bronchioles, or bronchi, perhaps surrounded by eosinophils. In more chronic cases, larvae are within eosinophilic granulomas. Like all larval ascarids of mammals, *A. suum* have cuticular ridges known as lateral alae visible in section. In the liver there is eosinophilic inflammation and fibrosis of portal tracts, which becomes most obvious beginning ~10-14 days after infection. Inflammatory foci containing giant cells, macrophages, and eosinophils may center on trapped larval nematode remnants. Hepatic inflammation in animals exposed to larval ascarids may become severe and generalized; this is reflected in the gross appearance of the liver, which usually has prominent definition of lobules and extensive white "milk spots." Where pigs are raised intensively, it is now rare to encounter extreme fibrosis of the liver associated with ascarid migration.

A. suum also infects animals other than swine. In sheep, and occasionally cattle, immature ascarids may be found in the intestine. Dyspnea and coughing associated with eosinophilic pneumonia, and focal eosinophilic hepatitis, may occur in lambs exposed to *A. suis*; mortality rarely occurs. Liver lesions in lambs are usually too small to be significant at slaughter inspection.

The nematode of cattle (*Toxocara vitulorum*) rarely causes clinical disease in cattle, but calves can be sporadic and aberrant hosts for various ascarids, when exposed to feces contaminated with eggs (*A. suum*, *T. vitulorum*, *Ascaris* spp.), and as larva mature and migrate through the lung. Signs of dyspnea, tachypnea, coughing, and increased expiratory effort are usually first seen ~7-10 days after exposure when large numbers of larvae are present in the lungs. The lungs can have variably severe gross lesions, but are usually moderately consolidated with alveolar, interstitial, and interlobular emphysema and edema. Microscopically, there is thickening of alveolar septa, and effusion of fibrin, hemorrhage, proteinaceous edema fluid, and macrophages into alveolar spaces. Larvae are present in alveoli and bronchioles and provoke acute neutrophilic-to-eosinophilic bronchiolitis. In addition to being usually observed readily in tissue sections, larvae may be recovered from the airways by washing with saline, or from minced lung in saline or digestion fluid, by use of the Baermann apparatus. Molecular techniques have been used to definitively identify the specific nematode.

Parascaris equorum is the ascarid of horses and is widespread and common in young horses. It may contribute to ill-thrift and occasionally causes death by intestinal obstruction by many adults. *P. equorum* is a large nematode; the females are up to 50 cm long. The life cycle resembles that of *A. suum*, although the prepatent period is slightly longer, ~10-15 weeks. Hepatic and pulmonary lesions are associated with larval migration, and coughing may occur at the time larvae are in the lungs, particularly if infections are heavy. The lesions in the lungs of foals with migrating *P. equorum* larvae 2 weeks after infection are similar to those described in swine with *A. suum*. It is possible to establish heavy infections of *P. equorum* in the intestine of foals a few months old, but not in yearlings because larvae appear to be killed during hepatopulmonary migration. In heavily infected foals, many worms are lost from the intestine before patency, suggesting an effect of crowding on the population of maturing adult nematodes. A heavy burden of intestinal ascarids may reduce weight gain and lead to inappetence and decreased protein intake in growing foals.

Ascarid infection reduces intestinal transit rate, and heavy burdens can cause luminal obstruction, intussusception or, rarely, perforation of the intestine.

Ascarids of small animals. ***Toxascaris leonina, Toxocara canis***, and ***Toxocara cati*** are the ascarids of small animals and affect both cats and dogs, dog only, and cat only, respectively. All occur in the *small intestine*, mainly in young animals.

Toxascaris leonina has a life cycle that may be direct but can involve a paratenic host. In the definitive host, larvae ingested in infective ova enter the wall of the intestine, where they remain for several weeks, molting to the fourth stage and emerging to the intestinal lumen to molt again and mature. The prepatent period is 10-11 weeks; clinical disease attributed to *T. leonina* is rare.

Toxocara canis has a complex life cycle, and dogs can be infected by ingestion of embryonated eggs from the environment, by ingestion of larvae from paratenic hosts including rodents and rabbits, or by vertical transmission including either intrauterine or transmammary routes. After ingestion of embryonated ova, larvae penetrate the intestinal mucosa, and migrate via the liver to arrive in the lungs 24-36 hours postinfection. From the lung, larvae follow 1 of 2 pathways. Depending on the age and immune status of the host, larvae may penetrate alveoli, and migrate via bronchioles and trachea, where they are swallowed and mature into adults in the intestine. Alternatively, larvae penetrate alveoli but are distributed by the circulatory system throughout the body where they encyst (larva migrans), rather than undergoing development and tracheal migration; this is more common in older animals. Most migrating larvae end up in the kidneys, skeletal muscle, liver, and CNS. Probably the most important route in young dogs is transplacental transmission, which occurs in the pregnant dam when encysted larvae in tissues are mobilized and cross the placenta to infect the fetus after day 42 of gestation, where they remain in the fetal liver until they pass into the lungs within 2-3 days following birth. Mobilized larvae may also result in transmammary transmission.

In some abnormal hosts, including humans, the syndrome *visceral larva migrans* is caused by ingestion of embryonated *T. canis* or *T. cati* eggs from soil or infective larvae from undercooked meat. Various pathologic and clinical sequelae are associated with this syndrome, and the outcome depends on the tissue involved (eye, liver, lungs, CNS), the number of larvae migrating, and the age of the host.

Baylisascaris procyonis is the raccoon roundworm, which is known for the ability of its larvae to cause visceral larva migrans in many accidental or "dead-end" hosts, including humans who ingest eggs or infective larvae. Dogs can serve as alternative definitive hosts for *B. procyonis*, and this can lead to patent intestinal infections. This is of significant zoonotic risk for humans because the eggs of *B. procyonis* easily can be mistaken for *T. canis*. Furthermore, dogs have an indiscriminate defecation pattern compared with raccoons, and *B. procyonis* eggs are extremely hardy in the environment.

Toxocara cati may infect cats directly by the transmammary route, ingestion of larvated eggs, or ingestion of an infected paratenic host; the latter 2 routes are most important in cats. Prenatal infection apparently does not occur. Larvae hatching from ingested eggs migrate via the liver, lungs, and trachea; those ingested from milk or via a paratenic host exhibit direct development, often involving the gastric mucosa but without tracheal or extraintestinal migration. Mature *T. cati* are up to 10 cm long, and heavy infection may be associated with clinical disease, but usually not death, in kittens up to several months of age.

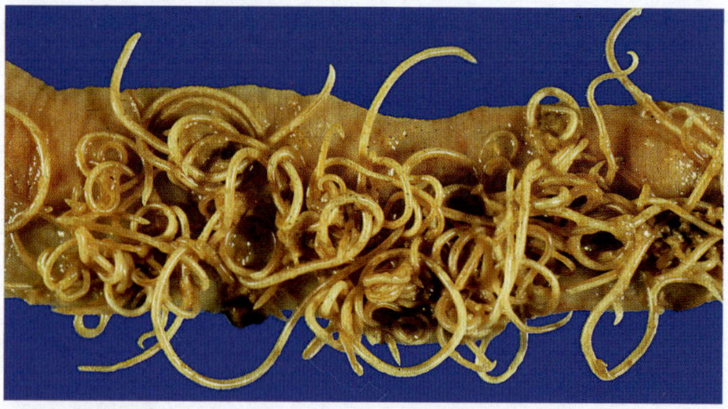

Figure 1-152 Tangled mass of ***Toxocara canis*** in the small intestine of a pup.

Lesions associated with ascariasis in dogs and cats are mostly secondary to larval migration, although in massive infections, adult parasites can cause intestinal obstruction (Fig. 1-152). Heavy infections of ascarids in puppies and kittens, often when reared in unhygienic communal environments, result in ill-thrift. The most significant effects are those caused by maturing *T. canis* in young puppies infected prenatally. Puppies may develop weakness, lethargy, and vomition that can be fatal. Gross lesions indicate poor growth relative to age, abdominal distension, cachexia, and masses of maturing adult nematodes in the intestine and perhaps stomach. Up to 20% of the body weight of young puppies may be accounted for by the worm burden. Mature *T. canis* are up to 18 cm long, and adult worms are often coiled or found free within the lumen; ascarids occasionally enter the bile or pancreatic ducts, and many perforate those structures or the intestine. Migrating *T. canis* larvae can cause focal hemorrhages in the lungs of puppies, and inflammatory foci are commonly seen grossly in the liver or kidney, as white, elevated, 1-2-mm spots in the cortex beneath the capsule. Ocular larva migrans has been described in dogs but not cats infected with *T. canis*. Histologic lesions include aggregates of mixed inflammatory cells, including eosinophils and macrophages in a variety of tissues, most commonly in the liver, kidney, and lung; some nodules may contain larvae of *T. canis*, although considering the large numbers of larvae that migrate through tissues, relatively few are encountered. *T. cati* larvae developing in the mucosa of the stomach and intestine may provoke a mild granulomatous response.

Toxocara (Neoascaris) vitulorum infects the small intestine of young calves of domestic cattle, mainly in the tropics and subtropics and rarely in North America; it is especially significant in water buffalo. The life cycle involves transmammary transmission of third-stage larvae mobilized from the tissues of the dam within a few days of parturition. The larvae reach the liver of the calf and undergo tracheal migration. Patency occurs within the calf ~1-month-old, but worms are expelled within a short time, and by 2-3 months of age, none are present. Signs of infection include foul-smelling diarrhea and ill-thrift. Immature and mature worms contribute to the signs. Heavily infected calves may die in an emaciated state, with burdens of up to 400-500 worms up to 30 cm long in the intestine. Occasionally, migration up the bile duct or perforation of the gut may occur.

***Trichuris* spp.** are the *whipworms*, so called because of their long thin cephalic end and shorter stouter caudal portion. They inhabit the cecum and occasionally the colon of all the domestic animals considered here, except the horse. The host-parasite relationships include: in dogs, *T. vulpis*; in cats, *T. campanula* and *T. serrata*; in swine, *T. suis*; in sheep and goats, *T. ovis*, *T. globulosa*, *T. skrjabini*; and in cattle, *T. discolor* and, less commonly, *T. ovis* and *T. globulosa*.

The life cycle is direct, and larvated ova may remain viable and infective for years in the environment. Ingestion of larvated eggs leads to release of third-stage larvae, which enter the mucosal glands of the proximal small intestine before returning to the lumen and passing into the cecum where they mature as adults. The prepatent period is 6-7 weeks for *T. suis* and 11-12 weeks for *T. vulpis*. In rare instances, disease may occur during the prepatent period, although ova will not be in the feces.

In all species, the filamentous cranial end of the worm is embedded at least partially in tunnels within the superficial mucosa of the cecum and colon; the caudal end lies freely within the intestinal lumen (Fig. 1-153). *Trichuris* sp. ingest blood, but disease is usually related more to localized tissue damage at attachment sites. Light infections cause minimal morphologic alteration; however, heavy infection with *Trichuris* sp. is associated with *severe and often hemorrhagic typhlitis or typhlocolitis in all species*. In the dog, large populations of worms can extend into the ascending colon and rectum. Clinical signs may include chronic diarrhea, dysentery, and weight loss; blood and foul odor of feces are due to hemorrhage and effusion of tissue fluid from the mucosal surface damaged by the embedded worms. Grossly, the mucosa is thickened, red, and edematous, and colonic content is often watery and contains blood or mucus, with masses of tangled worms visible on the mucosal surface. Microscopically, the mucosal surface is widely eroded or mildly ulcerated with effusion of proteinaceous fluid, inflammatory exudate, and hemorrhage. The glandular epithelium is hyperplastic. Occasionally, *T. vulpis* infection may be associated with more severe localized granulomatous inflammation and fibroplasia in deeper layers of the mucosa, although ova or worms are rarely identified in such lesions.

If enough *T. suis* worms are present in **swine**, they may cause mucohemorrhagic typhlocolitis associated clinically with anorexia, diarrhea, dysentery, dehydration, ill-thrift, and in some cases death. The disease is most common in animals exposed to dirt yards contaminated with infective *T. suis* ova. Clinical signs of the disease are due to loss of colonic absorptive function and effusion of protein into the lumen, with erythrocyte loss as a minor component of the pathogenesis. Typical gross lesions are similar to those described in dogs with thickened, edematous, reddened, and eroded mucosa with increased mucus secretion. *Gross lesions may resemble those of swine dysentery*; however, careful examination reveals characteristic nematodes on the mucosa, which may resemble *Oesophagostomum* sp. at first glance, but the distinct elongate threadlike cephalic end and thicker caudal end confirms these as *Trichuris* sp.

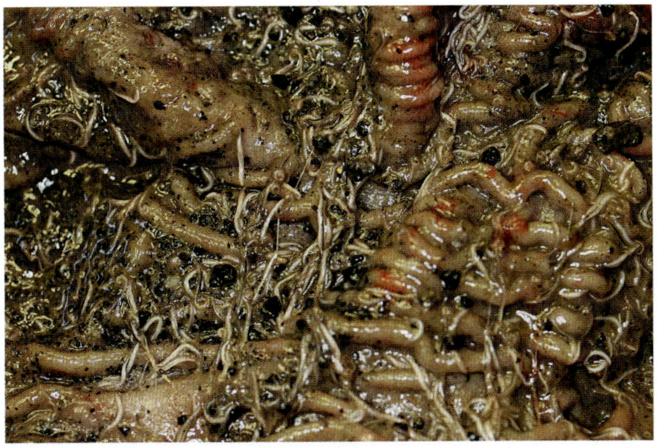

Figure 1-153 **Hemorrhagic typhlocolitis** in a pig caused by *Trichuris suis*.

Histologic lesions include hyperplasia of glandular epithelium, mucosal erosion, and surface effusion of proteinaceous fluid, inflammatory cells, and blood. Lesions are more severe in swine with conventional intestinal flora compared with germ-free swine, suggesting that *T. suis* suppresses mucosal immunity to resident bacteria.

Trichurosis in **sheep** and **cattle** usually occurs in animals that are concentrated in areas contaminated by ova, and immunocompromise has been suggested to increase susceptibility. Heavily infected animals develop chronic diarrhea, dysentery, and/or loss of condition. The gross lesions are nonspecific and may include cachexia and hypoproteinemia associated with catarrhal typhlocolitis; large numbers of parasites are usually observed (eFig. 1-15).

A **diagnosis** of trichurosis in all species is usually readily made during postmortem examination by identifying adult worms with their characteristic morphology. Histologically, the filamentous cephalic end of the adults is embedded in tunnels in the surface epithelium and contains the stichosome esophagus and single bacillary band typical of members of the *Trichuroidea*. The barrel-shaped thick-walled ova have polar plugs and may be seen histologically in the body cavity of adult worms, free within the host intestinal lumen, or occasionally in tissue. *Capillaria* spp. and their ova may appear similar in tissue section but are not expected in the cecum and colon.

Cestodes in 2 orders are of importance to veterinarians. *Pseudophyllidea* include the genera *Diphyllobothrium* and *Spirometra* and are associated with aquatic food chains and require 2 intermediate hosts: The first is a copepod and the second may be a fish, amphibian, or reptile. The order *Cyclophyllidae* contains several families of interest such as *Taeniidae*, *Mesocestoididae*, *Anoplocephalidae*, *Dipylidiidae*, and *Hymenolepididae*. Most cyclophyllideans require only one intermediate host, which may be a mammal or an arthropod. Adult tapeworms inhabit the GI tract or the hepatic, biliary, or pancreatic ducts, where they are generally of minor significance. They are flattened and segmented organisms with sequentially maturing hermaphroditic reproductive units, or proglottids, forming an elongate strobila a few millimeters to many meters long. Cestodes attach to the host by a specialized scolex (holdfast organ), which usually has 4 suckers, and perhaps a rostellum, sometimes armed with hooks. Cestodes lack an alimentary tract and absorb nutrients through the specialized absorptive surface or tegument of the proglottids.

The life cycle of tapeworms is complex and often specific to a particular species. The definitive host is infected by ingestion of the intermediate or paratenic host containing infective larvae. Carnivores tend be infected by tapeworms that use prey species as intermediate hosts. Larval cestodes use some species of domestic animals as intermediate hosts, and humans can serve as accidental hosts. Metacestodes, or larval cestodes within their intermediate or paratenic hosts, in domestic animals may cause disease, result in economic loss because of condemnation of tissues or organs at slaughter inspection, or can have zoonotic significance.

Adult cestodes have flattened solid parenchymatous bodies segmented into proglottids, and internal organs are embedded within the parenchymatous matrix and contain male and female reproductive organs but lack a digestive tract. Other features that may be observed histologically include anterior muscular suckers and hooks. Calcareous corpuscles are basophilic round-to-oval structures that may have concentric rings and are embedded within the outer parenchyma; corpuscles are more numerous in the head and neck region of adult and larval cestodes.

Intestinal tapeworms in ruminants include the widely distributed *Moniezia expansa*, *M. benedeni*, and *Thysaniezia (Helictometra) giardi*, as well as some less common species. *Stilesia globipunctata* is found in the small intestine of sheep and goats in Europe, Asia, and Africa, *S. hepatica* occurs in bile ducts of ruminants in Africa and Asia, *Thysanosoma actinioides* occurs in the small intestine, pancreatic and bile ducts of ruminants in North and South America, and *Avitellina* spp. occur in the small intestine of sheep and other ruminants in parts of Europe and Asia. The intermediate hosts of these tapeworms are oribatid mites or psocids (book lice).Heavy infestations of the small intestine by *Moniezia*, *Thysaniezia*, and *Avitellina* have been associated with diarrhea and ill-thrift in young lambs and calves; however, the pathogenicity of *Moniezia* spp. is considered very low.

The scolex of *S. globipunctata* may be embedded in 6-10-mm mucosal nodules in the upper small intestine, with their threadlike strobila streaming into the intestinal lumen. A chronic inflammatory reaction occurs around the embedded scolex; glands in the vicinity are hyperplastic, and together with the inflammatory cells cause nodule formation. The presence of many adults is associated with edema, diarrhea, and wasting in small ruminants.

S. hepatica and *T. actinioides* may cause mild fibrosis and ectasia of the bile ducts, and adults cestodes are often concentrated in the segmented saccular dilations of bile ducts. In areas where infection is common, these worms cause significant economic loss through condemnation of infected livers at slaughter inspection.

Anoplocephala perfoliata is the major cestode found in horses, and this cestode attaches to the intestinal mucosa in the region of the ileocecal junction; *Anoplocephala magna* and *Equinia (Paranoplocephala) mamillana* colonize the small intestine and occasionally the stomach. *A. magna* tends to live in the lower small intestine, where it can reach a length of up to 80 cm, and a width of 2.5 cm; *E. mamillana* is smaller, <5 cm long, and is rarely associated with disease or lesions. All use oribatid mites as intermediate hosts.

A. perfoliata is the most common cestode in horses and has a worldwide distribution. *A. perfoliata* does not invade the mucosa of the intestine, its attachment via 4 suckers on its scolex causes a localized inflammatory response. In heavy infections, *A. perfoliata* attach in clusters of up to several hundred at the ileocecal junction and cause erosion and ulceration of the mucosal epithelium. The surface may be covered by fibrin, hemorrhage, or localized granulation tissue. Histologic lesions at the site of attachment of adult cestodes include large numbers of eosinophils and lymphocytes with edema, mucosal ulceration, and fibrosis. Villus atrophy of ileal mucosa, hyperplasia of the ileal, colonic, and cecal epithelium, goblet cell hyperplasia, and hypertrophy of the muscular layers of the intestine may all be observed. Changes in the myenteric ganglia, including loss and degeneration of neurons, edema, and inflammation, have been described. The risk of spasmodic colic increases with parasite burden, which may be at least partially explained by the histologic lesions described. Ileal muscular hypertrophy, impaction, partial obstruction of the ileocecal orifice, and ileocecal and cecocecal intussusception (Fig. 1-154) are also associated with large numbers of *A. perfoliata*. Although histologic lesions are well correlated with the parasite burden, whether the development of colic, obstruction, muscular hypertrophy, or intussusception is the result of altered peristaltic waves or mucosal and submucosal lesions remains unclear.

***Diphyllobothrium* spp.** parasitize **dogs** primarily, although aberrant hosts can include humans, **cats, swine**, and other fish-eating mammals. The adults can reach lengths of up to 12-15 m in humans, although in animals they tend to be shorter. The adult cestode is ~2 cm wide and histologically has a central uterus containing dark operculate eggs. Intermediate stages occur in copepods and fish, and the adult worm matures in the intestine of piscivorous mammals. Infection by *Diphyllobothrium* spp. is rarely associated with clinical disease in animals.

Spirometra spp. are, like *Diphyllobothrium* spp., members of the order *Pseudophyllidea*, and their life cycle is similar. The taxonomy of the genus is difficult, recognized species include *Spirometra mansonoides*, which infects dogs, cats, and raccoons in North and South America; *S. mansoni* infects dogs and cats in East Asia and South America; and *S. erinacei* infects cats and dogs in Australia and the Far East. The definitive host must ingest the third larval form, or *plerocercoid*, usually via predation of an infected intermediate or paratenic host. Several animal species that are not definitive hosts can serve as paratenic or transport hosts when they ingest the plerocercoid (*spargana*) found in the body cavity, muscle, or subcutaneous tissues of the second intermediate host, usually an amphibian or reptile. Spargana are white and ribbon-like larvae that may be up to several centimeters long and usually found free or encysted in a thin fibrous capsule within the peritoneal cavity, muscle, or subcutaneous tissue. A chronic inflammatory reaction may occur around dead

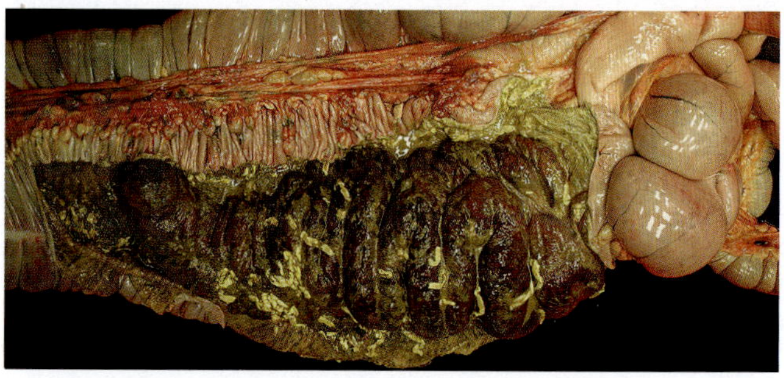

Figure 1-154 ***Anoplocephala perfoliata*** at the ileocecal junction of a horse with a cecocolic intussusception.

spargana, although the adult worms are nonpathogenic. Infection with third-stage plerocercoid spargana (*sparganosis*) occurs in carnivores, swine, or even humans if the first intermediate host *Cyclops* copepod containing the second larval stage (procercoid) is ingested, usually via contaminated drinking water. Sparganosis is a significant disease in humans, in which the plerocercoids migrate mainly in subcutaneous tissues or rarely in other organs.

Mesocestoides spp. occasionally infect dogs, as well as other mammals and some birds, in North America, Europe, Asia, and Africa. These cyclophyllidean tapeworms have a complex life cycle involving an insect or mite, and a vertebrate as second intermediate host. Infective tetrathyridia are found in the body cavities, liver, and lung of mammals, reptiles, or birds; ingestion of tetrathyridia causes infection of the definitive host. In the intestine of definitive hosts, *Mesocestoides* spp. adults may also replicate asexually, and heavy infections or continual re-infection may occur as a result of this, or from the consumption of large numbers of tetrathyridia in an intermediate host. Animals infected with intestinal *Mesocestoides* spp. may develop diarrhea. Tetrathyridia replicating in the intestine of the dog may also penetrate the gut wall, and proliferate in the peritoneal cavity, resulting in *peritoneal larval cestodosis*. Tetrathyridia in the abdominal cavity of dogs and cats may cause peritoneal effusion (*parasitic ascites*), perhaps with the development of pyogranulomatous peritonitis and adhesions. Tetrathyridia 1-2 mm in diameter are scattered in abundant exudate, along with small white cyst-like structures, composed of necrotic parasite tegument and host cellular debris. Mild infections may be discovered incidentally at autopsy. *Mesocestoides* spp. infection of the abdominal cavity must be differentiated from peritoneal infections by cysticerci of several *Taenia* spp., which occur very rarely in carnivores.

Dipylidium caninum is ubiquitous and occurs in dogs, cats, foxes, and, occasionally, children. The narrow adult cestodes are up to 0.5 m long, have distinctive cucumber seed–like segments, and are often encountered in the small intestine at autopsy; they are of no pathologic significance. Cysticercoids develop in fleas and perhaps in the dog louse *Trichodectes canis*. Infection in the normal definitive hosts or in accidental ones such as humans is by ingestion of fleas containing cysticercoids.

Taeniid cestodes are the most important tapeworms in domestic animals, not because of the effects of the adult worm in the carnivorous definitive host, but rather because of the *metacestode larval forms* in intermediate or paratenic hosts. Gravid taeniid segments exit from the definitive host and shed their eggs. When ingested by an appropriate intermediate vertebrate host, the egg hatches and the embryo enters the intestinal wall, then migrates to the organ of predilection, often the liver, peritoneum, or muscle, where they differentiate into second-stage larvae or metacestode stage. These have a distinctive fluid-filled bladder with one or more scolices (*bladder worm*), which is infective to the definitive host. Once the second-stage larva is ingested by the definitive host, the scolex embeds into the small intestinal mucosa, where it begins to bud segments to form strobila. Metacestodes occasionally may be found in organs other than the site of predilection.

Taeniid metacestodes assume 4 basic forms. The **cysticercus** is a fluid-filled, thin-walled muscular cyst into which the scolex and neck of a single larval tapeworm are invaginated. The **strobilocercus** is a modification of this theme: late in larval development the scolex evaginates, elongates, and segments while still in the intermediate host, so that it resembles a tapeworm up to several centimeters long. The **coenurus** is a single or loculated fluid-filled cyst, in which many scolices are present in clusters on the inner wall. Each scolex is capable of developing into a single adult cestode in the intestine of the definitive host. The **hydatid cyst** is formed by members of the genus *Echinococcus* spp. and is of unilocular or multilocular structure, on the inner germinal membrane of which brood capsules develop. Within the brood capsules, invaginated protoscolices form. Brood capsules may float free in the cyst fluid, where they are termed *hydatid sand*. Release of brood capsules or protoscolices into tissues following rupture of the hydatid cyst may lead to development of new cysts.

Taenia taeniaeformis infects the intestine of domestic cats and some wild felids, and the strobilocercus, *Cysticercus fasciolaris*, is found in the liver of small rodents. Formation of hepatic fibrosarcomas has been associated with chronic inflammation resulting from *C. fasciolaris*. The adults are up to 60 cm long and caudal segments are bell-shaped, so this species is readily differentiated from the other cestodes found in the feline small intestine. Usually, only a few adult cestodes are present in the cat, and they are of no consequence.

Taenia pisiformis is common in the small intestine in dogs and some wild canids, which prey on rabbits and hares. *Cysticercus pisiformis* migrates in the liver of the intermediate host, causing hemorrhagic tracks that are infiltrated by a mixed inflammatory reaction, and ultimately heal by scarring. The 3-5 mm diameter cysticerci encyst in a thin fibrous capsule on the mesentery, omentum, or on the ligaments of the bladder. Occasionally, cysticerci persist beneath the hepatic capsule. Burdens of up to 20-30 worms, sometimes more, may be present in the intestine of the dog.

Taenia hydatigena infects the dog, and its metacestode, *Cysticercus tenuicollis* (the long-necked bladder worm) is found in the peritoneal cavity of sheep, cattle, swine, and occasionally other species. Immature cysticerci in the liver migrate through the parenchyma for several weeks as they develop, before emerging to encyst on the peritoneum anywhere in the abdominal cavity. Immature cysticerci are <1 cm long, ovoid, and translucent. They cause tortuous hemorrhagic tracks similar to those produced by immature liver flukes, and if large numbers are present, they may cause a syndrome of depression and icterus. Heavily infected livers, with 4,000-5,000 actively migrating cysticerci, are mottled because of the subcapsular and parenchymal hemorrhagic tracks. Cysticerci up to 6-8 mm long may be present beneath or breaching the capsule by ~3 weeks after infection. Rarely, animals may exsanguinate into the abdominal cavity, or the hepatic necrosis may predispose to the development of black disease or bacillary hemoglobinuria. Cysticerci in the liver or along the diaphragmatic surface are evident in individual thin-walled fluid-filled cysts; they may be destroyed by eosinophilic granulomatous inflammation and mineralization, or they may persist within a thin fibrous capsule. Hepatic migration by *C. tenuicollis* may, at any stage, cause condemnation of lamb and swine livers at slaughter inspection.

Taenia ovis infects the intestine of dogs; the metacestode *Cysticercus ovis* is found in the muscle of sheep where it causes *cysticercosis* or *sheep measles*. Cysticercosis of muscle caused by *C. ovis*; by *C. bovis* in cattle; and by *C. cellulosae* in swine and other species, including dogs, is considered in Vol. 1, Muscle and Tendon. The adult stages of the latter 2 cysticerci, *Taenia* *saginata* and *T. solium*, respectively, occur in the small intestine of humans.

Taenia multiceps occurs in the intestine of dogs and wild canids, but the metacestode *Coenurus cerebralis* develops in the brain and spinal cord of sheep and other ungulates, and rarely in humans. In the goat, coenuri may also occur in other organs, including the subcutaneous space or skeletal muscle. Migration of small metacestodes in the CNS may cause tortuous red or yellow-gray tracks in the brain because of hemorrhage and malacia, and central nervous signs or death may occur. More commonly, signs of CNS disease termed "sturdy" or "gid" do not develop until coenuri enlarge up to 4-5 cm in diameter and develop more fully, usually 4-8 months after infection. Cysts may be present at any level and depth in the brain and spinal cord, and projecting into the cerebral ventricles, but they are most common near the surface of the parietal cortex in the cerebrum. They cause increased intracranial pressure, hydrocephalus, and necrosis of adjacent brain parenchyma that may extend to the overlying skull. Coenuri developing in the spinal cord may cause paresis or paralysis. ***Taenia serialis*** infects dogs and foxes throughout the world. The larval coenurus is found in the subcutaneous and intermuscular connective tissue of lagomorphs. Cerebral coenurosis has been reported in cats.

Cysticerci and coenuri are recognized histologically as cystic structures with an eosinophilic outer layer or tegument, which may appear fibrillar on the outermost surface. Beneath the tegument, a less cellular area, which may contain calcareous corpuscles, transitions to a web-like lightly cellular matrix and the central open fluid-filled portion of the cyst lacking internal organs. Muscular scolices with suckers and hooks on the rostellum (except *C. bovis*) may be encountered extending into the center of the metacestode. The size and shape of hooks may assist in a specific diagnosis if they are fully developed. Immature migrating metacestodes lack organized scolices. Other sources should be consulted for details on the taxonomy and specific identification of adult and larval taeniid tapeworms.

Echinococcus spp. tapeworms occur in the small intestine of several carnivores, predominantly canids. In enzootic areas, the distinctive metacestodes or *hydatid cysts* are commonly found in normal or accidental intermediate hosts. Humans may accidentally become infected with the metacestode, and echinococcosis or hydatidosis is a significant public health problem where carnivores shedding *Echinococcus* spp. eggs come in close contact with humans. The important species are *Echinococcus granulosus*, *E. multilocularis*, *E. oligarthus*, and *E. vogeli*. The latter 2 involve sylvatic cycles in Central and South America, with felids and canids as definitive hosts, respectively, and rodents as intermediate hosts in which polycystic hydatidosis occurs; *E. vogeli* may infect humans. The other 2 species may use domestic animals as definitive hosts and are considered further here.

The definitive host for ***E. granulosus*** is the dog and some other canids. The most widespread strain or genotype uses a sheep-dog cycle and has been disseminated wherever there is pastoral husbandry of sheep. It is significant as a potential zoonosis in many parts of Eurasia and the Mediterranean region, some parts of the United Kingdom, North America, South America, continental Australia, and Africa. Eradication has been accomplished, or virtually so, in Iceland, New Zealand, and Tasmania. Other cycles affecting domestic animals include horse-; cattle-; camel-; pig-; water buffalo-; goat-; and human-dog. Sylvatic cycles include: in Eurasia and North America, cervid-wolf; in Argentina, hare-fox; in Sri Lanka, deer-jackal; and in Australia, macropod-dingo. Not all cycles represent different genotypes.

In the small intestine of the definitive host, protoscolices evaginate and establish between villi and in the intestinal crypts. The scolex distends the crypt and the epithelium is gripped by the suckers and may become eroded, but there is little or no inflammatory response. The worms that develop are short, usually <6-7 mm long; they commonly have only 3-5 proglottids, the caudal gravid one making up almost half the length of the worm. Burdens of *E. granulosus* are often heavy, likely because many protoscolices are ingested at a meal containing one or more hydatid cysts. The heavily infected intestine is carpeted by the tiny white blunt projections, partially obscured between the villi and resembling lymphangiectasia; enteric signs are not normally observed. Eggs shed from adults are ingested by the intermediate host; oncospheres released from eggs in the intestine of the intermediate host migrate via subepithelial capillaries or lacteals to the liver, lungs, and general circulation. Hydatid cysts occur most commonly in the liver and lung, with some strain and host species variation in the relative prevalence in these organs. In sheep, they may be more common in lungs; in cattle and horses the liver is the usual site of establishment. Less common sites in domestic animals include the brain, heart, bone, and subcutaneous tissue. One to several hundred cysts may be present displacing tissue in infected organs. Disease is rarely attributed to hydatidosis in animals, even if heavily infected. However, strategic location of one or more cysts may lead to heart failure, bloat, or central nervous signs because of space occupation. Condemnation of infected organs at slaughter inspection may cause significant economic loss.

Grossly, hydatid cysts are spherical, turgid, and fluid filled. They usually measure 5-10 cm in diameter in domestic animals; rarely, cysts in animals may be larger, but in humans hydatid cysts can become huge. In contrast, fertile cysts in equine livers may be as small as 2-3 mm diameter. The lining of fertile cysts is studded with small granular brood capsules, which contain protoscolices. Hydatid sand is composed of free brood capsules and protoscolices and is typically present within the fluid; smooth-lined cysts are sterile. Although the potential exists for development of daughter cysts and exogenous budding by herniated cysts, most hydatid cysts in domestic animals are unilocular. They may be irregular or distorted in shape because of the tissue they are in, and variable resistance of parenchyma and portal tracts or bronchi and by the profiles of bone or other resistant tissues.

Microscopically, immature hydatid cysts are surrounded by an infiltrate of mixed inflammatory cells, including giant cells and eosinophils. As they develop, a layer of granulation tissue surrounds the cyst, and this matures so that in aged lesions the inner portion of the fibrous capsule is composed of acellular mature collagenous connective tissue. In close apposition is a PAS-positive acellular lamellar hyaline outer layer of the hydatid cyst wall, composed of a polysaccharide-protein complex that may become hundreds of micrometers thick. The cyst is lined by the thin syncytial germinal layer from which the brood capsules form on fine pedicles. If the cyst is ruptured and protoscolices are released into tissue, secondary cysts may form from them. If hydatid cysts degenerate, the inner structures collapse and the mass becomes filled with necrotic debris and may mineralize; these resemble tuberculous lesions grossly and histologically.

E. multilocularis has a holarctic distribution; adults occur mainly in foxes, and the metacestodes in small rodents, especially voles and lemmings. Dogs and cats may also become infected with adult *E. multilocularis* in enzootic areas. Although the parasite is principally arctic, the cycle is found in the northern prairie area of North America and in eastern and central Europe and is moving progressively southward with increasing cases reported. The mature cestodes in the intestine are similar to but smaller than *E. granulosus*. In the intermediate host, the *metacestode or multilocular alveolar hydatid* mainly infects the liver by forming a cystic structure with internal brood capsules and many protoscolices. The alveolar hydatid is capable of external budding that continuously proliferates and infiltrates surrounding tissue. They may metastasize via the bloodstream to the lungs or bone, or implant in the peritoneal cavity. The inflammatory reaction to alveolar hydatids is composed of macrophages, giant cells, lymphocytes, and plasma cells within a fibrous capsular stroma. The metacestodes are rarely found in domestic animals but may infect humans who ingest eggs shed by infected carnivores.

Digenetic trematode, or fluke, infections of the intestine of domestic animals are uncommon. Dogs and cats in many parts of the world may be infected with *Alaria* spp., the second intermediate hosts for which are frogs or other amphibia. *Heterophyes heterophyes*, *Metagonimus yokagawai*, *Echinochasmus perfoliatus*, and *Ascocotyle (Phagicola) longa* may infect dogs and cats fed fish that contain metacercariae. The former 2 occur in the Mediterranean area and the Far East; the latter in Eurasia. *Cryptocotyle* spp., most commonly parasitic in piscivorous birds, also may be found in dogs, cats, and mink fed infected marine fish.

Enteritis has been attributed to ***Alaria***, ***Echinochasmus***, and ***Cryptocotyle***. The flukes attach to the mucosa by suckers, and perhaps cause their effects by local irritation, erosion, and ulceration when present in large numbers. Excessive intestinal mucus production, hemorrhagic enteritis, vomiting, and ill-thrift have been associated with intestinal fluke infection in small animals. The flukes involved are small, <4-5 mm long, and thus can be easily overlooked at autopsy.

The digenean trematode ***Nanophyetus salmincola*** is the vector of salmon poisoning disease, which occurs in the small intestine of dogs, cats, and humans, and in various fish-eating wild mammals and birds in the northwestern United States; Vancouver Island, Canada; and eastern Siberia. The disease has been thought to be restricted to North America; however, similar organisms have been recognized in dogs with lesions compatible with salmon poisoning disease in southern Brazil. Its distribution is determined by that of the snails that are the first intermediate hosts. The second intermediate hosts are fish, especially salmonids. Adult flukes inhabit the small intestine, where they penetrate and attach to the mucosa and release large numbers of ova, which infect the snail. Mature cercariae, or free-swimming larvae, are released into water and penetrate the abdominal region of the second intermediate host. Metacercariae locate in the kidneys, liver, and intestine via the circulation of the fish. Adult trematodes attach deeply and develop in the intestine of the definitive host that has ingested metacercariae-infected fish. *N. salmincola* transmits ***Neorickettsia helminthoeca***, the etiologic agent of salmon poisoning disease, which is released from the trematode and is disseminated via the circulatory and lymphatic system in the definitive host. *N. helminthoeca* is nonpathogenic to either the first or second intermediate host; *N. salmincola* in high numbers can be pathogenic to both intermediate hosts.

Salmon poisoning disease has an incubation period of ~5-7 days and is characterized clinically by pyrexia, anorexia, depression, weakness, and weight loss. There may be serous nasal discharge, lymphadenopathy, and mucopurulent conjunctivitis. Diarrhea with tenesmus develops; feces are scant yellow and mucoid or watery, often with some blood. The condition is usually fatal; if untreated, only 5-10% of infected dogs survive, but they are immune to reinfection.

Gross lesions are most consistently found in the lymphoid tissues and include generalized enlargement of lymph nodes, especially in the abdominal cavity. Prominent enlarged tonsils are everted from their fossae, and Peyer patches and other intestinal lymphoid aggregates are elevated above the mucosal surface. There may be petechiae on the intestinal mucosa, pleura, gallbladder, and urinary bladder. In some cases, there is ulceration and hemorrhage of the intestine and hepatomegaly. *Microscopic changes* in lymph nodes, thymus, and spleen include depletion of lymphocytes with histiocytic infiltration in the cortex and medulla. Intracytoplasmic elementary bodies of *N. helminthoeca* may be demonstrated in reticuloendothelial cells of lymphoid tissue and other visceral organs by Giemsa or Macchiavello stains, or IHC. Small intestinal flukes may be embedded deep in the mucosa, although usually little reaction to them is present. Additional microscopic lesions may include lymphocytic and histiocytic leptomeningitis or meningitis, which may be most consistent over the cerebellum. Similar inflammatory cells may surround small- and medium-sized vessels throughout the neuroparenchyma; focal gliosis is relatively sparsely distributed but seems most common in the brainstem. Elementary bodies are also demonstrable in reticuloendothelial cells of the CNS, which confirms the diagnosis. The organisms can be isolated and grown on primary canine monocyte cultures and in several other cell culture systems, but this is not a routine procedure.

Paramphistome, or rumen fluke, infections may cause significant intestinal disease in ruminants. Adults of the genera *Paramphistomum*, *Cotylophoron*, *Calicophoron*, *Ceylonocotyle*, *Gastrothylax*, *Fischoederius*, and *Carmyerius* occur in the forestomachs of ruminants in various areas around the world. The species involved vary with the host and geographic area. In cattle, water buffalo, and American bison, the species incriminated in disease include *Paramphistomum cervi*, *P. microbothrium*, *P. explanatum*, *Calicophoron calicophorum*, and various species of *Cotylophoron*, *Gastrothylax, and Fischoederius*. In sheep and goats, *P. microbothrium*, *P. ichikawai*, *P. cervi*, *P. explanatum*, *Gastrothylax crumenifer*, *Cotylophoron cotylophorum*, and *Fischoederius cobboldi* have been associated with disease. *Skrjabinema ovis* has been associated with catarrhal enteritis in sheep in Eurasia.

Infection is most common in warm-temperate to tropical climates. In the rumen, the tan-to-red pear-shaped adult flukes with their characteristic cranial and caudal suckers are considered innocuous, although some papillae may become atrophic. When ingested, metacercariae encysted on herbage give rise to immature flukes that inhabit the duodenum, and in heavy infections may cause severe hemorrhagic enteritis. After 3-5 weeks in the small intestine, they migrate through the abomasum to establish and mature in the reticulorumen (see Fig. 1-31). With massive infections, growth of the organisms in the small intestine is slowed, and flukes may persist for months in the duodenum, prolonging the course of disease.

Calves and lambs with severe intestinal paramphistomosis are depressed and inappetent. Fetid diarrhea usually develops within several weeks of infection and may contain immature flukes. Hypoproteinemia is reflected in submandibular edema in some animals, and anemia is reported to occur occasionally. Morbidity and mortality can be substantial, and survivors may suffer considerable loss in condition. Chronic inappetence and protein loss into the gut probably accounts for the most important pathophysiologic consequences.

Gross lesions are nonspecific and include cachexia depending on the duration of the disease, edema of subcutaneous tissues, abomasal folds, and mesentery, and multicavitary effusion caused by hypoproteinemia. The proximal small intestine may be congested, and the mucosal surface is edematous, thickened, corrugated, and covered with mucus. Myriad immature pink or brown paramphistomes a few millimeters long are observed firmly attached and embedded in the proximal intestinal wall and may be visible through the serosa. Occasionally, the organisms perforate the intestinal wall and are found free in the abdominal cavity.

Histologically, larval paramphistomes are found deep in the lamina propria, occasionally in the submucosa, and sometimes in Brunner glands. Larger immature forms are attached to the surface of the mucosa by a plug of tissue taken into the oral sucker, or acetabulum (see Fig. 1-31B). There is atrophy of villi, elongation of crypts, erosion or ulceration of the mucosa, and potentially fibroplasia in heavily infected areas.

In swine, the paramphistomes *Gastrodiscoides* and *Gastrodiscus* may be found in the colon, where they are of little significance. *Fasciolopsis buski* and *Artyfechinosomum malayanum* may infect the small intestine of swine as well as humans. They are of little importance in pigs other than as potential reservoirs for human infection.

In horses in Africa and India, the paramphistomes *Gastrodiscus aegyptiacus* and *Pseudodiscus collinsi* occur in the large bowel. Larvae of the former species have been associated with severe colitis in horses, but they are generally nonpathogenic.

Intestinal schistosomosis is due mainly to *Schistosoma* spp. in ruminants and ***Heterobilharzia americanum*** in dogs. *H. americanum* has been located primarily in the southern Atlantic or Gulf coast states in the United States; however, naturally occurring disease has been reported in southcentral, western, and midwestern states. *H. americanum* has a complex life cycle involving both snail and mammalian hosts, such as raccoon and domestic canids. Dogs are infected while swimming or wading in water harboring the intermediate host lymnaeid snails, and then contaminated with infective free-swimming cercariae, which penetrate the skin and migrate hematogenously to the liver and lung. Immature flukes can be found in the liver within several days of infecting the mammalian definitive host; this is where most of their growth and development occurs. Mature adults migrate to mesenteric veins where sexual reproduction occurs; eggs then penetrate the serosal surface of the intestine and migrate through the intestinal wall, which incites a severe inflammatory response. Fertilized eggs can exit the body in feces, and in fresh water the miracidia emerge from the eggs and infect snails to complete their life cycle. Alternatively, eggs migrate to the liver and are carried by the portal circulation to various other organs, the most common of which include the pancreas and kidneys. Eggs embedded in these organs elicit a granulomatous inflammatory response; the number of embedded eggs determines the degree of organic dysfunction in these cases.

Clinical signs include intermittent hemorrhagic diarrhea with excess mucus production, tenesmus, vomiting, anorexia, and weight loss; involvement of the GI system is common. Gross intestinal lesions are nonspecific but may include a reddened thickened intestinal wall; intestinal intussusception has been associated with this syndrome in a small number of dogs. Histologic lesions in the intestine are typically *multifocal-to-diffuse granulomatous enterocolitis*; eggs may be present within the mucosa, submucosa, and muscular layers of affected dogs. Granulomas surrounding eggs embedded in other organs are also often observed. For additional information on syndromes caused by *H. americanum*, see Vol. 3, Cardiovascular System.

Adult flukes in tissue section are generally somewhat flattened or globose, with a loose mesenchymal parenchyma in which the internal structures are embedded. The tegument is eosinophilic and may contain spines. Muscular oral and acetabular suckers and pharynx may be encountered in sections. Ceca are usually present, and elements of the male and female reproductive systems in these typically hermaphroditic adult worms (excepting the schistosomes) may be seen. The uterus may contain ova with a tan-yellow or brown shell, perhaps with an operculum, and ova are often seen in the intestinal lumen or in tissue. The developing miracidium may be present in ova. Schistosomes are recognized by their intravascular location and sexual dimorphism, the leaflike male perhaps enveloping the slender cylindrical female within the gynecophoric canal.

Acanthocephalan infections are uncommon in animals. *Acanthocephala* is a phylum of parasitic worms known commonly as *thorny- or spiny-headed worms* that have an elongate saclike body, no internal alimentary canal, and use a spiny protrusible proboscis to attach to the intestinal wall. The life cycle typically involves obligate development in an intermediate host, usually an arthropod, and perhaps the use of a paratenic host to facilitate transmission. The acanthocephala of concern in domestic animals are in the genera *Macracanthorhynchus* and *Oncicola*. ***Macracanthorhynchus hirudinaceus*** is the thorny-headed worm that infects the small intestine of **swine**. The life cycle involves dung beetles or other *Scarabaeidae*, and foraging or rooting swine are prone to infection. Adult males are 10 cm long; females are up to 30-40 cm long, slightly pink, curved, and taper caudally. The proboscis has ~6 rows of hooks and is used to penetrate deeply the intestinal wall. Attachment incites a local granulomatous nodule that has been called a strawberry mark, which may be visible from the serosal surface as a gray or yellow 1-cm nodule surrounded by a hyperemic rim. The proboscis may penetrate the tunica muscularis and cause peritonitis. Heavily infected pigs may suffer ill-thrift and perhaps anemia, probably related partly to plasma protein loss and hemorrhage from numerous small ulcers.

Macracanthorhynchus catalinus and *M. ingens* are smaller but similar thorny-headed worms that inhabit the intestine of a variety of wild carnivores, and occasionally the dog.

Oncicola canis occurs in the small intestine of wild carnivores, and occasionally in dogs and cats, but rarely causes disease. Intermediate hosts are presumably arthropods, with insectivorous vertebrates acting as paratenic hosts. Up to several hundred worms, 0.5-1.5 cm long and dark gray, may infest the small intestine; infections are usually light. The proboscis is embedded to the subserosal level, and a focal nodular lesion develops about it.

Protistan diseases

Coccidiosis. The coccidia are members of the protistan phylum *Apicomplexa*, intracellular parasites characterized at some stage of the life cycle by a typical "apical complex" of organelles at one end of the organism. Members of the subclass *Coccidiasina* or *Coccidia*, which are considered together under coccidiosis, all have a similar basic life cycle. It begins with infection of a cell, often, but not always, in the intestinal mucosa, by a **sporozoite** released from a **sporocyst**, which is in turn contained within an oocyst, in the lumen of the gut. One or more cycles of asexual division, termed **schizogony** or **merogony**, follow, and the **merozoites** produced infect other cells, forming another generation of **meronts**, or transforming to sexual stages, termed **gamonts**. Gamonts subsequently develop into nonmotile female **macrogametes**, and motile male forms or **microgametes**. A nonmotile zygote produced by union of microgametes and macrogametes forms an **oocyst**. Oocysts are released in feces to the environment. **Sporogony**, which is the production of sporocysts containing infectious sporozoites within the oocyst, may occur in the host, or more commonly, after the resistant oocysts are passed in feces.

Members of the genus ***Eimeria*** and ***Isospora*** are **homoxenous**, with sexual and asexual development taking place in a single host. *Cystoisospora* (formerly *Isospora* spp.) and the genera *Toxoplasma, Sarcocystis, Hammondia, Besnoitia, Frenkelia, Neospora*, and *Caryospora* are all **heteroxenous**, in which case asexual stages occur in an intermediate host. There are, however, exceptions to this rule; for instance, *Toxoplasma* utilizes felids as both definitive and intermediate hosts with asexual and sexual replication. The heteroxenous genera exploit natural prey-predator relationships. In general, sexual development takes place in the intestinal mucosa of a definitive host predator; at least one generation of asexual replication, often several, occurs in the tissues of one or more species of prey.

The endogenous stages of coccidia are all intracellular, except, temporarily, the merozoite and microgamete. Mature developmental stages are usually readily recognized; immature forms may not be easily identifiable. **Trophozoites**, small undifferentiated, rounded, basophilic forms with a single nucleus, usually within a parasitophorous vacuole in the host cell, are found at 3 stages of the life cycle. They occur after invasion by the infective sporozoite, before merogony; after invasion by a merozoite, before a subsequent generation of merogony; and after invasion by a merozoite, before differentiation into a recognizable gamont. Developing meronts are multinucleate. Merogony may involve **endopolygeny**, which is multiple fission or apparent "budding" of merozoites from the periphery of the meront or from infoldings of it. A single residual body, surrounded by slightly curved, fusiform, or banana-shaped uninucleate merozoites, or many spherical clusters of merozoites with a central residuum, may be present. A second form of replication, termed **endodyogeny**, occurs in meronts of many of the heteroxenous coccidia. Two daughter organisms develop within a mother organism, which is destroyed when they are released. The location of a meront, and the number of merozoites it contains, vary with the species and the generation of merogony. A very few, or up to tens or hundreds of thousands of merozoites, may be released from a single meront.

Microgamonts mature in 2 steps. The first involves enlargement of the gamont and proliferation of nuclei. During the second phase, the microgametes differentiate about the periphery of the gamont, which may become deeply folded or fissured by invaginations. Immature microgametocytes during these stages may resemble developing schizonts. However, *fully differentiated microgametes* differ from merozoites in being small, densely basophilic, and comma-shaped, with 2-3 flagella. They may be present in swirling masses, perhaps with some residual bodies, in mature microgametocytes. Macrogametes, the female stage, have a large nucleus with a prominent nucleolus, and with time they usually enlarge to contain refractile eosinophilic "plastic granules" or wall-forming bodies, which give rise to the layers of the oocyst wall. *Mature macrogametes* typically have prominent wall-forming bodies, and contain clear or PAS-positive amylopectin granules, and a large nucleus and nucleolus.

Fertilization of the macrogamete by the microgamete leads to the development of the zygote, and subsequent formation of the oocyst wall. The contained *sporont* is spherical, with nucleus and nucleolus, and amylopectin granules in the cytoplasm. Sporulation usually occurs outside the host, but in *Sarcocystis* and *Frenkelia* it occurs in the tissue of the definitive host; in *Caryospora*, sporulated oocysts develop in tissues of the prey host. Sporozoites are enclosed within sporocysts, which in turn are contained within the oocyst wall. Oocysts of most coccidia, or sporocysts of *Sarcocystis* and *Frenkelia*, are passed in the feces.

Coccidia of domestic animals are relatively host, organ, and tissue specific. Asexual stages of *Toxoplasma* and *Neospora* are the obvious exception to this generalization. Species of *Eimeria* and *Cystoisospora* rarely occur in more than one genus of definitive host. Similar coccidia occurring in related genera of hosts, when tested, usually prove incapable of cross-infection.

The economic cost of coccidiosis in the mammalian food-animal species is considerable, in terms of mortality, morbidity, subclinical disease, and the cost of prevention and treatment. It is even more so in chickens. Coccidiosis is a very common cause of diarrhea in kittens and puppies, and it is almost always part of welfare kitten and puppy examinations and subsequent treatment.

Virulence reflects a number of factors. Among these are the species of coccidia, location and type of cell infected by various stages of the organism, the function of infected cells, and the degree of host reaction stimulated by infection. The effects of infection on the host cell are several and vary somewhat with the infecting species. Infected cells may be functionally compromised. They may hypertrophy; nuclei may enlarge or a considerable amount of cytoplasm may be displaced; and the outer membrane of infected cells may be highly modified, perhaps to facilitate metabolic exchange. The intercellular relationships may be affected. The rate of movement of infected epithelial cells up villi is altered. *Eimeria bovis* also induces apoptosis by interfering with both the receptor-mediated and inner pathways of apoptosis. Necrosis is also likely to occur. *Immune reactions* may be incited by coccidial infection. In experimental systems, resistance to coccidial infection is thymus dependent and is largely mediated by T-cell–driven intracellular killing directed mainly against asexual stages in the life cycle.

In mammals, acute inflammatory reactions in intestinal coccidiosis are most commonly associated with heavy infection and destruction of cells by the sexual stages and oocysts, rather than in response to asexual stages. In toxoplasmosis and neosporosis, necrosis and focal acute or chronic inflammatory reactions may be incited by actively replicating asexual stages in many organs. A hemorrhagic syndrome occurs in some species infected with asexual stages of *Sarcocystis*, about the time that merogony occurs in vascular endothelium.

The effects of *intestinal coccidiosis* in mammals vary with the host-parasite system. They are mainly related to malabsorption induced by *villus atrophy*, or to anemia, hypoproteinemia, and dehydration caused by exudative enteritis and colitis caused by *epithelial erosion and ulceration*. A not yet fully characterized heat-labile *neurotoxin* has been associated with the development of nervous disorders in cattle with coccidiosis. Many species of coccidia appear to have little pathogenic effect under normal circumstances.

Coccidiosis is typically a disease of *intensively managed animals*. It is especially important in naive young animals exposed to a high level of infection. This is predisposed to by high contamination rates associated with crowding, yarding, or high stocking rates on pasture. A damp substrate promotes oocyst sporulation and survival, and practices such as feeding on the ground or the natural propensity of young animals to nibble or perhaps indulge in coprophagy may promote infection. Oocysts are very hardy in the environment, making disinfection challenging. Although infections may not proceed to patency, chronic ingestion of oocysts may cause an intestinal immune response, villus atrophy, and in some situations perhaps ill-thrift. Immune reactions may only halt development of, but not kill, endogenous asexual stages. Epidemiologic evidence suggests that under some circumstances there may be relaxation of resistance and resumption of development of the organisms, ultimately expressed in disease. This seems the likely explanation for outbreaks of bovine coccidiosis occurring during midwinter in freezing climates, or in postparturient stabled dairy cattle.

Coccidiosis caused by members of the genus *Eimeria* in the various species are considered further here. The heteroxenous organisms, including *Cystoisospora*, *Toxoplasma*, *Neospora*, and *Sarcocystis*, are considered subsequently, as is *Cryptosporidium*.

Coccidiosis in cattle. Thirteen species of *Eimeria* parasitize cattle; of these, ***Eimeria zuernii*** and ***E. bovis*** are the most pathogenic; several others, notably *E. ellipsoidalis*, *E. alabamensis*, and *E. auburnensis* may cause diarrhea but probably not death (Table 1-3). *Coccidial infection is common*, and it usually comprises several species. Once *Eimeria* is present in a confinement operation, almost half the calves and yearlings shed oocysts, with calves shedding high numbers, whereas a much smaller proportion of cows shed low numbers of oocysts.

Disease occurs mainly in calves or weaned feeder cattle <1-year-old, when one or both of the potentially pathogenic species produce heavy infection. It may occur in animals at pasture or on range, concentrated at water holes, but is most common in animals in feedlots or yards where the level of sanitation is not high. The stress of shipping, cold weather, or intercurrent disease may be associated with outbreaks, which can occur in midwinter when oocyst transmission is expected to be poor. Bovine parvoviral infections have been associated with outbreaks of coccidiosis in a dry environment in northern Australia. Reactivation of latent schizonts in tissue may explain coccidiosis in stressed animals, or at a time when transmission is unlikely.

Table • 1-3

Recognized* Eimeria *species of domestic ruminants

PATHOGENICITY	CATTLE	SHEEP	GOAT
+++	*Eimeria bovis* *Eimeria zuernii*	*Eimeria ovinoidalis*	*Eimeria ninakohlyakimovae* *Eimeria caprina*
++	*Eimeria alabamensis*	*Eimeria ahsata* *Eimeria bakuensis* (*Eimeria ovina*) *Eimeria crandallis* *Eimeria gilruthi*[a]	
+	*Eimeria auburnensis* *Eimeria ellipsoidalis*	*Eimeria faurei*	*Eimeria alijevi* *Eimeria arloingi* *Eimeria aspheronica*
–	*Eimeria brasiliensis* *Eimeria bukidnonensis* *Eimeria canadensis* *Eimeria cylindrica* *Eimeria illinoisensis* *Eimeria pellita* *Eimeria subspherica* *Eimeria wyomingensis*	*Eimeria granulosa* *Eimeria intricata* *Eimeria marsica* *Eimeria pallida* *Eimeria parva* *Eimeria punctata* *Eimeria weybridgensis*	*Eimeria caprovina* *Eimeria christenseni* *Eimeria hirci* *Eimeria jolchijevi* *Eimeria kocharli*

[a]The meronts are observed in ovine abomasum. The species is suspected to be invalid, and is probably the developmental stage of a nonidentified *Eimeria* sp.
+++ = highly pathogenic; ++ = moderately pathogenic; + = mildly pathogenic; – = nonpathogenic.
From Bangoura B, Bradsley KD. Ruminant coccidiosis. Vet Clin North Am Food Anim Pract 2020;36:187–203.

In coccidiosis, *diarrhea that may progress to dysentery* with mucus, and tenesmus, perhaps causing rectal prolapse. Animals dehydrate and become hyponatremic and sometimes anemic. Morbidity may be high, but mortality is usually low. The duration of severe disease is ~3-10 days, after which most cases recover, because infection is essentially self-limiting. Some animals develop concurrent nervous signs, including tremors, nystagmus, opisthotonos, and convulsions, and many of these die within a few days.

The signs in bovine coccidiosis resulting from *E. zuernii* and *E. bovis* occur when the epithelium in the glands of the cecum and colon is infected by second-generation schizonts and gametocytes. In heavily infected animals, disease and sometimes death can occur before many oocysts are passed in the feces. The life cycles of both agents are similar, 2 schizogonous generations preceding gametogony. The first-generation schizont of ***E. bovis*** infects hypertrophic endothelial cells in lacteals on the upper part of villi in the *lower small intestine*, several meters proximal to the ileocecal valve. These schizonts may be large, up to ~300 µm in diameter, and are visible to the naked eye as *pinpoint white nodules in the mucosa*. They contain tens of thousands of merozoites but are invested by only a narrow rim of mononuclear inflammatory cells, unless they degenerate, when a marked local mixed reaction develops, including neutrophils and macrophages. Merozoites released from these schizonts ~14-18 days after infection enter cells deep in cecal and colonic glands. In heavy infections, intestinal crypts in the terminal ileum also may be infected. Here they produce small second-generation schizonts, which in turn release merozoites, infecting other cells in the gland. Gametogony may begin as early as 15 days after infection, and oocyst production peaks ~19-21 days after infection.

The first-generation schizonts of ***E. zuernii*** may be about the same size as those of *E. bovis*. However, they are most common in the *terminal meter of the ileum* and are located in the lamina propria below the crypt-villus junction, often deep near the muscularis mucosa, rather than in the endothelium of the lacteal. Hence, they are not so readily visible grossly as those of *E. bovis*. The second-generation schizonts and gamonts of *E. zuernii* also occur in glands of the cecum and colon, but not the terminal ileum. The merozoites tend to be somewhat longer (up to 15 µm) and schizonts more numerous and of greater diameter (~14 µm) than those of *E. bovis*. The timing of the development of *E. zuernii* infection is similar to that of *E. bovis*. First-generation schizonts of *E. bovis* occasionally reach the mesenteric lymph node, where they may mature, with no significance.

Animals dying of coccidiosis have fecal staining of the hindquarters, and may be somewhat cachectic and anemic. The **gross** enteric lesions in severe cases are those of *hemorrhagic or fibrinohemorrhagic typhlocolitis*, which may extend to the rectum (Fig. 1-155A); if *E. bovis* is involved, the terminal ileum also may be affected and sometimes a few schizonts are visible in the ileal villi. The contents of the large bowel are usually abnormally fluid and may vary from brown to black to overtly red, possibly with flecks of mucus or fibrin. The mucosa is edematous, with exaggerated longitudinal and perhaps transverse folds, which may be congested. Submucosal edema is also marked. Fibrin strands or a patchy diphtheritic membrane may be present on the mucosa, and fibrin casts can form. In milder cases, lesions are limited to congestion and edema of the mucosa.

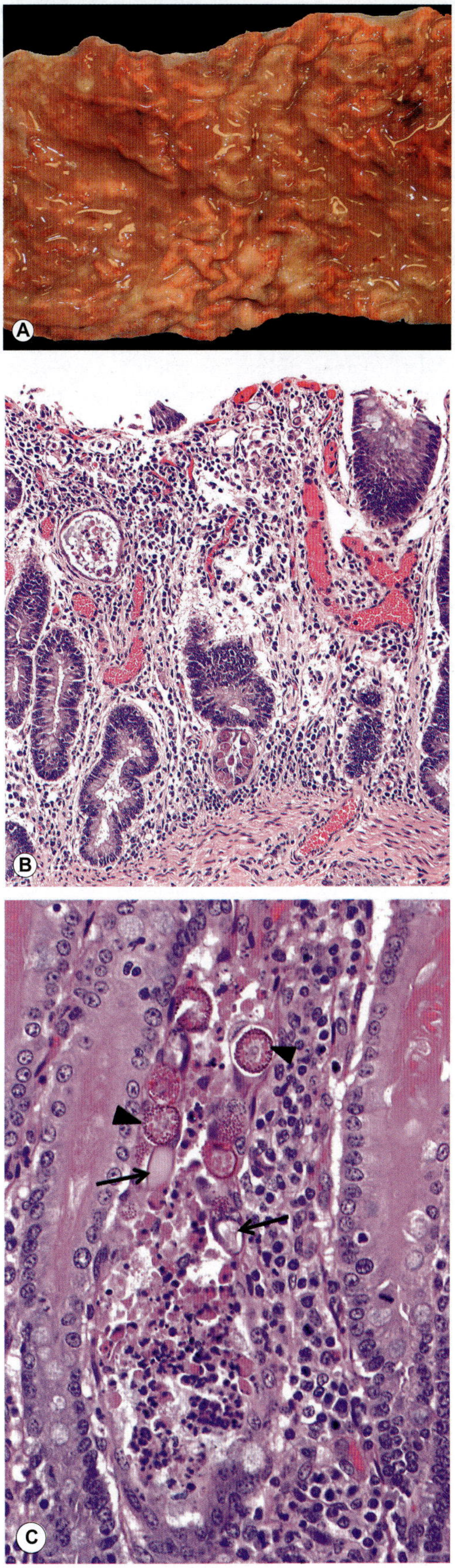

Figure 1-155 Enteric coccidiosis. **A.** Acute necrohemorrhagic colitis in a bovid. (Courtesy R. Moeller.) **B.** Heavy infection and destruction of colonic glands by gamonts. **C.** Destruction of colonic glands by developing gamonts (arrowheads). Oocysts (arrows) are in the lumen of a necrotic gland.

Microscopically, in animals dying at the peak of infection, virtually all cells lining cecal and colonic glands in many areas are infected by small schizonts, gamonts, or developing oocysts. Cells infected by *E. bovis* tend to dissociate and project into the lumen of the gland. As cells are disrupted and oocysts are released into the lumen of glands, the remaining glandular epithelium becomes extremely attenuated, or the gland collapses (see Fig. 1-155B and C). Concurrently, the surface epithelium becomes squamous, or the mucosa is eroded, and effusion of fibrin, neutrophils, and hemorrhage occurs from dilated, congested superficial vessels. Oocysts released into the glands and lumen of the colon may be seen in the exudate. At the same time, the mucosa begins to collapse, and the lamina propria is infiltrated by neutrophils, eosinophils, lymphocytes, macrophages, and plasma cells. Oocysts trapped in denuded glands in the collapsed mucosa may be surrounded by small giant cells.

If destruction is widespread, and the animal survives sufficiently long, the *mucosa may ulcerate* to the level of the muscularis mucosa and begin to granulate. In areas where the lesion is patchy, glands that have been relatively spared may become lined with hyperplastic epithelium, making an attempt to regenerate the mucosa. Flattened epithelial cells spread from these glands across the denuded surface, beneath the diphtheritic exudate. A few crenated oocysts in small giant cells in the stromal remnants of the mucosa may be the only evidence of coccidiosis found in lesions in animals surviving for 7-10 days.

Malabsorption caused by mucosal damage in the cecum and colon, and inflammatory effusion and hemorrhage explain the enteric signs of coccidiosis. The nervous signs in bovine coccidiosis are not associated with recognized lesions in the brain; they have been related to a not yet fully characterized neurotoxin found in the blood of affected animals.

The gross lesions of coccidiosis in cattle must be differentiated from those in salmonellosis, BVD, MCF, and bovine adenoviral and coronaviral infection, all of which may cause colitis or typhlocolitis. Coccidiosis often can be confirmed simply at autopsy by finding large numbers of developing stages in mucosal scrapings observed in wet-mount preparations. Oocysts of *E. bovis* are ovoid, smooth, and ~28 × 21 μm; those of *E. zuernii* are subspherical-to-ovoid, smooth, and ~18 × 15 μm.

Although other coccidia are unlikely to be the primary cause of diarrhea or death in cattle, several have distinctive endogenous stages that may be recognized in tissue section. ***E. auburnensis*** has a giant first-generation schizont that may be confused with those of *E. bovis* and *E. zuernii*. However, they are present usually 6-12 m cranial to the ileocecal valve and form in the epithelium deep in intestinal crypts, although this may not be apparent because of plane of section, or following their migration into the lamina propria. Second-generation schizonts and gamonts of *E. auburnensis* develop in the lamina propria in the ileum, small schizonts in villi, and gamonts in the deeper lamina propria. Microgametocytes may be several hundred micrometers across. Oocysts are ~38 × 23 μm.

The other bovine coccidian with gamonts apparently developing in the lamina propria is ***Eimeria bukidnonensis***. Oocysts of this species are large, ~48 × 35 μm, and thick-walled, with a micropyle, and have been found in the lamina propria. ***E. alabamensis*** develops in vacuoles within the nucleus of epithelial cells in the small intestine and, in heavy infections, the large bowel. Both schizonts and gamonts may be found together within the same nucleus. Gamonts of ***Eimeria kosti*** have been described in the epithelium deep in the abomasal glands. None of these organisms is particularly pathogenic.

Eimeria bareillyi is associated with clinical coccidiosis in water buffalo calves. The serosal vessels in the distal half of the small intestine are congested, and the lumen of the lower small bowel contains creamy or yellow fluid content in which some mucus, fibrin, or blood may be present. Focal-to-coalescent pale raised plaques or polypoid masses may be present on the mucosa, or the surface may appear granular and necrotic, with petechial hemorrhages. The gross changes are caused by hypertrophy of crypts and villi, upon which virtually every cell is infected with developing gamonts or oocysts. *E. bareillyi* will not cross-transmit to domestic cattle, although *E. ellipsoidalis* and *E. zuernii* of bubaline origin will. *E. zuernii* is pathogenic in water buffalo.

Coccidiosis in sheep and goats. *Coccidial infection is universal in sheep and goats*, and coccidiosis can be a significant problem in the young of both species. The etiology of coccidiosis in these species is complicated by the morphologic similarity of the coccidia infecting sheep and goats (see Table 1-3). Assumptions on the potential for cross-infection of coccidia between sheep and goats, and of the species found in each host, have been revised as new taxonomic and biologic information has come to light.

About a dozen species of coccidia are found in each of sheep and goats (see Table 1-3). Of these, three (*Eimeria pallida, E. caprovina, E. punctata*) may occur in both sheep and goats, although the validity of *E. punctata* as a species is questioned. Eight species pairs of *Eimeria* occur, in which the coccidia look and behave similarly in sheep and goats, but do not cross-infect. Listing the sheep-adapted species of each pair first, these are: *E. ahsata-E. christenseni; E. ovinoidalis-E. ninakohlyakimovae; E. bakuensis (=ovina)-E. arloingi; E. granulosa-E. jolchijevi; E. crandallis-E. hirci; E. faurei-E. apsheronica; E. parva-E. alijevi; E. intricata-E. kochrii.* Two *Eimeria* species are unique to sheep, *E. weybridgensis* (formerly *E. arloingi* "B") and *E. marsica;* in goats, one species, *E. caprina*, is unique. In addition, giant schizonts of an unknown coccidian, termed *E. (formerly Globidium) gilruthi*, are seen incidentally as pinpoint white foci in the abomasum of sheep and goats. *E. gilruthi* is assumed to be a stage of another intestinal *Eimeria* species rather than an individual species. An individual case of proliferative abomasitis associated with this parasite was described in a sheep. The taxonomic confusion has been carried over into descriptions of the natural or experimental disease, because many infections were of mixed species, resulted from inocula of poorly defined species of coccidia, or occurred under circumstances in which the oocysts associated were not described. However, although the taxonomic picture has changed, the syndromes associated with coccidiosis in sheep and goats have not.

Coccidiosis in sheep and goats is a disease of young animals. Under conditions of intensive pastoral husbandry or confinement, lambs and kids are exposed to oocysts of many species of coccidia within the first few days of life. Weaned lambs, presumably exposed to only light infections while at range, are also prone to coccidiosis when brought into feedlots. In young suckled animals and those in feedlots exposed to large numbers of oocysts, signs may occur before oocysts are passed. Suckling lambs, ~4-8-weeks-old, reared at pasture at relatively heavy stocking rates, may also develop signs and occasionally die. Under these conditions, the disease needs to be differentiated from GI helminthosis, which may be concurrent.

Outbreaks of coccidiosis in confined lambs and kids are usually acute, with moderate morbidity and low mortality; there is green or yellow watery *diarrhea*, occasionally with blood or mucus. Yarded and grazing animals may also suffer weight loss, or subclinical ill-thrift. Signs are usually associated with lesions in the lower small intestine, caused by *E. ahsata* and *E. bakuensis* in lambs, and their analogues in goats, *E. christenseni*, and *E. arloingi*, or with typhlocolitis, caused by *E. ovinoidalis* in sheep, and *E. ninakohlyakimovae* in goats. Some pathogenicity is also ascribed to *E. faurei*, *E. intricata*, *E. parva*, and *E. crandallis* in sheep, and presumably to their analogues in goats. Infections may be mixed, and gross and microscopic lesions may reflect this.

E. ovinoidalis in sheep and ***E. ninakohlyakimovae*** in goats presumably have similar endogenous development. In the sheep, giant schizonts up to 300 µm in diameter develop in cells deep in the lamina propria, in the terminal ileum. They release merozoites that enter epithelium in the glands of the cecum and colon, and sometimes distal ileum. Here, small second-generation schizonts evolve, and other cells in glands in the same area subsequently become infected by the gametocytes. These species are considered highly pathogenic and *E. ovinoidalis* often is associated with disease in feedlot lambs. Lesions other than those related to diarrhea, dehydration, and hypoproteinemia are limited to the terminal ileum, and especially the cecum and proximal colon, and are associated with second-generation schizogony and gametogony. Affected areas of gut are edematous and thickened. The most significant microscopic lesions are those in the cecum and colon, which resemble those in cattle caused by *E. bovis* and *E. zuernii*. ***E. caprina*** in goats also seems to have pathogenic potential. Like *E. ninakohlyakimovae*, it causes typhlocolitis; the small intestine is not involved.

E. christenseni and *E. arloingi* in goats and their analogues, *E. ahsata* and *E. bakuensis* in sheep, are also associated with serious disease. They seem to have somewhat similar developmental cycles and lesions, although interpretation of the literature is clouded by confusion among these species. Many cases of coccidiosis in lambs attributed to *E. bakuensis* (as *E. arloingi*) may in fact have been due to *E. ahsata* because the unsporulated oocysts, although of differing sizes, can be confused.

E. christenseni has a developmental cycle that involves giant schizonts up to nearly 300 µm across in the endothelium of the lacteal in villi in the middle small intestine. In heavy infections, every cell in a number of contiguous crypt-villus units may be infected. Although there may be an acute local reaction around ruptured primary schizonts, clinical disease is associated with the subsequent stages of development, diarrhea occurring during the late prepatent and patent periods. Affected intestine may be congested and edematous. Numerous pale white-or-yellow foci from a few millimeters to up to a centimeter in diameter, often visible from the serosa, are present as slightly raised plaques on the mucosa of the small bowel. These foci are areas of intense infection of cryptal and villus epithelium by gamonts and developing oocysts, and have been dubbed "*oocyst patches*."

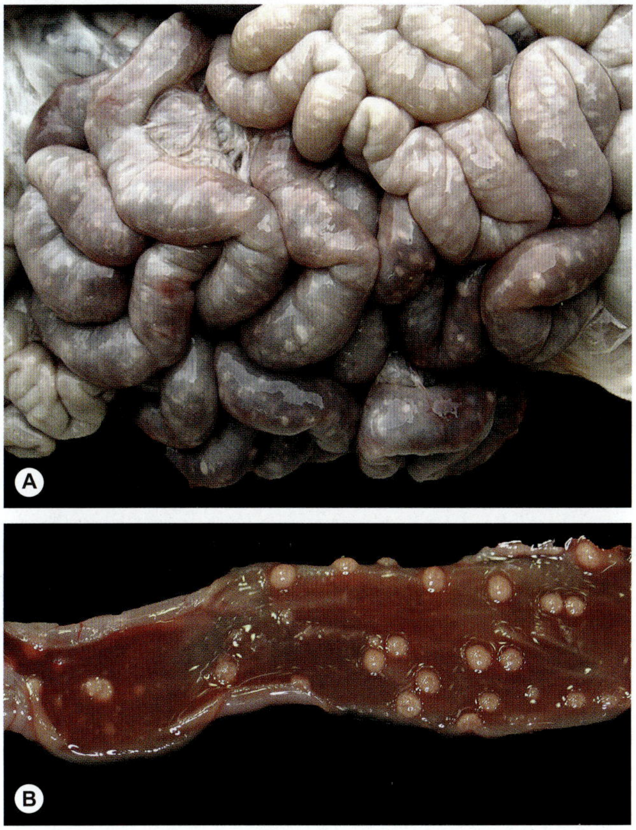

Figure 1-156 Enteric coccidiosis. A. White nodules can be seen through the serosa of the small intestine in a goat. (Courtesy V. Psychas.) **B.** White nodules present in the mucosa of the intestine in a goat. (Courtesy F. Giannitti.)

There may be some hemorrhage into the intestine, but the feces are rarely bloody.

E. arloingi undergoes a development similar to that of *E. christenseni* and causes similar gross and microscopic lesions in goats, with minor differences. First-generation schizonts are most numerous in the lacteals of villi in the lower jejunum, gamonts are mainly above the host cell nucleus. The associated gross lesions consist of nodules in the mucosa that also can be seen from the serosa (Fig. 1-156A and B); they tend to be more distal in the small intestine, and occasionally involve the large bowel. ***E. ahsata*** and ***E. bakuensis*** in sheep are similar.

Nodular polypoid structures, sometimes pedunculate, and ~0.3-1.5 cm in diameter, are encountered in the small intestinal mucosa of sheep and goats, usually as an incidental finding. These masses are hypertrophic crypt-villus units, in which virtually every epithelial cell is infected by mainly gametocytic stages of coccidia, which, in sheep, are probably *E. bakuensis* and *E. ahsata* (Fig. 1-157A and B).

Adjacent mucosa appears normal and is uninfected. The term "pseudoadenomatous" has been used to describe these polypoid lesions, and the oocyst patches or plaques was discussed earlier in the section on coccidian-infected sheep and goats. The infected epithelial cells appear somewhat hypertrophic, with eosinophilic cytoplasm and prominent brush borders. Often these coccidia-infected cells do not slough rapidly postmortem, in contrast with their uninfected fellows.

Why masses of infected cells apparently persist in chronically infected animals without clinical disease is unclear.

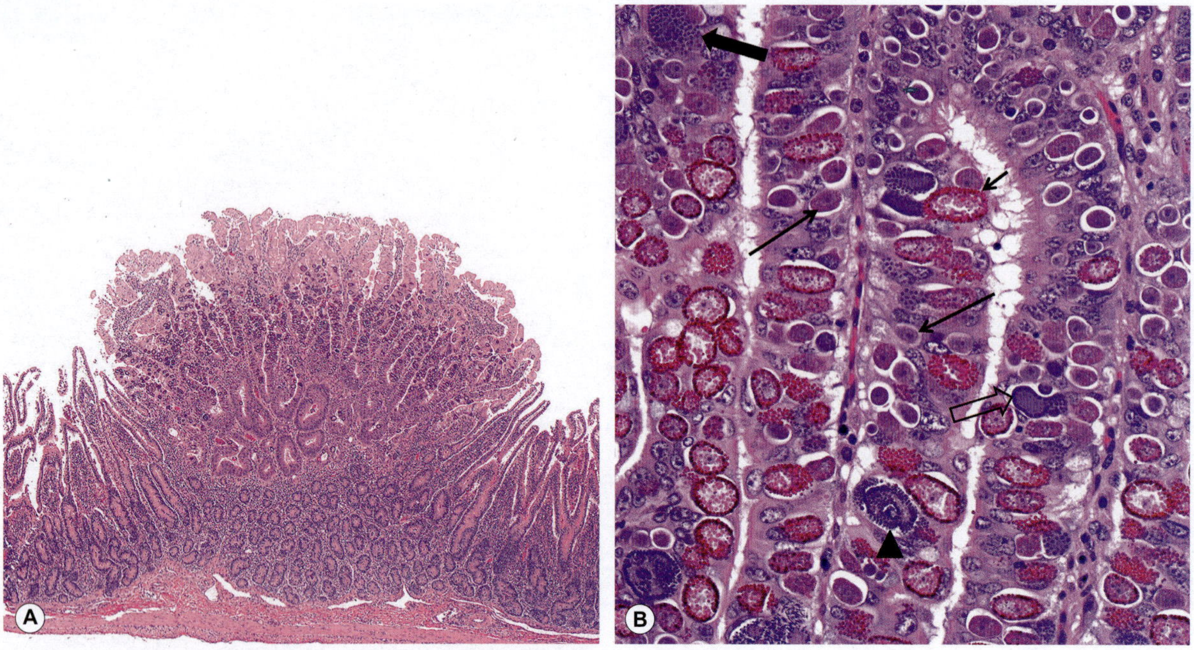

Figure 1-157 Enteric coccidiosis. A. Mucosal polyp with coccidial forms within many epithelial cells. **B**. Undifferentiated gamonts (long arrows), macrogametocytes (short arrow), microgametocytes (arrowhead), large schizonts (thick arrow), and developing oocysts (hollow arrow) in epithelium of ileal crypts and villi in a goat.

However, the plaques and polyps may be the result of mitogenic stimuli from progamonts, the immature stages in crypt epithelium, which appear to divide by binary fission in synchrony with the infected host cell.

Coccidiosis may also cause ill-thrift and diarrhea in suckling or weanling lambs 5-6-weeks-old heavily stocked on pasture. In the United Kingdom, ***E. crandallis***, which develops largely in the ileum, and ***E. ovinoidalis*** are mainly associated with this syndrome. ***E. weybridgensis*** (*E. arloingi* "B"), which infects most of the length of the small intestine, may also contribute. The only gross lesion in affected lambs is congestion and thickening of the mucosa of the lower small intestine.

Under some circumstances, probably sudden exposure to large doses of oocysts, ***E. crandallis***, at least, causes *villus atrophy* in infected areas of intestine. Giant first-generation schizonts develop in crypt cells that after infection migrate into the lamina propria. As the infection progresses, villi become stumpy or disappear, and in small bowel and cecum, crypts are straight, hypertrophic, and contain proliferative epithelium. Asexual or, more commonly, sexual stages of coccidia are present in epithelium on the surface of the mucosa. In hyperplastic crypts, epithelial cells are infected by progamonts, which seem to be dividing in synchrony with host cells. Masses of macrophages may invest and invade the base of infected crypts, and apoptosis of infected and uninfected cells may occur, resulting in attenuation of surviving crypt epithelium. In heavy infections, there also may be thickening of the cecal mucosa by hyperplastic coccidia-infected cells. Occasionally, areas of small intestine and cecum, in which there has been severe damage to crypts, may become eroded. Such lesions, if widespread, may cause malabsorption or perhaps PLE. It is unclear whether atrophy of villi is the result of excess loss of epithelium directly because of the effects of coccidial infection, or whether it is mediated by an immune response.

E. apsheronica in the goat has minor pathogenic potential. Giant schizonts develop in the lamina propria of villi throughout the small intestine and in the cecum; second-generation schizonts are in the epithelium on villi in the small intestine, and in the cecum, but not the colon. Gametocytes have the same distribution. Pale foci in the mucosa, where gametocytes are concentrated, and focal areas of erosion and hemorrhage, may occur in heavily infected animals.

Large schizonts are often encountered incidentally in submucosal lymphatics, or in the subcortical or medullary sinusoids of mesenteric lymph nodes in sheep and goats. Sometimes they may be visible grossly in these locations as pinpoint white foci. Occasionally, coccidial gametocytes or oocysts may also develop in intestinal lymphoid aggregates and mesenteric lymph nodes, where they may provoke a mild granulomatous reaction. Stages in lymph nodes probably result from establishment of sporozoites or primary merozoites swept from the lacteal into the lymphatic drainage early in infection. Development in such sites is not uncommon, but aberrant and likely dead-end. The species involved appear mainly to be those considered in the previous section, with a giant primary schizont developing in the lacteal.

In coccidiosis, *oocysts are usually numerous in feces*, but this is neither constant in, nor necessarily indicative of, disease. Mucosal scrapings or tissue sections of mucosa containing large numbers of asexual and gametogenous coccidial forms, in association with diarrhea, and perhaps some hemorrhage into the intestine, support the diagnosis, in the absence of other syndromes such as GI helminthosis.

Coccidiosis in horses. The only coccidian of horses reported with any frequency is ***Eimeria leuckarti***, which is found in horses and donkeys the world over. The complete mitochondrial genome of *E. leuckarti* has been determined. This is considered to be the only valid *Eimeria* species of equids, and it infects a range of both domestic and wild horses. In one survey of foals in Germany, it was found in 100% of animals, but prevalence elsewhere is usually very low. In a survey of horses in Iran, *E. leuckarti* was found in <1% of healthy horses. Although the infection by *E. leuckarti* is most common in foals, it also occasionally has been seen in adult animals. Its reputation for pathogenicity rests largely on the *distinctive large gamonts* found in the lamina propria of the small intestine in animals dead of enteric disease of undetermined etiology. However, implication of *E. leuckarti* in the disease process is rarely, if ever, convincing, and this parasite is encountered incidentally in the intestine of horses dead of other clearly defined conditions. Furthermore, heavy experimental inoculations, producing many gamonts in the gut and heavy oocyst passage, have failed to elicit clinical signs.

The stages present in the lamina propria of villi are giant microgametocytes and macrogametes, developing in markedly hypertrophic host cells, probably of epithelial origin (Fig. 1-158). The microgametocytes are up to ~250 µm in diameter, and when mature they contain swirling masses of microgametes. Immature microgametocytes very much resemble some of the giant schizonts of other species of coccidia and have frequently been referred to as such; this stimulated the application of the term *Globidium* to the organism. However, the only schizont containing merozoites that has been recognized in horses was very small (12.5 µm in diameter), and in the epithelium of the ileum. The macrogametes have distinctive large eosinophilic or PAS-positive granules that may be individual or confluent. The host cells are markedly hypertrophic with a fibrillar periphery, and the enlarged nucleus forms a crescent along one side of the parasitophorous vacuole. There is no inflammatory response to the gamonts, and only a mild reaction to degenerate stages in the lamina propria.

Coccidiosis in swine. At least 8-10 species of *Eimeria* are thought to occur in swine, along with a single species of *Cystoisospora*. The latter, ***Cystoisospora* (*Isospora*) *suis***, is the most important; it causes *porcine neonatal coccidiosis*, a disease of piglets ~5-6-days- to ~2-3-weeks-old. This disease is recognized in the United States, Canada, the United Kingdom,

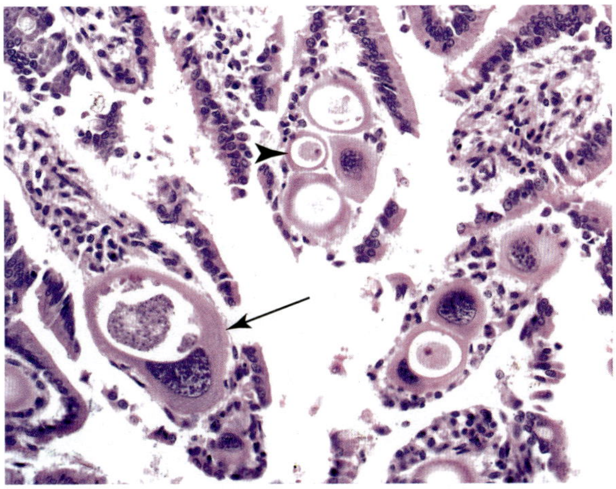

Figure 1-158 ***Eimeria leuckarti*** infection in a horse. Microgametocyte (arrow) and developing oocyst (arrowhead) in the intestinal lamina propria.

and western Europe; it also occurs in Australia, and probably wherever swine are reared intensively. The condition is most severe in herds in which continuous farrowing and total confinement are practiced, and some laboratories report a prevalence of 10-50% among scouring baby pigs. Rapid sporulation (12 hours) and short prepatent period (5 days) promote rapid buildup of coccidia in a farrowing house.

Porcine neonatal coccidiosis has high morbidity, and usually low but variable mortality. It causes yellow watery diarrhea, dehydration, loss of condition, and death, or at least a temporary check in growth. Some animals may runt severely. Illness usually begins at ~7-10 days of age. Piglets continue to nurse but may vomit clotted milk. At autopsy, many piglets have the typical appearance of undifferentiated neonatal diarrhea, with no specific gross findings in the GI tract other than fluid yellow content. However, the intestine in some animals with coccidiosis may look turgid, rather than flaccid, and in a minority of animals fibrinous or fibrinonecrotic exudate is present in the lower portion of the small intestine. Occasionally, casts form.

C. suis replicates in the epithelium on the *distal third of villi*, mainly in the *jejunum and ileum*, although infected cells may be found in the duodenum and colon in a few animals. Piglets usually become infected within the first day or two of life, perhaps by ingestion of the sow's feces. Merogony occurs in vacuoles in the cytoplasm, usually beneath the nucleus of the host cell. Infection of host cells is maximal 4-5 days after infection, and by 5 days gametogony is evident. Thick- and thin-walled sporulated oocysts have been observed in feces of infected pigs, but either form may cause disease. The onset of lesions and clinical signs corresponds with this period of heavy infection of cells, which undergo lysis. Villi may become markedly atrophic. The lumen contains massive numbers of exfoliated epithelial cells, inflammatory cells, and coccidial stages. The surface epithelium that remains is cuboidal-to-squamous, and infected epithelial cells may be seen degenerating or exfoliating. Erosions may develop at the tips of villi, through which there is effusion of neutrophils and fibrin. In the remnant of the villus, neutrophil infiltration, a moderate increase in mononuclear leukocytes and eosinophilic proteinaceous material, probably collagen, may be present in the lamina propria. Effusion of neutrophils and fibrin from the eroded tips of villi contributes to the fibrinonecrotic membrane seen in some animals, and ulceration can occur (Fig. 1-159A). Gram-positive bacilli are often present in the exudate. In animals surviving for a few days, the cryptal epithelium may be markedly hyperplastic.

The severity of the lesions is a function of the size of the inoculum and the age of the pigs. Heavier inocula, within limits, produce more cellular damage and villus atrophy; fibrinonecrotic enteritis indicates ingestion of a large dose of oocysts. However, severe lesions may not be associated with heavy shedding of oocysts because relatively few gamonts are able to develop in the reduced population of epithelial cells remaining on villi. The severity of lesions and signs is much greater in piglets a few days old in comparison with those 2-weeks-old. This is partly related to the lower rate of replication of epithelium in the crypts of young piglets, and therefore the development of more severe villus atrophy. The smaller size of young piglets also makes them more susceptible to the effects of malabsorption and diarrhea. Animals previously exposed to *C. suis* have relatively strong resistance to challenge.

A **diagnosis** of coccidiosis must be considered in scouring neonatal piglets and is strongly suggested by *fibrinonecrotic enteritis in the distal small bowel*. Atrophy of villi may be recognized at autopsy using a hand lens or stereomicroscope, or in tissue section. Asexual or sexual stages may be found in smears of mucosal scrapings. The distinctive binucleate type I meronts and pairs of large (12-18 µm in smears, 8-13 µm in sections) type I merozoites may be found in jejunal mucosa in the early phase of diarrheal disease. Multinucleate type II meronts and numerous small type II merozoites are the predominant stage during the clinical phase of disease. In section, these form clusters of 2-16 organisms such as bunches of bananas, perhaps with a small residual body, in the parasitophorous vacuole in the enterocyte (see Fig. 1-159B).

Macrogamonts and microgamonts are present in moderate numbers by day 5 of infection, and a few oocysts also may be seen. Microgametocytes are ~9-16 µm in diameter and are multinucleate. Oocysts in tissue sections are oval, ~15 × 12 µm; those in smears are ~18 × 16 µm. Coccidial stages may be difficult to find in animals that have been ill for several days. Oocysts may not be found in feces because the infection is not yet patent, the patent period has passed, or the lesions are very severe, reducing the number of oocysts produced.

Coccidiosis in older swine caused by several *Eimeria* species is uncommon; speciation can be accomplished. It typically occurs in animals with access to yards or pasture contaminated with oocysts. Weaners and growing pigs are affected. The species considered potentially pathogenic include ***Eimeria scabra, E. debliecki***, and ***E. spinosa***. It is difficult to produce disease in experimentally inoculated pigs; *E. scabra* is probably the most pathogenic. Coccidiosis in older swine is usually sporadic or affects a few pigs in a group. Typically, it causes diarrhea of a few days' duration, loss of appetite, and perhaps transient ill-thrift, or, in severe cases, emaciation. Occasionally animals die.

Lesions are usually limited to the lower small intestine, which may be congested or hemorrhagic, although overt blood is rarely found in the feces. Large numbers of schizonts, gamonts, and developing oocysts are in epithelial cells on villi and sometimes in crypts. Atrophy of villi, or erosion and local hemorrhage or inflammatory effusion may be evident, the lamina propria is edematous, and desquamated epithelium and oocysts are in the lumen of the gut. Rarely, heavily infected animals may have lesions in the large intestine. The species involved are diagnosed on the basis of the morphology of oocysts in feces or mucosal scrapings.

Coccidial gamonts and oocysts of a species resembling *E. debliecki* have been found infecting epithelium on the papilliform mucosa of cystic bile ducts in porcine liver. This is probably an aberrant site of development.

Coccidiosis in dogs and cats. Although several species of *Eimeria* have been reported from dogs and cats, their status as genuine parasites of these hosts is in doubt. The significant coccidia of dogs and cats are members of the genus *Cystoisospora*, considered here, and of the genera *Toxoplasma*, *Sarcocystis*, *Hammondia*, *Besnoitia*, and *Neospora*, dealt with subsequently. *Caryospora* spp. may occasionally produce dermal coccidiosis in immunosuppressed dogs.

Cystoisospora spp. oocysts are passed unsporulated in feces, and, when sporulated, have 2 sporocysts lacking a Stieda body, each with 4 sporozoites. Following ingestion of sporulated oocysts of heteroxenous species, transport hosts, usually prey species such as mice and other small rodents, but sometimes other hosts, are infected by large sporozoite-like "hypnozoites" in phagocytic cells in lymph nodes and other tissues. These, when ingested by the predator, resume development in the intestine, and lead to asexual and sexual development in the definitive host. Heteroxenous passage is not obligatory, and sporulated oocysts are also directly infective to the definitive host.

In **dogs**, 4 species of *Cystoisospora* are recognized. Meronts of ***Cystoisospora canis*** develop in the subepithelial lamina propria of the villi in the distal small intestine and, to a lesser extent, in the large bowel. Gamonts occur beneath and within the epithelium of the ileum and large intestine, and the oocyst is the largest among *Cystoisospora* spp. of dogs, being ~38 ×

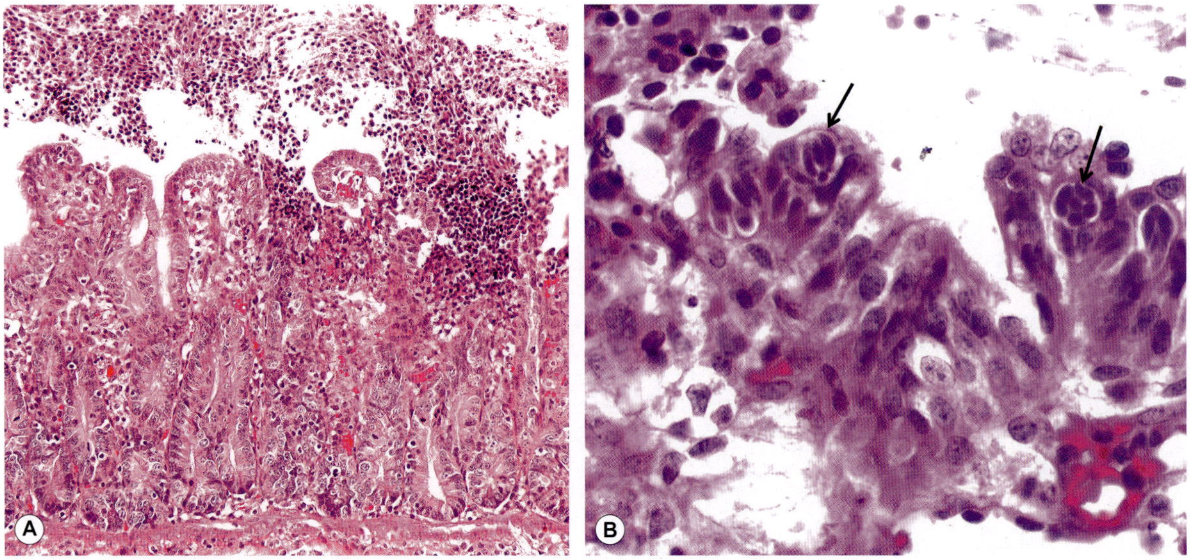

Figure 1-159 **Porcine coccidiosis** by *Cystoisospora suis*. **A.** Blunting and atrophy of villi. Erosions are present at the tip of villi, and there is effusion of neutrophils and fibrin into the lumen. **B.** Meronts containing merozoites (arrows) in epithelial cells.

30 µm. The other 3 are members of the "*Cystoisospora ohioensis* complex." **C. *ohioensis*** develops exclusively in epithelial cells, mainly in the distal portions of villi along the length of the small bowel, especially in the ileum, and occasionally in the large bowel. It may be the most pathogenic species in dogs. The oocysts of C. *burrowsi*, C. *ohioensis*, and C. *neorivolta* are similar. Original literature should be consulted for details that will permit differentiation of these species in tissue. Endogenous stages of ***C. burrowsi*** occur in epithelial cells, and in the lamina propria of the tips of villi in the distal two-thirds of the small intestine. ***C. neorivolta*** mainly develops in proprial cells beneath the epithelium in the tips of villi in the distal half of the small intestine, and rarely in the cecum and colon. Occasional stages may be in the epithelium. C. *canis* and C. *ohioensis* are known to be heteroxenous. Meronts of an unknown coccidian, probably a *Cystoisospora* sp., have been found in the intrahepatic bile ducts of a dog, associated with severe neutrophilic cholangiohepatitis.

In **cats**, 2 species of *Cystoisospora* occur. Meronts and gamonts of ***C. felis*** develop in epithelium of villi in the small intestine, and occasionally in epithelium in the large bowel. The oocyst is large, ~43 × 33 µm. ***C. rivolta*** also develops in epithelium on villi and in crypts and glands in the small and large intestine. Oocysts are ovoid, ~25 × 23 µm. Subepithelial schizonts and gamonts of an unknown coccidian, possibly a *Cystoisospora* species, have been associated with fatal enteritis in a cat.

Coccidiosis in the dog and cat is largely a clinical entity, *usually nonfatal*. The lesions of coccidiosis in small animals are poorly defined, and care must be taken not to ascribe disease to these organisms simply by finding endogenous stages in the mucosa of animals dead of enteric disease. Rotavirus and coronavirus might be expected to produce similar signs. However, genuine cases of fatal coccidiosis do occur, although few are recorded in the literature. Affected animals are young, and usually from environments such as pet shops, animal shelters, or kennels in which standards of sanitation may not be high. There is a history of diarrhea of several days' duration, and the animal is dehydrated. Other than mild hyperemia of the mucosa and excessively fluid content of the small intestine and colon, gross lesions in the gut may not be evident. Microscopically, there may be moderate atrophy of villi, with attenuation of surface enterocytes, and perhaps effusion of acute inflammatory exudate from the tips of some eroded villi. Asexual and sexual stages of coccidia are evident in moderate-to-large numbers in the epithelium or lamina propria of villi. In some cases, the large bowel may be infected, with exfoliation of surface epithelium, and accumulation of necrotic debris in some dilated glands.

Heteroxenous apicomplexan infection. *Toxoplasma, Neospora, Hammondia, Sarcocystis, Besnoitia*, and ***Frenkelia*** comprise this group of protists. All of these heteroxenous members of the *Apicomplexa* are known to *use carnivores as definitive hosts and* have one or more generations of merogony in the tissues of various species of prey. *Frenkelia*, which some would place in the genus *Sarcocystis*, as far as is known, uses only raptorial birds as definitive hosts and small rodents as intermediate hosts. It is not considered further.

Toxoplasmosis. Toxoplasma gondii uses felids as definitive hosts. It is optionally heteroxenous; cats may be infected directly by ingestion of oocysts, but probably most commonly by ingestion of asexual stages in the tissues of prey species. Cats excrete oocysts 3-10 days after ingesting *bradyzoites*, ~13 days after ingesting tachyzoites, and 18 days after ingesting oocysts. Transmission efficacy varies and cats can become infected after ingestion of one bradyzoite; ingestion of 1,000 oocysts is required to establish infection. Intermediate hosts are infected by oocysts shed in the feces of cats or by a variety of other routes considered later. Five stages of asexual development are recognized in the intestinal epithelium of cats infected with tissue cysts from intermediate hosts. The gametocytes also develop in epithelium on villi, especially in the *ileum*. Most cats will shed oocytes once; however, in cases of immunosuppression, repeated oocyte shedding may occur. In heavy infections, exfoliation of infected epithelium from villi is associated with the development of *villus atrophy*, and occasional spontaneous cases of diarrhea in kittens seem to be caused by *Toxoplasma*-induced atrophy of villi and malabsorption.

In intermediate hosts and in cats, extraintestinal asexual development occurs in a variety of organs and tissues. Rapidly dividing forms (*tachyzoites*) may by endodyogeny proliferate in cells in many sites for an indefinite number of generations and are the stage associated with acute toxoplasmosis in cats and other species. Eventually, tachyzoites induce the formation of a cyst wall in a host cell and divide slowly, forming bradyzoites, which reside in quiescent tissue cysts.

T. gondii, with *Neospora caninum*, is unique among protists in its ability to parasitize a wide range of hosts and tissues. *It is one of the most ubiquitous of organisms;* experimentally, essentially all homeothermic animals can be infected, and natural infections occur in birds, nonhuman primates, rodents, insectivores, herbivores, and carnivores, including domestic species and humans. Serologic surveys indicate that infection is widespread in most species of domestic animals; however, except for abortions in sheep and goats, overt disease is sporadic and rare.

Transmission may occur by a number of different routes. The shedding of oocysts in the feces of cats and wild felids has been mentioned earlier. Transplacental infection occurs commonly in sheep and goats and sporadically in swine and humans. Carnivorous animals and humans may become infected by ingesting oocysts from cats, or more commonly from cysts containing bradyzoites in tissues of infected animals, implying that the cycle of infection can be maintained by means of facultative homoxenous transmission, without a definitive host. It has been shown that infected rodents will lose avoidance behaviors to feline odor, and instead become attracted to areas where cats are present. This may favor transmission to the definitive host.

Systemic toxoplasmosis occurs most often in young animals, especially immunologically immature neonates and in immunocompromised hosts. *T. gondii* infection leads to alterations of proinflammatory and anti-inflammatory cytokine production, which includes the production of IL10, which is a negative regulator of IL12 and interferon gamma. Low levels of interferon gamma and the associated inability to activate macrophages are predisposing factors for systemic toxoplasmosis. In dogs, canine distemper, ehrlichiosis, and lymphoma are commonly concomitant with toxoplasmosis. The infection in juveniles may be acquired prenatally or postnatally. After ingestion, *Toxoplasma* organisms penetrate the intestinal mucosa. In cats, the enterointestinal cycle and systemic infection occur almost simultaneously. In other animals, the tachyzoites are the first stage of infection, after invasion of the lamina propria by sporozoites released from the oocyst, or by bradyzoites released from the tissue cyst digested from food in the intestine.

Dissemination of *Toxoplasma* occurs in lymphocytes, macrophages, granulocytes, and as free forms in plasma. From the intestine, the organism may follow 2 routes. It may spread via lymphocytes to the regional nodes and from there in the lymph to the bloodstream, or it may pass in the portal circulation to the liver and from there to the systemic circulation. Further dissemination occurs to a wide variety of organs. Tachyzoites actively invade or are phagocytosed by host cells and are surrounded in a parasitophorous vacuole formed of host cell membrane. Tachyzoites proliferate, destroying the host cell, and cell-to-cell transmission may occur within infected organs.

Focal necrosis is common and appears to be directly related to the rapid replication of tachyzoites. The outcome of infection is determined by a number of factors, including the number and strain of *Toxoplasma* in the infecting dose, and the species, age, and immune status of the host. Lesions in visceral organs are usually evident within 1-2 weeks after oral infection. Variable numbers of tachyzoites are usually found in the vicinity of the necrotic areas.

Specific immunity develops within a few days after infection; the cell-mediated arm is most significant in toxoplasmosis, mediated in large part by IL12 and interferon gamma production. This reduces the severity of infection but usually does not terminate it. Infection by *Toxoplasma* interferes with the cell-mediated immune response but does not completely inhibit it. The remaining cell-mediated immune capacity may control pathogen proliferation and promote progression to chronic disease. In experimental models lacking cytokines associated with cell-mediated immunity, including γ-interferon, *Toxoplasma* infection is nearly always fatal. In the *chronic or dormant form* of *Toxoplasma* infection, bradyzoite-containing *cysts* form mainly in the brain, skeletal muscle, and myocardium. Cysts may form as early as 1-2 weeks after infection, and they may persist for months, possibly years. Intracellular encystment protects the bradyzoites from both cellular and humoral immune mechanisms. *Inflammation is usually not associated with cysts*. When the level of resistance drops below a critical level, for example, because of treatment with immunosuppressive drugs, intercurrent disease, or other factors that depress immunity, particularly decreased levels of γ-interferon, *a chronic infection may become reactivated*. The cysts rupture and cause severe local inflammation. In experimental murine models, bradyzoites have been shown to revert to tachyzoites in the absence of γ-interferon.

The **clinical signs** of toxoplasmosis vary considerably, depending on the organs affected. The most consistent signs reported are fever, lethargy, anorexia, ocular and nasal discharges, and respiratory distress. Neurologic signs include incoordination, circling, tremors, opisthotonos, convulsions, and paresis. Paresis is often associated with radiculitis and myositis. In the dog, signs may coexist with those of canine distemper and are not sufficiently distinctive to allow ready differentiation.

Systemic toxoplasmosis has been reported in most species of domestic animals. The hallmarks are *interstitial pneumonia, focal hepatic necrosis, lymphadenitis, myocarditis,* and *mononuclear meningoencephalitis*. Pulmonary lesions are probably most consistently found, followed by CNS lesions. The lesions in the various organs are morphologically similar in most species, varying mainly in degree.

Macroscopic lesions in the lung vary from irregular gray foci of necrosis on the pleural surface to hemorrhagic pneumonia with confluent involvement of the ventral portions. Careful examination of the liver usually reveals either areas of focal necrosis or irregular mottling, and edema of the gallbladder. The spleen is enlarged, as are lymph nodes, which are wet and often red. Pleural, pericardial, and peritoneal effusions occur irregularly. Pale areas may be evident in the myocardium and skeletal muscle. Occasionally, the pancreas is the most severely affected organ, in which case an acute hemorrhagic reaction may involve the entire organ. Yellow, small, superficial intestinal ulcers with a hyperemic border have been reported in piglets. Large pale areas of necrosis may be present in the renal cortices, mainly in goats and kittens.

Microscopically, the early pulmonary lesions are *diffuse interstitial pneumonia;* the alveolar septa are thickened by a predominantly mononuclear inflammatory cell reaction with a few neutrophils and eosinophils. Macrophages and fibrinous exudate fill the alveoli. Foci of necrosis involving the alveolar septa, bronchiolar epithelial cells, and blood vessels are scattered throughout the lobules. These lesions are soon followed by regenerative changes of hyperplasia and hypertrophy of alveolar lining cells, mainly type II pneumocytes: so-called *epithelialization of alveoli*. In some areas, this may be so marked as to give the affected areas an adenomatous appearance. Tachyzoites are usually evident in alveolar macrophages and also may be found in bronchiolar epithelial cells and the walls of blood vessels.

In the *liver*, irregular foci of coagulative necrosis are scattered at random throughout the lobules. There is usually little evidence of inflammation associated with the necrotic areas. Variable numbers of tachyzoites may be present in hepatocytes and Kupffer cells, usually at the periphery of the lesions, but often at some distance. If the *pancreas* is involved, there is extensive peripancreatic fat necrosis, with areas of coagulative necrosis in parenchyma. Numerous tachyzoites usually are evident in both ductal and acinar cells.

Lesions in *lymph nodes* often are associated with infection in the corresponding organ. They are irregular areas of coagulative necrosis, mainly in the cortex. A moderate inflammatory reaction may be evident at the periphery of the necrotic areas. There may be necrosis and depletion of lymphocytes in the follicles. In more chronic cases, the changes are those of nonspecific hyperplasia of lymphoid cells in cortical and paracortical areas, with a large macrophage population in the medullary sinusoids. Tachyzoites may be seen in phagocytic cells in sinusoids. Similar lesions may occur in the *spleen;* necrotic areas are mainly located in the red pulp.

In the *heart and skeletal muscle,* foci of necrosis and mononuclear cell inflammation may be part of toxoplasmosis. There is often some difficulty in distinguishing between tachyzoites and mineralization of mitochondria in myocytes but, at some distance from areas of acute reaction, inert cysts usually can be identified in healthy fibers.

Brain lesions may vary in appearance. In the most fulminant cases, cerebral lesions may be relatively inconspicuous. They consist of mononuclear meningoencephalitis with multifocal areas of necrosis and often malacia. There is swelling of endothelial cells, necrosis of vessel walls, and vasculitis. There may be marked perivascular edema and hyperplasia of perithelial cells. Tachyzoites and occasionally cysts may be found in vessel walls and in necrotic areas in both the gray and white matter at all levels of the brain. If survival is prolonged, residual cerebral lesions consist of *microglial nodules* along with more extensive hyperplasia of perithelial cells and perivascular fibrosis that tends to make the vessels very obvious. At this stage tachyzoites are rare, and cysts 30 µm in diameter with a wall of amorphous acidophilic material ~0.5 µm thick, located in areas away from the lesions, may be the only form seen. Spinal cord lesions resemble those seen in the brain.

Systemic toxoplasmosis is reported from **cats** but is certainly seen less commonly in this species than in some others. Lesions are similar to those described for other species. Chronic granulomatous toxoplasmosis may involve the intestine in older cats and produce annular areas of thickening. The mucosa overlying the granulomas may be ulcerated.

The finding of tachyzoites and/or cysts in association with areas of coagulative necrosis in one or more organs is highly suggestive of toxoplasmosis. Often the *Toxoplasma* organisms are difficult to distinguish within the necrotic foci, and immunohistochemical techniques are very useful in highlighting their presence. Serologic tests are of limited value in the diagnosis of disease associated with *T. gondii* infection.

The placental and fetal lesions associated with *Toxoplasma* infection and abortion are described in Vol. 3, Female Genital System, and ocular lesions in Vol. 1, Special Senses.

Neosporosis. ***Neospora caninum*** causes disease in *dogs and ruminants* over much of the world. *Dogs, Australian dingoes, and coyotes are definitive hosts*; cattle, water buffalo, and white-tailed deer can act as intermediate hosts. *Neospora* has been associated with systemic and CNS disease in dogs, and with abortion and CNS disease in neonatal ruminants. Tachyzoites undergoing endodyogeny and cysts containing bradyzoites are found in the tissues of affected animals. Transplacental transmission occurs in ruminants and dogs. Infection may be maintained in lines of cattle in this manner; some subclinically infected dams have given birth to successive litters of pups that became affected within the first few months of life. Transmission may also occur by ingestion of infected tissue, as in toxoplasmosis.

Dogs of all ages may be affected, but disease seems most characteristic as *encephalomyelitis, polyradiculoneuritis*, and *polymyositis* in puppies older than ~5 weeks of age, and perhaps involving several animals in a litter. Ascending paralysis, muscle contraction causing hyperextension of the limbs, cervical weakness, and dysphagia may progress to death, or animals stabilize with caudal paralysis. In adult dogs, there are signs of widespread involvement of the CNS, and disseminated disease may be evident, with polymyositis, myocarditis, and dermatitis associated with parasite infection. Although disease may be precipitated or exacerbated by glucocorticoid administration, *Neospora* is regarded as a *primary pathogen*. Cell-mediated immunity including production of IL12 and γ-interferon may be related to immune resistance.

In acute systemic infections, there may be hepatic enlargement with coalescing areas of pallor related to widespread necrosis of hepatocytes; streaky pallor of muscles resulting from myonecrosis, mineralization, and mononuclear myositis; and pulmonary congestion and edema resulting from subacute alveolitis. Tachyzoites are common in affected tissues.

Mononuclear encephalomyelitis is associated with tachyzoites and tissue cysts in neurons and neuropil; the degree of necrosis, gliosis, neovascularization, and demyelination presumably depends to some extent on the duration of the lesion. Retinitis is also reported in association with *Neospora*, as is pyogranulomatous ulcerative dermatitis, occasionally.

In **ruminant abortion**, *Neospora* may be associated with *necrotizing placentitis*, and with *myositis* and *mononuclear encephalomyelitis* of the fetus after ~90 days of gestation. Gestation may lead to diminished γ-interferon production and this may promote dissemination of parasites to the fetus. Although a well-documented etiologic agent of abortion in cattle, the extent of natural *Neospora*-induced abortions in sheep and goats is unknown. Experimentally, sheep and pigs experience placental infection and necrotizing encephalitis in the fetuses. *N. caninum* also has been reported from a case of equine protozoal myelitis. *Neospora* has been isolated from wildlife including white-tailed deer and water buffalo.

Tachyzoites are ovoid, ~5-7 µm long, and are found in small groups or large clusters, free in the cytoplasm or in parasitophorous vacuoles in many types of cells throughout the body. Tissue cysts are found in only the brain and spinal cord. They are spherical or slightly elongate, up to ~110 µm in greatest dimension. The cyst wall is ~1–4 µm thick, usually greater than the width of the bradyzoites, which are slender (1.5 × 7 µm), slightly curved, with an obvious nucleus; they stain weakly PAS positive.

Neospora must be distinguished from *Toxoplasma* in all species, and from *Sarcocystis* in aborted fetuses. *Neospora* tachyzoites resemble those of *Toxoplasma* in tissue section. Ultrastructurally, *Neospora* tachyzoites have >11 rhoptries; there are few in *Toxoplasma*. *Toxoplasma* is always found in a membrane-bound vacuole in the cytoplasm; *Neospora* tachyzoites are often not within a parasitophorous vacuole. *Neospora* tissue cysts are relatively uncommonly encountered, especially in acute cases. They are distinguished from *Toxoplasma* by the thicker wall (<0.5 µm in *Toxoplasma*). Perhaps the most common method of distinction is by IHC using specific antibodies; PCR is also useful. *Sarcocystis* meronts divide by endopolygony in endothelium in domestic animals; they are not in a parasitophorous vacuole; and merozoites lack rhoptries. Sarcocysts in muscle cells are within a parasitophorous vacuole; they have a distinct wall; and they are usually subdivided internally by septa. Diagnosis may be challenging because some fetuses with *Neospora* infection and lesions may reach the end of gestation, so lesions alone do not confirm that *Neospora* infection was the cause of abortion.

Hammondia **infection.** ***Hammondia*** spp. are obligatorily heteroxenous organisms, with the cat (***Hammondia hammondi***) and dog (***H. heydorni***) as definitive hosts. They also have been known as *Toxoplasma hammondi* and *Isospora bahiensis*, respectively. *Toxoplasma*-like oocysts are shed in the feces of the definitive host and are infectious to intermediate hosts, mammals and birds (*H. hammondi*), and ruminants (*H. heydorni*). Here, bradyzoites develop in cysts in striated muscle, which are infective when ingested by the carnivore. Disease is not associated with infection of intermediate hosts; diarrhea may occur in heavily infected dogs.

Sarcocystis **infection.** ***Sarcocystis*** is composed of ~200 obligatorily heteroxenous species. Inconspicuous sexual stages occur in the epithelium at the tips of villi in the small intestine, and oocysts sporulate in the subepithelial lamina propria, producing 2 sporocysts within a thin oocyst wall. Sporocysts containing 4 sporozoites are shed in feces. These are infective to intermediate hosts, in which 3 generations of merogony occur in vascular endothelium, and a final cyst containing first *metrocytes* (mother cells), which produce *merozoites* (bradyzoites), is formed in myocytes and occasionally other cells. Ingestion of tissue cysts containing bradyzoites initiates gametogony in the definitive host. There is apparently no resistance to the development of gamonts, and no disease is associated with them in the definitive host.

Many species of *Sarcocystis* are recognized, based on prey-predator cycles, for instance, between cattle and dogs, and cattle and cats. Sporogony of a given species usually occurs in only one or a few genera of carnivores. The number of species capable of acting as intermediate hosts may be narrow or wide, depending on the species of *Sarcocystis*.

Sarcocystis cysts in ovine and, occasionally, bovine muscle may be grossly visible, causing losses at meat inspection. *Eosinophilic myositis* can result from granulomas caused by *Sarcocystis* infection of muscle. However, studies have shown that unaffected muscle often harbors more of these organisms than the inflamed portions. *Sarcocystis* infection in cattle (***Sarcocystis cruzi***), sheep (***Sarcocystis tenella***), and swine (***S. miescheriana***), and, experimentally, in goats (***S. capracanis***), may cause acute fatal disease, with anemia and widespread hemorrhage, which is associated with clotting disorders. As the disease progresses, cattle may develop inappetence, weight loss, reduced milk yield, hyperexcitability, hair loss, and in some animals, nervous signs. Ill-thrift associated with *Sarcocystis* infection may also occur in other species. Both syndromes are initiated during the *endothelial phase* of the infection. As well, abortion occurs during this phase in some species. Abortion associated with the acute disease is the result of the systemic illness, and the fetus is usually not infected. However, in cattle, some abortions, seen in otherwise clinically normal animals, are associated with meronts of *Sarcocystis* in the placenta and in vascular endothelium of the fetus, especially in the brain, and with mononuclear encephalitis. Encephalitis is occasionally associated with *Sarcocystis* infection in sheep, and in horses ***S. neurona*** is the cause of protozoal myeloencephalitis. Details of these syndromes are discussed in Vol. 1, Muscle and Tendon; Vol. 3, Female Genital System; Vol. 1, Nervous System.

Sarcocystis spp. have been identified as causing rare incidents of severe myositis in dogs and encephalomyelitis in cats. A *Sarcocystis*-like agent also has been implicated in mortality of Rottweiler dogs with hepatitis, encephalitis, and dermatitis.

***Besnoitia* infection. *Besnoitia* spp**. are also obligatorily heteroxenous, but the definitive host for many species has not been identified. Some stages of merogony and gametogony occur in the intestine of the only definitive host yet known, the cat, where they are not known to be pathogenic. Oocysts are shed unsporulated, and resemble those of *Toxoplasma* and *Hammondia* when sporulated. Meronts in the intermediate host develop in mesenchymal cells, probably fibroblasts, which become massively hypertrophic, forming cysts containing many clusters of merozoites (bradyzoites) in the host cell cytoplasm. Among domestic animals, cysts of *Besnoitia besnoiti* may assume some significance in the skin of cattle and goats (Vol. 1, Integumentary System), and *Besnoitia* cysts have been reported in association with laryngeal polyps in a horse.

Cryptosporidiosis. *Cryptosporidium* is a small apicomplexan protist, found on the surface of epithelium in the GI, biliary, and respiratory tracts of mammals, birds, reptiles, and fish. Disease in mammals is generally enteric; respiratory infection is most significant in birds.

Although its taxonomic position in relation to other apicomplexan protists, and its species nomenclature, are in a state of flux, on molecular genetic grounds ~15 morphologically similar species of *Cryptosporidium* are recognized. Five of these occur in domestic animals: 1) ***Cryptosporidium parvum***, small, and initially described in the mouse intestine, but parasitic in cattle, other ruminants, and humans; 2) **C. *andersoni*** in cattle; 3) **C. *suis*** in pigs; 4) **C. *felis*** in cats; and 5) **C. *canis*** in dogs. C. *parvum* is zoonotic, as are C. *suis*, C. *felis*, and C. *canis* to a lesser extent, and disease in humans has been associated with contamination of water sources, food, and milk products, as well as close contact with infected animals. However, humans also have a primate-adapted species, ***C. hominis***, which is probably responsible for most outbreaks of cryptosporidiosis not associated with direct animal contact.

All 3 stages of the *Cryptosporidium* life cycle—merogony, gametogony, and sporogony—occur extracytoplasmically in a vacuole within the apical region of epithelial cells, protruding above the cell surface (Fig. 1-160A and B). The prepatent period of C. *parvum* in calves is ~7 days and infections usually persist for weeks or, if the animal is immunocompromised, perhaps months. Type I merozoites recycle in a new host cell to produce another meront generation; type II merozoites differentiate to gamonts. Thin-walled oocysts excyst in the gut of the same host, resulting in autoinfection by the sporozoites released; thick-walled oocysts are excreted to the external environment and are responsible for transmission to another host. Various generations of merogony, and autoinfection by excystment of thin-walled oocysts, result in a large biotic potential and promote heavy colonization of the gut.

The organisms are enclosed within a parasitophorous vacuole formed by apposition of 2 unit membranes of the host cell, probably caused by inversion of a microvillus by the infecting sporozoite or merozoite (see Fig. 1-160C). A specialized "feeder" organelle is present at the attachment zone in the base of the vacuole, between the infecting organism and the cytoplasm of the host cell.

The frequently used expression "intracellular but extracytoplasmic location" for the location of *Cryptosporidium* spp. is a misnomer that should be abandoned as, by definition, if a structure is intracellular but is not in the nucleus, as in the case of *Cryptosporidium* spp., it must be in the cytoplasm. Developmental stages are small, in most cases ~2-6 µm in diameter. Undifferentiated meronts and gamonts are recognized as small basophilic trophozoites. Mature schizonts contain small falciform merozoites. Macrogamonts are ~5 µm in diameter and contain small granules. Oocysts in tissue sections are often collapsed into a crescent shape. The various stages may be recognized in wax- or plastic-embedded sections under the light microscope but are best studied with the electron microscope. Oocysts containing 4 sporozoites may be demonstrated by fecal flotation, or in fecal smears stained with Giemsa, by a modified Ziehl-Neelsen technique, or with auramine O or fluorescein-labeled antibody and examined with ultraviolet light.

Cryptosporidia are found in many circumstances, and, in some species, infection appears to be subclinical. Neonates are particularly susceptible to intestinal infections, and this is especially so among ruminants (calves, lambs, kids, red deer

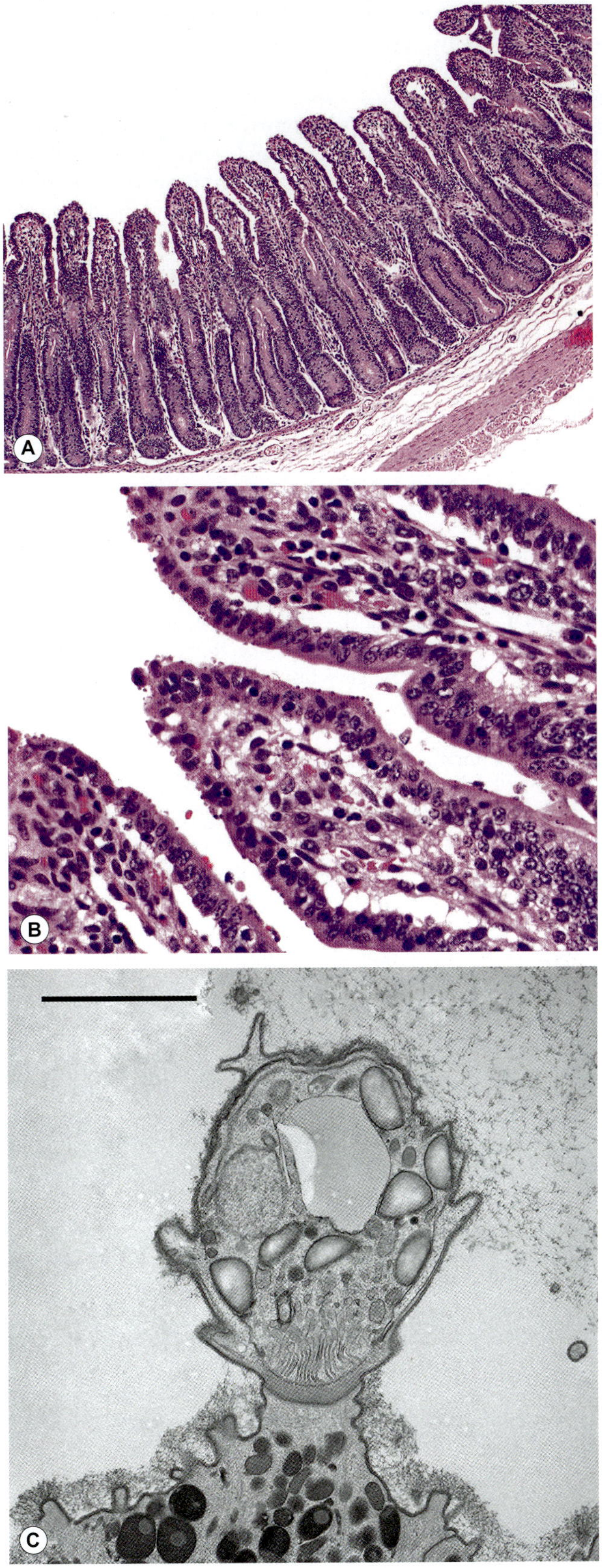

Figure 1-160 Cryptosporidiosis. A. Villus atrophy of the small intestine in a calf due to severe *Cryptosporidium parvum* infection. B. *C. parvum* organisms appear as 4-5 µm basophilic structures on the brush border of enterocytes. C. *Cryptosporidium* attached to apex of an enterocyte within a parasitophorous vacuole along the disrupted brush border in the small intestine. (Courtesy A. Armien.)

calves) infected with C. *parvum*. Diarrhea, anorexia, and depression in calves usually occur between ~1 and 4 weeks of age, and in lambs ~5-14-days-old. However, naive calves up to 3-months-old are susceptible to infection and may develop diarrhea.

Cryptosporidial infections are mainly eliminated by cell-mediated immune responses, including γ-interferon production by CD4 T lymphocytes, but the humoral arm also contributes. Immunosuppression is contributory to, but not essential for, the development of disease. Heavy infections are reported in Arabian foals with combined immunodeficiency, and cryptosporidiosis has occurred in cats with FeLV infection, and in dogs with canine distemper. In immunocompromised individuals, organisms may be present at any level of the GI tract, from the esophagus to colon. Liver, gallbladder, pancreas, and their ducts also may be involved, as may the respiratory tract. Cryptosporidia frequently occur concurrently with ETEC, rotaviral, or coronaviral infection in neonatal ruminants, but can be primary pathogens.

In all species, *intestinal cryptosporidiosis is associated with villus atrophy of variable severity*, blunting and some fusion of villi, and hypertrophy of intestinal crypts. Surface epithelium is usually cuboidal, rounded, or low-columnar, and sometimes exfoliating or forming irregular projections at tips of villi. *Large numbers of cryptosporidia are usually visible in the microvillus border of cells on the villi* (see Fig. 1-160A and B), and not in intestinal crypts, although occasionally, the reverse is true. Organisms typically are most heavily distributed in the distal half of the small intestine, especially in ileum, although occasionally cryptosporidia may occur in the cecum and colon. Mild proprial infiltrates of neutrophils and mixed mononuclear cells are present, probably attracted by proinflammatory cytokines released from infected epithelium. An increase in intraepithelial T lymphocytes has been documented in the intestine of infected calves.

Diarrhea in cryptosporidiosis is mainly attributable to malabsorption associated with villus atrophy and a population of immature enterocytes, and perhaps to the occupation of a large proportion of the surface area of absorptive cells by the organisms. Release of inflammatory mediators, principally prostaglandins, may stimulate mucosal secretion, and an increase in epithelial cell permeability to macromolecules has been demonstrated in vitro.

C. *parvum* is most significant in **calves**, as a cause of undifferentiated neonatal diarrhea, in which it must be differentiated particularly from coronaviral and rotaviral infection. Frequently, it is concurrent with other agents causing this syndrome; it tends to be most prevalent in animals ~2-weeks-old. A similar situation occurs in **lambs**, although disease does not appear to be as common or well recognized in that species. It is a sporadic or minor cause of sometimes fatal diarrhea in other species of ruminants.

Several species are susceptible to *Cryptosporidium* infection; however, many infections are subclinical. Although cryptosporidiosis can be induced experimentally in **piglets**, it is a very rare cause of spontaneous disease in swine. It is only occasionally associated with disease of carnivores, and then often in probably immunocompromised animals. Although infection of **foals** is not uncommon, *Cryptosporidium* has been associated with disease mainly in animals with combined immunodeficiency, complicated by adenoviral infection. Disease has not occurred in successful experimental infections in foals, and the role of cryptosporidia in the etiology of neonatal diarrhea in foals is poorly defined, although occasional outbreaks attributable to C. *parvum* may occur.

The **diagnosis** is based on finding large numbers of cryptosporidia in sections of freshly fixed lower small intestine, preferably in association with villus atrophy. Examination of smears of ileal mucosa stained with Giemsa may allow a rapid diagnosis, or permit a diagnosis on tissue from an animal dead for some hours.

C. andersoni, in the *abomasum of weaned calves and older cattle*, is not associated with diarrhea, but plasma pepsinogen levels rise, and weight gains of some growing animals may be adversely affected. There is mucous metaplasia/hyperplasia in the fundic glands, which are dilated, with attenuation of the lining epithelium, on which cryptosporidia are numerous. Infections have been associated with decreased milk production.

Rarely, cryptosporidia are seen in gastric biopsies from **cats**, sometimes associated with mild gastritis. There is some indication that concurrent infection with *H. felis* will precipitate disease because of cryptosporidia. A mixed infection of C. *muris* (stomach) and C. *felis* (small intestine) was identified in an adult cat with diarrhea that was refractory to therapy.

Amebiasis. *Entamoeba histolytica* is the cause of amebiasis in humans, nonhuman primates, and, rarely, in other species, including dogs and cattle; cats are susceptible to experimental infection. Infection in **dogs** is sporadic, probably acquired by exposure to cysts in feces from infected humans. Dogs tend not to pass encysted amebae; hence it has been suggested that they present little public health hazard and are unlikely to support spread from dog to dog. However, under some circumstances, cysts may be shed, and fecal material containing motile trophozoites has been used to transmit infection orally to other dogs.

Amebae are usually nonpathogenic inhabitants of the lumen of the large bowel, but sometimes they cause colitis. The diet and immune status of the host, and virulence attributes of various strains of the organism, seem to influence pathogenicity. Adhesion to mucus by specific lectins, enzymatic degradation of mucus, and lectin-mediated adherence of amebae to host epithelium are essential steps leading to tissue damage. Cysteine proteinases produced by *E. histolytica* contribute to epithelial cell damage and to induction of inflammation, both of which are involved in initiation of mucosal lesions. Cytolysis is induced by in-contact amebae.

Amebiasis in dogs is associated with diarrheic or mucoid feces, perhaps with some blood, or with dysentery. *Erosive mucosal colitis or ulcerative colitis* occurs in dogs with amebiasis, and disease seems more common or severe in animals with concomitant *Trichuris* or *Ancylostoma* infection.

Early lesions in human amebiasis seem to be diffuse acute mucosal colitis, with focal erosions or ulcerations. Amebae, although scarce, may be found in mucus on the colonic surface, but are most numerous in the fibrinocellular exudate over erosions or superficial ulcers. Ulcers advance as an area of necrosis and predominantly neutrophilic infiltrate, causing loss of glands, and extending for the full depth of the mucosa. Initial lesions consist of tiny erosions of the surface epithelium that evolve to deeper, more extensive ulcers. Established ulcerative amebic colitis classically has a flask-shaped ulcer, the narrow neck through the mucosa, and the broad base in the submucosa. There amebae, and necrosis, expand laterally, apparently less constrained by the architecture of the tissue. Intestinal perforations and intramural abscesses may form.

Amebae may be present, commonly in small clusters, in necrotic debris or in adjacent viable tissue, frequently not involved in an inflammatory reaction. Amebae in tissue, often surrounded by a clear halo, may be spherical or irregular, with extended pseudopodia, and are ~6-50 µm in diameter. The nucleus has a central dense karyosome and peripheral chromatin clumps. The cytoplasm may appear foamy, can contain remnants of erythrocytes in phagolysosomes, and contains glycogen, which makes the cytoplasm PAS positive. The lesions of established amebiasis in the colon of dogs resemble those in humans; the early lesions may as well.

Although dissemination of amebae, with abscessation in other organs, especially in the liver, lung, and brain, is a relatively common complication in humans, it seems rare in dogs. One such case occurred in an animal with canine distemper.

Giardiasis and trichomoniasis. Giardia spp. *are flagellate protists that inhabit the small intestine of a wide range of vertebrates*. The taxonomy of the genus is difficult. It appears that 4 or 5 morphologically distinct "species" exist, each with a relatively wide host range within amphibians, birds, rodents, and other mammals. ***Giardia duodenalis*** (= G. *lamblia*) infection is common in humans, and it also occurs in a wide array of mammals. Although morphologically similar, molecular genetic investigations have identified at least 7 genotypes within G. *duodenalis*, several of which (assemblages A and B) infect humans. Hoofed animals are infected by assemblages A and E, the former being potentially zoonotic, dogs by assemblages C and D, and cats by assemblage F. *Giardia* infection has been associated with disease, with various degrees of credibility, in most of these hosts. In an experimental model, genotypes A and B appear to be more infectious and cause more severe mucosal injury.

Giardia trophozoites are pyriform, ~10-20 µm long by 5-15 µm wide and 2-4 µm thick, and convex on the dorsal surface. The concave ventral surface is modified by a disk that functions in attachment. Nutrient absorption seems to occur through the dorsal surface. A pair of nuclei, 2 axonemes, 2 medial bodies, and 4 pairs of flagella are present, and the organisms multiply by binary fission in the gut lumen. They apply their ventral aspect to the microvillus surface of enterocytes, usually between villi, in folds on the villus surface, or occasionally in intestinal crypts. *Giardia* have been demonstrated in the mucosa, but this is an unusual and probably aberrant location. Relatively resistant oval cysts are passed in the feces, and transmission is by the fecal-oral route.

The significance of *Giardia* as a pathogen in humans and other species has been controversial because *subclinical infection is the rule*. However, under some circumstances, *Giardia* may cause disease. How the host-parasite relationship is modified, and the pathogenesis of the disease, are still unclear.

In *young dogs and cats*, in which giardiosis is most important, although still uncommon, the main sign is intermittent or chronic *diarrhea*, which may persist for several months. The stool is soft, pale, mucoid, and greasy. Although appetite is not usually impaired, there may be a reduced growth rate or weight loss, suggesting malabsorption. A poor haircoat is attributed to deficiency of fat-soluble vitamins. Among animals other than dogs and cats, *Giardia* seems most convincingly to be associated with *enteric signs in neonatal calves*, which may pass soft mucoid feces, and have a reduced growth rate.

GI dysfunction has not been extensively documented in domestic animals. However, in a variety of experimental systems, deficiencies in microvillus-associated digestive enzymes, electrolyte and glucose malabsorption, and microvillus shortening or injury have been documented, although not consistently. Some humans with *Giardia* infection have malabsorption of D-xylose and vitamin B_{12}, with steatorrhea and hypocarotinemia. Excess fecal fat has been found in infected cats, but was not demonstrated in experimentally infected rats. Also, D-xylose malabsorption was not demonstrated in a dog with giardiosis.

Selective deficiencies in some brush-border enzymes occur in humans with giardiosis, and in *Giardia*-infected calves. Possibly, these are related to the direct effects of *Giardia* on microvilli, which may be deformed adjacent to adherent organisms or diffusely shortened. *Giardia* may also inhibit the activity of pancreatic lipase, causing fat malabsorption. However, bacterial overgrowth of the small intestine may occur with *Giardia* infection, and associated bile salt deconjugation could explain steatorrhea in giardiosis.

Several mechanisms have been proposed to explain these findings. Although villus atrophy may occur in humans with giardiosis, this mainly occurs in a subgroup of patients with hypogammaglobulinemia. Marked histologic abnormality is not found in many cases of giardiosis in humans, and this also seems to be true for dogs, cats, and calves. In experimental murine giardiosis, infection is associated with hypertrophy of crypts and increased production of cells, combined with an increased rate of movement of enterocytes along villi, with an increased crypt:villus ratio. Deficiencies in brush border form and function may be attributable to incomplete differentiation of enterocytes in this circumstance, or perhaps to damage mediated by mucosal T cells. IELs are common in infected intestine, and altered epithelial kinetics may be related to cell-mediated immune reactions in the mucosa. Infection may lead to increased enterocyte apoptosis, and alterations in epithelial barrier function. Infection has been shown in experimental models to interfere with tight junctions in the epithelium. Atrophy of villi has been associated with restoration of cell-mediated immune competence in *Giardia*-infected athymic mice, reinforcing the notion that immune phenomena may be involved in the pathogenesis of giardiosis.

Giardiosis is usually *diagnosed clinically* on the basis of typical cysts in fecal flotations, or trophozoites in intestinal aspirates or fecal smears, coupled with remission of clinical signs following therapy, and an inability to identify other potential causes of the signs. Sometimes a diagnosis is based on findings in biopsies of the small intestine or at autopsy.

In all species, morphologic changes in the mucosa are not well defined in spontaneous cases of giardiosis. The mucosa may appear normal, but there may be equivocal blunting of villi, perhaps associated with a moderate infiltrate of mononuclear cells into the core of the villus, or a heavy population of IELs. *Giardia* should be sought in animals with malabsorption syndromes. They lie between villi and are usually evident as crescent shapes, applied by their concave surface to the brush border of epithelial cells. In favorable sections through the level of the nuclei, they may appear to have a pair of "eyes." Trophozoites oriented along the plane of section may look as they do in smears, the paired nuclei giving the organism a "face-like" appearance. An abnormal number of bacteria, suggestive of overgrowth, may be present in the mucus and content in the vicinity in symptomatic animals. A diagnosis of giardiosis always should be reserved for those cases in which no other explanation for the syndrome can be identified. Giardiosis has been associated with colitis in dogs, but the association is not clearly causal.

Trichomonads, small flagellate protists that reproduce by binary fission, and are transmitted directly between hosts, are sometimes encountered in the feces of horses, cattle, pigs, dogs, and cats with diarrhea. Only in cats is there a known causal association with disease (trichomonosis). ***Tritrichomonas foetus*** is associated with *persistent large-bowel diarrhea*, refractory to treatment, in **cats** <1-year-old, and the syndrome has been reproduced experimentally. The microscopic lesions are typical of chronic mucosal colitis, most severe in areas colonized by the organisms. The diagnosis is confirmed in section by detection of pyriform or crescent-shaped organisms, ~5 × 7 µm in size, with a faint nucleus and eosinophilic cytoplasm, applied to the surface epithelium, or in the lumen of colonic glands, usually in large numbers. However, the organisms are present in only a little more than half the sections examined from infected cats, and various samples may be necessary to have a high probability of detecting them. In some cases, trichomonads appear to disrupt the epithelium, attaining the subepithelial lamina propria around crypts, or they are associated with ulceration and foci of necrosis and pyogranulomatous inflammation that are distributed transmurally in the affected areas of colon, and in draining lymph nodes.

Balantiosis/balantidiasis. Balantioides (Balantidium) is a large oval protist ~50-60 µm or more long, and ~25-45 µm wide, with a macronucleus and micronucleus, and covered by many cilia arrayed in rows; reinstatement of the genus name *Balantioides* has been proposed. ***Balantioides (Balantidium) coli*** occurs in the large bowel of swine, humans, and nonhuman primates. It is very common in pigs, and many infected humans live in close contact with swine. Enteric disease by *B. coli* has been reported from a horse (eFig. 1-16) and from several dogs with access to swine yards, as a complication of trichurosis. Definitive role in enteric disease of horses and pigs is, however, controversial.

Balantioides spp. are normally present as commensals in the lumen of the cecum and colon but are capable of opportunistic invasion of tissues injured by other diseases. On rare occasions, it may be a primary pathogen, although definitive evidence of this is lacking. In swine, in which the organisms are most commonly encountered by veterinary pathologists, *Balantioides* spp. may be found at the leading edge of the crateriform necrotizing or ulcerative lesions of the large intestine that develop secondary to intestinal adenomatosis (Fig. 1-161), swine dysentery, or perhaps salmonellosis. *B. coli* was associated with enteritis in pigs infected with PCV2, although the role of the parasite in enteric disease was not confirmed. *Balantioides* spp. are recognized in tissue by large size, ovoid shape, the dense curved or kidney-shaped macronucleus, and cilia (which may be accentuated by silver stains) in rows on the surface.

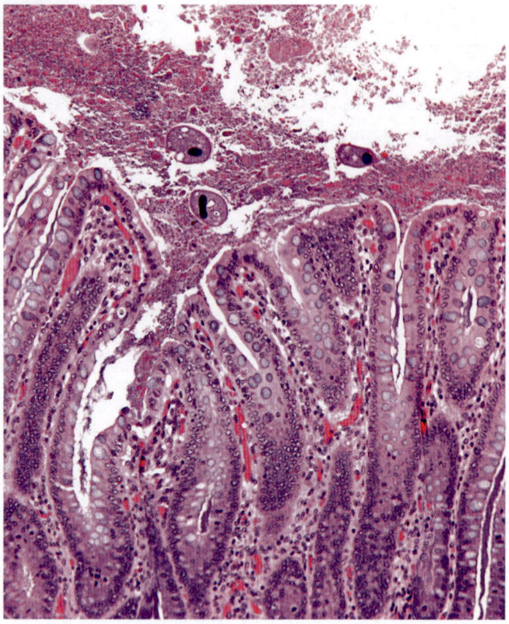

Figure 1-161 ***Balantioides coli*** in the colon of a pig.

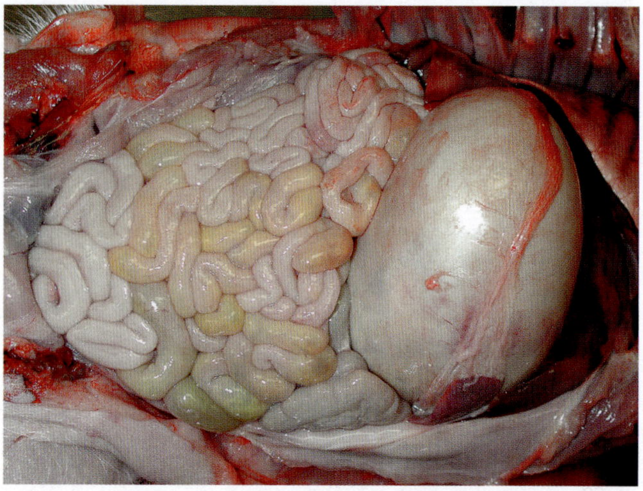

Figure 1-162 Undifferentiated neonatal diarrhea in a piglet. The small intestine is flaccid and filled by fluid content, with no gross evidence of inflammation. (Courtesy G. Andrews, Kansas State University Diagnostic Laboratory.)

DIFFERENTIAL DIAGNOSIS OF DIARRHEA

The diagnosis of GI disease is facilitated by knowledge of the entities that may be expected in a particular species and age group, and the clinicopathologic syndromes with which they are associated. *In this section, etiologic entities associated with diarrhea syndromes and their salient gross and histologic diagnostic features in domestic species are briefly summarized.*

Diarrhea in ruminants, swine, and horses

Diarrhea causing dehydration, metabolic acidosis, and electrolyte depletion is an important cause of morbidity and mortality in neonatal calves, lambs, goat kids, piglets, and to a lesser extent in foals. Several classes of agents occur in most species of large animals, and mixed infections often occur, such as *E. coli*, coronavirus, rotavirus, and *Cryptosporidium parvum* in calves. These and some other less common agents produce diarrhea in neonatal animals, the etiology of which cannot be readily differentiated on clinical grounds or on the basis of gross postmortem examination.

Diarrhea of neonatal animals requires etiologic diagnosis if appropriate advice is to be rendered regarding the prevention and management of the disease. Many of the agents involved are either transiently present or produce lesions such as villus atrophy that is easily obscured by autolysis, which significantly hinders accurate diagnosis. To overcome these obstacles, *one or more live untreated animals in the early phase of clinical disease and representative of the herd problem should be examined if available*. They should be euthanized and examined immediately using an autopsy procedure modified so that specimens of the small intestine are formalin fixed within a few minutes of death, and so that appropriate samples of tissue and content are quickly collected to facilitate a complete etiologic investigation.

The prevalence of diarrhea and potentially associated agents in neonates is expected to vary considerably on the basis of locality, climate, season, and the management system, as well as by species. Specific microscopic lesions and their distribution within the intestine may suggest an etiology. Bacterial culture, rapid immunologic and/or molecular methods using gut content, formalin-fixed, or frozen tissues may identify a bacterial or viral agent. Some agents, such as cryptosporidia and coccidia, may be identified in H&E- and/or Giemsa-stained mucosal scrapings or tissue sections. In each species, undifferentiated neonatal diarrhea may be caused by other less common agents; therefore, care is required to establish an accurate diagnosis and to distinguish from other potential diseases that may occur in each species.

In all species, neonates succumbing to the effects of undifferentiated diarrhea are overtly *dehydrated*. The eyes are sunken in the orbits, the skin lacks elasticity, and the subcutis and mucous membranes are tacky. There is usually fecal staining on the perineum, but rare acute cases may have signs of dehydration without significant diarrhea. Animals with diarrhea may continue to suckle during the early phase of their illness; therefore, a milk clot or curd may be present in the stomach and internal fat depots may be adequate. Animals that lose interest in feed because of more chronic disease and those taken off nutrients may have serous atrophy of fat and appear cachectic. The small intestine is flaccid and dilated with thin walls, and increased fluid content is present throughout the full intestinal length (Fig. 1-162). The content is usually watery and clear green-yellow and often separates into 2 phases, the more solid of which appears to consist of small masses of clotted milk or mucus. Sometimes the content is more homogeneous and creamy; however, in animals examined sometime after death, this appearance is due to postmortem autolysis of the epithelium. The large intestine also contains fluid, creamy or pasty content, usually white or yellow. The mucosa of the small intestine may appear glistening and mildly congested; that in the large intestine is usually unremarkable. The forestomachs in ruminants that have been tube fed, or in which the ruminoreticular groove has apparently failed to close, may contain sour fermented milk or milk replacer, and the mucosa may be mildly reddened. The abomasal mucosa of some calves may contain scattered focal stress-associated hemorrhages. In piglets, urates may precipitate in the renal medulla and pelvis as a result of dehydration.

Diarrhea of older animals shares many of the features mentioned above for neonatal individuals, although compared with neonates, adults are generally less susceptible to the negative effects of infection including dehydration, and have greater capacity for epithelial renewal and response to injury. Major features of diseases causing **diarrhea in cattle, small ruminants, pigs, and horses** of all ages were discussed in previous sections of this chapter and are summarized in Tables 1-4 and 1-5, 1-6 and 1-7, 1-8 and 1-9, and 1-10 and 1-11, respectively.

Diarrhea in dogs and cats

Many infectious pathogens can cause diarrhea in dogs and cats of all ages; in general, these infections are less common in cats than in dogs. In many diagnostic laboratories, the detection of various common and uncommon agents associated with various diarrhea syndromes in dogs and cats is attempted by individual or multiplex PCR assays (especially in puppies and kittens); however, caution is strongly advised when interpreting results because many of these agents can be identified in normal canine and feline feces. Significant causes of diarrhea in dogs and cats were previously discussed in detail in this chapter and are summarized in Tables 1-12 and 1-13, respectively.

PERITONEUM AND RETROPERITONEUM

Structure, function, and response to injury

Peritoneal and retroperitoneal diseases usually occur secondary to processes involving the organs covered by the peritoneum or arise within the retroperitoneum itself. The peritoneum lines the abdominal cavity, which is incompletely divided into compartments by the mesentery, omentum, and ligaments, with a total surface area greater than that of the skin. During organogenesis, the celomic space is partitioned into peritoneal, pleural, and pericardial cavities lined by mesothelial cells that become the peritoneum, pleura, and pericardium, respectively. *The normal peritoneum is a smooth shiny membrane that is semipermeable to the movement of water and small solute molecules. There is normally just enough fluid present in the cavity to keep it moist.* Peritoneal fluid is normally clear and watery, but, in neonatal pigs and lambs, normal peritoneal fluid may contain strands of mucinous coagulum lying on the intact serosal surfaces of abdominal viscera. The fluid is in osmotic equilibrium with plasma but does not contain fibrinogen or other high–molecular-weight proteins, and generally does not clot, except in pigs.

Table • 1-4

Causes of diarrhea in neonatal cattle

CAUSE	GROSS AND MICROSCOPIC DIAGNOSTIC FEATURES
Enterotoxigenic *E. coli*	Nonspecific diarrhea; myriad bacteria covering intact villi
Enteropathogenic *E. coli*	Nonspecific diarrhea; attaching-effacing bacteria in the small intestine and colon
Salmonella enterica	Fibrinonecrotizing enterocolitis
Clostridium perfringens type B	Necrohemorrhagic or fibrinonecrotizing enterocolitis
Clostridium perfringens type C	Necrohemorrhagic or fibrinonecrotizing enterocolitis
Bovine rotavirus A and B	Nonspecific diarrhea; villus atrophy in the small intestine
Bovine coronavirus	Nonspecific diarrhea; villus atrophy in the small intestine; crypt dilation in the colon
Bovine alphaherpesvirus 1	Multifocal necrotizing lesions throughout the GI tract; intranuclear inclusion bodies
Bovine viral diarrhea virus	Multifocal ulcerative lesions throughout the GI tract; vasculitis; lymphoid necrosis
Cryptosporidium parvum	Nonspecific diarrhea; cryptosporidia along brush border in the small intestine
Bovine adenovirus 7	Necrohemorrhagic enteritis; intranuclear inclusion bodies
Bovine torovirus	Nonspecific diarrhea; villus atrophy in the small intestine; crypt dilation in the small intestine and colon
Bovine astrovirus, parvovirus, calicivirus, enterovirus, birnavirus, kobuvirus[a]	Nonspecific diarrhea
Chlamydia pecorum	Nonspecific diarrhea
Strongyloides papillosus	Nonspecific diarrhea; villus atrophy in the small intestine
Bacillus fragilis[a]	Nonspecific diarrhea
Giardia sp.[a]	Nonspecific diarrhea

[a]The role of these pathogens in calf diarrhea has been suggested, but it is unproven.
GI = gastrointestinal.

Table • 1-5

Causes of diarrhea in cattle >3-weeks-old

CAUSE	GROSS AND MICROSCOPIC DIAGNOSTIC FEATURES
Enteropathogenic *E. coli*	Nonspecific diarrhea; attaching-effacing bacteria in small intestine and colon
Salmonella enterica	Fibrinonecrotizing enterocolitis
Mycobacterium avium subsp. *paratuberculosis*	Granulomatous enteritis; lymphadenitis; hepatitis; intralesional acid-fast bacteria
Listeria monocytogenes	Neutrophilic enteritis; inflammation of muscularis mucosa
Yersinia pseudotuberculosis	Necrotizing enterocolitis; lymphadenitis, hepatitis; intralesional bacterial colonies
Bovine viral diarrhea virus	Multifocal ulcerative lesions throughout the GI tract; vasculitis; lymphoid necrosis
Ovine gammaherpesvirus 2	Erosions throughout the GI system; lymphoid proliferation; vasculitis
Bovine adenovirus 7	Necrohemorrhagic enteritis; intranuclear inclusion bodies
Bovine coronavirus	Necrohemorrhagic colitis; villus atrophy in the small intestine; crypt dilation in the colon
Cryptosporidium parvum	Nonspecific diarrhea; cryptosporidia along brush border in the small intestine
Eimeria spp.	Fibrinohemorrhagic typhlocolitis; intralesional protozoa
Ostertagia spp.	Abomasitis; mucous gland metaplasia and hyperplasia
Strongyloides papillosus	Villus atrophy in the small intestine
Other nematodes (*Nematodirus, Trichostrongylus, Haemonchus, Bunostomum, Oesophagostomum, Trichuris*)	Nonspecific diarrhea; adult nematodes in the small and/or large intestine; submucosal nodules (*Oesophagostomum*)
Toxocara vitulorum	Necrotizing gastroenteritis; intralesional protozoa
Toxins (arsenic, oak, oleander, mustard seed, superphosphate, others)	Hemorrhagic or ulcerative gastroenteritis
Astylus atromaculatus	Fibrinonecrotizing gastroenteritis; insect parts in GI content
Ruminal acidosis	Rumen content pH <5.5; congestion of the forestomachs, abomasum, and intestine; neutrophilic rumenitis
Copper deficiency	Nonspecific diarrhea
Congestive heart failure	Nonspecific diarrhea

GI = gastrointestinal.

Table • 1-6

Causes of diarrhea in neonatal sheep and goats

CAUSE	GROSS AND MICROSCOPIC DIAGNOSTIC FEATURES
Enterotoxigenic *E. coli*	Nonspecific diarrhea; myriad bacteria lining intact villi
Rotavirus A and B	Nonspecific diarrhea; villus atrophy in the small intestine
Cryptosporidium parvum	Nonspecific diarrhea; cryptosporidia along brush border in the small intestine
Clostridium perfringens type B	Necrohemorrhagic or fibrinonecrotizing enterocolitis; focal symmetrical encephalomalacia
Clostridium perfringens type C	Necrohemorrhagic or fibrinonecrotizing enterocolitis
Clostridium perfringens type D (goats only)	Fibrinonecrotizing enterocolitis
Eimeria spp.	Proliferative enteritis; intralesional protozoa
Salmonella enterica	Fibrinonecrotizing enterocolitis
Strongyloides sp.	Nonspecific diarrhea; villus atrophy in the small intestine
Astrovirus (lambs only)	Nonspecific diarrhea
Adenovirus (goats only)	Nonspecific diarrhea
Giardia sp.[a]	Nonspecific diarrhea
Bacillus fragilis[a]	Nonspecific diarrhea

[a]The role of these pathogens in diarrhea of small ruminants has been suggested, but it is unproven.

Table • 1-7

Causes of diarrhea in sheep and goats >3-weeks-old

CAUSE	GROSS AND MICROSCOPIC DIAGNOSTIC FEATURES
Mycobacterium avium subsp. *paratuberculosis*	Granulomatous enteritis; lymphadenitis; hepatitis; intralesional acid-fast bacteria
Clostridium perfringens type D (only goats)	Fibrinonecrotizing enterocolitis
Yersinia pseudotuberculosis	Necrotizing enterocolitis; lymphadenitis, hepatitis; intralesional bacterial colonies
Peste-des-petitsruminants virus	Erosions in the upper alimentary tract; necrotizing enteritis; syncytial cells; intracytoplasmic inclusion bodies
Ostertagia spp.	Abomasitis; mucous gland metaplasia and hyperplasia
Other nematodes (*Nematodirus, Trichostrongylus, Haemonchus, Oesophagostomum, Trichuris*)	Nonspecific diarrhea; adult nematodes in the small and/or large intestine; submucosal nodules (*Oesophagostomum*)
Strongyloides sp.	Nonspecific diarrhea; villus atrophy in the small intestine
Eimeria spp.	Proliferative enteritis; intralesional protozoa
Schistosoma sp.	Nonspecific diarrhea
Terminal ileitis (sheep only)	Thickened ileum; enlarged small intestinal mesenteric lymph nodes
Ruminal acidosis	Rumen content pH <5.5; congestion of the forestomachs, abomasum and intestine; neutrophilic rumenitis

Table • 1-8

Causes of diarrhea in neonatal swine

CAUSE	GROSS AND MICROSCOPIC DIAGNOSTIC FEATURES
Enterotoxigenic *E. coli*	Nonspecific diarrhea; numerous bacteria covering intact villi of piglets <1-week-old
Coronavirus (including TGEV, PEDV, deltacoronavirus); rotavirus	Nonspecific diarrhea; villus atrophy
Coccidia *(Cystoisospora suis)*	Nonspecific diarrhea due to villus atrophy in piglets >5-6-days-old; meronts or gamonts in intestinal smears or within epithelial cells; fibrinonecrotic enteritis in severe cases
Clostridium perfringens type C	Hemorrhagic and necrotizing enteritis in piglets <7-days-old
Clostridioides difficile	Fibrinonecrotizing enteritis and mesocolonic edema in piglets <7-days-old
Adenovirus	Nonspecific undifferentiated diarrhea (but usually subclinical); villus atrophy distal small intestine; epithelial intranuclear inclusion bodies
Cryptosporidium; Giardia	Frequently present (likely as co-pathogens); villus atrophy with heavy infestations; organisms visible along brush border or in lumen, respectively
Other bacteria (*Salmonella, Klebsiella, Bacteroides fragilis*)	Nonspecific undifferentiated diarrhea; villus atrophy
Other viruses (enterovirus, astrovirus, calicivirus)	Villus atrophy; often of unclear clinical significance
Strongyloides ransomi	Villus atrophy; adult nematodes embedded along the base of the small intestinal epithelium

TGEV = transmissible gastroenteritis virus; PEDV = Porcine epidemic diarrhea virus.

Table • 1-9

Causes of diarrhea in swine >3-weeks-old

CAUSE	GROSS AND MICROSCOPIC DIAGNOSTIC FEATURES
Rotavirus; coronavirus (including TGEV, PEDV, deltacoronavirus)	Nonspecific diarrhea; villus atrophy
E. coli (postweaning)	Nonspecific diarrhea; villus atrophy; bacteria adhered to the brush border of villi
E. coli (edema disease)	Multisystemic edema (mesocolonic, GI, brain, etc.); usually no evidence of GI-specific disease
Salmonella sp.	Fibrinonecrotizing enterocolitis
Lawsonia intracellularis	3 forms: acute hemorrhagic enteritis; proliferative enteropathy (distal small intestine and colon); fibrinonecrotizing enteropathy (distal small intestine and colon)
Brachyspira sp.	Fibrinohemorrhagic colitis
Trichuris suis	Fibrinohemorrhagic colitis; characteristic adult nematodes within lumen of colon
Porcine circovirus 2	Histiocytic-to-lymphoplasmacytic enteritis (distal small intestine) and lymphadenitis; intracytoplasmic botryoid basophilic inclusion bodies in macrophages; most affected animals have lesions in other organs (lung, skin, liver, kidney)
Coccidia (*Cystoisospora suis*)	Fibrinonecrotizing enteritis; meronts or gamonts in intestinal smear or within epithelial cells; rare in older pigs
Nematodes (*Ascaris, Macracanthorhynchus, Oesophagostomum*)	Adult nematodes evident; submucosal nodules (*Oesophagostomum*)

PEDV = porcine epidemic diarrhea virus; TGEV = transmissible gastroenteritis virus.

Table • 1-10

Causes of diarrhea in neonatal horses

CAUSE	GROSS AND MICROSCOPIC DIAGNOSTIC FEATURES
Coronavirus	Nonspecific diarrhea; necrotizing enteritis; intracytoplasmic inclusion bodies
Rotavirus	Nonspecific diarrhea; villus atrophy
Cryptosporidium parvum	Nonspecific diarrhea; cryptosporidia along brush border in the small intestine
Parascaris equorum	Nonspecific diarrhea; nematodes in the small intestine
Strongyloides westeri	Nonspecific diarrhea; villus atrophy in the small intestine
Clostridium perfringens type C	Necrohemorrhagic or fibrinonecrotizing enterocolitis
Clostridium perfringens type B	Necrohemorrhagic or fibrinonecrotizing enterocolitis
Clostridioides difficile	Fibrinonecrotizing enterocolitis
Salmonella enterica	Fibrinonecrotizing enterocolitis
Rhodococcus equi	Pyogranulomatous enteritis and/or colitis; lymphadenitis
Actinobacillus equuli	Neutrophilic enterocolitis; intralesional bacterial colonies
Klebsiella pneumoniae	Neutrophilic enterocolitis; intralesional bacterial colonies
Enterococcus durans	Nonspecific diarrhea; villus atrophy; intralesional gram-positive cocci
Clostridium piliforme	Necrotizing colitis; intracytoplasmic filamentous rods
Enterotoxigenic *E. coli*[a]	Nonspecific diarrhea

[a]The role of this pathogen in diarrhea of foals has been suggested, but it is unproven.

Table • 1-11

Causes of diarrhea in horses >3-weeks-old

CAUSE	GROSS AND MICROSCOPIC DIAGNOSTIC FEATURES
Coronavirus	Nonspecific diarrhea; necrotizing enteritis; intracytoplasmic inclusion bodies
Clostridioides difficile	Fibrinonecrotizing enterocolitis
Salmonella enterica	Fibrinonecrotizing enterocolitis
Rhodococcus equi	Pyogranulomatous enteritis and/or colitis; lymphadenitis
Actinobacillus equuli	Neutrophilic enterocolitis; intralesional bacterial colonies
Klebsiella pneumoniae	Neutrophilic enterocolitis; intralesional bacterial colonies
Enterococcus durans	Nonspecific diarrhea; villus atrophy; intralesional gram-positive cocci
Clostridium piliforme	Necrotizing colitis; intracytoplasmic filamentous rods
Lawsonia intracellularis	Proliferative enteropathy
Neorickettsia spp.	Lymphoplasmacytic colitis
Large and small strongyle	Nonspecific diarrhea; intralesional nematodes
Parascaris equorum	Nonspecific diarrhea; nematodes in the small intestine
Various displacements	Intestinal displacements
Inflammatory bowel disease	Nonspecific lymphocytic, plasmacytic, eosinophilic-to-ulcerative chronic enterocolitis
Various toxicants (NSAIDs, cantharidin, others)	Ulcerative enterocolitis

NSAIDs = nonsteroidal anti-inflammatory drugs.

Table • 1-12

Causes of diarrhea in dogs

CAUSE	GROSS AND MICROSCOPIC DIAGNOSTIC FEATURES
Parvovirus 2	Segmental fibrinonecrotizing and hemorrhagic enteritis; cryptal necrosis; lymphoid and hematopoietic necrosis
Rotavirus and coronavirus	Villus atrophy; agents commonly identified in puppies but are rare causes of clinically significant disease
Enteroinvasive *E. coli*	Histiocytic colitis, mostly in adult Boxers, French bulldogs; PAS-positive macrophages
Gastrointestinal hemorrhage syndrome (netF-positive *Clostridium perfringens*)	Gastrointestinal hemorrhage and possibly villar necrosis; bacterial rods are associated with intestinal surface
Idiopathic inflammatory bowel disease	Nonspecific variably severe gastric, intestinal, or colonic inflammation (lymphoplasmacytic, eosinophilic); a diagnosis by exclusion (rule out other causes, especially dietary or antibiotic-responsive enteropathies)
Intestinal lymphoma	Monomorphic round-cell infiltration in lamina propria ± epitheliotropism
Lymphangiectasia	Dilation of villar lacteals and submucosal or mural lymphatics with associated histiocytic-to-neutrophilic inflammation
Canine distemper virus	Nonspecific lesions, poorlyl understood
Circovirus	Necrotizing hemorrhagic enteritis, vasculitis, lymphadenitis; some dogs also have necrohemorrhagic pneumonia
Other viruses (astrovirus, adenovirus, paramyxovirus, calicivirus, herpesvirus)	Nonspecific lesions, poorly understood
Bacteria (*Salmonella, Yersinia, Enterococcus, Campylobacter,* pathogenic *E. coli, Brachyspira*)	Nonspecific lesions

(Continued)

Table • 1-12

Causes of diarrhea in dogs—cont'd

CAUSE	GROSS AND MICROSCOPIC DIAGNOSTIC FEATURES
Neorickettsia helminthoeca (salmon poisoning)	Generalized histiocytic inflammation of lymph nodes and GALT; necrohemorrhagic enteritis; intracytoplasmic organisms
Clostridium piliforme (Tyzzer disease)	Enterocolitis, myocarditis, hepatitis
Castor beans	Nonspecific gastroenteritis
Ascarids (roundworms, hookworms, whipworms)	Adult parasites can be found in the lumen of the small intestine (roundworms, hookworms), or colon (whipworms); hemorrhagic enterocolitis
Coccidia (*Cystisospora* sp.)	Mild necrotizing or atrophic enteritis; organisms in epithelial cells
Fungal, oomycotic, or algal infection	Granulomatous-to-pyogranulomatous mural-to-transmural enteritis; characteristic organisms demonstrated by appropriate special stains
Entamoeba histolytica	Ulcerative colitis

Table • 1-13

Causes of diarrhea in cats

CAUSE	GROSS AND MICROSCOPIC DIAGNOSTIC FEATURES
Parvovirus (panleukopenia)	Segmental necrotizing and hemorrhagic enteritis (mostly kittens); cryptal necrosis; lymphoid and hematopoietic necrosis
Feline infectious peritonitis virus	Granulomatous-to-pyogranulomatous perivascular enterocolitis
Histoplasma sp.	Granulomatous mural-to-transmural enterocolitis, almost always part of multisystemic disseminated disease
Tritrichomonas foetus	Necrotizing colitis; many organisms are typically observed filling colonic glands
Intestinal lymphoma	Monomorphic round cell infiltration in lamina propria ± epitheliotropism
Feline leukemia virus	Cryptal necrosis (resembles panleukopenia but without lymphoid or hematopoietic necrosis)
Other viruses (astrovirus, enteric coronavirus, calicivirus, rotavirus, torovirus)	Nonspecific; these agents can be present but are rarely associated with clinical signs or GI lesions
Bacteria (*Salmonella, Shigella, Yersinia, Campylobacter, Anaerobiospirillum, Helicobacter, Clostridium piliforme*)	Nonspecific
Ascarids (roundworms, hookworms, whipworms)	Adult parasites can be found in the lumen; most are incidental and not associated with lesions or disease
Cryptosporidium, Cystoisospora, Toxoplasma, Giardia, Entamoeba	Mild necrotizing or nonspecific enterocolitis; organisms may be found in (coccidia) or along the epithelial surface (cryptosporidia, *Giardia*)
Enteroinvasive *E. coli*	Histiocytic, or pyogranulomatous colitis; PAS-positive macrophage contents
Fungal infections	Hemorrhagic ulcerative colitis; fungal elements present

The peritoneum consists of a single serosal lining layer of **mesothelial cells** on a basement membrane supported by submesothelial connective tissue containing a mixture of resident inflammatory cells, fibroblasts, blood vessels, and lymphatics. The submesothelial layer is inapparent in tissues such as the liver, and prominent in other places such as the mesenteries. Mesothelial cells vary in appearance from squamous to low-cuboidal with a single small round nucleus and can share histomorphologic features of both epithelial and mesenchymal cells. Surface microvilli play a role in retention of hyaluronate-based secretions and are more abundant on the visceral than parietal pleural surfaces. Tight junctions and desmosomes are discontinuous in the mesothelial layer, allowing for diffusion of water and small molecules across the membrane. Mesothelial cells are fragile and are readily injured after exposure to such mild insults as air, physiologic saline, intestinal dilation, and transient ischemia. Mesothelial wounds heal rapidly, however, and although cell division and migration of adjacent mesothelium is important, free-floating serosal progenitor cells are capable of mesothelial differentiation.

The *function of the peritoneum* has historically been considered to provide a protective nonadhesive surface in the abdominal cavity; however, it is clear that these cells are a dynamic membrane with several physiologic functions, including fluid and solute transport, immune surveillance, and production of extracellular matrix, cytokines, growth factors, and other molecules. Both parietal and visceral peritoneum are continuously involved in transport of fluid in both directions. Normal fluid contains only traces of protein and secreted macromolecules that reduce permeability, and the electronegativity of the endothelium relative to mesothelium inhibits transfer of plasma proteins from capillaries into the cavity, so net hydraulic forces favor movement of fluid into the abdominal cavity. *Several pathways contribute to the drainage of peritoneal fluid.* Direct transfer through stomata in the membrane to subserosal lymphatics is the main mechanism, from which fluid is transferred into lymphatics of the ventral diaphragm, through the sternal lymph nodes and then to the right lymphatic duct, or via mediastinal lymph nodes to the thoracic duct. Respiratory diaphragmatic movements assist transfer through the diaphragm to ventral mediastinal lymphatics. Less fluid is taken up through the omentum, abdominal viscera, and pelvic serosa, which then drains via visceral lymphatics and lymph nodes to the thoracic duct. Transfer of peritoneal fluid through and between mesothelial cells also occurs but is a minor contributor to overall fluid movement.

Mesothelial cells secrete glycosaminoglycans, proteoglycans, and surface lubricants to provide a nonadhesive surface. They also produce many cytokines and growth factors, which regulate inflammatory processes, leukocyte trafficking into and out of serosal cavities, and tissue repair. They produce fibrinolytic mediators, which aid in fibrin clearance and protect against formation of adhesions. Mesothelial cells have been implicated in both the spread and inhibition of tumor growth in serosal cavities.

Peritoneal milky spots, also known as omentum-associated lymphoid tissue, are small pale semitransparent *nests of lymphocytes, macrophages, and plasma cells* located on the omentum, as well as the peritoneal, pericardial, pleural, and mediastinal parietal membranes. Milky spots were first described in rabbits and are considered specialized structures that play an important role in transfer of particulate matter from peritoneal cavity to lymphatics, peritoneal defense, leukocyte trafficking, and neoplastic cell trafficking and metastasis. They are often assumed to be present in all species, although studies in healthy young dogs did not identify these structures.

The **retroperitoneum** is the adipose and connective tissue immediately beneath the peritoneal lining of the abdominal cavity. The concept of retroperitoneum properly includes the lymphatics and draining lymph nodes in addition to connective tissues, blood vessels, nerves, and the fixed and migratory mononuclear cell populations, most significant along the dorsum from the diaphragm to the anus. Its volume is small, except when adipose tissue accumulates, commonly around the kidneys, pelvic cavity, omentum, and mesenteries. With emaciation, fat stores of the retroperitoneum undergo *serous atrophy*, as do fat deposits in subcutaneous tissues, the thorax, and bone marrow cavities. Movement of fluid or exudates within the retroperitoneal space of dogs may occur in the fascia around the dorsal and ventral aspects of the sublumbar, abdominal, and iliopsoas muscles, and then through the lumbodorsal triangle, cranioventral to the tuber coxae. Antemortem and postmortem effusions and discoloration in the peritoneal cavity should be distinguished. Fluid accumulates in the peritoneal and other serous cavities after death and becomes stained with hemoglobin after erythrocyte lysis (hemoglobin imbibition); such fluid does not clot. Diffusion of bile pigments through the wall of the gallbladder, the bile ducts, or the duodenum will also stain adjacent peritoneum and viscera (bile imbibition).

Response and consequences of injury. Even minor injuries to the peritoneum or retroperitoneum cause rapid loss of mesothelial cells. The denuded area is quickly covered by a layer of fibrin, neutrophils, and macrophages. If the injury is minor, the mesothelial layer is soon regenerated; however, regeneration may be delayed if the injury is severe or prolonged, and submesothelial or retroperitoneal tissues are damaged. Under normal conditions, the mesothelium is a slowly renewing tissue. Restoration of the mesothelial surface may not be provided solely by proliferation and migration of adjacent mesothelial cells; current experimental evidence favors involvement of multipotent mesenchymal stem cells either lying in the immediate subserosa or free-floating in the peritoneum. Therefore unlike other epithelial-like surfaces, in which wounds heal only from the edges, mesothelial healing occurs more rapidly and diffusely across the denuded surface.

Mesothelial hyperplasia is a common response to various types of injury, including trauma, migrating foreign material, accumulation of fluid or exudate, or infection and inflammation. When injured, mesothelial cells proliferate and can become cuboidal or columnar; if the stimulus persists, nodules, plaques, or papillary projections of hyperplastic mesothelial cells can be observed grossly as roughened irregular regions involving either visceral or parietal peritoneal surfaces. Prominent and widespread hyperplasia of mesothelium is frequent following chronic or persistent injury including various forms of peritonitis. Proliferative mesothelial cells can exhibit atypical features that mimic neoplasia and can be difficult to differentiate from mesothelioma or carcinoma on cytologic or histologic examination.

Mesothelial papillary hyperplasia of the epicardium (i.e., epicardial fronds) is a common incidental finding in humans; this condition has also been described in dogs and cattle and is also thought to be an incidental lesion in these species. The prevalence in dogs is estimated to be 17%; in cattle, up to 97% may be affected. The lesions in both species are characterized grossly by firmly adhered irregular pale-tan to dark-red villous plaques or papillary fronds located on the epicardial surfaces of the right or left atria (dogs) or overlying the great vessels (cattle); however, any area can apparently be affected. Although dogs typically have papillary lesions, cattle are more similar to humans and have both papillary and plaque-like lesions; this may be a function of the location of the lesions and potential space between affected epicardium and pericardium. *Histologic features* include papillary fronds or plaques of variably dense fibrovascular-to-collagenous tissue covered by a single layer of proliferative mesothelial cells, along with variable numbers of mixed, mostly mononuclear, inflammatory cells.

An association of bovine epicardial mesothelial hyperplasia has been suggested with lymphoma and BLV infection; however, this association has not been confirmed. In both dogs and cattle, the lesions appear instead to be incidental and possibly the result of resolved epicardial inflammation, or secondary to chronic and persistent trauma or friction between the epicardium and pericardium. The lesions should be differentiated from other more significant causes of epicarditis and pericarditis, and from neoplasia. IHC can be helpful to identify mesothelial cells, and they often usually exhibit immunoreactivity for cytokeratin and vimentin. Wilms tumor protein 1 is considered a reliable marker for human mesothelial cells; it also has been used in dogs, but is not helpful in differentiating hyperplasia from neoplasia.

Aggregates of proliferative mesothelial cells are occasionally observed in lymph nodes where they can be confused with metastatic neoplasia; this phenomenon, known as **benign epithelial inclusions** in humans, has been described in the lymph nodes of cattle.

Mesothelial metaplasia to a cuboidal or columnar epithelium is occasionally observed and is probably the mildest response of the peritoneum to irritation but also may be associated with estrogens. Inflammatory metaplasia leading to ossification may even occur in peritoneal scars, especially in swine. It also may be found in the mesenteries and the dorsal retroperitoneum without obvious cause, although ossification may occur following fat necrosis as well. Ossified areas are discoid, of variable size and shape, and are usually found in adipose tissue.

Diseases of the peritoneum and retroperitoneum

Congenital and developmental anomalies

Congenital abnormalities affecting the peritoneal membranes are associated most frequently with retention of effete embryonic structures or defective partitioning of the celomic cavity.

Persistent vitelline or omphalomesenteric ducts *may form a fibrous ligament between the intestine or Meckel diverticulum and the umbilicus.* The remnant may be partial and not reach the umbilicus, or it may be attached to the mesentery or to a loop of intestine. These structures may become involved in herniation and obstruction or strangulation of the intestine; persisting ducts may become cystic.

A **mesodiverticular band** is the result of a **persistent vitelline artery**. The band is a fold of mesentery, occasionally carrying a patent vitelline artery in its free edge, which extends from the cranial mesenteric artery, or from a spot partway down the mesenteric veil, to the antimesenteric side of the intestine (the site of a Meckel diverticulum). The pocket formed between this fold and the normal mesentery *may entrap and permit strangulation of intestine*. Both left and right mesodiverticular bands have been rarely described, and fibrous cords of mesenteric tissue may be observed that do not appear to be part of embryonic remnants of vitelline structures.

The **falciform ligament** is a fold of peritoneum containing a remnant of the embryonic ventral mesentery and umbilical vein, which varies in size among species and individuals; it is typically largest in young animals. There is potential for entrapment or strangulation of bowel by a large persistent falciform ligament.

Retroperitoneal lymphatic malformations are rare, with only a few described in dogs. Historically, these lesions may have been misdiagnosed as lymphangioma, but they are likely not true neoplastic lesions; histologic differentiation though can be challenging, and malformations are not expected to exhibit infiltrative or progressive behavior. While most vascular malformation are of blood vessel origin, lymphatic vessel malformation has been described in the skin, intestine, liver, and mammary gland. These are described as multicystic dilation of lymphatic vessels, which result in distension of the retroperitoneal space, obstruction of lymphatic flow, and accumulation of lymphatic fluid in several body cavities. Histologically, numerous variably dilated vascular spaces are lined by well-differentiated flattened endothelial cells and supported by collagenous-to-fibrovascular connective tissue fronds. The lining cells lack immunoreactivity for cytokeratin (ruling out mesothelial origin) and exhibit positive immunoreactivity for vascular endothelial [platelet endothelial cell adhesion molecule (PECAM1/CD31) and von Willebrand factor antigen] and lymphatic endothelial [lymphatic vessel endothelial hyaluronic acid receptor 1 (LYVE1) and prospero homeobox protein 1 (PROX1)], which confirms their lymphatic endothelial origin.

Congenital peritoneal hernias in several species are not uncommon. *Partitioning of the celom* to separate the thoracic cavity from the developing GI tract begins embryologically with the formation of the *septum transversum* from the ventral body wall, eventually forming the ventral part of the diaphragm. The dorsal part of the diaphragm is provided by downgrowth from the dorsal body wall of the paired *pleuroperitoneal and pleuropericardial folds*. **Congenital pleuroperitoneal diaphragmatic hernias** are most commonly observed in dogs, but are observed occasionally in herd animals. *They usually involve a defect in the left dorsal quadrant of the diaphragm, presumably from failure of the left pleuroperitoneal fold to fuse with the septum transversum;* the reason for the particular susceptibility for the left side is unknown. The lesion in some breeds of dogs may have an autosomal recessive mode of inheritance. Some congenital pleuroperitoneal defects in small animals may be more extensive, where much of the diaphragm is missing. The margins of the diaphragmatic defect are smooth, and a large mass of abdominal viscera may pass into the thoracic cavity through the opening; large defects result in respiratory difficulties, abdominal pain, and bloating if incarceration of herniated viscera occurs. Most small animals born with these defects die at or shortly after birth. In large animals, the lesions may be clinically silent, especially when only a small portion of the liver is present in the hernia.

Peritoneopericardial diaphragmatic hernias *are triangular and ventral, and presumably result from abnormal development or fusion of the septum transversum*. They are more commonly diagnosed than pleuroperitoneal hernias in small animals, perhaps because the animals live longer. They can be associated with cardiac anomalies, malformations of the sternum and costochondral junctions, or umbilical hernias. Although various portions of the liver, spleen, omentum, and small intestine may herniate into the pericardial sac and cause cardiac tamponade, compromised respiratory function, or GI tract obstruction, these lesions also can be clinically silent.

External hernias are the result of abnormal openings in the abdominal wall that permit passage of the abdominal contents and may be congenital or acquired. Congenital defects resulting in hernias are of several types and include abnormally increased size of normal openings, such as the inguinal canal; persistence of fetal openings, as in umbilical hernias; and defects in closure of the abdominal cavity, as in schistosomus reflexus and diaphragmatic hernias.

Traumatic lesions of the abdomen and peritoneum

Physical trauma to the abdomen is common, and *sequelae* include hemorrhage, peritoneal sepsis, uremia caused by the escape of urine into the abdomen, and dysfunction of traumatized organs. Blunt trauma to the abdomen may result in contusion of abdominal viscera; avulsion of organs from supporting mesenteries or ligaments, and from their vascular supply; and perhaps laceration of the capsule of solid organs such as the liver, spleen, and kidney. Hollow organs, including the stomach, gallbladder, and urinary bladder, may rupture and release their contents into the abdominal cavity. Sudden increase in intra-abdominal pressure resulting from such trauma may cause acquired hernias by forcing viscera through natural apertures such as the inguinal canal, weak points such as the perineum, or through lacerations in the diaphragm or the abdominal wall, resulting in eventration.

Following abdominal trauma, contusions, lacerations, or perforation may be evident on the underside of the skin or in subcutaneous tissues; these lesions are often in apposition to internal lesions. Lacerations of the liver or spleen may result in internal hemorrhage and diffuse pallor of the animal. Contusion or laceration of the kidney results in subcapsular, retroperitoneal, or peritoneal hemorrhage. The source of hemorrhage may be subtle slits or crevasses in the capsule of the organ involved, or the laceration may be more obvious. In animals that die of exsanguination, the spleen is often contracted. Following splenic rupture, portions of spleen may implant and persist ectopically elsewhere in the abdomen (splenosis) and may be encountered as an incidental finding. Urine in the abdominal cavity may be easily mistaken for ascitic fluid; uroperitoneum should be confirmed by comparing creatinine concentration of the abdominal fluid to that of serum. Lacerations of the urinary bladder may be small and difficult to detect, particularly because the bladder contracts as urine is lost through the laceration or rupture. If the pregnant uterus is ruptured, fetuses may be free in the abdomen. They will die and cause peritonitis if the dam survives and they are not removed.

Acquired diaphragmatic hernia can also occur secondary to penetrating or blunt trauma; the latter is more common. The diaphragm is weaker than the abdominal wall, so during blunt trauma, a large pressure differential is generated between the abdominal and thoracic sides of the diaphragm, and this is relieved by rupture of the diaphragm and herniation of abdominal contents into the thoracic cavity (Fig. 1-163). In small animals, the diaphragmatic muscle usually ruptures before the tendinous part; in general, the location and orientation of the lesion are the result of the type of trauma and the location or direction of impact. Due to the initial trauma, ~50% of patients also have concurrent orthopedic or soft tissue injuries. Almost any of the abdominal viscera may herniate into the thoracic cavity through the defect, but the liver and small bowel are most commonly involved. The lesion may be clinically silent for a considerable period, but eventually typically causes respiratory difficulty, hydrothorax, ascites, chylothorax, gastric tympany, or intestinal obstruction. At surgery or autopsy, acute diaphragmatic laceration is readily observed. If chronic, the margin of laceration is usually thickened by fibroplasia, and may even be adhered to the viscera. Differentiation from congenital hernias is based on the age, clinical history, and any evidence of scarring or adhesions at the margin of the diaphragmatic defect.

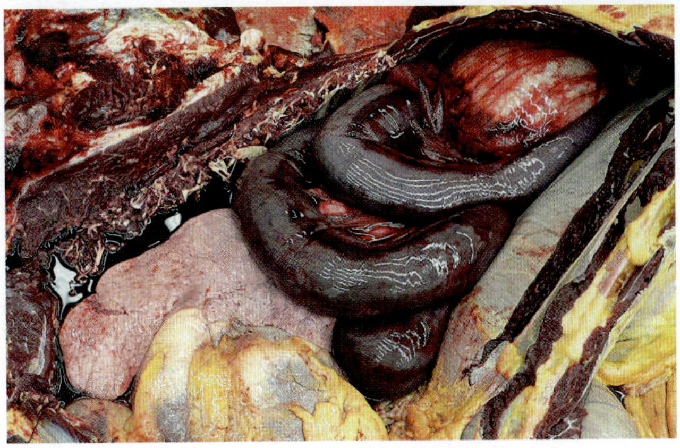

Figure 1-163 **Acquired diaphragmatic hernia** in a horse. Loops of the small intestine and stomach have passed through the diaphragmatic laceration into the thoracic cavity, compressing the lung.

In horses, acquired lesions usually involve the area where the tendinous portion meets the pars costalis; artifactual postmortem laceration of the diaphragm in the horse is most common at the ventral midline, near the xiphoid process. Most horses with acquired diaphragmatic hernias develop acute severe abdominal pain and signs of colic; respiratory signs are less common.

Endogenous forces may also result in herniation. The additional weight of intestinal contents during pregnancy, especially when complicated by an event such as hydrops amnios, may cause ventral hernia. Straining during defecation or parturition may also cause herniation; the former is associated with perineal hernias in dogs; the latter, with acquired diaphragmatic hernias in horses. Tympany of the large bowel in horses or the forestomachs in ruminants may also cause herniation involving the abdominal wall or diaphragm. Antemortem lesions must be differentiated from postmortem tears resulting from bloating of viscera during postmortem autolysis. *Hemorrhage, fibrin deposits, and acute inflammation in torn muscle, or strangulation of herniated gut, are usually sufficient evidence for an antemortem condition*.

Abnormal contents in the peritoneal cavity

Foreign materials within the peritoneal cavity, such as urine, ingesta, blood, or air, indicate an abnormality of another organ.

Ingesta or digesta in the peritoneal cavity caused by bowel rupture or perforation occurs in horses and cattle, less frequently in swine, sheep, and goats, and rarely in dogs and cats. The site of perforation or rupture is usually easy to find, especially when the animal dies before peritonitis develops; once adhesions develop between intestines and mesenteries, the primary site of perforation may be very difficult to identify. Ingesta may leak from any devitalized segment of small or large bowel as a consequence of impaction and pressure necrosis, tympany and rupture, or perforation either from sharp objects or deep mucosal ulceration. Cecal rupture in cattle following overload or impaction is reported, as well as in foals postsurgery. Rectal perforation can cause contamination of the abdomen with feces, and these lesions also may be difficult to document during autopsy.

Rectal perforation in horses occurs most commonly secondary to accidental iatrogenic injury during rectal palpation, but can also occur secondary to dystocia. Most tears occur 25-30 cm orad from the anus on the dorsal aspect of the rectum. Deep tears that involve the tunica muscularis have potential for contamination of the peritoneal cavity and secondary peritonitis. If the serosa remains intact, potential exists for development of subserosal or rectal diverticula, perineal abscessation or fistula, pelvic cellulitis, or other complications; these lesions can progress and eventually perforate the mesorectum, resulting in fecal contamination of the peritoneum.

Any portion of the bowel may rupture as a postmortem artifact; therefore, **postmortem rupture of a viscus** must be differentiated from an antemortem rupture or perforation. In contrast to antemortem loss of bowel wall integrity, the margins of a postmortem defect lack hemorrhage and exudate, and peritoneal surfaces have no evidence of mesothelial hyperplasia, inflammation, or exudate.

Pneumoperitoneum is air in the peritoneal cavity and arises from traumatic perforation of the abdominal wall (including surgery), from diaphragmatic tears in horses with concurrent pneumothorax, or from leakage of gas and liquid contents from a GI perforation. Rarely, pneumoperitoneum can develop secondary to rupture of the urinary bladder or the female reproductive tract.

Hemoperitoneum is blood or hemorrhagic effusion in the peritoneal cavity; hemorrhage can also occur in the retroperitoneal space and is usually trauma associated. The amount present at death is not necessarily an indication of the volume of bleeding during life because the blood may be removed quite rapidly via diaphragmatic lymphatics. Blood in the cavity may be partially clotted. Hemoperitoneum can be traumatic or atraumatic (spontaneous) and is seen most commonly in the dog and cat as a result of blunt or penetrating trauma. Spontaneous hemoperitoneum usually is associated with one of many pathologic processes, including hepatic or splenic torsion or rupture, gastric dilation and volvulus, coagulopathies, and neoplastic processes involving the liver, spleen, kidney, or other abdominal organs. When traumatic in origin, the liver and spleen are most commonly involved. Splenic nodular lesions, including a wide variety of benign and malignant lesions including hyperplasia and neoplasia, all can lead to hematoma formation and subsequent hemorrhage into the abdomen. These are the most common causes of spontaneous hemoperitoneum in middle-aged to older dogs. Enlargement of the liver or spleen because of infiltrating neoplastic cells, fat, or amyloid increases parenchymal friability and predisposes these organs to fracture and rupture. Fine fissures in the capsule of the liver resulting in hemorrhage have been reported in infectious canine hepatitis.

In several species, acquired coagulopathies following ingestion of *anticoagulant rodenticides* cause hemorrhage leading to unclotted blood in the abdomen. Calves born of cows that have been fed moldy sweet-clover hay hemorrhage from the umbilical vessels into the peritoneal cavity and elsewhere. Manual ablation of a corpus luteum by rectal palpation can be a source of peritoneal hemorrhage in cattle. In cattle and horses, laceration of the uterus or rupture of a uterine artery at parturition can result in massive fatal peritoneal or retroperitoneal hemorrhage. In horses, hemoperitoneum may be due to hemorrhage from granulosa-thecal cell tumor of the ovary, and in all species any friable intra-abdominal or retroperitoneal neoplasm may occasionally rupture and hemorrhage if traumatized. Hemoperitoneum has been associated with anaphylaxis in dogs, and although the mechanisms remain uncharacterized, likely involves various vasoactive chemical mediators including heparin, bradykinin, tryptase, histamine, or metabolic alteration of the normal coagulation cascade or complement system; affected dogs typically have concurrent or recent historical evidence of systemic anaphylaxis.

Hemorrhage on or beneath the peritoneal surface without free blood in the cavity may occur in acute bacterial toxemias and in other conditions that interfere with vascular integrity or hemostasis. *Peritoneal hemorrhage must be differentiated from hemorrhagic peritonitis*, which is an important lesion in some diseases. Subserosal hemorrhage and *hemomelasma ilei* occasionally occur on the intestine of the horse; this lesion has long been attributed to (but likely not pathognomonic for) the migration of strongyles. Subserosal hematomas may rarely cause intestinal obstruction. Hemorrhage into an omental or mesenteric cyst can cause sudden abdominal enlargement without free blood in the abdomen.

Uroperitoneum is urine in the peritoneal cavity, and in adults usually results from rupture of the urinary bladder, urethra, or ureters. Urine can also accumulate in the retroperitoneal space (urinoma), which is mostly associated with trauma. In ruminants, this occurs most frequently as a consequence of urethral obstruction due to urolithiasis. Uroperitoneum in neonates is associated with sepsis and is described as a frequent consequence of inflammation or congenital abnormalities involving the urachus or urethra. Effusion of fluid into body cavities (ascites) is part of the postmortem picture in sheep and cattle that die of *urethral obstruction*, and the fluid has a distinct uriniferous odor. The pathogenesis of this fluid accumulation is uncertain. In some cases, there is a rupture of the lower urinary tract that might permit overt uroperitoneum, although in many cases this cannot be definitively demonstrated.

Hydroperitoneum, or **ascites**, *is excess fluid, usually a modified transudate, in the peritoneal cavity*. Ascites occurs because of reduced removal or overproduction of fluid in the abdominal cavity. Ascitic fluid is generally watery and clear or straw-colored and contains few leukocytes but possibly numerous mesothelial cells. The serosal lining is normal and glistening but may become slightly opaque as a result of subserosal edema.

Reduced removal of fluid from the peritoneal cavity *is mainly caused by the obstruction of lymphatic drainage through the diaphragm*. The limited area for direct-to-lymphatic absorption and the small size of stomata on the diaphragmatic and pelvic serosa explain the ease and rapidity with which peritoneal drainage can be blocked. An example is peritoneal carcinomatosis, in which neoplastic cells implant throughout the abdomen; when they implant on the diaphragm in the region of the lymphatic stomata, obstruction of lymphatic drainage occurs. Ascites may also develop if there is obstruction to sternal lymphatic flow cranial to the diaphragm. This may occur with sclerosing lymphadenitis or space-occupying lesions in the ventral or cranial mediastinum and is common in lymphoma of adult cattle.

Overproduction of peritoneal lymph *is mainly related to altered hydrostatic pressure gradients in the hepatic and portal circulation*, except for **chylous ascites**, which results when the cisterna chyli leak triglyceride-rich milky fluid into the abdomen. Increased prehepatic portal venous pressure alone does not usually lead to ascites, although if present, such fluid is low protein, being derived from intestinal and mesenteric interstitial fluid. Acute portal vein obstruction causes intestinal infarction and death, but not ascites. Slowly developing portal hypertension of prehepatic, hepatic, or hepatic venous origin may cause transient ascites, which resolves with the development of acquired collateral portal-postcaval venous shunts within a few weeks. However, portal hypertension of cardiac origin does not usually result in portocaval shunts because the elevation in central venous pressure permits no pressure gradient between the portal and postcaval systems. *The sine qua non of hepatic ascites is increased resistance in the intrahepatic or posthepatic circulation*. The exception is when increased portal blood flow occurs due to hepatic arteriovenous fistulas or anastomoses; in this circumstance, hydrostatic pressure at the level of the hepatic sinusoids is elevated by the arterialization of the portal flow.

The usual conditions causing increased hepatic or posthepatic resistance to blood flow are fibrosis of the liver and congestive heart failure, respectively. Intrahepatic resistance due to hepatic fibrosis may be compounded by the development of arteriovenous anastomoses in the fibrous septa around regenerative hepatocellular nodules; these arterialize the hepatic portal circulation, further elevating hydrostatic pressure. Additional causes of portal hypertension include: primary neoplasms of the liver, especially cholangiocellular carcinomas, which tend to be diffuse and infiltrative; secondary tumors, especially lymphomas, which widely infiltrate the liver; extensive infestation with hydatid cysts; and chronic biliary trematodosis, or other causes of chronic cholangiohepatitis and portal fibrosis. Tumors or abscesses compressing the hepatic vein as it leaves the liver, or obstructions in the caudal vena cava cranial to the entry of the hepatic vein, may also cause posthepatic obstruction.

When the liver is congested, there is increased flow of high-protein hepatic lymph from the perisinusoidal space, which is separated from the sinusoidal lumen by fenestrated endothelium that is freely permeable to plasma constituents, including large protein molecules. Hence, the formation of hepatic lymph is not regulated by plasma oncotic pressure but is sensitive to small changes in hydrostatic pressure in the sinusoids. This accounts for the frequency with which ascites is associated with diseases causing increased central and hepatic venous pressure or increased intrahepatic resistance to blood flow.

Hypoproteinemia caused by reduced hepatic synthesis may occur in severe liver disease, and once advanced capillarization of sinusoids occurs, the free permeability of the hepatic vascular system to the flow of large molecules is reduced. In this circumstance, reduced plasma oncotic pressure caused by hypoalbuminemia promotes continued hepatic lymph formation and ascites.

Hypoproteinemia of nonhepatic origin is most commonly associated with PLE, such as paratuberculosis in ruminants, with protein-losing nephropathy, such as glomerular amyloidosis, or with severe parasitism. Severe hypoproteinemia reduces plasma oncotic pressure, promoting edema and permitting transudate to accumulate in serous spaces, including the peritoneal cavity.

Vascular injury in the portal circulation allows increased permeability to plasma protein and substantially favors development of ascites. Mild ascites may occur in a variety of systemic illnesses altering vascular permeability, such as the clostridial intoxications, endotoxemia, acute uremic syndromes in ruminants and pigs, and in exudative diathesis of pigs with vitamin E deficiency. Effusion of fluid into body cavities occurs with urethral obstruction, often without overt uroperitoneum due to rupture of urinary bladder, urethra, or ureters. Renal uremia, especially that caused by acute toxic nephrosis, also may be accompanied by significant abdominal effusions.

Necrosis of mesenteric or other abdominal or retroperitoneal fat occurs either as a consequence of acute pancreatic necrosis or pancreatitis (in several species), or as a poorly understood condition affecting the abdominal fat (predominantly ruminants).

Acute pancreatic necrosis occurs secondary to enzymatic digestion and necrosis of pancreatic parenchyma, and the peripancreatic adipose tissue is almost always involved; this may in fact be the initial or more severe morphologic lesion. In acute pancreatic necrosis, discrete foci or confluent masses of white necrotic adipose tissue are surrounded by a zone of intense hyperemia with fibrin deposited on the surface. Such lesions may be limited to the pancreas and peripancreatic fat, or they may be distributed more broadly throughout the abdominal cavity. Histologically, there is coagulative necrosis of adipocytes that appear eosinophilic and opaque with karyorrhectic or absent nuclei; there is frequent deposition of basophilic fibrillar-to-granular mineralized material, and depending on the duration, inflammation dominated by neutrophils. The necrosis is attributed to the release of proteolytic and lipolytic enzymes from damaged pancreatic acini and to degeneration of neutrophils recruited to the area.

Massive abdominal fat necrosis in cattle is reported most frequently in Channel Island breeds and occurs in older animals with increased body fat stores. Masses of necrotic fat of various sizes form and may coalesce to involve significant portions of the abdominal cavity. Although it is *often an incidental finding*, it can cause clinical signs and even death if there is compression or obstruction of abdominal viscera. Necrosis may occur in any portion of the omental, mesenteric, and retroperitoneal fat and has been observed in intermuscular and subcutaneous fat. Initially, there is acute inflammation, and the hard necrotic masses are surrounded by a zone of hyperemia; the overlying peritoneum may be necrotic, perhaps with adhesions to adjacent viscera. On cut section, these masses are firm, dry, and chalky, or sometimes moist, oily, and deep-yellow. Because of the unusual bulk of the necrotic tissue in some cases, and because necrotic fat is sometimes found in abnormal locations, such as under the serosa of the intestine, the condition has been called *lipomatosis*, but the lesions are not considered to be hyperplastic or neoplastic. The hard lumps of fat may be confused with fetal structures, lymphoid tumors, or other masses on abdominal palpation. Clinical signs, although uncommon, are most commonly caused by *intestinal obstruction* if the necrotic fat nodules surround and incorporate various intestinal segments (Fig. 1-164). Bovine obesity has been linked to fatty pancreas, pancreatitis, and subsequent abdominal fat necrosis.

Histologically, the lesions are a mixture of acute and chronic fat necrosis with infiltration of many macrophages and multinucleate giant cells, as well as fewer neutrophils, lymphocytes, and plasma cells. There is variable fibrosis and mineralization. The pathogenesis remains unclear, although it has been linked to alterations in lipid metabolism; there may be a genetic component. Abdominal fat necrosis may be related to dietary factors including ingestion of feeds high in long-chain saturated fatty acids. In several ruminant species, including cattle, sheep, goats, and deer, the condition also has been linked to grazing of endophyte-infested tall fescue pastures.

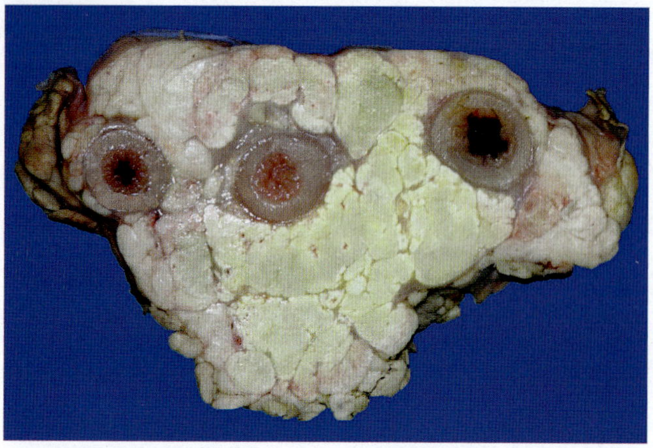

Figure 1-164 Abdominal fat necrosis in a cow. Abundant necrotic adipose tissue surrounds and encases intestinal loops in the abdomen.

Massive necrosis of abdominal fat is reported infrequently in **cats**; some cases are subsequent to trauma or pancreatitis; in other cases the cause was not determined. Nodular necrosis of abdominal fat (so-called Bates body or floater) is an incidental finding in aged dogs and cats.

Steatitis (*yellow-fat disease*) occurs in many species affecting the abdominal and peritoneal fat, along with other adipose tissue. It is associated with diets high in polyunsaturated fat and low in tocopherols, favoring oxidation of fatty acids. Peroxidation of susceptible lipids and membranes creates free radicals that provoke the characteristic inflammatory reaction in response to formation of irritant soaps, cholesterol deposits, and ceroid-lipofuscin (see section on Panniculitis in Vol. 1, Integumentary System).

Peritonitis, retroperitonitis, and their consequences

Peritonitis, inflammation of the serosa of the peritoneal lining, is very common in large domestic animals, and less common in dogs and cats. *Peritonitis may be classified as primary or secondary; as acute or chronic; as localized or diffuse; as septic or nonseptic; and on the basis of the type of exudate, which may be serofibrinous, fibrinopurulent, purulent, hemorrhagic, or granulomatous*. Most cases of peritonitis in domestic animals are secondary and arise as complications of other events in the abdomen, but primary serositis in systemic infections is of much importance for agricultural livestock. *The causes of peritonitis are numerous and varied*, and the more common and important of them are considered here.

Chemical peritonitis may be induced by a variety of chemicals, and intraperitoneal instillation of a number of therapeutic agents causes mild and usually inconsequential peritonitis; however, abdominal lavage has been associated with more severe serosal injury and formation of adhesions. Surgical glove powders, including *talc* or *starch*, provoke granulomatous peritonitis; starch granules have a characteristic Maltese cross appearance in polarized light and are PAS -positive. Accidental leakage of *barium sulfate* into the abdomen during contrast studies causes potentially severe and fatal hemorrhagic peritonitis that progresses over several days to severe granulomatous and fibrosing peritonitis. Leakage of barium is often concurrent with leakage of ingesta and thus is frequently complicated by intercurrent sepsis.

The most devastating forms of chemical peritonitis are endogenous and are caused by *bile* or *pancreatic enzymes*. **Bile peritonitis** occurs when bile leaks into the peritoneal cavity, usually from the gallbladder proper or from the biliary ductular tree, though leakage can also occur from the duodenum or stomach, all following rupture or perforation. The most common cause of bile peritonitis in domestic animals occurs as a complication of gallbladder mucocele in dogs; however, other causes of gallbladder rupture include neoplasia, trauma, choleliths, and cholecystitis. Bile is toxic to tissue parenchyma and causes endothelial dysfunction, altered permeability, increased production of proinflammatory cytokines, localized coagulative necrosis of tissue, and possibly systemic effects such as hypotension, abdominal pain and distension, and fever; these effects are exacerbated in cases with intercurrent sepsis. Bile peritonitis is recognized by yellow-green staining of visceral and parietal peritoneal surfaces.

Peritonitis associated with acute pancreatic necrosis is also common in dogs. The reaction occurs within and adjacent to the pancreas and consists of acute coagulative necrosis and neutrophilic inflammation; there is often adhesion of the lesser omentum to the pancreas, adjacent liver, and other organs. This localized peritoneal reaction resolves completely if the animal survives, and only very minor adhesions of the mesentery and pancreas persist due to fibrosis. Depending on the duration and severity of disease, persistence of neutrophilic peritoneal exudate may be mild, but often contains droplets of fats and soaps released from the adipose tissue by the pancreatic enzymes. Though rare, accumulation of chylous effusion within the peritoneal space can occur secondary to acute pancreatic necrosis, and this causes a peritoneal reaction referred to as **chylous peritonitis**.

Bacterial peritonitis may occur if bacteria reach the peritoneum by direct implantation after traumatic perforation of a contaminated external surface. It most commonly originates with peritoneal contamination by ingesta following perforation or rupture of the GI tract; however, bacteria also can be introduced from the skin (e.g., migrating plant awn) or in females via the reproductive tract. Endometritis caused by tuberculosis or brucellosis in cows, and brucellosis in sows, may extend to the peritoneum through the uterine tubes. Cystitis and rupture of the urinary bladder may also cause peritonitis. Bacterial peritonitis can occur as an extension from localized inflammation in other organs, including the umbilicus, via mural extension of bacteria through the GI wall damaged by inflammation or ischemic necrosis, or as a component of bacteremia or septicemia. For example, acute serofibrinous peritonitis may occur by extension through the wall of an intestine or uterus with localized inflammation or ischemic necrosis before overt rupture or perforation is evident. Secondary peritonitis occasionally results by extension from retroperitoneal infection, or in ruminants from omental bursitis. When peritonitis develops by direct extension, there is little difficulty in ascertaining its origin, even when the process becomes diffuse.

Retroperitonitis may arise from sepsis involving the pelvic or abdominal urogenital tract, or the mesenteric root; from penetrating wounds; from rectal tears in horses; and from migrating grass awns or other foreign bodies. Frequently, it evolves to form a fluctuant abscess or draining fistula in the flank, based on the path of least resistance in the soft tissue of the region. The lesion is usually a poorly encapsulated sinus or abscess containing purulent exudate, with a wall of granulation tissue. It may extend to involve adjacent vertebrae as periostitis or osteomyelitis. A foreign body may be encountered on exploration, or the lesion may be traced back to a primary septic focus in the abdomen, perhaps a renal or perirenal abscess; an ovarian stump with a remnant of unresorbed suture; or an abscess or pyogranuloma in the root of the mesentery. These are typically associated with mixed bacterial flora. Chronic lesions in this region due to previous injury may resolve as retroperitoneal fibrosis.

The consequences of peritonitis in individual cases can vary from insignificant to catastrophic. Acute generalized peritonitis can be a catastrophic sequel of many localized diseases of the abdominal cavity, but it may also be a relatively insignificant secondary event in generalized infections, such as *E. coli* septicemia. Within the first few hours of generalized peritonitis, there may be intestinal hypermotility; however, *paralytic ileus* mediated by autonomic innervation typically follows. Long-term development of fibrinous adhesions between loops of intestine can be significant and eventually produce fibrous adhesions and their sequelae.

The systemic effects of generalized peritonitis are related to detrimental effects on cardiovascular function, circulatory homeostasis, and acid-base balance, resulting at least partially from sequestration of fluid and plasma proteins in the peritoneal exudate; sequestration of fluids and electrolytes in the lumen of immotile intestine; and loss of intestinal absorptive function. Toxins generated in the intestinal lumen by bacteria (including endotoxins) may be absorbed through the peritoneum or via the lymphatic drainage, causing increased vascular permeability, shock, and other detrimental cardiovascular effects; death from toxemia may result before overt peritonitis develops. Bacteria may spread via the lymphatics to the pleura and the sternal or mediastinal nodes, or may reach the general circulation, causing septicemia.

Not all cases of generalized peritonitis are immediately fatal. Depending on the severity and distribution of the inflammation, the lesions may persist locally, mature into fibrous adhesions, or resolve completely. Peritoneal lesions are debrided by phagocytes; fibroplasia neovascularization and collagen deposition occur within days, and mesothelial restoration is accomplished by 5-8 days after the insult. Because the mesothelium differentiates from mesenchymal elements in the subserosa or from free-floating peritoneal stem cells, reconstitution of the mesothelium is not affected by the size of the defect. Fibrin along serosal surfaces persisting beyond 3-4 days after the original insult becomes progressively organized and mature, resulting in formation of **fibrous serosal adhesions** that have various downstream effects resulting in impaired motility or obstruction. *Formation of adhesions seems to be promoted by ischemia, increasing severity of tissue necrosis, foreign material such as sutures on the serosa, and by sepsis; all these increase and prolong the inflammatory response.* Determining the duration of peritonitis may be important in cases such as iatrogenic rectal perforation, and its assessment requires careful gross and microscopic examination of the serosal surface and the adherent exudates. Proliferation, degree of differentiation of fibroblasts and mesothelial cells within and along the margins of any wound, and thickness of serosal granulation tissue will give some indication of the age of the lesion.

Sclerosing encapsulating peritonitis is an unusual, unique, and characteristic form of chronic peritonitis that occurs in humans and has been described in dogs and cats. This condition is mostly due to extensive fibrosis and thickening of both visceral and parietal peritoneum with widespread adhesions between abdominal organs that is usually associated with underlying or concurrent diseases, including peritoneal dialysis, previous abdominal surgery, foreign body migration, and abdominal neoplasia such as pancreatic adenocarcinoma; some cases have been considered idiopathic. Histologic lesions include progressively mature granulation tissue, fibrosis, and collagenous tissue deposition involving the parietal and visceral peritoneal surfaces, which may be variably infiltrated with lymphocytes, plasma cells, and neutrophils. Only a few cases in dogs are described, and the prognosis is poor due to the concurrent conditions, and to the severity of lesions at the time of diagnosis.

Peritonitis in horses *(especially if diffuse) is usually acute and fatal*; this is perhaps due to a small omentum and a poor capacity to heal contaminated areas. In most cases, peritonitis is secondary to rupture or perforation of the stomach or intestine, which may be associated with verminous lesions of *Habronema*, *Anoplocephala*, or *Gasterophilus* infestation, and subsequent leakage of ingesta into the abdominal cavity; however, primary idiopathic peritonitis is also described in horses.

When not clearly secondary to bowel leakage, hypotheses for the pathogenesis of apparently primary idiopathic peritonitis include leakage of GI organisms from the lumen, by migration of parasites or foreign bodies, via mucosal erosions associated with NSAIDs, or associated with nonstrangulating intestinal infarctions. Horses often have fever, lethargy, and abdominal pain; bacterial culture for *Actinobacillus* spp. (or other bacteria such as *C. perfringens*, *Bacillus* spp., *Bacteroides* spp., etc.) will be positive in at least a proportion of cases. Antemortem cytologic evaluation and culture of peritoneal fluid is often helpful to confirm the diagnosis and guide medical therapy. Most cases respond well to antimicrobial therapy, also supporting the idea that many of these are associated with bacteria, although the specific bacterial source is not readily identified. Parasitic migration, including by *S. vulgaris* and cyathostomes, has also been proposed to be a significant factor in the development of idiopathic peritonitis of horses, although this remains definitively unproven.

Peritoneal lavage may cause severe diffuse chemical peritonitis. Seminoperitoneum caused by laceration of the vagina at breeding is an unusual cause of acute diffuse nonseptic peritonitis; sperm are present in the cytoplasm of neutrophils. Chronic diffuse peritonitis is virtually never recorded in horses, other than rare cases of nocardiosis. Acute or chronic local peritonitis does occasionally occur after castration, and the colon may adhere to the inner inguinal area; from penetrating wounds originating from the skin; and from streptococcal abscesses in the mesentery. Migrating *S. equinus* or *S. edentatus* larvae are thought to cause retroperitoneal lesions in the flank, perirenal fat, and diaphragm; fibrous tags on the liver capsule; and chronic diffuse thickening and inflammation in the mesentery, omentum, and hepatorenal ligament. Large strongyles returning to the gut may cause focal peritoneal lesions on the ileum, cecum, and colon, and migration of large strongyles in the wall of the small intestine is thought to be a cause of hemomelasma ilei.

Acute diffuse fibrinopurulent ***peritonitis in cattle*** *is common and* is usually the result of perforation of a viscus (Fig. 1-165), including the GI or reproductive tracts. Perforation initially results in localized acute disease, which is then typically

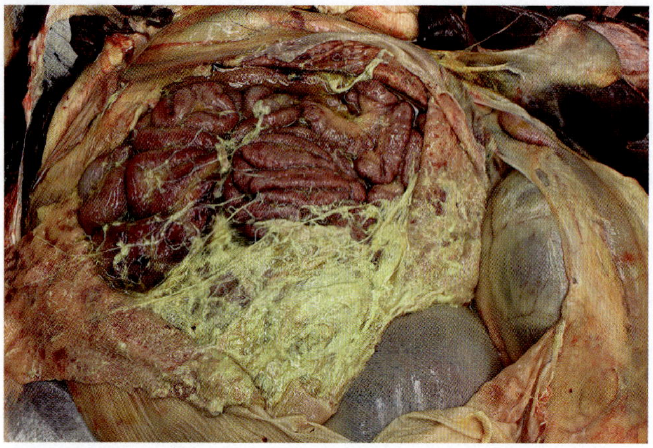

Figure 1-165 **Acute diffuse fibrinous peritonitis** in a cow.

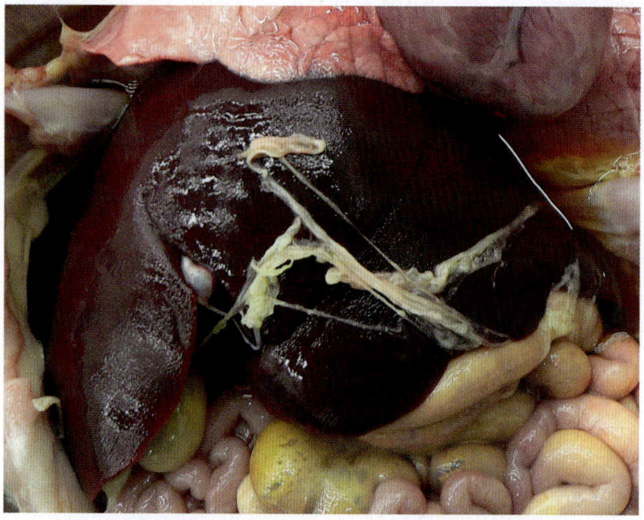

Figure 1-166 **Strands of fibrin** overlying the liver in a pig.

followed by diffuse chronic peritonitis with adhesions. Diffuse fibrinous **traumatic reticuloperitonitis** (hardware disease) may evolve to include septic **reticulopericarditis** if the offending foreign body migrates as far as the pericardial sac. Disordered motility of the forestomachs manifests clinically as vagus indigestion and may follow peritoneal scarring that interferes with function of the vagus nerve or esophagus.

Cattle seem to have a relatively high capacity to localize and limit septic foci through fibrous tissue encapsulation within the peritoneal cavity, and abscesses frequently develop. Sometimes these may become quite large; mixed bacterial flora is most commonly isolated. Perforation of the abomasum or intestine is more likely to cause diffuse fibrinous or fibrinohemorrhagic peritonitis, but, depending on the precise location of the perforation, occasionally causes local chronic peritonitis and abscessation.

In neonates, extension of inflammation following infection of the umbilicus and associated structures produces fibrinopurulent peritonitis, which tends to be most severe along the ventral abdominal wall, adjacent to concurrent liver abscesses, or extending along the urachus to the urinary bladder. Fibrinous peritonitis may be an expression of *polyserositis* in neonatal calves with septicemic colibacillosis and neonatal streptococcal infection. Copious serofibrinous peritonitis (with similar lesions on other serous membranes) is typical of sporadic bovine encephalomyelitis. Diffuse fibrinohemorrhagic peritonitis occurs in most cases of clostridial hemoglobinuria, and in some cases of blackleg and septicemic pasteurellosis, a more localized peritonitis of this type occurs in clostridial enteritis and abomasitis of calves caused by *C. perfringens* type B and type C, and *C. septicum*, respectively.

Tuberculosis, actinobacillosis, and infection with green algae are rarely reported causes of inflammatory lesions in the peritoneum of cattle.

Peritonitis in sheep of specific cause is uncommon. A local inflammatory reaction accompanies penetration of the intestine by the larvae of *O. columbianum*. Rare cases of peritonitis in sheep with caseous lymphadenitis are described, caused by rupture of caseous lesions in internal organs. The postpartum uterus is probably the most common site in adults from which bacteria and exudate spread into the peritoneum. Outbreaks of peritonitis in lamb flocks are frequently ascribed to coliform infection.

Mycoplasma mycoides may cause acute fibrinous **peritonitis in goats**, although acute deaths from septicemia, or arthritis and mastitis are more common. Paratuberculosis frequently produces nodular granulomatous lymphangitis in the mesentery, and sometimes caseous or mineralized lymphadenitis.

Peritonitis in swine is a well-recognized part of several defined infectious syndromes. A few filmy strands of mucin with appearances of fibrin frequently overlie the intestine, mesentery, and liver in many acute infectious diseases of swine, and in conditions that result in vascular damage, such as edema disease and vitamin E/selenium-responsive disease; this does not qualify as peritonitis (Fig. 1-166).

Diffuse fibrinopurulent peritonitis is common in pigs. Acute diffuse serofibrinous peritonitis with fibrinous arthritis and meningitis is characteristic of Glasser disease, caused by *Glaesserella* (formerly *Haemophilus*) *parasuis*. In chronic infections, pigs have a reduced growth rate because of severe polyserositis and arthritis. Similar clinical signs and lesions can also be associated with several other septicemic bacterial infections, especially *S. suis* and *Mesomycoplasma* (*Mycoplasma*) *hyorhinis*. Small firm nodules and flattened disks of inspissated fibrin are often found free in the peritoneal cavity in chronic *Mycoplasma* infections. Further testing using bacteriology or molecular methods is required to differentiate specific causes and diseases.

A variety of other bacterial organisms can be isolated from cases of peritonitis in pigs, including *T. pyogenes*, *E. coli*, or possibly several organisms simultaneously. In some cases, the cause can be traced to castration or other wounds, especially when peritonitis is localized to the inguinal and pelvic regions; alternatively, there is no apparent cause at autopsy because the intestines are extensively adhered together with fibrin and they cannot be separated. Occasionally, *T. pyogenes* produces discrete abscesses on both visceral and parietal peritoneum.

Tuberculosis in swine may cause lymphadenitis or peritonitis and induce adhesions in the peritoneum. In cases of rectal stricture, there is marked dilation of the colon and cecum, and the serosa may be covered with fibrin, similar to other causes of infectious serositis. Peritonitis also can occur in pigs with perforating gastric ulcers, but many pigs die from acute gastric hemorrhage before perforation is possible.

Stephanurus dentatus larvae cause subserosal focal hepatitis and a mild reaction with edema in the perirenal fat and retroperitoneal tissue, and sometimes in the mesentery and local lymph nodes, as they migrate to the kidney.

Septic peritonitis in dogs is uncommon and occurs secondary to microbial contamination in a variety of scenarios, including perforation or rupture of the GI tract, reproductive tract, urinary bladder or other viscera, or bacteremia; microorganisms are varied and typically reflect the source of contamination. Septic peritonitis involving a variety of agents, including *E. coli* and anaerobes, may follow surgical contamination of the abdomen; a percutaneous penetrating wound; rupture or perforation of the bowel; rupture of the urinary bladder; rupture of the uterus, occasionally as a result of pyometra; or rupture of pancreatic, umbilical, hepatic, or prostatic abscesses. Peritonitis also occurs when the uterus ruptures, either as a result of pyometra or septic metritis with fetal putrefaction. Mild *fibrinohemorrhagic peritonitis and serositis* associated with canine parvoviral enteritis, infectious canine hepatitis, and toxoplasmosis can be easily overlooked.

A distinctive pyogranulomatous variant of peritonitis with copious brown odoriferous exudate occurs in dogs and cats, and is usually associated with Actinomyces spp., most commonly *A. viscosus*, or bacteria of the *Nocardia asteroides* complex. The exudate often contains small yellow sulfur granules free in the exudate or within granulomas adhered to serosal surfaces, including omentum, mesenteries, and mesenteric lymph nodes.

Chronic pyogranulomatous or granulomatous peritonitis occurs with rare cases of eumycotic mycetoma and mucormycosis that can involve the abdominal cavity. There is usually serosal thickening and fibrosis of affected segments of the intestine with formation of adhesions, and the development of firm granulomatous masses on the intestinal wall, in the mesenteries, and in the omentum. *Mycobacterium microti* (llama-type), the vole bacillus, has been reported as a rare cause of severe diffuse granulomatous peritonitis.

Retroperitoneal inflammation or abscesses occurs in dogs and are diagnostically challenging antemortem due to the vague clinical signs. Various aerobic or anerobic bacteria, including *Actinomyces* spp., *E. coli*, *Bacillus* spp., *Pasteurella multocida*, *Prevotella* spp., have been implicated, although in many cases, a cause cannot be definitively identified. They are often assumed to be due to migrating foreign material, such as plant or suture.

Body cavity parasitism by larval stages of some tapeworms, including *Mesocestoides* and *Spirometra*, causes proliferative-to-granulomatous peritonitis with cysts containing cestode larvae and occurs mostly in dogs who act as intermediate hosts for these parasites (see later the Parasitic Diseases of the Peritoneum and Retroperitoneum section).

Peritonitis in cats is generally uncommon but occurs when the uterus ruptures because of pyometra or fetal putrefaction. Peritonitis also occurs from penetrating wounds or by extension from retroperitoneal tissues, and occasionally, septic peritonitis is caused by anaerobes such as those associated with cat-bite abscesses. Actinomycotic peritonitis similar in appearance to the disease in dogs may complicate FeLV infection in cats and the other myeloproliferative diseases.

Feline infectious peritonitis (FIP) is caused by feline infectious peritonitis virus (FIPV; *Coronaviridae, Alphacoronavirus 1*), a mutated variant of feline enteric coronavirus (FECV). FCoVs can be divided into 2 antigenically distinct serotypes (I and II) based on cell culture CP effect and other features; both FIPV and FECV strains are represented among FCoV types I and II, although type I FCoV induce higher antibody titers and are more frequently associated with FIP than type II FCoV. In domestic and wild felids, the various FCoV strains have a spectrum of virulence that ranges from subclinical enteric infection and healthy lifelong carrier status, through clinical enteric infection, to virulent systemic infection expressed as FIP.

FCoVs are ubiquitous in cats, but the disease FIP is sporadic with a low prevalence that *predominantly affects young intact male cats*. Purebred cats appear to be more susceptible to FCoV. FECV is transmitted by the fecal-oral route, and the virus initially infects enterocytes but soon becomes restricted to the cecum and colon. Some cats become persistently infected and, although they remain clinically healthy, continue to shed virus in their feces. FECV is generally regarded as the avirulent pathotype of FCoV, although some cats may develop catarrhal-to-hemorrhagic enteritis. Enteric infection with FCoV may produce mild subclinical blunting and fusion of villi, and possibly failure to gain weight or thrive, but rarely results in clinical signs.

FIPV was initially thought to have evolved as a deletion mutation of FECV; however, analysis of the viruses has revealed a much more complex picture of several genes and proteins involved in mediating virulence. There is strong evidence that FIPV is not transmitted horizontally but emerges within each cat that eventually develops FIP, individually. A requirement for development of FIP is likely the capacity of the virus to replicate within monocytes of the host. In comparison to FECV, FIPV strains have a distinct shift in tropism from intestinal epithelium to monocytes. *FIPV replicates in macrophages*, and it is thought that macrophages from the intestine acquire virus from the intestinal epithelium for transit to regional lymph nodes and dissemination to many parts of the body; this is central to their virulence. Mutation and transformation of FECV to FIPV may also take place within macrophages; however, this has not been definitively demonstrated. Incidence of the disease is apparently not higher in cats infected with FeLV or FIV; however, FCoV replicates 10-100-fold more in macrophages of cats infected with FIV, thus enhancing the probability of spontaneous mutations.

Resistance to FIPV infection is cell mediated, and systemic clinical disease probably only occurs if the cell-mediated response is ineffective; the lack of cell-mediated immunity may allow viral persistence or more pronounced virus production within macrophages. The cytokine response appears to be important in the response to FIPV infection, and immunity against FIPV may be associated with low tumor necrosis factor/high interferon-γ responses, whereas high tumor necrosis factor/low interferon-γ responses favor disease. There is also evidence that type III and type IV immune reactions play a role in vasculitis and CD4+ cell-heavy granulomatous inflammation of FIPV-infected cats, respectively. Cats that recover from FIP have dominant humoral immune responses and immune complexes that are demonstrable in blood, and although viral clearance eventually occurs, persistence and fecal shedding may extend for several months.

Cats that do not clear FIPV appear to develop either the dry or wet clinical forms of disease depending on whether ineffective cell-mediated or humoral immunity dominates the clinical disease. Although often described as distinct entities, *the effusive (wet) and noneffusive (dry) forms of FIP are best thought of as extremes of a continuum of syndromes, with hallmarks of* ***vasculitis*** *and* ***pyogranulomatous inflammation***. Effusive disease is more common than the noneffusive form, and mixed forms are probably common.

Cats with the **effusive form of FIP** often develop severe abdominal distension. Pleural effusion is present in ~25%

of cases and may cause dyspnea. Cardiac tamponade caused by pericardial effusion is rare, although significant amounts of abdominal exudate may be present in cats with effusive FIP. The fluid is usually viscous, clear, and pale to deep-yellow, although it may be flocculent and contain strands of fibrin. The serosal surfaces may be covered with fibrin, giving them a granular appearance; fragile adhesions may be present between viscera. There are foci of necrosis, raised plaques, or nodular cellular infiltrates that vary from a few millimeters to a centimeter in diameter on serosal surfaces and that extend into the parenchyma of organs. The mesentery is often thickened and opaque; the omentum may be seen as a contracted mass in the cranial abdomen and adhered to other abdominal surfaces (Fig. 1-167A). Fibrin is usually less prominent in the thoracic cavity, but firm white nodules may be present under the pleura, and the lungs may be dark and rubbery. *The effusive form of FIP may appear grossly similar to bacterial peritonitis.* Abdominal and thoracic lymph nodes may be enlarged. Some cats with FIP are lame because of generalized synovitis caused by migration of macrophages into the synovium. Ocular and central nervous signs are rare in this form. The cats are hypergammaglobulinemic and may have leukocytosis and neutrophilia. The clinical course for effusive FIP is rapid, and most cats die within a few weeks.

Cats with the **noneffusive form of FIP** have chronic disease of insidious onset and frequently develop signs specific to organs severely affected by vascular-oriented lesions. These may include ocular disease; central nervous disorders such as ataxia, paraparesis, head tilt; specific nerve palsies, nystagmus, and behavioral changes; renal failure; hepatic or pancreatic insufficiency; and diarrhea caused by ulcerative colitis.

Peritonitis is present in most cats, although marked effusion is not found in those with the noneffusive form of FIP. In cats with *noneffusive FIP*, there may be aggregates of inflammatory cells in the abdominal or thoracic organs, or lesions may be restricted to the eyes and nervous system. Diffuse uveitis, chorioretinitis, and sometimes panophthalmitis are observed; fibrin is often present in the anterior chamber. Lesions in the CNS can involve the leptomeninges, spinal cord, or brain, but usually are subtle grossly and easily overlooked. Occasionally, hydrocephalus, hydromyelia, and syringomyelia may result from ependymitis and obstruction of cerebrospinal fluid flow. The kidneys may be enlarged with perivascular, variably sized, firm, white-to-tan nodules protruding from the cortical surface. Hepatitis and pancreatitis of variable degree may also be present, with small, white foci of inflammation. The tunica vaginalis may be affected, resulting in periorchitis in intact males. There may be marked thickening of the small and large intestine by firm, white inflammatory nodules extending through the wall of the affected bowel; there is often adhesion to the adjacent enlarged lymph nodes.

The characteristic microscopic lesion is generalized vasculitis and perivasculitis, especially of small- to medium-sized venules of the leptomeninges, renal cortex, eyes, abdominal serosa/peritoneal surfaces, and less frequently the lungs and liver (see Fig. 1-167B). Macrophages predominate and probably mediate lesion development; however, variable numbers of neutrophils, lymphocytes, and plasma cells also accumulate in and around the affected vessels. The endothelium swells, and medial vascular necrosis may be evident in some cases; narrowed vascular lumina may predispose to thrombosis and infarction. The proportion of neutrophils in the reaction varies, and some lesions may be composed mainly of a mixture of macrophages and lymphoid cells. Fibroplasia is variable; occasionally, adventitial fibrosis occurs with little cellular infiltrate. The vascular lesion results in the serofibrinous and cellular exudate on the serosal surfaces, and the nodules visible on the surfaces and deeper in solid organs.

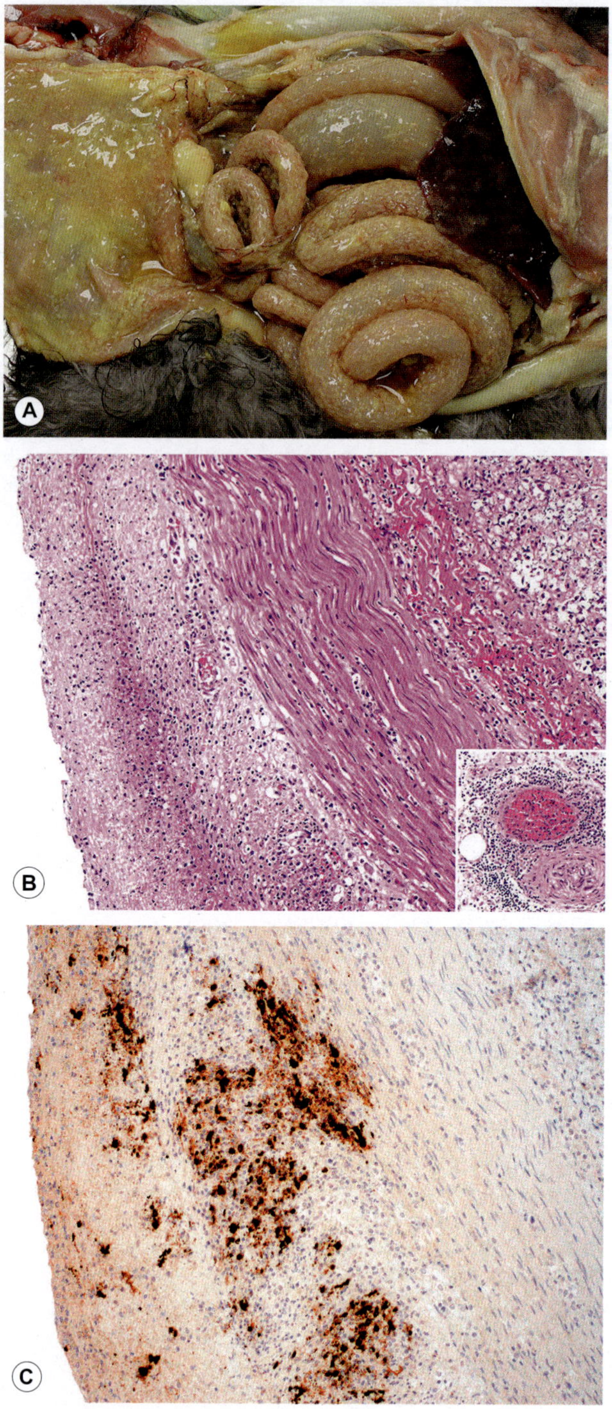

Figure 1-167 Feline infectious peritonitis in a cat. **A.** Fibrin and pyogranulomatous inflammation covering the visceral and parietal peritoneal surfaces of the abdomen. **B.** Abundant fibrin intermixed with neutrophils, macrophages, and karyorrhectic cellular debris expands the visceral peritoneal surface and extends into the underlying muscle and submucosal layers of the small intestine. Inset: perivascular orientation of inflammation is characteristic. **C.** IHC (feline enteric coronavirus) confirms abundant viral antigen within macrophages of the peritoneal inflammation.

The microscopic changes in the *omentum, mesentery*, and *serosal tissues* vary in severity. Mild changes include proliferation of mesothelial cells, fibrin accumulation, fibroblast proliferation, and scattered neutrophils and mononuclear cells. More severe changes include dense fibrin accumulation on serosal surfaces, with necrosis and/or mesothelial hyperplasia, and large numbers of neutrophils, mononuclear cells, and necrotic debris may be embedded in the fibrin. Serosal inflammation may extend into the intestinal wall, affecting the tunica muscularis, myenteric ganglia, the submucosa, and the mucosa, which may be segmentally infarcted.

Lesions in various organs, including the kidney, liver, lung, and pancreas, are largely caused by the vascular damage that occurs because of inflammatory cellular infiltrates in the capsule and stromal connective tissue. Severe multifocal lymphoplasmacytic interstitial nephritis may develop. In addition to focal lung lesions, there may be diffuse interstitial pneumonia, sometimes most severe close to the visceral pleura. Degenerative and necrotic lesions in the parenchyma of the CNS, including the meninges, choroid plexus, and ependyma, also appear to be related to vasculitis. The ependyma may be visibly roughened due to proliferation, inflammation, and syncytia formation of lining cells. Ocular lesions are common, but usually subclinical (see Vol. 1, Special Senses). While the *effusive form of FIP must be differentiated from bacterial peritonitis, noneffusive forms of FIP will appear grossly similar to lymphoma, steatitis, mycotic infections, and toxoplasmosis*. With thorough postmortem examination, the constellation of lesions is usually sufficiently distinctive to allow a gross diagnosis with a high degree of accuracy.

Serologic tests such as enzyme-linked immunosorbent assay or immunofluorescence may be useful in supporting a diagnosis of FIP or managing the disease in cat populations; however, histopathologic examination of tissues with identification of viral antigen in lesions using IHC (see Fig. 1-167C) or PCR remains the most conclusive means of diagnosis of FIP.

Parasitic diseases of the peritoneum and retroperitoneum

Most parasites found in the peritoneal cavity are in the normal course of migration to another site, or as an aberrant or accidental migratory pathway; only a few larval and adult helminths use the abdominal cavity as their normal habitat.

Cysticerci (*Cysticercus tenuicollis* in ruminants; *C. pisiformis* in lagomorphs) may be found on the peritoneal surface during their normal development; they are nonpathogenic and induce virtually no tissue response beyond their thin bland fibrous capsule. Rarely, cysticerci have been encountered in the abdomen of carnivores, which are considered abnormal or aberrant hosts. **Spargana** are elongate larval forms of *Spirometra* spp. that may be found encysted in a bland fibrous capsule in the peritoneal cavity of carnivores and swine. **Tetrathyridia**, the larvae of the tapeworm *Mesocestoides*, may proliferate extensively in the abdominal cavity of carnivores, where they cause a characteristic pyogranulomatous and proliferative peritonitis known as *parasitic ascites*.

Fasciola hepatica larvae can cause acute and chronic peritonitis in cattle and sheep; inflammation involves the parietal peritoneum and sometimes the visceral peritoneum, especially that of the liver, spleen, and omentum. The lesions may consist of many fibrin tags, or more diffuse thickening of the peritoneum; young flukes may be found in the inflammatory lesions both on and beneath the peritoneum.

Dioctophyma renale seems to be better adapted to dogs than to cats. In most cases in dogs, the large adult worms are located in the right kidney; however, they have been observed in the abdominal cavity, suggesting that they did not complete their normal migration pathway from the small intestine to the kidney. Migration of the worm or its ova may initiate chronic perihepatitis or peritonitis.

Stephanurus dentatus migrates through the liver and peritoneal cavity to the kidneys in pigs and may cause local hemorrhage, peritonitis, and perihepatitis. ***Strongylus edentatus*** and ***S. equinus*** normally migrate through the liver, and the ligaments and lumen of the peritoneal cavity. Fibrous tags on the liver, particularly the diaphragmatic aspect, are thought to be sequelae of *S. edentatus* migration, although this remains unproven. The larvae of both species may be found in the retroperitoneal tissues of the dorsal abdomen in horses, and in the mesenteries and omentum, where they may incite eosinophilic inflammatory response.

Ascarids of all species may occasionally cause obstruction and rupture of the small intestine or bile duct, such that they may be found in the abdomen as a terminal event.

Some parasites use the peritoneal cavity as their final habitat. ***Setaria*** spp. are onchocercid filariid nematodes that inhabit the peritoneal cavity of many wild and domestic ungulates, including horses, cattle, sheep, goats, and swine. They are commonly found during postmortem examination or during surgery of cattle and horses in endemic areas. Some species of *Setaria* have a cosmopolitan distribution and may be found in several species of wild and domestic ungulates (***Setaria equina*** in equids; ***S. labiatopapillosa*** in cattle, buffalo, and perhaps deer and antelope); others are restricted geographically (***S. digitata***, Asia; ***S. marshalli***, Asia) perhaps by the distribution of intermediate hosts.

Adult *Setaria* do not usually cause significant peritoneal lesions in their normal host. There are rare reports of occlusion of the uterine tube by *S. labiatopapillosa* in cattle. Adult *S. labiatopapillosa* in the peritoneal cavity, or in the tunica vaginalis around the testis, may incite granulomatous peritonitis or periorchitis if they die; remnants of the dead nematode may be detected in sections of the granulomatous reaction. Adult *S. digitata* rarely may be found in abnormal locations, such as the heart, lungs, and mesenteric lymph nodes, where they incite eosinophilic granulomatous inflammation. The larval form of *S. digitata* can produce mild peritonitis and granulomas in the retroperitoneum and bladder of cattle. The larvae of *S. equina, S. digitata*, and perhaps others that normally spend part of their time in the CNS, may occasionally penetrate the neural parenchyma and cause lesions. The sheathed microfilariae deposited by adult females in the peritoneal cavity are found in the blood. The intermediate host may be a mosquito, or for some *Setaria* spp., biting flies (*Haematobia* and *Stomoxys* spp.). The microfilariae develop into infective larvae in 2-3 weeks. They are released from the feeding arthropod and enter the final host.

S. digitata is normally found as an adult in the peritoneal cavity of cattle and buffalo in Asia, but its larvae can cause *cerebrospinal nematodiasis* in aberrant hosts (see Vol. 1, Nervous System). *Setaria* species that may occur normally in cervids have been reported to cause CNS lesions in deer; however, *Elaphostrongylus* larvae produce similar signs and lesions, and differentiation may be difficult.

S. digitata larvae may invade the eye of horses, via the optic nerve to cause endo-ophthalmitis, as do the microfilariae of *S. equina*.

Proliferative and neoplastic lesions of the peritoneum and retroperitoneum

Reactive mesothelial hyperplasia and metaplasia were discussed earlier in this chapter. **Nonneoplastic peritoneal or retroperitoneal masses** may include hematomas or accumulations of urine that often follow trauma to the caudal abdominal or pelvic area. Hemorrhage may dissect widely in this area, and the origin may be difficult to detect. Rupture of retroperitoneal hematomas may be fatal. Retroperitoneal hemorrhage in newborn calves is often an indication of fracture of the spinal column caused by inappropriate rotation during assisted calving or dystocia. Sublumbar hemorrhage is frequent in male lambs castrated by traction of the testis. Renal and perirenal cysts, and pseudocysts or capsular cysts, also may be encountered, and are usually incidental.

Primary neoplasms of the peritoneum and retroperitoneum in all domestic animal species are quite rare. They may arise from the serosal lining (the peritoneum proper, including of the pleura, peritoneum, pericardium, or the tunica vaginalis testis), or from the subserosal connective tissues including adipose tissue, nerves, nerve sheaths, and lymphatic and blood vessels (the retroperitoneum). Secondary neoplasms of the peritoneum and retroperitoneum originate in a wide variety of tissues elsewhere in the body and metastasize or infiltrate the peritoneal or retroperitoneal tissues. Distinguishing reactive from neoplastic mesothelial cells is a significant diagnostic dilemma; it is probably an impossible antemortem task, although cytologic and nuclear atypia of the cells support a diagnosis of neoplasia, *especially in cats*. Furthermore, because mesothelial cells can have either epithelial or mesenchymal differentiation (which leads to their varied histomorphologic subtypes), histologic confirmation of mesothelioma and differentiation of mesothelial reactive hyperplasia from mesothelioma is also challenging, especially when only small or superficial samples are available for evaluation.

Neoplasms arising specifically from the serosal layer or the peritoneum proper are **mesotheliomas**. The term *malignant* is typically applied to mesotheliomas in which there is evidence of localized tissue infiltrative growth, invasion into lymphatic vessels, or evidence of nodal or distant metastasis; however, the terminology of distant metastasis in the context of mesothelioma is controversial and practically without meaning because *virtually all mesotheliomas can readily metastasize by implantation*.

Mesotheliomas are rare. They occur with greatest frequency in cattle and dogs but are occasionally reported in horses, cats, pigs, and other species; congenital mesotheliomas have been described in calves. Interest in mesotheliomas has increased following the discovery of the association between asbestos fiber and mesothelioma in humans. This association has not been confirmed in animals, although ferruginous bodies, which are suggestive of asbestos exposure, have been described in the lungs of some urban dogs with mesothelioma and in peritoneal mesothelioma of dogs, and an association has been made between mesothelioma in dogs and exposure of their owner to asbestos. *Many fiber types other than asbestos are capable of causing mesotheliomas, and this ability seems to be related mostly to fiber size and solubility*. In domestic animals, mesothelioma is notable because it occurs most frequently as a *congenital neoplasm* in fetal or young cattle.

Patients with mesothelioma usually have tachypnea and dyspnea due to pleural effusion, or abdominal distension due to ascites, which is due to peritoneal implantation of neoplastic cells and lymphatic obstruction. The prognosis of mesothelioma is considered poor in the long term, despite draining of the effusion and chemotherapy.

Mesotheliomas arise from the cells of the serous linings of pericardial, pleural, peritoneal cavities, or the tunica vaginalis testis; they may involve various locations simultaneously. They are typically pleural in pigs, and peritoneal in calves. They can occur as a single distinct mass, but usually appear as *multiple firm sessile or pedunculated nodules, from* a few millimeters to 6-10 cm in diameter; *as villus projections* on a thickened mesentery or serosal surface; or as plaque-like *fibrous or sclerosing forms* (Fig. 1-168A). In sclerosing tumors in which adhesions more often occur, mesothelioma might resemble chronic granulomatous or sclerosing encapsulating peritonitis. The tumor is frequently associated with ascites or a milky to blood-tinged effusion as the result of blocked lymphatics.

Mesotheliomas of the pleura, pericardium, or peritoneum are often classified based on their major histologic patterns as *solid* type (with neoplastic cells in solid sheets, nests, or

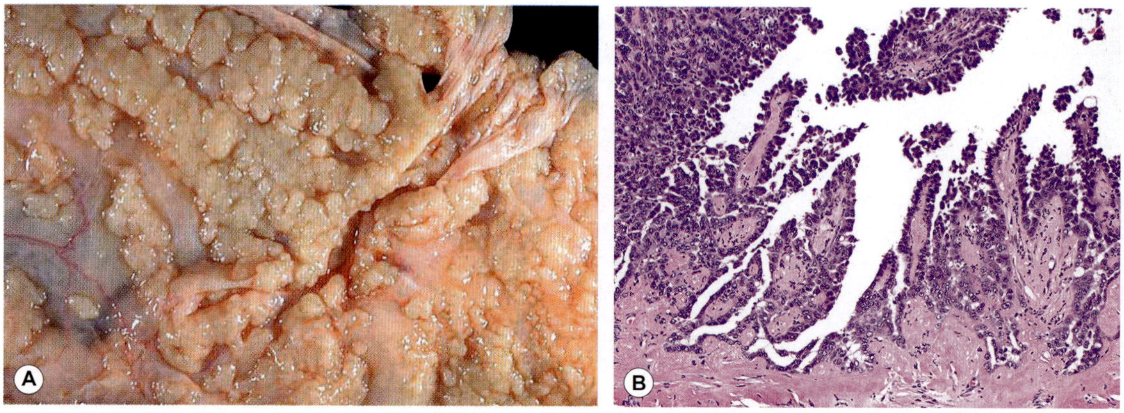

Figure 1-168 Abdominal mesothelioma in a dog. **A**. The peritoneal surface is thickened by plaque-like to nodular accumulations of proliferative mesothelial cells. **B**. Proliferative mesothelial cells form papillary projections and nodules, and although there is widespread transabdominal spread, there is minimal infiltrative growth of the mesothelial cells into the underlying tissue.

trabeculae), *papillary* type (with central cores of connective tissue covered by numerous branching fronds of neoplastic mesothelial cells, see Fig. 1-168B), *tubular* type (with formation of tubules supported by fibrovascular stroma), *cystic* type (with neoplastic cells forming variably sized cystic structures filled with serous fluid), *sclerosing* type (with neoplastic cells embedded in or surrounded by dense nonneoplastic fibrous connective tissue, or desmoplasia), *deciduoid* type (with enlarged eosinophilic neoplastic cells resembling decidual cells), *sarcomatoid* type (with plump spindle neoplastic cells arranged in interwoven bundles, or whorls), or *mixed* type (with biphasic differentiation including areas of both epithelioid and sarcomatoid morphology). The epithelial types are composed of single layers of dark plump cuboidal, columnar, or rounded, epithelial cells with a distinct border and abundant pink cytoplasm supported by a thin fibrovascular stroma. Mitotic figures are typically not numerous. Some tumors have atypical cells with marked anisokaryosis and prominent nucleoli, or large multinucleate cells. Epithelioid types can resemble carcinomas and mimic implantation and lymphatic metastasis; the sarcomatous types resemble fibrosarcomas; therefore, careful evaluation of various sections of tissue, careful exclusion of a primary malignant carcinoma or sarcoma elsewhere, and additional immunohistochemical testing is often required for definitive diagnosis.

IHC is useful for the diagnosis of mesotheliomas in humans, but the markers most reported in the human literature are unreliable in animals (calretinin, keratin-5, Wilms tumor protein, E-cadherin, and carcinoembryonic antigen); however, Wilms tumor protein (cats), calretinin (dogs), and E-cadherin (dogs) do show promise. Mesothelial cells, including epithelioid and sarcomatoid variants, are well known for expressing both cytokeratin and vimentin, and because dual expression is unusual in most other carcinomas and sarcoma, these IHC assays are usually helpful. Transmission electron microscopy to detect the characteristic mesothelial cell apical microvilli (absent in carcinomas and sarcomas) can be useful, although it is infrequently performed and some subtypes of mesothelial cells lack microvilli.

Lipomas are the most frequently encountered retroperitoneal neoplasm of domestic species. These benign tumors are well known in horses, in which they usually originate in the mesenteries. They may reach enormous size, but their greatest significance is when they become pedunculated and cause acute strangulation obstruction because the pedicle wraps around and entraps a loop of intestine. The core of many lipomas is friable and necrotic, probably from ischemia; in many lipomas, only the superficial centimeter or so remains viable, perhaps nourished by diffusion from the peritoneal environment (Fig. 1-169). In the dog, lipomas more commonly arise in the omentum rather than the mesenteries and settle on the abdominal floor. They may become very large but tend not to become pedunculated and therefore do not cause acute strangulation of bowel as they do in horses. Lipomas are benign lesions that do not metastasize.

Other retroperitoneal neoplasms are rare, but include myxomas, fibromas/fibrosarcomas, lymphomas, osteosarcomas, and extra-adrenal paragangliomas (due to concentration of sympathetic paraganglionic tissue in this location in dogs); many of these are discovered incidentally, or as part of more widespread disease. Neurofibromatosis of cattle may involve the abdominal nerves and plexuses, and ganglioneuromas are also observed in this species.

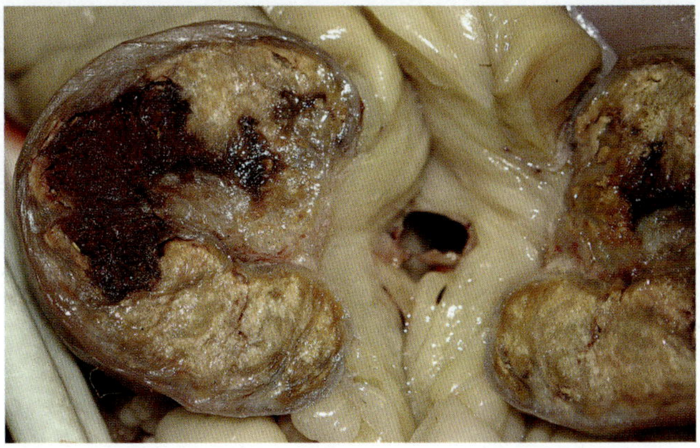

Figure 1-169 **Pedunculated lipoma** (transected) with necrotic core and thin capsule of viable tissue, from the mesentery of a horse.

Secondary or metastatic neoplastic diseases of the peritoneum and retroperitoneum are not common but may occur with almost any abdominal neoplasia, and typically occur by direct implantation in the peritoneum, or by direct implantation, extension, or lymphatic and hematogenous metastasis in the retroperitoneal space. Various metastatic neoplasms are described including lymphoma and many carcinomas (urothelial, prostatic, colonic). Neoplasms of the kidney, adrenal glands, or of the anal sac apocrine glands may extend into the retroperitoneal space. Carcinomas occur much more commonly than sarcomas. They may induce a robust scirrhous response, and when accompanied by ascites may resemble chronic peritonitis. The relative or complete absence of adhesions can be a helpful distinguishing feature grossly.

Ovarian carcinomas are a cause of significant ascites and may be difficult to differentiate from mesothelioma; implants of ovarian carcinoma tend to be papillary. Bile duct carcinomas and pancreatic adenocarcinomas tend to be scirrhous, as do intestinal adenocarcinomas in cattle and sheep. Prostatic carcinomas may form discrete firm white nodules on the peritoneum and resemble other carcinomas. SCCs of the equine stomach form rather discrete implants that may resemble nodules of mesothelioma or granulomas; they typically produce keratin, and this may be recognizable during gross inspection. Urothelial tumors that develop in cattle with enzootic hematuria can implant locally on the pelvic surfaces; implants from rectal adenocarcinoma in dogs also tend to be confined to the pelvic peritoneum. Malignant melanomas of perineal origin in horses produce pigmented plaques on the peritoneum or in the mesenteries, as may occasional metastatic melanomas in dogs.

Visit Elsevier eBooks+ (eBooks.Health.Elsevier.com) for eFigures and further readings.

CHAPTER 2

Liver and Biliary System

John M. Cullen • Arnaud J. Van Wettere

ACKNOWLEDGMENTS

The authors acknowledge the major contributions of Dr. W. Roger Kelly, Dr. M.A. (Tony) Hayes, and Dr. Margaret Stalker as previous authors of this section. In addition, the authors thank Drs. W. Roger Kelly and Jeremy Allen for critical review, discussions, and provision of images.

GENERAL CONSIDERATIONS

From a contemporary perspective, the liver is a marvel of biology. It is the guardian of homeostasis, the epicenter of the body's metabolic capability, a massive filter detoxifying the portal blood releasing cleansed blood to the systemic circulation, and a lymphoid organ protecting against infection. However high our regard for the liver is, it is dwarfed by the perspective of ancient civilizations that regarded the liver as the seat of life and window to the future. In ancient Mesopotamia and Babylonia, the liver was used to divine the future using a technique termed hepatoscopy. This interest is captured in a Biblical quote from Ezekiel 21:21, *"For the king of Babylon stands at the parting of the way, at the head of the two ways, to use divination; he shakes the arrows, he consults the household idols, he looks at the liver."* Hepatoscopy was continued by the Greeks, Etruscans, and the Romans. The practice is continued in fashion today. Liver injury or neoplasia foretells a poor future for many pharmaceuticals in development.

The liver plays a central role in processing dietary carbohydrates, lipids, amino acids, and vitamins; in the synthesis and turnover of most plasma proteins; and in the detoxification and biliary excretion of endogenous wastes and xenobiotic compounds. The liver also functions as an important organ of the innate immune system, integrated into the complex system of defense against foreign macromolecules. As such, hepatic disorders have far-reaching consequences, given the dependence of other organs on the metabolic function of the liver.

Origin, structure, and function

The embryonic origin of the liver is an outpouching of the embryonic endoderm forming the duodenum, termed the *hepatic diverticulum* or the *liver bud*. Primitive epithelial cells of the hepatic diverticulum extend into the adjacent mesenchymal stroma of the septum transversum, a sheet of cells that incompletely separates the pericardial and peritoneal cavity and that will develop into the connective tissue of the liver. The primitive epithelial cells are arranged in close approximation with the vessels that form the vitelline venous plexus, a complex of vessels that drain the yolk sac. Thus, the essential sinusoidal arrangement of the liver is established very early in development. The gallbladder and the cystic duct arise from the caudal part of the hepatic diverticulum.

The hepatic diverticulum is also the origin of the *biliary epithelium*. Development of the biliary tree begins at the hilus and spreads outward to reach the subcapsular zone over time. Intrahepatic bile ducts develop from the **ductal plate**, a structure that is composed initially of a single row of bipotent hepatoblasts that surround the portal vein branches and ensheath the mesenchyme of the primitive portal tract. The development of the bipotent hepatoblasts next to the portal tract mesenchyme is altered by interactions with the mesenchyme. The cells of the ductal plate can be identified by expression of cytokeratin (CK) 7, differentiating them from the hepatoblasts that will differentiate into hepatocytes (Fig. 2-1). A second discontinuous outer layer of cells forms subsequently, and the 2-cell–thick regions remodel into tubules. Most undergo apoptosis, but 1 or 2 ducts become incorporated in the developing portal tract. At about the time the bile ducts are forming, the hepatic artery branches appear in the developing portal tract. Nerves and lymphatics eventually invest the portal tracts as well, completing the mature portal tract. The *periportal space (space of Mall)* is found between

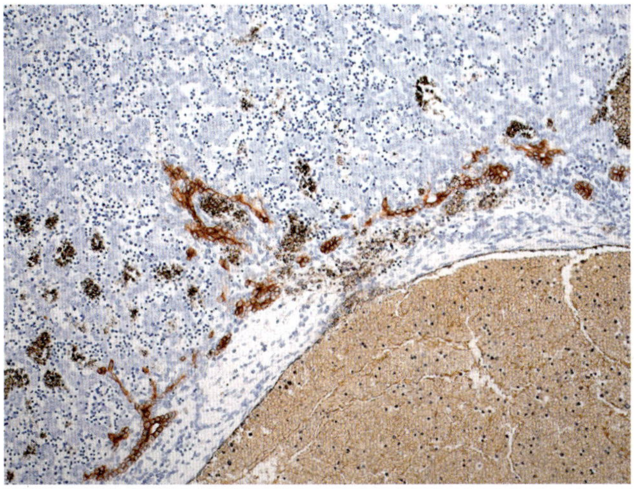

Figure 2-1 Immunohistochemical stain of the **ductal plate** of a fetal dog with 2-cell–thick rows of cytokeratin-7–positive cells formed at the edge of the developing portal tract.

the limiting plate, the first row of hepatocytes that border the portal tract connective tissue, and the portal connective tissue. The periportal space likely functions as a prelymphatic channel leading fluid toward the lymphatic vessels and the perisinusoidal space (space of Disse). The wave of development from the hilus to the subcapsular region is imperfect, as the veins, arteries, and bile ducts reach their terminal ends separately. Consequently, in human liver, up to 30% of subcapsular portal tracts are "dyads" containing only bile duct and artery profiles. Sinusoidal lining cells other than the endothelium likely arise in the bone marrow and populate the liver via a hematogenous route.

The liver is the largest internal organ in the body. In adult carnivores, the liver constitutes ~3% of body weight. In adult omnivores, it is ~2% of body weight, and ~1% of body weight in adult herbivores. In neonates of all species, the liver is a larger percentage of body weight than in the adult. The liver has a smooth capsular surface, and the parenchyma consists of friable red-brown tissue that is divided into *lobes*. The number and shape of the liver lobes of the major domestic mammals vary among species. In monogastric animals, the liver abuts the diaphragm and occupies the central area of the cranial abdomen. In ruminants, and to a lesser extent in horses, the liver is displaced to the right side of the cranial abdominal cavity. A series of ligaments maintain the liver in its position. The *coronary ligament* attaches the liver to the diaphragm near the esophagus. The *falciform ligament* attaches the midline of the liver to the ventral midline of the abdomen. The *round ligament*, a remnant of the umbilical vein, is embedded within the falciform ligament. The hepatoduodenal and hepatogastric ligaments connect to the transverse fissure, or hilum, of the liver (porta hepatis).

The liver receives ~25% of the cardiac output via the hepatic artery but is also supplied by the **portal vein**. The valveless portal vein drains the digestive tract, as well as the spleen, gallbladder, and pancreas. Portal vein flow supplies 70-80% of the total afferent hepatic blood flow and ~50% of the oxygen supply. The **hepatic artery** supplies the remainder of the hepatic blood flow. While portal blood flow is not regulated, hepatic arterial flow is regulated by several mechanisms, but primarily by the hepatic arterial buffer response.

When portal blood flow is reduced, there is a compensatory increase in hepatic arterial flow. It is believed that the *hepatic arterial buffer response* can be accounted for by the *adenosine washout hypothesis*. Adenosine is released at a constant rate into fluid in the periportal space, where hepatic lymph is collected, sandwiched between the connective tissue of the outer limits of the portal tract and the hepatocytes. It surrounds the hepatic resistance vessels and portal venules. The concentration of adenosine is regulated by washout into the portal vein and the hepatic artery. As portal blood flow is reduced, less adenosine is washed away from the periportal space, and the elevation in adenosine level leads to dilation of the hepatic artery with a subsequent increase in hepatic arterial flow. The liver normally has more oxygen than needed and can sustain significant reductions in flow without affecting hepatocyte function. However, age-related decreases in hepatic blood flow can alter the rate of clearance of endogenous and exogenous substances.

Portal blood flow is important for the rapid clearance of nutrients, xenobiotics, microorganisms, and potentially immunogenic materials that enter the circulation from the gastrointestinal tract. Hepatic arterioles disperse into a peribiliary capillary plexus, a perivenous plexus surrounding the portal vein, or join terminal hepatic arterioles before entering the sinusoids, lowering pressure, and preventing reversal of portal venous inflow. Portal and arterial blood eventually mix in the *low-pressure hepatic sinusoids*. Both terminal portal venules and hepatic arterioles flow into the sinusoids, but flow is tightly regulated by a series of inlet sphincters formed by endothelial cells for the venules and smooth muscle for the arterioles. Thus, at any time, sinusoidal blood could be entirely venous, mixed arterial and venous, or arterial. This blood flow pattern may account for the interlobular and intralobular heterogeneity of lesions following various toxicities. Blood leaves the liver via the **hepatic vein**, which is very short, and enters the caudal vena cava.

Hepatic sinusoids have an average diameter of 10 μm but can expand up to 30 μm. The periportal sinusoids are more tortuous than those in the centrilobular region. Hepatic sinusoids are lined by specialized endothelial cells. Hepatic sinusoids differ from vascular structures elsewhere in that they lack a typical basement membrane and are supported by a specialized, discontinuous or loose extracellular matrix (ECM). Hepatic **sinusoidal endothelial cells** are fenestrated, and these 100-200-nm sievelike pores control fluid, solute, and particulate interchange between blood and the perisinusoidal space, regulated by the action of the cellular cytoskeleton. Sinusoidal endothelial cells are actively pinocytotic and internalize and degrade various endogenous glycoproteins, glycosaminoglycans, and immune complexes.

Kupffer cells are macrophages attached to the inner sinusoidal wall in direct contact with blood moving at a relatively low velocity. This arrangement facilitates phagocytic removal of particulates, especially bacteria that enter the portal blood via the lower alimentary tract. Kupffer cells also take part in the regulation of inflammatory and repair responses by secretion of various cytokines into the circulation and perisinusoidal space. **Natural killer** (NK) **cells** (formerly referred to as *pit cells*) are *large granular lymphocytes* with NK activity that adhere to the sinusoidal endothelium, where they are also well situated to participate in various innate immune defenses, for example, targeting infected cells that enter the liver via the blood. **Invariant natural killer T** (iNKT) **cells** also inhabit sinusoids and patrol the liver by crawling along sinusoids. Both NK and iNKT cells can directly kill target cells and produce various cytokines with roles in liver injury, fibrosis, regeneration, and hepatocarcinogenesis.

The sinusoids are separated from the adjacent hepatocellular plates by an extracellular space, the **perisinusoidal space**, that contains **hepatic stellate cells (HSCs)** (also termed *lipocytes* or *Ito cells*), reticulin fibers, and nerves. The perisinusoidal space is not readily visible by light microscopy unless there is fluid retention, such as can occur with impediments to venous outflow. Although hepatic sinusoids in the normal liver lack a conventional basement membrane, the perisinusoidal space contains a low-density ECM consisting of collagen type IV; laminin; fibronectin; minor amounts of collagen types I, III, V, and VI; nonfibrillar collagen XVIII; tenascin; and various proteoglycans. A conventional ECM composed of fibrillar collagen types I, III, and V, and fibronectin is found in the **hepatic (Glisson) capsule**, septa, and around portal tracts and central veins. **Reticulin fibers** are the components of the ECM that are stainable by silver impregnation techniques, consisting mainly of collagen type III with attached fibronectin and other glycoproteins. The fenestrated sinusoidal endothelium, coupled with the loose subendothelial matrix, allows for exchange of various macromolecules between hepatocytes and the sinusoidal blood. After hepatic injury, a denser, less-permeable matrix resembling a true basement membrane may form, and sinusoidal endothelial cells may lose their fenestrae (so-called **capillarization of sinusoids**), reducing uptake and secretion of plasma proteins and other metabolically important substances.

The **terminal hepatic venules** *(central veins)* collect the outflow blood from the sinusoids and converge into the larger **hepatic veins** that empty into the caudal vena cava. In most species, increased pressure in the vena cava during right-sided heart failure or hepatic vein thrombosis causes passive congestion and distension of the hepatic veins and sinusoids. However, the large and small hepatic veins in dogs have prominent spiral circumferential smooth muscle that can also affect the central venous pressure on the sinusoids. Fluids from the perisinusoidal space drain into **lymphatics** in the extracellular connective tissue spaces of the liver capsule, the portal tracts, and the connective tissue of the terminal veins. These flow out the portal hilus to the hepatic lymph nodes and eventually enter the thoracic duct. In species such as the dog, lymphatics around the larger hepatic veins cross the diaphragm into the mediastinum. The liver is the largest lymph producer in the body, contributing substantially to the thoracic duct flow (15-20% in humans). Hepatic lymph is high in protein, containing 85-95% of the protein of plasma and a high cell count composed of lymphocytes and macrophages. In sheep, more lymphocytes pass through the liver than any typical lymphoid organ, and ~2×10^8 macrophages leave the liver in lymph daily.

Hepatic nerves contain both sympathetic and parasympathetic fibers. Autonomic and sensory nerve fibers modulate many aspects of liver function, repair, and cell proliferation and regeneration. Metabolic functions, including bile secretion, glycogen, and lipid metabolism, are also influenced. The fibers enter via the hilus and invest major blood vessels, the hepatic artery, portal veins, and bile ducts. In most species, sympathetic, but not parasympathetic nerves, form synapses with the hepatocytes. Nerve connections modulate functions of hepatocytes, endothelial cells, and HSCs in health and during injury.

The vasculature of the liver parenchyma defines its functional microanatomy, but *debate continues as to what best represents* ***the hepatic structural-functional unit***. Mammalian hepatocytes are organized in platelike monolayer arrays among the sinusoids and in 3 dimensions; *plates, sinusoids, and tracts anastomose in a complex pattern*. A somewhat baffling array of models exists, each with their own adherents. These include the well-known *lobular and acinar patterns* and several others. The Matsumoto primary lobule is based on detailed reconstructions of human liver sections and considers the penetrating venule extending from the portal tract as a "vascular septum" and the origin of the primary lobule's blood flow as it is a starting place for the radially arranged sinusoids flowing to the terminal hepatic vein. In this model, a series of branches is formed by the portal vein. The first branches supply a conducting portal flow, and the next level of branches drain directly into the sinusoids forming the distributing portal flow. The **choleohepaton**, related to the concept of the nephron, is composed of an isosceles triangle of hepatocytes with its apex in contact with the terminal hepatic venule and drained by a single bile ductule/intrahepatic bile ductule at the base of the triangle.

Arrangements of hepatocytes in the most-used nomenclature systems are referred to as either **acini** or **lobules**.

- The **classic hepatic lobule** is a 6-sided anatomic arrangement of hepatocytes centered on the **terminal hepatic venule**, also termed the "central vein" in this context. Peripherally, lobules are outlined by fibrovascular septa extending from the portal tracts. In the pig liver, septa form obvious lobular perimeters, but in most mammalian species, the lobules are less pronounced because connective tissue is restricted to portal tracts. The terms **periportal** and **centrilobular** are mainly used for pathologic conditions that are centered on the hepatocytes surrounding the *portal tracts* or the *central veins* of the classic lobule.
- The **hepatic acinus** of Rappaport is a functional diamond-shaped subunit divided into *zones* in relation to blood supply:
  - **Zone 1 (periportal)** hepatocytes are arranged around an axis formed by the portal tract and the distributing vascular branches that leave the portal tract and are closest to the oxygen- and nutrient-rich arterial and portal inflow.
  - **Zone 2** is the transitional midzone.
  - **Zone 3 (periacinar, centrilobular)** hepatocytes form the apex of the diamond-shaped acinus, are nearest the outflow (terminal hepatic venule), and are exposed to reduced oxygen and nutrients.

The functional activity of hepatocytes is heterogeneous, and virtually, all liver functions have a zonal gradient. Periportal hepatocytes, exposed to the blood with the highest concentration of oxygen, insulin, glucagon, and amino acids, are the principal site of gluconeogenesis, protein synthesis, aerobic metabolism, urea cycle, and lipid and cholesterol metabolism. In the centrilobular region, glycolysis, lipogenesis, and the major biotransformation functions are more active, including the expression of most cytochromes P450 (CYPs), glucuronyl transferases, glutathione S-transferases, and other biotransformation/detoxification enzymes. *Centrilobular hepatocytes are therefore more susceptible to hypoxic injury as well as injury by toxic substances that are metabolically activated by CYPs*. By comparison, *hepatocytes in periportal hepatocytes are more susceptible to direct-acting toxicants*, such as ingested metal salts, given their proximity to the vascular inflow. Under the influences of various inducers, the patterns of enzyme expression can extend beyond the resting limits. Lobular variation is not restricted to parenchymal cells but is also apparent in the structure and function of sinusoidal endothelial cells, Kupffer cells, perisinusoidal stellate cells, and the composition of the matrix in the perisinusoidal space.

The **portal tract**, or *portal triad*, is a well-defined structure *containing at least one small arterial branch, a portal vein branch, and a bile duct*, surrounded by connective tissue composed primarily of type I collagen (Fig. 2-2). Because of the pattern of progressive branching of the portal tract system, individual tracts exhibit a range of sizes and shapes, from round to triangular or branching. In larger portal tracts, lymphatic channels and autonomic nerve fibers may be seen. Thus, the mature portal tract is a collection of structures confined within the associated connective tissue. It should be recognized that each of the 3 main structures of the portal tract relate to one another in a manner termed a "menage a foie" by Dr. Ian Wanless, a human hepatic pathologist. This term indicates that since each of the main elements of the portal tract are in close proximity, an issue with one of the structures has an impact on the others. The hepatic artery sends branches that surround the bile ducts, and arterial injury has consequences for the biliary tree.

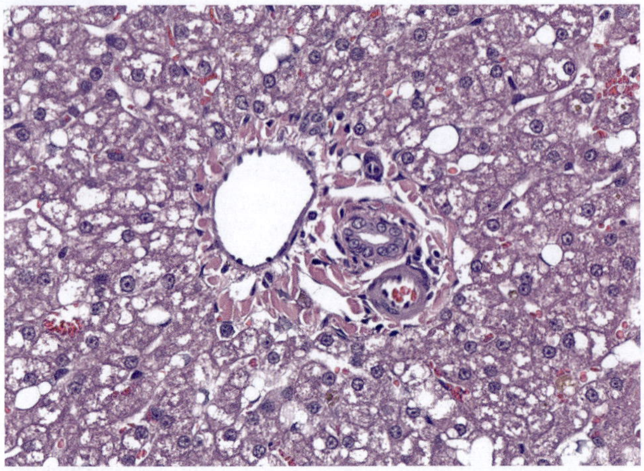

Figure 2-2 The **normal portal tract** contains branches of the portal vein and the hepatic artery, as well as a bile duct, lymphatic vessels, and nerves. The first row of hepatocytes adjacent to the portal tract connective tissue is termed the **limiting plate**.

Leakage of bile from the ducts can lead to vascular wall injury in the hepatic artery and the portal vein. Lack of portal flow stimulates hepatic arterial dilation and proliferation. Thus, there is an integrated relationship among these structures.

The **bile duct** system is a branching outflow that ultimately enters the proximal duodenum. Most species, apart from the horse, llama, deer, and rat, have a bile storage diverticulum **(gallbladder)**. Cats occasionally have divided or bipartite gallbladders. The bile duct joins the pancreatic duct before entry into the duodenum in some species and has a separate entry in others. Intrahepatic bile ducts range in size from the larger septal or trabecular ducts (internal diameter of >100 µm in humans) to the smaller interlobular ducts and tend to be adjacent to a hepatic artery branch of approximately the same size. Bile ducts are lined by cuboidal to low-columnar **bile duct epithelial cells**, subtended by a periodic acid-Schiff (PAS)–positive basement membrane. **Bile ductules** are smaller yet (lumen size of <20 µm) and are located at the periphery of portal tracts. Bile ductules are connected to **bile canaliculi** between hepatocytes by a short transitional segment partly lined by biliary epithelium and partly by hepatocytes at the level of the limiting plate, termed the **intrahepatic bile ductule** (canal of Hering).

Cells of the liver

Hepatocytes (referred to as **parenchymal cells**) constitute ~70-80% of the liver mass. However, >50% of liver DNA is found in smaller **nonparenchymal cells** (bile duct epithelium, HSCs, sinusoidal endothelium, Kupffer cells) and itinerant cells (e.g., leukocytes). The hepatocyte is a polygonal epithelial cell, ~30-40 µm in diameter, arranged in single-cell–thick anastomosing plates, separated by hepatic sinusoids. Each hepatocyte is therefore exposed to sinusoidal blood on 2 sides. A discontinuous line of hepatocytes, termed the **limiting plate**, is found at the interface with the collagenous ECM of the portal tract. Normal hepatocytes have abundant eosinophilic cytoplasm, and most have a single, round, centrally placed nucleus with finely dispersed chromatin and at least one nucleolus. Some binucleate hepatocytes are present normally in mammals and can become more numerous in response to various stimuli and injuries that induce or affect regeneration.

Hepatocytes are metabolically highly active cells, containing an array of organelles, including smooth endoplasmic reticulum (SER) and rough ER, mitochondria, lysosomes, peroxisomes, Golgi complexes, and transport vesicles. These organelles support a variety of hepatocellular functions, including the synthesis and secretion of plasma proteins, coagulation factors, and acute-phase proteins. Hepatocytes store nutrients in times of adequate energy and release glucose when needed. They are key modulators of lipid metabolism, and they synthesize and secrete lipoproteins. In addition, they are the only cells capable of bile acid synthesis, and they can absorb and secrete them into bile. Finally, hepatocytes detoxify most xenobiotics and secrete them into the bile. Because of this central role in metabolism, the liver is subject to a variety of nutritionally based insults as well as toxin-related damage. A greater proportion of the genome is expressed in the normal liver than has been observed in any other tissue, an indication that brief surveys of liver functions are necessarily oversimplified. However, those constituents that are most abundant have the most influence on the microscopic appearance of the liver. The normal hepatocyte contains abundant glycogen, which varies depending on food intake, and which can be demonstrated by PAS staining, as well as variable amounts of stored triglycerides and various proteins, such as ferritin, an iron-binding protein. The cytoplasm of the centrilobular hepatocytes may also contain golden-brown granules of **lipofuscin**, particularly in older cats. This "wear-and-tear" pigment becomes more prominent with age and progressively accumulates in midzonal and periportal hepatocytes. Hepatocytes have a cytoskeleton composed of microtubules, microfilaments, and intermediate filaments. Microtubules are found throughout the cytoplasm and are involved in the movement of secreted proteins into the extracellular perisinusoidal space; accordingly, microtubule inhibitors such as colchicine and *Vinca* alkaloids may reduce hepatic protein secretion. Microfilaments, composed of actin and myosin, are concentrated around the bile canaliculus, where they are involved in canalicular peristalsis and bile secretion; microfilament inhibitors result in cholestasis. Intermediate filaments (predominantly CK8 and CK18) form an irregular meshwork extending from the plasma membrane to the perinuclear zone and are responsible for spatial organization of the hepatocyte.

There are 3 morphologically and functionally distinct surfaces of the hepatocyte plasma membrane.

1. The **sinusoidal domain** faces the perisinusoidal space and has numerous irregular microvilli, increasing hepatocyte surface area by approximately 6-fold (considerably less than that seen in enterocytes). This specialized membrane is modified to facilitate an exchange of substances with the blood. Ultrastructurally evident pits between the villi, some of which represent secretory vacuoles in the process of exocytosis, send various products into the plasma; others are clathrin-coated pits involved in selective receptor–mediated endocytosis. Various membrane receptors for glycoproteins, asialoglycoproteins, peptides, hormones, growth factors, immunoglobulin (Ig) A, and other endocytotic or signaling ligands are found at the sinusoidal pole. In addition, transmembrane proteins involved in plasma exchange of small ionic substances with the sinusoidal plasma, and transmembrane proteins responsible for matrix recognition, are concentrated on the sinusoidal surface.
2. The **lateral domain** extends from the sinusoidal surface to the edge of the canaliculus. This portion of the cell membrane is specialized for adhesion via junctional complexes,

including desmosomes, tight junctions, and intermediate junctions, as well as for intercellular communication via gap junctions.

3. The **canalicular domain** is the beginning of the bile drainage system of the liver. *The canaliculus is an intercellular space between 2 adjacent hepatocytes, isolated by junctional complexes.* The canalicular surface is covered with an irregular array of microvilli. Canalicular diameter increases as it approaches the periportal region, enlarging from ~0.5 to 2.5 µm. Bile is propelled along the canaliculi by a web of contractile microfilaments. This specialized membrane contains various adenosine triphosphate (ATP)–dependent carriers that export many products, including leukotrienes, bile salts, xenobiotics, and their metabolites into the bile.

Cholangiocytes (biliary epithelium) account for ~3-5% of the liver cell population. Although derived from common embryologic progenitor cells, cholangiocytes differ from hepatocytes in both phenotype and function. They contain a strongly developed network of intermediate filaments, including CK7 and CK19. They also express marked heterogeneity along the anatomic course of the biliary system. Functionally, bile duct epithelial cells actively modify the composition of bile. Secretion is primarily under the control of secretin and somatostatin. Secretin released from the duodenum triggers secretion of bicarbonate-rich fluids that buffer acids released from the stomach. Cholangiocytes secrete IgA and IgM, but not IgG. Absorption involves the sodium-dependent glucose transporter and aquaporins responsible for glucose and water uptake, as in the renal proximal tubule. They express γ-glutamyltransferase (GGT), which removes glutamic acid from glutathione conjugates.

Given that hepatocytes and biliary epithelial cells originate from a common precursor, the hepatoblast, it is not surprising that transdifferentiation between hepatocytes and cholangiocytes occurs. A specific location where **hepatic progenitor cells** (HPCs), or oval cells in rodents, are found is not as well defined in the liver as in other organs such as the intestine. While studies have shown that all hepatocytes or cholangiocytes divide to replace cell loss following physiologic cell turnover or mild injury, pools of progenitor cells give rise to hepatocytes and cholangiocytes via transdifferentiation when replication of one cell type is impaired. Following injury causing severe hepatocellular loss or limiting hepatocellular proliferation, cholangiocytes residing in the intrahepatic bile ductule proliferate and transdifferentiate into hepatocytes. When the injury targets bile ducts, and cholangiocytes proliferation is insufficient to repair damage, periportal hepatocytes can transdifferentiate into cholangiocytes. HPCs in humans and rats contain both markers of hepatocyte phenotype (i.e., albumin) and biliary phenotype (i.e., CK7). Similar markers have been described in dogs and cats. Bone marrow–derived pluripotential stem cells also appear to have the ability to differentiate into hepatic cells (e.g., hepatocytes, Kupffer cells, endothelial cells).

Hepatic endothelial cells are specialized, perforated by numerous ~100-200-nm fenestrations, and often clustered together forming sieve plates. Larger, but less frequent, up to 1-µm fenestrations are more common at the periportal end of the sinusoid, but opening size is dynamic, responding to endogenous mediators and toxins. The endothelial cells rest on a very thin and discontinuous ECM. The fenestrations allow direct connection between the sinusoidal lumen and the perisinusoidal space. Only larger particles, such as chylomicrons, and cells are excluded. Sinusoidal endothelial cells differ from normal vascular endothelium in several additional ways, including the absence of factor VIII–related antigen (except in inflammatory conditions) and high endocytic activity. Endocytosis of immune complexes and some proteoglycans are major functions. They also synthesize molecules that affect vascular tone, such as nitric oxide, endothelins, and prostaglandins.

Kupffer cells *are specialized macrophages located in sinusoidal lumens*, mainly at branch points. Once thought to be "fixed," it is now known that they can migrate along the sinusoid and into areas of tissue injury (Fig. 2-3). Kupffer cells may have a dual origin as they are derived, at least in part, from blood-borne monocytes, but they are also capable of local proliferation, particularly in inflammation. They are not efficient antigen presenters, but they are proficient phagocytes of apoptotic and necrotic cells, particulates, and microorganisms; consequently, the liver is a major "filtering organ" for the body. There are species differences in the efficiency of this process. Clearance of particulates, and endotoxin in particular, is carried out more effectively by Kupffer cells in dogs, humans, and laboratory rodents than in ruminants, horse, pig, cats, and whales, species that have a significant population of intravascular macrophages in the pulmonary vasculature. Kupffer cells can phagocytose a variety of gut-derived materials, bacteria, various biologically active bacterial components, including lipopolysaccharides (LPSs), lipoteichoic acids, and peptidoglycans, without stimulating inflammation. Activated Kupffer cells can secrete tumor necrosis factor (TNF) and other cytokines, and nitric oxide; these contribute to peripheral vasodilation and hypotension in systemic inflammatory response syndromes started by bacterial components. Other secreted cytokines, such as interleukin 1 (IL1) and interleukin 6 (IL6), mediate the acute-phase response and some aspects of the immune and liver regenerative responses. However, there can be a balance in proinflammatory and anti-inflammatory signaling as there are distinct differences in the signaling repertoire of different Kupffer cells. Some Kupffer cells are more likely to secrete interleukin 10 (IL10), which can suppress macrophage activation and cytokine secretion. Cytokine responses of Kupffer cells are important in regulating the extent of the adaptive immune response or tolerance to potentially antigenic macromolecules that can reach the liver through the portal blood.

The liver contains large numbers of **lymphocytes**, making up ~5% of the entire cell population of the liver, with an organ-specific lymphocyte distribution characterized by the

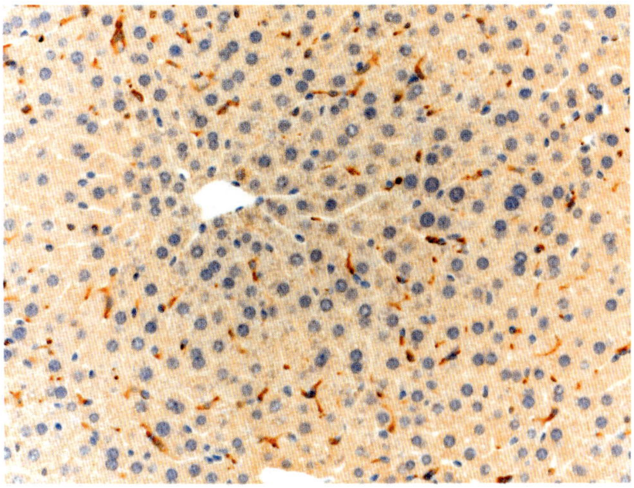

Figure 2-3 **Kupffer cells**, stained with antibodies against myeloperoxidase, line the sinusoids at regular intervals.

enrichment of elements of the innate immune system, including iNKT lymphocytes (iNKT cells), NK cells, and other innate lymphocytes, in addition to the Kupffer cells previously mentioned. The liver parenchyma is scattered with immune cells even during homeostasis. These cells are distributed throughout the parenchyma but enriched in periportal regions. The zonation of immune cells in the liver is organized by hepatic signals related to hepatocyte homeostasis and endothelial cell signals, as well as extrahepatic signals such as microbial metabolites from the gut-liver axis. Most intrahepatic lymphocytes are involved in innate immune responses rather than acquired immunity. Hepatic NK cells make up ~40% of hepatic lymphocytes and are distinct phenotypically and functionally from blood NK cells. Hepatic NK cells reside in the sinusoid, are considered large granular lymphocytes, and were previously referred to as pit cells. Intrahepatic NK cells have essential functions in defense against foreign antigens released from the gut, viral infections, metastatic tumors, hepatocellular carcinoma, and modulation of hepatic fibrosis. The liver also contains the largest population of γδ T cells in the body. Although much remains to be learned about the functions of these diverse lymphocyte types in the liver, they play a vital role in immunologic homeostasis and response to immunologic challenges. Elements of the acquired immune system, CD8+ T cells, are also increased compared with peripheral blood. The large number of lymphocytes in the liver indicates that *the liver can be considered a lymphoid organ*.

Hepatic dendritic cells play a significant role in the induction and regulation of immune responses by linking the innate and adaptive immune responses. There are several other antigen-presenting cells in the liver, including the sinusoidal endothelial cells, stellate cells, and Kupffer cells. Unlike cells that reside within the sinusoid, hepatic dendritic cells are found within the portal tract. Overall, the diverse phagocytic cells and lymphocytes in the liver play an essential role in homeostasis by balancing immune tolerance to foreign but harmless molecules (e.g., food antigens), and ability to mount a rapid response to infectious agents and cancer.

Hepatic stellate cells (HSCs), originally described by Boll and von Kupffer in 1876, were neglected until the 1950s, when they were described in detail by Ito. They have also been known as *lipocytes,* ***Ito cells****, or fat-storing cells*. HSCs reside in the perisinusoidal space, and there are other populations of similar cells with the ability to produce ECM and to transform into a myofibroblast phenotype within the connective tissue of the portal tract and centrilobular veins. There are 4 key functions of HSCs: 1) storage and homeostasis of retinoids, including vitamin A; 2) maintenance and remodeling of the sinusoidal ECM in health and disease; 3) contribution to regeneration and inflammatory reaction by production of growth factors (e.g., hepatocyte growth factor), various cytokines and chemokines, and antigen presentation once activated; and 4) regulation of sinusoidal diameter by contraction of cellular processes. This may be in response to adrenergic stimulation, as all HSCs are in contact with autonomic nerve fibers. HSCs can become greatly distended with lipid in carnivores on some diets.

Activation of HSCs has been studied extensively because of their importance in hepatic fibrosis. In the transdifferentiation from quiescence to activation, HSCs lose their characteristic lipid droplets, possibly catabolizing the lipid to support their activation. They then *develop a myofibroblast phenotype* characterized by the expression α–smooth muscle actin and increased proliferative ability. A broad variety of factors are involved in the activation of HSCs. Novel pathways and mediators, including autophagy, ER stress, oxidative stress, retinol and cholesterol metabolism, epigenetics, and receptor-mediated signals, reveal the complexity of HSC activation. In addition, extracellular signals from both resident and inflammatory cells modify HSC activation. Proinflammatory cytokines released primarily by Kupffer cells, such as transforming growth factor β (TGFβ) released in response to tissue injury, stimulate HSCs to transdifferentiate and increase the deposition of ECM, including collagen types I, III, and IV, and laminin. This new ECM transforms the sinusoid to a less permeable capillary, lined by a basement membrane–like layer and without fenestrations in the sinusoidal endothelium, reducing transfer of macromolecules between hepatocytes and the blood. The acquired contractility of the HSC during fibrogenesis is increased because of an increase in the contractile stimulus of endothelin-1 and a reduction in vasodilation driven by diminished nitric oxide generation. In severe chronic injury leading to cirrhosis, the increased expression of contractile proteins within activated stellate cells can further restrict sinusoidal blood flow as a primary effect, rather than a consequence of nodule formation and fibrosis. Peribiliary fibrosis arises from activation of the circumferential fibroblasts of the bile ducts that undergo a transdifferentiation similar to that of the HSCs along the sinusoids. Fibrosis of the portal tracts and the central vein connective tissue develops from activation of myofibroblasts resident in these areas as well. It is also possible that epithelial-mesenchymal transition of hepatocytes, biliary epithelial cells, or HSCs can contribute to hepatic fibrosis during chronic injury.

Mast cells are abundant in the liver, particularly in dogs. They typically occupy a perivenous location, where they may influence vascular tone and respond to various potentially injurious substances or organisms. Degranulation of mast cells in the liver leads to contraction of the spiral smooth muscle, restricting blood outflow from the canine liver. This is a feature of shock in dogs.

Hematopoiesis in the fetal life of mammals occurs in various locations during development including in the liver. Postnatally, hepatic hematopoiesis declines but can return as *extramedullary hematopoiesis* in conditions of increased

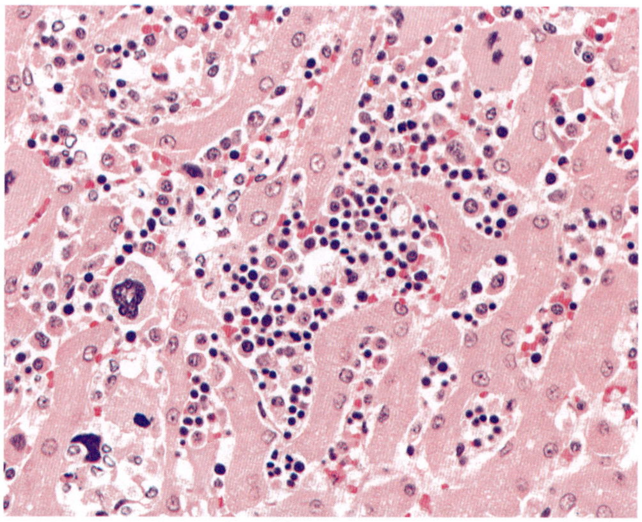

Figure 2-4 Extramedullary hematopoiesis in the liver of a dog.

demand (Fig. 2-4). Because the liver is an early site of hematopoiesis, the environmental conditions and cells, including resident populations of appropriate stromal cells and, possibly hematopoietic stem cells, remain supportive for the initiation or reactivation of a stem cell niche. The degree of hepatic extramedullary hematopoiesis in larger species can have diagnostic significance, but in laboratory rodents and other small animals, it can be an incidental observation.

DEVELOPMENTAL DISORDERS

Hepatic cysts

Serosal cysts are occasionally found attached to the capsule on the diaphragmatic surface in calves, lambs, and foals (Fig. 2-5). These cysts are generally small and multiple, but some are isolated and very large. Cyst walls are composed of connective tissue lined by flattened or cuboidal epithelium. The content is clear and serous. Their origin is not known, but it is postulated that they are serosal inclusion cysts. They do not contain bile. The declining incidence of these anomalies with age suggests that a substantial proportion of them involute or rupture in the early postnatal period.

Solitary biliary cysts—single round cysts lined by a flattened single layer of biliary epithelium—are uncommon and may be congenital or acquired. **Multiple hepatic peribiliary cysts** putatively arising from peribiliary glands have been reported in a 6-month-old pig.

Hamartomas

Von Meyenburg complexes (biliary hamartoma or microhamartomas) are developmental malformations arising from persistent embryonic ductal plate remnants. These are discrete, usually subcapsular, fibrotic areas containing small, irregularly shaped, often dilated, U-shaped or branching, bile duct–like structures lined by low cuboidal epithelium (Fig. 2-6).

Mesenchymal hamartomas, rare benign tumorlike lesions characterized by disorganized hepatocellular and/or biliary structures embedded in a mucinous primitive mesenchyme, have been reported in 2 equine fetuses.

Ductal plate malformations

Persistence and/or aberrant remodeling of the embryonic ductal plate can give rise to a spectrum of biliary diseases. **Congenital hepatic fibrocystic diseases**, part of the group of hepatorenal fibrocystic disease that includes the polycystic kidney diseases, *are a product of ductal plate malformations occurring at different levels of the biliary tree*. Analysis of the underlying genetic basis of human hepatorenal fibrocystic diseases has identified defective protein components in primary cilia and associated basal bodies. These mechanotransducer organelles are involved in environmental monitoring, signal transduction, and cell proliferation, and are important in the normal development of the biliary system in the liver, as well as renal tubules. As such, many of these diseases are now considered "ciliopathies."

In human hepatopathology, the hepatorenal fibrocystic diseases can be grouped into 3 descriptive categories: 1) **polycystic liver disease** (often seen in association with autosomal dominant polycystic kidney disease of adults), with isolated microscopic-to-macroscopic unilocular or multilocular cysts in a fibrous stroma, with no continuity with the intrahepatic biliary tree, thought to originate from von Meyenburg complexes in the most peripheral branches of the biliary tree; 2) **congenital hepatic fibrosis** (often seen in association with autosomal recessive polycystic kidney disease of childhood), with defective remodeling of the ductal plate at the level of interlobular ducts, with excess abnormally shaped embryonic bile ducts retained in the primitive ductal plate configuration, small or absent portal veins, and bridging fibrosis of the portal tracts; and 3) **Caroli disease**, with nonobstructive saccular or fusiform dilation of medium and large intrahepatic and extrahepatic bile ducts, with maintenance of continuity with the biliary system. Caroli syndrome refers to Caroli disease co-occurring with congenital hepatic fibrosis. In veterinary medicine, a similar classification of the liver lesions has been proposed: **adult polycystic disease** (including von Meyenburg complexes), **juvenile polycystic disease/congenital hepatic fibrosis**, and **congenital dilation of the large intrahepatic and extrahepatic bile ducts** (resembling Caroli disease).

Congenital cystic lesions involving the hepatic biliary system and kidneys have been reported in juvenile dogs, cats, pigs, goats, and foals, and have been compared with congenital hepatorenal fibrocystic disorders of humans. Cysts may also be formed in the pancreatic ducts. Animals may die from progressive renal insufficiency and/or from hepatic dysfunction and portal hypertension associated with hepatic fibrosis. Hepatic

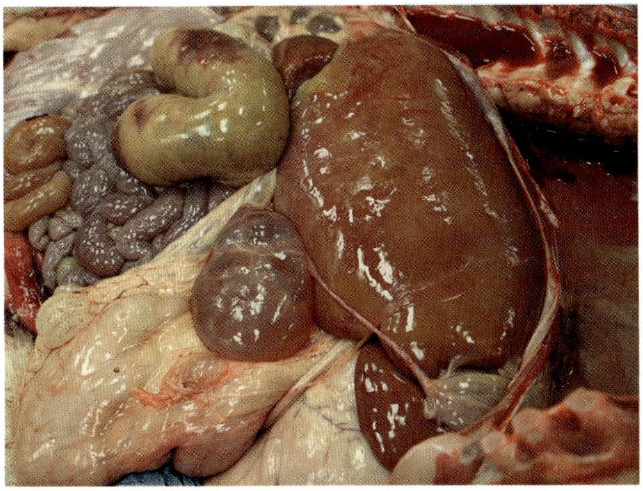

Figure 2-5 Serous cyst attached by a stalk to the hepatic capsule in a 3-day-old Holstein calf. (Courtesy J.L. Caswell.)

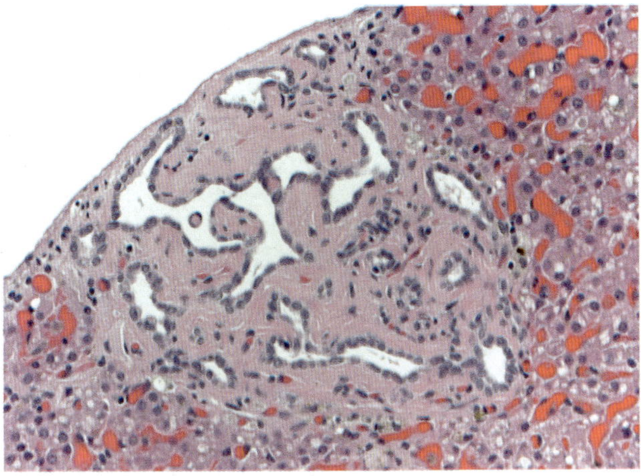

Figure 2-6 Von Meyenburg complex in a dog liver.

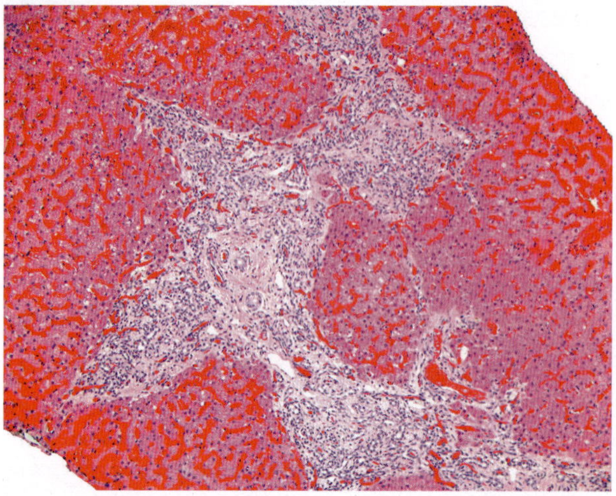

Figure 2-7 Congenital hepatic fibrosis in a dog. Porto-portal bridging fibrosis with numerous abnormal bile ducts.

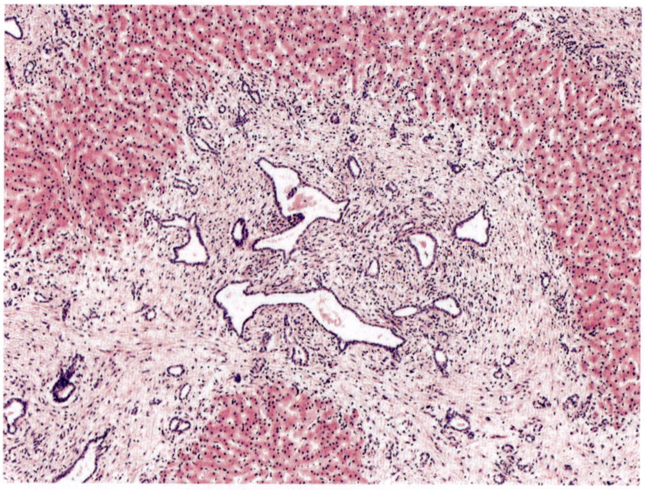

Figure 2-8 Congenital hepatic fibrosis in a Swiss Freiberger foal.

fibrosis and cysts are present in a significant proportion of cats with *polycystic kidney disease*, inherited in Persian cats, exotic shorthaired, and other related breeds as an autosomal dominant C→A transversion mutation in exon 29 of the feline *PKD1* gene, resembling the adult form of polycystic kidney disease in humans. The liver lesions have been more difficult to classify and may appear as numerous large cysts resembling adult-type polycystic disease, as congenital hepatic fibrosis characterized by portoportal bridging fibrosis with excess abnormally formed bile ductules (Fig. 2-7), or as combination of both lesions. Polycystic kidney and liver disease reported in West Highland White and Cairn Terrier litters resembles the autosomal recessive polycystic kidney disease of children.

Congenital hepatic fibrosis has been described in dogs. Affected animals are typically presented at or before a year of age with clinical signs of liver disease, including ascites, microhepatica, portal hypertension, and acquired *extrahepatic portosystemic shunts (PSSs)*. Histologically, these dogs had livers with extensive bands of portal bridging fibrosis containing numerous small, irregular, tortuous bile ducts, often accompanied by absent or hypoplastic portal veins and compensatory arteriolar proliferation, and with no evidence of nodular regeneration and minimal inflammation, allowing differentiation of this congenital condition from acquired chronic liver disease. Congenital hepatic fibrosis has also been reported in aborted and neonatal calves, in the latter case accompanied by cyst formation in the kidney and lung. Congenital hepatic fibrosis with cystic bile ducts has been described in Swiss Freiberger foals (Fig. 2-8) and is seen occasionally in other equine breeds, with generalized portal bridging fibrosis containing many small, irregularly formed and occasionally cystic bile ducts. Macroscopic congenital segmental dilation of the large bile ducts and diffuse cystic kidney disease, resembling *Caroli disease*, has been reported in dogs.

Extrahepatic biliary anomalies

Cats occasionally have **divided or bipartite gallbladders**. Reduplication of the gallbladder has also been reported in swine. Other, uncommon, anomalies of the extrahepatic biliary system include **agenesis of the gallbladder** reported in dogs and cats, and *the absence or atresia of one or more ducts*, reported in lambs, calves (eFig. 2-1), foals, a cat, a dog, and a pig. In carnivores, **bile duct atresia** may lead not only to jaundice but also to vitamin D deficiency rickets, because of their inability to absorb fat-soluble vitamins. Congenital atresia may be associated with defects in the developmental morphogenesis of bile ducts, or in utero vascular, inflammatory, or toxic insults to the biliary tree that culminate in the obliteration of the lumen.

Choledochal cysts arising from the cystic or common bile duct have been observed in cats and dogs.

Congenital vascular anomalies

Congenital vascular anomalies include congenital portal vein aneurysms, hepatic arteriovenous malformations, congenital portosystemic shunts (PSSs) between the portal vein and other systemic veins, and primary hypoplasia of the portal vein. Most congenital vascular anomalies lead to hypoperfusion of the parenchyma and a relatively stereotypic response of the liver to hypoperfusion, namely, small or absent portal veins, proliferation of hepatic artery branches, some duct proliferation, and centrilobular or subcapsular hepatocyte atrophy. Thus, there can be similar histologic patterns seen in each of the anomalies, and clinical data are often needed to decide the correct diagnosis.

Extrahepatic congenital PSSs are readily distinguished from shunts that are acquired during portal hypertension, as acquired shunts are typically various, thin-walled, tortuous collateral venous connections between the portal vein or its tributaries and caudal vena cava, renal vein, or azygos vein (Fig. 2-9). Although various acquired shunts do not develop in the presence of congenital PSSs, they can arise with other congenital abnormalities, such as arteriovenous malformations, ductal plate developmental malformations, or hypoplasia or dysplasia of portal veins, because of portal hypertension. Acquired shunts resulting from portal hypertension secondary to liver injury and repair are discussed later in the Vascular Factors in Hepatic Injury and Circulatory Disorders section.

Portal vein aneurysms, both congenital and acquired because of concurrent liver disease, have been described in dogs. Extrahepatic aneurysms were always located at the level of the gastroduodenal vein insertion. All were asymptomatic, although predisposed to portal vein thrombosis.

Hepatic arteriovenous malformations have been reported in dogs and cats, and a calf. These are congenital or, in some instances, acquired communications between branches of the

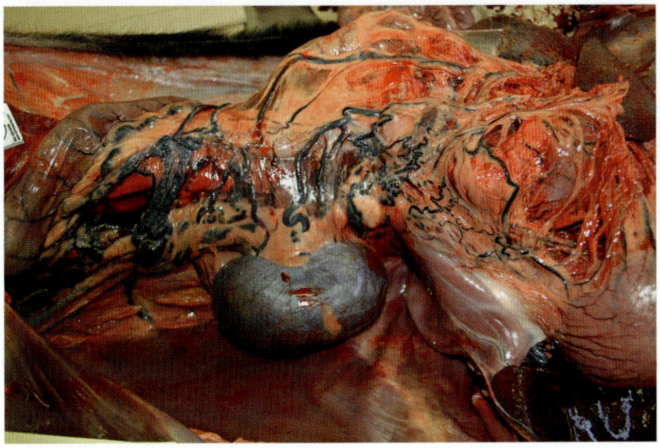

Figure 2-9 **Acquired portosystemic vascular shunts** in a dog with chronic liver disease.

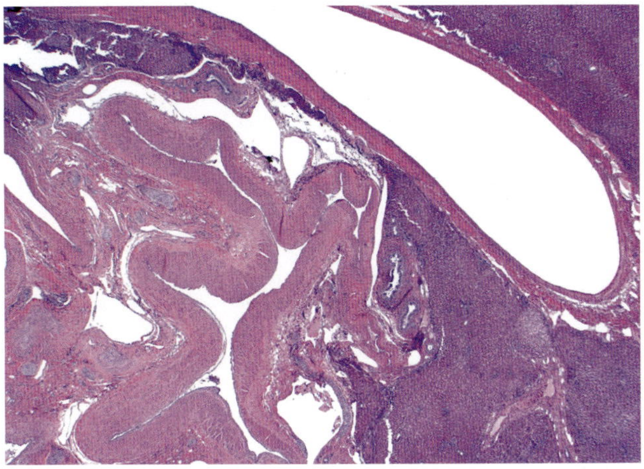

Figure 2-10 **Congenital intrahepatic arterioportal fistulae** with thick-walled anastomosing vessels and atrophy of adjacent parenchyma in a dog.

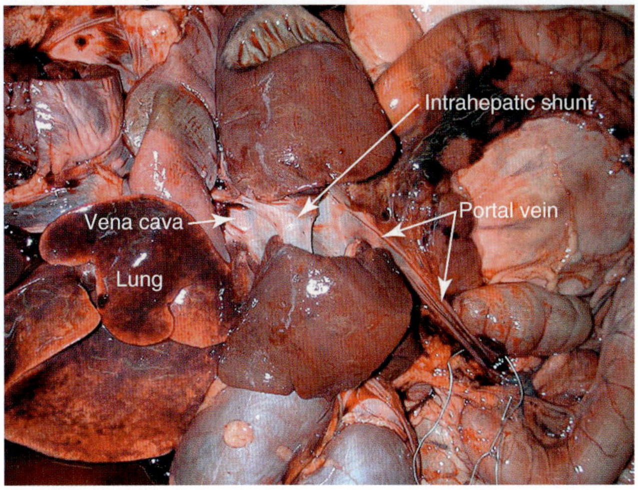

Figure 2-11 Congenital intrahepatic shunt, **persistent patent ductus venosus** in a dog. (Courtesy J.L. Caswell.)

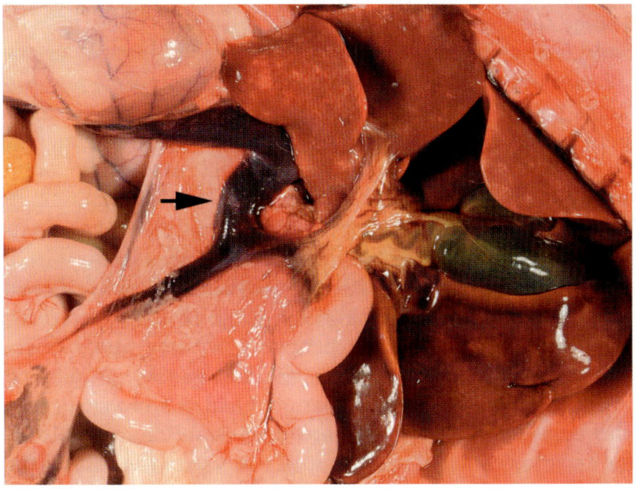

Figure 2-12 Congenital extrahepatic **portocaval shunt** (arrow) in a cat.

hepatic artery, and more rarely, the gastroduodenal artery and left gastric artery and portal vein. Mixing of higher pressure arterial blood with venous blood results in retrograde flow into the portal vein, arterialization of the portal circulation, and development of portal hypertension, with the opening of vestigial, low-resistance, collateral, extrahepatic portosystemic communications (acquired extrahepatic shunts). The fistulae may be macroscopic or microscopic, are typically multiple, and may involve one or more lobes of the liver. The hepatic parenchyma of affected lobes may be atrophied, with dilated, tortuous, pulsatile vessels visible on the capsular surface. Histopathologic findings include hyperplasia and anastomoses of arterioles and venules (Fig. 2-10). Affected vessels have irregularly thickened walls with intimal hyperplasia consisting of smooth muscle proliferation and deposition of elastin fibers, focal subintimal fibromuscular proliferation, and smooth muscle hyperplasia of the tunica media. Degenerative changes characterized by deposition of mucinous material and mineral in the intima and media of arterioles, as well as thrombosis and recanalization of portal veins, are also observed. Adjacent hepatic parenchyma may be atrophic, with periportal fibrosis, bile duct proliferation, arteriolar proliferation, and relative collapse of portal vein branches within portal tracts.

Arteriovenous fistulae may also be acquired, developing after abdominal trauma, rupture of hepatic artery aneurysms, and secondary to hepatic vein obstruction.

Congenital PSSs *are typically single anomalous vessels that directly connect the portal venous system with the systemic venous circulation, bypassing the hepatic sinusoids and hepatic parenchyma*. They occur in dogs and cats, and, rarely, in pigs, foals, goats, and calves. These PSSs may be either intrahepatic or extrahepatic. In dogs, the most common *intrahepatic shunt*, located in the left hepatic division, is a **persistent patent ductus venosus** (Fig. 2-11). Central and right divisional intrahepatic shunts have also been described in dogs and cats. The major types of *extrahepatic shunts* in dogs include direct shunting from the portal vein or major tributary (typically left gastric or splenic veins, less commonly the gastroduodenal or mesenteric veins) to the caudal vena cava (**portocaval shunt**) (Fig. 2-12, eFig. 2-2) or to the azygos vein (**portoazygos shunt**), or connection of the portal vein to the caudal vena cava, which itself shunts to the azygos vein. In cats, most PSSs originate from the left gastric vein and connect to the vena cava. Extrahepatic PSSs may also have hypoplasia of the portal vein distal to the origin of the shunt. Large-breed dogs typically have intrahepatic shunts, usually a patent ductus venosus, but sometimes other large intrahepatic communications. Small-breed dogs and cats usually have single large extrahepatic shunts between the portal vein and vena cava or azygos vein. An inherited basis is suspected in several breeds, including Irish Wolfhounds, Maltese, Yorkshire Terriers, and Australian Cattle Dogs.

Affected dogs are usually presented in adolescence with failure to thrive or with the neurobehavioral manifestations of hepatic encephalopathy (HE). Often, there is a clinical history of depression, convulsions, and other nervous signs that are exacerbated by a high protein diet and may be alleviated by dietary control. *Because there is no portal hypertension, these dogs do not develop ascites.*

The liver that has been bypassed by a congenital PSS is hypoplastic, largely because of diversion of hepatotrophic factors, including insulin, glucagon, and epidermal growth factor (EGF), that originate in the intestine and pancreas. Affected livers may be smooth surfaced with normal color and texture. Histologically, hepatocytes and hepatic lobules are small with close and irregular spacing of portal tracts. Larger portal veins may be inapparent or appear collapsed and empty of circulating blood elements; portal veins in smaller tracts may be small, collapsed, absent, or indistinguishable. Hepatic arterioles are often more prominent and may be multiple and tortuous (Fig. 2-13), related to increased compensatory arterial perfusion. Numbers of arteriolar structures within tracts may also appear increased, as small caliber and usually inapparent arterioles become evident histologically after compensatory hypertrophy. A proliferation of small caliber bile ducts (ductular reaction) has been confirmed in some cases by CK19 immunohistochemistry. Dilated vascular structures devoid of blood, presumably small- and large-caliber lymphatics, are often prominent in the periphery of some portal tracts. The disproportionate arterial inflow may increase local blood pressure favoring lymph formation. Dilated lymphatics may also be present in the connective tissue surrounding sublobular hepatic veins. The spiral smooth muscle in the wall of the sublobular veins may be more prominent in dogs with shunts than normal dogs. Release of endothelins 1 and 3 from sinusoidal endothelial cells and to a greater extent, HSCs, can lead to contraction of the spiral smooth muscle surrounding canine sublobular veins leading to impeded outflow of blood and increased interstitial pressure. Low serum protein also contributes to lymph formation. There may be increased deposition of fibrous connective tissue surrounding portal tracts and hepatic veins. Hepatocytes may contain cytoplasmic lipid droplets, and small lipogranulomatous foci with hemosiderin and ceroid in Kupffer cells; macrophages are typically present throughout the liver, especially in animals >1-year-old.

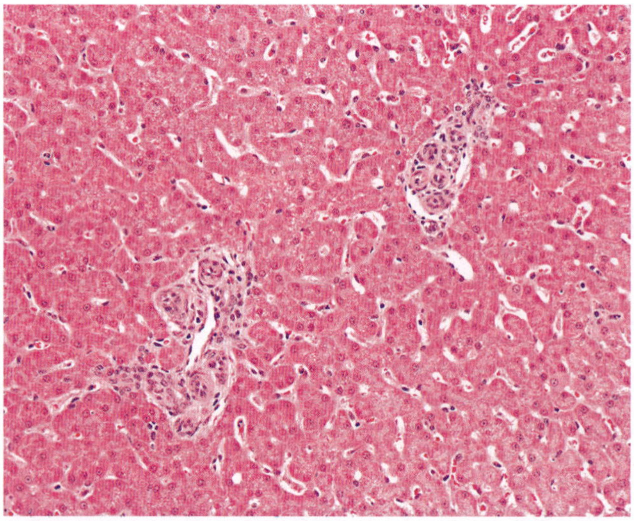

Figure 2-13 Histology of the liver of a dog with a **congenital portocaval shunt**. Closely spaced portal tracts contain various sections of hepatic arterioles and lack discernable portal veins.

Primary portal vein hypoplasia (PVH) has been reported in dogs, particularly Cairn and Yorkshire Terriers, and occasionally in cats, affecting either the extrahepatic or intrahepatic portal vein, or both. Intrahepatic PVH is considered to be the underlying lesion in conditions previously described as *microvascular dysplasia, hepatoportal fibrosis,* and *idiopathic noncirrhotic portal hypertension* in some young dogs. Depending on the level of the abnormality and extent of involvement of the lobes of liver, *PVH may be accompanied by portal hypertension, ascites, and the development of various collateral PSSs.* Histologically, there is hypoplasia or absence of portal vein radicles, secondary arteriolar proliferation, and atrophy of hepatocytes. Moderate-to-marked portal fibrosis may also be present, with ductular reaction (biliary hyperplasia). These changes represent stereotypic sequelae to underperfusion and thus can be indistinguishable histologically from congenital PSSs; however, development of portal hypertension is a distinguishing feature of PVH.

Macroscopic PSSs and microscopic portosystemic vascular anomalies may co-occur in dogs, as evidenced by a lack of resolution of clinical signs, and persistence of histologic changes in additional liver biopsies after macroscopic shunt ligation. Decreased tolerance of complete surgical shunt attenuation has been associated with lack of identifiable portal veins and a ductular reaction found in biopsies taken during the initial surgical shunt attenuation procedure, although an earlier study showed no association of severity of several histologic findings, such as arteriolar proliferation, ductular reaction, and fibrosis, with survival time after shunt attenuation.

Ductal plate developmental anomalies are also characterized by small or absent portal veins and have the potential to lead to portal hypertension. Typically, the anomalies have extensive biliary epithelial proliferation, along with excessive abnormal ECM deposition. The anomalies can be difficult to separate histologically from cases of PVH in some instances.

DISPLACEMENT, TORSION, AND RUPTURE

The position of the liver should be observed as soon as the abdomen is opened at postmortem examination. *Caudal displacements* resulting in extension of the margins of the liver beyond the costal arch may be the result of hepatic enlargement or of displacement of the diaphragm secondary to pleural effusion or other space-occupying lesions in the thorax. Congenital or acquired displacements associated with ventral and *diaphragmatic hernias* are common. Individual lobes or the entire organ may be displaced into the subcutis, pleural cavity, or pericardial sac, often along with other viscera; lobar blood supply may not always be compromised; however, individual displaced lobes may be severely congested and may rupture, or, given time, become indurated.

Partial or complete **liver lobe torsions** have been reported in pigs, dogs, cats, and horses. The left lateral lobe may be predisposed because of its mobility, large size, and relative separation from other lobes; however, torsions of other lobes, particularly the left medial lobe, as well as double-lobe torsions have been reported in dogs and horses. Other predisposing causes include the absence of or damage to the ligamentous attachments that provide spatial support for the liver, trauma, or a mass lesion in the affected lobe. Torsed lobes undergo various degrees of ischemia, culminating in infarction caused by venous occlusion or venous and/or arterial thrombosis, and affected animals may die because of shock, hemorrhage, or development of septic peritonitis. Ischemia may favor overgrowth of *Clostridium* spp. with the development of necrosis and emphysema. Subacute cases may develop hepatic abscessation, and if the animal survives, fibrosis and chronic inflammation.

Rupture *of the liver occurs commonly as the result of trauma because the organ is fragile relative to its mass.* Fatal liver rupture may be produced by the sudden accelerations and pressures of vehicle collisions without much evidence of trauma to other parts of the body. Large tears may be obvious in the liver capsule and hepatic parenchyma after trauma; however, anastomosing linear patterns of fine shallow capsular fissures may be concealed in part by clotted blood. Liver rupture is often clinically occult because quite large ruptures may not disturb liver function unless severe enough to cause rapid exsanguination, or unless the biliary tract is involved. *Intrahepatic bile duct rupture* results in bile extravasation into the hepatic parenchyma or beneath the hepatic capsule, forming bile lakes or bile infarcts, areas of hepatocyte degeneration, and necrosis surrounded by reactive macrophages; larger accumulations of bile may be walled off by a pseudocapsule, forming biliary pseudocysts. Rupture of major bile ducts or the gallbladder results in yellow-stained *bile peritonitis*, which may remain sterile and become chronic, or may be fatal, particularly if infected by enterohepatic circulation of bacteria such as clostridia.

The liver is more likely to rupture after trauma in young animals. Fatal ruptures occur in foals during parturition, sometimes concurrently with costal fractures, and in the smaller species subjected to energetic emergency resuscitation. Diffuse hepatic conditions with enlarged friable parenchyma (e.g., acute hepatitis, amyloidosis, severe congestion, severe lipidosis, and infiltrating neoplasms) are more likely to rupture, sometimes spontaneously, and the clinical consequences are related to the extent of hemorrhage. Parasites that penetrate the capsule cause numerous small ruptures but seldom lead to significant hemorrhage.

HEPATOCELLULAR ADAPTATIONS, INTRACELLULAR AND EXTRACELLULAR ACCUMULATION

The liver must be highly adaptable to balance function with changing demand. Increases in the size of hepatocytes *(hypertrophy)* and their numbers *(hyperplasia)* collectively bring a larger mass of hepatocytes into service. Such adaptations in hepatic volume and function result from alterations in the expression of many genes. These responses are more evident in smaller species, notably in laboratory rodents that have a very pronounced liver growth response after exposure to various xenobiotics. The liver can also adapt to reduced demand or oxygen supply by a combination of *cellular atrophy* and *apoptosis*. Hepatocytes can be lost by apoptosis in substantial numbers, with minimal elevation in activities of serum enzymes of hepatic origin, such as alanine aminotransferase.

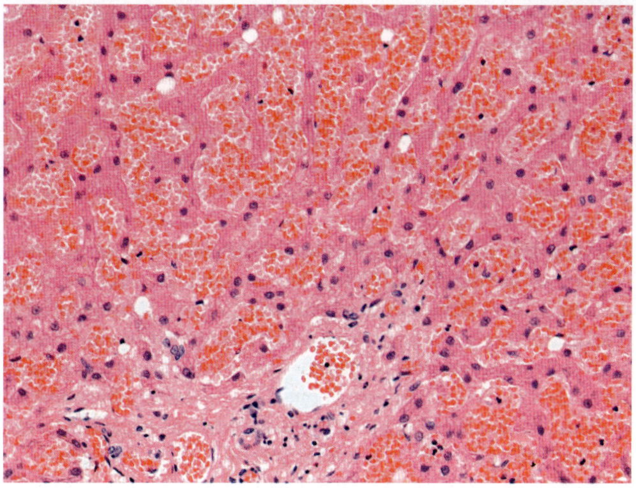

Figure 2-14 **Hepatocellular atrophy** and marked sinusoidal congestion in a dog with chronic right-sided heart failure.

Hepatocellular atrophy

Hepatic mass readily adapts to metabolic demands, and *the liver can undergo marked atrophy during illness and/or starvation without much evidence of impaired hepatic function*. During prolonged starvation, some hepatocytes are removed by apoptosis without replacement, but most of the atrophy is explained by the loss of cytoplasmic mass. Atrophic livers, as seen, for example, in old grazing herbivores with poor teeth, are dark and small, and the capsule may appear too large for the organ, showing fine wrinkles on handling. These livers may even appear to be firmer than normal because of condensation of normal stroma. Histologically, portal tracts and hepatic venules are closer together, and lobules contain increased numbers of smaller hepatocytes with scanty cytoplasm (Fig. 2-14). *Hepatocellular mass can be rapidly lost by autophagy and apoptosis* (see later the Types and Patterns of Cell Injury and Death in the Liver section).

Hepatic atrophy, rather than hepatocellular atrophy, can also result from impaired replication of hepatocytes. Adult hepatocytes are replicatively competent, although mitotic figures are infrequent because healthy hepatocytes have a relatively long lifespan of several months. Diminished portal blood flow limits not only oxygen but also trophic factors that act to regulate replication and mass of the liver. These trophic factors include several polypeptide growth factors, including hepatocyte growth factor and insulin-like growth factors, and many hormones, including insulin, glucagon, and catecholamines.

Atrophy of only a part of the liver may be a response to pressure or to impairment of blood or bile flow. The histologic features of this atrophy are like those of starvation atrophy. However, the functional consequences of focal hepatic atrophy are minor because the remaining liver can compensate and adapt by a process that involves replication and enlargement of hepatocytes. Local pressure atrophy occurs next to space-occupying lesions in the liver, or because of chronic pressures from neighboring organs, such as distended rumen in the ox. It has been suggested that *right hepatic lobe atrophy*, reported in horses, results from long-term compression from abnormal distension of the right dorsal colon and base of the cecum (eFig. 2-3). Chronic diffuse diseases of the biliary tract, such as sporidesmin poisoning and fascioliasis, are likely to cause atrophy of the left lobe in ruminants, possibly because of the greater difficulty in maintaining adequate biliary drainage from this lobe, whose bile ducts are longer than those of the right in these species. The atrophy of biliary obstruction is complicated by some degree of superimposed inflammation and fibrosis.

Hepatocellular hypertrophy

Hypertrophy is the term used for the *increase in liver size caused by an increase in hepatocyte volume* that may result from expansion of one or more organellar components of the hepatocytes. Exposure to various xenobiotics can induce the expression of many genes, leading to expansion of the SER, resulting in hepatocyte hypertrophy. Agents that elicit this response act via nuclear receptors, such as the arylhydrocarbon-activated receptor (AHR), the constitutive androstane receptor (CAR), or the pregnane X receptor (PXR). Phenobarbital, for example, is a potent inducer of the various enzyme systems of the SER, including several CYPs. Hypertrophy may occur in defined lobular regions, typically the centrilobular region, or may affect the entire lobule in more advanced cases, depending on the activity and dose level of the xenobiotic (Fig. 2-15). Even when it is restricted to the centrilobular region, hypertrophy usually enlarges the entire liver. Although hepatocellular hypertrophy is most often associated with preferential increase in SER, proliferation of peroxisomes, or mitochondria can also cause hepatocellular hypertrophy. The light microscopic appearance of hypertrophy upon routine H&E staining will sometimes suggest the selective involvement of one organelle. If total SER volume is increased, the cytoplasm will typically have an *eosinophilic ground glass appearance* upon light microscopy. If total peroxisomal volume is increased, the cytoplasm is often noted to have an *eosinophilic granular appearance*. The response can be seen within a few days after exposure to various drugs and other xenobiotic compounds. Accordingly, the liver becomes grossly enlarged. This induction of SER or peroxisomes is reversible, and after discontinuation of exposure to the inducing agent, the expanded SER or excess peroxisomes are removed by autophagy, and many hepatocytes undergo apoptosis. Although these changes are considered physiologic adaptations, there are potential adverse sequelae; accordingly, this response has toxicologic significance and will be dealt later in the Toxic Hepatic Disease section.

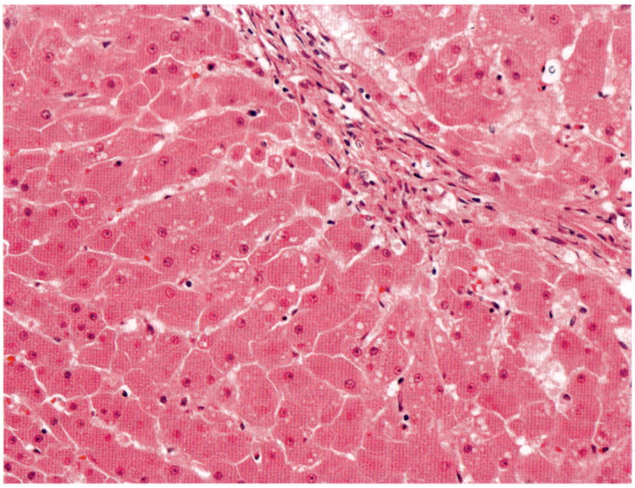

Figure 2-15 Increased hepatocellular cytoplasmic volume resulting from **smooth endoplasmic reticulum induction** in a dog treated chronically with phenobarbital.

Polyploidy and multinucleation

Most mature mammalian hepatocytes are *tetraploid or octaploid*; many immature and replicating hepatocytes are *diploid*. The relative proportion of polyploid hepatocytes varies among species, and polyploidy increases with age. Polyploidy is more common in rodents and is believed to result from asynchrony of cell division in which binucleate diploid cells undergo a second round of DNA replication, giving rise to 2 tetraploid daughter cells. Impaired replication can also increase the number of polyploid cells. The term **megalocytosis** was first used to describe the changes of liver cell cytoplasm and nucleus that occur in pyrrolizidine alkaloid poisoning. This form of megalocytosis has some specific features and is described later in the Chronic hepatotoxicity: plant-derived and environmental toxins section. Impaired regeneration, atrophy, and >4N polyploidy can also be produced by other DNA-damaging agents, such as aflatoxins. A feature of these patterns of atrophy with polyploidy is the persistence of larger replication-impaired polyploid hepatocytes amid regenerating smaller diploid hepatocytes, hepatocellular nodules, and hyperplastic bile ductules.

Most hepatocytes are mononuclear, but a variable proportion is binucleate, especially in young or regenerating livers of small animals. Multinucleation by >2 nuclei of non-neoplastic hepatocytes is a rare phenomenon in domestic mammals, and its diagnostic or pathogenetic significance is usually unclear. Multinucleation can result from incomplete cell division or cell fusion, but this distinction is difficult to determine. Hepatocytes can fuse during severe steatosis, but the degree of multinucleation in fatty livers is hard to discern because the plasma membrane perimeters of fatty hepatocytes are ill defined. *Syncytial multinucleation* of hepatocytes has been observed in various degenerative and regenerative conditions. In protoporphyria of Limousin cattle, small clusters of hepatocytes contain 4-10 or more closely packed nuclei, but it is not clear whether this represents fusion or numerous nuclear divisions. Syncytial hepatocytes are a characteristic of postinfantile giant-cell hepatitis of children, and similar hepatocyte multinucleation can be seen in association with some forms of hepatitis in newborn cats, foals, and piglets (see the Inflammatory Diseases of the Liver and Biliary Tract section). Multinucleate hepatocytes have been described in young cats with thymic lymphomas, and in cats with experimental dioxin poisoning.

Intranuclear inclusions and pseudoinclusions

In addition to the various nuclear inclusions associated with some viral infections, 3 types of inclusions or pseudoinclusions may be found in hepatocyte nuclei.

1. Spherical, apparently hollow globules within the body of the nucleus are *membrane-bound entrapped nuclear membrane invaginations* that ultrastructurally contain cytoplasmic components, such as glycogen and mitochondria. These **pseudoinclusions** are infrequent in otherwise normal livers but are more often seen in chronically injured livers, especially in chronic pyrrolizidine alkaloid poisoning, in which polyploid nuclei are more likely to indent and invaginate.
2. Eosinophilic blocklike intranuclear inclusions with a regular crystal lattice (**"brick inclusions"**) are common in hepatocytes and renal proximal tubular epithelium. They are more numerous in old animals, specifically dogs. Their composition and pathogenesis are unknown, but they evidently have a negligible effect on the health of the cells in which they occur, even when they are large enough to distort the nucleus. They do not contain heavy metals and can

be distinguished from the acid-fast, noncrystalline intranuclear inclusions seen in renal epithelial cells and occasionally in hepatocytes in lead poisoning.

3. **Lead inclusions** consist of a lead-protein complex and have a characteristic furry electron-dense ultrastructure.

Pigmentation

Congenital melanosis occurs in calves and occasionally in lambs and swine. The melanin deposits may be numerous and vary in size from flecks, to irregular, blue-black areas 2 cm or more in diameter. The melanin is confined to the capsule and the stroma. These deposits are sharply defined in young animals but become more diffuse and fade with age (eFig. 2-4).

Acquired melanosis is the massive accumulation of black pigment (not melanin) in hepatocytes and Kupffer cells of mature sheep and, less often cattle, after prolonged grazing on extensive unimproved pastures in inland eastern Australia, the Falkland Islands, and Scandinavia. The condition in Norway has also been described as *hepatic lipofuscinosis*. The color of the affected livers ranges from dull-gray to uniform black, and there is usually a prominent lobular pattern. In severe cases, there is also pigmentation of the hepatic lymph nodes, lungs, and renal cortex. Histologically, the pigment is present as granules in lysosomes in periportal and midzonal hepatocytes and macrophages of the liver, the proximal tubular epithelium of the kidneys, and in alveolar and interstitial macrophages in the lung. There is no evidence of liver dysfunction, even in the blackest livers. The source of this pigment is not known, but the epidemiologic features of its occurrence indicate that it is derived from a component of the diet that is sequestered within lysosomes.

Bile pigmentation may impart an olive-green color to the liver in diffuse or segmental obstructive biliary disease or intrahepatic cholestasis. Histologically, conjugated bile pigments may distend bile canaliculi, visible microscopically as golden-brown linear streaks arrayed in a chicken wirelike pattern between the hepatocytes (Fig. 2-16). In this case, the identity of the pigment is obvious, but when it is present in granular form in Kupffer cell cytoplasm, it may easily be confused with hemosiderin or hematin. Bile pigment is encountered infrequently in hepatocyte cytoplasm, almost never in dogs, except in rare cases with dramatic cholestasis. Death of individual hepatocytes releases the canalicular plugs into the perisinusoidal space and the sinusoids, where they may be phagocytosed by Kupffer cells.

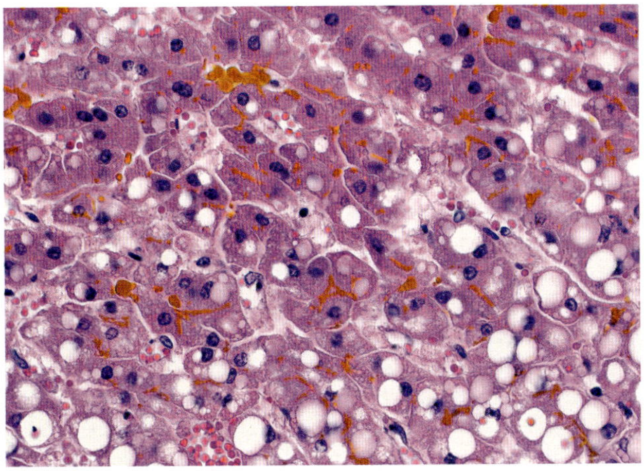

Figure 2-16 Bile plugs distend bile canaliculi in a cow with high-altitude pulmonary hypertension and hepatic chronic passive congestion.

Lipofuscin is the term given to small, golden, granular cytoplasmic deposits *derived from the lipid component of membranous organelles*. Lipofuscin accumulates in hepatocellular lysosomes and indicates senility, atrophy, or increased turnover of membrane lipids. The pigment is particularly common in the centrilobular regions of the liver of cats after they reach maturity.

Ceroid is a colorless or yellow pigment similar to lipofuscin and is associated with *peroxidation of fat deposits*. This material is only slightly soluble in lipid solvents and is PAS positive, diastase resistant, variably acid fast, and autofluorescent.

Black pigment also accumulates in hepatocellular lysosomes of mutant Corriedale sheep with hyperbilirubinemia. These sheep have a condition resembling the human Dubin-Johnson syndrome, in which there is mutation in the canalicular transporter in the organic anion-transporting polypeptide (OATP) family. This suggests that retention of the pigment might be a sequel to a hepatic excretory defect.

Congenital erythrocytic protoporphyria (ferrochelatase deficiency) manifests as a photoreactive dermatopathy and has been described in cattle, sheep, pigs, cats, and dogs. A dark golden-brown lipofuscin-like lysosomal material accumulates in macrophages, Kupffer cells, hepatocytes, cholangiocytes, biliary canaliculi, and sinusoidal endothelial cells. The pigment has a unique yellow-to-green birefringence, and an orange-red Maltese cross can be seen in pigment aggregates under polarized light (Fig. 2-17A and B).

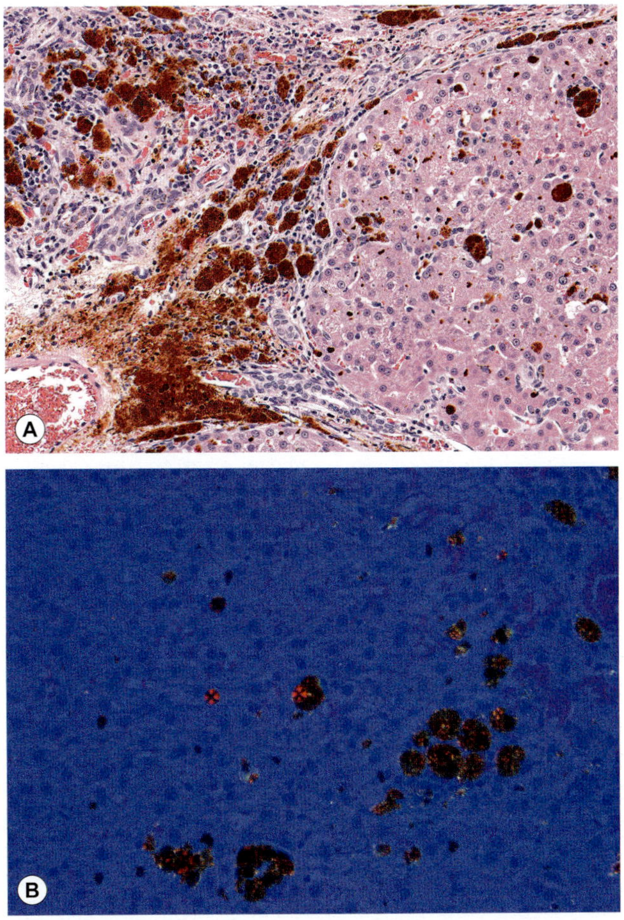

Figure 2-17 A. Dark golden-brown **protoporphyrin crystals** in the fibrotic, inflamed liver of a dog. **B**. Protoporphyrin crystals with bright red **Maltese cross** birefringence when viewed under polarized light. (Courtesy E. Choi.)

Acquired protoporphyria with liver injury has been described in a cohort of German Shepherd dogs presumed to have been exposed to an unknown toxicant and in Beagle dogs exposed to 2 experimental drugs. Grossly, affected German Shepherd dogs had dark livers that had numerous regenerative nodules. Histologically, there was abundant bridging portal fibrosis and typical orange birefringent protoporphyrin crystals in hepatocytes. Photosensitization was not evident. Hepatocellular vacuolation and nodule formation have also been described in a cat with porphyria.

Hemosiderin deposits are seldom sufficient to give gross discoloration, but when this occurs, the color is dark-brown. The pigment is detected microscopically as yellow or brown crystals chiefly in the Kupffer cells, although lesser amounts may be found in hepatocytes. The ferric iron component of this pigment can be shown by Prussian blue staining; otherwise, it can easily be confused with lipofuscin. *Most hemosiderin deposits are punctate Prussian blue staining aggregates in Kupffer cells* but can also be seen as finer particles in hepatocytes. Diffuse hemosiderin deposits in Kupffer cells occur quite commonly in all species and are usually *suggestive of excess hemolytic activity* relative to the rate of reutilization of iron. Thus, they are seen in hemolytic anemia, anemia of copper deficiency, in cachexia, after blood transfusions as well as iron injections, and following chronic hepatic injury. It may be seen in Kupffer cells of the centrilobular zones in severe chronic passive congestion of the liver. Localized hemosiderin deposition occurs in areas of hemorrhage. Hemosiderin is normally present in the liver in the early neonatal period when fetal hemoglobin is being replaced by mature hemoglobin.

Hemosiderin should be distinguished from **hematin**, which is produced by the action of acids on hemoglobin and is usually regarded as a *histologic artifact* following the use of improperly buffered formalin, or when the amount of blood exceeds the fixative solution buffering capacity. Hematin is also an iron-containing pigment, but the iron is in the reduced ferrous state and does not stain with ferricyanide. It takes the form of crystalline brown deposits that are birefringent under polarized light, mainly within hemoglobin-rich areas such as blood vessels. Hematin is darker than hemosiderin and occurs in irregular clumps, often extracellularly. Hematin may, however, be found in Kupffer cells and macrophages in small amounts.

Hepatic iron overload has previously been divided into **hemosiderosis** when there is only an excess accumulation of hepatocellular iron, and **hemochromatosis** when the excess iron storage has produced fibrosis and inflammation and hepatic injury, although this terminology is not used consistently. Hemochromatosis, an inherited disorder, is relatively common in humans with specific mutations. Iron overload is common in some birds, such as mynahs, and in lemurs, but rare in domestic mammals. A form resembling heritable hemochromatosis has been reported in Salers or Salers-cross cattle. Affected animals develop a wasting disease at ~1-2 years of age, have a 30-100-fold increase in liver iron content, with dark-brown discolored, firm livers, hemosiderin accumulation in hepatocytes, and periportal and perivenular bridging fibrosis. Hemosiderin also accumulates in Kupffer cells, lymph nodes, kidneys, pancreas, spleen, and other organs.

Iron overload from **dietary excess** has been seen in sheep and cattle exposed to *high levels of iron in pasture and water*. The liver is enlarged and brown with diffuse fine nodularity, and the hepatic and adjacent lymph nodes are also darkened. Large amounts of iron are present in the hepatic parenchyma, the biliary epithelium, and the cortex of lymph nodes, and lesser amounts are present in the broad fibrous septa. The iron is stored predominantly in lysosomes. Brown discoloration of bone marrow resembles the osseous pigmentation of porphyria. The pathogenesis of nutritional iron overload is unknown. Iron overload has also been described in horses, with animals displaying signs of liver failure and neurologic impairment. The microscopic lesions in the livers of these animals are similar to those of other species.

Brown crystalline deposits of **2,8-dihydroxyadenine** (2,8-DHA) have been described in hepatocytes and in other tissues in slaughtered cattle with no evidence of other disease. These accumulations are strongly birefringent under polarized light and are seen in the cytoplasm of hepatocytes and macrophages of hepatic lymph nodes and as extracellular deposits in portal stroma and renal tubular lumens. Grossly, the portal stroma stands out as a green network; affected lymph nodes were enlarged, and the medullary sinusoids were distended with green pasty material. The crystals were identified as 2,8-DHA by a panel of crystallographic methods and mass spectrometry. The pathogenesis is unknown. A genetic deficiency of the enzyme adenine phosphoribosyltransferase or exposure to a toxin affecting the same metabolic pathway was speculated.

Pigments of parasitic origin are particularly associated with *flukes*. Heavy deposits of *black iron-porphyrin compound* are formed around the cysts and migratory pathways of *Fascioloides magna*. Lesser amounts of similar pigment are deposited in bile ducts infected by *Fasciola hepatica* (see later the Helminthic Infections section). Finding this pigment in the hilar nodes should suggest otherwise inapparent infections by flukes. In schistosomiasis, the liver may be gray because of the accumulation of black pigment in Kupffer cells.

Hepatocyte swelling: vacuolation and cytoplasmic rarefaction

The term **"vacuolar hepatopathy"** has been used to denote multifocal or diffuse zonal hepatocellular swelling due to *cytoplasmic unstained open spaces* in histologic sections before a more specific term can be applied, for example, before contents of the open spaces are identified. However, due to the different causes and clinical significance of different types of hepatocyte swelling, specific terminology is favored. Specific forms of hepatocyte swelling include hydropic swelling, cytoplasmic rarefaction (glycogenosis), steatosis (lipidosis), and some storage disorders. **Hydropic degeneration** can only be appreciated in carefully controlled experimental circumstances and is an early cytoplasmic ballooning seen after various toxic and metabolic insults, hypoxia, and cholestasis. Water and sodium ion influx expands membranous compartments of mitochondria, lysosomes, and ER. Ultrastructural changes include plasma membrane alterations (blebbing, blunting, and distortion of microvilli, formation of myelin figures, and loosening of intercellular attachments), mitochondrial changes (swelling, rarefaction, and appearance of amorphous densities), dilation of the ER with detachment and disaggregation of polysomes, and nuclear alterations.

The term **feathery degeneration** is applied to the type of cytoplasmic rarefaction that occurs in hepatocytes in which there has been prolonged cholate stasis. The cells are swollen with open spaces and crisscrossed by a fine network of cytoplasmic constituents with a small amount of brown bile pigments (Fig. 2-18). This change is uncommon in cats and dogs and seen more often in horses.

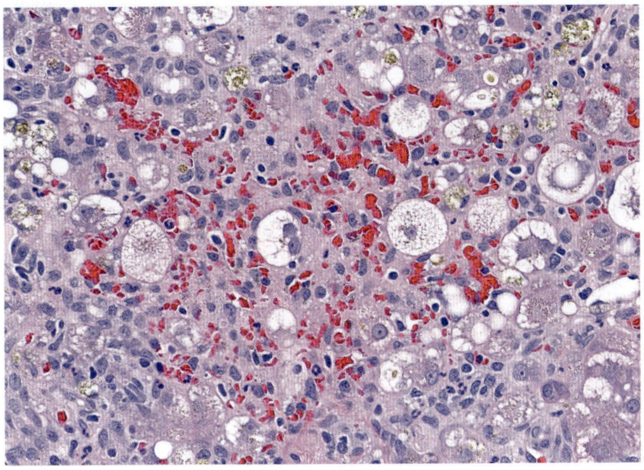

Figure 2-18 **Feathery degeneration** in a dog with cholestasis.

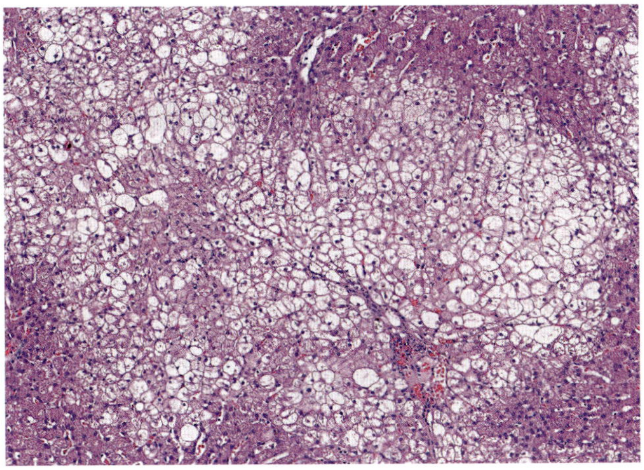

Figure 2-19 Prominent vacuolation of hepatocytes following **glucocorticoid administration** in a dog.

Hepatic glycogenosis or **glucocorticoid hepatopathy**, often referred to as **steroid-induced hepatopathy**, involves *glycogen accumulation*, because of *either functional adrenocortical or pituitary tumors, or treatment with glucocorticoids*. The liver is enlarged and pale-tan. Hepatocytes are swollen, and the cytoplasm appears as fine, diaphanous strands that enclose several spaces with poorly demarcated edges. Vacuolar change has been used to describe the cytoplasmic change, but *cytoplasmic rarefaction* is a better terminology. Glycogen, unlike lipid and abnormal storage products, does not form vacuoles in the cytoplasm. Removal of glycogen in fixation and processing of histologic slides leads to ragged open spaces. **Cell swelling** may range from mild to severe, with enlargement of hepatocytes from 2 to 10 times normal size and displacement of the nucleus and organelles to the cellular periphery in more affected instances (Fig. 2-19). The zonal distribution may be variable and may become diffuse in long-standing cases or with higher doses. Single-cell dropout, small aggregates of neutrophils along sinusoids, and scattered small foci of extramedullary hematopoiesis are also commonly observed. The ill-defined boundaries of excess glycogen in steroid hepatopathy are readily distinguishable from spherical lipid vacuoles in hepatic steatosis (eFig. 2-5). *The pathogenesis of this condition is* uncertain because glycogen storage alone does not fully explain the influx of fluid, and possible perturbations in hepatocellular ion channels or aquaporins have not been assessed. The amount of glycogen remaining in affected cells is widely variable, a function of the original glycogen concentration, recent catabolism, and postmortem dissolution. Glycogen content can best be demonstrated in *frozen section*, followed by staining with *PAS*, and can be confirmed as glycogen by its sensitivity to *digestion with diastase*. Livers affected by glucocorticoid hepatopathy maintain normal hepatocyte functions, but the condition can be confirmed by the induction and *serum increase of glucocorticoid-inducible alkaline phosphatase*, with minor or negligible increases in alanine aminotransferase. Similar **cell swelling and cytoplasmic rarefaction** may be created by other adrenocortical steroids, predominantly progestins, as occasionally seen in older, female dogs that appear to have overproduction of adrenocortical hormones other than cortisol, and alkaline phosphatase elevation, although the specific pathogenesis is unknown. Intact female dogs accumulate abundant hepatocellular cytoplasmic glycogen in diestrus and possibly during pseudopregnancy, further supporting a role for progesterone. Some drugs, such as the chelator D-penicillamine, can produce similar cytoplasmic rarefaction.

Loss-of-function mutations in hepatic and renal glucose-6-phosphatase resulting in increased hepatic glycogen storage have been reported in Maltese puppies or related crossbred dogs, and these dogs serve as an animal model of **glycogen storage disease (glycogenosis) type Ia**. These dogs have severely debilitating problems in maintaining their blood glucose because dephosphorylation of glucose-6-phosphate is a key step in both glycogenolysis and gluconeogenesis. The condition is typified by severe hepatocellular glycogenosis. Livers are markedly enlarged, pale, and have diffuse hepatocellular cytoplasmic rarefaction with substantial amounts of glycogen and small amounts of lipid. Hepatic fibrosis and nodular regeneration can develop with time. Renal tubular epithelium is also vacuolated. Glycogen storage disease **type II** is reported in Lapphund dogs, and Shorthorn and Brahman cattle. Glycogen storage disease **type III**, with hepatic glycogen storage, has been reported in German Shepherd dogs and Curly-Coated Retrievers. **Type IV** glycogenosis has been reported in Norwegian Forest cats and American Quarter Horses, although this disorder causes pale-blue granules in hepatocellular cytoplasm rather than clear cytoplasmic rarefaction.

Characteristic hepatocellular vacuolation is also described in dogs with end-stage nodular livers presented clinically with *superficial necrolytic dermatitis* (*hepatocutaneous syndrome*).

Hepatocellular steatosis (lipidosis)

Hepatocellular steatosis is the term used to describe *fatty livers of animals*. However, *the terms steatosis, lipidosis, and fatty change tend to be used interchangeably*. Hepatocellular steatosis represents a true vacuole formation as there is a limiting membrane around the lipid, unlike cytoplasmic glycogen or water in other forms of cell swelling. All these terms refer to the *visible accumulation of triglycerides (triacylglycerols) as round globules in the cytoplasm of hepatocytes*. The threshold for application of these terms is vague because triglyceride storage and transport are normal hepatic functions, but they are appropriate when the amounts are greater than would normally be seen. Hepatocellular steatosis can be *physiologic or pathologic*. Any circumstance in which hepatic uptake of lipids exceeds oxidation or secretion can lead to hepatocellular steatosis. Increased mobilization of triglycerides during *late pregnancy or heavy lactation in ruminants* is associated with hepatocellular steatosis. The lipid represents increased transit of triglycerides in an otherwise healthy liver, so there is little diagnostic significance in mild degrees of hepatocellular steatosis in lactating cows. In some of these animals, severe energy deficiency can also lead to clinical ketosis with metabolic acidosis. In addition, severe steatosis occurs in high-producing dairy cows fed diets in which either the mix of available fatty acids is incorrect, or lipids are oxidized and rancid.

Hepatocellular steatosis is *common in injured hepatocytes* because the normal high throughput of fatty acids and triglycerides can be readily impeded at various points in the complex pathway of hepatic lipid metabolism and secretion of very low–density lipoproteins (VLDLs). Hepatocytes obtain some fatty acids from albumin and other carrier proteins in the portal blood, but most is hydrolyzed by sinusoidal endothelial hepatic lipase from triglyceride in chylomicrons or VLDL in plasma. Very long–chain fatty acids are initially oxidized by acyl-coenzyme A oxidase in peroxisomes to shorter acyl-coenzyme A that can be transported via a carnitine-dependent process into mitochondria for further oxidation. Although some fatty acid is used for energy in hepatic mitochondria, most from dietary or adipose sources is converted to triglycerides that are further processed into lipoproteins in the hepatocyte ER and actively secreted into the plasma as VLDL. Endothelial lipoprotein lipase in muscle and adipose tissue hydrolyzes triglycerides in the VLDL, and the fatty acids released are used locally by β-oxidation in mitochondria of muscle or re-esterified into triglyceride in adipocytes. The depleted VLDLs are returned by receptor-mediated endocytosis to hepatocytes, where their constituents are catabolized and recycled.

The synthesis and export of VLDL in hepatocytes are energy and resource dependent, so any disturbance of the supply of apoproteins (apoprotein B primarily), phospholipids, cholesterol, or ATP, or physical disruption of the organelles involved in synthesis, assembly, and secretion, has the potential to inhibit lipoprotein synthesis or secretion. Fatty acids can continue to enter hepatocytes, allowing triglyceride globules to accumulate in the hepatocyte cytoplasm. In some species, damage to peroxisomes reduces the initial peroxisomal oxidation step for catabolism of long-chain fatty acids and upregulates various genes regulated by peroxisome proliferator–activated receptor–α (PPAR-α). Lipoproteins in the ER, Golgi, and membrane-bound secretory vesicles can also accumulate if there is selective damage to the distal secretory apparatus. Damage by various toxic and hypoxic insults will not lead to triglyceride accumulation in hepatocytes if supplies of mobile triglycerides from adipose tissue or the diet are low.

The microscopic appearance of triglyceride globules in hepatocytes ranges from small discrete microvesicles to large coalescing macrovesicles. Lipid is evident as clear, round, empty spaces in the cytoplasm in routine formalin-fixed paraffin-embedded tissue as lipid is removed during routine processing. Lipid can be demonstrated in frozen sections using Oil Red O or Sudan black, or in tissue that has been postfixed in osmium tetroxide. Microvesicular lipid vacuoles are smaller than the nucleus and tend not to displace the nucleus (Fig. 2-20). **Microvesicular steatosis** can be a hallmark of more severe hepatic dysfunction than macrovesicular steatosis. This pattern can occur in several toxic hepatopathies causing mitochondrial injury, including some human drug toxicities, such as antiviral nucleosides, aspirin in Reye syndrome, and excessive tetracycline administration, all of which can be fatal. These toxicities target mitochondria, disrupting energy production; the normal electron transfer chain, causing oxidative injury; and interfere with β-oxidation of lipids. Partially oxidized lipids typically have a lower surface tension than triglycerides and therefore form smaller vesicles in the aqueous medium of the cytoplasm. Uncontrolled diabetes mellitus, fading puppy syndrome, and feline fatty liver syndrome can produce microvesicular hepatic steatosis or a mixture of microvesicular and macrovesicular steatosis. Acute steatosis with predominantly microvesicular accumulation tends to result in a modestly enlarged pale liver without much change in texture, while macrovesicular hepatic steatosis more often produces an enlarged liver.

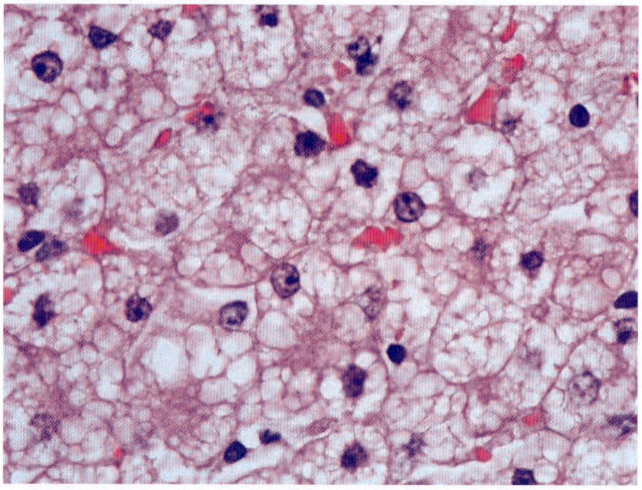

Figure 2-20 Microvesicular lipid is characterized by numerous round, clear vacuoles that are smaller than the nucleus and do not displace the nucleus.

In some more protracted toxic injuries, smaller lipid globules can coalesce into large central **macrovesicles** that displace the nucleus. The pathogenesis of the larger globules is not well understood, but it involves some alteration of the globule-cytoplasm interface that normally prevents coalescence of the small micellar globules, possibly the greater hydrophobicity of the triglycerides. These fatty livers tend to be more yellow and enlarged, and the texture is more friable than livers with microvesicular steatosis. Each hepatocyte usually contains one large globule (macrovesicle) that alters the contour of the cell and displaces the nucleus (Fig. 2-21). The sinusoids are compressed and appear underperfused, and the tissue at low magnification resembles adipose tissue. In severe degeneration, the liver is moderately or greatly enlarged, with a uniform light-yellow color. The edges are rounded, and the surface is smooth (eFig. 2-6). The cut surface has a diffuse greasy appearance or a red and yellow lobular pattern if there is also hepatic congestion or zonal necrosis. *In severe diffuse hepatic steatosis, the parenchyma is less dense, and portions will float in water or fixative*.

Assessment of the functional significance of steatosis depends on the differentiation of physiologic steatosis caused by increased mobilization by otherwise normal hepatocytes from pathologic changes that represent some degenerative change in hepatocytes. However, *fat accumulation is a sensitive response to hepatocellular injury and can occur in the absence of other obvious alterations in hepatic structure or function*. The triglyceride globules themselves are not harmful to hepatocytes, so the amount of fat present is more an indicator of the duration of insult and triglyceride supply than of the severity

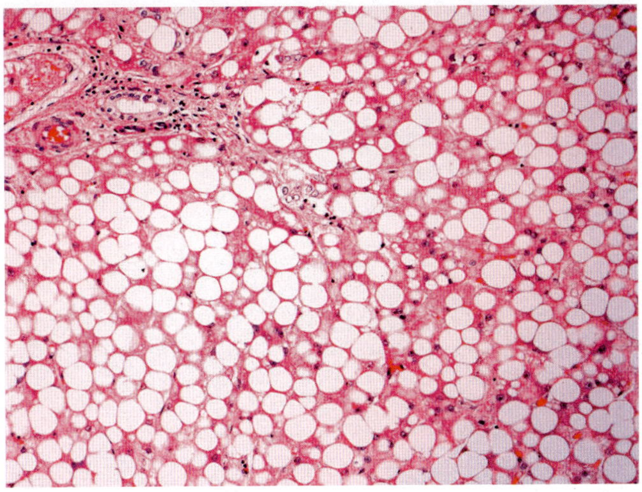

Figure 2-21 Macrovesicular lipid vacuoles in the liver of a donkey. Vacuoles are larger than the nuclei and tend to displace nuclei to the periphery of the cell.

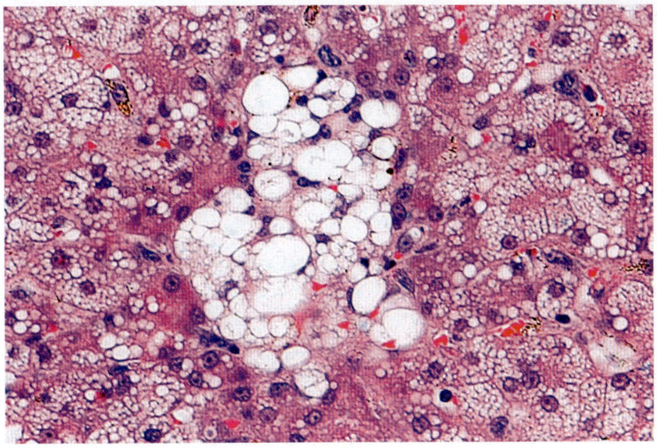

Figure 2-22 Lipogranuloma in the liver of a dog.

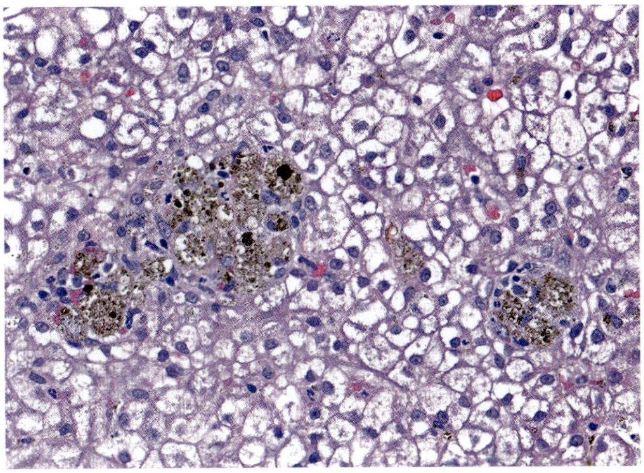

Figure 2-23 Pigment granuloma in the liver of a dog.

of hepatic injury. Steatosis is usually reversible, although a liver that has been fatty for some time is more likely to have concurrent damage, including fibrosis, pigment accumulation, and nodular hyperplasia, mostly attributable to ongoing peroxidative damage, cell turnover, and activation of stellate cells.

Hepatocellular steatosis is now recognized as a more significant indicator of potential, more severe liver injury than previously appreciated. In ruminants, the association between hepatic steatosis, ketosis, and displaced abomasum are well recognized. Infectious diseases, such as metritis and mastitis, may be more likely or prolonged. Neutrophil function is suppressed, as is interferon production by lymphocytes, and endotoxin clearance is also reduced. Hepatocytes become more sensitive to injury following exposure to cytokines, such as TNF, or endotoxin as well. Consequently, *fatty livers are more vulnerable to a wide range of toxic and nutritional insults*, so other necrogenic insults and responses can be concurrent. Increased levels of fatty acids in the liver increase the oxidative stress and contribute to membrane lipid peroxidation, reduced hepatocyte lifespan, and some local repair responses. Hepatocyte enlargement compromises biliary canalicular function resulting in cholestasis. Cholestasis due to hepatic lipidosis is most commonly observed in cats.

When lipid accumulates in substantial amounts, there is a tendency for *groups of the fat-laden cells to rupture* (Fig. 2-22). The released lipid is picked up by macrophages that form aggregates in sinusoids, and in the stroma of portal tracts, and hepatic venules. Such an aggregate of foamy and variably pigmented macrophages is termed a **lipogranuloma**. Subsequent peroxidation of the less-saturated fatty acids and covalent modification and polymerization of oxidized lipids form a complex of lysosomal residues known collectively as **ceroid**. When granulomas are composed of nonvacuolated or minimally vacuolated macrophages containing a mixture of hemosiderin, lipofuscin, and/or ceroid, they are termed a **pigment granuloma** (Fig. 2-23). A few lymphocytes and/or plasma cells are often present within lipogranulomas and pigment granulomas. These granulomas accumulate with age and hepatocellular turnover. They have no known clinical significance, but they indicate increased cell turnover and are typically present in some diseases such as congenital PSS in dogs. Some chronic changes commonly seen in the *livers of old dogs* can be associated with fatty liver; these include lipogranulomas, and ceroid accumulation.

Physiologic steatosis (fatty liver) *occurs in late pregnancy and heavy lactation, particularly in ruminants and llamas*. In this circumstance, the lipid is typically macrovesicular, with large, round, clear vacuoles that tend to displace the nucleus. Obvious steatosis is also seen in neonates, especially in those species whose milk is relatively rich in fat. The high rate of mobilization of triglycerides from body fat stores is mainly responsible for fatty liver in lactating ruminants. However, fatty liver is a concern because lipid mobilization also increases when the dietary energy intake is insufficient relative to the production demands that are greatest in early lactation of high-producing cows. Insufficient dietary intake by an animal with adequate fat reserves depletes hepatocellular glycogen and initiates a heavy demand for triglycerides from adipose tissue. When hepatic triglyceride concentrations exceed 10% on a wet weight basis, severe or clinical fatty liver ensues. At this time, urinary ketones are elevated, and body weight loss and appetite depression can occur. In severe cases, cattle can suffer from *hepatic encephalopathy*. It is estimated that in the first month after parturition 5-10% of high-producing dairy cattle develop severe fatty liver, and 30-40% have moderate fatty liver (5-10% liver triglyceride by wet weight basis). The liver depends primarily on fatty acid oxidation for its own energy needs. It must also synthesize a large amount of protein and phospholipids for lipoprotein export to other tissues, and this process can be rate limiting, resulting in accumulation of triglyceride in the cytoplasm. In starvation, the reduced availability of protein and lipotrope cofactors, such as choline, can exacerbate the bottleneck. The liver is the main supplier of glucose for the brain and milk saccharides, and it adapts by converting fatty acid metabolites to glucose (gluconeogenesis) and ketones.

Acute **ketosis** of lactating dairy cows with intake insufficiency or secondary to abomasal displacement is usually associated with fatty liver with a predominantly diffuse macrovesicular pattern. *Cows are more tolerant of ketosis associated with lactation than are pregnant ewes that can die from undernutrition-induced* **pregnancy toxemia** *and ketoacidosis*. In cows, hepatic steatosis is predominantly centrilobular, while it is most severe in the periportal zone in pregnancy toxemia of sheep. The hepatic changes reflect increased mobilization of triglycerides from adipose tissue rather than hepatic disease per se. In cows and ewes with increased mobilization of triglycerides, there may be indistinct foci of white discoloration of abdominal fat that tend to be obscured when adipose tissue solidifies postmortem.

Fatty liver of ***diabetes*** *occurs when insulin is deficient or inactive* because of *lack of functioning receptors*. Reduced insulin-dependent glucose uptake by cells leads to accelerated lipolysis from adipose tissue in much the same way as when energy intake is limiting. The liver is thus presented with a large load of fatty acids, and the rate at which lipid moves through the liver can be impeded in many ways. Insulin deficiency alone will produce fatty liver. Some cases in carnivores are also complicated by concurrent exocrine pancreatic insufficiency, so protein malabsorption can be a contributing influence on diabetic hepatic steatosis. The centrilobular hepatocytes usually show the greatest degree of steatosis, but in advanced long-standing diabetes, the change is often diffuse and marked.

Lipoprotein synthesis and transport are dependent on oxidative metabolism, so **hypoxia** of hepatocytes leads to triglyceride accumulation. The 2 most common causes of hepatocellular hypoxia are *anemia* and reduced sinusoidal perfusion in *passive venous congestion*. In these situations, hepatic steatosis is most severe in the centrilobular zone, provided that the adipose and dietary supply of triglyceride is sufficient. Hepatic steatosis can be grossly visible as a yellow zonal pattern in chronic passive congestion of the bovid but is less obvious in carnivores with passive hepatic congestion.

Local hypoxia is probably the basis for another example of fatty liver. Small, sharply demarcated patches of intense fatty infiltration are often seen in bovine livers at or adjacent to sites of capsular fibrous adhesions—so-called **"tension lipidosis."** These patches are neither swollen nor shrunken, usually extend <1 cm into the parenchyma, and are of the same consistency as normal liver (Fig. 2-24). The lobular structure of these lesions is undisturbed, but the hepatocytes have pronounced steatosis, presumably related to interference with local perfusion caused by tensions transmitted to the parenchyma by the adhesion.

Hepatic steatosis caused by **intoxication** is common. There are several stages of the cycle of hepatic lipid metabolism that can be affected selectively by various toxins to produce fatty liver. For example, it is possible experimentally to cause triglyceride accumulation by interfering with mitochondrial fatty acid oxidation with sublethal doses of

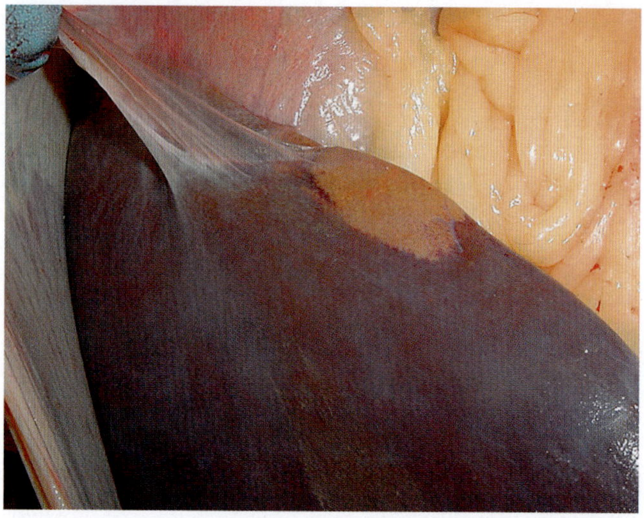

Figure 2-24 Subcapsular focal fatty change **("tension lipidosis")** associated with capsular ligamentous attachment in an ox. (Courtesy A.P. Loretti.)

cyanide, or by inhibiting apolipoprotein synthesis by administration of orotic acid. Most toxins that cause fatty liver in naturally occurring situations, however, also produce a greater or lesser degree of hepatocellular necrosis. Fatty liver occurring as a manifestation of toxic hepatic disease will be further discussed in the Toxic Hepatic Disease section, but the generalization may be made here that most important veterinary hepatic intoxications cause widespread membrane damage and/or disturbance of protein synthesis. These cause lipid accumulation in the hepatocyte by interfering with lipoprotein synthesis and export, as well as with fatty acid oxidation. *Steatosis requires time to develop, so it is more likely to occur in toxicoses with a longer clinical course*. However, if adipose reserves are depleted, there is less lipid available to accumulate in the liver.

Although fatty liver in domestic animals is more often associated with generalized interferences with energy metabolism, there are some specific **nutritional deficiencies** that will produce fatty liver. These have usually been defined under experimental conditions. *Choline deficiency*, in conjunction with deficiency of other lipotropic factors, such as *L-methionine* and *vitamin* B_{12}, rapidly produces fatty liver, largely because of reduced synthesis of phosphatidylcholine, a component of secreted lipoproteins. Fatty liver in experimental choline deficiency involves lipid peroxidation and increased hepatocellular turnover, leading to cirrhosis and neoplasia. It is unlikely that primary choline deficiency occurs in domestic animals, but other lipotrope deficiencies have been reported.

Ovine white-liver disease, first described in lambs in New Zealand, also occurs in southern Australia, the United Kingdom, and continental Europe. Goats are also susceptible. Ovine white-liver disease is a syndrome of ill-thrift to emaciation, anorexia, and mild normocytic normochromic anemia, occasionally with photosensitization and icterus. The condition is associated with low liver cobalt levels and low plasma concentrations of vitamin B_{12}, and the disease has been shown to be *cobalt and vitamin* B_{12} *responsive*. Lambs up to 1 year of age are more commonly affected than ewes, and pastures are likely to be adequate at the times of peak incidence in late spring and early summer.

In the first stages, the liver changes consist of vacuolar accumulation of triglyceride in hepatocytes, usually most severe in the centrilobular zones. In addition, ceroid pigment is present in all cases, early in hepatocytes and later also in sinusoidal cells and macrophages. The fatty change may be very severe in the early stage, the liver being grossly swollen. A moderate degree of *bile ductular proliferation* is also a consistent feature, and the epithelium of the smaller ductules in the tracts is dysplastic. Spongy degeneration of cerebral white matter, typical of the *hyperammonemia* of hepatic failure, is present in some cases.

Experimental feeding of a diet low in cobalt to sheep resulted in reduced growth rate, anorexia, lacrimation, alopecia, emaciation, and marked reduction in plasma and liver vitamin B_{12} concentrations. At autopsy, livers were pale, swollen, and fatty. Histologically, livers with severe fatty degeneration had widespread hepatocyte disassociation, accumulation of lipid droplets, eosinophilic inclusions and lipofuscin in hepatocyte and Kupffer cell cytoplasm, nuclear lipid pseudo-inclusions, ductular proliferation, and hepatocyte apoptosis. These lesions are characteristic of spontaneous cases of ovine white-liver disease. Ultrastructurally, degeneration of mitochondria and proliferation of the SER are evident. The disease can be produced in cobalt-deficient sheep fed diets high in propionate precursors, which may help explain the explosive nature of outbreaks on lush pasture.

Hepatic lesions, such as nutritional cirrhosis induced by experimental choline methionine deficiency, have been reported in sheep, goats, cattle, deer, and pronghorn antelope from Texas, New Mexico, and northeastern Mexico. **Hard yellow-liver disease**, or **hepatic fatty cirrhosis**, *is a progressive, chronic disease characterized by weight loss and HE* (eFig. 2-7). The disease typically appears in years following above-average winter rains, followed by drought conditions in the summer months. Grossly visible liver lesions in sheep begin in the subcapsular hepatic parenchyma along the porta hepatis as pale-yellow, firm areas, spreading peripherally to involve ~80% of the liver in the final stages of the disease. Microscopic changes include the accumulation of fine cytoplasmic lipid droplets in centrilobular hepatocytes, later involving the entire lobule, with rupture and formation of fatty cysts. Centrilobular fibrosis accompanies the ruptured fatty cysts, progressing to widespread bridging centrilobular fibrosis, with islands of regenerating hepatocytes. Kupffer cells and macrophages in regional lymph nodes, spleen, and lung contain abundant ceroid. Ascites and acquired extrahepatic shunts may be present. The etiology of this condition is unknown, although unidentified hepatotoxins, possibly altering lipoprotein synthesis and secretion, combined with nutritional stress, have been postulated.

Equine hyperlipemia *is almost exclusively a disease of donkeys, miniature horses, and ponies*, and among these, the Shetland breed predominates. There is marked elevation of the serum triglyceride concentration, predominantly of VLDLs, but other lipid fractions are also elevated, with visibly prominent lipemia and hepatic steatosis. The condition is usually fatal after about a week. A negative energy balance is a key feature. Pregnant or lactating mares are most likely to develop the disease, particularly if they are older, excessively fat, and have recently suffered reduced feed intake because of the onset of parturition, conditions such as laminitis or parasitism, or other causes of stress. The clinical course is marked by somnolence, complete anorexia, and colic, progressing to mania in some cases, although most simply become progressively more depressed. Some ponies develop ventral subcutaneous edema and most develop moderate diarrhea. Metabolic acidosis is a consistent feature in animals that die.

The liver at autopsy is severely fatty and may have ruptured; steatosis also extends to the heart and skeletal muscle, kidney, and adrenal cortex. *Hepatic steatosis is remarkable only by its severity;* there may be some focal hepatocellular necrosis, and there is consistent prolongation of bromsulfthalein retention times and elevation of serum alkaline phosphatase activity. Evidence of disseminated intravascular coagulation is seen as serosal hemorrhages and microscopic thrombi in various organs, and even gross infarction of myocardium and kidney. *Small lipid emboli* may be detected in frozen sections of the lung, myocardium, and brain in these animals; their relationship to the microthrombosis is uncertain.

The pathogenesis of this disease is not entirely understood. Because the excess lipid in the liver and blood is in the form of triglyceride, the implication is that the liver is capable of esterifying fatty acid mobilized from depot fat. The triglyceride thus formed is presumably then exported to the plasma as VLDL. It is believed that the primary cause of hyperlipemia is increased production via an increased rate of adipocyte lipolysis, leading to fatty acids and glycerol being released into the bloodstream and the increased hepatic synthesis of triglyceride as VLDL, rather than reduced clearance of VLDL from the serum. Another possibility is that there is an inability on the part of all tissues other than the liver to use fatty acids from VLDL at the normal rate; triglyceride synthesis from fatty acids continues in the liver. In any event, at this stage, lipids begin to accumulate in hepatocytes.

It has been proposed that an underlying cause of pony hyperlipemia is a *comparative resistance to insulin* in susceptible animals and that this is compounded in stressful episodes by *increased levels of circulating cortisol.* Various steroid hormones, including glucocorticoids, have been shown to interfere with insulin action, and hyperlipemic ponies often have elevated plasma insulin levels, which suggests reduced function of insulin receptors. However, plasma ketones are much less consistently elevated, which appears to be characteristic of equids; this suggests that the increased ketogenesis that one might expect in insulin resistance is not a typical feature in horses.

Hepatic steatosis is common in **companion animals**. Following periods of stress or fasting, puppies from toy-breed dogs can develop profound hypoglycemia and a striking microvesicular hepatic steatosis (*fading puppy syndrome*). This may be the result of poor homeostasis of blood glucose levels. Most often, affected pups die from cerebral complications of hypoglycemia, but significant liver dysfunction also occurs. Dogs eating diets deficient in vitamin E may develop severe hepatic steatosis, but there are many circumstances in companion animals in which the exact cause for individual cases of steatosis cannot be determined.

The syndrome of **feline hepatic steatosis** most commonly occurs in obese, nutritionally stressed female cats, seen as vomiting, anorexia, weakness and weight loss, icterus, and hepatomegaly (Fig. 2-25). Neurobehavioral signs indicative of HE, other than drooling and depression, are rarely reported. Affected cats typically have hyperbilirubinemia, and a significant increase in serum alkaline phosphatase activity, in the face of normal or modest increases in GGT activity, a key diagnostic feature of this syndrome. Untreated, the mortality rate is high. The liver has diffuse, macrovesicular with microvesicular steatosis, by definition affecting >50% of hepatocytes. Focal or zonal lipid accumulation in <50% of the parenchyma

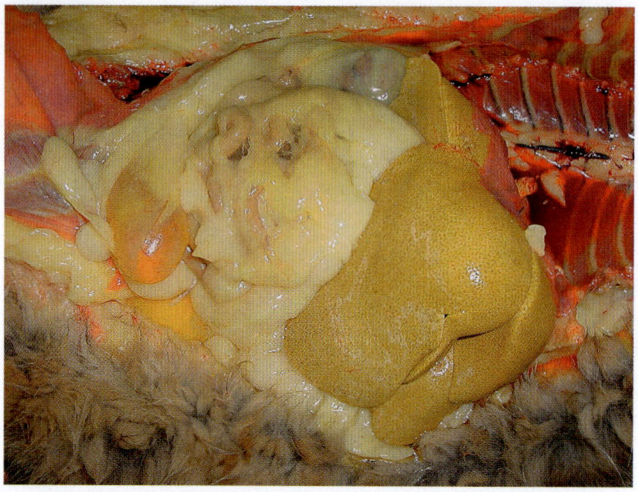

Figure 2-25 Hepatomegaly resulting from **hepatic steatosis** in an obese cat. (Courtesy A.P. Loretti.)

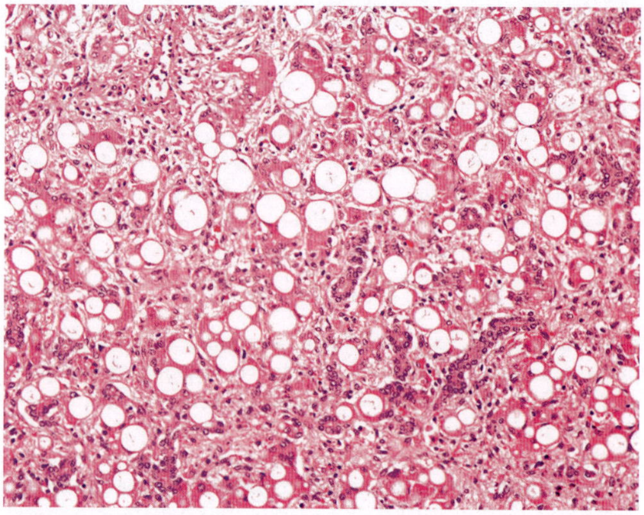

Figure 2-26 Hepatic steatosis, portal fibrosis, and bile duct hyperplasia resulting from **hepatic lipodystrophy** in a Galloway calf. (Courtesy M.J. Hazlett.)

is considered more likely to be physiologic, or associated with other systemic abnormalities, rather than feline hepatic steatosis. Bile pigment accumulates in canaliculi or Kupffer cells and can be confused with lipofuscin and ceroid.

The pathogenesis of hepatocellular triglyceride accumulation in this disease is complex and likely multifactorial, involving increased mobilization and uptake of nonesterified fatty acids by the liver, alterations in formation and release of VLDL, and impaired oxidation of fatty acids within hepatocytes. Ultrastructural studies have demonstrated decreased numbers and abnormal morphology of hepatic peroxisomes as well as mitochondria, both of which are important in the oxidization of fatty acids, but whether these changes are significant or simply adaptive responses is unknown. Starvation may reduce the availability of proteins, choline, and other precursors necessary for lipoprotein synthesis.

Severe hepatic steatosis can also develop in cats, *concurrent with or secondary to other major medical problems* such as diabetes mellitus, which alters the metabolism of fat. *Acute pancreatitis* appears to be an important predisposing disease to secondary hepatic steatosis in cats—an association with clinical significance as it has a poorer prognosis than uncomplicated idiopathic hepatic steatosis. Secondary hepatic steatosis has also been reported with concurrent inflammatory liver disease, such as cholangitis, renal disease, small intestinal disease, neoplasia, and hyperthyroidism.

Familial hyperlipoproteinemia has been described in cats, associated with *congenital lipoprotein lipase deficiency*. The condition is characterized by lipid vacuoles and ceroid accumulation in the liver, spleen, lymph nodes, kidneys and adrenal glands, xanthomas, and focal arterial degenerative changes. An autosomal recessive mode of inheritance is suspected. **Primary idiopathic hyperlipidemia** has also been reported in Miniature Schnauzer dogs and Beagles, although the metabolic defect has not been identified. Affected dogs have fasting hypertriglyceridemia with or without hypercholesterolemia, elevated plasma VLDL, and may have hyperchylomicronemia. Affected animals may develop severe vacuolar hepatopathy associated with both glycogen and triglyceride accumulation, with eventual stromal collapse and regenerative nodule formation. There is also an association between hyperlipidemia and gallbladder mucocele.

An incompletely characterized condition known as **hepatic lipodystrophy** has been recognized in pedigree Galloway calves since 1965. Calves initially appear normal but develop lethargy, tremors, and opisthotonos, and die by 5 months of age. On postmortem examination, affected calves have an enlarged, tan-yellow liver. Histologically, there is marked hepatic steatosis with portal fibrosis and ductular reaction (Fig. 2-26). Vacuolar changes in the white matter of the brain are consistent with *HE*. A metabolic defect has been proposed.

Lysosomal storage diseases and other enzyme deficiencies

In common with other tissues in animals with a heritable deficiency of specific lysosomal enzymes, liver cells may accumulate substrates normally catabolized by the missing enzyme. These lysosomal stores can be less obvious in the liver than in other tissues such as the central nervous system, and although they are unlikely to affect hepatic function, they can sometimes be recognized in liver biopsies (eFig. 2-8). However, *hydropic and fatty changes in hepatocytes can obscure or lead to misidentification of lysosomal storage vacuoles*. Kupffer cells and bile duct epithelium may be more severely affected than hepatocytes, which have additional catabolic and excretory pathways, including the ability for lysosomal exocytosis into the bile canaliculi. In animals with ceroid lipofuscinosis, lysosomal storage is minimal in Kupffer cells compared with that in the brain. Examples of storage disorders associated with hepatomegaly and abnormal hepatic or Kupffer cell lysosomal inclusions in dogs and cats include *GM1 gangliosidosis* (β-1-galactosidase deficiency), *mucopolysaccharidosis type I* (α-L-iduronidase deficiency), and α-mannosidosis. These and others are discussed in more detail in Vol. 1, Nervous System.

Hepatic **phospholipidosis** is an excessive accumulation of phospholipids within the cytoplasm of hepatocytes, Kupffer cells, and macrophages. This condition is an acquired storage disorder caused by some therapeutic drugs and chemicals, including amiodarone and chlorphentermine. Despite the diversity of agents capable of causing phospholipidosis, most of these are cationic amphipathic molecules. Mechanistically, phospholipidosis is caused by cationic amphipathic molecules binding to cellular phospholipids and inhibiting complete digestion by lysosomal phospholipase A1, A2, or C within lysosomes; although less often, direct inhibition of phospholipase can occur, as in the case of gentamicin. This leads to an accumulation of lysosomal phospholipids that can develop acutely or only following long-term drug administration. The histologic appearance of phospholipidosis can be quite variable, but typically, hepatocellular and Kupffer cell cytoplasm contains many round clear vacuoles that are smaller than the diameter of the nucleus or larger, imparting a *foamy appearance to the cytoplasm*. Fine vacuoles are most often apparent adjacent to canaliculi. Zonal distribution can vary depending on the type of drug or chemical. Biliary epithelium can also be affected, with or without hepatocellular involvement. The clear vacuoles can be confused with microvesicular steatosis; LAMP2 (lysosome-associated membrane protein 2) immunohistochemistry and ultrastructural examination are needed to identify phospholipidosis. At the ultrastructural level, there is a characteristic multilaminated whorl of material with a "fingerprint" pattern, termed *myeloid bodies*, within affected lysosomes.

Cobalamin deficiency has been described in several dog breeds, with several reports of deficiency in young Beagles and Border Collies due to a mutation in the *CUBN* gene. Deficiency produced pups that were weak and failed to thrive. Histologically, the liver had irregularly distended hepatocytes with rarefied cytoplasm affecting all zones of the lobule. Hematologic issues also occur. This mutation can be fatal if untreated. Other enzyme deficiencies affecting hepatocytes are discussed in the Hepatocyte Swellin: Vacuolation and Cytoplasmic Rarefaction section.

Amyloidosis

In most species, *hepatic amyloidosis is usually part of generalized amyloidosis*. **Systemic amyloidosis** of domestic animals is typically associated with overproduction of amyloid A (AA), an amino-terminal fragment of serum amyloid A, a highly inducible acute-phase protein in most species. In humans, AA amyloidosis occurs either as a familial trait (familial Mediterranean fever) or secondary to a sustained acute-phase reaction in chronic inflammatory or neoplastic diseases. Amyloid infiltration of the liver occurs sporadically in cattle, sheep, goats, horses, dogs, and cats as a secondary response to chronic disease or tissue-destructive process. In horses, hepatic amyloidosis occurs chiefly because of chronic inflammation and has been well recognized in horses used to produce hyperimmune serum. Horses may develop icterus and other signs of hepatic failure, but cattle die first of the primary disease or from uremia resulting from concurrent renal amyloidosis. Dogs and cats typically develop signs of renal dysfunction, although cats may be presented with spontaneous hepatic rupture. **Familial AA amyloidosis** is recognized in Chinese Shar-Pei dogs. The condition resembles familial Mediterranean fever in humans and is characterized by febrile episodes, swelling of the tibiotarsal joint, and the development of renal and sometimes hepatic amyloidosis. Familial AA amyloidosis is also recognized in Abyssinian and Siamese and oriental cats.

Affected livers in horses are pale, enlarged with rounded edges, friable, and prone to fracture; in cattle, affected livers may be firm. Affected livers in all species are predisposed to rupture and bleeding (eFig. 2-9). Amyloid is deposited in perisinusoidal spaces and leads to atrophy of hepatocellular cords. Amyloid is sometimes also found in the walls of the afferent vessels. On H&E staining, amyloid appears as *homogeneous eosinophilic amorphous extracellular material* (Fig. 2-27).

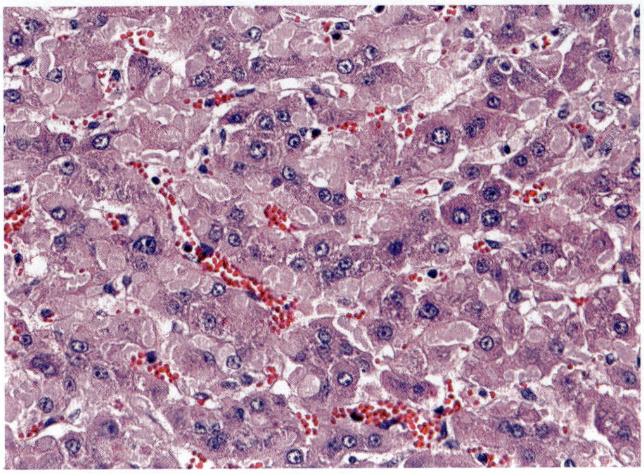

Figure 2-27 Amyloid in perisinusoidal spaces compressing hepatocytes in a bighorn sheep.

Staining with Congo red results in apple-green birefringence when viewed with polarized light. Thioflavin T stain produces yellow-green fluorescent staining of amyloid when viewed under ultraviolet light.

TYPES AND PATTERNS OF CELL INJURY AND DEATH IN THE LIVER

Reversible injury

Reversible hepatocytic injury includes hepatocellular swelling, steroid-induced cytoplasmic rarefaction, and steatosis (syn. lipidosis, fatty change). These lesions are discussed in more detail in the Hepatocyte swelling: vacuolation and cytoplasmic rarefaction, and Hepatocellular steatosis (lipidosis) sections. Reversible injury is a form of damage to the hepatocyte that does not necessarily lead to death and that may resolve leading to normal hepatocytes once the inciting insult is eliminated. A common feature of reversible injury is the *formation of membranous blebs that are released into the circulation*. Blebbing is a particularly relevant feature because it is the released blebs with entrapped cytoplasm that are the source of transaminase elevations following hepatocyte injury. Transaminases are high–molecular-weight molecules and any openings in the cell membranes large enough to allow these molecules to exit the cells directly would be so large that the influx of calcium would trigger cell death.

Hepatocellular swelling (also termed cloudy swelling or hydropic degeneration) is the first form of injury to cells resulting from altered membrane permeability and osmotic cell edema with an influx of sodium and water. Mechanistically, damaged cells are unable to maintain ionic and fluid homeostasis due to membrane damage or reduced energy production. This change is easier to conceptualize than to recognize by light microscopy. In carefully controlled environments, subtle changes in the cytoplasm can be identified, but in most biopsy and particularly autopsy samples, the change is challenging to identify correctly. In more severe instances, the hepatocytes have marked swelling and pale-staining cytoplasm arranged in thin strands.

Feathery degeneration is a form of hydropic degeneration of hepatocytes associated with cholestasis and likely caused by the detergent action of an intracellular accumulation of bile acids, which imparts a diffuse, foamy, reticular appearance to swollen hepatocytes (see Fig. 2-18). Feathery degeneration is most evident in severe extrahepatic cholestasis and in destructive cholangitis.

Steroid-induced cytoplasmic rarefaction (steroid hepatopathy) is limited to dogs primarily and involves excessive hepatocellular glycogen accumulation. Affected hepatocytes are swollen with clear cytoplasm and strands of eosinophilic cytoplasm and nondisplaced, central nuclei (see Fig. 2-19). The lesion varies markedly in extent and distribution. Cytoplasmic rarefaction can be diffuse, zonal, or affect small groups or even individual cells. While frozen sections yield the best assessment of the presence of glycogen, PAS staining with or without diastase may be useful. This lesion is usually induced by either exogenous or endogenous glucocorticoids.

Hepatocellular steatosis (lipidosis, fatty change) is the presence of lipid-containing vacuoles within the cytoplasm of hepatocytes. Lipid is evident as clear, round, empty spaces in the cytoplasm in routine formalin-fixed paraffin-embedded tissue as lipid is removed during routine processing. Hepatocellular steatosis is a nonspecific reversible form of cellular injury, and different mechanisms account for triglyceride (triacylglycerol) accumulation in the liver. Two major patterns of steatosis are recognized by light microscopy: microvesicular and macrovesicular steatosis (see Figs. 2-20 and 2-21).

Irreversible damage leads to **cell death** that is evident histologically if the affected animal survives for a sufficient period, usually hours. Although all cells in the liver are susceptible, most interest and evaluation has been directed toward hepatocytes, biliary epithelium, and sinusoidal endothelium. The 2 predominant types of cell death are **necrosis**, also termed **oncotic necrosis**, and **apoptosis**, although there are other less common forms of cell death. These types of cell death can be separated mechanistically and histologically to a certain extent.

Types of cell death

In routine diagnostic settings, the terms apoptosis and necrosis can frequently be based on descriptive criteria recognized in routine H&E-stained sections of the liver. There have been attempts to refine the terminology and criteria for cell death in the liver, but this is still hindered by our incomplete understanding of different cell death pathways and cellular responses in various diseases.

Apoptosis

Apoptosis *is a form of programmed cell death* that permits the removal of cell debris without much leakage of cell contents or inflammation. *Key features of apoptosis include retention of plasma membrane integrity until the later stages of the process; proteolysis of intracellular cytoskeletal proteins by aspartate-specific proteases, leading to collapse of subcellular components; chromatin condensation and marginalization; nuclear fragmentation; plasma membrane bleb formation; and eventual cell fragmentation into smaller apoptotic bodies bound by intact plasma membrane* (Fig. 2-28). These bodies are rapidly phagocytosed and degraded by neighboring hepatocytes or Kupffer cells. The rapid disappearance of these fragments means that very few apoptotic bodies in a section can indicate a rapid rate of hepatocellular death and turnover. Biochemically, apoptotic cells have phosphatidylserine on the outer surface of the cell membrane, and increased mitochondrial permeability with release of internal proteins and activation of caspases.

Apoptosis is the main means of physiologic removal of damaged or aged cells and for remodeling of tissue. Liver mass is maintained by a balance of mitosis and apoptosis.

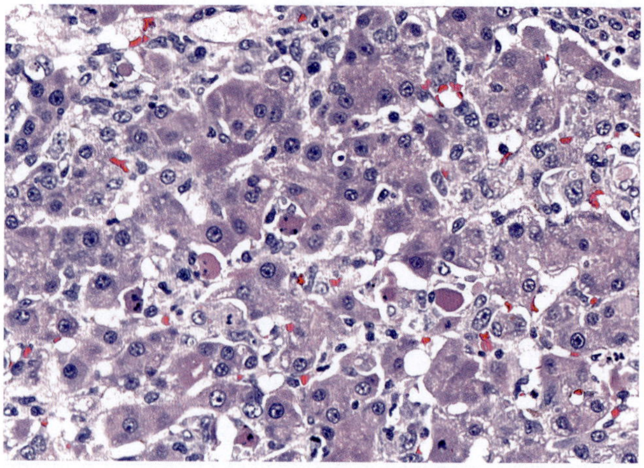

Figure 2-28 Apoptotic hepatocytes in a region of injury in the liver of a dog.

Experimental support for the importance of this balance comes from studies of mutant mice deficient in the principal mediator of apoptosis, the receptor Fas (Fas/CD95), which develop prominent hepatocellular hyperplasia over time.

Functional classification of cell death has been developed based on chemical rather than the histologic-morphologic criteria because different pathways can lead to similar morphologies.

Injury to the ER via oxidative stress, hypoxia, calcium depletion, inflammation, and altered glycosylation, among other mechanisms, leads to the *"unfolded protein response (UPR)"* that can also activate the distal caspase pathway by a separate mechanism. Hepatocytes are also susceptible to an intrinsic mechanism of apoptosis that is active after removal of hepatotrophic influences, including those that function via the constitutive androstane receptor, and other nuclear receptors. In addition, lysosomes can undergo selective membrane permeabilization, leading to a partial release of their contents in response to death signaling mediated by oxidative stress, some lipid mediators, and by Bcl2 family members. Release of lysosomal proteases can cooperate with the caspase cascade or act in a caspase-independent manner.

An important feature of apoptosis is the requirement for ATP to initiate the execution phase. If the degree of mitochondrial damage is sufficient to exhaust ATP stores, membrane ion homeostasis deteriorates and leads to a mechanism of cell death more consistent with necrosis. For example, although mild-to-moderate oxidative stress may start intrinsic pathways of apoptotic cell death, processes leading to marked oxidative stress typically cause cell death by necrosis, not only resulting from the severity of mitochondrial damage but also by direct inhibition of the proapoptotic caspase cascade.

Loss of cell anchorage to the ECM can activate a form of programmed cell death related to apoptosis that is termed **anoikis**. Detached cells can die intact, as in exfoliation, or undergo typical fragmentation into apoptotic bodies. Hepatocyte survival in vitro depends on their integrins that adhere to the ECM, but it is still unknown how loss of these contributes to cell death of hepatocytes in the intact liver.

Phagocytosis of apoptotic fragments follows flipping of phosphatidylserine from the inner leaflet of the plasma membrane to the outer leaf, where it can then be recognized by the phosphatidylserine scavenger receptor. Various assays can be used to detect portions of these pathways in hepatocytes;

caspase-cleaved CK18 can be recognized by antibodies to an internal domain, while chromatin fragmented by a calcium-activated endonuclease generates double-strand breaks that can be tagged by the terminal deoxynucleotide transferase-mediated dUTP nick-end labeling (TUNEL) technique. However, there are still few diagnostic situations in which these indicators have been shown to be useful. Increased numbers of apoptotic hepatocytes can be more readily assessed with a suitable cytologic marker in routine diagnostic pathology. *In sections, a previous increase in apoptosis can be suggested by increased amounts of lysosomal debris and pigment in Kupffer cells, but this is not specific for apoptosis.*

Rapid phagocytic removal of apoptotic hepatocyte fragments can minimize secondary inflammation in cases of minor injury. However, phagocytosis of apoptotic bodies by Kupffer cells and HSCs is not innocuous and can engender inflammation and fibrosis. Kupffer cells and resident macrophages express several ligands (TNF, TRAIL, and Fas ligand) that lead to increased hepatocyte apoptosis. Similarly, HSCs are stimulated to release profibrotic cytokines and type 1 collagen following phagocytosis of apoptotic bodies. In addition, apoptotic cells release nucleotides, ATP, and uridine triphosphate, which can bind to purinergic receptors on macrophages and HSCs and which may provide added stimulus for fibrosis and inflammation. Excessive apoptosis is viewed as a driver of hepatic inflammation and fibrosis.

Necrosis

Necrosis *is morphologically recognizable by initial cell swelling and subsequent loss of plasma membrane integrity, leading to large organelle-free blebs and cell lysis.* Some authors prefer the term **"oncosis"** to emphasize the cell swelling response in necrosis to contrast with cell shrinkage in apoptosis (Fig. 2-29). Necrosis occurs when cells are depleted of ATP and lack sufficient energy to maintain membrane-associated ionic pumps, leading to swelling and gross calcium influxes that result in disruption of the mitochondrial and plasma membranes, including release of lysosomal enzymes. Oncosis *is generally regarded as a severe injury to cell membrane integrity or other vital functions,* leading to enzyme leakage, inflammation, and tissue repair. *Release of cellular contents typically elicits a secondary inflammatory response and provides the serum enzymes that are useful clinically to detect liver necrosis.* However, these sequelae can also occur after hepatocyte apoptosis, either because the capacity for phagocytic removal of dead cells is exceeded, or because the insult worsens such that necrosis may supervene.

Necrosis is often a consequence of profound loss of mitochondrial function involving the opening of the membrane permeability transition pore, a megachannel composed of inner and outer membrane proteins. This results in mitochondrial depolarization and ATP depletion because of inhibited oxidative phosphorylation. Poly-ADP-ribose polymerase (PARP) is a DNA repair enzyme that can deplete injured cells of available ATP when it is activated to repair the multitude of DNA strand breaks induced by cell damage. Conversely, PARP is swiftly cleaved in apoptosis to maintain ATP levels. Much of the ATP in hepatocytes is used for membrane homeostasis of Na^+, K^+, and Ca^{2+} ions. ATP depletion or physical damage to membranes of the cell surface, mitochondria, and ER leads to loss of ion homeostasis, altered cellular volume regulation, and increased intracellular calcium ion concentrations. Activation of calcium-dependent endonucleases, proteases (e.g., calpains), and phospholipases is responsible for the terminal events in necrosis. The source of calcium may influence the type of cell death, as calcium influx from the plasma membrane is associated with necrosis, but calcium released from the ER is more likely to trigger apoptosis. Necrosis may not be entirely a passive process. For example, necrosis can be initiated via cell surface receptor–driven processes when TNF is present in high concentrations.

The term **coagulative necrosis** *may be applied to groups or zones of intact, but dead hepatocytes that have shrunken slightly, stain intensely with eosin, and may have visible but distorted nuclei* (Fig. 2-30). These cells may also be dehydrated, but, unlike apoptosis, the removal of water is not an active process, and the affected cells do not undergo spontaneous fragmentation. It seems that coagulative necrosis, which is often seen in acute hepatotoxicity, is the *result of sudden and catastrophic denaturation of cytosolic protein,* which imparts a rather dense, rigid texture to the dead cells, somewhat preserving their shape. *The term* **lytic necrosis** *has been used for areas of necrosis in which the hepatocytes are disintegrating, usually in the presence of infiltrating phagocytes, especially neutrophils.* This is consistent with the later stages of postnecrotic inflammation that follow necrosis rather than apoptosis.

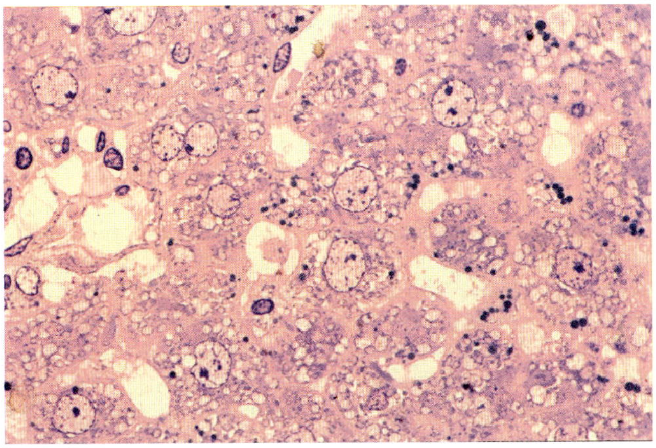

Figure 2-29 Necrosis of hepatocytes is initiated by cell swelling evident in this toluidine blue–stained section of the liver. (Courtesy V. Meador.)

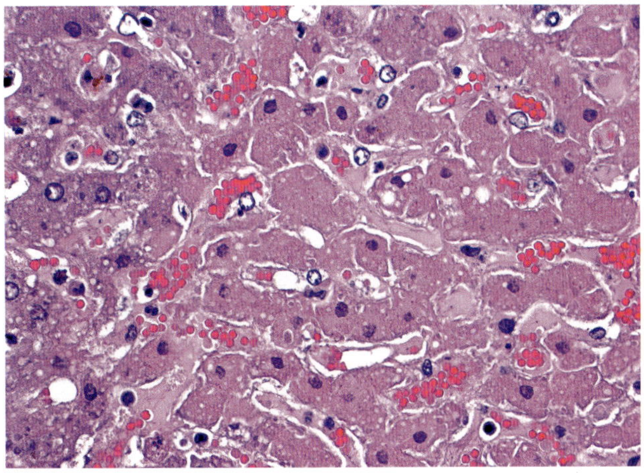

Figure 2-30 Coagulative necrosis of hepatocytes in a horse resulting from anemia.

One might expect that the distinct types of cell death might be informative in relation to causes and pathogenesis. However, apoptosis, necrosis, and mixed responses are common in liver injury in vivo. *Many insults can initiate either necrosis or apoptosis of hepatocytes*; these include hypoxia, reactive oxygen metabolites, hepatotoxic chemicals, viral infections, bacterial toxins, and inflammation. Some of the molecular events are common to both. Mitochondrial damage and several other activation responses are common to apoptosis and necrosis, and programmed cell death responses can be activated before they are overwhelmed by more intense injury responsible for necrosis. Susceptibility therefore depends on many factors, including the level and duration of insults, replication status, and integrity of the various homeostatic and cytoprotective functions. Indeed, review of caspase-cleaved substrates reveals that different toxic drugs do not cause a uniform pattern of caspase activation and that it is likely that there are distinct pathophysiologic pathways of apoptosis. Clearly, apoptosis is not a consistent and stereotypic response.

There are important misconceptions regarding differences between apoptosis and necrosis and their effects on the liver. It is often assumed that apoptosis, unlike necrosis, leads to a "clean" death that does not provoke inflammation or elevation of transaminases and other markers of inflammation. However, phagocytosis of apoptotic bodies, termed *efferocytosis*, particularly by Kupffer cells, can, in fact, activate the Kupffer cells and stimulate additional cell death. Various inflammatory markers are elevated in both acute and chronic apoptosis. The view that apoptosis, because it involves release of intact membrane bodies, does not lead to transaminase elevation has been shown in several studies to be incorrect. Injection of Fas ligands has been shown to produce significant increases in serum transaminases within hours and that this response is blocked in Bcl2 transgenic mice. In addition, deletion of antiapoptotic proteins results in elevated transaminase levels.

Other forms of cell death

There are several other forms of cell death. These include autophagy, pyroptosis, necroptosis, entosis, netosis, parthanatos, and cuproptosis (discussed in the Chronic Hepatitis in Dogs section), which can be identified by biochemical means and specific forms of inhibition. A complete description of each is beyond the scope of this text.

Tissue patterns of cell death

Focal necrosis

Focal necrosis is quite common in autopsy material. The lesions are microscopic or barely visible to the naked eye and are usually numerous. Their designation as focal depends on their size and on a random distribution relative to the lobules. There may be a tendency for focal necrosis to occur nearer the portal vessels than to the periphery of the circulatory fields, and to be concentrated in some lobular agglomerates rather than others.

Focal necrosis occurs in many infections, parasitic migrations, and instances of biliary obstruction, and in these, the designation **focal hepatitis** will often be more appropriate, because most are attended by some degree of focal inflammation. The infectious causes may be viral (Fig. 2-31) or bacterial. Many septicemic bacterial infections consistently produce focal hepatic lesions; examples are salmonellosis, tularemia, pseudotuberculosis, listeriosis in the fetus and newborn, and *Mannheimia haemolytica* septicemia in lambs. Focal necrosis may be the outcome of a Kupffer cell reaction, as in salmonellosis, or of bacterial embolism. The cause can usually be determined by histologic examination.

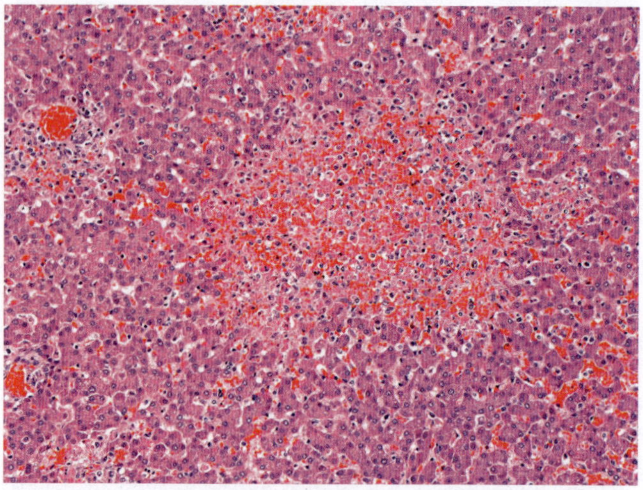

Figure 2-31 **Focal necrosis** caused by canid alphaherpesvirus 1 in a dog.

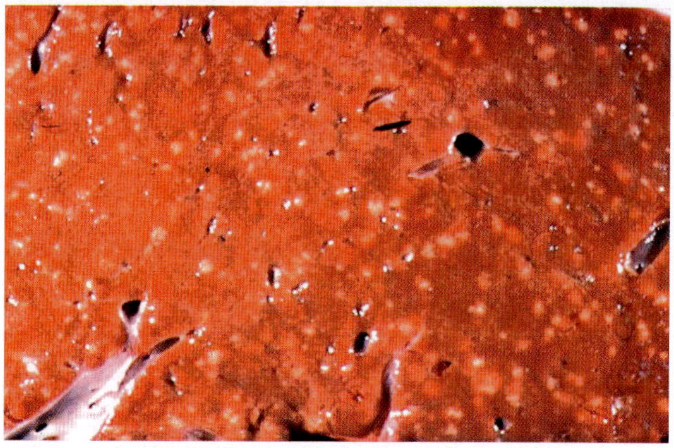

Figure 2-32 **Mulifocal hepatitis**—the so-called **"sawdust liver"** of cattle.

In cattle, focal necrosis in a few or many visible foci is common at autopsy and is common enough to be important at slaughter; it is responsible for the descriptive appellation *"sawdust liver"* (Fig. 2-32). The pathogenesis is not known and probably varies, but it may be caused by organisms from the gut that reach the liver in the portal blood. *The lesion is not specific and consists of focal parenchymal necrosis with disruption of reticulin fibers and infiltration of neutrophils and lymphocytes*; frank suppuration does not occur. This lesion is said to be more frequent in livers from feedlot-fattened cattle.

Focal necrosis in biliary obstruction follows rupture of distended canaliculi or smaller cholangioles, with the formation of small bile lakes. Necrosis of larger bile ducts caused by neutrophilic cholangitis or destructive cholangitis can also release bile. The yellow pigment is readily visible microscopically and provokes small granulomas with giant cells.

Focal necrosis is of very little functional significance for the liver, even when numerous. The lesions heal with some scarring, but this too probably disappears in time. They are of diagnostic importance in some diseases as indicators of possible bacteremia, such as salmonellosis.

Lobular necrosis

Although various terms are used, the simplest way to visualize these patterns of necrosis is by using the hepatic lobule concept.

The time-honored designation "centrilobular necrosis" is a common lesion in response to intoxication or hypoxia. **Centrilobular (zone 3) necrosis** *is the most common form of zonal necrosis in domestic animals*. The hepatocytes in the centrilobular zone are particularly vulnerable to necrosis, in part because they are farthest from incoming arterial and portal venous blood bearing oxygen and essential nutrients. They also contain the greatest concentration of cytochromes P450 (CYPs) that activate various exogenous compounds into reactive metabolites capable of injuring or killing hepatocytes (see later the Toxic Hepatic Disease section).

Severe viral infections, such as canine adenovirus 1 (CAdV1) and Rift Valley fever virus (RVFV), can produce centrilobular necrosis, and the reasons for the increased susceptibility of the hepatocytes of this zone in these diseases are not established. Plausible explanations include zonal expression of entry receptors used by viruses to infect hepatocytes or ischemia-related hepatocellular swelling and sinusoidal damage because of virus-induced endothelial injury that reduce effective perfusion of the centrilobular hepatocytes.

Centrilobular degeneration and necrosis are seen commonly in animals that have died rather slowly. It is assumed that, in the agonal period, the hepatocytes in this zone are disproportionately affected by tissue hypoxia because of the failing circulation. This necrosis is more extensive if the animal is anemic. Centrilobular necrosis is also seen in passive venous congestion of the liver, most often in cases of acute and dramatic decompensation of cardiac function, as atrophy of hepatocytes is a more common outcome.

In the liver with centrilobular necrosis, there is usually a prominent zonal pattern, which takes the form of a fine, regular, pallid network of surviving, often fatty, hepatocytes in the periportal zone, which stands up above the red, collapsed areas adjacent to the hepatic venules (Fig. 2-33). The zonal necrotic insult frequently affects the sinusoidal endothelium, allowing erythrocytes to enter perisinusoidal spaces and contribute to the redness of the necrotic zones. Histologically, necrosis is confined to the centrilobular region (Fig. 2-34), although bridging can occur in more severe cases (Fig. 2-35). Necrotic cells that are removed can be replaced by stagnant blood, at least in the acute phase. This red-on-yellow zonal pattern is difficult to interpret because hepatic steatosis may also have a zonal distribution without having significant necrosis.

However, vascular influences on the susceptibility to necrosis mean that segments of the lobule can be differentially affected. Frequently, the areas of necrosis are joined to one another, thus cutting the conventional lobules into segments, and at the same time, outlining the periphery of the circulatory fields of the hepatic lobules. Some of these areas of necrosis extend up to larger portal tracts because the periphery of some lobules may lie against the larger portal tracts. Often, the hepatocytes between the necrotic and more normal zones have hydropic degeneration or fatty change.

If the insult is of short duration, quite extensive centrilobular necrosis may be followed by phagocytic infiltration and hepatocellular proliferation and complete restoration of normal structure and function within a few days. Severe centrilobular necrosis may be followed shortly by proliferation of hepatocytes, bipotential progenitor cells found near cholangioles, and mature bile duct epithelia that also respond to the regenerative stimulus. With restitution of the normal complement of hepatocytes, the proliferative response in the progenitor cells and

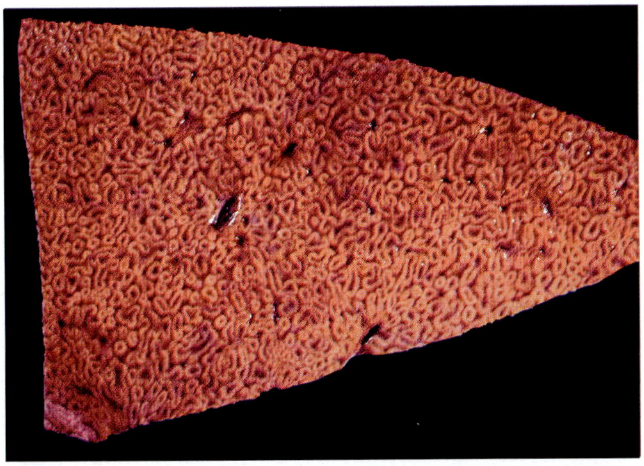

Figure 2-33 **Enhanced centrilobular zonal pattern** of hepatocellular necrosis in a horse. (Courtesy R. Panciera.)

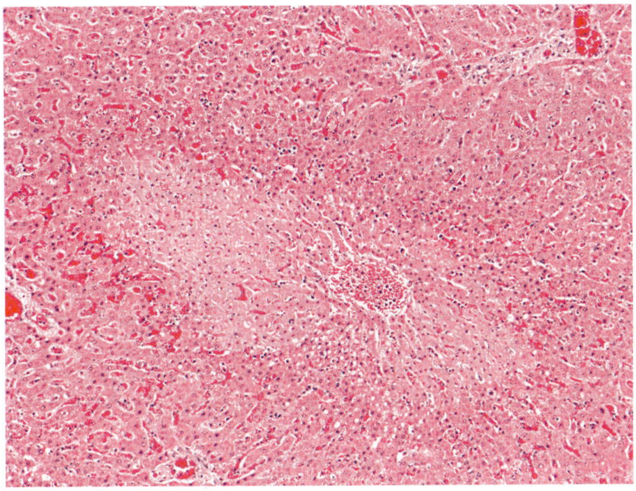

Figure 2-34 **Acute centrilobular necrosis** in an ox.

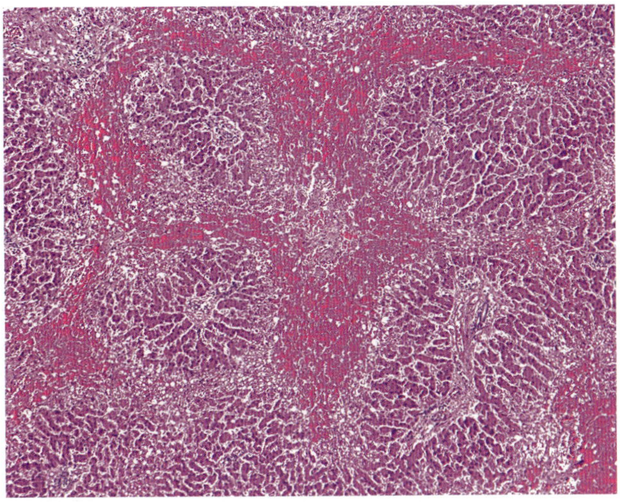

Figure 2-35 Bridging centrilobular **hemorrhagic necrosis** in a dog.

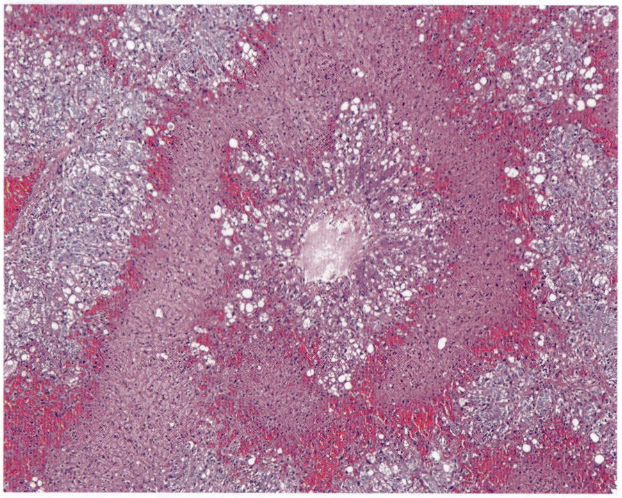

Figure 2-36 Acute **midzonal necrosis** in a horse.

biliary tract subsides unless the original insult is continuous or repeated.

Some intoxications can produce selective **midzonal (zone 2) necrosis**, affecting only a narrow, sharply defined band of hepatocytes (Fig. 2-36). It may be more diffuse within the lobule, so that periportal or centrilobular degeneration may be superimposed on the more severe midzonal lesion.

Periportal (zone 1) necrosis *is also an uncommon lesion*, perhaps seen more often than midzonal necrosis, and can be caused by direct-acting hepatotoxins that do not require metabolism by the CYPs to produce toxic moieties. More than one pattern of zonal necrosis can be found in the same liver. The various forms of zonal necrosis cannot reliably be distinguished from one another grossly, but one may expect to see in periportal necrosis a reversal of the pattern seen in centrilobular necrosis; that is, in periportal necrosis, the surviving hepatocytes about the hepatic venules may appear as pale, raised islands within a regular network of red, collapsed periportal tissue. Scrutiny may reveal the smallest hepatic venules at the center of the pale islands.

Paracentral necrosis, *a form of coagulative necrosis, occurs when an isolated portion of the centrilobular region of the lobule (or complete hepatic acinus of Rappaport—perhaps visualized more easily as an entire acinus) dies and is viewed in transverse section* (Fig. 2-37). It is possibly an ischemic lesion or infarct produced by occlusion of a terminal portal venule, such as may occur in disseminated intravascular coagulation. Its appearance in certain of the acute hepatotoxicities probably represents the death of a single complete acinus because of local vascular insufficiency, although, theoretically, high local microsomal enzyme activity or local deficiency of hepatocellular protective factors may play a part. Occlusion and rupture of a bile ductule or cholangiole are other potential causes of paracentral necrosis.

Panlobular (massive) necrosis

The terminology used to describe necrosis of an entire lobule is confusing. The terms massive and submassive necrosis have been used by some authors to describe necrosis of an entire lobule microscopically or a large part of the liver grossly. Because of these inconsistent definitions, the use of the descriptive term **panlobular necrosis** to describe necrosis of an entire lobule is preferred (Fig. 2-38). Without surviving

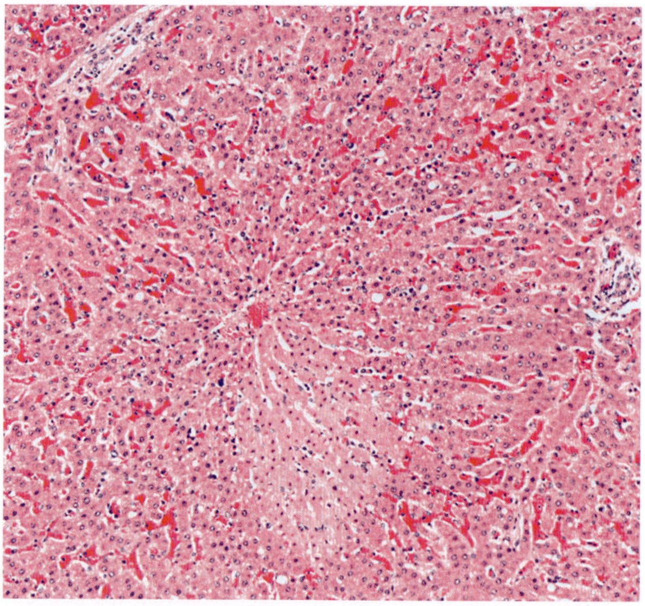

Figure 2-37 Paracentral necrosis.

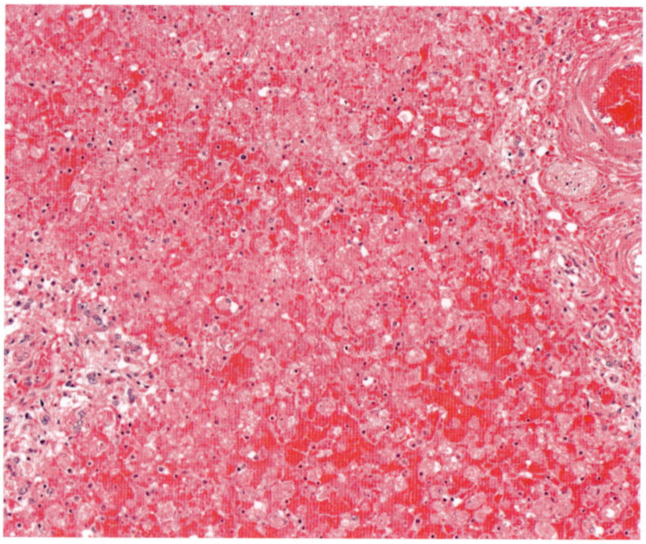

Figure 2-38 Panlobular necrosis with destruction of the periportal limiting plate and ductular reaction caused by *Amanita* poisoning in a cat.

parenchyma to support regeneration, affected lobules collapse, portal areas and hepatic venules are approximated, and the intervening stroma is condensed. Such a liver must regenerate from surviving hepatocytes in other, less severely affected lobules or by proliferation of progenitor cells that mature into hepatocytes. The distribution of massive hepatic necrosis is often related to the distribution of larger vessels. Collapse, condensation, and subsequent scarring are characteristic, the result being known as **postnecrotic scarring**. The liver is not uniformly involved typically. Large areas of parenchyma remain intact, and these enlarge amid scarring areas during compensatory regeneration.

A liver that is the seat of panlobular necrosis may be of normal size or smaller. Fine red threads of fibrin may be present on the surface, especially in the grooves between lobes. There is a surface mosaic appearance of red, gray, or yellow areas intermingled with areas of dark-red. The gray or yellow areas of parenchyma, representing surviving tissue, form irregular, coalescing patches that may be <1.0 cm in diameter. *The intermingled red areas represent areas of necrosis, hemorrhage, and collapse, and these are depressed a few millimeters below the surface*. In the healing stage, the depressed areas of hemorrhage and necrosis are condensed, shrunken, and scarified so that the surface of the liver is traversed by fine or heavy scars that separate large nodules of regenerative hyperplasia. Further acute episodes may be superimposed so that the presented lesion may be a mixture of acute panlobular necrosis and postnecrotic scarring.

Hepatosis dietetica *of swine is a now uncommon syndrome of severe hepatic necrosis in association with its immediate or late effects, namely, "yellow-fat disease," degeneration of skeletal and cardiac muscle, serous effusions, ulceration of the squamous mucosa of the stomach, and fibrinoid necrosis of arterioles*. These lesions may occur alone or in any combination, although all seldom occur in one animal. They are known to be of nutritional origin, and the fact that the various lesions can occur separately indicates the complexity of the pathogenesis. Experimental observations have revealed the *need for concurrent deficiencies of sulfur-containing amino acids, tocopherols, and trace amounts of selenium if hepatic necrosis is to develop*. Selenium protects efficiently against hepatic necrosis and massive effusions, and tocopherols are probably protective against other lesions that occur as part of the syndrome. The pathogenesis is incompletely understood but is in part related to the generation of free radicals, exacerbated by deficiency of free-radical scavengers, such as vitamin E, and selenium, protective against reactive oxygen radicals through its role in glutathione peroxidase and some other selenoproteins. Hepatosis dietetica occurs in rapidly growing pigs fed diets largely of grain and containing protein supplements lacking in either quality or quantity. There is some evidence that, in pigs that, are nutritionally predisposed, a cold and damp environment or some other stress may precipitate the disease. Death usually occurs without signs of illness or after a brief period of dullness. Melena, dyspnea, weakness, and trembling may be seen in some cases. Jaundice is indicative of a relapsing course.

Affected pigs are usually in good condition. The carcass may be anemic if ulceration of the gastric mucosa has occurred, and, in these cases, free and digested blood may be found in the stomach and intestine. Jaundice is not common, but *yellow staining of adipose tissues* (*yellow-fat disease*) is. In relapsing cases, hemorrhagic diathesis may occur, manifested mainly by hemorrhage into and about joints. Protein-rich fluid collects in the serous cavities in small volume. Fine strands of fibrin are present in the peritoneal cavity.

Pulmonary edema accompanies the myocardial lesions of intramural and subendocardial hemorrhages with focal areas of hyaline degeneration. The changes in the liver dominate the autopsy findings. Hepatic necrosis is of the typical appearance described earlier, and in several cases, both acute and chronic lesions are found (Fig. 2-39). The sites of severest injury are the dorsal parts on the diaphragmatic surface. The right lobe may escape and later undergo marked hypertrophy. The gallbladder is often edematous.

The histologic changes that occur in this syndrome are described elsewhere with the organs involved. Briefly, *centrilobular necrosis of the liver is typical* (eFig. 2-10). Additionally, fibrinoid degeneration of small arteries occurs in some cases. Arterial degeneration may occur in any organ or in most organs but is relatively common in only the small vessels of

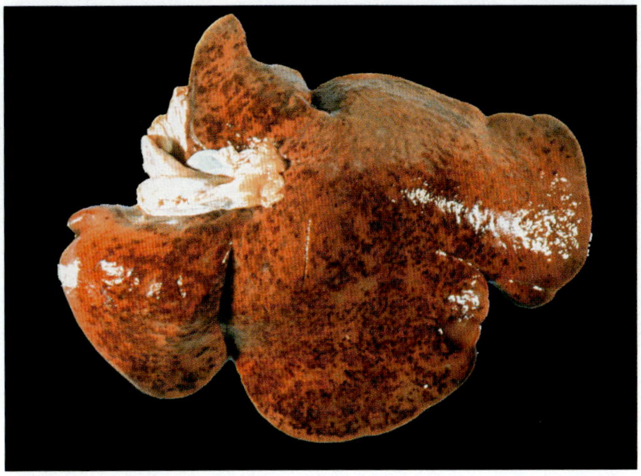

Figure 2-39 **Hepatosis dietetica** in a pig. (Courtesy University of Guelph.)

the mesentery, gut, and heart (see Mulberry Heart Disease in Vol. 3, Cardiovascular System).

Interface hepatitis (piecemeal necrosis)

Interface hepatitis (previously termed piecemeal necrosis) refers to a pattern on inflammation and hepatocellular necrosis in which *inflammation within the portal tract extends to and penetrates the limiting plate of hepatocytes* immediately adjacent to the edge of the portal tract. A second feature is *death of hepatocytes* in this region. This type of liver injury, in which inflammation characteristically disrupts the limiting plate, giving an irregular appearance to the periportal zone, is discussed further in the Chronic Hepatitis section.

Necrosis of sinusoidal lining cells

Injury to the endothelium of hepatic sinusoids can develop in a variety of forms. The sinusoidal endothelial cells may lose their typical fenestrae or pores, limiting contact between plasma and hepatocellular microvilli, and, if there is increased deposition of ECM beneath the altered endothelium, causing capillarization of sinusoids leading to reduced hepatic function. Sinusoidal endothelial cells may relax their connections to the fine meshwork of the hepatic "reticulin" or detach completely forming microemboli in the sinusoid downstream. In addition, the residual, exposed perisinusoidal space has an increased risk of sinusoidal thrombosis. Acute endothelial injury can occur because of ischemia-reperfusion injury, toxicant exposure (e.g., acetaminophen, pyrrolizidine), and effects of endotoxin, all of which can lead to localized ischemia and necrosis. Other endothelial toxins include ngaione poisoning and microcystin-LR, a highly toxic cyclic heptapeptide produced by *Microcystis aeruginosa* and other aquatic cyanobacteria (blue-green algae). Microcystin-LR is injurious to hepatic sinusoidal endothelial cells by inhibiting protein phosphatases causing hyperphosphorylation of cytoskeletal proteins and redistribution of actin filaments. Cytoskeletal collapse leads to apoptosis in endothelial cells and hemorrhagic necrosis.

Some forms of hepatic sinusoidal angiectasis (peliosis hepatis) may develop following endothelial necrosis. More chronic injury can produce fibrosis, leading to diminished or disrupted sinusoidal blood flow. Alteration of the sinusoidal blood flow can be a primary event leading to hepatocyte hypoxia with liver dysfunction and disruption of the portal circulation. Secondary

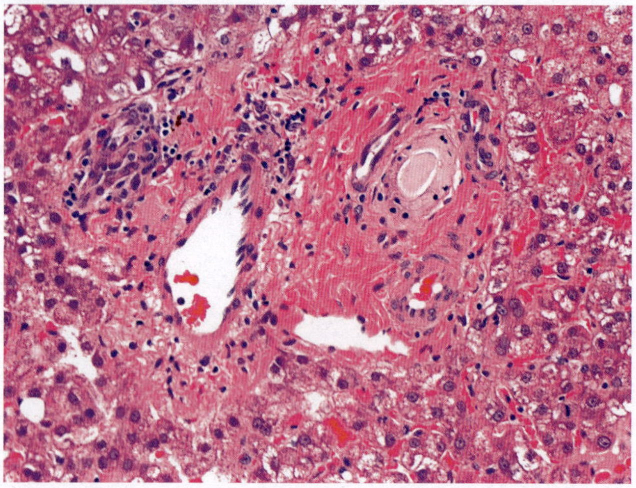

Figure 2-40 **Acute necrosis of biliary epithelium** in a dog following exposure to trimethoprim-sulfa.

endothelial cell injury can result when hepatocytes are being destroyed by the elaboration of toxic molecules within their cytoplasm; it is to be expected that the *sinusoidal-lining cells may also suffer should the products of these biotransformations spill into the perisinusoidal space*. Erythrocytes increase in the perisinusoidal space and, when endothelial damage is severe, the regions of necrosis are hemorrhagic. Necrosis of sinusoidal endothelial cells is seen very early during many hepatotoxicities.

Sinusoidal phagocytes are sometimes vulnerable to necrosis by virtue of their role in clearing the portal blood of particulate or colloidal material; should these particles be toxic or infectious, Kupffer cell necrosis may occur alone, but more usually, there is damage to surrounding hepatocytes as well.

Necrosis of bile duct epithelium

It is unusual for the bile duct epithelium to be singled out by specific lethal insults, but this is seen in intoxication by *sporidesmin* (see the Toxic Hepatic Disease section). Usually, there is accompanying portal inflammation. Some experimental toxicants, such as α-naphthyl isothiocyanate, are lethal to bile duct epithelia and elicit local cholangitis. Idiosyncratic drug-induced destructive cholangitis can lead to acute cholangiolar injury as well as chronic cholestasis with damage and loss of bile ducts *(destructive cholangitis)*. Treatment with sulfonamides, other drugs, and viral infection have been linked to this response (Fig. 2-40).

RESPONSES OF THE LIVER TO INJURY

The liver is a remarkably versatile organ. Given its central position in the body, supplied by blood draining the gastrointestinal tract, pancreas, spleen, and gallbladder, and the fact that it is the key organ involved in detoxification of exogenous (xenobiotics) and endogenous (endobiotics) compounds, the liver must respond to insults, including metabolic, infectious, and hemodynamic. The sequential concept seen as injury followed by inflammation and ending in fibrosis is oversimplified. These processes are intertwined rather than hierarchical. A plethora of pathogenic mediators: cytokines, danger signals, microbial metabolites, and bile acids, all simultaneously affect metabolism, injury, inflammation, and fibrosis. In addition, the cellular composition of parenchymal, nonparenchymal, and immune cells in the liver is much more heterogeneous than previously anticipated and can change rapidly. Cellular interactions and adaptations of cellular functions are clearly complex during hepatic injury, and our understanding is evolving. In this section, we describe the 2 main categories of liver response to injury: regeneration, including transdifferentiation, and fibrosis.

Hepatic regeneration

Acute injury involving the hepatocytes, biliary epithelium, endothelial cells, and mesenchymal elements typically is resolved quickly through regeneration. The liver is the only solid organ that can maintain a constant organ to body-weight ratio. This is particularly true in younger animals, as the vigor of regeneration diminishes modestly with age. Even in cases of severe hepatocellular necrosis, complete recovery is possible if the reticulin framework of the liver persists and surviving hepatocytes and/or biliary epithelial cells have sufficient time to regenerate or transdifferentiate and replace the lost hepatic mass.

In adulthood, the liver is a stable organ with limited replication of mature hepatocytes, biliary epithelium, and other cells in the liver. However, loss of hepatic mass through injury, such as infections, toxic insult, or surgical removal, will transform the mature hepatocytes, biliary epithelium, as well as HSCs, Kupffer cells, and endothelial cells, into actively proliferating cells until normal functional mass has been replaced. *As much as 70% of the normal liver can be removed surgically without clinical insufficiency, and over a few weeks, it is back to its normal mass*. In cases of mild-to-moderate acute injury, cell loss is replaced by proliferation of mature hepatocytes or biliary epithelium, providing swift replacement of parenchymal loss. Hepatocytes and cholangiocytes are typically characterized by phenotypic fidelity during regeneration. Regeneration of mature hepatocytes following surgical removal is well known. An example from Greek mythology is Prometheus, punished for giving fire to the mortals, had his liver partially eaten daily by an eagle (a symbol of Zeus), only to regrow and be eaten again. Although the mythical *daily* regrowth of hepatic mass is more prodigious than the real-world response, hepatic regeneration is nonetheless remarkable. In rodents, partial hepatectomies can be repeated more than 10 times, followed by restoration of normal hepatic mass. *Individual hepatocytes can replicate indefinitely*. Simple replacement of missing hepatocytes alone does not truly constitute regeneration because normal liver ultrastructural and microscopic architecture is essential to maintain normal hepatic function. Although new lobes are not regenerated following hepatectomy, the remaining lobes enlarge, and the proliferated hepatocytes and other cellular elements progress through a series of steps that involve interaction of hepatocytes and angiogenic processes to restore the normal relationships between hepatocytes and sinusoids.

Regeneration of mature hepatocytes is stimulated by several factors. These include polypeptide growth factors and their receptors; hepatocyte growth factor and its receptor (MET) and ligands of the EGF receptor; EGF, transforming growth factor–α (TGF-α), heparin-binding EGF-like growth factor, and amphiregulin. There are many auxiliary signals that can delay hepatocyte regeneration in their absence, but that do not directly simulate hepatocyte mitosis. These include IL6, bile acids, TNF, vascular endothelial growth factor (VEGF), and insulin. Within minutes following partial hepatectomy, hepatocyte growth factor is released from the ECM of the liver through the action of urokinase-type plasminogen activator, which converts plasminogen to plasmin, in turn activating metalloproteinases. Various blood-borne (i.e., EGF) and local signals affect regeneration. HSCs and sinusoidal endothelial cells also produce hepatocyte growth factor during regeneration. Hepatic regeneration is also enhanced by nutrition; fasting slows regeneration and dietary protein promotes regeneration. The autonomic nervous system also plays a role in hepatic regeneration, as denervation of the liver can significantly limit hepatic regeneration. *Following hepatocyte proliferation, normal liver architecture must be preserved to support hepatic function.* Several cell types are involved in this process. Following partial hepatectomy, the initial proliferation creates aggregates of hepatocytes 10-14 cells thick. These aggregates are penetrated by endothelial buds that eventually establish sinusoidal channels. Ingrowth of the endothelial cells is driven by regulators of angiogenesis, such as VEGF and platelet-derived growth factor (PDGF). HSCs replicate and synthesize ECM within ~4 days of partial hepatectomy and help establish normal hepatocyte-matrix interactions.

Once the needed hepatic mass has been replaced, the regenerative process must be regulated to terminate cell proliferation. TGF-β and related family members, including *activin*, are the best known mediators responsible for curtailing hepatocyte proliferation. These mediators are produced primarily by the HSCs. Mediators can increase ECM production as well as suppress hepatocellular replication, are downregulated during proliferation, and increase once appropriate hepatic mass has been achieved.

Ductular reaction (biliary hyperplasia)

In cases of more severe injury, or conditions that inhibit replication of mature cells, particularly if one lineage is disproportionately affected, transdifferentiation of either hepatocytes or biliary epithelium into facultative stem cells can replace the affected cell type. There does not appear to be a liver "stem cell" per se. At the interface of the portal tract connective tissue and the hepatic parenchyma, biliary cells in the intrahepatic bile ductules can form progenitor cell populations that can differentiate into mature hepatocytes and cholangiocytes. Periportal hepatocytes also have the capacity to form progenitor cell populations giving rise to hepatocytes and biliary epithelium. In many, often chronic, liver diseases, hepatocyte proliferation is impaired and expansion of progenitor cells differentiating toward cholangiocytes occurs. This process is termed a **ductular reaction** and recognized histologically as small, basophilic cells that form single-cell arrays or ductules with narrow lumens (Fig. 2-41A).

The "oval cells" described in rodents and the ductular reaction likely involve the same cell types. Immunohistochemical staining of these progenitor cells in humans and rodents reflects their common embryologic origin as hepatoblasts since they contain CK markers of biliary epithelium and, simultaneously, hepatocyte markers such as albumin (see Fig. 2-41B). The ability of these transdifferentiated cells in the ductular reaction to form mature biliary or hepatocellular phenotypes is well established. Ductular reaction can be observed in various circumstances. Both cholestasis and hypoxia can drive the ductular reaction causing proliferation in the periportal region for the former, and in the centrilobular region in the latter, instance.

Biliary obstruction leads to proliferation of bile duct epithelium, creating a rapid increase in bile duct surface area. Biliary epithelium proliferation can protect hepatocytes from bile

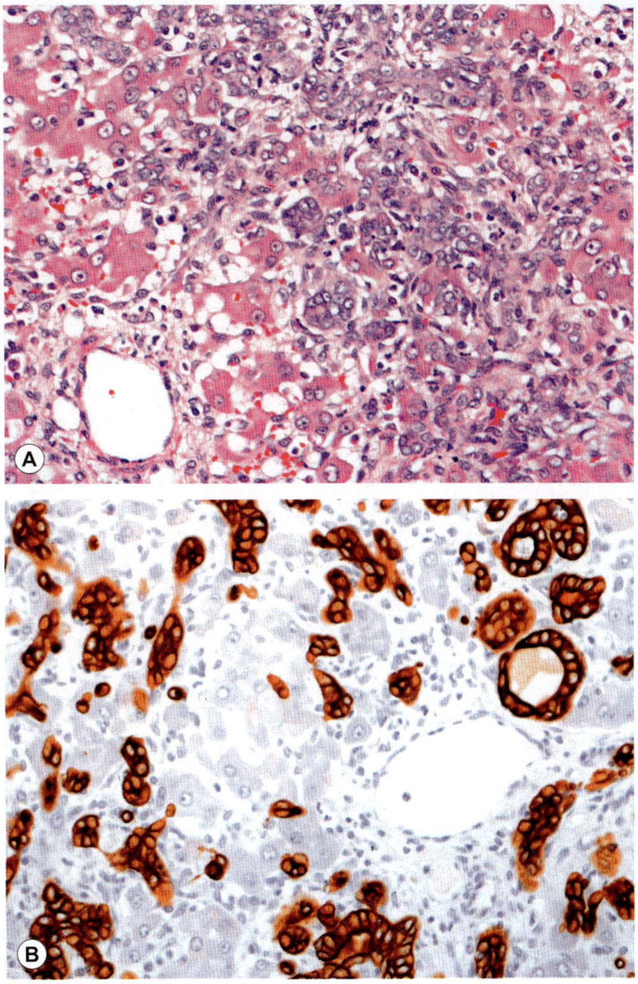

Figure 2-41 **A. Ductular reaction** in an injured liver. **B.** Cytokeratin-7 stain.

acid buildup through a recirculation process termed *cholehepatic recirculation*. Following panlobular necrosis, all remaining hepatocytes are likely to start a replicative response; random focal necrosis will engender a local proliferation of hepatocytes. Scattered individual cell necrosis is repaired almost imperceptibly. In the more common pattern of centrilobular necrosis, seen in many acute toxic insults, complete repair is usually evident with 24-48 hours. There are several circumstances that can trigger the ductular reaction other than necrosis, although this is the best recognized form.

In cases of severe injury to hepatocytes, particularly when mature hepatocytes are not able to replicate, prominent ductular formation occurs through transdifferentiation of biliary epithelial cells. A dramatic presentation of ductular proliferation is often evident in animals that succumb several days after a fatal hepatic intoxication or in horses with equine serum hepatitis. Ductular reaction may also develop secondarily *to chronic portal inflammation and fibrosis*. Ductular formation can also occur in areas of *hypoxia*. Such ducts formed by transdifferentiation of mature hepatocytes can be found in centrilobular areas in animals with chronic heart failure and passive congestion, for example.

Of course, in most clinical circumstances, hepatic regeneration is a less orderly process than that which occurs in healthy experimental animals. *Regeneration requires normal arterial and venous inflow as well as venous and biliary drainage.* Without a supportive environment, regeneration of hepatocytes, biliary epithelium, and nonparenchymal cells may be quite variable within different regions of the liver.

With persistence, the ductular reaction can contribute to *portal and periportal fibrosis* as the ductular cells secrete profibrogenic growth factors, cytokines, and chemokines. Illustrative examples from natural disease are provided by the toxicoses of phomopsin, pyrrolizidine alkaloids, and aflatoxin, and by equine serum hepatitis and ovine white-liver disease. Chronic or repetitive injury often results in *regenerative nodule formation*.

Fibrosis

Hepatic fibrosis is a potentially reversible form of wound healing in which there is an accumulation of various ECM components in response to various toxic, infectious, metabolic, and immune-mediated injury. In cases of acute or self-limited injury, *fibrosis may resolve completely*, and normal liver architecture can be restored. Elimination of the inciting cause can permit significant restoration of hepatic architecture. Anti-inflammatory mediators are released by phagocytes that clean up the debris when inflammation subsides and this engenders the atiraction of endothelial cells, blood vessel growth, and activation of tissue macrophages and myofibroblasts to rebuild and reform the ECM, eventually closing the wound. *However, if the injury is persistent or damage disrupts the normal ECM, a process leading to the "final common pathway" and ending in fibrosis and cirrhosis can develop.*

In normal liver, the ECM exists in a state of dynamic balance, with synthesis and degradation occurring in balance to maintain normal levels of all constituents. Various combinations of ECM are found in the portal tracts, along the perisinusoidal spaces, around the central vein, and in the hepatic capsule. Normally, the hepatic ECM constitutes only 3% of the relative areas on a tissue section and only 0.5% of the total liver wet weight. The main constituents of the hepatic ECM are collagens of different types, proteoglycans, laminin, fibronectin, and matricellular proteins. In the perisinusoidal space, the matrix is composed primarily of collagens IV and VI. Following injury, however, fibrillar collagens I and III, as well as fibronectin, are deposited. These deposits disrupt the normal structure and function of the sinusoids, leading to *capillarization of sinusoids*. The ECM is not merely scaffolding for the liver. It also functions as a repository for various growth factors and metalloproteinases in latent form, and it can bind a variety of survival factors, such as hepatocyte growth factor and TNF, that may protect the growth factors and inhibit hepatocyte apoptosis. In addition, interactions between cells and the ECM can affect the phenotype of the hepatocytes and stellate cells and the composition of the ECM. Thus, the process of hepatic fibrosis is distinct from the condensation of the hepatic reticular framework that can be seen following hepatocyte loss.

ECM production in the injured liver involves the ***hepatic stellate cell (HSC)*** *as the major fibrogenic cell following its transdifferentiation into an activated, myofibroblast-like cell type*. The activated phenotype of HSCs results from a broad variety of intracellular events and signals in all cellular compartments. Various inflammatory mediators can activate HSCs, resulting in excessive ECM deposition as a wound healing or scarring response. In turn, proinflammatory mediators released by activated HSCs and inflammatory cells lead to a chronic cycle of inflammation and formation of scar tissue, ultimately resulting in organ failure. While the best recognized *cell type* in this family is the *HSC*, there are other important cell *populations* in this family, including portal fibroblasts, bone marrow–derived cells, and, possibly via epithelial-mesenchymal transition, hepatocytes that can acquire a mesenchymal phenotype. *Portal fibroblasts*, particularly those surrounding the bile ducts, are an important source of ECM formation in the portal tracts. This is particularly clear in cases of biliary tree injury. Portal fibroblasts/myofibroblasts are distinct from stellate cells based on distinct protein markers.

Hepatic blood flow can be significantly modified by activated HSCs. Blood flow through sinusoids can be restricted by the contraction of the HSCs that extend processes around the sinusoidal endothelial cells. In health, there is a balance between nitric oxide–stimulated vasodilation and endothelin-1–driven vasoconstriction. During active fibrosis and cirrhosis, endothelin-1, produced by sinusoidal endothelial cells, increases, causing contraction of the HSC-derived myofibroblasts.

Fibrosis can occur within portal tracts expanding their area, or as septa extending into the parenchyma and eventually bridging between portal tracts or central veins. Fibrosis in the portal tracts is primarily generated by the activity of portal fibroblasts, rather than HSCs. Biliary injury leads to rapid proliferation of periductular myofibroblasts derived from portal fibroblasts and ECM production. The volume of the portal tracts is increased by the generation of the ECM, ductular proliferation, myofibroblast proliferation, and edema.

Fibrosis can be less florid and more insidious when it lines the perisinusoidal spaces, disrupting the normal exchange between the plasma and hepatocyte microvilli. The essential microvascular unit of the liver is the sinusoid, lined by fenestrated endothelial cells, and separated from hepatocytes by the perisinusoidal space. A porous basal membrane–like matrix in the perisinusoidal space helps to maintain the differentiated states of the hepatocytes and HSCs that inhabit that space. When there is excess ECM in the perisinusoidal space, the adjacent sinusoidal endothelial cells lose their characteristic fenestrations, and *the sinusoids are transformed functionally into capillaries*. This process is known as **capillarization** and leads to significantly impaired exchange between the hepatocytes and the plasma. This causes diminished hepatic function when the lesion is extensive. The cells responsible for the ECM deposition are primarily in the myofibroblast family, including HSCs.

Because collagen has a finite half-life, and as hepatic fibrosis exists in a balance of synthesis and removal, it is potentially reversible. Elimination of the source of injury or successful therapy can lead to HSC apoptosis, reversion, and senescence. Studies in mice show that half of the activated HSCs escape from apoptosis during regression of liver fibrosis and acquire a phenotype like, but distinct from, quiescent HSCs. These reverted HSCs stay in a primed state with enhanced capacity to reactivate in response to fibrogenic stimuli. There is a commensurate reduction in the synthesis of inhibitors of the enzymes responsible for degradation of the collagen and other ECM elements, primarily matrix metalloproteinases. This has been demonstrated in rodent models of hepatic fibrosis produced by bile duct ligation, and models using carbon tetrachloride.

However, over time, collagen can mature, and fibrils can cross-link and become resistant to enzymatic degradation, leading to permanent fibrosis. Long-term or permanent fibrotic changes can also be caused by severe acute injury that leads to an initial focus of fibrosis and is so severe that it affects local vascular supply.

The **distribution of fibrosis** in the liver can reflect the pathogenesis of the injury responsible.

- Inflammatory disorders that produce interface hepatitis (piecemeal necrosis) of hepatocytes, typically viral hepatitis in humans and often an idiopathic disorder or possibly immune-mediated hepatitis in veterinary species, can evolve to form portal-to-portal, or portal-to-central, **fibrous septa**.
- In the event of *inflammation or obstruction involving the bile ducts*, proliferation of periductular myofibroblasts and prominent ductular reaction can lead to **biliary fibrosis** or a pattern of portal-to-portal bridging termed **biliary cirrhosis** when accompanied by nodular regenerative proliferation of hepatocytes (Fig. 2-42).
- **Postnecrotic scarring** *occurs after severe necrosis*, where large areas of parenchyma are destroyed. The reticulin network collapses and condenses and portal areas converge, resulting in broad, irregular bands of scar tissue with variable irregular areas of parenchymal regeneration interspersed (Fig. 2-43).
- **Diffuse hepatic fibrosis** is the outcome of *chronic parenchymal injury*, such as prolonged inflammation or several episodes of zonal necrosis. The fibrosis throughout the lobules bridges connective tissue tracts in portal areas and hepatic venules to produce *pseudolobulation*, in which small areas of parenchyma are separated by a pattern of fibrosis on the scale of true lobules. This pattern of fibrosis can lead to capillarization of sinusoids, or intrahepatic bypass of portal and arterial blood, both of which can reduce the influences of growth factors and nutrients on liver regeneration. The accompanying hypoxia is important in the genesis of the hepatocellular atrophy that is almost always concomitant with diffuse hepatic fibrosis.
- **Centrilobular (periacinar) fibrosis** is the most common pattern *following zonal necrosis in hypoxic and toxic injury*. Good examples are seen in animals with prolonged passive venous congestion of the liver, especially when this is caused by extracardiac sources of increased venous pressure, rather than congestive heart failure (Fig. 2-44). Otherwise, this pattern of fibrosis is a response to toxic injury; and extraordinary development of centrilobular fibrosis may follow accidental exposure to nitrosamines in several species.

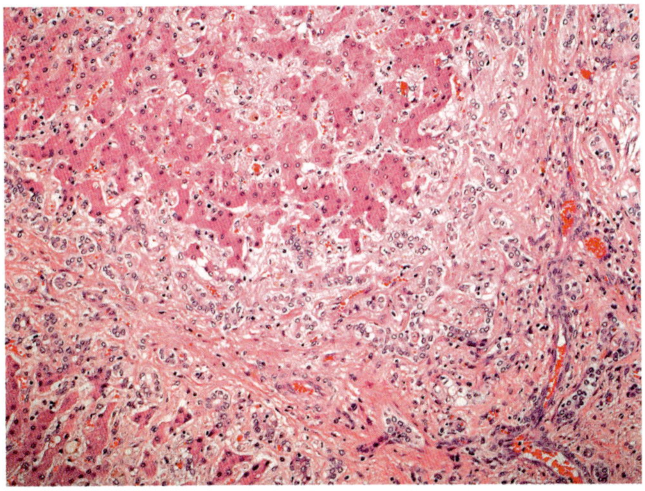

Figure 2-42 Bridging portal fibrosis and bile duct hyperplasia secondary to bile duct obstruction in a horse.

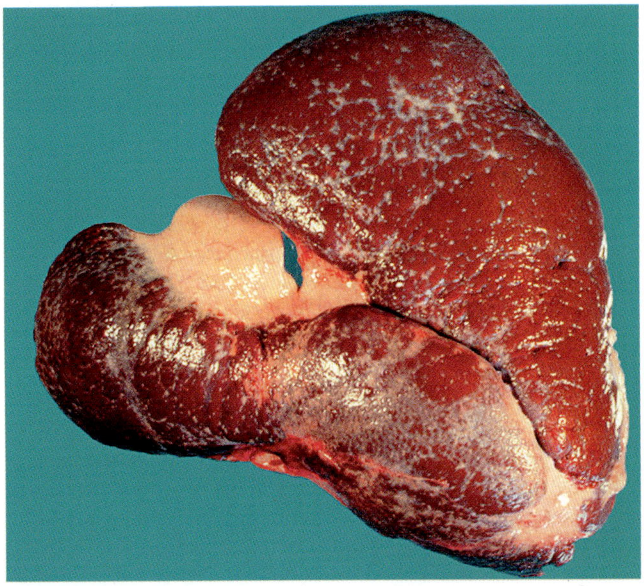

Figure 2-43 Postnecrotic scarring in the liver of a sheep. (Courtesy P. Stromberg.)

Cirrhosis

Cirrhosis has several definitions, and consensus regarding the essential features is difficult to obtain. In general, it is agreed that cirrhosis is not merely an end stage of ECM accumulation in the liver, but, in fact, is a multifaceted distortion of hepatic parenchymal architecture and hepatic vascular anatomy. By one definition, cirrhosis is defined anatomically by "the presence throughout the liver of fibrous septa that subdivide the parenchyma into nodules." Functionally, the *key features* are distortion of the hepatic architecture with regenerative nodule formation and fibrous septa associated with abnormal blood flow and eventually portal hypertension. These changes arise in a background of cell death, deposition of abnormal ECM, and vascular reorganization. Other than dogs, most veterinary species develop diffuse hepatic fibrosis following chronic injury, but only infrequently develop regenerative nodules. *Chronically injured canine livers often have robust formation of regenerative nodules separated by fibrous septa typical of cirrhosis*

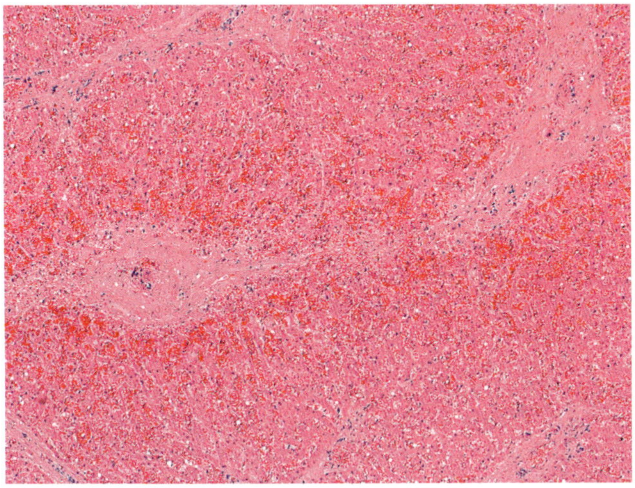

Figure 2-44 Centrilobular fibrosis (cardiac fibrosis), most severe at the center of the lobe in chronic passive congestion in a dog.

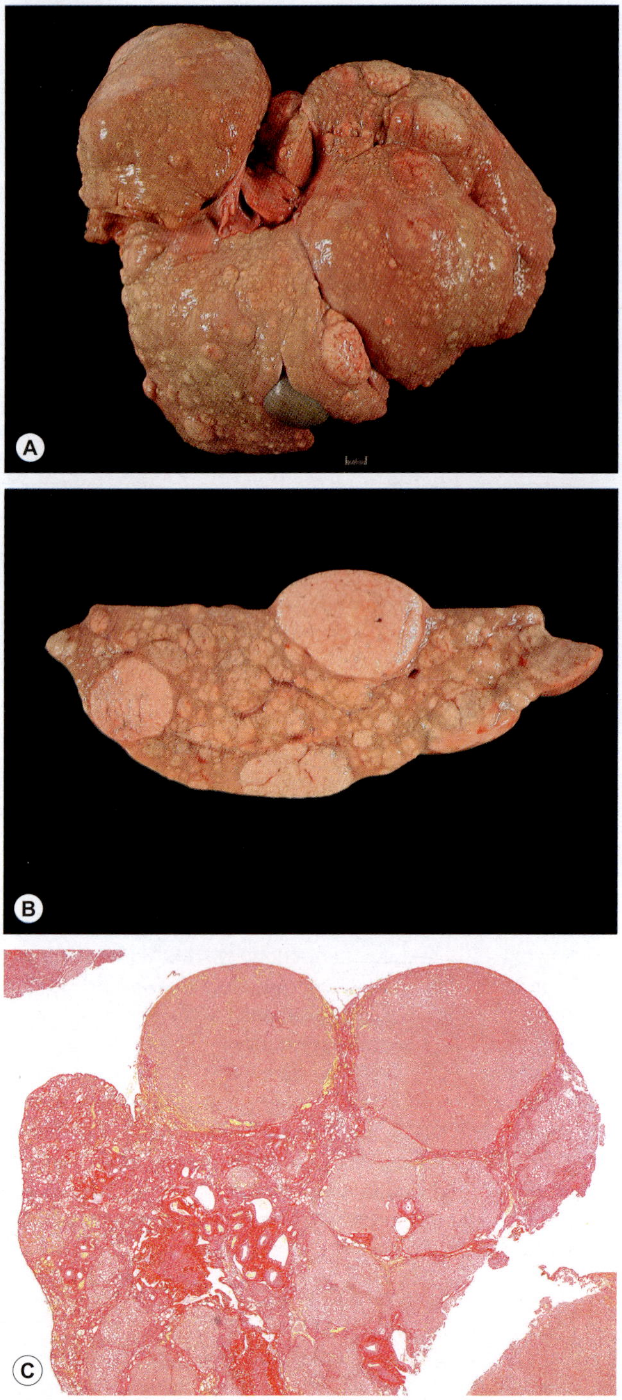

Figure 2-45 **A. Regenerative nodules** in the liver of a dog. **B.** Cut surface of the liver. **C.** Microscopic appearance of the regenerative nodules and adjacent septa (picrosirius red stain).

(Fig. 2-45A-C). Venous occlusion may result, interfering with hepatic function, driving portal hypertension, and acquiring PSSs. *Note that not all nodular livers are cirrhotic.* Clinically, *cirrhosis results in hepatic insufficiency*, mainly in the form of ascites and hypoproteinemia rather than excretory dysfunction and icterus, although, in advanced cases, all manifestations of fatal liver failure can occur. The **hallmarks of cirrhosis** are as follows:

1. *Bridging fibrous septa*, ranging from delicate bands to broad scars that replace adjacent lobules. These fibrous septa contain vascular channels, originating from sinusoids in collapsed parenchyma or angiogenesis that allow a considerable portion of blood to bypass hepatocytes. These microvascular channels in fibrous septa resist flow more than normal sinusoids. This factor, as well as the relative increase in flow in these vessels shunting around the nodules, *contributes to portal hypertension*.
2. *Impaired exchange* between hepatocytes and sinusoidal blood because of the increase in perisinusoidal ECM.
3. *Parenchymal nodules*, created by the regenerative attempts of entrapped hepatocytes, and of <3 mm (*micronodular*) up to several centimeters in diameter (*macronodular*). These nodules are composed of trabeculae that are typically 2 or more cells thick, with relative reduction of sinusoidal space. Some expanding nodules may compress the vessels within fibrous septa, contributing to portal hypertension. Nodule formation is prominent in dogs, but significantly less so in most other domestic species.
4. *Ongoing damage and reorganization* of the hepatic connective tissue, sometimes with areas of portal vein and arterial thrombosis and segmental ischemia is typical, but not always present.

Cirrhosis is usually the result of several pathogenic processes, namely, cell death (necrosis or apoptosis) and inflammation with fibrosis. Cirrhosis is not a synonym for chronic hepatic fibrosis, although some insults that cause chronic diffuse fibrosis in the liver can lead to cirrhosis. The nodular pattern of regeneration in cirrhosis is caused by expanding islands of surviving parenchyma entrapped between bands of scar tissue. At the point of liver failure, these regenerative attempts are insufficient to restore function. Despite the increased hepatocellular mass, the inability to restore normal function is attributed to altered circulation through the bridging scar tissue, portal hypertension and shunting, deposition of ECM in the perisinusoidal space, inhibition of ECM degradation, reduced supply of portal growth factors, and toxic inhibition of hepatocellular proliferation. The characteristic fibrovascular septa that bridge portal and central vascular tracts are readily seen in liver sections, but the portal-hepatic shunting therein can be difficult to identify. Clinical evidence for portosystemic shunting, such as impaired ammonia or bile acid clearance, can reflect acquired portocaval shunts that often develop because of portal hypertension from chronic hepatic fibrosis.

Studies in humans indicate that reversal or significant repair of cirrhosis can occur when the inciting cause, such as copper or immune-mediated inflammation, is removed.

Acquired portosystemic shunts

Any chronic liver disease that causes sufficient fibrosis or atrophy to restrict portal blood flow significantly and produce portal hypertension has the potential to cause the development of collateral PSSs. These are described later in the Vascular Factors in Hepatic Injury and Circulatory Disorders section.

HEPATIC DYSFUNCTION

***Hepatic failure** is a syndrome that results from inadequate hepatic function.* The liver provides many essential processes, and liver failure can affect metabolic, synthetic, catabolic (detoxification), and immune functions. There is no specific point at which diminished function can clearly be defined as "failure," given the various functions of the liver, but it is best understood as the point at which liver function is not capable of sustaining life. The liver is an organ with a large functional capacity and regenerative potential. Signs of insufficiency do not develop until the reserves in production, supply, and recovery are exhausted. *The central role of the liver in many systemic functions means that liver disease can be manifest as lesions or dysfunctions elsewhere, for example, in the brain, skin, blood, and gut.* Failure may develop suddenly, often following exposure to toxic compounds, or failure may develop in a slow inexorable manner as a chronic disease process. Hepatic failure, particularly chronic liver failure, may not affect all processes equally, and one or more features of liver failure may predominate in individual cases.

Acute liver failure is uncommon and is clinically evidenced as a severe and rapid liver injury. There are several causes. The consequences are also multiple and varied, including abrupt loss of normal metabolic and immunologic functions, as well as HE, coagulopathy, jaundice, photosensitization (in herbivores), and possibly dysfunction of other organs. In humans, recognized viral infections can cause acute liver failure, but there are currently no known domestic animal viruses capable of causing this syndrome. Equine serum hepatitis is caused by an *equine parvovirus*; however, the infection is chronic despite the acute clinical presentation of liver failure. Bacterial infection, such as *leptospirosis*, can occasionally cause acute liver failure. *Toxicant-induced* acute liver failure is likely the most common form in veterinary medicine. The toxic injury may come from natural sources, such as those found in plants and fungi, or from overdose of, or idiosyncratic reactions to, therapeutic drugs. *Hyperthermia* from environmental heating or prolonged seizure activity can also cause acute hepatic failure. *Acute ischemic injury* from profound hypotension secondary to sepsis or cardiac failure may also occur.

Chronic liver failure results from progressive destructive processes, such as fibrosis or inflammation, or a combination of the two. The hallmarks of chronic liver failure in dogs are *fibrosis and nodular regeneration*, but other species are more prone to a fibrotic response alone. The progressive loss of critical functional hepatic mass caused by ongoing hepatocyte injury, shunting of portal blood within fibrous septa bypassing hepatocytes, and abnormal bile drainage, lead to a terminal stage of hepatic insufficiency.

Chronic liver failure can be subdivided into 2 forms: *end-stage liver*, the typical fibrotic liver with progressive loss of functional hepatic mass, and *"acute-on-chronic failure,"* a circumstance in which a patient with compensated chronic liver disease develops failure acutely. The causes for the acute transition to failure are not certain, but the buildup of various toxins, such as aromatic amino acids and ammonia, among others, may be involved. Other theories include increased bacterial or fungal translocation from the gut, leading to hepatic infection and sepsis.

Liver failure, whether acute or chronic, affects several critical processes. These disturbances include HE, cholestasis and jaundice, hepatogenous photosensitization, hemorrhagic diathesis, hepatorenal syndrome, ascites, and hepatocutaneous syndrome.

Hepatic encephalopathy

The neurologic manifestations of hepatic failure are variable and nonspecific; they range from dullness, through complete unawareness and compulsive aimless movement, to mania and generalized convulsions. There is considerable variation in the clinical signs of hepatic encephalopathy (HE) between different species. Sheep rarely show more than dullness and central blindness, with perhaps some compulsive chewing movements and tremor. The picture in cattle is similar, but mania and aggression may also be seen; frenzy is more often recorded in horses. The closer clinical observation of cats and dogs may reveal more subtle behavioral changes; inappetence and vomiting are commonly reported in carnivores with PSSs. Drooling is common in cats with HE.

The clinical context in which HE occurs can be important. *In animals with acute hepatic disease, HE is a serious sign, usually indicating imminent death.* However, in animals with more chronic conditions, such as portosystemic shunting or deficiency of a urea cycle enzyme, neurologic signs can be intermittent for many months and may disappear after appropriate dietary modification. The pathogenesis of HE involves more than just neurons, as glial cell responses are evident. Older literature, particularly in vitro studies, which did not take all these features into account, will likely need reinterpretation.

Ammonia toxicity *is regarded as the major part of the clinical signs and the brain lesions; however, there are several other factors that may play a role.* Blood ammonia is largely of dietary origin, derived from protein and urea by microflora in the large bowel. Ammonia is also derived from hepatic deamination of amino acids and from metabolism of glutamine in peripheral tissues. Ammonia is normally removed in the first pass of portal blood through the liver, wherein it is incorporated with carbon dioxide into carbamoyl phosphate that enters the urea cycle. In shunting or hepatic failure, ammonia that bypasses hepatic clearance accumulates in the circulation. Ammonia can cross the blood-brain barrier, and initially, this influx leads to astrocyte injury. Astrocytes are the site of ammonia detoxification in the brain, and they eliminate ammonia by the synthesis of glutamine through amidation of glutamate by the enzyme glutamine synthetase. Elevated blood ammonia increases the accumulation of glutamine in astrocytes, resulting in osmotic stress and astrocyte swelling caused by cytotoxic edema. Affected astrocytes that are adjacent to endothelium cannot maintain the blood-brain barrier, and this permits increased ammonia entry into the brain. Direct ammonia-induced effects on brain endothelial cells are also possible. Briefly, the consequences of increased ammonia in the brain include a net decrease in energy metabolism within the brain, increased edema formation because of astrocyte dysfunction, and injury to neurons, leading to an imbalance in neurotransmitters that emphasizes neural inhibition.

The pathogenesis of HE may vary depending on the type of liver failure—acute or chronic—that produces the cerebral injury. Also, not all parts of the brain are affected in a similar manner. In acute hepatic failure, cerebral edema may be the leading cause of death because of increased intracerebral pressure with possible herniation. The increase in intracranial pressure is, however, linked to brain ammonia levels. It is thought that swollen astrocytes release vasogenic factors, such as nitric oxide, causing intracerebral hyperemia, and that this leads to edema formation. Systemic inflammatory responses can enhance the severity of HE. Neuroinflammation, mediated by microglia, is evident in acute liver failure and tends to increase with increasing duration of HE. Synergetic interactions between increased ammonia and systemic or neuroinflammation can increase the severity of HE. However, the specific mechanisms by which systemic inflammation triggers neuroinflammation are not known.

In chronic hepatic failure, ***ammonia and neuroinflammation*** *are likely to contribute synergistically to HE.* Ammonia plays a role as a directly neurotoxic agent, altering neurotransmission, and potentially contributing to cerebral energy failure through inhibition of α-ketoglutarate dehydrogenase, a rate-limiting enzyme in the tricarboxylic acid (TCA) cycle. Chronic increase in brain ammonia is associated with disrupted neural transmission involving all the different neurotransmitter systems of the brain. The main neurotransmitter systems affected involve neuropeptides, with evolution toward an increase in the inhibitory γ-aminobutyric acid (GABA)ergic system, and downregulation of the excitatory glutaminergic system. Increased intracerebral ammonia leads to an increase in extracellular glutamate, which will initially drive upregulation of N-methyl-D-aspartate (NMDA) receptors, causing neuronal damage, but eventually, there is a reduction in NMDA receptors and glutaminergic signaling, leading to neuroinhibition. In addition, increased ammonia alone has been linked to neuroinflammation, possibly through direct activation of microglia, which also interferes with normal neural transmission.

Studies in animal models have demonstrated that agents acting on specific targets in the brain, including phosphodiesterase 5, type A GABA receptors, and mitogen-activated kinase (p38), can improve cognitive function in mild forms of experimental HE. Survival can be increased by treatment with NMDA receptor agonists. Studies have also implicated alterations in inhibitory and excitatory neurotransmitters, including endogenous benzodiazepines, and serotonin, as well as their receptors. Although infusion of ammonia, or hyperammonemia caused by deficiency of urea cycle enzymes, reproduces similar neurologic signs and vacuolar lesions, other noxious substances in the alimentary tract are also believed to contribute to HE resulting from liver failure. These include *variably toxic amines, captans, thiols, and short-chain fatty acids (SCFAs)*, which are normally removed from the portal blood in one passage through the liver after production in the large bowel. The significant role of the gut microbiome in the gut-liver-brain axis is a newly recognized pathogenic feature of HE. Altered gut microbiota may lead to a variety of effects, such as reduced production of SCFAs, reduced production of bile acids, increased intestinal barrier permeability, and bacterial translocation, all of which can contribute to impaired neural function. Thus, there are many factors to consider in the pathogenesis of HE.

The microscopic lesions of HE are subtle and variable, likely because postmortem examinations of the brain are performed at various stages of chronicity and clinical severity. There are also significant differences in the microscopic lesions between species. In humans, *the hallmark of HE is Alzheimer type II astrocytosis, in which astrocytes are enlarged with swollen nuclei, margination of chromatin, and prominent nucleoli.* These Alzheimer type II astrocytes can be found in large animals, particularly horses. *In dogs, Alzheimer type II changes are rare if they occur at all*, but *vacuoles in the gray matter*, particularly in brainstem nuclei, predominate. Lesions in cats have features of both the dog and the horse (see Vol. 1, Nervous System). These changes can be observed best in animals with chronic liver disease and PSSs; the brain lesions can be minimal in animals with acute liver failure.

Cholestasis and jaundice

Cholestasis is the term for impaired bile secretion and flow as well as a failure to secrete organic and inorganic components of bile, with accumulation of these elements in blood. Normal bile formation and flow is dependent on the activity of a series of membrane transporters found in enterocytes, hepatocytes, and biliary epithelium. In rare cases, hereditary mutations can lead to cholestasis, but more often, cholestasis is caused by exposure to injurious drugs, hormones, proinflammatory cytokines, or obstruction. Clinically, cholestasis leads to increased levels of bilirubin and bile acids in the blood because of retention. Injury to the biliary tree leads to increases in serum alkaline phosphatase activity. Disturbance of bile flow can originate from altered function of hepatocytes, termed hepatocellular cholestasis, or because of obstruction of the biliary tree, termed obstructive cholestasis. *Hepatocellular cholestasis* can be attributed to impaired uptake, metabolism, secretion, or transport of bile constituents. *Obstructive cholestasis* is related to obstruction of bile flow at the level of the major bile ducts or gallbladder.

Jaundice (icterus) occurs when the tissues, particularly the sclerae, are pigmented yellow because of an excess of bile pigments, primarily bilirubin, in the plasma. Jaundice can arise from *hepatocellular cholestasis* or *obstructive cholestasis* and, in addition, from *prehepatic causes*, such as an overproduction of bilirubin from heme catabolism in hemolytic diseases (Fig. 2-46). The associated hypoxia caused by anemia may facilitate cholestasis in hemolytic diseases.

Histologically, both forms of cholestasis share common features, but there are additional lesions associated with **duct obstruction** in the portal tracts and bile ducts. The main histologic manifestation of cholestasis is the accumulation of homogeneous waxy brown bile pigment in bile canaliculi. Bile regurgitated from hepatocytes can also be found in Kupffer cells following phagocytosis. Bilirubin can be found in the hepatocellular cytoplasm in most species, especially if frozen sections are examined, but it is quite rare for bile to be evident in canine hepatocytes. Bile accumulation is more severe in the centrilobular regions of the lobules but can extend to the periportal regions in severe cases. With time, canalicular plugs are cleared, and they may not be evident in more chronic cases of cholestasis. *Hepatocyte rosettes*, collections of 2 or more hepatocytes surrounding a dilated

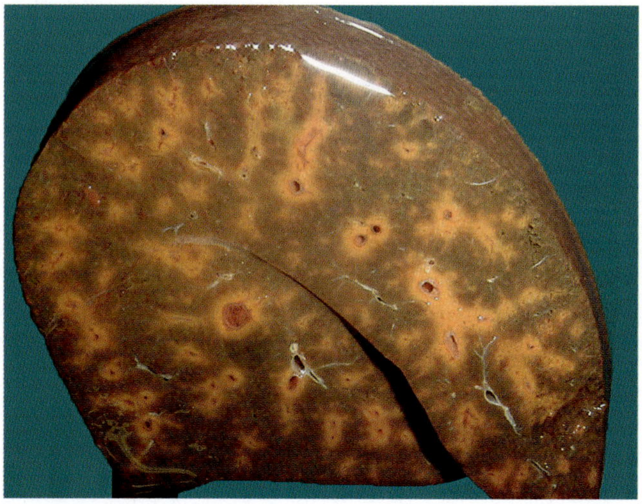

Figure 2-46 Deeply bile-stained liver from a jaundiced dog with immune hemolytic anemia and cholecystitis. (Courtesy A.P. Loretti.)

canaliculus are common. *Hepatocellular degeneration* may also be evident, sometimes with bile staining of the cytoplasm of injured hepatocytes. Scattered apoptotic cells may be present, although significant necrosis is not usually a feature of cholestasis. In severe cases of obstructive cholestasis, confluent areas of bile-stained hepatocellular necrosis, termed **bile infarcts**, can develop. Bile infarcts are rare in dogs and cats but can be found in other species. **Cholate stasis** refers to hepatocellular degeneration in the periportal region, often accompanied by a proliferation of small-caliber bile ducts (ductular reaction). Affected hepatocytes have swollen pale cytoplasm, and they may contain copper granules. This lesion is most common in horses with obstruction and rare in dogs. In hepatocellular cholestasis, there are no distinctive lesions in the portal tracts. However, in obstructive cholestasis, there are several distinctive changes. Initially, there is edema in the portal tract and an inflammatory infiltrate that is most often predominantly neutrophilic. There is an accompanying proliferation of small-caliber bile ducts arranged in an apparently haphazard manner (ductular reaction). There may be degeneration or proliferative changes in pre-existing interlobular bile ducts, often associated with inflammation, depending on the cause of the obstruction. Ductal ectasia may also be present. With time, fibrosis expands the portal tract outline and can bridge between portal tracts in cases of severe obstruction. In addition, concentric fibrosis surrounds the bile ducts. Mixed inflammatory cells, usually with fewer neutrophils than seen in acute cholestasis, as well as macrophages containing pigment, are found in portal tracts.

Hepatocellular cholestasis arises when there is a disturbance in 1 or more of the 3 main steps involved in bile excretion. They include failure 1) to take up bilirubin, bile acids, or other bile constituents; 2) to conjugate bilirubin, bile acids, or other constituents; and 3) to transport and excrete conjugated bilirubin, bile acids, or other bile constituents into canaliculi. Most of these bile metabolism issues are mediated by a series of hepatobiliary transporters, molecular pumps involved in the transport of bilirubin, bile acids, and other organic ions in hepatocytes, canaliculi, and biliary epithelium, although some pumps serve to export substances as well. Hepatocellular uptake of unconjugated and conjugated bilirubin, such as other organic ions, is mediated by members of the OATP family found on the basolateral aspects of hepatocytes. Bilirubin is conjugated by uridine diphosphate (UDP)–glucuronyl transferase in the ER of hepatocytes. From there it is transported into the bile. Bile acids are imported from the plasma by the Na^+-taurocholate cotransporting polypeptide (NTCP). Transport of bile acids, the main osmotic driving force for bile formation (bile acid–dependent flow), into the canaliculus is performed by the bile salt export pump (BSEP). Aquaporin channels facilitate the movement of water into the canaliculus in response to the osmotic forces produced by the bile acids. Movement of bilirubin into the canaliculus for excretion is accomplished by the multidrug resistance–associated protein–2 (MRP2). Reduced glutathione is also a substrate for MRP2, and it is reduced glutathione and bicarbonate that are the main elements of the bile acid–independent portion of bile flow, the second most significant force in bile flow. Bile is continually modified by transporter-driven processes of secretion and absorption during its transit to the duodenum.

In hepatocellular cholestasis, drugs or endotoxin-induced proinflammatory cytokines interfere with the activities of molecular pumps or inhibit their synthesis. Endotoxin exposure not only reduces the activity of OATP and NCTP but also interferes with the activity of BSEP and MRP2.

Hepatocellular cholestasis can also occur through disruption of the structural integrity of the canaliculi, as discussed later for *Lantana camara* toxicity. Poisons such as phalloidin and cytochalasin, which disrupt the polymerization cycle of pericanalicular actin microfilaments, are cholestatic because these contractile filaments are required for propelling bile along the canaliculi. In horses, fasting can cause an increase in plasma bilirubin and jaundice. The mechanism may be the impaired uptake of bilirubin from plasma or possibly impaired conjugation of bilirubin when energy supplies are low. Rarely, cholestasis and its indicators can occur in the absence of significant hepatocellular damage and other signs of liver failure. This can occur in toxicity by *L. camara* in ruminants and as an idiosyncratic reaction to some drugs.

In **obstructive cholestasis**, the activities of NTCP and OATP transporters are reduced, causing bile acids and bilirubin to accumulate in the blood. Transport of bile acids out of the hepatocyte and into the canaliculus is maintained by BSEP. The regulation of transcription of the various transporters in hepatocellular or obstructive cholestasis is controlled by the interaction of bilirubin or bile acids with several nuclear receptors, primarily PXR and, to a lesser extent, others, such as CAR and farnesoid X receptor. During cholestasis, nuclear receptors orchestrate protection of hepatocytes from injury by reducing the expression of basolateral uptake transporters and increasing the expression of basolateral export pumps, as well as reducing new bile acid synthesis and increasing the rate of intrahepatic metabolism of bile acids. However, these adaptive responses are not always sufficient to prevent cholate-induced hepatotoxicity.

Biliary canalicular function can be compromised during severe hepatic lipidosis leading to cholestasis, which is observed most commonly in cats. Jaundice may be present. Segmental duct obstructions that spare some parts of the liver can lead to cholestasis but not jaundice. This can occur in anorexic or dehydrated cats, in which bile may become dehydrated and viscous, causing ductal obstruction.

Severe diffuse liver necrosis obviously impairs bile excretion at various levels, but *the severity of cholestasis or of jaundice depends on the amount of liver affected, the chronicity, the supply of heme for catabolism, and nonhepatic routes of bilirubin excretion*. Focal liver injury can cause substantial local cholestasis, but clinically detectable cholestasis does not occur because bilirubin can be cleared by unaffected parts of the liver.

Various transporters and conjugating enzymes involved in bilirubin excretion can be genetically defective. *Congenital hyperbilirubinemia in mutant Southdown sheep* is the result of impaired hepatic uptake of unconjugated bilirubin. These animals have few liver lesions, but eventually develop chronic renal disease, the reason for which is not clear. Unconjugated bilirubin levels in the plasma are consistently elevated, but sufficient excretion takes place to prevent them from becoming icteric. They become photosensitized, indicating that excretion of phylloerythrin (phytoporphyrin) is less efficient than that of bilirubin.

Hyperbilirubinemia in mutant Corriedale sheep is a defect in excretion of conjugated bilirubin, as in Dubin-Johnson syndrome in humans and mutant rat strains. In humans and rats, there is a mutation in *Mrp2* causing hypofunction, and a similar mutation is likely in affected sheep. Affected sheep have an elevation of plasma bilirubin (just over half of which is conjugated), but there is no obvious jaundice. Nevertheless, phylloerythrin (phytoporphyrin) excretion in these Corriedale sheep is also sufficiently impaired to produce photosensitization. There is impaired excretion of other conjugated metabolites, and there is dark pigmentation of the liver by polymerized residues of retained catecholamine metabolites. This pigment, resembling lipofuscin, accumulates in lysosomes in the pericanalicular cytoplasm.

The recognition of jaundice at postmortem sometimes involves differentiation of bile staining of tissues from the yellow staining caused by the accumulation of carotenoid pigments. These latter are limited to fat depots and are to be expected in certain species such as horses; sometimes, there are breed influences, as seen in the yellow fat of Channel Island breeds of dairy cattle. The yellow discoloration of fat depots of older cats is less well understood. In animals fed ox liver, carotenoids may again be responsible, and in others, there may be some contribution by ceroid-type pigments. The distinction of the fatty pigments from bile depends on the absence of the former from pale, nonfatty tissues, such as periosteum and dermal collagen.

Photosensitization

Photosensitization is the term applied to inflammation of the skin (usually unpigmented) because of the action of ultraviolet light of wavelengths 290-400 nm on photodynamic compounds that have become bound to dermal cells. In **primary photosensitization**, these compounds may have been deposited unchanged in the skin after ingestion before the normal liver can excrete the native compound. This is seen, for example, after ingestion of hypericin in St. John wort *(Hypericum perforatum)*. Photodynamic agents may also be produced by aberrant endogenous metabolism. This can occur, for example, in congenital erythropoietic protoporphyria caused by ferrochelatase deficiency in Limousin and Blonde d'Aquitaine calves.

Hepatogenous photosensitization almost always accompanies cholestasis of more than a few days' duration in herbivores that are kept in sunlight and that have been eating green feed. *Phytoporphyrins* (formerly termed phylloerythrins) are green photoactive catabolites of plant porphyrins (mainly chlorophyll) that are generated by the alimentary microflora of herbivores. Some phytoporphyrin is absorbed and normally excreted in the bile by the transporters that eliminate bilirubin. Cholestasis in herbivores can increase retention of phytoporphyrin in the blood, and it can result in photosensitive dermatitis of unpigmented areas of skin exposed to sunlight for several days (Fig. 2-47). It is possible, however, for mild photosensitization to appear in the absence of gross or microscopic evidence of cholestasis in animals grazing alfalfa, *Paspalum*, pangola, or *Panicum* grasses; however, it is unclear if these are related to phytoporphyrin or other photoactive products of these forages. The absence of serum biochemical evidence for cholestasis or liver damage is used to differentiate primary from secondary photosensitization in these circumstances.

If no hepatic changes can be discerned in photosensitized animals, the possibility of primary photosensitization must be considered, but hepatogenous photosensitization cannot be excluded unless adequate liver function tests are performed.

Hemorrhage and liver failure

Hemorrhagic diathesis characterized by widespread ecchymoses and petechiae can occur when the liver is injured and becomes the site of significant clotting factor consumption. However, investigations suggest that clinically significant hemorrhage is not common in acute liver failure. The liver is the source of plasma proteins involved in the clotting cascade, but these are normally supplied in substantial excess, and can be induced as part of the acute-phase response to inflammation. Thus, *coagulopathy with hemorrhage is most likely to occur when there is acute liver necrosis*, for example, in acute canine infectious hepatitis or xylitol toxicity. Under these conditions, there is significant intrahepatic consumption of clotting factors at sites of endothelial necrosis in the damaged liver. Although the damaged liver also fails to resupply the clotting factors, consumption is probably a minor contributing influence. *In more chronic liver diseases with hypoproteinemia, coagulation tests may be prolonged, but hemorrhagic diathesis is unlikely*, unless there is an added demand for hemostasis, for example, during the trauma of surgery. Although the production of clotting factors is often reduced in liver failure, there is a commensurate reduction in anticoagulant synthesis as well. Portal hypertension and endothelial cell dysfunction may also be a contributing cause of bleeding in chronic liver disease. Overall, the pathogenesis of hemorrhagic tendencies in chronic liver disease is complex, multifactorial, and incompletely understood. Consumption of clotting factors can also occur in septic diseases that affect the liver and other tissues.

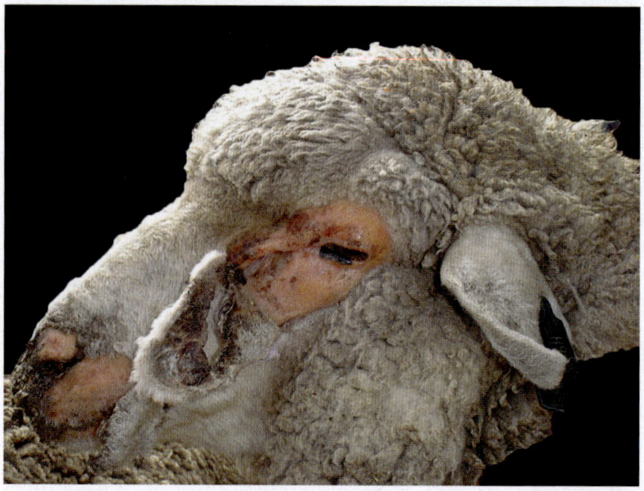

Figure 2-47 Hepatogenous photosensitization caused by *Panicum miliaceum* (French millet) in a sheep. (Courtesy P. Hoskin.)

Nephropathy

Acute liver failure may be accompanied by oliguria and biochemical indications of renal failure. **Hepatorenal syndrome** is a complication of advanced cirrhosis in humans, characterized by renal failure in which there are no intrinsic renal morphologic or functional causes. The pathogenesis of hepatorenal syndrome is related to *deterioration in effective arterial blood volume because of splanchnic arterial vasodilation and reduced venous return and cardiac output*. Intense compensatory vasoconstriction of the renal circulation results in decreased glomerular filtration and resultant renal failure. In addition, some hepatic toxins, such as acetaminophen, may injure the nephrons as well.

Edema and ascites

Ascites (retention of excess low-protein peritoneal fluid) is a feature of chronic liver failure but is more often associated with systemic venous congestion (e.g., right-sided heart failure) or hypoproteinemia secondary to protein-losing renal or alimentary tract conditions. *It is likely that ascites in advanced liver disease is influenced by both mechanical and dynamic influences on blood flow through a damaged liver.* Reduced synthesis of albumin and globulins by the failing liver can reduce vascular oncotic pressure, but edema resulting from this mechanism is generalized. Experimentally, restriction of blood flow from the liver leads to a swift increase in sinusoidal plasma within the perisinusoidal space, leading to increased lymph flow into the thoracic duct and through the hepatic capsule. This explains the rapid formation of ascites in cases of hepatic outflow obstruction or veno-occlusive diseases.

Several theories explain the complicated process of ascites formation in chronic liver disease. The theory that best encompasses the known circulatory changes is the *peripheral arteriolar vasodilation hypothesis.* In end-stage livers, there is progressive sinusoidal and portal vein hypertension with collateral vein formation and acquisition of shunting vessels to the systemic vasculature. Sinusoidal hypertension appears to be an important feature as ascites rarely develop with prehepatic portal hypertension. *The main factor leading to ascites formation is splanchnic vasodilation.* In chronic liver failure, there is increasing portal vein hypertension and a local release of vasodilators, such as nitric oxide, leading to splanchnic arterial dilation. With progression, the extent of the arterial vasodilation increases to the point that effective arterial volume and pressure drops, leading to activation of vasoconstrictor and antinatriuretic factors, including activation of the renin-angiotensin-aldosterone system and the sympathetic nervous system, promoting retention of sodium and fluid. In addition, reduction in clearance of hormones such as aldosterone by the diseased liver contributes to fluid retention. Intestinal capillary pressure and permeability are increased because of the increased portal vein hypertension, promoting excess fluid transit to the abdominal cavity. Over time, sodium retention by the kidneys is insufficient to compensate for the progressive arteriolar vasodilation as well as the movement of sodium and fluid to the extracellular space of the abdomen. This movement is enhanced by hypoproteinemia caused by reduced synthesis by the liver and dilution secondary to fluid retention. Consequently, there is persistent activation of antinatriuretic systems, and fluid continues to accumulate. Increased venous return caused by reduced peripheral arterial vasodilation stimulates endogenous natriuretic substances, but this response is insufficient to counteract the more significant release of antinatriuretic signals.

Retention of peritoneal fluid can also sometimes result from mechanical obstructions to mesenteric and peritoneal lymphatics by inflammatory or neoplastic lesions. Peritoneal fluids with a higher protein and cell content that accumulate in various abdominal inflammatory conditions are considered exudates (see the Peritonitis section in Vol. 2, Alimentary System).

Hepatocutaneous syndrome

An *idiopathic vacuolar hepatopathy with parenchymal collapse and nodular regeneration* has been reported in dogs and cats that have been presented clinically with hepatocutaneous syndrome *(necrolytic migratory erythema, superficial necrolytic dermatitis).* The skin disease resembles necrolytic migratory erythema in humans, a well-defined paraneoplastic syndrome typically associated with hyperglucagonemia secondary to glucagon-secreting pancreatic neoplasia, but also reported in individuals with hepatitis, cirrhosis, celiac disease, chronic malabsorption, and inflammatory bowel disease. *In dogs, hepatocutaneous syndrome is mostly associated with liver disease,* including severe vacuolar hepatopathy, idiopathic hepatocellular loss and stromal collapse, hepatopathy secondary to anticonvulsant drug administration, and, more rarely, with glucagonoma and gastric carcinoma.

Clinical presentation is typically because of dermatitis; skin lesions include erythema, crusting, exudation, ulceration, and alopecia, affecting footpads, periocular, perioral, anogenital regions, and pressure points. The dermatologic lesions are described more fully in Vol. 1, Integumentary System. Affected dogs have depressed plasma amino acid concentrations, inconsistent elevations of plasma glucagon levels, and may also become diabetic. The liver of affected dogs is usually grossly nodular, resembling cirrhosis (eFig. 2-11A); however, histologically, there is typically moderate-to-severe vacuolation of hepatocytes, with parenchymal collapse accompanied by nodular regeneration (see eFig. 2-11B). Inflammation, necrosis, and fibrosis are not usually prominent. Although some studies report fibrosis typical of cirrhosis, more characteristically, a network of reticulin and fine collagen fibers represents the remnants of collapsed hepatic lobules, with proliferation of bile ductules. The vacuolated hepatocytes stain with Oil Red O for lipids. *The hepatic lesions have been suggested to support an underlying metabolic, hormonal, or toxic etiology.* In humans, persistent hyperglucagonemia stimulates prolonged gluconeogenesis, resulting in secondary hypoaminoacidemia. Although hepatic insufficiency can increase glucagon levels in animal models, in dogs, the link between liver disease and hypoaminoacidemia is still unclear. A hypermetabolic state with exaggerated amino acid catabolism has, however, been suggested. Other biologically active molecules that are normally cleared by the normal liver or generated by a damaged liver should also be considered.

POSTMORTEM AND AGONAL CHANGES IN THE LIVER

The liver, rich in nutrients for bacteria and freely exposed to agonal invaders from the intestine, *undergoes postmortem decomposition very rapidly.* Gas bubbles generated by anaerobic saprophytes form first in the hepatic blood vessels, but soon suffuse large portions of the organ. The vessels and adjacent parenchyma are stained by hemoglobin. The substance of the organ becomes soft and claylike, and the formation of putrefactive gases may make it foamy. On the capsular surface, irregular, pale foci are visible; they superficially may resemble infarcts or fatty areas but can be observed to increase in size during the postmortem interval, and microscopically are without cellular reaction. Bacilli are present in large numbers in such foci. Green-black pigmentation of the capsule and superficial parenchyma occurs where the liver is in contact with gut, and the lobes surrounding the gallbladder become stained by bile.

Microscopic structural changes occur in the liver, approaching and immediately following death. Shrinkage of liver cells, possibly because of a period of anaerobic catabolism of glycogen, and widening of centrilobular (periacinar) sinusoids because of hepatic congestion, are seen after death. *Dissociation of liver cells* may be complete, with every cell in every cord separated and free from adjacent cells, so architectural patterns are lost. The early expression of this change affects centrilobular cells, which become detached, rounded, condensed, and hyperchromatic. The dissociation is particularly evident in feline panleukopenia and leptospirosis, related in part to antemortem changes.

VASCULAR FACTORS IN HEPATIC INJURY AND CIRCULATORY DISORDERS

Hepatic artery

The hepatic artery delivers ~20-30% of the afferent hepatic blood supply, but ~40-50% of the oxygen. Hepatic artery flow responds to alterations in portal vein flow to sustain overall perfusion of the liver at a nearly consistent level via what is termed the *hepatic arterial buffer response*. Hepatic arterial flow is believed to be regulated via adenosine levels in the periportal space. Adenosine is produced at a constant level, but with decreased portal flow less adenosine is washed out, raising local concentrations and causing the hepatic artery to dilate and increase arterial flow. Other mediators of arterial flow are recognized and include hydrogen sulfide, nitric oxide, and the autonomic nervous system.

Complete loss of arterial flow can be, after a brief period of injury, compensated for via the portal flow because the liver normally only extracts ~40% of the oxygen supplied by the portal vein. Within the liver, branches of the hepatic artery form several patterns, including 1) a peribiliary plexus, 2) a vasa vasorum for the portal vein, or 3) an array of terminal hepatic arterioles that drain directly into the sinusoids. In addition, the hepatic artery provides branches to supply the liver capsule and vasa vasorum for the sublobular veins. The peribiliary plexus surrounds intrahepatic bile ducts and plays a role in the exchange of bile constituents and vasoactive factors. Hepatic arterial occlusions may occur in animals but usually involve small intrahepatic branches and are of little consequence. Large segments of the liver may be necrotic in cats because of thrombosis of the aorta and hepatic artery. Verminous arteritis may occlude the hepatic artery in horses. The extent of necrosis depends on how completely the obstruction excludes collateral circulation and on the oxygen tension of the portal blood. Ischemic areas of the liver can be sequestered, but in some instances, bacteria such as clostridia and other anaerobes can flourish and release potent toxins with systemic effects.

Portal vein

The portal vein drains the large and small intestine, stomach, pancreas, gallbladder, and spleen, and normally contributes 70-80% of hepatic blood flow. Because the portal vein collects blood from the abdominal viscera, the rate of flow is variable, depending on physiologic factors, such as eating, which increases, or stress, which decreases, portal flow. Portal venous blood has considerably more oxygen than most systemic venous blood and contributes ~60% of the liver's oxygen needs. The portal vein branches successively until the finest branches, the terminal portal venules, drain into the sinusoids via side branches, the inlet venules. The entry of blood into the sinusoids is regulated via sphincters in the terminal inlet venules. Portal blood flow is likely streamlined, rather than turbulent, but there is little agreement about the existence of specific patterns of flow. Streamlining may account for the different regional distributions sometimes observed with metastatic tumors and infections. The umbilical vein usually drains to the left lobe, so hematogenous umbilical infections tend to localize in the left lobe.

The liver cannot regulate portal venous flow, so hepatic blood flow is largely balanced by arterial supply that varies with the portal venous supply to maintain relatively consistent hepatic perfusion. Hepatic microcirculation is well regulated at the level of inflow by sphincters in the finest branches of the portal venules, the inlet venules, as well as the terminal branches of the hepatic arterioles, and at the level of outflow by sphincters that regulate the passage of blood from the sinusoids to the terminal hepatic venules. In dogs, the spiral smooth muscle that invests the wall of sublobular hepatic veins can contract and alter hepatic venous outflow in various conditions, particularly in shock, in which contraction leads to acute congestion and pooling of blood in the liver and the organs that drain into the portal vein. Hepatic blood thus flows evenly through the sinusoids under a very-low–pressure gradient with minor flow adjustment made by stellate cells. The liver receives ~25% of the cardiac output, even though it is only ~2.5% of body mass. Approximately 25% of the weight of the liver in situ is blood. *Obstruction of the portal vein*, if sudden and complete, can produce a condition akin to strangulation of the gut, and death occurs quickly.

Portal hypertension is defined as increased blood pressure within the portal vein caused by resistance to normal flow rates. Portal hypertension can arise from disturbances of venous blood flow in any of the following 3 sites: *prehepatic, intrahepatic, and posthepatic.*

Prehepatic portal hypertension is relatively uncommon and occurs when blood flow through the portal vein is impaired before it enters the liver. The most common cause is portal vein thrombosis. *Portal vein thrombosis* may be caused by damage to the portal vein by local inflammatory processes or be associated with states of hypercoagulability or intravascular growth of portal vein wall or hepatic neoplasms. In dogs, thrombosis of the portal vein has been associated with distant neoplasia, immune-mediated hemolytic anemia, protein-losing nephropathy and enteropathy, pancreatitis, peritonitis, and corticosteroid administration (Fig. 2-48). External compression may occur because of adjacent abscesses or neoplasms. Portal vein obstructions of slow development are expected to lead to portal hypertension and its consequences. Atresia or hypoplasia of the extrahepatic portal vein can be demonstrated in some cases of primary portal vein hypoplasia (PVH) (discussed in the Developmental Disorders section).

Intrahepatic portal hypertension arises from increased resistance to blood flow at the level of the hepatic

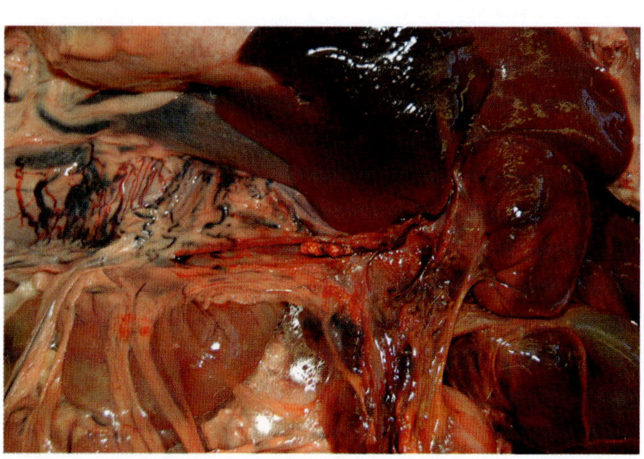

Figure 2-48 **Portal vein thrombosis** in a dog.

parenchyma. Intrahepatic portal hypertension can be subdivided into 3 forms: *presinusoidal, sinusoidal, and postsinusoidal. Presinusoidal forms* include intrahepatic PVH (discussed in the Developmental Disorders section), intrahepatic arterioportal fistulae, periportal neoplastic or inflammatory infiltrates, and periportal fibrosis. Obstruction of many small portal radicles is common, with necrosis of many lobules. If a collateral supply develops and oxygenation remains adequate, obstruction of portal radicles will have no immediate effect on the hepatic parenchyma, save perhaps to make it more sensitive to toxic injury. The parenchyma in the affected lobe, deprived of hepatotrophic factors, loses much of its regenerative power and atrophies rapidly, allowing condensation and scarification of the stromal tissues. *Obstruction of intrahepatic portal vessels* can be a consequence of progressive fibrosing lesions of primary hepatic disease centered on the portal tracts. The small portal vessels may be obliterated in the proliferative portal lesions, and new connections may be established, including small functional arteriovenous communications. Regenerative hepatic nodules and neoplasms may deform and compress portal vessels in some locations. The *sinusoidal* form occurs in cases of cirrhosis or long-term inflammatory disease with fibrosis and capillarization of sinusoids with sinusoidal constriction due to HSCs. Other causes include sinusoidal amyloidosis and neoplastic infiltration. The *postsinusoidal* form arises from the sinusoidal occlusion syndrome (veno-occlusive disease) or forms of perivenous fibrosis.

Posthepatic portal hypertension is uncommon and is discussed in the Efferent hepatic vessels section. *Acute increases in pressure in the portal vein* may occur in any severe episode of widespread acute hepatic necrosis; the cause appears to be simple obstruction of the sinusoidal flow by thrombosis and actual sinusoidal disruption. In such animals, there is severe acute congestion of the liver, slight ascites, free fibrin accumulations in the abdomen (not the firm capsular adhesions seen in passive congestion), and distended portal lymphatics; however, surgical diversion of the portal vein into the vena cava produces only transient injury to the liver. Obstruction of a large branch of the portal vein in cattle, sheep, and cats leads to acute ischemia of a wedge of tissue in which necrosis may be zonal or panlobular. Loss of portal venous inflow and obstruction of hepatic venous outflow, a double-hit insult, can lead to complete infarction of the liver as seen in hepatic lobe torsion. Arterial supply can be obstructed as well in this situation.

Regardless of cause, *persistent portal hypertension can lead to acquired PSSs* (discussed later), except for passive congestion, which rarely, if ever, results in the development of shunts. These shunts are usually numerous and composed of distended thin-walled veins, which may connect the mesenteric veins and the caudal vena cava. Ascites is common in conditions that develop acquired shunts because of the associated portal hypertension.

Efferent hepatic vessels

Efferent flow begins in the sinusoids and passes through terminal hepatic venules and larger hepatic veins to the vena cava. In the sinusoidal network, flow is interconnected in many directions. However, in normal conditions, lobule outflow is closely matched to inflow. In dogs, sublobular hepatic veins have substantial spiral smooth muscle sphincters that regulate outflow, but these are not evident in other domestic species. Splanchnic engorgement during anesthesia and anaphylaxis is an indication that these smooth muscles control canine hepatic outflow in a dynamic manner. Obstruction at the level of the large hepatic veins can occasionally occur because of neutrophilic phlebitis, hepatic abscesses, neoplasms, or other physical obstacles that impinge on the hepatic veins. Similar space-occupying lesions in or around the vena cava in the diaphragm or mediastinum can also affect hepatic outflow, along with systemic venous return.

The amount and arrangement of conventional connective tissue around the terminal hepatic veins and larger hepatic veins influence the patterns of fibrosis seen in various patterns of centrilobular injury. Hypoxia from anemia, heart failure, or shock can cause centrilobular necrosis, as can many toxic agents that are preferentially injurious to zone 3 hepatocytes. Necrosis at this level elicits a tissue repair response involving the fibrous connective tissue along the terminal hepatic venules. Tissue fibrosis can increase the resistance of hepatic parenchyma and slow local outflow. This can redirect sinusoidal blood to alternative less affected venules unless the necrosis is extensive.

Sinusoidal obstruction syndrome (SOS) previously termed *hepatic veno-occlusive disease is the obliteration of small intrahepatic veins that may begin with damage to the sinusoidal endothelium, accumulation of red cells and fibrin in the subintimal space, and subsequent subendothelial fibrosis*. This pattern of postnecrotic fibrosis can contribute to the development of portal hypertension. SOS is a feature of pyrrolizidine toxicosis in humans ingesting these alkaloids in the so-called *bush tea*. In domestic animals, occlusive changes in terminal venules are notable in poisoning by ragwort *(Senecio jacobaea)* in cattle and in dogs treated experimentally with the pyrrolizidine alkaloid monocrotaline. SOS has also been reported because of prolonged chemotherapy, radiotherapy, and bone marrow transplantation in humans, and similarly in dogs treated with irradiation or busulfan. Idiopathic SOS with perivenular fibrosis around central and sublobular veins, causing *Budd-Chiari–like syndrome* (see later), has also been reported as a rare occurrence in the dog and cat. Total or subtotal obliteration of central hepatic or sublobular veins by subintimal accumulation of collagen and fibrous tissue has also been reported in captive snow leopards and cheetahs.

Passive congestion of the liver develops when the blood pressure in the hepatic veins increases compared with that of the hepatic portal veins and can occur in any species. *It is almost always the consequence of cardiac dysfunction*, including acute and chronic heart failure, pericardial disease, and processes that obstruct the flow of blood into or out of the heart, such as abscesses, heartworm disease, and local neoplasia. Right-sided heart failure produces elevated pressure within the caudal vena cava that later involves the hepatic vein and its tributaries.

Acute passive congestion of the liver occurs when there is sudden cardiac decompensation, particularly on the right side of the heart, or shock. Grossly, there is slight enlargement of the liver, which is typically dark-red, and blood flows freely from any cut surface (Fig. 2-49). The intrinsic lobular pattern of the liver may be slightly more pronounced, particularly on the cut surface, because centrilobular areas are congested (dark-red) in contrast to the more normal color of the rest of the lobule. The microscopic picture in acute passive congestion is initially characterized by distension of central veins

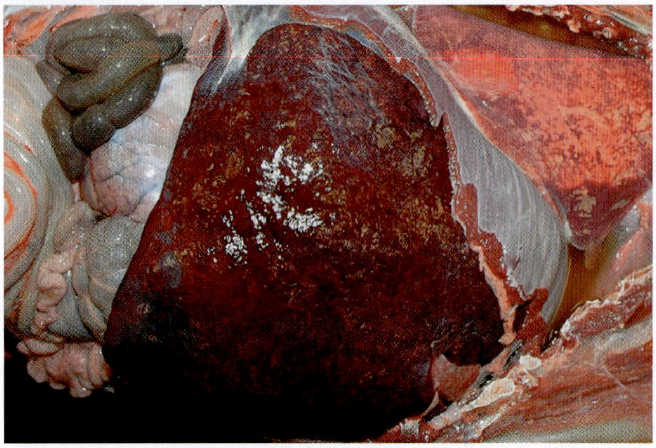

Figure 2-49 **Acute passive congestion** of the liver in a cria with a congenital heart defect.

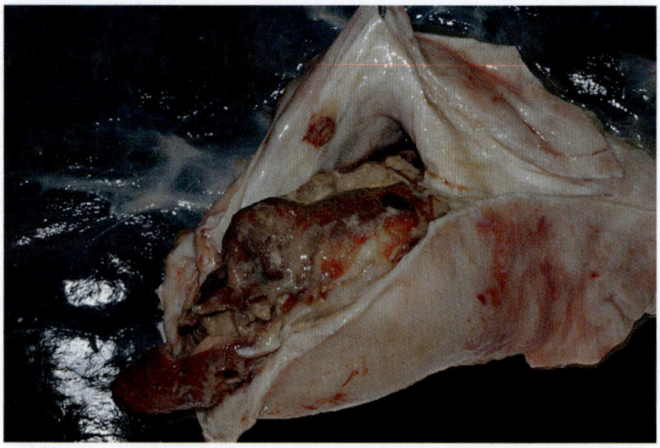

Figure 2-50 **Thromboembolism of the caudal vena cava** in an ox. (Courtesy K.G. Thompson.)

and adjacent sinusoids, with accompanying distension of lymphatics in the stroma of hepatic veins, portal tracts, and the capsule. The appearance of the liver differs with the duration and severity of the congestion. Fatty change, trabecular atrophy, and necrosis of centrilobular hepatocytes with retention of the perisinusoidal reticulum framework develop quickly. Erythrocytes tend to move into the perisinusoidal spaces left by the lost hepatocytes and may be seen trapped there when blood drains from sinusoids and veins in freshly fixed sections. The intrahepatic network of lymphatics at this stage becomes very distended and may form extensive cavernous channels about hepatic veins and venules, in portal tracts, and just beneath the capsule. With increased venous pressure, transudation of red blood cells and high protein–content edema can develop, leading to polymerization of released fibrinogen on the capsular surface that yields a fibrin coating of the capsule and blood-tinged abdominal fluid. Distension of the perisinusoidal spaces may be seen, but rarely, if ever, in tissue well fixed soon after death, and is best regarded as a postmortem artifact. By comparison, perisinusoidal edema is more obvious in hepatic congestion associated with shock or inflammatory conditions.

In **chronic passive congestion**, the amounts of fibrous connective tissue in the liver increase in various patterns that differ among species. The capsular surface becomes thicker and more opaque and can develop a finely nodular texture with the formation of capsular plaques (eFig. 2-12A). In dogs and cats, the edges of the central lobes become rounded; the margins of lateral and caudate lobes are sharpened by peripheral atrophy and fibrosis. If the cause of the congestion is still present, there is usually copious ascites at this stage. In species in which fibrosis is more pronounced, a chronically congested liver has a distinct reticulated lobular pattern, often more obvious beneath the capsule than in deeper parenchyma. This pattern is known as **"nutmeg liver"** and is *the result of the contrast of red centrilobular zones of congestion with loss of hepatocytes, among pale swollen periportal parenchyma composed of viable hepatocytes that are fatty* (see eFig. 2-12B). This classic pattern of chronic passive congestion is most obvious in ruminants and horses. The "nutmeg" pattern can be mimicked by some forms of toxic periacinar necrosis or fatty change but should always be distinguishable from them by the fibrous plaques in the hepatic capsule in the passively congested liver. The pale lobular pattern is less obvious in carnivores and should not be expected in animals that have insufficient adipose reserves for mobilization. Over longer periods, *centrilobular fibrosis links terminal hepatic venules with one another and with the larger portal tracts in a pattern known as* ***cardiac fibrosis***.

Inflammatory changes in the outflow veins are sometimes seen. Acute inflammation and thrombosis of sublobular veins are typical of acute salmonellosis in many species, but these changes are terminal and not associated with hepatic dysfunction. Inflammatory cell infiltration is occasionally observed in the larger hepatic veins and has been described in dogs with parvoviral myocarditis. Muscular hypertrophy of walls of hepatic veins has been described in dogs with arteriovenous fistulae. Fibrous remodeling of these veins has been associated with nitrosamine intoxication in domestic animals.

The term **Budd-Chiari syndrome** is used to describe the clinical features associated with hepatic venous outflow obstruction caused by thrombosis of the main hepatic veins in humans. **Hepatic vein thrombosis** is a rare occurrence in dogs and cats. In veterinary medicine, it is more appropriate to use specific morphologic diagnostic terms to describe pathologic changes that develop in response to various mechanical causes of postsinusoidal obstruction of hepatic venous flow, resulting in the development of *hepatomegaly, postsinusoidal portal hypertension, high-protein ascites, and acquired portosystemic collateral shunting*. Causes include obstruction of flow caused by tumors (e.g., intraluminal leiomyosarcoma or other vascular wall sarcomas, adrenal pheochromocytoma with extensive invasion into the caudal vena cava in the dog) or abscesses in the liver or caudal vena cava, hepatic venous or vena caval thrombosis, congenital malformation (fibrous web), kink or acquired stricture occluding the lumen of the vena cava or hepatic veins, or cardiac abnormalities impairing right atrial function (cor triatrium dexter, neoplasia). Histologic changes include distension of the hepatic veins and perivenous sinusoidal congestion, which, with chronicity, leads to perivenous fibrosis typical of chronic passive congestion.

Thrombosis of the caudal vena cava has been described in detail in cattle, in which rupture of a hepatic abscess into the caudal vena cava is the most common etiology (Fig. 2-50). Sequelae include pulmonary emboli, endoarteritis, multifocal pulmonary abscessation, and chronic neutrophilic bronchopneumonia.

Acquired portosystemic shunts

Congenital shunts have been described previously in the Developmental Disorders section. *Acquired portosystemic shunts (PSSs) within and external to the liver can develop in association with various chronic liver diseases that lead to portal hypertension. These shunts tend to be multiple, small, and tortuous* (see Fig. 2-9). They may be difficult to identify postmortem when they are collapsed. They are easily destroyed by routine dissection, so they must be noted before removal of the abdominal viscera. Acquired shunts can be associated with evidence of portal hypertension, such as distension of the portal veins and ascites, but when shunts are multiple and well established, portal hypertension is somewhat relieved. *It is important to distinguish these varicose dilations that develop in response to portal hypertension from true congenital PSSs.* Acquired PSSs arise in vestigial nonfunctional portosystemic communications that dilate and become functional in response to portal hypertension. They tend to develop between mesenteric veins and the caudal vena cava, right renal vein, or gonadal veins, and are multiple, taking the form of *a plexus of tortuous, thin-walled vessels*. Esophageal shunts and varicosities are common in humans with cirrhosis but are much less important in domestic animals. This may be related to postural differences such that shunts are more likely to enter the vena cava, where central venous pressure is least. In dogs, acquired PSSs are most numerous along the caudal mesentery.

In cats, mostly spayed females, there is an unusual condition characterized by a large shunting vessel that courses within the abdominal cavity and connects the splenic vein to the vena cava, termed the "*spaghetti sign*" by radiologists. This structure is thought to presage shunting due to hypertension in some instances and may be incidental in others. It is not clear if they are congenital or acquired.

Hepatic sinusoidal angiectasis (peliosis hepatis)

Hepatic sinusoidal angiectasis *(peliosis hepatis, also known as "telangiectasis") is a disorder of cystic, blood-filled spaces in the liver.* The terminology used to describe sinusoidal lesions unfortunately varies between authors, and the pathogenesis of hepatic angiectasis is speculative. Hepatic sinusoidal angiectasis should not be confused with **cystic degeneration** (spongiosis hepatis, eFig 2-13A) in which cystic spaces are filled with acidophilic material rather than blood. Hepatic angiectasis has been reported in humans, cattle, dogs, and cats, but the pathogenesis is unknown. *Two forms of angiectasis occur* in the liver, and both can appear in the same animal. Presumptive perturbation of sinusoidal outflow and/or intrinsic weakness of the sinusoidal wall lead to hemodynamic imbalance and cystic sinusoidal dilation in the *phlebectatic (cystic) form* of angiectasis. The *parenchymal (cavernous) form* is presumed to result from primary loss of hepatocytes and sinusoidal ectasia. The angiectatic lesions occur throughout the liver as dark-red areas, irregular in shape but well circumscribed, and range from pinpoint to many centimeters in size (Fig. 2-51, eFig 2-13B). Sectioned or capsular surfaces are depressed after death, and on cutting, blood drains from the cavities to reveal a delicate network of residual stroma. Histologically, the dilated, blood-filled spaces are sometimes surrounded by fibromyxoid stroma and may or may not be lined by endothelium.

Hepatic sinusoidal angiectasis is quite common in older cats, cattle, and dogs (Fig. 2-52). There is no evidence clinically of related liver dysfunction. The cavities in cats are more frequent in the subcapsular zone and rarely exceed 2-3 mm. Other senile changes in these livers are frequent and include chronic fatty change, nodular hyperplasia, and chronic hepatitis. In humans, hepatic angiectasis has an idiosyncratic association with administration of various drugs, including anabolic and contraceptive steroids. Infectious angiectasis caused by *Bartonella henselae* or *B. quintana* infection has also been described in immunosuppressed human patients. Hepatic angiectasis in cats has not been found to be associated with *B. henselae* infection.

A specific condition termed *"peliosis"* develops in cattle poisoned by *Pimelea* spp. plants. This form begins as *diffuse periportal sinusoidal dilation*. Because these changes are also found in these animals in the spleen and in other organs with sinusoidal microcirculation, it seems that the lesions may be adaptive to progressive and dramatic increases in total blood volume. In the late stages of the intoxication by *Pimelea*, the liver may resemble a huge, blood-filled sponge (Fig. 2-53). The animals eventually die of a combination of hemodilutional anemia and circulatory failure.

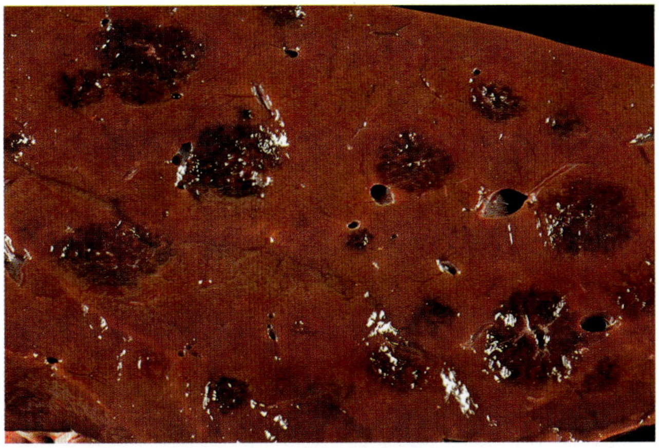

Figure 2-51 **Hepatic sinusoidal angiectasis** (peliosis hepatis, telangiectasis) in an ox. (Courtesy K.G. Thompson.)

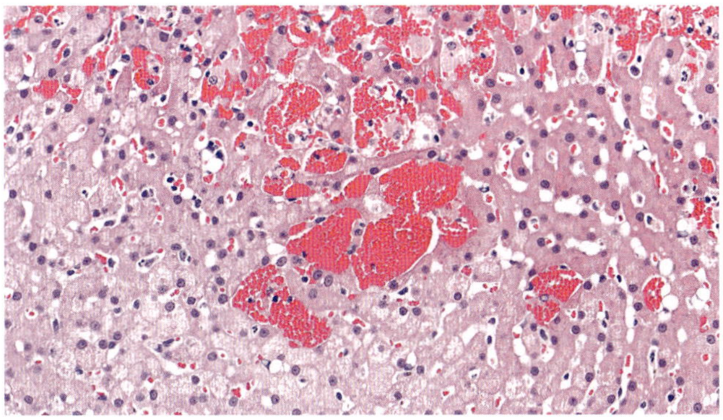

Figure 2-52 Histologic appearance of **hepatic sinusoidal angiectasis** (peliosis hepatis) in a dog.

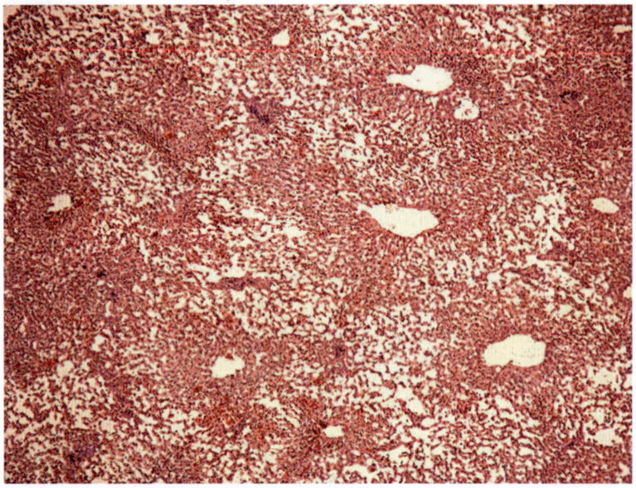

Figure 2-53 Periportal sinusoidal dilation ("peliosis") resulting from chronic *Pimelea* poisoning in an ox. (Courtesy R. Kelly.)

INFLAMMATORY DISEASES OF THE LIVER AND BILIARY TRACT

The inflammatory response in the liver is unusual for 3 main reasons. First, ***hepatic microvasculature*** *is structurally and functionally different from tissues with capillary vasculature.* Microvascular permeability to plasma proteins, a hallmark of acute inflammation in most tissues, is a normal property of the fenestrated sinusoidal endothelium of the liver. Thus, sinusoidal edema is not a prominent feature of acute parenchymal inflammation, although edema can be seen in the capsule, portal tracts, connective tissue of the terminal and sublobular hepatic veins (particularly in dogs), and in the wall of the gallbladder. Microvascular blood flow in hepatic sinusoids is also less responsive to the actions of various vasoactive mediators that alter blood flow in most other acutely inflamed tissues.

Second, resident ***Kupffer cells*** *play an important and complex role in liver inflammation, injury, and repair.* Kupffer cells function in the innate immune response, acting as the final component of the gut barrier by phagocytosing pathogens, immunoreactive material, and endotoxin entering the liver via the portal circulation. However, Kupffer cells also show a range of activated phenotypes, depending on the local metabolic and immune environment. Classically activated macrophages secrete proinflammatory cytokines, including TNF, IL1, IL6, IL12, and inducible nitric oxide synthase, influencing cell populations in the liver and elsewhere; alternatively, activated macrophages express anti-inflammatory mediators, including IL10, and contribute to resolution of inflammation and promote repair. Dysregulation of the complex control of inflammatory responses in Kupffer cells can contribute to chronic inflammation in the liver.

Third, *the liver has* ***central regulatory influences*** *on many proinflammatory insults and inflammatory mediators.* As the major source of acute-phase proteins, including secreted pathogen recognition receptors, short pentraxins, components of the complement system, and regulators of iron metabolism, hepatocytes are essential constituents of innate immunity and contribute importantly to the control of a systemic inflammatory response. The liver is also the site of degradation of most soluble plasma proteins, and Kupffer cells are the main site of clearance of immune complexes from the circulation, playing an important role in the development of immunotolerance to potential antigenic substances absorbed from the intestine. A full discussion of immune surveillance, and the complex innate and adaptive immune responses involved in initiation and regulation of liver inflammation, is beyond the scope of this chapter, and readers are directed to current review articles on the subject.

These unusual aspects of the inflammatory response in the liver can make it more difficult to differentiate certain degenerative and inflammatory conditions in this organ. Ongoing cell death and repair can appear inflammatory, and acute leukocytic responses can cause necrosis and apoptosis in the liver. *The term* **"necroinflammatory"** *is convenient when the underlying pathogenetic mechanisms of necrosis and inflammation are unknown.*

Increased numbers of leukocytes **(sinusoidal leukocytosis)** are seen in hepatic sinusoids in many acute or subacute bacteremias, as well as in conditions of steroid excess in dogs. This change can be diagnostically useful but does not constitute evidence of hepatitis unless there is obvious infiltration of granulocytes, monocytes, or lymphocytes into the perisinusoidal space. **Extramedullary hematopoiesis** can also appear as focal aggregates of myeloid cells in the sinusoidal compartment. This change can be distinguished from inflammatory infiltrates by the presence of immature myeloid cells and lack of evidence of cell injury. Occasionally, hematopoietic cells from the splenic red pulp can be artifactually extruded into the portal vasculature and appear in the liver, usually as nucleated cell aggregates in the larger portal veins.

Infectious agents capable of causing hepatitis include viruses, bacteria, fungi, protozoa, and helminths. Autoimmune and idiosyncratic drug responses also occur, but often the etiology of acute or chronic hepatitis cannot be determined.

Hepatic inflammation

The liver is subject to infectious and degenerative insults that elicit inflammatory responses in various patterns, for which the general term *hepatitis* is appropriate. Unlike many organs, the liver harbors a dense network of phagocytes that maintain tolerance under noninflammatory conditions. These cells quickly sense hepatocyte stress and injury signals leading to the activation of proinflammatory cascades. The term **hepatitis** is used for *focal or diffuse hepatic conditions that are either caused by infectious agents or characterized by a leukocytic infiltrative inflammatory response, irrespective of the cause.* These leukocytes swiftly infiltrate the liver parenchyma, contributing to inflammation and fibrogenesis by producing soluble mediators that activate nonparenchymal cell population and other immune cells. This definition allows inclusion of viral infections that are hepatotropic, even though the lesions are mainly characterized by hepatocellular necrosis or apoptosis rather than by the inflammatory response to the agent. The term hepatitis is also used for responses to some hepatic toxicants, metals, or drug metabolic idiosyncrasies in which there is a prominent leukocytic response to damaged cells. However, in responses in which single necrotic hepatocytes elicit a mild neutrophilic or histiocytic response, the term hepatitis is less appropriate because the pattern of injury is primarily degenerative. **Cholangitis** *refers to inflammation of the biliary tree.* More specifically, **choledochitis** refers to inflammation of the bile ducts, and **cholecystitis** refers to inflammation of the gallbladder. **Cholangiohepatitis** *applies to hepatic inflammation centered on the biliary tract and extending into adjacent hepatic parenchyma.*

Patterns and character of inflammation in hepatitis vary according to causative agent, severity and stage of disease, the route of entry into the liver, and pathogenesis of liver injury. Some viral pathogens, such as canine adenovirus 1, can cause acute and diffuse hepatitis, with centrilobular-to-widespread hepatocellular necrosis, mixed leukocyte infiltrates, sinusoidal congestion, and edema. By comparison, most infectious causes of hepatitis, for example, toxoplasmosis, various herpesviruses, and various bacteria, produce a random pattern of inflammation with focally intense leukocyte and Kupffer cell responses in the vicinity of areas of necrosis. The distribution, character, and chronicity of these focal lesions are important diagnostically, but they typically do not damage enough functional hepatic parenchyma, ducts, or vasculature to produce systemic signs of liver failure. Foci of hepatitis with necrosis are common incidental findings, and these are assumed to reflect localized responses to bacteria that arrive via the portal system. Occasionally, such focal necroinflammatory lesions are large and numerous, for example, in cattle with rumenitis.

Acute hepatitis

Hallmarks of acute hepatitis typically include a combination of inflammation, usually a granulocytic inflammatory cell infiltrate, foci of hepatocellular apoptosis and necrosis, and, in some instances, evidence of regeneration. Leukocyte infiltrates in acute diffuse hepatitis tend to accumulate mainly in the vicinity of the portal tracts, around major bile ducts, or sometimes in the capsule and around the central veins. Small but important numbers of neutrophils and mononuclear cells, including lymphocytes, are usually seen in the perisinusoidal space and among hepatocytes and are often focally concentrated in sites of necrosis, or adjacent to infectious organisms. Edema is an unusual feature of acute hepatitis but is seen in severe injury, for example, in infectious canine hepatitis (ICH). Grossly, hepatic edema is most obvious in the gallbladder, large extrahepatic bile ducts, hepatic lymph nodes, and sometimes in the capsule. Microscopically, edema is also evident in the portal tracts, in the connective tissue of the terminal and sublobular veins, and sometimes by an increase in the perisinusoidal space.

Kupffer cells are key participants in the acute inflammatory responses in the liver. They can enlarge and accumulate vacuoles and lysosomal debris during regular phagocytic removal of microorganisms, cell debris, and extravascular erythrocytes. They can also be activated to secretory histiocytes that release various cytokines and other mediators that induce hypertrophic or proliferative responses of hepatocytes, stellate cells, and endothelium. Activated Kupffer cells are larger and more prominent or numerous in sections, their nuclei are larger and vesicular, and their cytoplasm is basophilic and may contain vacuoles or ingested particulate matter. In overwhelming infections, many of the Kupffer cells and adjacent sinusoidal endothelial cells and hepatocytes undergo necrosis.

Chronic hepatitis

Chronic liver disease in domestic animals has historically been classified into several different entities based on morphologic criteria, but *fibrosis is a consistent feature*. In human medicine, classification of chronic hepatitis has been simplified, and morphologic divisions such as chronic active hepatitis and chronic persistent hepatitis, originally defined in specific clinical contexts, have been abandoned because of problems of evolving definitions and application, and lack of correspondence with prognosis. The single designation **"chronic hepatitis"** is now used for *chronic necroinflammatory disease*. Chronic hepatitis is characterized by hepatocellular death either by apoptosis or necrosis, a variable inflammatory infiltrate of either mononuclear or mixed inflammatory cells, along with fibrosis and often regeneration. The extent and distribution of these components vary widely. Consequently, it is necessary to include the activity and stage of the disease in the diagnosis as well as the possible etiology. The *activity* of the disease is determined by the quantity of inflammation and extent of hepatocellular death, which can be seen as interface hepatitis as well as random focal or a confluent pattern within the lobule.

Interface hepatitis, previously referred to as *"piecemeal necrosis,"* often occurs in chronic hepatitis (Fig. 2-54). Interface hepatitis is characterized by an *inflammatory infiltrate that penetrates the limiting plate of periportal hepatocytes over a portion or the entirety of the circumference of the limiting plate and causes hepatocyte death*. This process may continue to erode into the hepatic parenchyma, expanding the portal areas. Portal inflammation is variable in intensity and includes infiltration by lymphocytes and plasma cells primarily. The mechanisms may involve either direct damage to hepatocytes by the uptake of antigen-antibody complexes or cooperation between macrophages and T lymphocytes. These may cause cell-mediated destruction of hepatocytes that have taken up these complexes or, perhaps, native antigen or virus. Whatever the agency, the mode of cell removal in this sort of injury often takes the form of *single-cell necrosis or apoptosis*, which may be directly triggered by immunologically competent cells. Bridging necrosis, with tracts of necrosis dissecting across the hepatic lobule between portal tracts or between portal areas and central veins, may also develop. Degenerative changes affecting hepatocytes in areas of interface hepatitis include cell swelling and apoptosis. Bile duct degeneration, multifocal necrosis, and hepatocellular regeneration, in the form of 2-cell–thick hepatic plates and mitotic figures, may also be seen. Single or small groups of hepatocytes may be isolated and entrapped in expanded portal areas.

The *stage* of the disease, and thus the possible prognosis, is determined by the extent and pattern of fibrosis and

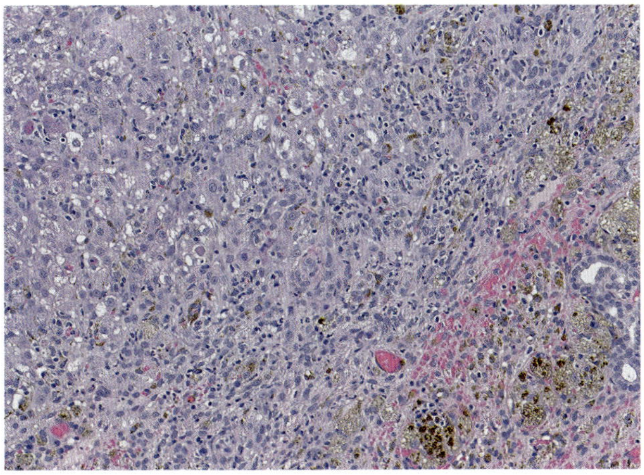

Figure 2-54 Periportal interface hepatitis in chronic hepatitis in a dog.

the possible architectural distortion. Fibrosis may occur as porto-portal, porto-central, and centro-central fibrosis or lobular dissecting, following collapse and condensation of the reticulin network or by direct activation of HSCs with perisinusoidal deposition of collagen. Deposition of collagen and basement membrane material in the perisinusoidal space leads to capillarization of hepatic sinusoids. Regeneration and, in dogs, regenerative nodules of hepatocytes are often seen as well as proliferation of ductular structures at the periphery of the parenchyma and within fibrous septa. Numerous systems for *grading and staging chronic hepatitis* have been developed.

In human medicine, chronic hepatitis is usually the result of chronic infection with hepatotropic viruses, and, less commonly, autoimmune, drug-induced, or associated with inherited metabolic diseases, such as Wilson disease. In veterinary medicine, chronic liver disease may develop following chronic bile duct obstruction, familial or hereditary metabolic diseases, or may be toxicant-, drug-induced, or possibly autoimmune in origin. Infectious etiologies are rare in domestic animals except for domestic cat hepadnavirus. However, *most of the chronic liver disease in dogs and cats is idiopathic*, reflecting deficiencies in our current level of understanding of the etiologic, pathophysiologic, and clinical implications of the patterns of inflammation and necrosis.

Regardless of the etiology, *initial acute liver damage will not progress to fibrosis or cirrhosis unless the inflammation and damage are protracted*, for example, by ongoing hepatocellular injury mediated by immunologic mechanisms, including antibody- and lymphocyte-mediated cytotoxicity, or ongoing oxidative damage. Clinical signs are nonspecific in the early stages, but as the disease progresses to involve more of the liver and impair regeneration, icterus, ascites, and HE may develop as typical correlates with hepatic insufficiency.

Chronic hepatitis in dogs

Chronic hepatitis is a relatively common diagnosis in dogs, characterized by hepatocellular apoptosis or necrosis, a variable mononuclear or mixed inflammatory cell infiltrate, evidence of regenerative attempts, and fibrosis of variable extent and pattern. Although various infectious etiologies and drug- and toxicant-induced chronic hepatic disease have been described, *most remain idiopathic, although excess hepatic copper accumulation is the best characterized cause of chronic hepatitis in the dog. Disease grade* in the dog is correlated with increasing hepatocellular apoptosis, proliferation, expression of nitric oxide synthase isoforms, and total hepatic iron; *disease stage* is correlated with increasing α–smooth muscle actin–labeled periductular myofibroblasts and perisinusoidal stellate cells, CK7-positive ductular cells, the ECM protein tenascin-C, and expression of genes important in the production and regulation of hepatic fibrosis, including platelet-derived growth factors (PDGFB and PDGFD), thrombospondin 1, transforming growth factors β1 and β2 (TGF-β1 and TGF-β2), matrix metalloproteinase 2 and tissue inhibitor of matrix metalloproteinase 1, and the collagen genes *COL1A1* and *COL3A1*.

Breeds of dogs reported to be at increased risk for chronic hepatitis include the Bedlington Terrier, Doberman Pinscher, West Highland White Terrier, Labrador Retriever, American and English Cocker Spaniel, Skye Terrier, Standard Poodle, Dalmatian, and English Springer Spaniel. Hepatic copper accumulation in association with chronic hepatitis has been documented in most of these breeds, but chronic hepatitis may be present without copper excess.

The mechanism and role of **hepatic copper** accumulation in dogs continue to generate interest. The heavy metal copper is an essential trace element that plays a significant role in many essential biologic processes, including mitochondrial respiration (cytochrome C oxidase), connective tissue maturation cross-linking (lysyl oxidase), antioxidant defense (superoxide dismutase), melanin synthesis (tyrosinase), iron metabolism (ceruloplasmin), and neurotransmitter biosynthesis (dopamine β-hydroxylase). However, *copper is toxic at excess concentrations because of its 2 redox states that can mediate free-radical production, resulting in direct oxidation of cellular components*. The liver is the major organ involved in the regulation of copper levels, and homeostasis is maintained by the balance of dietary intake and copper excretion via the bile. Dietary copper is taken up by the enterocytes of the small intestine by dedicated transporters, divalent metal transporter (DMT1) and copper transporter 1 (Ctr1), conveyed in the portal blood bound to carrier proteins ceruloplasmin and transcuprein, or in a nonspecific manner to albumin, to the liver for uptake. In the hepatocyte, copper is sequestered in metallothionein or glutathione. Excretion into the bile or blood is regulated by a series of specific chaperone proteins, such as COMMD1 and the copper-transporting ATPases ATP7A and ATP7B. Excess copper is stored in lysosomes. Copper-induced cell death is termed **cuproptosis**, a process by which excess Cu^{2+} causes mitochondrial stress, especially via copper binding to lipoylated enzymes in the TCA cycle in the mitochondria, which leads to subsequent lipoylated protein aggregation, and the loss of iron-sulfur (Fe-S) cluster protein, essential cofactors most commonly known for their role mediating electron transfer within the mitochondrial respiratory chain. Cellular metabolism, structural integrity, and energy generation are affected.

Hepatic copper accumulation can arise 1) as the result of a primary metabolic defect in hepatic copper metabolism, 2) as a consequence of excess dietary copper intake, or 3) possibly secondary to cholestasis and altered biliary copper excretion. While it is recognized that copper is excreted through the bile and cats develop histochemically detectable copper with cholestasis, there is little evidence to suggest that dogs accumulate enough copper to be detected by typical stains due to cholestasis, based on experimental studies following ligation of the common bile duct.

In the dog, the relationship between liver copper concentration and hepatitis is not well understood. The reference interval for hepatic copper is generally considered to be ≤400 µg/g dry weight (DW); concentrations >1,800-2,000 µg/g DW are considered pathogenic. Individual variation in the copper levels and the degree of hepatic injury is common, suggesting that additional factors, such as the antioxidant status of the dog, medications, diet, and microbiome, may contribute to a multifactorial pathogenesis. *In primary genetic copper storage disorders and excess copper intake, copper accumulation appears at least initially to be primarily centrilobular, extending throughout the lobule as the condition progresses*, with hepatic copper concentrations usually >2,000 µg/g DW. When the hepatic concentration of copper surpasses ~400 µg/g DW, the excess begins to accumulate within lysosomes. These copper-laden lysosomes become consistently demonstrable by the histochemical stains rubeanic acid and rhodanine at copper concentrations >400 µg/g DW (Fig. 2-55), although some studies

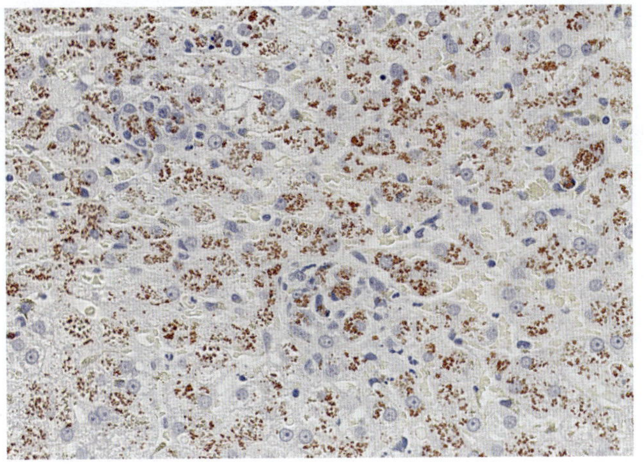

Figure 2-55 **Copper staining** (rhodanine) in the liver of a Dalmatian.

note visible copper granules at hepatic copper concentrations as low as 200 µg/g DW. A reasonable estimate of copper burden can be made from stained sections; however, biochemical determination of copper is more reliable and can be useful to follow the effectiveness of copper chelation therapy. Care should be taken when collecting liver for copper levels, as once the normal lobular architecture is lost because of injury and regenerative nodule formation, copper distribution within the liver becomes heterogeneous. Hepatocytes in regenerative nodules often have relatively low levels of copper, possibly as an adaptation that facilitates their ability to proliferate and form nodules, or as a function of inadequate time for significant copper accumulation in the hepatocytes forming nodules. The intervening areas of parenchymal collapse may contain an abundance of copper. Because of this regional variation, small samples, such as those taken from needle biopsies, are often inaccurate, and larger samples are needed.

Regardless of the reasons for copper accumulation, lysosomal copper can exceed a threshold or be released when hepatocytes die, and thereby contribute to the development of hepatitis. The relationship between liver copper levels and inflammation appear complex as relatively high values can be found in some dogs with normal liver histology, and other factors, such as antioxidant levels and other oxidative stress from drugs or other factors, may influence the relationship between copper concentration and injury.

A hereditary, *autosomal recessive copper-associated hepatopathy* associated with impaired biliary copper excretion and progressive accumulation of copper within hepatocytes has been well documented in ***Bedlington Terriers***. Most affected Bedlington Terriers have been found deficient in a protein, COMMD1 (copper metabolism MURR1 domain protein–1), caused by deletion of exon 2 in the *COMMD1* gene, although there are other less common mutations that can also occur. Although its function is not fully understood, the COMMD1 protein has been shown to interact with the copper transporter ATP7B, important in Wilson disease, a copper storage disorder in humans, and its absence in affected dogs may impair ATP7B-mediated copper export from hepatocytes into the canaliculus. Homozygous affected dogs have the highest copper levels. *Bedlington Terriers are the only breed to date shown to accumulate copper continuously throughout life*, and hepatic copper concentrations in these animals may be exceedingly high; as much as 12,000 µg/g DW has been recorded, and levels >5,000 µg/g are common. Affected dogs usually have signs of progressive liver failure, including ill-thrift, wasting, ascites, and signs of encephalopathy. An acute form may occur in some dogs, with acute hepatic necrosis and release of copper into the systemic circulation, where it provokes a hemolytic crisis and rapidly developing anemia and icterus (eFig. 2-14). The initial histologic lesion is multifocal centrilobular hepatitis, with foci of macrophages, lymphocytes, plasma cells, and neutrophils among the copper-laden hepatocytes in zone 3. Apoptotic hepatocytes, some containing copper granules, appear at the periphery of some foci. Copper levels >3,000 µg/g DW result in widespread necrosis in some dogs. Survivors may progress to develop postnecrotic cirrhosis. Grossly, the livers in later stages are fibrotic, pale, and finely nodular.

Copper-associated chronic hepatitis can develop in ***Labrador Retrievers***, with centrilobular hepatocytes and infiltrates of macrophages containing intracytoplasmic copper and hemosiderin, fewer neutrophils, mononuclear inflammatory cells, as well as scattered foci of hepatocellular necrosis, lobular collapse, portal and centrilobular-to-bridging fibrosis, nodular regeneration, and in some cases cirrhosis. Mutations in the copper chaperones *ATP7A* and *ATP7B* have been shown in this breed. Hepatic copper concentrations in one study were typically >2,000 µg/g; the mean hepatic copper concentrations in a separate study were also found to be significantly higher in affected dogs (614 µg/g, range 104-4,234 µg/g) compared with age- and sex-matched control dogs (299 µg/g, range 93-3,810 µg/g). A concurrent general increase in hepatic copper concentrations in a study population of Labrador Retrievers spanning 30 years was postulated to be associated with increased dietary copper availability, the result of a change in the form and bioavailability of supplemental copper added to commercially produced dog foods. A positive association between dietary copper levels and hepatic copper concentrations has been demonstrated, and high dietary copper has been suggested as a risk factor for development of copper-associated hepatitis in susceptible animals within the breed. Concurrent renal proximal tubular dysfunction with glucosuria and increased renal copper has been described in some Labrador Retrievers with copper-associated hepatitis, and sporadically in other breeds.

Chronic hepatitis is well documented in ***Doberman Pinschers***. The disease is more common in middle-aged female dogs. Histologic changes in the livers of dogs with clinical signs of advanced hepatic disease include interface hepatitis of periportal hepatocytes, with a mixed inflammatory cell infiltrate, as well as necrosis of centrilobular hepatocytes with bridging necrosis crossing the lobule (Fig. 2-56). Copper accumulation is evident in centrilobular hepatocytes, with various degrees of portal fibrosis, ductular reaction, bridging fibrosis, and development of cirrhosis in the most severely affected dogs. Intracanalicular bile stasis can be present, along with iron accumulation in Kupffer cells and macrophages.

Elevated concentrations of hepatic copper have been reported in many, but not all, Doberman Pinschers with chronic hepatitis, and *the significance of increased hepatic copper concentration in this breed remains controversial*. An investigation into the possibility of impaired copper excretion in affected Doberman Pinschers reported that 5 dogs with elevated liver copper and persistent subclinical hepatitis but without demonstrable cholestasis had comparable rates of plasma copper clearance to control dogs, but reduced rates of biliary excretion of ^{64}Cu, suggesting that impaired copper

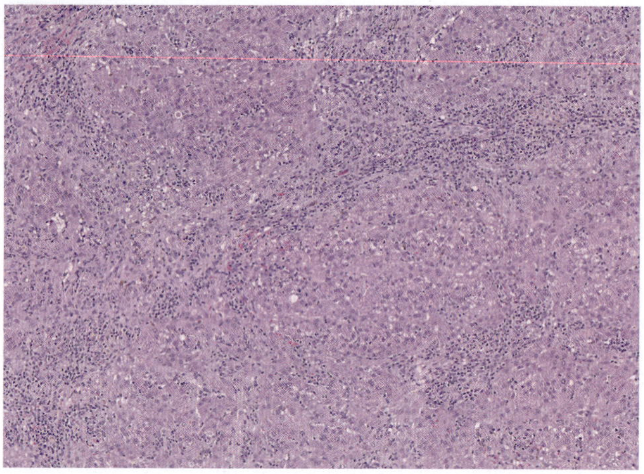

Figure 2-56 Chronic hepatitis with mixed inflammatory cell infiltrates in a Doberman Pinscher dog.

excretion may play a role in disease in this breed. Significantly reduced levels of mRNA of various proteins involved in copper binding, transport, and excretion, including ATP7A, ATP7B, ceruloplasmin, and metallothionein, have been documented in Dobermans with clinical hepatitis with high hepatic copper concentrations, along with a reduction in gene expression of components of the antioxidant defense system, including SOD1, catalase, as well as reduced levels of glutathione. Continued investigations are needed to further clarify the pathogenesis of chronic hepatitis in Dobermans.

***West Highland White Terriers** are at increased risk of developing chronic hepatitis and cirrhosis*. There is evidence to support *familial* hepatic copper accumulation in some West Highland White Terriers, although the mode of inheritance is not completely understood. Hepatic copper accumulates in centrilobular hepatocytes but appears to plateau and does not appear to progressively accumulate as they age, with concentrations rarely >2,000 µg/g DW. Clinical illness directly attributable to copper hepatotoxicity (concentrations >2,000 µg/g DW) in West Highland White Terriers is, however, apparently uncommon. *Idiopathic chronic hepatitis progressing to cirrhosis* does also occur in this breed and may be distinguished because of a different zonal location and morphology of the inflammatory lesions. In idiopathic disease, inflammatory foci are smaller, composed of a single apoptotic hepatocyte or fragments of cells accompanied by a few lymphocytes and plasma cells, and are commonly localized to periportal areas, or may be random in distribution. In dogs with copper toxicosis, foci of inflammation and necrosis were larger, always found around the central vein among copper-laden hepatocytes, and were composed of debris-filled macrophages, lymphocytes, plasma cells, and scattered neutrophils, with occasional apoptotic hepatocytes around the periphery. *Distinguishing between copper toxicosis and idiopathic chronic hepatic disease may be difficult in cirrhotic livers*, which, irrespective of the underlying cause, may have reduced copper burdens because of connective tissue displacement of hepatic parenchyma, and typically lower concentrations of copper in regenerative nodules.

*Chronic hepatitis occurs in related **Skye Terriers***, accompanied by modest and somewhat inconsistent hepatic copper accumulation. Lesions ranged from hepatocellular degeneration and necrosis with mild inflammation in centrilobular areas to chronic hepatitis and cirrhosis with marked

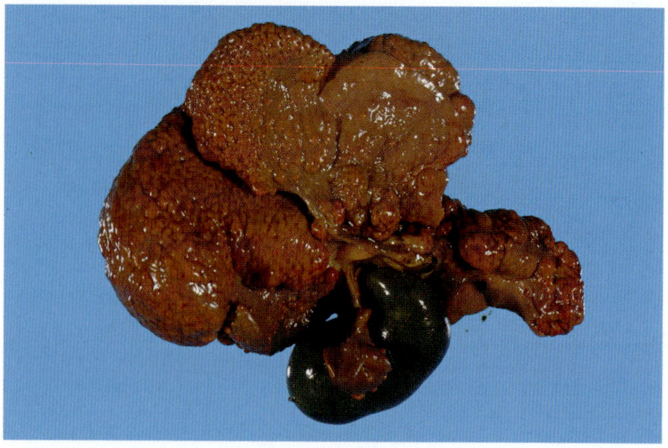

Figure 2-57 Chronic hepatitis in an American Cocker Spaniel.

intracanalicular cholestasis. Hepatic copper concentrations of to 800-2,200 µg/g DW and copper-containing hepatocytes were found predominantly in centrilobular areas.

*Chronic liver disease associated with elevated hepatic copper concentrations has also been reported in **Dalmatians***. A range of necroinflammatory changes has been reported, including multifocal, interface, centrilobular-to-panlobular hepatic necrosis, and cirrhosis, although, in one study of 10 dogs, various degrees of interface hepatitis and bridging fibrosis were the most common histologic change, with either primarily lymphocytic or neutrophilic inflammatory infiltrates. Morphologic or biochemical evidence of cholestatic liver disease was not prominent. Hepatic copper concentrations were 745-8,390 µg/g DW (mean 3,197 µg/g) in one report of 10 dogs, aged 2-10 years. Three previous cases in young Dalmatians reported hepatic copper concentrations of 7,940 µg/g DW, 1,916 µg/g wet weight, and 2,356 µg/g wet weight, and 2 of these reports describe diffuse positive staining for copper in all hepatocytes, with the strongest staining seen in centrilobular hepatocytes.

*Chronic hepatitis of unknown etiology has been reported in **American and English Cocker Spaniels** and **English Springer Spaniels***, expressed clinically in the later stages as ascites, weight loss, and icterus. Affected dogs develop chronic hepatitis and cirrhosis, and, at postmortem, livers are typically small and firm, with numerous small regenerative nodules (Fig. 2-57). Histologically, there is moderate-to-severe portal hepatitis, with inflammatory infiltrates of predominantly lymphocytes, plasma cells, and fewer neutrophils, and variable degrees of portal fibrosis and bridging fibrosis. One study of American Cocker Spaniels reported diffuse fibrosis typical of lobular dissecting hepatitis in 7 of 13 affected dogs, in addition to patterns of fibrosis more typical of cirrhosis. Interface hepatitis and limiting plate destruction have been reported in Cocker Spaniels; in English Springer Spaniels, hepatocyte necrosis and apoptosis in areas of inflammatory infiltrates in both portal areas and scattered throughout the hepatic parenchyma was more typical. Marked ductular reaction was noted in affected Cocker Spaniels. Hepatic copper staining is variable, and hepatic copper accumulation is not a consistent feature.

Immune-mediated hepatitis. Several studies have suggested that there is an immune-mediated hepatitis in dogs and, given the unexplained pathogenesis for two-thirds of chronic hepatitis cases in dogs and the importance of autoimmune hepatitis in human medicine, this seems probable. Several lines of evidence support this form of hepatitis, including abnormal MHC class II protein expression on hepatocytes, autoantibodies in serum, lymphocytic infiltrates in the liver, association with other autoimmune diseases, female sex, and breed predispositions. Treatment with immunosuppressive drugs such as cyclosporin is reported to yield significant clinical improvement, and some response to corticosteroids may also occur. Upregulation of MHC class II antigen expression in hepatocytes has been shown in Doberman hepatitis in association with lymphocyte infiltration, and it has been proposed that hepatocytes with a putative MHC class II molecule–associated autoantigen could be targets for T cell–mediated immune attack. An association with specific MHC DLA class II haplotypes has been described in Doberman Pinschers and English Springer Spaniels with subclinical or clinical hepatitis, and it has been suggested that the highly polymorphic *DLA* genes may be involved in altered susceptibility to chronic hepatitis. Histologically, specific criteria for diagnosis are not yet formulated, but the interface hepatitis and parenchymal infiltration with lymphocytes along with hepatocyte apoptosis are possibly useful features to suggest an immune-mediated pathogenesis. However, a primary autoimmune pathogenesis has yet to be shown.

α1-Antitrypsin (α1-AT) **deficiency** *has been suggested to play a role in chronic hepatitis in some dog breeds, including English Cocker Spaniels,* although whether this is an epiphenomenon or a cause of chronic liver disease has not yet been proven.

Lobular dissecting hepatitis*, associated with predominantly sinusoidal inflammation and fibrosis, has been described in young dogs with ascites and acquired PSSs.* The liver is usually small, pale with a predominantly smooth surface, and occasional hyperplastic nodules (eFig. 2-15). The histologic lesion is dissection of lobular parenchyma by reticulin and fine collagen fibers into individual and small groups of hepatocytes, accompanied by a variable, mixed inflammatory infiltrate of lymphocytes, plasma cells, and lesser numbers of neutrophils and macrophages (Fig. 2-58A and B). Activated fibroblastic cells, likely HSCs, may also be prominent along sinusoids. Hepatocytes form rosettes or pseudoductular structures, and regenerative nodules may be present. Portal inflammation and periportal fibrosis are not conspicuous features of this disease. The etiology of this disorder remains unknown.

A form of chronic hepatitis in dogs termed **histiocytic hepatitis (granulomatous hepatitis)** is characterized by small aggregates ranging into sheets of macrophages with variable numbers of infiltrating lymphocytes or intact neutrophils. The infiltrating cells are space-occupying foci, and there is necrosis of hepatocytes in the interface with hepatic parenchyma (Fig. 2-59). The pathogenesis is unknown. Advanced cases can be fatal, but response to immunosuppressive medication with or without antibiotics can occur.

Chronic hepatitis in other species

Chronic hepatitis in cats induced by **excess copper** may be more common than previously thought. As in dogs, it is characterized by copper deposition in hepatocytes, starting in the centrilobular region, with subsequent inflammation and hepatocyte death, copper-containing macrophages and fibrosis, and in more severe cases cirrhosis. An initial description of copper-associated hepatitis, with reported excess hepatic copper (4,074 µg/g DW) in a Siamese cat, was characterized by enlarged, finely vacuolated, and individual necrotic hepatocytes with centrilobular and midzonal copper accumulation.

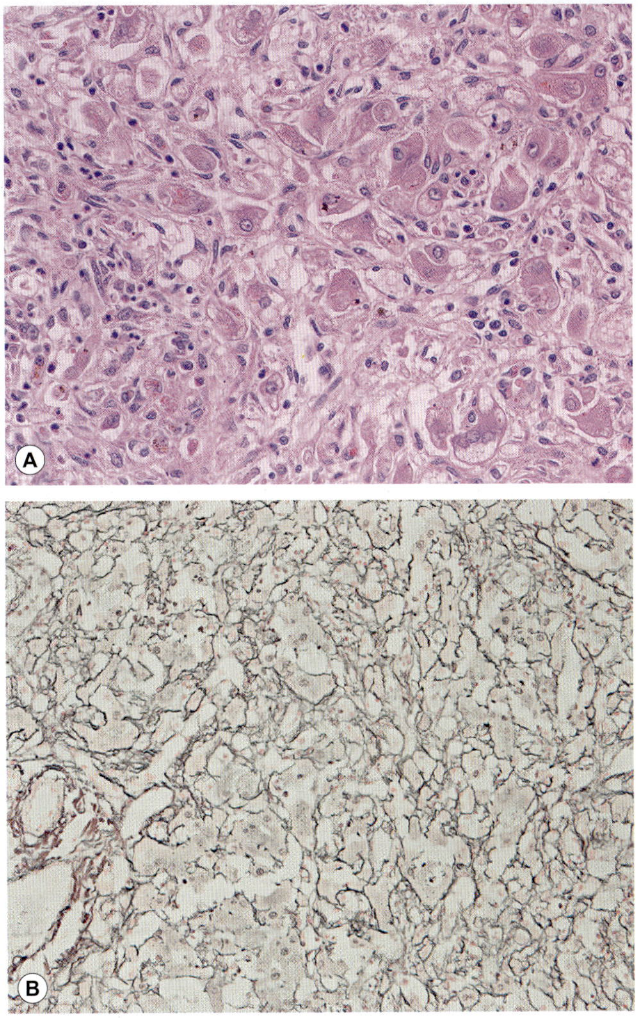

Figure 2-58 A. **Lobular dissecting hepatitis** with diffuse fine interstitial fibrosis isolating hepatocytes in a juvenile Golden Retriever dog. **B.** Reticulin stain demonstrating the pattern of lobular dissection and disruption of lobular architecture.

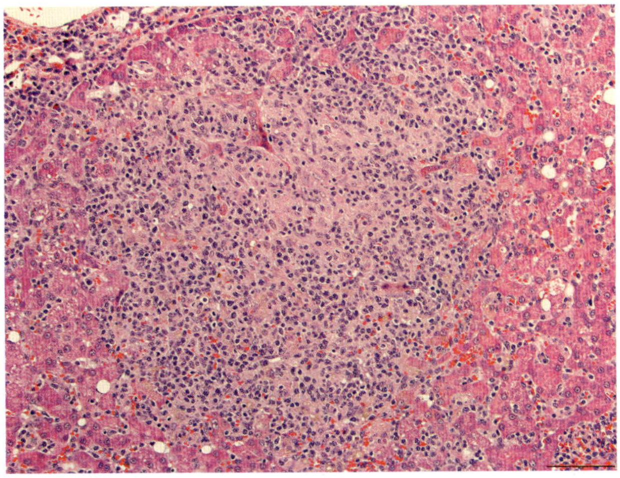

Figure 2-59 Histiocytic (granulomatous) hepatitis in a dog.

Chronic hepatitis and cirrhosis, with marked accumulation of stainable copper in macrophages in fibrous septa and with sparser staining in regenerative nodules, were reported in a European Shorthair cat with similarly elevated liver copper concentrations (4,170 µg/g DW; the upper reference interval limit for hepatic copper concentration in cats is <180 µg/g DW). A retrospective study described an additional 11 cats with presumed primary copper-associated hepatopathy, characterized by elevated hepatic copper concentrations (>700 µg/g DW), diffuse or centrilobular and intermediate zone copper staining, without any other co-occurring cholestatic disorders. Affected cats had hepatocyte vacuolation consistent with glycogen accumulation, fibrillar collagen in the perivenular region, and variable mild parenchymal collapse, with bridging fibrosis in one cat. Single-nucleotide variations in the *ATP7B* gene indicating loss of function of the ATB7B protein in some cats have been described, suggesting a cause of feline primary copper-associated hepatitis. Cats also accumulate copper in the liver secondary to cholestatic hepatobiliary disorders, such as chronic cholangitis/cholangiohepatitis, or extrahepatic bile duct obstruction, although copper staining in these cases is principally in hepatocytes in portal and intermediate zones. Cats may also develop chronic hepatitis during prolonged *domestic cat hepadnavirus infection*.

Chronic hepatitis sometimes seen as end-stage livers occurs in **horses** (eFig. 2-16) and ruminants, particularly **cattle**, and is often assumed to be associated with ingestion of hepatotoxins, such as pyrrolizidine alkaloids in forage, or a consequence of prolonged administration of hepatotoxic therapeutics, although in the absence of specific histologic lesions and/or a corroborative clinical history, the underlying causes are rarely discovered.

Miscellaneous inflammatory liver disease

Nonspecific reactive hepatitis refers to hepatic inflammation characterized by light inflammatory infiltrates, primarily in the portal tracts, without hepatocellular necrosis. It is often observed during inflammation of the splanchnic organs or oral cavity and is a reactive response to systemic inflammation, rather than primary inflammation of the liver.

Giant cell hepatitis *is an uncommon lesion in animals, but is recorded in cats, calves, and foals* (Fig. 2-60). There is evidence for maternal leptospirosis as a cause in some cases reported in foals. Two cases are reported in young cats with concurrent thymic lymphomas. Histologically, the lobular structure is effaced, and the blood vessels engorged. Hepatocytes are large and syncytial and may contain 10 or more nuclei. The pale or ballooned cytoplasm contains bile pigments, and cytoplasmic invaginations into hepatocyte nuclei are common. Inflammatory cells may be conspicuous. Liver parenchymal giant cell transformation occurs in humans in a wide variety of congenital and neonatal liver disorders, including bile duct obstruction associated with biliary atresia, viral and bacterial infections, some metabolic disorders such as galactosemia, some cases of Down syndrome and other genetic disorders, as well as in idiopathic neonatal hepatitis, a cholestatic condition of undetermined cause. Although giant cells were originally suggested to be a marker of infantile obstructive cholangiopathy in humans, their association with a wide range of disorders supports an *alternative conclusion that giant cell formation represents a nonspecific reaction of the infant's hepatocytes to various types of injury*.

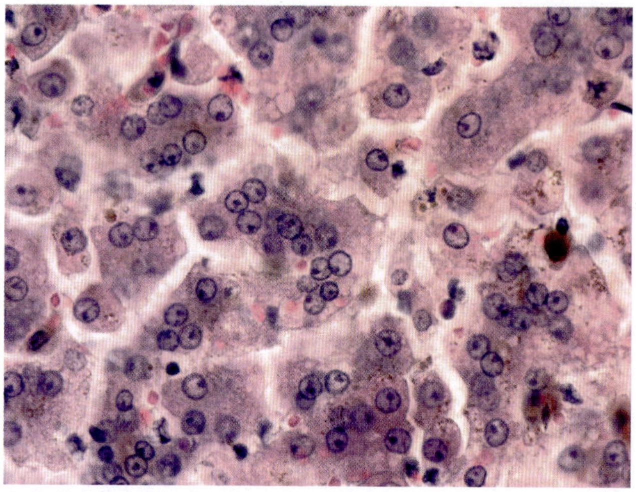

Figure 2-60 **Giant cell hepatitis** in a cat.

Systemic granulomatous disease has been reported in cattle grazing *hairy vetch (Vicia villosa)*. Clinical signs include dermatitis, pruritus, diarrhea, wasting, and high mortality. Histologic lesions include infiltration of the skin and internal organs, including portal areas of the liver, by monocytes, lymphocytes, plasma cells, eosinophils, and multinucleate giant cells. The pathogenesis is unknown, although the inflammatory reaction has characteristics of a type IV hypersensitivity reaction. Alternatively, vetch lectin may activate T lymphocytes directly to initiate the cellular response.

Inflammatory diseases of the biliary tract

Inflammation of the gallbladder is termed **cholecystitis**. *Inflammation of the large bile ducts is* **cholangitis;** *inflammation of the smallest bile ductules is termed* **cholangiolitis**. Cholangiolitis is uncommon in animals and occurs mainly in conjunction with inflammation of larger ducts. Destructive cholangiolitis has been observed in dogs and is likely associated with adverse drug reactions, as it is in humans.

Cholecystitis

Isolated cholecystitis is uncommon or possibly under-recognized and is often associated with concurrent cholelithiasis, although acalculous cholecystitis is reported in the dog, with a solitary case report in a pig. Cholecystitis in cattle is often associated with *Salmonella* spp. (*Salmonella* Dublin or *Salmonella* Typhimurium), but the pathway to the gallbladder is unclear. *Cholecystitis is thought to be caused by reflux of intestinal bacteria into the gallbladder via the bile ducts, or hematogenous entry of bacteria from the adjacent hepatic circulation*. Enteric aerobic gram-negative bacteria are the most frequent isolates from canine cases, although occasionally anaerobic bacteria such as clostridia have been cultured. *Campylobacter jejuni* has been isolated from 2 dogs with bacteremia and cholecystitis. Occasionally, parasites, such as flukes that colonize the bile ducts, can enter the gallbladder and cause cholecystitis. Canine cholecystitis has been associated with various systemic disorders, including diabetes mellitus, severe enteritis, biliary stasis, septicemia, as well as with the use of immunosuppressive drugs, each of which may promote bacterial colonization of the gallbladder. In the acute lesion, histologic changes include neutrophilic inflammatory infiltrates in the wall and lumen of the gallbladder, with focal erosion or ulceration, fibrin, and edema. Occasionally, the infiltrate may be predominantly lymphoplasmacytic, with the formation of lymphoid follicles within the mucosa. More chronic stages develop typical mixed inflammatory infiltrates, with fibrosis. With chronicity, prominent mucosal hyperplasia can develop.

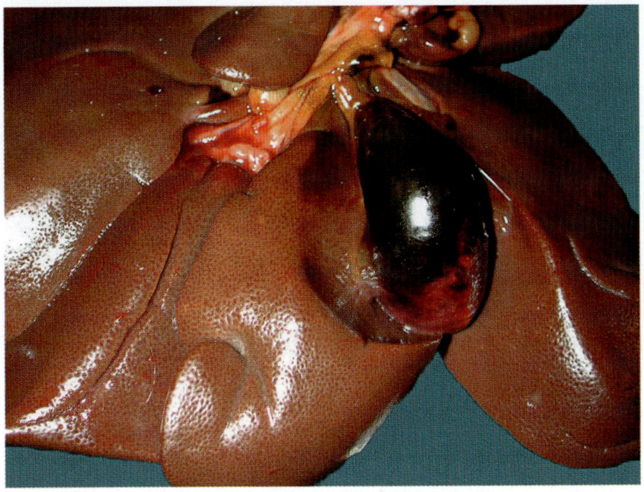

Figure 2-61 **Infarcted gallbladder** in a dog.

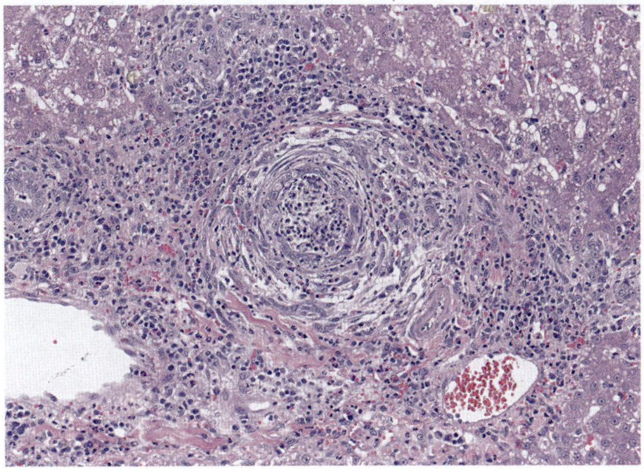

Figure 2-62 Neutrophilic bile duct inflammation with portal edema, early fibrosis, and a mixed infiltrate of neutrophils, lymphocytes, and plasma cells in a case of **subacute cholangitis** in a cat.

Gallbladder infarction, which is transmural coagulative necrosis of the gallbladder wall with intravascular fibrin thrombi, has been reported in dogs (Fig. 2-61). The arterial blood supply to the gallbladder is the cystic artery, a branch of the hepatic artery, and occlusion may cause partial or complete infarction. Predisposing factors have not been identified; however, the lack of significant concurrent inflammatory response suggests that this is not simply a sequela to underlying cholecystitis.

Cholangitis/cholangiohepatitis

Cholangitis—inflammation of the bile ducts—occurs in neutrophilic, lymphocytic, and destructive forms in animals. Extension of inflammation from the ducts into the adjacent hepatic parenchyma can occur, and such lesions can quite accurately be regarded as *cholangiohepatitis*.

Neutrophilic cholangitis (neutrophilic or exudative cholangitis/cholangiohepatitis) *is a relatively common disorder of cats and, much less commonly, dogs*. Bile contains various antimicrobial factors, including IgA, β-defensins, and bile acids, that are inhospitable to most bacteria, except for some species with capsule adaptations. Bacterial infection of the bile ducts is usually caused by common opportunists of enteric origin that give rise to neutrophilic cholangitis. In cats, the condition often occurs in conjunction with other disorders, including *acute extrahepatic bile duct obstruction, pancreatitis, or inflammatory bowel disease*. In the cat, the biliary and pancreatic ducts share a common entry to the duodenum, and simultaneous infectious inflammation of these systems is common. *Escherichia coli* is the most frequent bacterial isolate; however, *Bacteroides, Klebsiella*, hemolytic *Streptococcus*, and clostridia have also been reported. Some bacteremic organisms, including some *Salmonella*, can be cultured from the bile, but the mechanism by which they get there is unknown, possibly via a hematogenous route. Salmonellosis is a distinctive cause of fibrinous cholecystitis in cattle, especially calves.

The *pathogenesis of neutrophilic cholangitis/cholangiohepatitis* depends on various predisposing conditions, such as those involved in the pathogenesis of pyelonephritis. These include infection by bacteria that reach the ducts hematogenously, facilitated by localization in the peribiliary plexus or by extension from Kupffer cells or foci of necrosis. Descending cholangitis is occasionally seen in cattle with neutrophilic hepatitis with extension from abscesses directly into the ducts or via the portal lymphatics. Cholangitis/cholangiohepatitis of this origin may be restricted in its distribution to biliary fields, but in some cases, it does become quite diffuse in the biliary system. Alternatively, and more frequently than other routes, bacteria can ascend the ducts from the intestine, facilitated by bile stasis caused by mechanical or functional obstructions. The inflammatory and proliferative responses in cholangitis further interfere with bile flow and exacerbate the ductular spread of bacterial infections once they are established. The distribution of these lesions can be variable and may be missed on hepatic biopsy if only small areas are sampled.

The course and pathologic changes in neutrophilic cholangitis/cholangiohepatitis vary greatly, from fulminating neutrophilic infection to chronic neutrophilic cholangitis with persistent mild inflammation that, over a period of months or years, leads to hepatic fibrosis paralleling biliary proliferation. Severe neutrophilic cholangitis/cholangiohepatitis may follow a short course to death, the effects being those of the infection itself, which may become septicemic following rupture of ducts, rather than of hepatic injury. At autopsy, the liver may be swollen, soft, and pale. Few or many neutrophilic foci may be visible beneath the capsule and on the cut surface. They are small, sometimes miliary in distribution, and not encapsulated. Lesions in other organs may be those of septicemia and jaundice. Microscopically, the acute stage is characterized by edema and neutrophilic portal infiltrates, inflammation, and degeneration of bile ducts with neutrophils in ductular lumens and emigrating through the ductular epithelium. Bile plugs may be found in the canaliculi during the acute phase. Some cases may progress to cholangiohepatitis, with infiltration of inflammatory cells into hepatic lobules and periportal hepatocellular necrosis. Areas of suppuration and hepatic abscessation may occur. Cholangitis or cholangiohepatitis, with neutrophils, lymphocytes, and plasma cells infiltrating portal areas accompanied by bile duct proliferation, biliary epithelial degeneration, and various degrees of periportal to bridging fibrosis, may represent the subacute stage (Fig. 2-62), with concentric portal fibrosis surrounding bile ducts in the chronic stage.

In *subacute and chronic cholangitis/cholangiohepatitis*, inflammation is more proliferative than exudative, with mononuclear inflammatory cells predominating against a background of fewer neutrophils. The liver is enlarged and may be of normal shape or distorted because of irregular areas of atrophy and regenerative hyperplasia. Its surface may be smooth or finely granular; the capsule is thickened and may bear fibrous tags or may adhere to adjacent viscera. Within areas of duct obstruction, retention of bile pigments can be found in the regions served by the occluded ducts, but systemic icterus (or photosensitization in herbivores) is unlikely unless a substantial portion of liver is affected. On cut surface, the enlarged portal tracts are easily visible and accentuate the architecture of the organ. Eventually, the new fibrous tissue replaces the parenchyma, and in diffuse cases, continuous fibroplasia may produce hepatic enlargement. These gross liver changes resemble changes seen with alsike clover poisoning ("big-liver disease") in horses (discussed later in the Toxic Hepatic Disease section). Alternatively, chronic fibrosis may occur in wedge-shaped areas oriented to a small bile duct. The enlarged interlobular ducts may be readily visible and often contain plugs of inspissated secretion and debris.

Microscopically, the reaction remains centered on portal tracts. These are expanded in subacute cases by infiltration of leukocytes and the proliferation of small ducts and, in chronic cases, chiefly by organizing fibrous tissue and proliferating bile ducts. Bridging fibrosis can develop with chronicity. Blood flow in the hepatic venules and sublobular veins can be impaired by fibrosis leading to congestion and potentially increasing the risk of portal hypertension. Regenerative nodules are not a prominent feature of cholangitis/cholangiohepatitis unless large areas of parenchyma have been destroyed, in which case the least damaged lobes are expanded by coarse nodules.

A distinct condition of cats, **lymphocytic cholangitis** (lymphocytic portal hepatitis, mononuclear cholangitis/cholangiohepatitis) is a slowly progressive disease characterized by lymphocytic infiltrates within the portal area, with variable degrees of ductular reaction and peribiliary, portal-to-bridging fibrosis (Fig. 2-63). An immune-mediated pathogenesis has been proposed, and most cats with lymphocytic cholangitis have T cell–predominant portal infiltrates, often with accompanying portal B-cell aggregates. The various degrees of lymphocytic targeting and infiltration of bile ductules with concurrent degenerative changes in ductular epithelium, destructive lymphocytic cholangitis leading to ductopenia, and portal lipogranulomas may be useful in distinguishing this condition from hepatic lymphoma in the cat, along with T-cell receptor clonality assays. The lymphocytes around central veins or extension along the sinusoids suggest lymphoma rather than lymphocytic cholangitis.

Destructive cholangitis is rare, but has been described in dogs, and can also occur in cats. Destruction and loss of bile ducts occurs in the large and small portal tracts or only interlobular or smaller bile ducts, with inflammation composed of pigment-laden macrophages, neutrophils, and/or eosinophils, and in some instances, fibrosis. Often, there is no duct proliferation, suggesting continued injury during the attempts to repair the damage. The extent of injury may be sufficient to cause marked icterus and acholic feces because of marked intrahepatic cholestasis. The pathogenesis of this lesion is unclear; however, toxic injury, idiosyncratic drug reactions (see Fig. 2-40), and infection by canine distemper virus (CDV; *Paramyxoviridae, Morbillivirus canis*) have been implicated in some cases. Recovery can occur, but severe cases are fatal.

Biliary tract obstruction

Cholelithiasis (gallstone formation) is seldom seen in animals. The choleliths usually form in the gallbladder and are composed of a *mixture of cholesterols, bile pigments, salts of bile acids, calcium salts, and proteinaceous matrix*. Choleliths of mixed composition are yellow-black or green-black and are friable. *Pigment stones*, composed of calcium bilirubinate, and *cholesterol stones* have also been reported in dogs. There may be hundreds of small stones or a few large ones, which are usually faceted. The origin of these mixed gallstones is uncertain, but their development is probably secondary to chronic mild cholecystitis and related to disturbances of the resorptive activities of the gallbladder, whereby the bile salts are removed faster than the stone-forming compounds. Gallstones are usually subclinical. Occasionally, they lodge in and obstruct bile ducts and cause jaundice. The larger stones may cause pressure necrosis and ulceration of the mucosa, local dilations of the bile ducts, and saccular diverticula of the gallbladder. Calculi seldom form in the ducts, although calcareous deposits often do so in fascioliasis of cattle. Calcium bilirubinate calculi have been reported in the bile ducts of horses (Fig. 2-64), associated with intermittent jaundice.

Occasionally, particles of solid ingesta may find their way into the gallbladder; sand has been seen in sheep, and seeds in pigs.

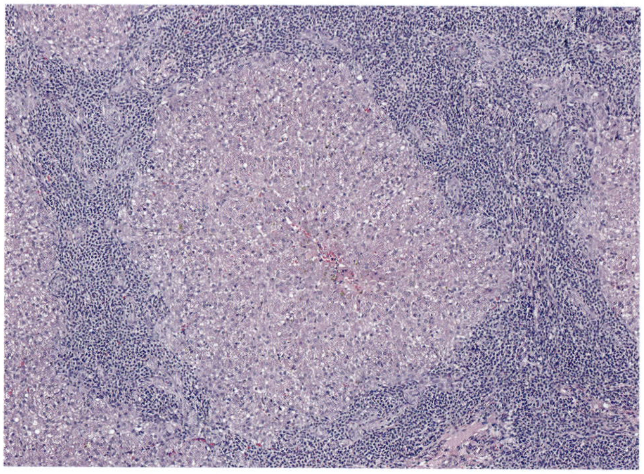

Figure 2-63 **Lymphocytic cholangitis** in a cat.

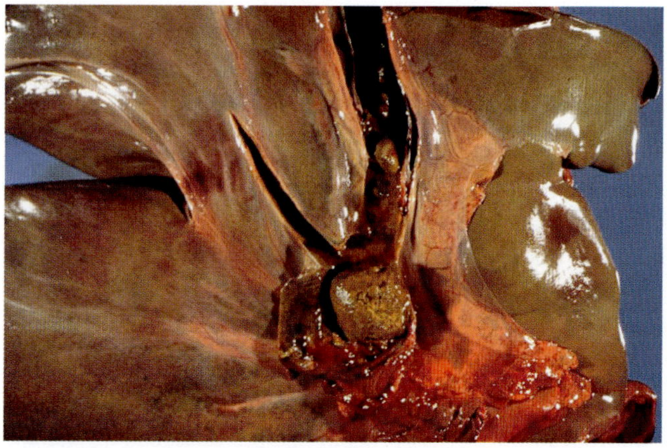

Figure 2-64 **Cholelith** obstructing the bile duct in a horse.

Biliary obstruction is rarely caused by impacted gallstones. Usually, it is *the result of cholangitis or cholecystitis*, the obstruction being produced by masses of detritus and biliary constituents, parasites, or cicatricial stenosis of the ducts. Adult ascarids may cause mechanical obstruction. Inspissated bile-stained friable plugs are occasionally responsible for obstructions in segments of the liver in horses. Edematous swelling of the papilla in enteritis may also be of significance, as well as compression due to edema associated with acute pancreatitis or fibrosis associated with chronic pancreatitis. Tumors of the pancreas and duodenum, and tumors and abscesses of the hilus of the liver and portal nodes, may cause compression stenosis of the ducts. Biliary obstruction by abnormal intraluminal mucoid secretion *(gallbladder mucocele)* has been reported in dogs (see later the Ectopic, Metaplastic, and Hyperplastic Lesions section).

The consequences of biliary obstruction depend on the site and duration of the obstruction. When the common bile duct is involved, there is jaundice. When one of the hepatic ducts is involved, there is no jaundice, and depending on the efficiency of biliary collaterals, there may be no pigmentation of the obstructed segments of the liver. Increases in serum GGT and alkaline phosphatase activities usually occur when a sufficiently large amount of the duct system is affected. Histologically, there is a characteristic response to acute obstruction. Affected portal tracts are edematous, often with a neutrophilic infiltrate that can be due to bile acids or bacteria. Neutrophils may be restricted to the portal tract connective tissue or may be found between biliary epithelial cells or within the lumen of the ducts. The ducts undergo progressive cylindrical dilation, which may be extreme. The smallest interlobular ducts and the cholangioles proliferate (ductular reaction). These infections may be acute and purulent, or low grade; in these cases, bacteria may not be easily cultured. The cholangitis/cholangiohepatitis that almost inevitably follows has been described previously.

Rupture of the biliary tract or the gallbladder causes steady leakage of bile into the peritoneal cavity, the omentum being unable to seal even small defects. The bile salts are very irritating and may cause *acute chemical peritonitis*. The peritoneal effusion that follows may remain sterile; more often, it is infected by enteric bacteria, and severe diffuse peritonitis ensues. This may be rapidly fatal, particularly if clostridia are involved. Many perforations of the biliary tract are traumatic in origin; however, in dogs, cholecystitis, gallbladder necrosis/infarction, and gallbladder mucocele have all been associated with gallbladder rupture.

INFECTIOUS DISEASES OF THE LIVER

Viral infections

Various systemic viral diseases may affect the liver. *Adenoviral infections* of lambs, calves, and goat kids can cause multifocal hepatic necrosis and cholangitis, in addition to pneumonia. While mild-to-moderate, periportal, lymphohistiocytic hepatitis is common with porcine circovirus 2 (PCV2; *Circoviridae, Circovirus porcine2*) infection in pigs, severe hepatitis with hepatocellular necrosis/apoptosis, vacuolation, karyomegaly, disorganization of hepatic plates, and perilobular stromal condensation occurs only sporadically. Bile stasis and icterus may also be present in such instances. The morphology of the hepatic lesions alone may resemble a toxic hepatic injury on histology, especially if typical circoviral botryoid inclusions are absent (Fig. 2-65A and B). Canid alphaherpesvirus 1 (canine herpesvirus, CaAHV1; *Orthoherpesviridae, Varicellovirus canidalpha1*) infection in puppies and juveniles and, more rarely, in adult dogs causes disseminated focal necrosis and hemorrhages in parenchymal organs, including the liver, with the formation of amphophilic intranuclear inclusion bodies in epithelial cells of the kidney, lung, and liver. Similar microfoci of hepatic necrosis sometimes occur in aborted or newborn foals with congenital equid alphaherpesvirus 1 (equine herpesvirus, equine abortion virus, EqAHV1; *Orthoherpesviridae, Varicellovirus equidalpha1*) infections (Fig. 2-66), in neonatal calves infected with bovine alphaherpesvirus 1 (infectious bovine rhinotracheitis virus, BoAHV1; *Orthoherpesviridae, Varicellovirus bovinealpha1*), in piglets with suid alphaherpesvirus 1 (pseudorabies virus, Aujeszky disease virus, SuAHV1; *Orthoherpesviridae, Varicellovirus suidalpha1*) infections, and in feline fetuses following intravenous felid alphaherpesvirus 1 (felid herpesvirus 1, FeAHV1; *Orthoherpesviridae; Varicellovirus felidalpha1*) inoculation of the pregnant female cat. Feline coronavirus (FCoV; *Coronaviridae, Alphacoronavirus 1*) infection can cause lymphohistiocytic or granulomatous hepatitis in some infected cats, as part of feline infectious peritonitis (Fig. 2-67). Multifocal hepatic necrosis has been described in large felids and domestic cats infected with *highly pathogenic influenza A*

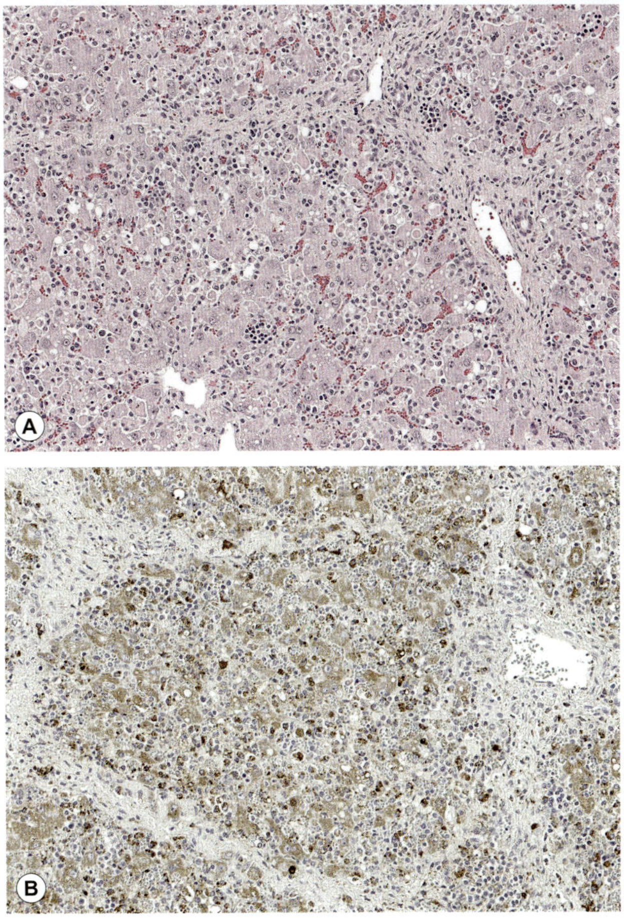

Figure 2-65 A. Hepatitis caused by **porcine circovirus 2 (PCV2)** infection in a pig. **B.** Immunohistochemical stain for PCV2 antigen. (Courtesy Dr. Marta Mainenti, Iowa State University Veterinary Diagnostic Laboratory.)

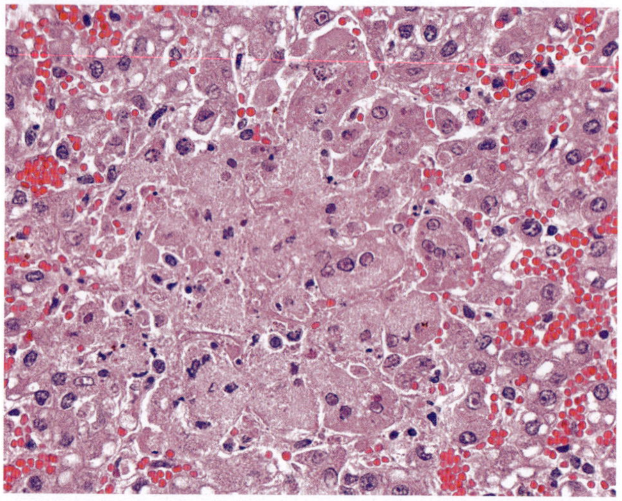

Figure 2-66 Focal hepatic necrosis with intranuclear inclusion bodies and syncytial cells in **congenital equid alphaherpesvirus 1 infection** in a foal.

virus H5N1. Hepatocellular and Kupffer cell necrosis with mild mononuclear portal inflammation was reported in outbreaks caused by virulent systemic strains of feline calicivirus (FCV; *Caliciviridae*; *Vesivirus*) in cats in the United States and the United Kingdom. Systemic cowpox virus (CPV; *Poxviridae, Orthopoxvirus*) infection with foci of hepatic necrosis containing immunoreactive cowpox viral antigen has been reported in a cat. Canine minute virus (carnivore bocaparvovirus 1, CnMV; *Parvoviridae, Bocaparvovirus carnivoran1*) has been identified in one fatality due to liver injury. Infection with severe fever with thrombocytopenia syndrome virus (SFTSV; *Phenuiviridae, Bandavirus dabieense*), a novel zoonotic phlebovirus that is lethal in humans, dogs, and cats, targets mainly lymphoid organs but can cause small foci of hepatic necrosis.

The viral diseases discussed in more detail later are those in which the liver is the major target organ, causing substantial hepatic injury that sometimes culminates in hepatic failure. Unlike humans, in which several pathogenic hepatitis viruses from various families are well described, few viruses that specifically target the liver have been identified in the major domestic mammals. Hepadnaviruses, found in members of the squirrel family, including woodchucks and various species of ground squirrels and arctic ground squirrels, as well as in some species of birds, have been reported in domestic cats. Infection with hepatitis E virus (HEV) genotypes 3 and 4 is common in domestic and wild pigs, and although clinical disease is not apparent in infected swine, they may serve as reservoirs for this potentially zoonotic pathogen. Lesions of mild multifocal lymphoplasmacytic hepatitis with focal hepatocellular necrosis have been reported in pigs experimentally inoculated with HEV, but lesions in natural infections are not recognized. Three *Flaviviridae* members have been found in horses. Two of these infect hepatocytes: non-primate hepacivirus (equine hepacivirus, NPHV; *Flaviviridae, Hepacivirus equi*) and Theiler disease–associated virus (TDAV; *Flaviviridae, Pegivirus equi*), although their clinical significance is modest. A third virus, equine pegivirus (EPgV; *Flaviviridae, Pegivirus caballi*), is not hepatocytotropic. A novel parvovirus of horses identified as the likely cause of equine serum hepatitis is described in more detail later.

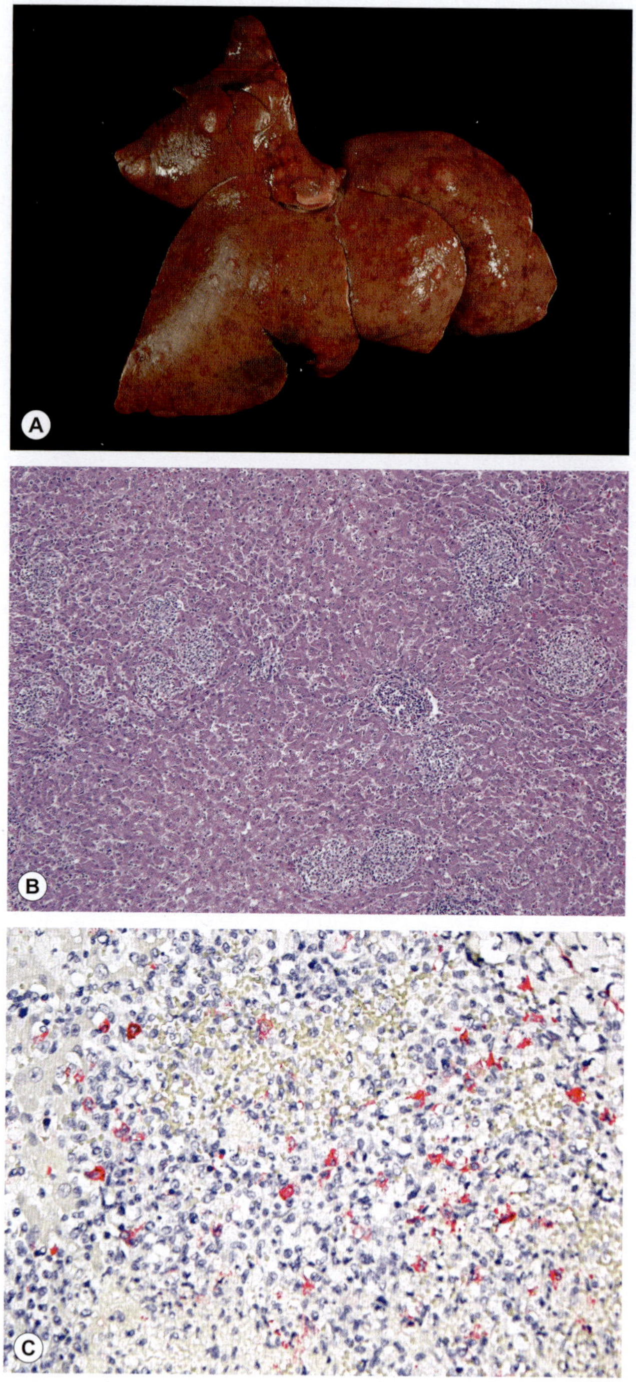

Figure 2-67 A. and B. Pyogranulomatous hepatitis caused by **feline infectious peritonitis virus** infection. C. Immunohistochemical stain for feline coronavirus antigen.

Infectious canine hepatitis

Canine adenovirus 1 (CAdV1; *Adenoviridae, Canine mastadenovirus A*) infection is the cause of infectious canine hepatitis (ICH), a severe liver disease in dogs; other canids, including coyotes, foxes, and wolves; and in bears. Vaccination has made the disease rare in many countries in which it was endemic. Deaths from ICH are usually sporadic, although small outbreaks can occur among young dogs in kennels. Fatalities seldom occur among dogs >2-years-old. In areas where ICH is not controlled by vaccination, it is probable that most dogs in the general population contact CAdV1 in the first 2 years of life and suffer either inapparent infection or mild febrile illness with pharyngitis and tonsillitis.

In more severe cases, there is vomiting, melena, high fever, and abdominal pain. There may be gingival petechiae; the mucous membranes are pale and occasionally slightly jaundiced. Nonspecific nervous signs occur in a few cases. There is also a peracute form of the disease in which the animal is found dead without signs of illness, or after an illness of only a few hours. In convalescence, there may be unilateral or bilateral opacity of the cornea caused by corneal edema (so-called *blue eye*, a type III hypersensitivity reaction with immune complex–mediated corneal injury; Fig. 2-68), which typically disappears spontaneously.

CAdV1 has special tropism for endothelium, mesothelium, and hepatic parenchyma, and it is injury to these that is responsible for the pathologic features of edema, serosal hemorrhage, and hepatic necrosis. The histologic specificity of the lesions depends on the demonstration of large, solid intranuclear inclusion bodies in endothelium or hepatic parenchyma (Fig. 2-69). Inclusions are occasionally observed in other differentiated cells but always have the same morphologic and tinctorial features, being deeply acidophilic with a blue tint.

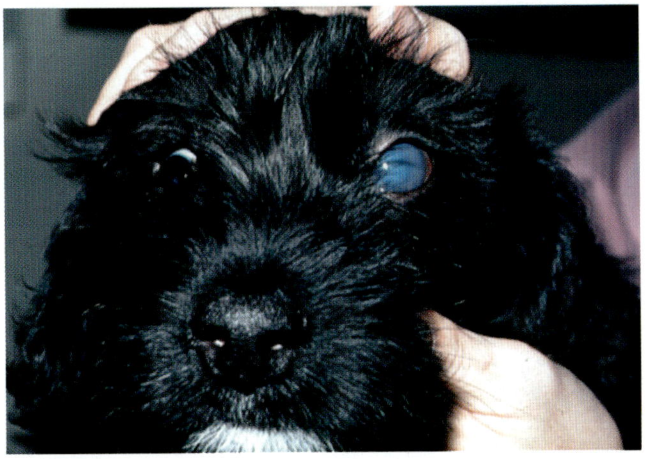

Figure 2-68 Infectious canine hepatitis. Corneal edema or "blue-eye." (Courtesy North Carolina State University CVM.)

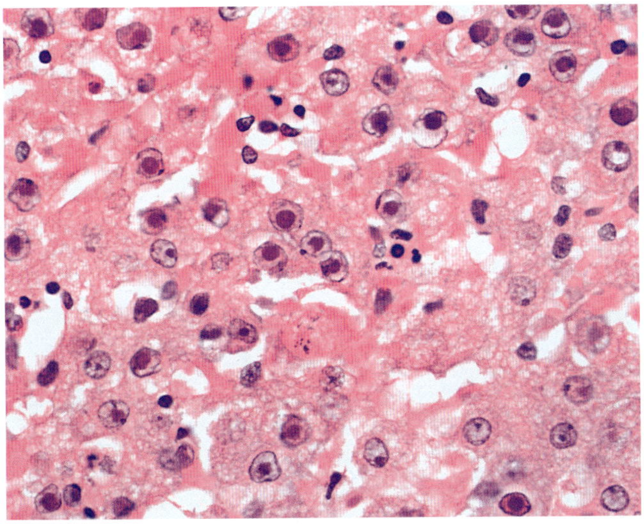

Figure 2-69 Infectious canine hepatitis (canine adenovirus 1 infection). Intranuclear viral inclusion bodies in numerous hepatocytes. (Courtesy University of Guelph.)

The morbid picture of spontaneously fatal cases of ICH is usually distinct enough to allow a diagnosis to be made at autopsy. Superficial lymph nodes are edematous, slightly congested, and often hemorrhagic. Blotchy or paintbrush hemorrhages may be present on intestinal and gastric serosae, and there is usually a small quantity of clear or blood-stained fluid in the abdomen. Jaundice, if present, is slight. The liver is slightly enlarged, with sharp edges, and is turgid and friable, sometimes congested, with a fine, uniform, yellow mottling (eFig. 2-17A). Red strands of fibrin can be found on its capsule, especially between the lobes. In most cases, the wall of the gallbladder is edematous (see eFig. 2-17B) and may have intramural hemorrhages; when edema is mild, it may be detected only in the attachments of the gallbladder.

Gross lesions in other organs are inconstant. Small hemorrhagic infarcts may be found in the renal cortices of young puppies. Hemorrhages may occur in the lungs, and occasionally, there are irregular areas of hemorrhagic consolidation in the caudal lobes. Hemorrhages in the brain occur in a small percentage of cases, typically only grossly visible in the midbrain and brainstem. Hemorrhagic necrosis of medullary and endosteal elements occurs in the metaphyses of long bones in young dogs, and the hemorrhages are readily visible through the thin cortex of the distal ends of the ribs.

At low magnification, the histologic changes in the liver are of *centrilobular (periacinar) zonal necrosis*, resembling the zonal pattern of some acute hepatotoxicities. *The susceptibility of centrilobular parenchyma to necrosis in this disease is unexplained*. Close to the portal tracts, the hepatocytes may be nearly normal in appearance, except for loss of basophilia and a scattering of inclusion bodies. In spontaneously fatal cases, most of the parenchyma of the peripheral and central portions of the lobules (acini) is dead, the hepatocytes having undergone coagulative necrosis, and in some of these, ghosts of inclusion bodies may be detectable. The margin between necrotic parenchyma and viable tissue is usually quite sharp, although in the viable tissue, there are many individual hepatocytes undergoing apoptosis or necrosis, most of them without inclusion bodies. Fatty change is common. The dead cells do not remain long, so the sinusoids become dilated and filled with blood. The reticulin framework remains intact, an observation in keeping with the fact that, *in recovered cases, restitution of the liver is complete*. Panlobular necrosis with collapse does not occur. As is typical of severe centrilobular necrosis, the necrotic zones, initially eccentric areas about hepatic venules, extend and link to isolate portal units. Intranuclear inclusions can be found in Kupffer cells in variable numbers. Many of the Kupffer cells are dead, others are proliferating, and others are actively phagocytic in the removal of debris. Leukocytic reactions in the liver are mild and are directed against the necrotic tissue; mononuclear cells are present, but neutrophils, many degenerating, predominate. There is some collection of bile pigment, but it is moderate, in keeping with the short course of the disease.

Microscopic lesions in other organs are largely the result of injury to endothelium. Inclusion bodies in endothelial cells can be difficult to find and are looked for with most profit in renal glomeruli, where endothelium is concentrated. Occasionally, they are found in the epithelium of collecting tubules. When areas of hemorrhagic consolidation of the lungs are present, there is hemorrhage, edema, and fibrin formation in the alveoli, and in these consolidated areas, inclusions are often common in alveolar capillaries and even in dying cells of the bronchial epithelium. Changes in the brain are secondary to vascular injury. Hemorrhages, if present, are from capillaries and small venules, and inclusions in endothelial nuclei can usually be found in vessels that have bled. Other endothelial and adventitial cells are hyperplastic and mixed with a few lymphocytes. Small foci of softening or demyelination may be present in relation to the hemorrhages. Lymphoreticular tissues are congested, and inclusions may be found in reticulum cells of follicles, in the red pulp of the spleen, and in macrophages anywhere.

Following natural oronasal exposure, viral multiplication occurs in the tonsils and leads to tonsillitis, which may be quite severe with extensive edema of the throat and larynx. Fever accompanies the tonsillitis and precedes the viremic phase, which lasts 4-8 days, accompanied by leukopenia. Hepatic necrosis develops at about day 7 of experimental infection; however, an immune response with adequate neutralizing antibodies may clear the virus from the blood and limit the extent of hepatic damage. *In surviving animals, hepatic regeneration occurs rapidly, and there do not appear to be any significant residual lesions*. Small foci of hepatocellular necrosis may still be present at 2 weeks, and foci of proliferated Kupffer cells may be detectable for another week or 2. Progressive hepatic injury does not seem to follow the acute phase of the natural disease, although chronic hepatitis has been reproduced experimentally in partially immunized dogs challenged with the virus. Adenoviral antigen has been detected immunohistochemically in occasional Kupffer cells in 5 dogs with a range of chronic hepatic inflammatory lesions and in one dog with a patent ductus venosus; however, a retrospective study of formalin-fixed paraffin-embedded liver from 45 dogs with chronic hepatitis or cirrhosis failed to reveal CAdV1 by either PCR or immunohistochemistry, although the possibility that the virus initiates hepatic damage by provoking self-perpetuating hepatitis could not be excluded. Focal interstitial nephritis occurs commonly, and the cellular infiltrates are persistent but not functionally significant. They consist of interstitial lymphocytic accumulations, especially about the corticomedullary junction and in the stroma of the pelvis.

Corneal edema is a late development, corresponding temporally to increasing neutralizing antibody titer. It may occur as early as day 7 of infection but is usually delayed to between 14 and 21 days. Viral antigen can be detected in affected eyes by fluorescence techniques. Inflammatory edema is present in the iris, ciliary apparatus, and corneal propria, and inflammatory cells are abundant in the filtration angle and iris. The infiltrates are principally plasma cells, and there is evidence that the ocular lesion is a hypersensitivity reaction to circulating deposition of immune complexes, with complement fixation, inflammatory cell chemotaxis, and corneal endothelial damage resulting in an *anterior uveitis with corneal stromal edema*.

Originally, it was assumed that the widespread tendency to hemorrhage in ICH was because of leakage from damaged vascular endothelium, coupled with an inability on the part of the damaged liver to replace clotting factors. Although these effects play a role, *the exhaustion of clotting factors is in large part the result of their accelerated consumption, as the widespread endothelial damage is a potent initiator of the clotting cascade*.

Wesselsbron disease

This disease is caused by **Wesselsbron virus** (WESSV; *Flaviviridae, Orthoflavivirus wesselsbronense*), an arthropod-borne flavivirus that, according to serosurveys, is widespread in Africa in various species of animals and birds. Various *Aedes* mosquitoes are vectors. Humans are also susceptible to clinical and inapparent infection. *WESSV produces abortion and perinatal death in sheep*. Newborn goats are also susceptible. Adult sheep, goat, and cattle rarely show clinical signs but may have a biphasic febrile response to infection; other clinical signs, when present, are of hepatitis and jaundice. Congenital malformation of the CNS and arthrogryposis are also reported, mainly in lambs.

The lesions in lambs dying within 12 hours of birth consist mainly of widespread petechiae and gastrointestinal hemorrhage; longer survival allows jaundice to develop, and the liver becomes orange-yellow, enlarged, friable, and patchily congested. The bile in the gallbladder becomes thick and dark in some cases, but this may be due more to hemorrhage into the gallbladder than to hemolysis. Lymph nodes are rather constantly enlarged, congested, and edematous.

The most characteristic histologic changes are seen in the liver. The liver lesions vary from necrosis of scattered individual hepatocytes or small groups of hepatocytes throughout the liver to extensive necrosis (Fig. 2-70). Mononuclear cells and pigment-filled macrophages accumulate in the portal stroma as well as in the sinusoids. Ductular reaction may be present. A variable number of *hepatocyte nuclei may contain eosinophilic, irregular inclusions*. WESSV antigen can be demonstrated in necrotic acidophilic and degenerating hepatocytes and rarely in the inclusions. Canalicular cholestasis is often conspicuous. Hepatocellular proliferation is apparent in the less acute cases. Lymphoid follicles in lymph nodes and spleen have variable lymphocyte necrosis and stimulation of lymphoblasts.

Rift Valley fever

This is an *arthropod-borne viral infection of ruminants and humans*, in many respects similar to Wesselsbron disease. **Rift Valley fever virus** (RVFV; *Phenuiviridae, Phlebovirus riftense*) is, however, responsible for greater losses. Morbidity and mortality may occur in adult sheep; death sometimes occurs in adult cattle, but it is chiefly a disease of the young, causing

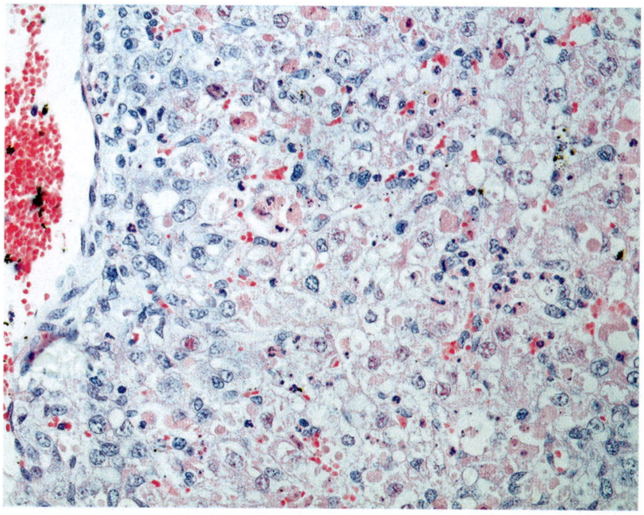

Figure 2-70 Focal necrosis and apoptosis in Wesselsbron disease in a lamb. (Courtesy S. Youssef.)

heavy mortality among lambs, kids, and calves, and abortion in ewes, does, and cows. Camelids can be affected. The infection in enzootic form is widespread in eastern and southern Africa, but it has extended to West Africa, Egypt, and the Arabian Peninsula. RVFV is transmitted by many species of mosquito of the genera *Culex, Aedes,* and *Anopheles,* in which transovarial passage can occur. Mosquitoes, once infected, remain so, and in them, the virus is not pathogenic. Elevated levels of viremia occur in sheep and cattle and are maintained for up to 5 days. During epizootics, the virus may be spread by fomites, aerosols, and mechanically by other biting insects.

In endemic situations, the disease in adults is usually mild, but in epidemics in sheep and goats, abortion unrelated to the period of gestation and illness with fever, mucopurulent nasal discharge, and dysentery occur. The mortality rate is then very high, reaching 90-100% in lambs and 10-30% in adults. The disease in cattle is less severe, but pregnant animals abort, and the mortality rate in adult animals is 5-10%, while in calves it may reach 70%.

As in Wesselsbron disease, *the gross postmortem picture is dominated by widespread hemorrhage, ranging from serosal and mucosal petechiae to occasional severe gastrointestinal bleeding.* The liver in the acute cases in neonatal lambs is similar to that in cases of Wesselsbron disease, being swollen, friable, and yellow to yellow-brown to dark-red when patchily congested or hemorrhagic. In older animals and in less acute cases, however, the liver tends to be darker and has scattered, pale, 1-2-mm foci of necrosis. Lesions suggestive of endothelial injury are often present: fibrinous perihepatitis, edema of the gallbladder wall and abomasum, and hydropericardium, hydrothorax, and ascites. Experimental infection of calves produced encephalomyelitis in an animal that survived the initial viremic stage.

In natural and experimental infections, the liver lesions start with single-cell and small foci of hepatocellular necrosis admixed with a few infiltrating neutrophils and macrophages within 12-24 hours of infection in lambs (eFig. 2-18). Within the next 24-48 hours, these primary foci enlarge and sometimes become almost confluent. In addition, the remaining parenchyma may rapidly undergo necrosis that spares only a small rim of degenerate periportal hepatocytes. The primary foci of necrosis undergo lysis more rapidly than the surrounding parenchyma resulting in randomly distributed foci of liquefactive necrosis on a background of diffuse hepatocellular degeneration and necrosis. The inflammatory infiltrate is mild and composed of degenerate neutrophils and macrophages. Where the expanding foci of necrosis include portal tracts, there may follow fibrinous vasculitis and thrombosis. *Eosinophilic intranuclear inclusion bodies,* fibrin deposition in sinusoids, and mineralization of necrotic hepatocytes are seen in variable numbers. Cholestasis is not a prominent feature as it is in Wesselsbron disease. RVFV antigen can be detected in hepatocytes by immunohistochemistry.

Equine serum hepatitis (Theiler disease)

Equine serum hepatitis is a common cause of acute hepatic failure in horses. The disease was originally described in 1919 by Arnold Theiler, in horses passively immunized with equine serum against African horse sickness and was later recognized in horses passively immunized against anthrax, tetanus, and equine encephalomyelitis. Various injectable biologics of equine origin have been associated with the disease, including *Clostridium perfringens* toxoids, antiserum against *Streptococcus equi,* tetanus antitoxin, and equine herpesviral vaccines prepared from equine fetal tissue, equine plasma, and pregnant mare serum. Equine serum hepatitis has a global distribution. The incidence of fulminant hepatitis among horses receiving antiserum in outbreaks of equine serum hepatitis has been reported to be 1.4-2.2%. The mortality rate is high among clinical horses, but some survive after transient illness with jaundice. Residual hepatic disease is not reported; some horses can survive with residual neurologic problems.

However, although such an association with exposure to equine biologics holds for most cases, there are many, usually sporadic, cases in horses that have not received any injections. One possible route is via ingestion as oral exposure to viremic serum is reported to transmit the infection. It is unknown how many exposed horses get subclinical disease because the condition is seldom diagnosed before the onset of hepatic failure. Initial studies found a previously unknown and highly divergent member of the *Flaviviridae* family, designated "*Theiler disease–associated virus*" (TDAV) as a putative cause of equine serum hepatitis. However, additional studies revealed that, in fact, an infection with a novel parvovirus, **equine parvovirus-hepatitis** (EqPV-H; *Parvoviridae, Copiparvovirus ungulate6*), is the actual etiologic agent of equine serum hepatitis. Infection does not necessarily lead to disease. The virus is relatively widespread, with 13% of horses surveyed viremic, but subclinical. Infections can be persistent. The factors that lead to disease following infection are unknown. The incubation period of disease is typically 42-60 days, sometimes up to 90 days. Onset of the typical clinical syndrome is sudden, with death occurring in 6-24 hours. Clinically, there is lethargy; jaundice; photosensitivity; hyperexcitability, often with mania; continuous walking and pushing; apparent blindness; and ataxia. Death occurs suddenly without a period of prostration.

At autopsy, icterus is present, with moderate ascites; the spleen is normal or congested, and there may be petechial hemorrhages on serous membranes and renal cortices, and some congestion of the intestine with hemorrhage into its lumen. Grossly, the liver usually appears atrophic, small, and flabby because of the acute loss of many hepatocytes (Fig. 2-71A). The liver may be stained by bile pigments, and its surface mottled with a few strands of fresh fibrin. The mottling is more evident on the cut surface, which may be severely congested with an apparent zonal pattern, and sometimes fatty (see Fig. 2-71B).

Microscopically, the hepatic lesion is considerably older than the clinical course would suggest. *There may be a few surviving swollen and vacuolated periportal hepatocytes or sometimes complete depletion of parenchymal cells in the section* (see Fig. 2-71C). In less affected regions in animals with adequate dietary or adipose reserves to mobilize, there is severe macrovesicular fatty change in most remaining hepatocytes. Acute necrosis is typically not seen, and there is no significant hemorrhage. Variable numbers of apoptotic hepatocytes are expected. In the centrilobular regions, severely ballooned cells undergo dissolution to leave either sinusoids that are dilated and filled with blood or a condensed and distorted reticulin framework. Extensive deposits of bile pigments are present in Kupffer cells and hepatocytes. Leukocytes, including lymphocytes, plasma cells, histiocytes, and a few neutrophils, may infiltrate diffusely, but not in large numbers. There is diffuse but very slight fibroplasia, especially in the portal units. In some livers, there is a ductular reaction, with small irregular clusters of proliferating ductular cells evident in the portal areas.

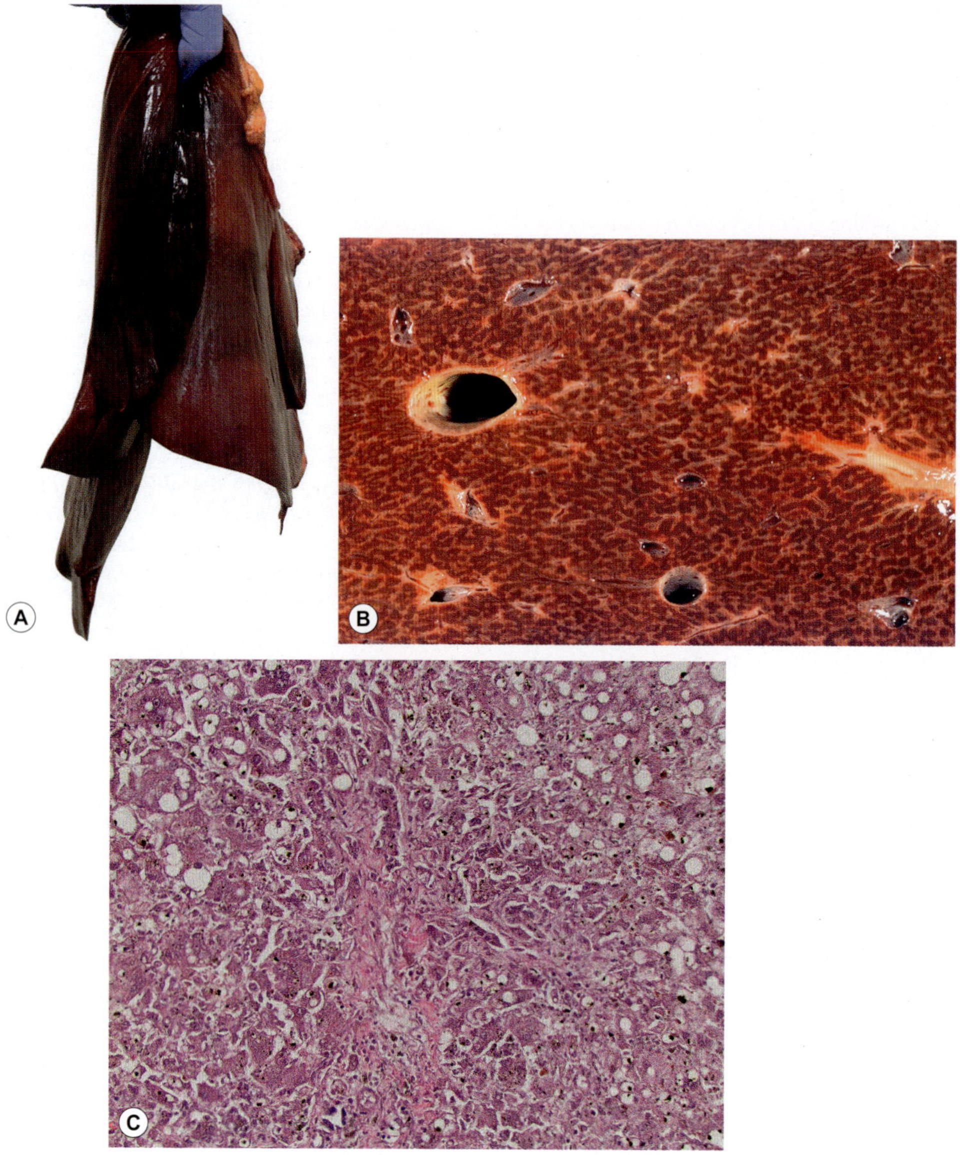

Figure 2-71 **Equine serum hepatitis** (Theiler disease). **A.** Small, limp, and flaccid "dishrag" liver. **B.** The reticular pattern in this slice of liver suggests zonal necrosis. **C.** Marked necrosis and loss of hepatocytes, parenchymal collapse, and macrovesicular fatty change in some remaining hepatocytes.

Bacterial infections

Bacterial hepatitis is common, but, with a few important exceptions, is usually focally distributed and of little clinical significance. Bacteria may gain entrance to the liver in numerous ways: by direct implantation, for example, by foreign body penetration from the reticulum; by invasion of the capsule from an adjacent focus of neutrophilic peritonitis; hematogenously via the hepatic artery or portal and umbilical veins; or via the bile ducts.

Excepting peracute septicemias, *there are few specific bacterial infections that have a sustained or repeated bacteremic phase without producing hepatic lesions*. There are, in addition, many cases of nonspecific bacteremia, especially those originating in the drainage field of the portal vein, in which focal hepatitis occurs. Because their differential diagnosis is of some importance, it is probably useful to list here those specific bacterial diseases in which focal hepatitis is expected or characteristic, but not constant. Specific infections may occur as fetal or perinatal infections. The list includes *Salmonella* spp. in all hosts (Fig. 2-72); *Listeria monocytogenes* in fetal and neonatal lambs, calves, foals, and piglets; *Campylobacter fetus* in fetal and neonatal lambs (Fig. 2-73); *Actinobacillus equuli* in foals; *Actinobacillus suis* in pigs; *Yersinia pseudotuberculosis* in lambs and occasionally in dogs and cats; *Francisella (Yersinia) tularensis* in lambs and cats; *Mannheimia haemolytica* and *Histophilus somni (Haemophilus agni)* in lambs; *Clostridium piliforme* (formerly *Bacillus piliformis*; Tyzzer disease) in foals, cats and dogs; *Nocardia asteroides* in dogs; and the mycobacteria in all hosts (Figs. 2-74 and 2-75A and B).

Hepatic abscess

Hepatic abscesses, quite apart from the lesions of the specific infections just given, *are common*, especially in cattle. They may arise by direct implantation of a foreign body from the reticulum or by direct invasion of the capsule from a neutrophilic

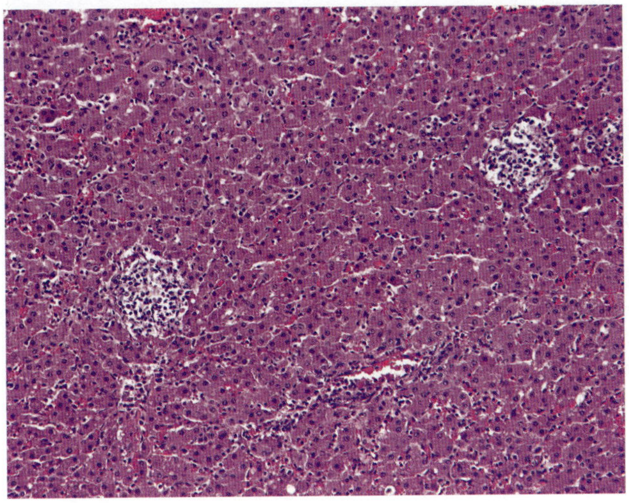

Figure 2-72 Multifocal hepatitis caused by ***Salmonella*** **sp.** infection in a calf.

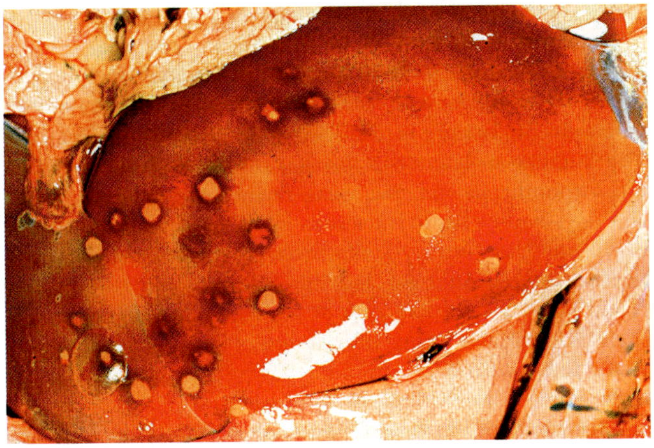

Figure 2-73 ***Campylobacter fetus*** infection in an ovine fetus. (Courtesy P. Stromberg.)

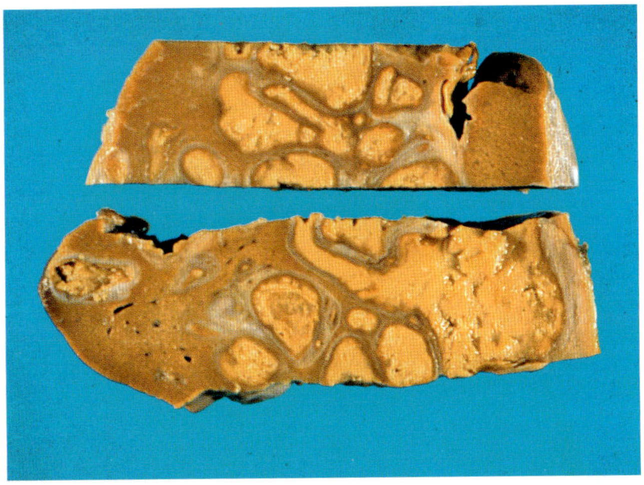

Figure 2-74 **Tuberculosis** in a bovine liver. (Courtesy University of Guelph.)

lesion of *traumatic reticulitis* and may be single or multiple, but in either case, they are often preferentially distributed to the left lobe. They may be hematogenous from *portal vein emboli*, or by direct extension of **omphalophlebitis**. Abscesses via the hepatic artery may occur but are quite uncommon.

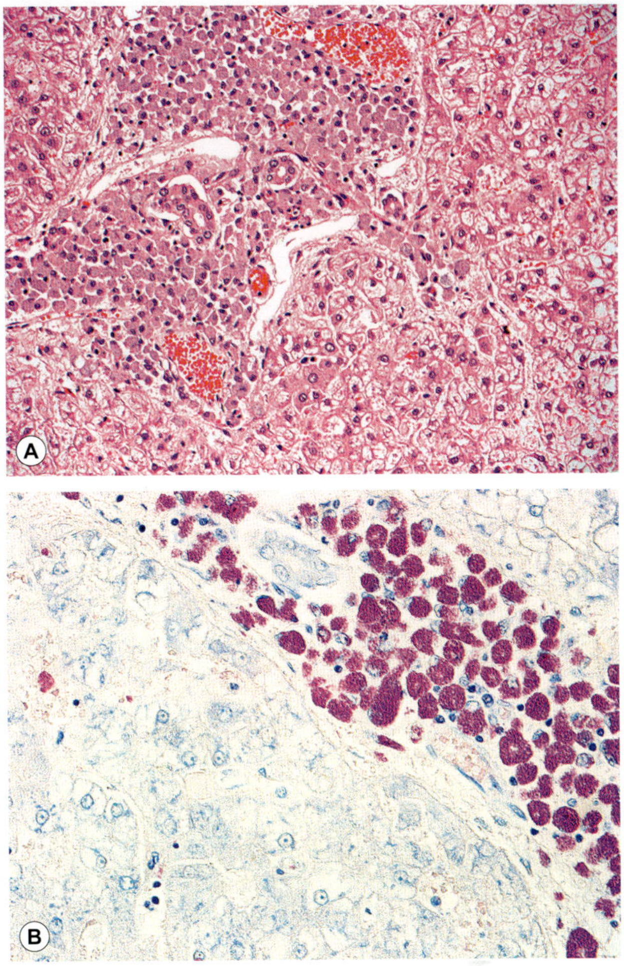

Figure 2-75 **Hepatic mycobacteriosis** in a Schnauzer dog **A**. H&E. **B**. Acid-fast stain. (Courtesy J.L. Caswell.)

Abscesses originating from the umbilicus are more common in calves than in other species but occur in all. The bacterial flora is often mixed, but *Trueperella pyogenes, Fusobacterium necrophorum*, streptococci, staphylococci, and *E. coli* usually predominate. Hepatic abscesses are not inevitable sequelae to omphalitis or even to omphalophlebitis, but they do not develop from navel infections in the absence of omphalophlebitis. As there is no flow of blood in these vessels after birth, involvement of the liver is by direct growth along the physiologic thrombus. Omphalophlebitis can be quite severe without extension to the liver. Hepatic abscesses of omphalogenic origin are often restricted to the left lobe (Fig. 2-76), but they may be restricted to the right or be generalized in their distribution.

Hepatic abscesses are also common and of economic importance in ***feedlot cattle***. They are usually found at slaughter but, when numerous, may be fatal after a few days of vague digestive illness. Their pathogenesis and character are discussed with rumenitis, to which they are a sequel (see Vol. 2, Alimentary System). Liver abscesses in *feedlot sheep* likely have a similar pathogenesis, with *F. necrophorum* as the primary isolate. A second category includes parasitic granulomas populated by various opportunistic bacteria.

Hepatic abscesses of biliary origin occur in all animals. They occur in pigs in which ascarids have migrated into the bile ducts. Cholangitic abscesses in horses, dogs, and cats are usually

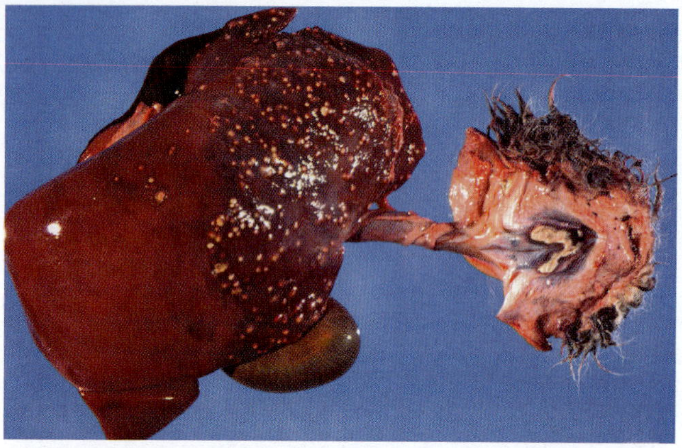

Figure 2-76 Omphalophlebitis with **miliary metastatic abscesses** in the left lobe of the liver in a calf.

caused by enterobacteria as part of a fulminating ascending cholangiohepatitis that is fatal after a short course.

The *sequelae* of hepatic abscessation are variable. Usually, they are insignificant and subclinical. Sterilization of the focus with either resorption and complete healing or encapsulation is common. Those near the surface of the liver regularly produce fibrinous and then fibrous inflammation of the capsule and adhesion to adjacent viscera. They seldom perforate the capsule but do *commonly break into hepatic veins* to produce any one or a combination of thrombophlebitis of the vena cava, endocarditis, or pulmonary abscesses or embolism. Acute extension of a hepatic abscess into the major hepatic vein can lead to pulmonary embolism that can be acutely fatal. In adults, death may occur if the hepatic abscesses are multiple and fresh, and especially if they are necrobacillary in origin; death is probably the result of toxemia.

Hepatic necrobacillosis

Occasionally, ***F. necrophorum*** infection of the liver is seen following *omphalophlebitis in lambs and calves*, or as a complication of *rumenitis in adult cattle*. In feedlot cattle, both *F. necrophorum* subsp. *necrophorum* (biotype A) and subsp. *funduliforme* (biotype B) have been isolated. The hepatic lesions are multiple, slightly elevated, rounded, dry areas of coagulative necrosis, sometimes a few centimeters in diameter (eFig. 2-19), and surrounded by a zone of intense hyperemia. Affected neonates seldom live long enough for the necrotic foci to liquefy and assume the appearance of ordinary abscesses, but this may be seen in adult cattle. *The histologic appearance of the foci in the stage of coagulative necrosis is quite characteristic.* The necrotic amorphous central area is bordered by a zone of wholesale destruction of leukocytes, whose nuclear chromatin is dissipated in a finely divided form, and among which the filamentous fusobacteria are mostly concentrated. Outside this zone, there is severe hyperemia and hemorrhage, and thrombosis of local vessels is common. The lesion in neonatal lambs is to be distinguished from that caused by *Campylobacter fetus*.

The pathogenic mechanisms of *F. necrophorum* involve various toxins, particularly a high–molecular-weight *leukotoxin* specifically toxic to ruminant neutrophils. This unique toxin activates neutrophils and induces their apoptosis, consistent with the remarkable abscess-inducing propensity of *F. necrophorum* in ruminants. However, other toxins, endotoxic LPS, and hemagglutinins are also implicated as virulence factors. Mixed infections are frequent, and synergism between *F. necrophorum* and other pathogens, such as *T. pyogenes*, may also play a role in the pathogenesis of liver necrosis and abscessation.

Necrotic hepatitis (black disease)

Organisms of the genus *Clostridium* are notably circuitous in their means of producing disease. This is true of ***Clostridium novyi;*** *type B strains, which produce potent exotoxins and are the cause of black disease (infectious necrotic hepatitis)*. The alpha toxin of *C. novyi* is related to the large clostridial cytotoxins produced by *Clostridioides difficile* and *Paraclostridium (Paeniclostridium) sordellii*. These toxins enter cells by receptor-mediated endocytosis and inhibit ras and rho guanosine triphosphatases by glycosylation. The beta toxin is a necrotizing and hemolytic phospholipase C (lecithinase). Black disease occurs in nonimmune animals when these exotoxins are released by *C. novyi* within an anaerobic focus in the liver. These anaerobic sites, which provide a suitable environment for germination of *C. novyi* spores, are most commonly a result of migrating liver flukes.

C. novyi is widely distributed in soil, and the spores are continually ingested by grazing animals in areas where black disease occurs. Some spores cross the mucous membranes, probably in phagocytes, and remain as latent infections in macrophages, mainly in the liver, spleen, and bone marrow. The duration of latency in tissue is not known, but it can be many months. In endemic areas, many healthy sheep, cattle, and dogs harbor latent infections in their livers. *Black disease is principally an acutely fatal disease of sheep in regions where the inciting helminths are endemic.* Sporadic cases have been reported in cattle, goats, pigs, and horses. The disease is *most commonly initiated by migrating larvae of the common liver fluke* ***Fasciola hepatica***. Sporadic cases may be related to *Cysticercus tenuicollis* infection or may be idiopathic.

Deaths in sheep from black disease occur rapidly and usually without warning signs. Illness, if seen, is brief and occurs as reluctance to move, drowsiness, rapid respiration, and quiet subsidence. Affected animals are usually in good nutritional condition. Postmortem decomposition occurs rapidly. *The name of the disease is derived from the appearance of flayed skin, the dark coloration being caused by an unusual degree of subcutaneous venous congestion.* Frequently, there is edema of the sternal subcutis, and airways contain stable foam. Serous cavities contain an abundance of fluid that clots on exposure to air. The fluid is usually straw colored, but that in the abdomen may be tinged with blood. The volume of fluid in the abdomen and thorax may vary from ~50 mL to 1.5 L. The pericardial sac is distended with similar fluid in amounts up to ~300 mL. Subendocardial hemorrhages in the left ventricle are almost constant. Patchy areas of congestion and hemorrhage may be present in the pyloric part of the abomasum and in the small intestine.

The *typical and diagnostic lesions* occur in the liver and are always present. They are usually clearly evident on the capsular surface, the diaphragmatic surface especially, but the organ may have to be sliced carefully to find them. The liver will be the seat of either the acute traumatic hemorrhagic lesions of acute fascioliasis, the cholangiohepatitis of the chronic disease, or both. *The lesions of black disease are several, or rarely single, yellow-gray, 2-3-cm areas of necrosis, surrounded by a broad zone of intense hyperemia, roughly circular in outline, and extending hemispherically into the substance of the organ.* There may be a coagulum of fibrin on the capsular surface overlying the necrotic area. Occasionally, the essential lesions are rectilinear in shape or very irregular. The lesions appear homogeneous on the cut surface, but some contain poorly defined centers of soft or caseous material. The microscopic lesions are similar to those of bacillary hemoglobinuria. Focal or multifocal coagulative necrosis of hepatocytes is surrounded by a rim of degenerate and viable neutrophils, sometimes admixed with a few lymphocytes, plasma cells, and macrophages. Large numbers of gram-positive rods, with sometimes visible subterminal spores, are within necrotic centers at the junction with inflammatory cells. Necrotic tracts associated with liver fluke migration and/or portal fibrosis, ductular reaction, and cholangitis due to chronic fascioliasis may occur concurrently.

Bacillary hemoglobinuria

Bacillary hemoglobinuria is a counterpart of black disease. The cause is ***Clostridium haemolyticum***, which is closely related to *C. novyi* type B. Both species produce the *beta toxin*, a necrotizing and hemolytic lecithinase (phospholipase C). The main difference between these 2 bacteria is that edema-inducing alpha toxin (TcnA) is produced by *C. novyi* type B, but not by *C. haemolyticum*. The pathogenesis of the 2 diseases is comparable, as both depend on a focus of hepatic injury within which latent spores can germinate. *Bacillary hemoglobinuria exists endemically only in areas where **F. hepatica** exists, and it is probable that flukes are the primary cause of the initiating lesion*. The disease does occur sporadically where there are no flukes and may be prompted by other parasites or other diverse focal lesions, which are smudged out in the expanding areas of necrosis. There is scant information on the ecology of the organism, but it is clear that it has its own environmental requirements, and the disease will not persist in areas where these requirements are not met. The spores will remain in the livers of cattle for several months after removal from pastures where the disease is endemic. Spores may persist in the bones of cadavers for 2 years. Spores of this and other sporulating anaerobes can often be demonstrated in the liver, where they are probably retained in Kupffer cells.

Bacillary hemoglobinuria occurs primarily in *cattle*. Sporadic cases have been reported in sheep, pigs, and horses. It is characterized clinically by *intravascular hemolysis with anemia and hemoglobinuria*, but perhaps reflecting the variety in exotoxins between strains of the organism, hemolysis may not be a feature. The gross and microscopic hepatic lesions are similar to those of black disease but much larger and usually single (Fig. 2-77). It has been described as an infarct secondary to portal thrombosis, and although this may occur in isolated cases, it is scarcely a credible pathogenesis for a disease of endemic occurrence. Thrombosis does occur in the affected areas but can be a result, rather than a cause, of the initial lesion and is found more often in the hepatic venules than in branches of the portal vein. The remainder of the liver is usually brown-tan and may have a prominent acinar pattern, due to centrilobular degeneration and necrosis, likely resulting from hypoxia. Severe anemia, variable jaundice, diffusely red or brown kidneys due to hemoglobin, and port-wine–colored urine are additional lesions. Peritoneal vessels are congested, and in some cases, there is severe, dry, fibrinohemorrhagic peritonitis.

Clostridium piliforme *infection*

C. piliforme (formerly *Bacillus piliformis*) infection has long been known as **Tyzzer disease**. The disease occurs in numerous animal species; however, **horses**, especially foals, and laboratory animals represent most of the cases. Sporadic cases have been reported in *calves, dogs, and cats*. The disease is probably initiated by ingestion of *C. piliforme* spores, an intestinal infection and subsequent hematogenous spread to the liver and other organs such as the heart. The lesions in the gut are less specific and constant than those in the liver, which consist of *focal hepatitis and necrosis*.

Affected foals usually die between the ages of 1 and 4 weeks; often they are found dead after a short illness. The

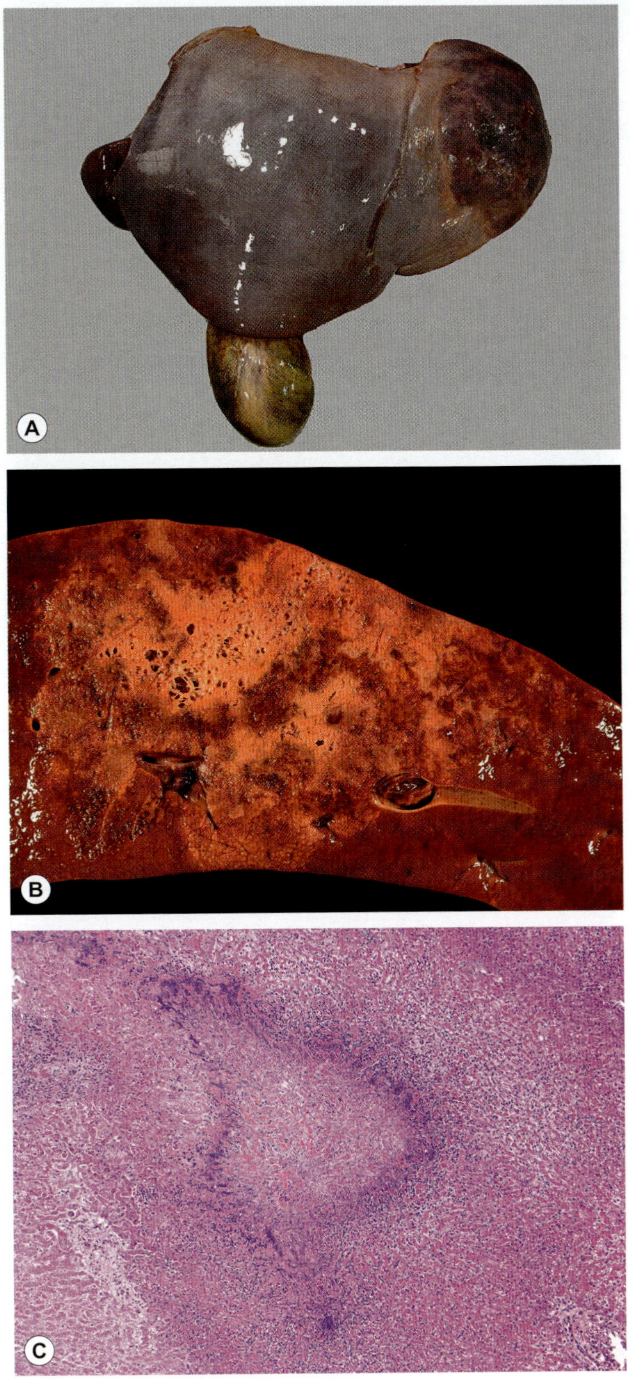

Figure 2-77 A. Large focus of hepatic necrosis in an ox with **bacillary hemoglobinuria.** B. Cross section of the focus of hepatic necrosis. C. Hepatic necrosis with peripheral bacterial colonies and neutrophilic inflammation.

gross liver lesions consist of an enlarged liver with variably visible, randomly distributed, pale foci up to a few millimeters across (Fig. 2-78). Microscopically, the lesions are randomly distributed foci of coagulative necrosis surrounded by viable and degenerate neutrophils (Fig. 2-79A). Aggregates of macrophages forming granulomas with occasional fibrosis and mineralization may occur in chronic cases. The lesion is not diagnostic in itself; its specificity depends on finding the causal organism in hepatocytes in the periphery of the necrotic zones. *C. piliforme* can only be isolated with difficulty on artificial media; hence, diagnosis is usually based on demonstration of the large, long bacilli in the cytoplasm of degenerate and otherwise apparently normal hepatocytes at the periphery of the necrotic zones. *The bacilli tend to lie in sheaves or bundles.* The organisms are gram-negative and are best delineated with silver impregnation techniques, such as Warthin-Starry, but they may be seen with routine stains, such as H&E, Giemsa, and PAS stains, particularly when the material is fresh (see Fig. 2-79B). Icterus is often present. There may also be *colitis* sufficiently severe to cause diarrhea, but not as severe as that seen in rabbits with this disease, as well as *myocarditis*. Lesions in the liver, intestine, and heart constitute a *triad of lesions diagnostic for Tyzzer disease*, but all 3 lesions are not always present.

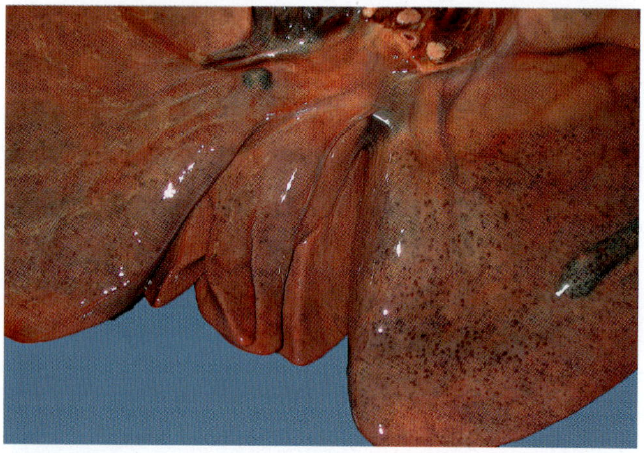

Figure 2-78 Foal liver with multifocal hepatitis in ***Clostridium piliforme*** infection (Tyzzer disease).

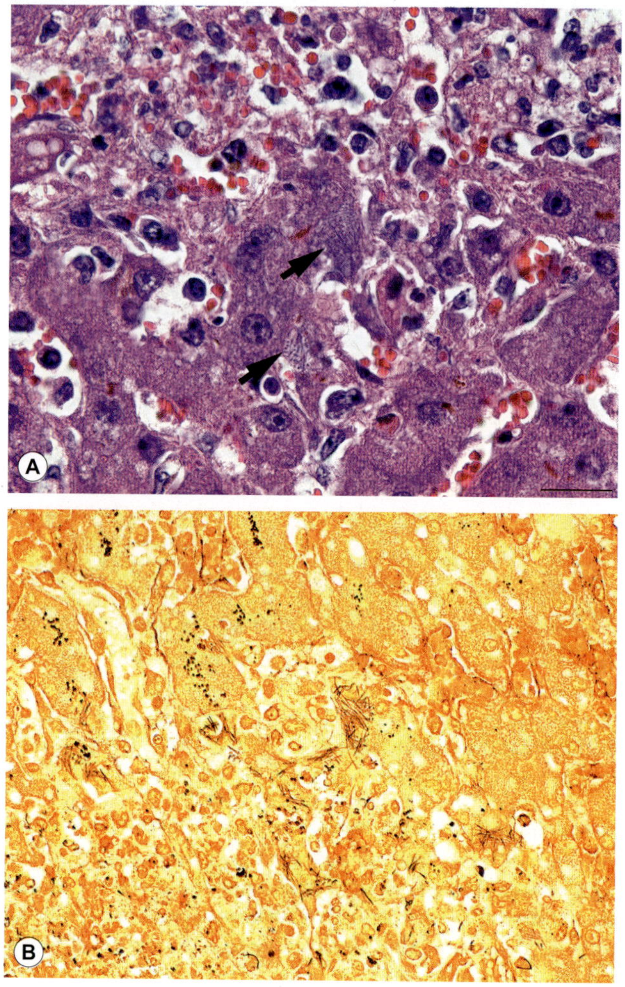

Figure 2-79 **Tyzzer disease** in a foal. **A.** Bundles of *Clostridium piliforme* bacilli in hepatocytes at the margin of lesion are sometimes visible on H&E-stained section (arrow). **B.** A Warthin-Starry silver stain highlights *C. piliforme* bacilli in hepatocytes. (B, Courtesy F. Uzal.)

Sporadic cases of Tyzzer disease have been reported in dogs and cats. The lesions are essentially the same as those in foals and rodents. Immunodeficiency predisposes to the disease because it occurs sporadically in dogs that have undergone immunosuppressive or anticancer therapy. Such cases may be complicated by concurrent viral, mycotic, or protozoal infections.

Leptospirosis

Leptospirosis is a systemic disease that results in acute jaundice, cholestatic liver injury, and renal failure in dogs, and is discussed in more detail in Vol. 2, Urinary System. The hepatic lesions described following acute experimental infection of dogs with *Leptospira kirschneri* serovar Grippotyphosa include mixed perivascular portal infiltrates of neutrophils, lymphocytes, and plasma cells, with mild hepatic lipidosis, dissociation of hepatocytes, and intracanalicular bile plugs evident by day 12 postinfection, along with increased hepatocellular mitotic activity. *Clinical icterus has been attributed to cholestasis caused by dissociation of hepatocytes* (eFig. 2-20). Dogs experimentally infected with *Leptospira interrogans* serovar Pomona developed pulmonary and renal petechial hemorrhages, and friable livers with multifocal 1-2-mm raised white foci corresponding to periportal inflammatory infiltrates of lymphocytes, plasma cells, neutrophils, and macrophages; small foci of hepatic necrosis; and bile plugs in canaliculi, in addition to renal, pulmonary, and cardiac lesions. Organisms were identified by immunohistochemistry at the brush borders of renal proximal convoluted tubules as well as at the luminal surface of bile duct epithelium. In a retrospective study of dogs with supportive clinical signs and microscopic agglutination test titers of ≥320 for one or more serovars tested, including Autumnalis, Bratislava, Canicola, Grippotyphosa, Icterohaemorrhagiae, and Pomona, histologic lesions in the liver were subtle, with sinusoidal neutrophil margination, Kupffer cell hypertrophy, and low levels of hepatocellular single-cell necrosis and mitoses. Some livers had diffuse interstitial lymphocytic hepatitis, with mitotic figures, anisokaryosis, binucleation, and some degree of lobular collapse. Chronic hepatitis has also been experimentally produced by leptospiral infection in dogs; however, clinical cases are rarely documented. Clinical disease in domestic cats is rare despite widespread serologic evidence of infection by *Leptospira* spp. Cats are considered disease resistant compared with other animal species.

Other bacteria

A sole case of clinical disease associated with ***Helicobacter canis*** has been reported in a 2-month-old puppy with peracute disease causing weakness and vomiting before death. Coalescing yellow foci in the liver of up to 1.5 cm diameter consisted of hepatocellular coagulative necrosis with infiltrating mononuclear cells and neutrophils. Spiral bacteria were visualized by Warthin-Starry silver stains in area of necrosis, within bile canaliculi, and occasionally in bile duct lumens. This organism has previously been found in the blood of diarrheic children, and in the feces of 4% of dogs in an epidemiologic study examining the incidence of *Campylobacter*-like organisms in 1,000 dogs.

Bartonella spp. infection has been associated with a wide variety of granulomatous syndromes and hepatic sinusoidal angiectasis in humans, often in association with immunosuppression. *B. henselae* and *B. clarridgeiae* are associated with self-limiting illness and persistent intravascular infection in cats; mild lymphocytic cholangitis/pericholangitis and lymphocytic hepatitis have been reported with experimental infection of cats with *B. henselae*. *B. henselae* has been shown in liver tissue by PCR from a single case of hepatic sinusoidal angiectasis in a Golden Retriever and in granulomatous hepatitis in a Basset Hound. *B. clarridgeiae* DNA was identified in liver tissue from a Doberman Pinscher with histologic lesions of Doberman hepatitis; however, the extent to which infection induces disease in dogs is currently unknown.

Helminthic infections

Various helminths, including cestodes, nematodes, and trematodes, as well as the larval pentastome *Linguatula serrata*, can produce inflammation of the liver and bile ducts. Those parasites that have the biliary system as their final habitat will be discussed in detail later. The others produce hepatic lesions during their natural or accidental migrations and are discussed under the organ (for most of them, the gut) that is their final habitat. It is useful, however, to describe briefly here the lesions produced by larvae in transit.

The initial lesion produced by wandering larvae is traumatic. Sinuous tunnels permeate the parenchyma and often breach the capsule. In the tunnels, there are free red cells, degenerating hepatocytes, and leukocytes, chiefly eosinophils, which react to the parasites. Bordering the tunnel is a narrow zone of coagulative necrosis of parenchyma with neutrophils at its margin. Eosinophils also infiltrate the portal tracts. The necrotic parasitic tracts heal by scarification, and the fibroblastic tissue, infiltrated with eosinophils, is eventually incorporated into the portal units. Most larvae escape from the liver, but some eventually become encapsulated in the liver in abscesses containing numerous eosinophils. The abscesses may caseate and come to resemble tubercles, and eventually many are heavily mineralized to form permanent pearly nodules. In sheep, the most common cause of this type of hepatitis (aside from liver fluke) is ***Cysticercus tenuicollis*** in its wandering phase. Lambs may die of severe hemorrhagic hepatitis (Fig. 2-80) caused by very heavy infections of this parasite, and in pigs, an aberrant host, *C. tenuicollis*, can produce a very intense inflammatory reaction.

In pigs, larvae of ***Ascaris suum*** and ***Stephanurus dentatus*** produce similar but distinct patterns of focal interstitial hepatitis. The ascarids produce their distinctive accentuation of the stroma (*"milk spots"*; Fig. 2-81) when quite small larvae are immobilized by the host's inflammatory reaction; thus, the foci are relatively small. The fibrotic lesion produced by *S. dentatus* larvae, on the contrary, is less focal and more in the nature of a track, and there are generally small, inflamed, capsular craters where the larvae have emerged from the liver to migrate to their preferred perirenal site. There will be obvious portal phlebitis at the hepatic hilum when infection by *S. dentatus* has been by the oral route, and in these livers, the parenchymal lesion is more severe in this vicinity.

Migration tracks left by **larval strongyles** can be found under the liver capsule in young horses, and historically, these have been thought to be related to the dense, discrete, capsular fibrous tags and plaques that are almost universally found on the diaphragmatic surface of the liver of mature horses. However, these hepatic fibrotic lesions remain common in horses even after the widespread use of effective anthelmintics, and their precise etiology remains unknown (Fig. 2-82).

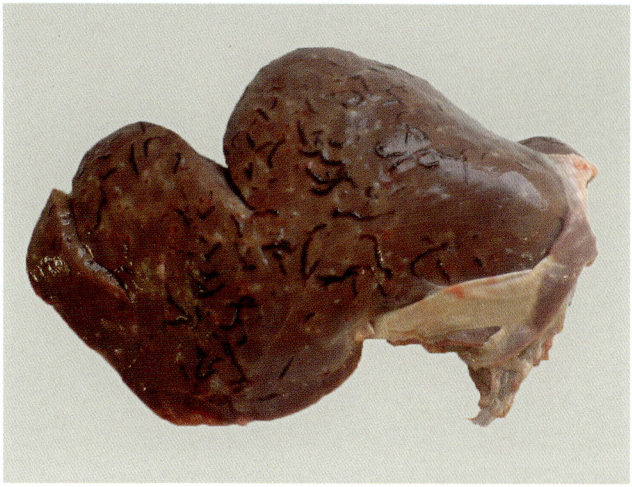

Figure 2-80 **Hemorrhagic subcapsular migration tracks** caused by *Cysticercus tenuicollis* in a lamb. (Courtesy A. Rehmtulla.)

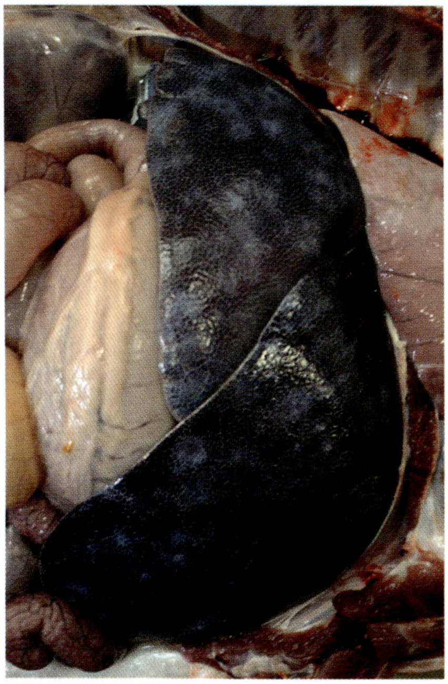

Figure 2-81 **Multifocal interstitial hepatitis** ("milk-spot liver") caused by *Ascaris suum* migration in a pig.

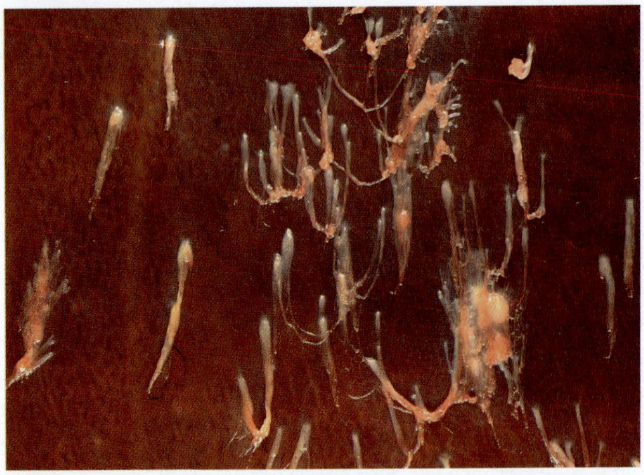

Figure 2-82 **Fibrous tags** on the diaphragmatic surface of an equine liver.

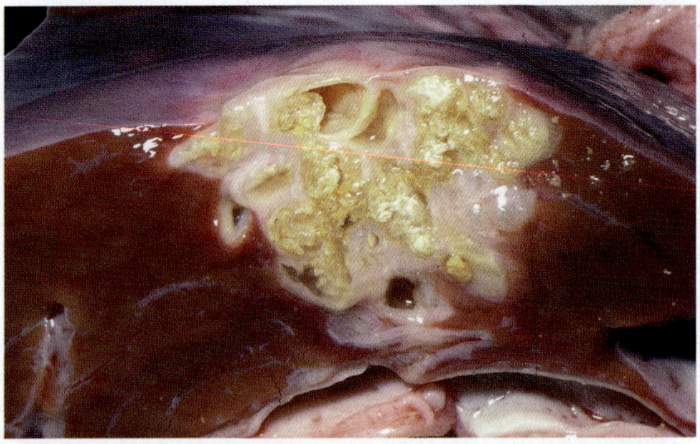

Figure 2-83 **Hydatid liver disease** (*Echinococcus granulosus* infection) in an ox. (Courtesy F. Uzal.)

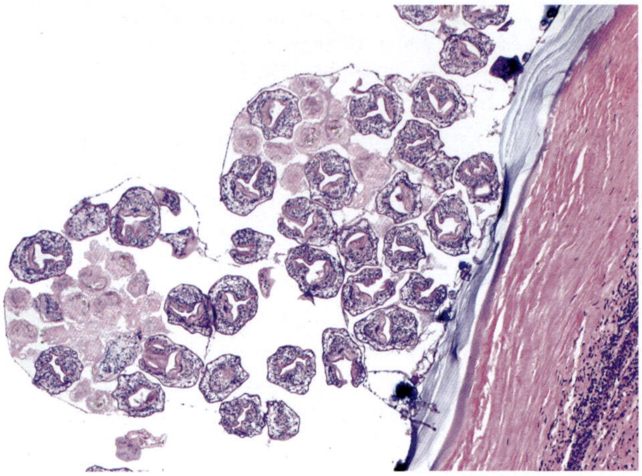

Figure 2-84 ***Echinococcus granulosus*** **cyst** with acellular laminated layer and brood capsules with protoscolices in the liver of a moose. (Courtesy J. Kurz.)

Parasites can produce hepatic lesions by other means. The hydatid intermediate stages of *Echinococcus* encyst in the liver and may destroy much of it; the larvae of *A. suum* in cattle add to the usual insult by causing portal phlebitis and small areas of infarction; the adults of *Ascaris* in all species, but especially in pigs, may migrate into the bile ducts; and the eggs of schistosomes enter in the portal blood to lodge in the intrahepatic portal vessels and provoke granulomatous inflammation.

Cestodes

Stilesia hepatica and ***Thysanosoma actinioides***, the "fringed tapeworm," are the only cestodes that inhabit the bile ducts. They are parasites of ruminants, *Stilesia* occurring in Africa, and *Thysanosoma* in North and South America. The life cycles of the parasites are not completely known but may involve oribatid mites as intermediate hosts. *T. actinioides* may also be found in the pancreatic ducts and small intestine. Usually, the infections are light but, even when heavy, are not of much significance (eFig. 2-21). Very heavy infections by *S. hepatica* occur without signs of illness, although the bile ducts may be nearly occluded, slightly thickened, and dilated. Saccular dilations of the ducts may occur and be filled with worms. The fringed tapeworm is perhaps more pathogenic, and unthriftiness may accompany heavy infections.

Echinococcus granulosus *hydatid cysts* occur most commonly in the liver of ruminants in endemic areas (Fig. 2-83) but have been reported as incidental postmortem findings in the liver of pigs and horses. The cysticerci and hydatids, which in the intermediate stages invade the liver, are discussed further in Vol. 2, Alimentary System.

Echinococcus multilocularis is found in Europe, parts of northern Asia, and North America, where it has a sylvatic life cycle. Red and arctic foxes are the most important definitive hosts, although coyotes, raccoon-dogs, and wolves can also be infected. In North America, there are increasing cases of intestinal infection by *E. multilocularis* tapeworms in domestic dogs; fewer in cats. The adult tapeworm is small, 5 mm, and infective eggs are shed in the feces to be ingested by intermediate hosts, which in temperate areas are typically various species of rodents, including voles, lemmings, and deer mice. The hexacanth embryo is released from the egg, travels through the intestinal wall, and migrates to the liver via the hepatic portal circulation. The metacestode stage is an *alveolar hydatid cyst*, composed of numerous small vesicles lined by a PAS-positive acellular laminated membrane or cuticle layer and a layer of germinal epithelium from which protoscolices develop. Some infections in dogs do not progress to form protoscolices and instead form irregular large cysts with a PAS-positive laminated membrane (Fig. 2-84). Additional exogenous budding results in the spread of the metacestodes to other internal locations. The life cycle is completed when the infected intermediate host is consumed by a definitive host, in which the protoscolices attach to the intestinal wall and mature. Other species can occasionally act as aberrant intermediate hosts, including pigs, horses, and humans; *human alveolar echinococcosis is a serious zoonosis*. Dogs can simultaneously act as definitive and aberrant intermediate hosts for this parasite. Cases of hepatic alveolar hydatid cysts have been reported in dogs from endemic areas. Affected dogs have progressive abdominal enlargement, intermittent inappetence, and vomiting, and the cysts may be found in the liver, omentum, abdominal cavity, or lungs.

Nematodes

Calodium hepaticum (syn. *Capillaria hepatica*) is the one nematode that in the adult phase inhabits the liver. It is a slender worm, morphologically resembling the whipworms, and it lives in the parenchyma rather than in the bile ducts. The usual hosts of the adult stage are rodents, but sporadic infections are observed in dogs. These worms are *not highly pathogenic*. The adults provoke some traumatic hepatitis, and the eggs, which are deposited in clusters, provoke the development of localized granulomas. The eggs are readily recognized by their ovoid shape and polar caps. The granulomas can be seen through the capsule or in the substance of the liver as yellow streaks or patches. The eggs cannot escape from the liver unless a predator eats them. Predators, however, act only as transport hosts, and the ingested eggs are passed in the feces. Larvae develop in the eggs only in the external environment, and the cycle is completed when a suitable host eats the mature larvae in the eggs.

Trematodes

Various trematodes (flukes) are parasitic in the livers of animals. They belong to the families ***Fasciolidae*** *(Fasciola hepatica, F. gigantica, Fascioloides magna)*, ***Dicrocoeliidae*** [*Dicrocoelium dendriticum, D. hospes, Platynosomum fastosum* (syn. *Platynosomum concinnum*)], ***Schistosomatidae*** *(Heterobilharzia americana)*, and ***Opisthorchiidae*** (including *Metorchis* spp., *Opisthorchis felineus, Clonorchis sinensis, Pseudamphistomum truncatum*). The diseases produced are known collectively as **distomatoses**.

Fasciola hepatica*, the common liver fluke of sheep and cattle, is the most widespread and important of the group*. Patent infections can develop in other wild and domestic animals and in humans. These flukes are leaf shaped and ~2.5 cm long in sheep and slightly larger in cattle. *They are found in the bile ducts*. Being hermaphroditic, only one fluke is necessary to establish a patent infection, and each adult may produce 20,000 eggs per day. The longevity of the adult flukes is amazing and is potentially as great as or greater than that of the host; they have been known to survive for 11 years, and it seems that they can produce eggs all this time. The eggs are eliminated in bile, and on pasture, in conditions of suitable warmth and moisture, hatch a larva (miracidium) in ~9 days. If the environmental temperature is low, the incubation period may be delayed for some months. The miracidium can survive only in moisture. It is actively motile and penetrates the tissues of the intermediate host, which is an aquatic snail. Different snails serve this purpose in different countries, but all of them belong to the genus *Lymnaea*.

Each *miracidium*, on penetrating a snail, develops into a mother *sporocyst* that reproduces, probably parthenogenetically, giving rise to a small number of the second generation, the *redia*. Each redia produces either rediae or *cercariae*, or the 2 successively. Cercariae, the larval stage of the third (sexual) generation, first appear 1-2 months after the miracidium penetrates. Cercariae continue to escape daily for the life of the snail, but even so, total cercarial production is only 500-1,000. They actively escape from the snail and are attracted to green plants, where they encyst and become infective metacercariae in 1 day. These can remain infective for 1 month in summer and up to 3 months in winter. The developmental events from egg to this stage take 1-2 months under favorable conditions.

Infection occurs by ingestion. Excystment occurs in the duodenum. The young flukes penetrate the intestinal wall and cross the peritoneal cavity, attaching here and there to suck blood and penetrate the liver through its capsule; a few no doubt pass in the portal vessels or migrate up the bile duct. They wander in the liver for a month or more before settling down in the bile ducts to mature, which they do in 2-3 months. Some may, by accident, enter the hepatic veins and systemic circulation to lodge in unusual sites; intrauterine infections are on record. *Lesions caused by aberrant flukes are quite common in bovine lung*. They consist of resilient nodules just under the pleura of the peripheral parts of the lung. They range in diameter from ~1 to many centimeters and consist of thinly encapsulated abscesses situated at the ends of bronchi. The content is slightly mucoid, unevenly coagulated brown fluid; in some lesions, the reaction is predominantly caseous. The location of the lesion suggests that it begins as a peripheral bronchiectasis that later becomes sealed off. The fluke persists in the debris but is small and hard to find.

The essential *lesions* produced by *F. hepatica* occur in the liver and may be described, first, as those produced by the migratory larvae, and second, as those produced by the mature flukes in the bile ducts; the two often intermingle (eFig. 2-22). There is further incidence of peritonitis, which is produced by the young flukes on their way to the liver and, perhaps also, by some that break out through the capsule.

Usually, there is no obvious reaction to the passage of young flukes through the intestinal wall and across the peritoneal cavity, except for small hemorrhagic foci on the peritoneum, where the flukes have been temporarily attached. Few or many parasites may be found in any ascitic fluid and attached to the peritoneum of the diaphragm and the mesenteries. When the infections are heavy and repeated, such as may be observed in sheep, cattle, and swine, *peritonitis* occurs. The young flukes at this stage are <1.0 mm long. Peritonitis may be acute and exudative or chronic and proliferative. It is usually concentrated on the hepatic capsule, especially its visceral surface, but may be restricted to the parietal peritoneum or to the visceral peritoneum, including the mesenteries of the gut. In acute cases, there are fibrinohemorrhagic deposits on the serous surfaces, and in chronic cases, there may be fibrous tags, with adhesions or a diffuse thickening by connective tissue. Many young flukes can be found microscopically in the fibrinous deposits, and in the diffuse peritoneal thickenings, there are tortuous migration tunnels containing blood, debris, and the young parasites. In cases with involvement of the visceral peritoneum, young flukes can be found in enlarged mesenteric lymph nodes.

The acute lesions in the liver caused by the wandering flukes are basically traumatic, but there is an element of coagulative necrosis, which is possibly related to toxic excretions of the flukes. The migratory pathways are tortuous tunnels that appear on cross section as hemorrhagic 2-3-mm foci. If a tunnel is followed, a young fluke <1.0-mm long can be found at the end. When the infection is heavy, the liver may appear to be permeated by dark hemorrhagic streaks and foci. Older tunnels from which the debris has been cleared may appear as light-yellow streaks because of infiltration of eosinophils. Microscopically, fresh tunnels are filled with blood and degenerate hepatocytes and are soon infiltrated by eosinophils. Later, macrophages and giant cells arrange themselves about the debris and remove it, and healing occurs by granulation tissue, which is rich in lymphocytes and eosinophils. In light infections, the scars may disappear, but in heavy infections, they may fuse with each other and with portal areas to produce moderate irregular fibrosis. There may, as yet, be no change in the bile ducts. Probably, *most of the young flukes reach the bile ducts, but some do not and become encysted in the parenchyma*. One or more flukes may be present in each cyst, which consists of a connective tissue capsule and a dirty brown content of blood, detritus, and excrement from flukes. The cysts ultimately caseate and may mineralize or are obliterated by fibrous tissue. These cysts are most frequent on the visceral surface, where they cause bulging of the capsule.

Heavy infections by immature flukes may cause death at the stage of acute hepatitis. Such an outcome is not common but occurs in sheep. It is estimated that 10,000 metacercariae ingested over a brief period are necessary to produce death in sheep. Death may occur suddenly or after a few days of fever, lassitude, inappetence, and abdominal tenderness. This is also the stage of parasitism in which *black disease* occurs.

Mature flukes are present in the larger bile ducts and cause cholangitis. The relative importance of varied factors in their pathogenicity is not known, but they cause mechanical irritation by the action of their suckers and scales, cause obstruction of the ducts with some degree of biliary retention, predispose to bacterial infections, suck blood, and probably produce toxic and irritative metabolic excretions.

The *biliary changes* occur in all lobes but are usually most severe in the left, and the right may be moderately hypertrophied. From the hilum, *the bile ducts on the visceral surface stand out as white, firm, branching cords* that in extreme instances may be 2 cm in diameter and allow detectable fluctuation over extended segments or in localized areas of ectasia. This dilation of the ducts in sheep, swine, and horses is largely mechanical and is caused by *distension by masses of flukes and bile*. It is permitted by the relative paucity of new connective tissue formation in the walls of the ducts in these species; this in turn is probably related to the rather mild catarrhal type of inflammation in the lumina of the ducts. In *cattle*, desquamative and ulcerative lesions in the large bile ducts are more severe than in other species, and there is a correspondingly greater proliferation of granulation tissue in and about the walls of the ducts (Fig. 2-85). The walls of the ducts in cattle are, in consequence, much thickened, and the lumen is irregularly stenotic and dilated and lined largely by granulation tissue. This contributes the typical *"pipestem"* appearance to the ducts in cattle; the connective tissue may be, in addition, mineralized, sometimes so heavily that it cannot be cut with a knife. The bile ducts contain dirty dark-brown fluid of a mucinous or tough consistency, formed from degenerate floccular bile, pus, desquamated cells and detritus, clumps of flukes, and small masses of eggs in dark-brown granular aggregates.

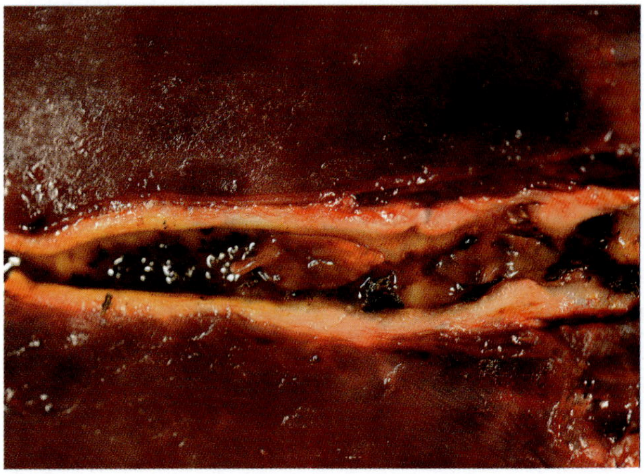

Figure 2-85 ***Fasciola hepatica*** in the lumen of thickened and dilated bile ducts in an ox.

Although the lesions are most obvious in ducts large enough to contain the flukes, there is, with time and severe or repeated infections, *progressive inflammation in the smaller portal units* because of direct irritation by the flukes, superimposed infections, and biliary stasis. The course of events is as described earlier for *subacute and chronic cholangitis*. The proliferating connective tissue and bile ductules in individual portal areas extend to join each other and the scars left over from the migratory phase, so that inflammatory fibrosis may obliterate parenchyma in many foci. In such livers, the left lobe, which is the one most severely affected, may be atrophied, indurated, and irregular.

The development of cholangitis to the degree described depends on long-standing or heavy infections. Lesions of lesser severity, or those less fully developed, are associated with light infections of short duration. They may then be recognized only by local dilations of the ducts, or even these may not be readily apparent. In such mild infections, the fact of past or present parasitism may only be suggested by the detection of characteristic black iron-porphyrin pigments, grossly visible in the hilar nodes. It also contributes to the character of the biliary contents.

Chronic debility with vague digestive disturbances is common in chronic fascioliasis, and deaths are common among sheep. Clinically and at postmortem, there are, in addition to the essential lesions, more or less severe anemia, moderate anasarca, and cachexia. Jaundice is seldom seen.

Fasciola gigantica displaces *F. hepatica* as the common liver fluke in many parts of Africa and in nearby countries, southeast Asia, and the Hawaiian Islands. It is 2 or 3 times as large as *F. hepatica*, but its life cycle and pathogenicity are comparable.

Fascioloides magna *is the large liver fluke of North America;* cervids are the definitive hosts. It is a parasite of *ruminants* and lives in the hepatic parenchyma, not in the bile ducts, although in tolerant hosts (cervids) the cysts in which it localizes communicate with the bile ducts to provide an exit for ova and excrement. The life cycle of this parasite generally parallels that of *F. hepatica*. The young flukes are very destructive as they wander in the liver. In cattle, they wander briefly, producing large necrotic tunnels before becoming encysted. The cysts, enclosed by connective tissue, do not communicate with bile ducts but form permanent enclosures for the flukes, their excreta, and ova. *The cysts, which may be 2-5 cm in diameter, are remarkable for the large deposits of jet black, sooty iron-porphyrin pigment they contain* (eFig. 2-23), and except for the flukes and soft contents, they superficially resemble heavily pigmented melanotic tumors. Commonly, these flukes pass from the liver to the lungs of cattle to produce lesions of similar character. In sheep, this parasite wanders continuously in the liver, producing black, tortuous tracts, which may be 2 cm in diameter, and extensive parenchymal destruction. Even a few flukes may kill a sheep. There is a case report of natural infection in a horse.

The **dicrocoelid flukes** inhabit both biliary and pancreatic ducts. *Eurytrema pancreaticum* prefers the pancreas (and is described with that organ) but in heavy infections can be found in the bile ducts. *Dicrocoelium* and *Platynosomum* prefer the bile ducts. These are small, narrow flukes, 0.5-1.0-cm long, and may easily be mistaken for small masses of inspissated bile pigment. They are not highly pathogenic, and even in heavy infections, there may be no signs of the toxemia observed in infections by *F. hepatica*. These flukes may occur as mixed infections.

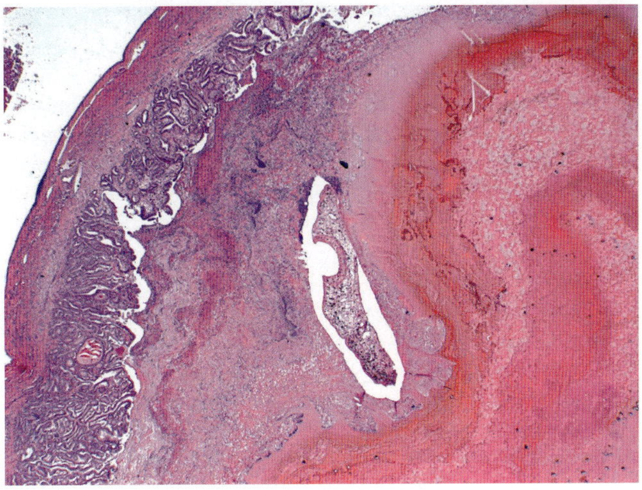

Figure 2-86 **Dicrocoelid fluke** in the gallbladder of a cat. (Courtesy Purdue University CVM.)

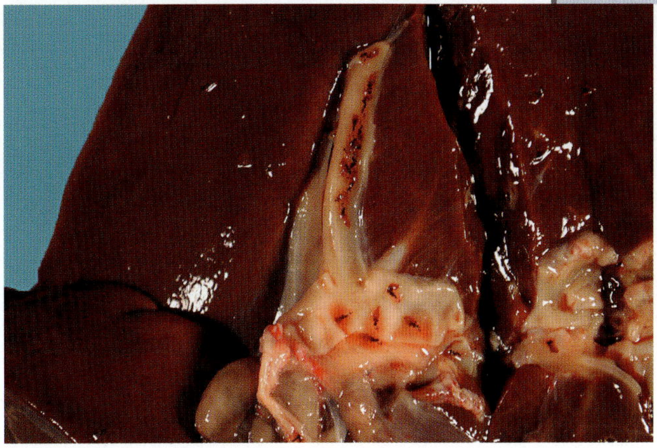

Figure 2-87 ***Dicrocoelium dendriticum***, the lancet fluke, in the bile ducts of a sheep.

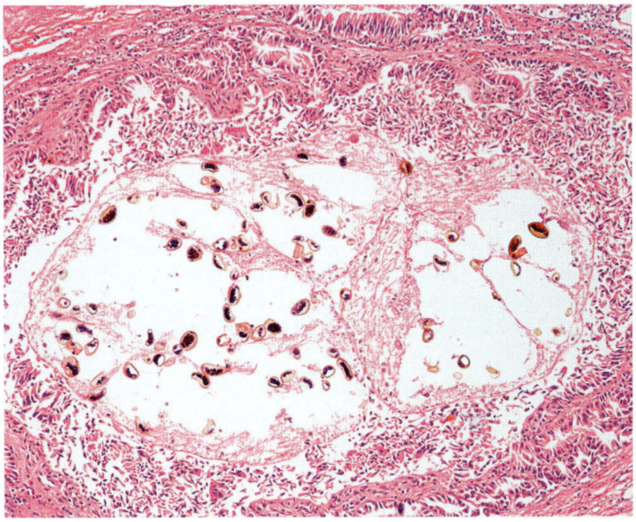

Figure 2-88 ***Dicrocoelium dendriticum*** **with embryonated eggs** in the bile duct of a sheep.

Platynosomum fastosum is a small fluke inhabiting the biliary ducts and gallbladder of *cats* from southern North America, Central and South America, Malaysia, and the Pacific Islands. The life cycle includes *Sublima octona* snails as the first intermediate host and *Anolis* spp. lizards, marine toads *(Bufo marinus)*, geckos, and various arthropods as second intermediate or paratenic hosts. Cats become infected after ingestion of the second intermediate or paratenic hosts, the cercariae are released into the upper digestive tract, enter the biliary tree, and complete their life cycle. Mature flukes are found in the gallbladder and bile ducts, and after 8-13 weeks, eggs are shed into the feces (Fig. 2-86). Although most infections are subclinical, heavy infections may cause anorexia, vomiting, lethargy, jaundice, and death. Severely affected livers are enlarged, friable, and may be bile stained, with thickened, distended gallbladders, dilated and/or thickened common bile ducts and cystic ducts, and dilated intrahepatic ducts. Histologically, there are various degrees of chronic cholangitis, fibrosing cholangiohepatitis, and cholecystitis, with dilated and hyperplastic ducts surrounded by lymphocytes, plasma cells, and eosinophils, and in some cases neutrophils, with fluke eggs within or adjacent to ducts. Eggs and adults may be difficult to find. Infection has been reported to co-occur with cholangiocarcinoma in some cats.

Dicrocoelium hospes is found in *cattle* in Africa south of the Sahara. Little is known of it, but it is presumed to be comparable in all respects to the better-known *D. dendriticum*, which is common in Europe and Asia and sparsely distributed in the Americas and North Africa. *Dicrocoelium* spp. are found in dry lowland or mountain pastures; *Fasciola* spp. occur in wetter habitats, so the prevalence of *Dicrocoelium* is increasing with desertification. This fluke is no more fastidious in its choice of final hosts than many other species of fluke, and, depending on opportunity, it can infest all domestic species, apart from cats. It is, however, of most importance as a parasite of sheep and cattle, in which it inhabits the bile ducts. Other domestic species and rodents are important as reservoirs.

The life cycle of ***Dicrocoelium dendriticum***, the lancet fluke or small liver fluke, differs in some details from that of *F. hepatica*. The eggs are embryonated when laid and do not hatch until swallowed by one of the many genera of land snails that are the first intermediate hosts. In the snails, the mother sporocyst produces a second generation of daughter sporocysts, which in turn produce cercariae. The cercariae leave the snail in damp weather and are expelled from the snail's lung, clumped together in slime balls. The slime balls are not infective until the cercariae are swallowed by, and encyst in, the ant *Formica fusca*; other ants may be involved in different countries. The cycle is completed when the definitive hosts swallow the ants. The route of migration of the larvae from the gut to the liver is probably via the bile ducts from the duodenum.

The pathologic changes in the liver produced by *D. dendriticum* are those of cholangitis that is less severe than that produced by *F. hepatica* (Fig. 2-87, eFig. 2-24). The severity and diffuseness of the hepatic lesion are determined by the number of lancet flukes present, and they may be in the thousands. The flukes and their eggs darken the dilated ducts. Even in early infections, there may be some scarring of the organ at its periphery. In heavy infections of long standing, there is *extensive biliary fibrosis*, producing an organ that is indurated, scarred, and lumpy and that at the margins may bear areas that are shrunken and completely sclerotic. The histologic changes are the same as those in fascioliasis, with perhaps more remarkable hyperplasia of the mucous glands of the large ducts (Fig. 2-88).

Heterobilharzia americana, a trematode in the family *Schistosomatidae*, is the causative agent of *canine schistosomiasis* in North America, primarily reported from the South Atlantic and Gulf Coast states. Raccoons are the most common definitive hosts, although in addition to dogs, several other mammalian species may become naturally infected, including domestic horses. Eggs shed in feces hatch in water and release motile miracidia, which penetrate the tissues of the intermediate host, lymnaeid freshwater snails. Larval stages multiply in the snail, and free-swimming cercariae are released into freshwater. These penetrate the intact epidermis of the definitive host, migrate to the lung, and finally the liver, where they mature, move to the mesenteric and intrahepatic portal veins to mate, and release eggs that migrate through mesenteric venules, crossing into the bowel lumen by means of proteolytic enzymes. Aberrant migration of eggs results in multifocal eosinophilic and granulomatous inflammation in the intestines, pancreas, and liver. Adult trematodes may occasionally be found in hepatic vessels. Clinical signs in affected dogs include diarrhea, vomiting, weight loss, and lethargy, and ~50% of cases in dogs are associated with hypercalcemia, thought to be the result of unregulated calcitriol synthesis by macrophages in the granulomatous lesions. In horses, small fibrosing granulomas scattered throughout the liver, with rare intact or fragmented eggs, are typical and are usually clinically inapparent (eFig. 2-25).

The **opisthorchid flukes** are parasites in the bile ducts of *carnivores*. They may also occur in swine and humans, and one species, *C. sinensis (Opisthorchis sinensis)*, is an important human parasite. The life cycles, where known, include mollusks as the first intermediate hosts and freshwater fish as the second.

Metorchis conjunctus *is the common liver fluke of cats and dogs in North America* and is important as a parasite of sled dogs in the Canadian Northwest Territories. The first intermediate host is the snail *Amnicola limosa porosa*, and the second is the common sucker-fish *Catostomus commersonii*. The cercariae actively burrow into the musculature of the fish to encyst and become infective. The immature flukes crawl into the bile ducts from the duodenum and mature in ~28 days. Infections may persist for >5 years. *Metorchis albidis* has been described in a dog from Alaska, *Parametorchis complexus* in cats in the United States, and *Amphimerus pseudofelineus* in cats and coyotes in the United States and Central and South America; the life cycles are not known but are presumed to include fish. *Metorchis bilis* has been reported in red foxes and occasionally in cats.

Opisthorchis felineus (*O. tenuicollis*) *is the lanceolate fluke of the bile ducts of cats, dogs, and foxes in Europe and Russia.* It is particularly common in eastern Europe and Siberia and is sparser in other areas. ***Clonorchis sinensis***, the Oriental or Chinese liver fluke, is an important human pathogen endemic in Japan, Korea, southern China, and southeast Asia; dogs, cats, and swine can act as reservoir hosts. There are additional, less well-known, species of *Opisthorchis* in humans and animals. The first intermediate hosts for the miracidia of *O. felineus* and *C. sinensis* are snails of the genus *Bithynia*, and several genera of cyprinid fishes can act as second intermediate hosts.

Pseudamphistomum truncatum occurs in carnivores and humans sporadically in Europe and Asia. Its life cycle is as for *Opisthorchis*.

The opisthorchid flukes, as far as is known, resemble *Dicrocoelium* in migrating up the bile ducts to their habitat. This may be the reason that they are more numerous in the left than in the right lobes of the liver. They can probably live in the liver for as long as the host lives. The pathologic effects are comparable to those of *D. dendriticum*. Light infections may be subclinical, and heavy infections may cause jaundice, chronic cholangiohepatitis, and severe biliary fibrosis. In both humans and animals, adenomatous and carcinomatous changes of the biliary glands have occurred in association with these parasites; the association is probably more than coincidental.

Protozoal infections

Protozoal hepatitis is due mainly to infection with *Toxoplasma* (Fig. 2-89), *Neospora*, and *Leishmania*. Granulomatous hepatitis has been described in dogs associated with systemic infections by *Hepatozoon canis*. Vascular occlusion by enlarged monocytes bearing *Cytauxzoon felis* merozoites can be found in the liver of infected cats. *Sarcocystis neurona* schizonts were reported in the liver of a few dogs with systemic, multiorgan infection, and schizonts from an unspeciated *Sarcocystis* were observed in hepatocytes in a horse with necrosuppurative hepatitis.

Hepatic coccidiosis causing acute cholangitis similar to that in mink and rabbits has been seen in isolated cases in the goat, calf, and dog (Fig. 2-90). These infections are usually

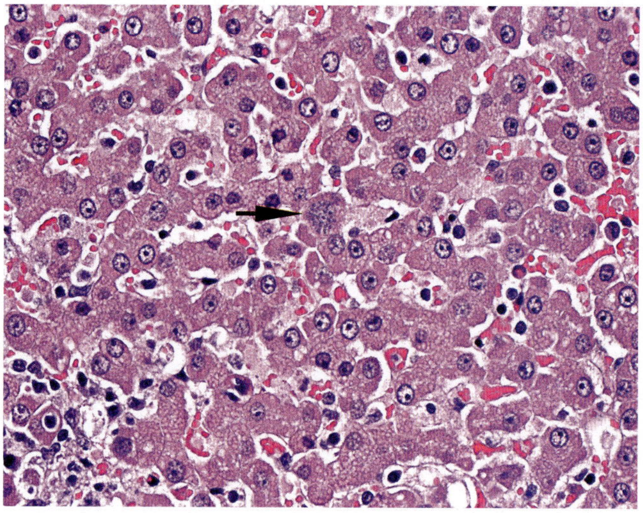

Figure 2-89 ***Toxoplasma gondii*** cyst (arrow) in the liver of a kitten.

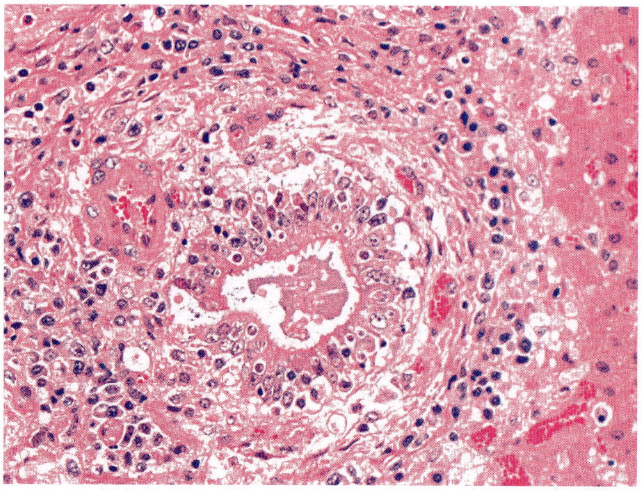

Figure 2-90 **Hepatic coccidiosis** in the bile duct of a pig.

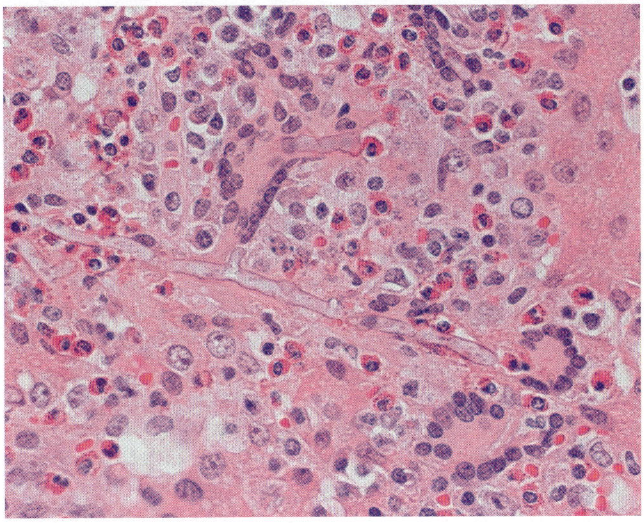

Figure 2-91 **Fungal hepatitis** in a pig.

considered aberrant and often coincide with intestinal coccidiosis. Coccidial meronts and, in some cases, gamonts are present within the cytoplasm of biliary epithelium. The organisms are presently unclassified.

Fungal infections

Fungal infections of the forestomachs with hematogenous dissemination to the liver occur occasionally in cattle and sheep, usually as a complication of rumenitis. Lesions in the liver are typically hemorrhagic infarcts initially, or granulomatous with chronicity, and are associated with infection by *Aspergillus fumigatus* and various members of the former phylum *Zygomycota*, or zygote fungi, and now part of 2 phyla, the *Mucoromycota* and *Zoopagomycota* (Fig. 2-91).

Granulomatous hepatitis associated with disseminated fungal or algal infections has also been reported in dogs and cats. The species involved include *Histoplasma capsulatum*, *Cryptococcus* spp., *Coccidioides immitis*, *Sporothrix schenckii*, *Aspergillus* spp., and *Prototheca* spp.

TOXIC HEPATIC DISEASE

Hepatic susceptibility

The liver is particularly vulnerable to toxic injury because it is exposed to virtually everything that is absorbed from the gastrointestinal tract. The portal vein drains the stomach and intestines, as well as the spleen, pancreas, and gallbladder, and flows directly to the liver. This facilitates high hepatic concentrations of ingested foreign chemicals or drugs termed **xenobiotics**, as well as many naturally occurring substances with toxic potential. Most xenobiotics are unable to directly enter the hepatocyte and require specific transporters to pass through the lipid bilayer of the hepatocyte membrane. The uptake of exogenous and endogenous compounds from the sinusoidal blood is facilitated by a variety of *transmembrane hepatocellular transport proteins* located on basolateral surfaces of hepatocytes. Similarly, transport into the bile and efflux from the hepatocytes is facilitated by related transporters. Because of its role as the primary site of biotransformation for many therapeutic agents and endogenous substances, the liver is exposed to highly reactive metabolites of toxic xenobiotics. Some metabolites may produce hepatocellular injury, and others may cause biliary injury once they are transported into the canaliculi. Certain drug metabolites may be reabsorbed in the enterohepatic recirculation in a manner similar to bile acids, facilitating repeated exposure to the drug metabolites in question. Some substances may be concentrated in hepatocytes to various degrees by mechanisms that remain obscure, but which are associated with upregulation of solute uptake transporters, special binding proteins of hepatocytes, attachment to enzymatic sites where metabolic conversions occur, and inhibition of export into the bile. In addition, many drug administration regimens may achieve relatively high intrahepatocytic concentrations, resulting in depletion of conjugating cofactors such as glutathione, leading to an imbalance of bioactivated metabolites and protective conjugating cofactors or antioxidants leading to a disruption of their cytoprotective roles and hepatocyte injury.

Role of hepatic biotransformation in hepatotoxicity

An understanding of hepatic biotransformation is essential for an appreciation of the hepatotoxic potential of xenobiotics and some endogenous substances. *Hepatocytes are the major site of metabolism of endogenous substances and xenobiotics, including plant- or fungal-derived secondary metabolites consumed in food, environmental chemicals, and drugs.* Given the numerous enzymes and the magnitude of their expression, the liver easily exceeds the metabolic capacity of all other organs. A major metabolic function of the liver is to transform lipophilic substances, including endogenous steroid hormones and most xenobiotics, into more water-soluble polar molecules to be excreted in bile or urine. Relevant stages of biotransformation and hepatic enzymes involved in biotransformation and their associated activities can be grouped into *3 major categories*.

- Phase 1 reactions promote oxidation, reduction, hydrolysis, cyclization, and decyclization of the parent compounds leading to a reactive metabolite. This is typically carried out through addition of oxygen or removal of hydrogen, by mixed-function oxidases that are usually CYP enzymes (i.e., cytochrome P450 monooxygenases), using NADPH and O_2. Most of these phase 1 enzymes are found in the *smooth endoplasmic reticulum* of the hepatocyte.
- Phase 2 reactions are typically *conjugation reactions* in which a polar molecule, such as glucuronic acid, sulfate, or glutathione, is added to carboxyl, hydroxyl, amino, or sulfhydryl groups on phase 1 metabolites, making them typically less toxic and more water soluble. Most of these enzymes are found in the *cytosol*.
- In phase 3 reactions, conjugated molecules are transported by various *transporter molecules* across the modified hepatocyte membrane that lines the canaliculus.

Phase 1 reactions may either increase (bioactivate) or eliminate the biologic activity of the xenobiotic substrate. However, bioactivation of molecules poses a potential risk. Although this step is necessary to prepare the substrate to form a covalent bond with polar compounds in phase 2, it creates, if only transiently, reactive intermediates, such as free radicals and epoxides. These reactive intermediates can bind to cellular macromolecules, such as the CYP enzymes, that produced them, other cellular enzymes or structural proteins, or RNA and DNA, leading to hepatocyte injury, death, or neoplastic transformation. The CYPs can be found in all parts of the hepatic lobule, but the centrilobular hepatocytes have a higher content than those of the periportal region, which apparently accounts for the *centrilobular predominance of injury produced* *by compounds metabolized by this system*, including carbon tetrachloride and acetaminophen. In contrast, *hepatocytes in the periportal zone are more susceptible to direct-acting toxicants, such as metal salts*, because of their proximity to incoming portal and arterial vascular flow.

So-called "drug-drug" interactions can arise when 2 drugs are metabolized by the same CYP, so that metabolism of one or both compounds is altered by competition or interference with the relevant CYP enzyme function leading to toxic increases in intracellular concentrations.

Phase 2 reactions inactivate the phase 1 metabolite through conjugation with a polar molecule and facilitate its export by transforming the lipophilic molecule into a water-soluble molecule that can be transported out of the hepatocyte and into the bile or the circulation for removal via the kidney. *Reduced glutathione is a major substrate for phase 2 reactions mediated by glutathione S-transferases*. Active metabolites of many compounds, including acetaminophen, are detoxified by conjugation with glutathione. Depletion of glutathione can greatly enhance the toxicity of many compounds. Hepatic glutathione is also important in the removal of various free radicals and reactive oxygen species generated by normal metabolic processes as well as detoxification pathways through the action of glutathione peroxidase. Different species and different breeds of animals possess a divergent array of phase 1 and phase 2 types with differing levels of activity and target substrates that contribute to the differences in metabolism and toxicity of xenobiotics observed in different species. Acetaminophen toxicity in the cat is a relevant example. Felids have limited phase 2 metabolism caused, in part, from diminished activity of UDP-glucuronosyl transferase, an enzyme involved in glucuronidation of bioactivated molecules. Limited glucuronidation of acetaminophen metabolites leads to saturation of other detoxification pathways and depletion of glutathione. The lack of glutathione then enables a highly toxic metabolite of acetaminophen, N-acetyl-para-benzoquinoneimine (NAPQI) to bind to cellular proteins and membranes, causing cell injury and death. NAPQI is also responsible for the prominent methemoglobinemia seen in intoxicated cats. *Toxic hepatic injury depends on the balance between the production of reactive metabolites and their detoxification by conjugation and other protective mechanisms*.

The enzyme complex involved in bioactivation is not limited to metabolism of foreign substances but is also involved in the metabolism or synthesis of several lipophilic endogenous substances. The principal endogenous substrates include arachidonic acid, eicosanoids, cholesterol, bile acids, steroids, and vitamin D.

Phase 3 reactions involve movement of conjugated substrates across the membrane of the canaliculus. As with the processes involved in uptake of substances from the plasma, several transporters embedded in the canalicular membrane are responsible for the movement of the water-soluble conjugated substrates from the hepatocellular cytoplasm into the lumen of the canaliculus. These transporters have a range of occasionally overlapping substrates, including bile acids and conjugates of glutathione, glucuronate, and sulfonate. These water-soluble metabolites are excreted in the bile via members of the ATP-binding cassette (ABC) superfamily of transport proteins, among others, found on the apical canalicular membrane. These include the most significant transporter in humans, the multidrug resistance protein–1. MRP2 is responsible for export of glutathione conjugates, such as bilirubin conjugates, and shows a striking species difference in expression, with low expression in the dog and high expression in the rat. This variation influences biliary excretion of drug conjugates from the liver and may influence toxicity in the liver or elsewhere.

The mechanism by which xenobiotics and some endogenous substances can cause CYP enzyme induction in the liver, as well as induction of phase 2 reactions, and hepatocellular hypertrophy is mediated by the activation of nuclear receptors that function as transcription factors. These **transcription factors** include aryl hydrocarbon hydroxylase receptor (AHR), constitutive androstane receptor (CAR), pregnane X receptor (PXR), and peroxisome proliferator–activated receptor-α (PPARα). These nuclear receptors are also important mediators of hepatocellular metabolism, including hepatic lipid metabolism, bile acid homeostasis, as well as liver regeneration, inflammation, fibrosis, cell differentiation, and tumor formation. Each of these receptors may be directly activated by the binding of the xenobiotic (or its metabolite) to the receptor, although some activators of CAR do not bind to the receptor but rather phosphorylate the receptor, which results in nuclear translocation. The nuclear receptor genes vary among species, and there are many species differences and gene polymorphisms that affect the receptors or the genes that they stimulate.

In summary, a broad variety of factors can influence the mechanisms and extent of **drug-induced liver injury** (DILI), the term for hepatic injury from xenobiotics. There are various alternative pathways for metabolism, supported by a variety of isoforms of different gene families, particularly the CYP enzymes and the many genetic polymorphisms within individual alleles that code for the different isoforms. Other factors such as age, nutritional status, sex, diet, microbiome, prior or concurrent exposure to environmental compounds, or intercurrent disease all influence the response to toxic injury. Some of these variables contribute to the variations seen in responses among species and individuals to liver injury.

Role of inflammation in hepatotoxicity

The extent of liver injury following exposure to xenobiotics is not, however, determined by the chemistry of drug metabolism alone. Following exposure to injurious compounds, the inflammatory response, particularly the innate immune response, can significantly influence the extent of hepatocellular injury. Studies using acetaminophen have provided most relevant information on this issue; however, the effects of inflammation are complex, and not all studies agree. Depending on the model studied, Kupffer cells or monocyte-derived macrophages can play the major role. Some clarification of this controversy has been facilitated by the identification of different phenotypes of intrahepatic macrophages following injury. Two major phenotypes of intrahepatic monocyte-derived macrophages and phenotype switching can occur. A population of monocyte-derived infiltrating macrophages can be detected quite soon (within 12 hours) after acetaminophen intoxication and are the predominant macrophage population present. Initially following injury, the monocyte-derived macrophages are *proinflammatory*, a source of TNF, interleukin-1β (IL1β), IL18, and nitric oxide, which stimulates hepatocellular injury. Appearing later, *anti-inflammatory* monocyte-derived macrophages, secreting matrix metalloproteinases, growth factors (hepatocyte growth factor, insulin-like growth factor), and phagocytosis-related genes [macrophage receptor with collagenous structure (MARCO)] IL10-, IL6- and IL18-binding proteins, modulate inflammation and initiate repair. The phenotype switch is engendered by phagocytosis of necrotic cells (*efferocytosis*) and interactions with other cell types. Stimulation of other members of the innate immune system, such as NK and NK T cells can accentuate acetaminophen toxicity. Neutrophils recruited to the liver by the release of damage-associated molecular pattern molecules from necrotic hepatocytes also augment tissue injury. Thus, altered *inflammation can influence drug-induced hepatic injury*, but the subtleties remain to be unraveled.

Mechanisms of injury

There are many mechanisms underlying hepatotoxicity. These include 1) covalent binding of cellular proteins by bioactivated metabolites, which leads to intracellular dysfunction manifested by loss of normal intracellular ionic gradients altering intracellular calcium homeostasis, by actin filament disruption, and by cell membrane damage, such as cell blebbing or swelling and total disruption. A consequence of actin filament disruption can be cholestasis because of the loss of pulsatile contractions that drive canalicular bile flow; 2) drug-induced disruption of canalicular transport pump function, leading to cholestasis and jaundice; 3) inhibition of cellular enzyme pathways of drug metabolism because of covalent binding of CYPs by bioactivated metabolites; 4) covalent binding of the drug to cell proteins, which creates new adducts that serve as immune targets for cytotoxic T-cell attack or antibody formation when transported to the cell surface in vesicles, inciting an immunologic reaction; 5) programmed cell death (apoptosis), occurring through TNF and Fas pathways; and 6) inhibition of mitochondrial function, limiting β-oxidation of fat and ATP generation, leading to accumulation of reactive oxygen species and lipid peroxidation, microvesicular fat accumulation, lactic acidosis, and inability to generate ATP. These are discussed in detail in other texts. The liver is composed of several cell types, not only hepatocytes, and similar types of injury can also affect the biliary epithelium and sinusoidal endothelium, and to a lesser extent, HSCs, Kupffer cells, and other immune cells.

Classification of hepatotoxicants

Hepatotoxicants can be classified as intrinsic or idiosyncratic, and these categories apply as well to the types of drug-induced hepatotoxicity that are observed in humans and animals. The effects of **intrinsic hepatotoxicants** *are dose related, predictable, and reproducible in experimental animals, and the underlying mechanisms are typically at least partially understood.* Intrinsic hepatotoxicants can cause liver injury in overdose situations in most normal recipients but are also capable of inducing similar liver damage at lower doses in individuals with genetic or acquired abnormalities in drug metabolism. Most intrinsic hepatotoxicants are converted to *reactive metabolites*, including lipoperoxidative free radicals.

Acetaminophen is a well-characterized example of an intrinsic hepatotoxicant, with species differences in metabolism and associated susceptibility to oxidative and hepatic injury. Dogs and cats can tolerate doses within therapeutic levels; however, higher doses may saturate the glucuronidation and sulfation detoxification pathways, resulting in increased formation of the reactive benzoquinone-imine metabolite NAPQI via a third CYP-mediated pathway. These can be scavenged by glutathione conjugation; however, massive doses can cause lethal acute hepatic failure, associated with overproduction of reactive metabolites, and depletion of hepatic and erythrocyte glutathione. As discussed previously, clinical toxicity occurs at lower doses and is more severe in cats because they express fewer hepatic isoforms of glucuronyltransferase as part of phase 2 hepatic metabolism and are unable to accelerate excretion of excess metabolites through glucuronide conjugation. This is compounded by a propensity for hemoglobin oxidation, resulting in methemoglobinemia. Toxicity results when reduced glutathione levels drop below a threshold level, resulting in marked oxidative stress, and allowing reactive metabolites to bind covalently to cellular macromolecules.

By comparison, **idiosyncratic hepatotoxicants** are typically *less dose related* (although there is likely a minimum threshold), *more unpredictable*, and importantly, idiosyncratic hepatotoxicities occur in only a *very small proportion of exposed individuals* (i.e., <1 in 10,000-100,000). The mechanisms of idiosyncratic hepatotoxicity are generally not known but reflect an unusual susceptibility of individual recipients to effects that are unrelated to the drug's therapeutic action or overdose toxicity. Idiosyncratic hepatotoxicity is more likely a series of rare drug-related toxicities with different forms of pathogenesis than a single entity. There are 2 main categories of idiosyncratic hepatotoxicity recognized in humans: *hypersensitivity-related DILI (drug allergy)* and *toxic metabolite-dependent DILI*.

Hypersensitivity-related idiosyncrasies are characterized by a latency period before toxicity is evident and reoccur promptly upon re-exposure. Typically, they involve immune-mediated hypersensitivity responses to the drug metabolites that covalently bind to liver proteins, forming neoantigens that may be recognized as foreign by the adaptive immune system, primarily CD8+ T cells. Components of the innate immune system likely play a role in engaging the adaptive immune system by activating antigen-presenting cells and through the release of cytokines necessary for priming T lymphocytes. In humans, a genetic component to hypersensitivity-related idiosyncratic hepatic toxicity is strongly suspected. Single nucleotide polymorphisms in the human leukocyte antigen (HLA) region or particular HLA haplotypes have been associated with idiosyncratic drug toxicity in humans for several drugs, reflecting the development of pharmacogenomics. Other possible triggers for idiosyncratic toxicity include the "danger hypothesis" that proposes that hepatocyte injury from the parent compound or metabolite can predispose the liver to an enhanced immune-mediated response in the context of inflammation- or damage-related signaling, leading to greater injury to the liver.

Toxic metabolite–dependent idiosyncrasies involve excessive generation of a regular toxic metabolite or altered metabolism to unusual hepatotoxic metabolites. Considerable genetic diversity (polymorphisms) exists in hepatic drug metabolism among individual humans and domestic animals, and these polymorphisms may explain many unusual responses to drugs. This variation could be qualitative, with the production of a toxic metabolite not normally produced, or quantitative, with overproduction of a normally minor hepatotoxic metabolite.

Morphology of toxic injury to the liver

The morphologic forms of hepatic injury produced by hepatotoxicants are varied. *Acute toxic injury to the liver can be cytotoxic (hepatocellular), cholestatic, or mixed.* **Cytotoxic hepatocellular injury** results in hepatic degeneration, zonal necrosis, focal and nonzonal necrosis (apoptosis, necroptosis, pyroptosis, cuproptosis), or lipidosis, accompanied by the clinicopathologic features of acute hepatic injury. In general, necrosis produced by intrinsic hepatotoxicants is zonal. *Acute cytotoxic injury is often initially manifested as steatosis (lipidosis)*, a result of impairment of movement of triglycerides through the liver, interference with VLDL synthesis or transport, or impaired hepatic consumption of fatty acids by mitochondrial oxidation. **Cholestatic injury** reflects failure of bile excretion associated with biliary epithelial or canalicular injury or other alteration of bile secretion and displays the features of intrahepatic or extrahepatic obstructive jaundice. The typical histologic manifestation consists initially of bile casts in canaliculi, with variable parenchymal injury. An exception to this pattern can be seen in some plant intoxications, such as those produced by steroidal sapogenins and *Lantana* spp., which can cause cholestasis with minimal evidence of canalicular plugging. **Mixed toxic insults** display the morphologic and clinical features of both hepatocellular and obstructive injury.

The histologic changes in **acute toxic hepatic injury** are rather stereotypic. They range from apoptosis, through confluent coagulative and zonal necrosis, to panlobular hemorrhagic destruction that includes sinusoidal-lining cells (see Fig. 2-38). The histology of these acute intoxications is often characterized by *centrilobular necrosis*, usually coagulative (see Fig. 2-34). Rarely, the pattern of necrosis may be periportal or midzonal, although dose-related expansion of the zones of injury occurs. Depending on the nutritional status of the animal, there may be variably severe fatty or hydropic change in hepatocytes adjacent to the necrotic zones. Necrotic cells may accumulate calcium. Variations on the general process of hepatocellular necrosis have little diagnostic or pathogenetic specificity. In sublethally injured cells, there may be prominent but nonspecific clumping of SER, particularly in the centrilobular zones.

The *clinical and gross characteristics of fatal acute intoxications* that destroy liver parenchyma are rather consistent, regardless of the origin of the toxin. The animal dies after a brief period of dullness, anorexia, colic, and various neurologic disturbances, including convulsions; these are attributed to HE. Postmortem examination reveals a slight excess of clear, yellow abdominal fluid, which contains sufficient fibrinogen to form a loose, nonadherent clot. The appearance of the liver depends on the severity and stage of the injury. Severe acute toxicity that destroys endothelium typically results in a hemorrhagic zonal pattern, in which case the liver may be deep red-purple and obviously swollen and turgid. In less severe injury without hemorrhage, the liver tends to be lighter brown because of a combination of edema (exclusion of sinusoidal blood), destruction of cytochrome pigments, and accumulation of bile pigments and/or fat. If the animal survives for several days, the liver develops a typical zonal yellow fatty change as triglyceride accumulates in sublethally injured hepatocytes.

In acute fatal hepatotoxicities, there may be widespread hemorrhage resulting from lack of coagulation factors. Petechiae and ecchymoses are seen most consistently on serous membranes, especially on the epicardium, endocardium, and abdominal viscera. Diffuse hemorrhage into the gut, particularly the duodenum in ruminants, is also common, as are hemorrhages into the wall of the gallbladder. Hemorrhages are largely the result of excessive consumption of clotting factors and platelets within the areas of necrosis in the liver, although the concurrent failure of the damaged liver to maintain a balance of pro- and anticoagulation factors undoubtedly becomes important. Gross lesions, such as icterus, and photosensitization, which reflect failure of biotransformation or excretion of endogenous materials, develop too slowly to be a feature of acutely fatal hepatotoxicities. However, the rate of accumulation of bilirubin increases when hemorrhage occurs in the necrotic liver or because of coagulopathy.

Chronic hepatotoxic injury *may manifest in many patterns*. These include areas of necrosis with primarily mononuclear inflammatory infiltrates, steatosis, fibrosis, cirrhosis, regenerative nodules, hepatic vein thrombosis, sinusoidal obstructive syndrome, hepatic sinusoidal angiectasis, cholangitis, ductular reaction (biliary hyperplasia), and carcinogenesis. In contrast to acute intoxications, chronic hepatotoxicities are more likely to display a mix of these responses, and this can provide more diagnostic specificity. For example, agents that impair hepatocellular regeneration might not be potent necrogens but tend to produce hepatic apoptosis and atrophy, fibrosis of various patterns, compensatory bile duct hyperplasia, nodular regeneration, some degree of cholestasis, and frequently megalocytosis (polyploidy). Such hepatotoxicants are potential carcinogens because they favor the selective growth of hepatocellular nodules that are resistant to mitoinhibitory effects.

Clinical signs of chronic hepatotoxicity usually result from inadequate detoxification and excretion; these include jaundice, photosensitization in ruminants, and HE, as well as sepsis from reduced bacterial clearance by Kupffer cells. Most of the toxins responsible for chronic hepatotoxicity may produce acute nonspecific zonal or massive necrosis if experimentally administered at dose rates higher than those to which animals are likely to be exposed in the field, although such acute toxicity is only occasionally seen in field cases of the diseases.

Toxic agents

The range of substances that can cause hepatotoxicity is so broad that it encompasses virtually all categories of natural and synthetic chemicals. These include metals (e.g., iron, copper), drugs (e.g., acetaminophen), plant components (phytotoxins), fungal metabolites (mycotoxins), bacterial products (e.g., cyanobacterial microcystin-LR), vitamin A, the trace element selenium, and various industrial products (especially aromatic solvents). Many drugs are also hepatotoxic. Differences in individual susceptibility to hepatotoxic responses likely occur for all classes of chemicals that are metabolized in the liver.

In the following sections, toxic hepatic disease will be separated into drug- or pharmaceutical-induced hepatotoxicity (so-called adverse drug reactions), and hepatotoxicity associated with exposure to plant or environmental toxins, including metals. The latter have been somewhat arbitrarily divided into acute and chronic, and although it is recognized that the difference between acute and chronic hepatotoxicity is often simply a matter of dose rate, it is convenient to categorize the sources according to the syndrome of liver damage that they most commonly produce. Various plants and moldy feeds are hepatotoxic, and some phytotoxins (e.g., pyrrolizidine alkaloids) and mycotoxins (e.g., aflatoxins) are notorious hepatotoxins and hepatocarcinogens. Many phytotoxins and mycotoxins target other organ systems or have physiologic rather than pathologic effects. Some of those that cause diagnostic lesions are discussed under the respective target tissues elsewhere. Generally, these areas of toxicology are better accessed in comprehensive references on phytotoxins or mycotoxins.

Adverse drug reactions: drug-induced liver injury

The definition of an adverse drug reaction is any injurious or unintended response to a drug that occurs at a normal dose for normal use. Drug-induced liver injury (DILI) is the most common form of adverse drug reaction in humans, and although hepatotoxic drug reactions are recognized in dogs and cats, the true prevalence of DILI in domestic animals is unknown. DILI should not be considered as a single disease, given the diverse array of drugs and mechanisms of toxicity that can trigger injury.

Acute hepatic disease has been attributed to adverse reactions to a wide variety of therapeutic drugs, particularly in companion animals. Zonal-to-panlobular hepatic necrosis and cholestatic hepatitis have been reported in dogs as an idiosyncratic reaction to **trimethoprim-sulfonamide** combination therapy and the related sulfonamide-based anticonvulsant drug **zonisamide**, although zonisamide, in a different chemical category, is less likely to form toxic adducts, and is not likely to share a similar pathogenesis of liver injury. Severe lobular-to-panlobular hepatic necrosis may occur in cats associated with repeated oral administration of **diazepam** at recommended doses. Severe centrilobular hepatic necrosis has been associated with the use of the anthelmintic **mebendazole** in dogs. Hepatotoxicity has been reported in dogs treated with **amiodarone**, a class III antiarrhythmic agent. Hepatic injury is one of the more commonly reported adverse effects of amiodarone in humans and is related to the drug's effect on lipid metabolism. Administration of the anabolic steroid **stanozolol** has also been associated with elevated alanine aminotransferase activity, coagulopathy, and development of hepatic lipidosis with cholestasis in cats. Adult beef cattle testing positive for stanozolol in urine also had hepatic changes, including cholestasis, periportal fibrosis and inflammation, and focal necrosis, although the changes could not conclusively be attributed to anabolic steroid administration. Other pharmacologic agents associated with acute hepatic injury include **thiacetarsemide, methoxyflurane, halothane, oil of pennyroyal**, intravenous injection of **manganese chloride**, **acetaminophen**, and inadvertent subcutaneous injection of intranasal *Bordetella bronchiseptica*/canine parainfluenza vaccine in dogs; **methimazole, glipizide**, and the photodynamic therapy agent **aluminum phthalocyanine tetrasulfonate** in cats.

Xylitol is an artificial sweetener used commonly in baked goods or chewing gum intended for use by dieters of those with diabetes. Although high doses can be tolerated by most species, dogs are particularly sensitive. Dogs that ingest >0.5 g/kg can be at risk to develop acute severe hepatic necrosis. Dogs exposed to fatal doses have centrilobular-to-panlobular lytic necrosis of hepatocytes and widespread hemorrhage. Affected dogs also develop hypoglycemia and hyperinsulinemia. There may be an element of idiosyncratic toxicity involved as dogs have tolerated higher doses in experimental settings; breed-related or other factors may influence acute toxicity. The mechanism of toxicity is not currently known, but intracellular ATP depletion and generation of reactive oxygen species have been suggested as possible mechanisms for hepatocyte injury.

Carprofen is a nonsteroidal anti-inflammatory drug used in the treatment of degenerative joint disease and management of pain in dogs primarily. Diffuse and panlobular hepatocellular injury, characterized by hepatocellular vacuolar change, lytic necrosis, apoptosis, and bridging necrosis, with mild secondary inflammation and cholestasis, has been reported in dogs administered therapeutic dosages of carprofen. The injurious response is likely to be idiosyncratic as a chronic experimental study did not produce injury. A related nonsteroidal anti-inflammatory drug, *diclofenac*, causes idiosyncratic liver injury in humans.

The anticonvulsant drugs **primidone, phenytoin**, and **phenobarbital** have been associated with the development of *chronic hepatic disease and cirrhosis in dogs*. These drugs, used either alone or in combination, can cause biochemical and clinical signs of hepatic dysfunction in up to 14% of dogs treated for >6 months, but only a small percentage of cases progress to cirrhosis and hepatic failure. Currently, monitoring blood levels and adjusting dosages of these drugs to a nontoxic level has significantly reduced the incidence of liver injury. The most consistent histologic finding in most dogs treated with phenobarbital is *proliferation of the hepatocellular SER resulting from induction of microsomal enzymes*, including various subfamilies of CYP. This results in hepatocellular swelling with fine diffuse granularity, a so-called "ground-glass" appearance to hepatocyte cytoplasm. This histologic change is an adaptive response, reflected clinically by increases in serum activities of alkaline phosphatase, alanine aminotransferase, and GGT, but is not indicative of hepatocellular injury. Actual hepatotoxicity may be an idiosyncratic reaction in a small percentage of treated dogs, although the possibility of dose-dependent intrinsic hepatotoxicity with long-term treatment has not been ruled out. It is also possible that the enzyme induction associated with anticonvulsant therapy may alter the ability of the liver to detoxify other nonspecified compounds that could be the effectors of liver damage. Certainly, enzyme induction can alter the pharmacokinetics of other coadministered drugs. *Chronic hepatitis associated with anticonvulsant therapy is characterized by bridging portal fibrosis, ductular reaction, nodular regeneration, and mild infiltrates of inflammatory cells*. A separate syndrome of *cholestatic hepatotoxic injury with jaundice* has also been described in dogs receiving high doses of phenytoin in combination with primidone or phenobarbital; pathologic changes are intrahepatic cholestasis, with hepatocellular swelling, vacuolation, and small multifocal areas of hepatocellular necrosis, which have been suggested to represent a metabolic disturbance rather than direct cytotoxic hepatocellular injury. ***Hepatocutaneous syndrome*** (*superficial necrolytic dermatitis*) associated with typical hepatic lesions of parenchymal collapse, vacuolation, and nodular regeneration has also been reported as a separate syndrome in dogs with a history of chronic phenobarbital therapy.

Acute and chronic hepatic disease, characterized by portal inflammatory infiltrates, periportal fibrosis, and ductular reaction, has been reported historically in dogs treated with **oxibendazole-diethylcarbamazine** combination therapy for prevention of hookworm and heartworm disease. Chronic hepatic disease has also been reported following the administration of **mibolerone, methotrexate**, and **CCNU** (1-(2-chloroethyl)-3-cyclohexyl-1-nitrosourea) in dogs, **ketoconazole** in dogs and cats, and **megestrol acetate** and **griseofulvin** in cats. **Vitamin A** in dietary excess can lead to hepatic fibrosis in cats.

Hepatotoxic plants

Hepatotoxic plants occur in botanical families as diverse as the relatively primitive *Cycadaceae* through the *Compositae* and *Solanaceae*. The evolutionary relationships between herbivores and toxic plants are complex; in some situations, consumption of plants by herbivores has competitive or neutral advantage for the plant, especially those that are lush and prolific, so toxicity is counterproductive or unnecessary. However, in arid or semiarid habitats, plants must put up more resistance to herbivores that could obliterate them. Indigenous herbivores are typically reluctant to do this and are either resistant or reluctant to graze some plants. Plants sometimes protect critical parts at particular stages of growth. For example, *Xanthium pungens* (Noogoora burr) concentrates its toxin in the cotyledons. The seeds are rarely eaten, even by cattle, but intoxications can occur when this plant is eaten shortly after germination. Phytotoxic liver disease is therefore more frequently encountered in animals grazing pastures at times of the year with limited choice or supply, or when hungry animals are introduced to plants for which their natural or induced resistance is low. The patterns of liver disease resulting from consumption of toxic plants are for the most part quite consistent compared with what is seen with exposure to other classes of hepatotoxins. An exhaustive review of the toxicity of all such plants would be repetitive. However, some plants that do produce more distinctive patterns of liver lesions will be discussed in more detail.

Acute hepatotoxicity: plant-derived and environmental toxins

Cyanobacteria (blue-green algae)

These highly toxic microorganisms can flourish as a seasonal bloom on lakes and ponds that have accumulated phosphates and nitrates as runoff from fertilized soils. Outbreaks of poisoning occur in many countries and may be responsible for heavy mortality among mammals or birds that drink from affected bodies of water. ***Microcystis aeruginosa*** is the most common hepatotoxic cyanobacterium involved. Other hepatotoxic species are included in the genera *Anabaena, Oscillatoria, Nostoc, Nodularia, Cylindospermopsis*, and *Aphanizomenon*. Some cyanobacteria produce neurotoxins such as anatoxin-a; there are no hepatic or other specific lesions in this form of toxicosis.

The most well-understood cyanobacterial hepatotoxin is ***microcystin-LR****, a highly potent cyclic heptapeptide protein phosphatase inhibitor* found in *M. aeruginosa, Anabaena, Oscillatoria*, and *Nostoc* spp. Other species of hepatotoxic cyanobacteria include *Nodularia spumigena*, which contain nodularin, and *Cylindospermopsis, Aphanizomenon*, and *Anabaena*, which contain cylindrospermopsin. Ruminants and dogs are most commonly poisoned, but poisoning has been reported in horses and sheep. The cyanobacterial toxin is released when the microorganisms disintegrate, which may occur spontaneously in bodies of water or after the application of copper sulfate for algae control, or in the rumen or stomach after ingestion. Microcystin-LR is very stable and persists in water at typical ambient conditions, with a 10-week half-life. It is stable following boiling as well. The toxin is taken into hepatocytes by OATP membrane transporters and causes cell damage by inhibiting cytoplasmic protein phosphatase 1 and 2A. This leads to disorganization of hepatocyte and endothelial cytoskeletal actin filaments, and disruption of their shape and integrity, leading to necrosis, apoptosis, and hemorrhage. The distribution of the necrosis is usually centrilobular to panlobular. The pattern may vary within the individual liver and from case to case. In subacute intoxications, the liver is severely fatty, and necrosis is limited to randomly distributed individual or small groups of hepatocytes, rather than being zonal. Pigments accumulate in the cytoplasm, and there is slight ductular reaction and fibrosis. Necrosis of the renal tubules can also occur. Diagnosis can be made by detection of microcystin in the gastrointestinal content, liver, or water.

Toxic fungi

Amatoxins are potent hepatotoxins found in several mushroom genera, including *Amanita, Galerina*, and *Lepiota*. The genus ***Amanita*** contains several species, including *Amanita phalloides, A. verna, A. virosa*, and *A. ocreata*, which are considered extremely toxic. These mushrooms are mycorrhizal with various species of deciduous and coniferous trees and may be found in urban, suburban, and rural areas. The amatoxins are *bicyclic octapeptides*, ingestion of which is responsible for gastroenteritis, hypoglycemia, and fulminant liver failure in humans, dogs, cats, cattle, and other animals. They are stable compounds and persist in the acid environment of the stomach and following cooking. Amanitin, one of the amatoxins, is transported from the systemic circulation to hepatocytes by a specific OATP transporter on the hepatocyte surface. Toxicity is accentuated by enterohepatic circulation of the toxin, causing repeated hepatic exposure. Amanitin inhibits nuclear RNA polymerase II, thus interfering with transcription and inhibiting protein synthesis, resulting in cell death. Dogs or cats dying after ingestion of *Amanita* spp. have *diffuse panlobular hepatocellular necrosis with hemorrhage* (see Fig. 2-38). Remaining periportal hepatocytes have vesicular nuclei with loss or fragmentation of nucleoli, consistent with ultrastructural reports of chromatin condensation, dissolution of the nucleolus, and decline in nucleolar RNA content. *Necrosis of the proximal convoluted tubules* often accompanies hepatic injury and can aid in the index of suspicion for amanitin intoxication. The histologic lesions are nonspecific, and a definitive diagnosis of amanitin intoxication requires detection of the toxin. The liver, gastrointestinal content, kidney, and urine are the preferred samples for testing.

Aflatoxins

The **aflatoxins** are a group of *bisfuranocoumarin compounds* produced as metabolites mainly by *Aspergillus flavus, A. parasiticus*, and *A. nomius*. Nevertheless, other *Aspergillus* and *Penicillium* species such as *P. puberulum* can produce aflatoxins. The metabolites are designated by the blue or green color that they fluoresce when viewed under ultraviolet light and migration patterns during chromatography; and the major ones are B1, B2, G1, and G2. A less toxic metabolite, M1, is found in milk and other dairy products from cattle that ingest B1. Many others may be produced in minor amounts in fungal colonies or as metabolic products of the major toxins in animals. *The most significant and best studied of the aflatoxins is B1* because of its relative abundance and its potency as a hepatotoxin.

Strains of ***Aspergillus*** differ in the varieties and amounts of individual toxins produced, indicating that the biosynthesis of the toxins is genetically determined. The production of toxins also varies under different conditions of fungal growth, which is influenced by the quality of the substrate, temperature, relative humidity, moisture content of the substrate, and microbial competition. Thus, the toxicity of moldy feedstuffs is impossible to assess without measurement of toxin production. Aflatoxins can be produced on growing crops in the field, but much greater levels are likely to accumulate in *stored or unharvested mature grains*, particularly if they are damaged by moisture. Various feeds other than grains, ranging from legume stubbles to bread, may be the substrate in outbreaks of aflatoxicosis. Contaminated grain has been incorporated into commercial dog food, leading to outbreaks of acute toxicity.

Aflatoxins are metabolized by the hepatic mixed-function oxidase system to various toxic and nontoxic metabolites, the proportions of which vary with the species and age of the animal involved. The most potent of these is the 8,9-epoxide metabolite of aflatoxin B1, which binds to a variety of cellular proteins causing acute toxicity; its carcinogenic activity derives primarily from adduct formation with guanine in nucleic acids in sensitive species that lack adequate glutathione S-transferase–mediated resistance. The mutational consequence is a G to T transversion. Acute toxicity is most evident in dogs, piglets, pregnant sow, calves, rats, and guinea pigs, and each species may be fatally intoxicated by a dose rate of <1.0 mg/kg body weight. Although cats are also sensitive, they rarely ingest contaminated food. Adult ruminants are most resistant. *Acute, fulminating liver necrosis* is sometimes seen in dogs that eat contaminated bread, dog food, or garbage, which may contain extremely high concentrations of the toxin. Younger animals of all species are much more susceptible and may die within a few hours. The gross postmortem picture is dominated by widespread hemorrhage and diffuse hepatic necrosis. *Centrilobular-to-panlobular necrosis and hemorrhage* are seen at the microscopic level, followed by hepatic fibrosis and lipidosis (eFig. 2-26), although midzonal necrosis can occur in pigs and horses.

Cycadales

Acute hepatotoxicity has been reported in dogs, cattle, and sheep that have eaten the seeds or young leaves of species of *Cycas* or *Zamiaceae*, often referred to as *sago palm*. Dogs are intoxicated by eating the seeds of *Cycas* spp. usually raised as ornamental plants in warmer climates. The toxin responsible is *methylazoxymethanol*, which is the aglycone of various nontoxic glycosides, including cycasin and macrozamin, in these plants. The toxin is split from the glycoside by bacterial metabolism in the gut, and its hepatotoxicity is the result of further metabolism by hepatic CYPs; the pattern of necrosis is thus centrilobular. The metabolites of the aglycone are apparently *potent alkylating agents*, and the chronic liver lesions reflect this; there is megalocytosis (which is not as persistent as that of pyrrolizidine alkaloid poisoning), nuclear hyperchromasia, cholestasis, fatty change, and various degrees of diffuse fibrosis. There is consistent acute renal tubular injury. Chronic exposure leads to the development of neoplasia in the liver, kidney, and intestinal tract of laboratory rodents.

In addition to chronic hepatotoxicity, neurotoxicity occurs in cattle and sheep. Cycads produce a *neurotoxic amino acid, β-N-methylamino-L-alanine* (BMAA). BMAA is excitotoxic, activating neurotransmission mediated by glutamate receptors, which in excess can lead to cytotoxic influx of calcium ions. Chronic cycad poisoning of cattle causes a chronic nervous disorder characterized by a progressive proprioceptive deficit. This is the result of axonopathy in upper spinocerebellar and lower corticospinal tracts. The axonopathy, morphologically subtle at first, may eventually progress to frank Wallerian degeneration.

Solanaceae

Toxic species of the genus ***Cestrum*** (jessamine) include *Cestrum diurnum*, a cause of enzootic calcinosis in ruminants attributed to active vitamin D analogs; the other known toxic species all produce similar hepatic disease. Speciation within the genus is uncertain, partly because of hybridization; however, the species reported as hepatotoxic include *Cestrum parqui*, *C. laevigatum*, *C. aurantiacum*, *C. intermedium* and *C. axillare*.

Cestrum spp. cause *acute hepatotoxicity* in the field in South America, southern and central Africa, and Australia. Cattle are more frequently poisoned than other species, but sheep and goats are susceptible, and fowl may be if they eat the fruit. The young leaves and unripened berries are the most toxic parts of the plant. In acute hepatoxicity, there is *marked centrilobular-to-panlobular necrosis, hemorrhage, and hepatocellular vacuolation at the periphery*. Gallbladder wall edema can also occur. Status spongiosus is often present in the brain. There are no records of chronic liver disease caused by this plant under natural exposure, and photosensitization is rarely seen. However, experimental chronic exposure results in chronic hepatitis. The toxins are water soluble and have been identified as a *carboxyatractyloside, atractyloside*, and *carboxyparquin*.

Compositae/Asteraceae

Xanthium pungens (Noogoora burr) in Australia and *X. strumarium* (rough cocklebur) in the United States, as well as *X. cavanillesii* (the cocklebur) in Brazil and South Africa, have been reported to be hepatotoxic while in the seedling stage because the toxins are concentrated in the cotyledons. The burrs are also toxic, and although usually too coarse to be grazed, they can be consumed if ground into feeds. Swine, cattle, and sheep are susceptible, and toxicosis typically occurs following a period of feed scarcity, after flooding, or rain has allowed germination. The clinical signs and lesions are not specific, being those described for acute hepatotoxins in general. The toxic principle is a *diterpenoid glycoside, carboxyatractyloside*, although there may be other closely related toxic glycosides in some plants. ***Wedelia glauca*** also contains atractyloside and causes acute hepatotoxicity in cattle and sheep in South America. The condition has been reproduced experimentally in sheep and cattle and rats.

Atractyloside toxins inhibit exchange of ATP from the mitochondria with adenosine diphosphate (ADP) in the cytosol, a process essential for oxidative phosphorylation. Atractylosides inhibit the ADP/ATP carriers (AACs), including the form expressed in the liver. Carboxyatractyloside blocks exchange by binding to a cationic functional domain of bovine AAC1. Lack of ATP and mitochondrial pore leakage lead to apoptosis and necrosis, with ion pump failure, lipid peroxidation, and glutathione depletion. The extent of necrosis depends on dosage. Gross lesions include hepatomegaly with lobular accentuation, hepatic congestion, gallbladder wall edema, and fluid accumulation in the body cavities. *Diffuse centrilobular necrosis and hemorrhage* with vacuolar degeneration of hepatocytes at the periphery of areas of necrosis are seen histologically. Acute renal tubular degeneration and necrosis, cerebral edema, and neuronal degeneration may be present.

Other plants produce similar lesions, but the toxins have not been identified. *Helichrysum blandowskianum* is hepatotoxic to cattle and sheep in southern Australia and has caused sudden deaths with centrilobular necrosis. The condition has been reproduced experimentally. High mortality with acute centrilobular liver necrosis has been reported in cattle grazing sprouting plants of *Vernonia rubricaulis* in Brazil. Similar lesions were reproduced with 3 g/kg of sprouting plants. Various species of *Asteraceae* in South Africa, including *Asaemia axillaris, Athanasia trifurcata, Lasiospermum bipinnatum, Hertia pallens,* and *Pteronia pallens*, have been associated with field outbreaks of acute hepatotoxicity in grazing sheep or cattle. Similar liver lesions have been reproduced experimentally. Experimental intoxications by all of these species have, in some animals, produced *centrilobular-to-midzonal necrosis*. *Asaemia axillaris*, *Athanasia trifurcata*, and *Lasiospermum bipinnatum* are associated with more chronic liver toxicity with photosensitivity.

Ulmaceae

Trema tomentosa *(T. aspera)*, the poison peach, has caused severe losses of cattle in Australia. Similar disease has been reported in goats and horses ingesting *Trema micrantha* in Brazil, and hepatotoxicity has been reproduced in rabbits. The syndrome is acute, there is no photosensitization, and mildly intoxicated animals may recover completely. The toxic principle is a glycoside, designated *trematoxin*. The pattern of necrosis is consistently *centrilobular* and is identical in appearance to that of *Cestrum* and *Xanthium* poisoning.

The gross and microscopic histopathology of experimental poisoning by *Trema*, *Xanthium pungens*, and *Cestrum parqui* has been shown to be identical in all morphologic respects in the same group of sheep.

Myoporaceae

Hepatotoxic species of *Myoporaceae* so far incriminated are ***Myoporum deserti***, *M. acuminatum*, *M. insulare*, and *M. tetrandum* of Australia, and *M. laetum* in New Zealand, southern Brazil, and Uruguay. The toxic oils are contained in the leaves and branchlets, but within the species, there is variation in the chemical characters and toxicity of the oils; not all strains of toxic species are toxic. There is some delay between ingestion and absorption of the *furanosesquiterpenoid oils*, the best known of which is *ngaione*, which are responsible for intoxication. Twenty-four to 48 hours may elapse before signs of toxicity appear. Gross lesions include widespread hemorrhage and a pale-yellow liver. Histologically, the pattern is unusual, as the injury to the hepatocytes is *mainly periportal*, although midzonal and centrilobular injury occur. Ductular reaction may be present (Fig. 2-92A and B). Some animals live long enough to become photosensitized; others may die much more rapidly, with pulmonary edema. The edema appears to be a direct effect of the toxin after its metabolism by the club cells (formerly Clara cells) of the airway.

Livers from intoxicated sheep may show a striking, broad pattern of variable congestion and even infarction, which is superimposed on the more regular lobular pattern of periportal necrosis. Sections of these livers have acute fibrinoid necrosis of portal vessels, which suggests that the coarser lesions may have a vascular basis.

Sawfly larvae

Sawfly larval poisoning is an acute hepatotoxicosis documented in cattle and to a lesser extent sheep and goats in various locations, including Australia, Denmark, and South America. Ingestion of the larval stage of the "sawfly," 1 of 3 insect species that are members of the order *Hymenoptera* and the suborder *Symphyta*, produces hepatic injury. In Australia, the insect species is *Lophyrotoma interrupta (Pergidae)* or *L. zonalis (Pergidae)*; in Denmark, the insect is *Arge pullata (Argidae)*, and in South America a third species, *Perreyia flavipes (Pergidae)*, is incriminated. In parts of northeastern Australia, the larvae are parasitic on the leaves of the tree *Eucalyptus melanophloia*, and heavy infections may occur.

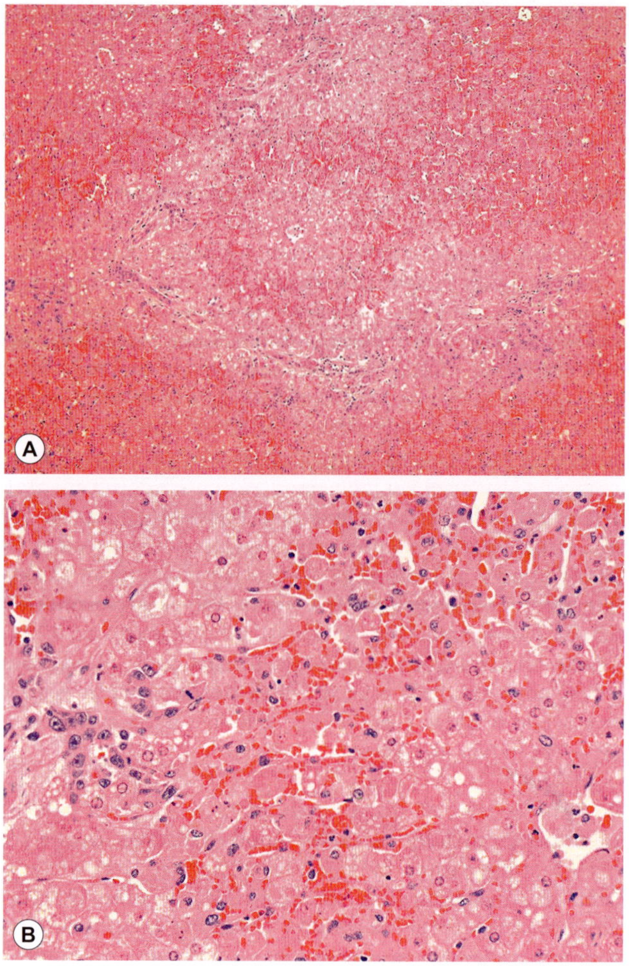

Figure 2-92 **Midzonal necrosis** caused by ingestion of ***Myoporum*** sp. in a donkey. **A**. Low-power view. **B**. Higher magnification. (Courtesy R. Kelly.)

L. zonalis has been introduced to Florida to control the spread of *Melaleuca quinquenervi*. In Denmark, sawfly larvae feed on birch trees. There is a short clinical course following ingestion, and affected cattle are often found dead. Animals that survive typically develop icterus and secondary photosensitization. At postmortem examination, ascites, petechiae, and ecchymoses are evident. The liver is enlarged with an accentuated lobular pattern. Mural edema of the gallbladder may be apparent. Sawfly larvae can be found in the rumen and, on occasion, through to the abomasum. Histologically, there is *centrilobular-to-panlobular acute hepatic necrosis*. Outbreaks tend to be seasonal, related to the life cycle of the insects. The toxic principle is believed to be D-amino acid–containing peptides. The major toxin is an octapeptide, *lophyrotomin*, present in the larvae of Australian and Danish sawflies. There is a different toxin in the South American sawflies, identified as the heptadecapeptide *pergidin*.

Halogenated hydrocarbons

Various halogenated hydrocarbons, such as *carbon tetrachloride* (used historically as a fasciolicide), *bromobenzene*, *hexachloroethane*, *tetrachloroethylene*, and *chloroform*, are activated by CYPs to hepatotoxic or nephrotoxic metabolites. They have similar hepatotoxic properties, but these agents are little used now, so few animals encounter them in toxic doses. However, some of these chemicals have been used experimentally to investigate the mechanisms of hepatotoxicity; hence, they warrant brief consideration here. Carbon tetrachloride is metabolized to trihalomethane, a necrogenic free-radical metabolite, and reactive oxygen radicals are concurrently generated. *Centrilobular hepatic necrosis with midzonal hydropic change* caused by membrane peroxidation occurs within 30 hours of experimental exposures, but lethal toxicity occurs later, when steatosis and the initial stages of tissue repair responses are manifest.

Phosphorus

White phosphorus has historically been used for vermin control and has been implicated in the accidental exposure and deaths of wild waterfowl. It may be present in some incendiary devices such as fireworks. As a rodenticide, it is mixed with fat to promote absorption, and much of the dose is transported to the liver shortly after ingestion. A small amount may be lost by vomition, as elemental phosphorus is directly irritating to the gastrointestinal tract. The mechanism of phosphorus hepatotoxicity is uncertain. It is apparent that metabolism to a toxic intermediate is not necessary, but there is some dispute about the involvement of lipoperoxidation in the hepatocellular injury. There is evidence that protein synthesis is impaired early and that this is responsible for the lipid accumulation that is a prominent feature. A few hours after ingestion of phosphorus, there is severe colic and vomition. If the animal survives this acute phase, there may be apparent recovery for a few days, followed by jaundice and other signs of liver failure, and death by about the fifth day. At postmortem, there is severe icterus and fatty liver, the latter sometimes being *predominantly periportal* in distribution. Hepatocellular necrosis is not often a prominent feature histologically, notwithstanding the evidence of liver failure. Fatty change is also seen in the myocardium and distal nephrons.

Iron

Iron-dextran complexes have been widely used in the prevention and treatment of anemia in suckling swine. Very occasionally, *severe losses may occur in animals with marginal vitamin E-selenium deficiency;* in these cases, there is, apparently, iron-catalyzed lipoperoxidation in hepatocytes and muscle. The result is *sudden panlobular hepatic necrosis* similar in many respects to that of hepatosis dietetica. Substantial amounts of potassium escape into the circulation from the liver and muscle, and sudden death may result from the cardiotoxicity of this ion. At postmortem, there is staining of subcutaneous tissues and lymph nodes near the site of injection, and there are lesions in the liver or skeletal muscles. The liver is of normal size and of normal color or pale, depending on whether the animal is anemic. The underlying necrosis may be indicated only by the numerous small or large hemorrhages present on the capsular and cut surface. Insoluble iron compounds with the staining reactions of hemosiderin are found in mesenchymal cells in many tissues, the largest amounts being in macrophages of the local lymph nodes and in Kupffer cells. Death in piglets from hepatic necrosis occurs ~10 hours after administration. Saccharated iron may produce acute widespread muscle necrosis at ~24 hours, rather than hepatic necrosis in piglets with marginal vitamin E-selenium status. The myocardium is not affected.

Acute hepatotoxicity was reported in young *foals* because of administration of a proprietary *paste of iron and yeast products*, given as a dietary supplement within a few hours of birth. Not all foals so treated became sick, but those that did develop severe acute centrilobular hepatocellular necrosis, resembling the disease in piglets, and dramatic ductular reaction (biliary hyperplasia).

Acute iron intoxication has also been reported in young *cattle* administered injectable hematinics containing elemental iron, and rarely in adult *horses* administered oral vitamin supplements containing ferrous fumarate or ferrous sulfate. Over-supplementation, low vitamin E or selenium concentrations, or concurrent disease may have contributed to these cases. Consumption of *elemental iron* produces a periportal or panlobular pattern of necrosis.

Chronic hepatotoxicity: plant-derived and environmental toxins

Aflatoxin

Large animal species rarely are exposed to sufficient doses of aflatoxin by normal dietary intake to develop acute toxicity. Sheep and adult cattle are quite resistant to the toxin. *Prolonged exposure to low concentrations of the toxin is a more frequent problem than acute toxicity* in large animal species and may merely produce reduced growth rates and moderate enlargement of the liver without any significant hepatic signs. The enlargement may be partly the result of hypertrophy of hepatocellular SER and some degree of fatty change. As the level of aflatoxin in the ration increases (in young pigs, to 1.0 mg/kg ration), the liver may have all or none of the following changes: pallor, enlargement, bile staining, increased firmness because of fibrogenesis, and fine nodular regenerative hyperplasia. There may also be edema of the gallbladder and bile-tinged ascites in more severe cases. Even under experimental conditions, some individuals may have minimal liver lesions, while others, under the same levels of exposure, die of liver failure. Histologically, affected livers have an obvious increase in size of some hepatocytes and their nuclei (megalocytosis) with focal necrosis or apoptosis. Bile ductules proliferate rapidly after exposure, and reticulin and collagen deposition occur throughout the lobule according to no distinct pattern (Fig. 2-93). Fatty change in affected livers is variable in extent and occurrence, and bile pigments accumulate in canaliculi and hepatocytes in more severely affected livers. Minor degrees of megalocytosis may be seen in proximal tubular epithelium in the kidney. *The changes*

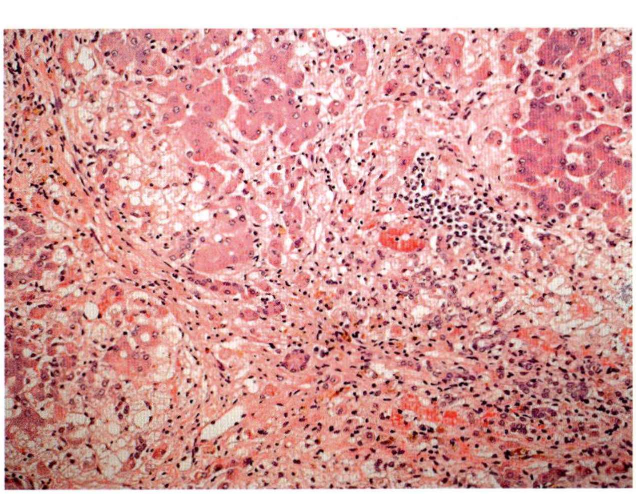

Figure 2-93 Hepatocellular steatosis, fibrosis, and ductular proliferation in canine **chronic aflatoxicosis**.

produced resemble those of pyrrolizidine alkaloid toxicosis. This can be attributed to the fact that aflatoxin and pyrrolizidine alkaloids *inhibit hepatocellular regeneration* such that nodules of resistant hepatocytes and ductules regenerate as the liver becomes atrophic. These are also *genotoxic* and *carcinogenic*, so they might be involved in the occurrence of liver neoplasms in animals, as they are in humans.

At higher dose rates of aflatoxin, most centrilobular hepatocytes disappear and are replaced by a mixture of inflammatory cells, fibroblasts, and primitive vascular channels. The liver may be much smaller than normal, particularly in young animals, presumably because of mitotic inhibition, and focal hepatocellular necrosis is more obvious or may be supplanted by zonal (centrilobular) necrosis. Fatty change in these livers may be severe and uniformly distributed.

Fumonisin

Fumonisin B1, a mycotoxin elaborated by certain strains of ***Fusarium verticillioides*** (previously *moniliforme*) and ***F. proliferatum*** in infected corn, induces a pulmonary edema syndrome in pigs, hepatocellular carcinomas in laboratory rats, and leukoencephalomalacia in horses. Three toxins produced by the fungi have been classified as fumonisin B1 (FB1), B2 (FB2), and B3 (FB3). FB1 and FB2 are of similar toxicity; FB3 is relatively nontoxic. Hepatotoxicity occurs in horses and swine. Hepatic toxicity has also been reported in sheep and baboons. In horses, hepatoxicity occurs less often than leukoencephalomalacia. The clinical course is relatively short, with death likely within 5-10 days of the onset of clinical signs, such as anorexia, depression, icterus, and edema of the head. Bilirubin and liver enzyme activities are typically elevated. At postmortem, the liver is typically firm, yellow, and small, with an accentuated lobular pattern. Histologic lesions include abundant apoptosis/necrosis that may progress from centrilobular to panlobular vacuolar degeneration and necrosis with variable amounts of fibrosis and ductular reaction in the portal tracts. Cardiotoxicity is also evident in swine and horses.

Fumonisin B1 is also a *primary hepatotoxin in pigs*. Experimental feeding trials with pigs have shown dose-related differences in pathology. Pigs intubated with a minimum of 16 mg fumonisin B1/kg body weight per day developed interlobular edema, variable hydrothorax, and pulmonary edema; pigs intubated with 8 mg/kg per day for 7-8 days or fed diets containing 200 mg fumonisin B1/kg of feed for 21 days developed marked icterus. Histologic changes included hepatocellular necrosis without a zonal distribution, depletion of centrilobular hepatocytes, lobular disarray, and megalocytosis characterized by large numbers of swollen hepatocytes with abundant granular eosinophilic cytoplasm and occasional large nuclei, randomly interspersed with small angular hepatocytes and scattered necrotic cells. These pigs had no evidence of pathologic changes in the lungs; pigs given higher doses had *hepatic necrosis in addition to pulmonary edema*. The liver changes appear to be reversible upon cessation of exposure. Gilts fed low levels of fumonisin B1 for 90 days developed regenerative nodules along with hyperkeratosis and parakeratosis and hyperplasia of the distal esophageal mucosa. Fumonisins are inhibitors of sphingosine and ceramide synthetase, leading to inhibition of sphingolipid biosynthesis. Consequently, bioactive intermediates of sphingolipid metabolism accumulate (sphinganine and other sphingoid bases and derivatives), as well as complex sphingolipids are depleted, which interferes with the function of some membrane proteins and may be involved in the toxic hepatic effects.

Phomopsin

There are 2 distinct manifestations of toxicity associated with *Lupinus* spp.; discussed here is the condition formerly known as *"lupinosis," which is a true mycotoxic liver disease*. The teratogenic and neurotoxic effects of some of the isoquinoline alkaloids from the plants themselves are discussed in Vol. 1, Bones and Joints and Vol. 1, Nervous System.

Phomopsin poisoning occurs mainly in sheep in Australia and South Africa but is also reported in Europe and New Zealand. Cattle and horses are occasionally affected, and pigs and goats are also susceptible. The fungus ***Diaporthe toxica*** (formerly *Phomopsis leptostromiformis)* is parasitic on green *Lupinus* plants, but it becomes saprophytic after the host plant dies. Phomopsins (A or B) are produced if the lupin stubble is moistened, and such stubbles may remain toxic for months. Additional toxins are suspected. Severe acute liver damage has been described in sheep on very toxic stubbles in Western Australia, but in many of these cases, it has been difficult to separate the toxicity of the lupins from that of copper, which in this area is often concentrated in ovine livers (see later the Copper section).

The usual syndrome of phomopsin poisoning is subacute to chronic. Inappetence occurs soon after experimental administration of the toxin is begun; liver damage is clinically inapparent for several days. The gross pathologic abnormalities of acutely intoxicated sheep include icterus and modest ascites. The main abnormalities are evident in the liver, which varies from a yellow discoloration because of lipidosis in more acute cases, to a variable ochre-to-orange discoloration with a firm texture with increasing chronicity (Fig. 2-94A). Histologically, there is early hepatocyte swelling and accelerated cell death among hepatocytes. Increased mitotic activity is soon apparent, although by this time, the liver has become smaller. The mitotic activity is in fact largely ineffectual, as close examination reveals that many mitotic figures are abnormal. There is either clumping or dispersal of chromatin, and *there appears to be mitotic arrest at late metaphase* (see Fig. 2-94B-D). Remaining hepatocytes swell, their cytoplasm becomes granular, and their nuclei become vesicular and may contain vesicular intranuclear pseudoinclusions. There is variably severe fatty change, dependent to a large degree on the fat reserves of the animal. There is also accumulation of complex pigment in macrophages in portal stroma and around hepatic venules; this granular material contains lipofuscin, ferric iron, and copper at least. Bile duct proliferation is also a prominent feature of chronic disease. With progression, hepatic fibrosis occurs, predominantly diffuse in distribution, and by this stage, there is usually clinical icterus and anorexia.

The liver continues to shrink, presumably because of *continued mitotic inhibition and progressive fibrosis*. The organ is small, tough, and has a finely granular surface and texture. It is pale gray-orange but usually retains its shape. Fibrosis is initially portal to periportal, but central areas can also become fibrotic. Bridging fibrosis between portal areas and portal to central regions can develop. In naturally occurring cases, however, discontinuous intake of the toxin may produce a liver grossly distorted by asymmetrical nodular regeneration and fibrosis. The atrophic changes are most severe in the left lobe.

Photosensitization occurs in phomopsin-poisoned sheep; it may be severe if the animals have access to green feed while under the influence of the toxin. Lupinosis in sheep has also

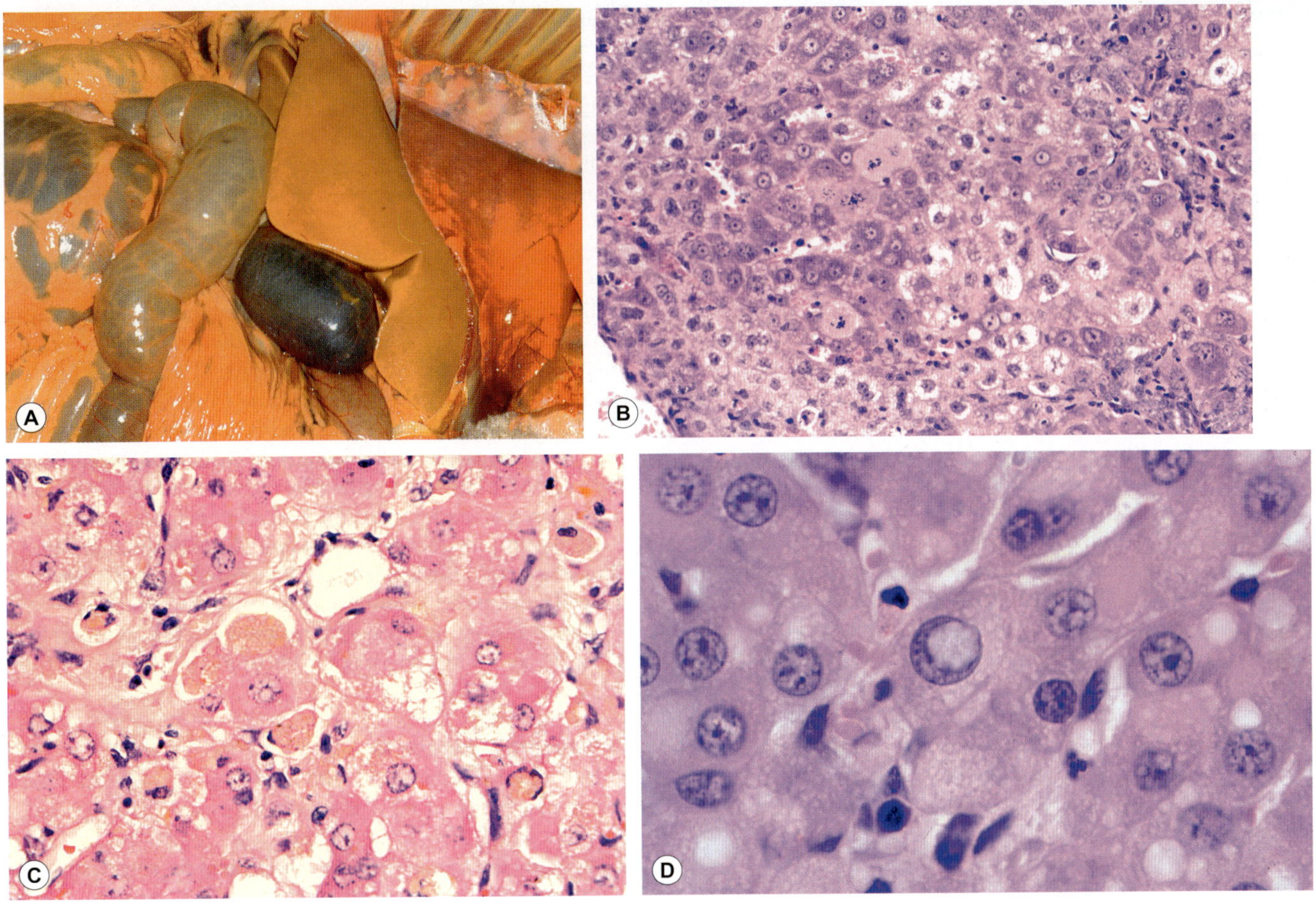

Figure 2-94 Phomopsin poisoning (lupinosis) in sheep. A. Affected sheep have pale livers and prominent icterus. B. Numerous, and **abnormal, mitotic figures** in subacute phomopsin poisoning. C. **Brown pigment** within Kupffer cells. D. Clear **intranuclear pseudoinclusions** can be found in affected hepatocytes. (Courtesy J.G. Allen.)

been experimentally observed to induce mild skeletal myopathy, resembling nutritional myopathy.

Phomopsin poisoning in cattle causes most losses when the animals are lactating or heavily pregnant; in these animals, the syndrome is essentially one of ketosis, to which such cows would be predisposed by the anorexia that is an obvious clinical feature of this intoxication. Pregnant sheep are less likely to have access to toxic lupin roughage during late gestation; otherwise, ketosis triggered by phomopsin would be expected just as often as in cattle.

Chronic hepatic fibrosis with fine, nodular regeneration may occur infrequently in cattle as the result of chronic phomopsin poisoning. Similar liver changes may also be seen in horses, in which there may also be hemolytic anemia of unknown pathogenesis.

Sporidesmin

The mycotoxin *sporidesmin* is produced by the fungus ***Pithomyces chartarum*** and concentrated in the conidia (spores); the most important substrate is dead perennial ryegrass *(Lolium perenne)* that has been moistened in warm weather. Intoxication causes *chronic liver damage and severe hepatogenous photosensitivity* ***("facial eczema")*** and is a serious cause of loss of sheep and, to a lesser extent, cattle, goats, and farmed deer on the North Island of New Zealand. Sporadic and subclinical intoxication occurs irregularly on the South Island, in southern Australia, Africa, Europe, and South America. Sporidesmin intake in conjunction with ingestion of *Tribulus terrestris* causes another hepatogenous photosensitivity *(geeldikkop)*; this is similar to, but distinct from, facial eczema and is described later.

Sporidesmin is concentrated in the fungal spores, and the toxigenicity of pasture is related to the density of the spores in it. Sporidesmin is not specifically hepatotoxic. Administration of the toxin does produce rapid disorganization of hepatocellular organelles and triglyceride accumulation, but these are mild and nonspecific changes. If administered in suitable dosage, the toxin causes permeability alterations in many tissues and will, for example, produce corneal edema on local application. The mechanism of toxicity is not entirely proven. *The hepatobiliary lesions may be caused by the excretion of unconjugated sporidesmin in bile, where its concentration may initiate oxidative injury*. Effect on cell adhesion affecting the integrity of epithelial and endothelial lining may also play a role. Sporidesmin is also excreted in urine, and if the dose is high enough, edema and mucosal hemorrhage occur in the urinary bladder. A high concentration of sporidesmin can injure biliary epithelium, allowing diffusion of the bile duct contents. Release of toxin, possibly accentuated by the release of bile acids as well, produces irritative lesions and necrosis in the adjacent blood vessels.

In acute forms of the disease, the carcass is jaundiced, and the liver is enlarged, with rounded edges, and is finely mottled and discolored yellow-green by retained bile pigments, although the discoloration may be blotchy. There is mild edema and congestion of the wall of the gallbladder, which may be distended with bile of normal quality or with mucin (white bile). The extrahepatic ducts are thickened and prominent, and there is edema of the adventitia. The ductal changes may extend to the **major duodenal papilla** (papilla of Vater) and can be traced by the naked eye deeply into the parenchyma. In more chronic cases, the liver is small, but alterations of size and pigmentation of the liver are variable. Pale areas of capsular thickening, which may be elevated or depressed, are visible. On cut surfaces, they extend deeply as wedge-shaped areas in which biliary fibrosis has produced an exaggerated acinar pattern, and the parenchyma is pale and atrophic; these areas are related to occluded bile ducts.

The liver is firm and cuts with increased resistance. The medium and large caliber intrahepatic ducts are conspicuous. There is irregular stenosis of their lumens, some are occluded by cellular debris and inspissated bile or mucin, and in some, cicatrization of the new fibrous tissue causes complete atresia. Occlusion of the ducts causes the parenchyma served by them to undergo atrophy, necrosis, and fibrosis (Fig. 2-95). The livers of animals that have survived an attack of cholangitis of this genesis are distorted in shape and size by large nodules of regeneration and persistent areas of atrophy and fibrosis. Atrophy and fibrosis may affect either lobe, but usually, the left is most severely affected. Gallbladders are large and contain biliary sludge and sometimes gallstones.

In acute cases, the histologic changes are those of *acute cholangitis or cholangiohepatitis* to which there is minimal leukocytic reaction. There is extensive necrosis of the lining of the intrahepatic ducts and the extrahepatic ducts, the epithelium being necrotic and cast off as debris mixed with a few leukocytes. There is edema of the adventitia of the ducts and portal tracts. Inflammatory cells are present, but not in large numbers, and they are chiefly lymphocytes and histiocytes. Injury to the smaller radicles of the bile ducts is less severe. Ductular reaction is at the periphery of portal tracts. Affected camelids appear to be susceptible to florid hyperplasia of the bile ducts. Changes in the hepatic parenchyma are secondary to those in the portal tracts. There is variable periportal fatty change, and hepatocellular and canalicular cholestasis in centrilobular regions. Hepatocyte degeneration and necrosis may also be observed. Small aggregates of neutrophils and macrophages, sometimes multinucleate, surround bile pigment ('bile lakes') in hepatic lobules.

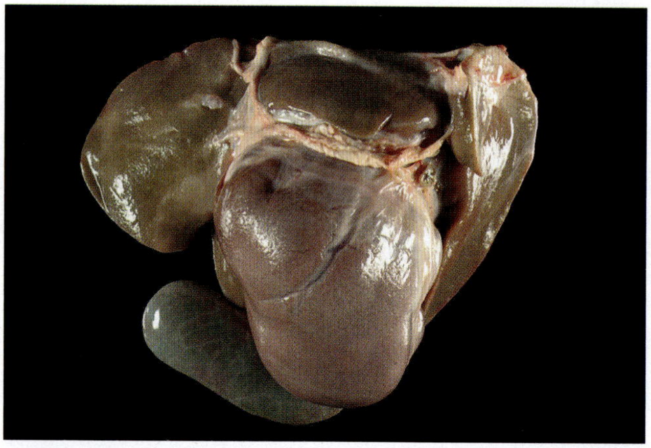

Figure 2-95 Chronic sporidesmin intoxication ("facial eczema") in a sheep. Liver lobe atrophy and fibrosis. (Courtesy K.G. Thompson.)

In chronic cases, biliary fibrosis with variable bridging and prominent ductular reaction is present (eFig. 2-27). The leukocytic portal inflammation is more intense and characterized by lymphocytes, plasma cells, and pigment-laden macrophages. The pigment is a mix of lipofuscin, hemosiderin, and copper.

In severe acute intoxications, there may be *coagulative necrosis of blood vessel walls in the portal tracts;* when this is incomplete, the most damaged segment of the vessel tends to be that adjacent to the nearest injured bile duct. Both arteries and veins may be affected, and it is possible that necrosis is related to vascular insufficiency as well as to impaired bile drainage. Myointimal proliferation is observed in extrahepatic and intrahepatic arteries, and sublobular veins near injured bile ducts. Lymphocytic phlebitis and phlebosclerosis consisting of fibrosis around central veins and fibromuscular hypertrophy of the walls of ectatic hepatic veins are also documented.

Other lesions include enlargement of the adrenals produced by cortical hypertrophy, cholemic nephrosis, and dermal lesions of photosensitization.

Pyrrolizidine alkaloids

Dehydropyrrolizidine alkaloids (DHPAs) have been identified in nearly 3% of all plant species, from >6,000 species of 3 families: the *Asteraceae (Compositae)*, *Leguminosae (Fabaceae)*, and *Boraginaceae*. The main genera responsible for plant toxicoses in domestic mammals are ***Senecio, Crotalaria, Heliotropium, Cynoglossum, Amsinckia, Echium***, and ***Trichodesma***, which are widely distributed around the world. Intoxication is relatively infrequent because most plants containing DHPAs are unpalatable. Contamination of baled or cubed forage with toxic plants is a common route of exposure. The seeds are also toxic, and the small seeds of *Amsinckia* and *Crotalaria* may, depending on harvesting technique, heavily contaminate other harvested grains used in prepared pig and poultry feeds. More than 350 DHPAs have been identified chemically, and most of the toxic plant species contain more than one of the alkaloids. So far, only a small proportion of the known DHPAs have well-characterized toxicity. DHPAs are chemically composed of a 2-ring base structure (necine) and 1 or 2 side chains. They can be classified as monoesters, diesters, or macrocyclic diesters based on the chemical composition of the side chains. The **retronecine group** includes *monocrotaline, retrorsine, retronecine, riddelliine, senecionine*, and *jacobine*, and the **heliotridine group** includes *lasiocarpine* and *heliotrine*. DHPAs are protoxins and require metabolic activation by CYPs to reactive intermediates for toxicity. Bioactivation occurs by hydroxylation of the necine bases at the C3 or C8 positions followed by spontaneous dehydration to the *highly reactive pyrrolic esters*. The toxic pyrrolic esters are potent electrophiles and can bind covalently to amino acids, proteins, and nucleic acids at guanine and adenine residues. Acute toxicity derives from damage to cellular proteins. Antimitotic effects occur and may result from damage to microtubules.

Carcinogenicity has been demonstrated in mice and rats. The DNA-binding activity of DHPAs is responsible for genotoxicity and carcinogenicity; DNA adducts with pyrrolic esters are a common pathway for carcinogenic activity of pyrrolizidine alkaloids. Pyrrolic esters can be detoxified by glutathione conjugation by glutathione S-transferases. Ester linkages at the C7 and C9 positions can be hydrolyzed by carboxylesterases to generate the necine or acid moieties; this is generally considered to be a detoxification pathway. CYPs enzymes can also mediate N-oxidation of the necine bases, resulting in a more water-soluble compound that can be excreted more easily.

The toxicity of a pyrrolizidine alkaloid–containing plant depends on many factors. The content of toxin varies by species of plant; the stage of growth, as new growth tends to have more toxin in general; and the time of year and environmental factors such as rainfall. For an individual DHPA, toxicity depends on the amount of alkaloid that can be converted to reactive metabolites, the rate of CYPs-mediated generation of pyrrolic esters, and the efficiency of detoxification by glutathione conjugation. Susceptibility to toxicosis depends on the species, age, and sex of the animal intoxicated, nutritional status, and the metabolic activity and the mitotic stage of its target cells. Young animals are generally much more susceptible than adults. Grazing animals are more likely to be exposed to plants that contain DHPAs, but because the toxins are produced by the plants to deter herbivores, it is unusual for an animal to consume substantial amounts. Ruminants, especially sheep and goats, are much less susceptible than pigs, in part because the toxins can be degraded in the rumen. However, sheep can graze out stands of *Senecio* that would be lethal to cattle. Horses and cattle have similar, intermediate susceptibilities. *Most DHPAs are hepatotoxic because they are metabolically activated to pyrrole esters in the liver.*

There are 2 common morphologic expressions of pyrrolizidine poisoning. First, *acute hepatic necrosis increasing to panlobular depending on exposure dose* occurs in animals ingesting substantial amounts of these alkaloids. Because the plants responsible are unpalatable, naturally occurring outbreaks of acute poisoning are generally restricted to circumstances in which animals face starvation, such as grazing pastures affected by prolonged drought. Ingested dosages in grazing circumstances are usually too low for acute effects; however, acute hemorrhagic centrilobular-to-panlobular necrosis has been described after experimental exposures to high doses of DHPAs. The centrilobular pattern of necrosis produced is similar to that caused by many other hepatotoxins that are bioactivated by hepatic CYPs, although other lobular patterns can occur. Second, phasic (usually seasonal) repetitive chronic exposure to these alkaloids leads to *hepatic atrophy and fibrosis* with possible formation of regenerative nodules depending on the species exposed. *This is the most common expression of field exposure to DHPAs, and affected livers have a characteristic pattern of fibrosis, ductular reaction, and hepatocellular polyploidy known as* ***megalocytosis*** (Fig. 2-96). If seasonal exposure to these toxic alkaloids declines, then a remarkable degree of recovery is possible.

DHPAs inhibit DNA synthesis and mitosis in hepatocytes, but some cells can replicate their DNA without undergoing mitosis, resulting in greatly enlarged hepatocytes with large convoluted polyploid nuclei. Some enlarged nuclei have cytoplasmic invaginations that can become entrapped as intranuclear inclusions. However, many hepatocytes in an affected liver do not become megalocytic. Those that are completely inhibited do not replicate DNA at all; those that are more resistant can replicate more normally and give rise to nodular populations of smaller, more normal hepatocytes. Inhibited hepatocytes and megalocytes are long lived but eventually many undergo apoptosis.

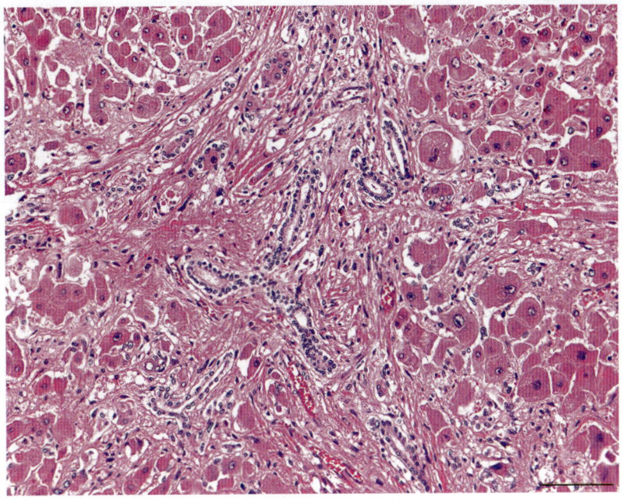

Figure 2-96 Fibrosis, ductular reaction, and megalocytosis in pyrrolizidine alkaloid poisoning in a horse.

In *chronic DHPA poisoning,* the liver can become atrophic as hepatocytes are lost faster than they can be replaced. The atrophy can be compensated to various degrees by megalocytosis and proliferation of small, less inhibited hepatocytes. Concurrently, there is usually proliferation of bile duct epithelial cells (*ductular reaction*) in the portal tracts. This is largely explained by the propensity of HPCs to proliferate forming ductules when adult hepatocytes cannot respond to the regenerative stimuli that prevail when liver mass is inadequate. There may also be some *portal fibrosis* that varies with species and exposure; typically, it is mild in sheep, moderate in horses, and may be marked in cattle (eFig. 2-28). In **cattle**, the fibrous stroma can infiltrate along sinusoids to dissect lobules, separate individual cells, and link up with the walls of efferent veins. In acute poisoning, in which there is centrilobular necrosis, fibrosis can also develop in a "veno-occlusive" pattern around and sometimes obliterating the hepatic venules. There is evidence that DHPA metabolite injury is not restricted to hepatocytes and that endothelial cells are also involved, leading to additional vascular insult and fibrosis in the liver. Direct endothelial injury from DHPAs may occur, but an alternative explanation proposes a form of "bystander" injury, in which toxic metabolites are formed in hepatocytes but are able to damage adjacent endothelial cells. This pattern of fibrosis may occur in some field cases in cattle but is more commonly seen in humans exposed to DHPAs in herbal preparations or "bush teas," and it can be produced experimentally after sublethal acute experimental hepatotoxicity. In fatal cases in cattle, the livers are very tough and nodular. Hepatic fibrosis can result in *portal hypertension* with ascites, severe mesenteric edema, and diarrhea. Excretory insufficiency with moderate jaundice and photosensitization can also occur.

The disease in **sheep** is always protracted because of the relative resistance of this species; indeed, clinical signs may not be seen until after several seasons of exposure. The plants most often implicated are *Heliotropium europaeum* and *Echium plantagineum*. The shape of these failed livers is normal, but they are small, gray-yellow, smooth, and toughened by condensation of normal stroma more than fibroplasia. If the liver copper content was high before intoxication, toxicity can culminate in copper release and an episode of intravascular hemolysis. In this case, the carcass will be intensely jaundiced, and the kidneys are stained with methemoglobin and bilirubin. The relationship of chronic copper poisoning to DHPA poisoning is discussed later.

Horses are susceptible to both acute and chronic toxicosis, and liver failure produced in horses by these alkaloids is like that seen in cattle. Horses are more likely to manifest signs of HE with head-pressing and compulsive walking; in some places, these nervous signs give rise to colloquial names such as "walkabout" and "walking disease." Administration of a high dose of *Cynoglossum officinale* resulted in severe liver disease within 7 days after dosing, with elevated serum enzyme activities, altered bile acid metabolism, and extensive hepatocellular necrosis with minimal periportal fibrosis and ductular reaction, and little or no megalocytosis. Edema and infarction of the cecum and colon were also present at postmortem. Administration of a low dose to horses for 14 days resulted in transient clinical depression and weight loss, transient elevations of serum enzymes and bile acids, and minimal periportal hepatocellular necrosis with fibrosis, developing extensive megalocytosis by week 14. The megalocytosis became the most prominent change 6 months after exposure.

Metabolites of DHPAs are formed by any cells with adequate CYP activity. Although the liver is the main site of bioactivation, other cells such as proximal convoluted renal tubules and club cells (formerly termed Clara cells) in the lung can generate metabolites that cause local injury. Death in some instances may be the result of renal damage and in others the result of pulmonary vascular and interstitial lesions. Variation in the source of the toxin and in the species-based metabolic differences in the affected animals accounts for the differences in susceptibility of the different tissues. Alkaloids from *Crotalaria* affect the widest range of tissues in most animals; most notably, monocrotaline causes diffuse lung injury, leading to pulmonary edema progressing to fibrosis. Respiratory difficulty has been described in horses eating *C. dura*, and *C. crispata* produces similar lesions. Sheep develop pulmonary signs after eating *C. globifera* and *C. dura*, and pigs after eating *S. jacobaea*. The experimental feeding of *C. spectabilis* to rats or the injection of monocrotaline, extracted from the plant, produces progressive pulmonary disease, pulmonary hypertension, and cor pulmonale, with necrotizing vasculitis of the pulmonary arterioles. Emphysema occurs in pigs and is an outstanding feature of the pulmonary disease of horses; the essential reactive lesion is diffuse fibrosis of alveolar and interlobular septa, with patchy epithelialization occurring more slowly.

Lantana camara

Lantana camara is an attractive ornamental shrub native to Central and South American tropics and Africa that grows readily in a wide variety of tropic, subtropical, and warm temperate habitats. The leaves, stems, roots, and unripe fruits contain various *toxic pentacyclic triterpenes*, the most abundant of which are lantadene A, B, C, and icterogenin, although metabolites may also be toxic. Lantadene A and B appear to be the most toxic. *Lantana* toxins cause intrahepatic cholestasis in addition to hepatocellular damage. Experimental lantana poisoning in sheep causes *acute periportal hepatocellular degeneration and necrosis*. The mechanism of toxicity is not known but may be related to the effects of the toxins on mitochondrial energetics. *L. camara* poisoning in grazing animals is manifested as *cholestasis, characterized by severe icterus and photosensitization*, mostly seen in cattle, but rarely in sheep, goats, and horses. Goats are quite susceptible to the toxin but are less likely to eat the plant. Neonatal ruminants appear resistant, suggesting that the rumen may retain the plants and provide longer exposure to the toxins.

Photosensitization is usually severe after 2 days, but jaundice is more severe in chronic cases. Heavily intoxicated cattle can die within 2 days, but most fatal cases run a course of ~2 weeks. Ruminal stasis and anorexia appear early, and the large bowel contains dark, dry feces. The rumen is a reservoir of toxin that remains active and can perpetuate the intoxication after access to the plant is curtailed. The liver is enlarged, pale, and stained yellow, orange, or green-gray by bile pigment. The gallbladder is greatly distended with pale, sometimes slightly mucoid, bile.

The severity of the liver changes may be much less than expected from the intensity of the icterus and photosensitization. The most consistent histologic finding in the liver is hepatocellular enlargement and fine cytoplasmic vacuolation, together with some degree of bile accumulation in canaliculi, hepatocyte cytoplasm, and Kupffer cells. The canalicular cholestasis is usually more severe in the centrilobular zones; the cytoplasmic vacuolation is often more pronounced in the periportal hepatocytes. There is usually some ductular reaction, and in some cases, there will be a high incidence of periportal apoptosis, focal coagulative necrosis, or hepatocellular dissociation.

Electron microscopy reveals an apparent increase in volume of SER and a quite characteristic form of collapse of many bile canaliculi. Other canaliculi are distended and have damaged microvilli. Because much of the bilirubin that accumulates in the plasma of such animals is conjugated, it seems that the cholestasis is due in large measure to direct interference with canalicular transport of bile. The mechanisms of cholestasis have not been determined, but damage to the contractile pericanalicular cytoskeleton or its associated cell adhesion molecules required for canalicular integrity are plausible targets (see the Cholestasis and Jaundice section).

Animals are usually polyuric because of *acute renal tubular injury*, resulting in severe dehydration, in part related to a disinclination to drink. The kidneys are slightly enlarged and wet on section, and, especially in the more chronic cases, the cortex is pale and the medulla is hyperemic. The renal lesion is a nonspecific acute tubular injury, ranging in severity from mild vacuolar change to patchy tubular necrosis and extensive tubular cast formation. The role of hyperbilirubinemia in the production of renal damage has not been assessed. Myocardial necrosis and pulmonary edema can be produced in sheep by *Lantana* poisoning and may be responsible for the early deaths in cattle.

Intoxication by steroidal sapogenins: tribulosis and related toxicoses

Consumption of ***Tribulus terrestris***, particularly by the grazing of young, wilted plants, or sometimes hay, causes cholangitis and photosensitization in sheep. This plant has caused enormous loss of sheep in South Africa, where the toxicosis is known as **geeldikkop** ("yellow bighead," because of icterus and marked edema of ears and face). The disease has been reproduced by oral administration of crude extracts of *steroidal sapogenins or their glycosides, saponins*, of *T. terrestris*, but which of the various saponins in the plant are responsible for the disease is unknown. The disease has also been reproduced experimentally by coadministration of sporidesmin and *T. terrestris*, but the liver lesions are histologically distinct from those produced by sporidesmin alone (facial eczema). In poisoning by sporidesmin alone, there is more obvious edema and fibrosis of bile ducts, and bile infarcts in the parenchyma are more common.

In geeldikkop, the most characteristic gross finding is a white, semifluid accumulation of fine, crystalline material that can be expressed from the cystic duct and larger intrahepatic ducts. The gallbladder mucosa is also partly covered with a fine, crystalline deposit. The gross lesions of geeldikkop are like those of facial eczema in that there is generalized icterus, and the liver is discolored by bile pigment and either slightly swollen or distorted, according to the duration of the disease.

The acute lesion consists of swelling and feathery vacuolation of hepatocytes, and marked hyperplasia of Kupffer cells that may show similar cytoplasmic changes. In these acute cases, the acicular crystals may be difficult to detect (Fig. 2-97A and B). *With more chronic intoxication, the most consistent histologic abnormality is the crystalline material in bile ducts* (see Fig. 2-97C). The crystals are fine, flat, and are deposited in affected ducts, and, less commonly, in hepatocytes themselves and in renal tubules. There may be associated bile ductular proliferation in severe cases, but often the degree of histologic hepatocellular damage is mild compared with the severity of the photosensitization. Cholestasis is not solely the result of mechanical obstruction by the crystals because photosensitization can occur in such outbreaks in animals whose livers have very little cholangitis and contain very few crystals. The severity of peribiliary fibrosis is more variable and probably depends on the relative contribution of sporidesmin to the intoxication. There is some hepatocellular degeneration and apoptosis, and there is uniform swelling of cytoplasm. Bile pigment accumulates in Kupffer cells and hepatocyte cytoplasm, but not to any marked extent in canaliculi. Focal necrosis of the gallbladder mucosa is often present. The severity of the hepatic lesion increases with the duration of exposure.

The biliary crystals from sheep with geeldikkop are composed principally of *calcium salts of steroidal sapogenins* present in *T. terrestris*. Plant saponins are metabolized in the rumen and liver to episapogenin glucuronides, which in the presence of calcium may precipitate, forming the characteristic biliary crystals. Cholestasis is likely related to reduce bile acid secretion into the lumen of the canaliculi, rather than biliary occlusion by these plant sapogenins. This explains the evidence of cholestasis before crystals can be seen histologically. Other unidentified plant components may also play a role in hepatocellular and biliary injury. It has also been suggested that the toxins responsible may act primarily on the membranes of the bile canaliculi, in a manner like that of *Lantana* poisoning. *Hepatocellular damage likely also plays a role in phytoporphyrin (phylloerythrin) retention.*

Switchgrass *(Panicum virgatum)*, Kleingrass *(P. coloratum)*, and other ***Panicum*** **sp.** are associated with *hepatogenous photosensitization* in grazing animals, including sheep, goats, and horses in the United States, Australia, and other areas of the world. The toxic agent(s) are *steroidal sapogenins*, and their type and concentration vary with the part of the plant (highest concentrations being in the young growing leaf) and with the environmental conditions. Hot and dry conditions have been associated with outbreaks. Younger animals appear to be more susceptible. Crystals may be produced in the biliary tree, hepatocytes, sinusoids, or Kupffer cells.

Crystal-associated cholangiohepatopathy is not specific for *Tribulus* or *Panicum* spp. intoxication. Similar changes occur in the hepatogenous photosensitivity disease, **alveld**, in sheep grazing pastures in Norway, the British Isles, and in the Faeroe Islands containing *Narthecium ossifragum*. Similar disease has been reported in ruminants intoxicated by *Agave lechuguilla*, *Nolina texana*, and the pasture species *Brachiaria decumbens* (signal grass) in Brazil. In New Zealand, crystal deposition in the biliary tree of cattle has been reported

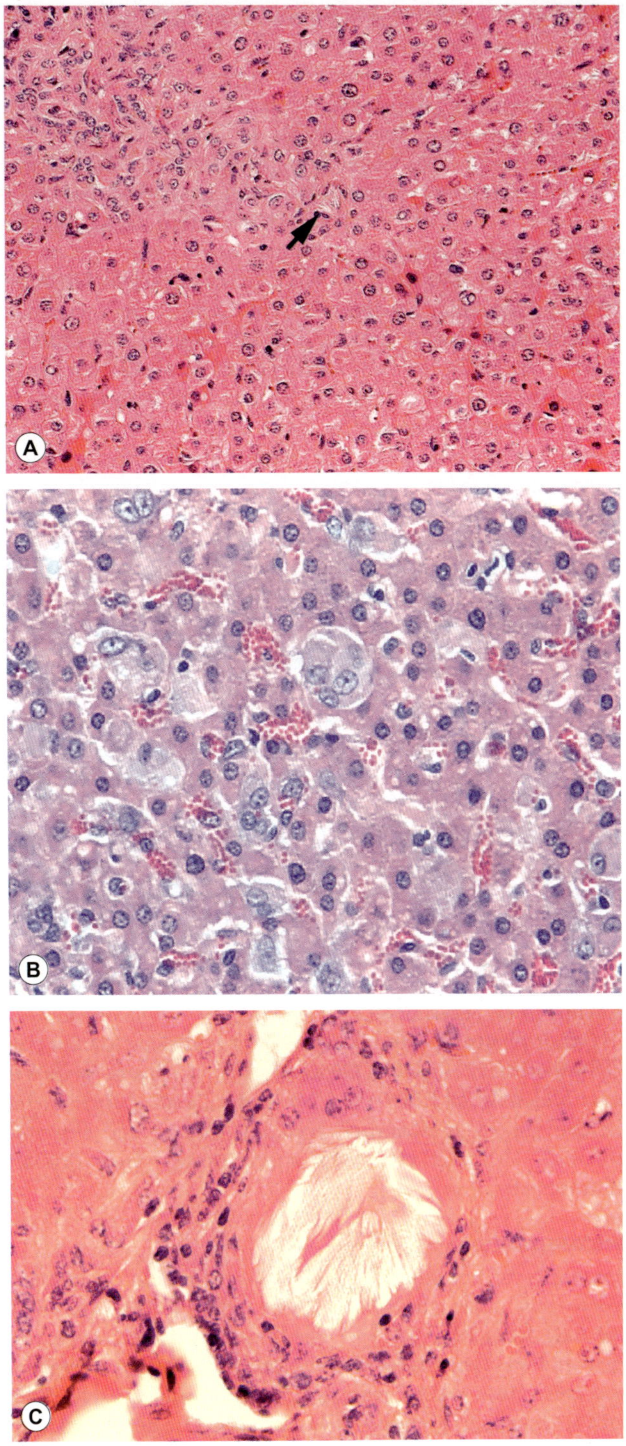

Figure 2-97 Crystal-associated cholangiohepatopathy. **A. Crystal deposition** (arrow) within bile duct epithelium in a goat grazing *Panicum* sp. **B. Foamy material within macrophages** in an ox ingesting *Brachiaria* sp. (Courtesy R. Kelly.) **C.** Fine crystalline material in **expanded Kupffer cells** in a goat grazing *Panicum* sp.

following ingestion of *Phytolacca octandra* (inkweed). The saponin-containing plants corn cockle (*Agrostemma githago*), cowcockle (*Vaccaria hispanica*), soapwort (*Saponaria* spp.), and broomweed (*Amphiachyris* spp.) are uncommon cause of poisonings in the United States. In those cases studied (*T. terrestris, Panicum dichotomiflorum, P. schinzii, N. ossifragum*), the characteristic crystalloid material deposited in the bile is principally composed of calcium salts of steroidal sapogenins. In some cases, crystal formation may not be apparent in bile ducts, and affected Kupffer cells and macrophages are more evident. There may be differences in the histologic responses of cattle and sheep grazing various sapogenin-containing plants. Foamy Kupffer cells and hepatocytes along with foamy macrophages in mesenteric and hepatic lymph nodes may be a more common response in cattle versus crystal formation within bile ducts in sheep. To complicate diagnostic efforts, foamy macrophages in the mesenteric and hepatic lymph nodes are also found in healthy cattle and sheep grazing *B. decumbens* in Brazil. Except for *N. texana*, steroidal sapogenins have been demonstrated in all these plants. As with *T. terrestris*, extracts of *B. decumbens* containing steroidal saponins produced typical lesions of cholangitis with crystal deposition when orally administered to lambs, with *P. chartarum* spore counts below detectable levels. Similarly, analysis of samples of *B. decumbens* and *P. dichotomiflorum* on which cattle and goats had recently been photosensitized showed only low levels of *P. chartarum* spores, and all isolates obtained failed to produce sporidesmin. Despite this, it is also apparent that neither *Tribulus* nor *Panicum* stands are always dangerous. Levels of saponins have been shown to vary greatly within a species from site to site, and with the age of the plant. Additionally, the role of sporadic environmental conditions, such as wilting, which might concentrate the saponins or other unidentified toxins, or the synergistic involvement of endophytic fungi, remains to be determined.

Other plants reported occasionally to produce unexpected photosensitivity include *Digitaria* spp., *Cooperia pedunculata*, *Nidorella foetida*, and *Chloris* spp., and such valuable pasture genera as *Medicago*, *Trifolium*, *Avena*, and *Biserrula pelecinus*, although the latter species may cause primary photosensitization.

Nitrosamines

Epizootics of poisoning by **dimethylnitrosamine** occurred in Norwegian cattle, sheep, and fur-bearing animals (i.e., **mink** and **fox**), from 1957 to 1962. The toxin was present in herring meal and was thought to be a *reaction product of trimethylamine and other lower amines with sodium nitrite*, added as a preservative, the reacting amines being products of decomposition. Animals consumed several pounds of the toxic meal each day before becoming ill. *This intoxication has little importance in livestock now that it is easily prevented*.

At postmortem, there was moderate anasarca and signs of hemorrhagic diathesis. Livers affected acutely were enlarged and firm, with mottled discoloration and sometimes a nutmeg appearance. In chronic intoxication, the liver was small, granular, and very firm. A few cases recovered after prolonged convalescence, and in these, there was atrophy and fibrosis of the left and caudate lobes, and the right lobe was hyperplastic and hemispheric. Histologically, in acute cases, there was widespread hemorrhagic centrilobular necrosis and an unusual degree of intimal and subendothelial reaction in sublobular and hepatic veins. The chronic lesion was dominated by extensive centrilobular fibrosis, with obliterative changes in many central and sublobular veins. Sporadic cases of portal hypertension in **Greyhound dogs** have been recognized in which hepatic veno-occlusive disease is the predominant lesion. In these cases, a history of feeding meat treated with substantial amounts of nitrites or sulfites to preserve the color of fresh meat is common, but a causal relationship has not been established.

The *hepatocellular changes are not specific* for dimethylnitrosamine or other hepatotoxic nitrosamines. Nitrosamines are metabolized in the liver and other tissues to reactive alkyl groups that bind covalently to various macromolecules, especially guanine in nucleic acids. Hepatotoxicity develops more slowly than in response to toxicants that induce membrane peroxidation, as many hepatocytes with DNA damage undergo apoptosis when stimulated to replicate. There is some megalocytosis, nuclear vesiculation and nucleolar prominence, cytoplasmic intranuclear inclusions, and variable fatty change and cytoplasmic bile accumulation. The typical effects of chronic experimental nitrosamine hepatotoxicity, such as hepatocellular fibrosis, nodules, and neoplasms, have not been evident in accidental poisonings. Dimethylnitrosamine-induced hepatotoxicosis in dogs has been proposed as a model of toxin-induced progressive hepatic disease in this species.

Indospicine

Legumes of the genus ***Indigofera*** have long been known to contain the toxic amino acid indospicine (6-amidino-2-hexanoic acid), which is a structural analogue of arginine, and which was shown in early experimental work to be hepatotoxic for rats and other species. The dose rates necessary to cause chronic liver injury in these species were, however, quite high, and field cases of intoxications were only seen in cattle grazing *Indigofera spicata*, which has the highest naturally occurring concentrations of indospicine. Indospicine has also caused toxicity in dogs following consumption of indospicine-contaminated meat. *Indigofera* plants are palatable legumes that are readily consumed by livestock; accumulation in the meat of cattle, camels, and horses has been documented. In Australia, a serious outbreak of fatal liver disease occurred in dogs that had been fed meat from horses that had been grazing *Indigofera linnaei*, a plant native to the arid zones of Australia that has been known to produce, in horses, a chronic neurologic disorder known as "Birdsville horse disease." The disease in horses is not associated with liver damage, although these animals do accumulate indospicine in most tissues, including the muscle. Dogs ingesting canned commercial camel meat have developed serious and sometimes fatal liver disease.

Dogs fed indospicine-contaminated meat for several weeks may develop *progressive liver damage*. Affected livers may be small, firm, and pale, or they may be nodular because of hypertrophy of surviving hepatocytes (eFig. 2-29A). Histologically, lesions begin as vacuolation of a narrow band of centrilobular hepatocytes, followed shortly by accumulation of mononuclear inflammatory cells in this zone and in the stoma of the hepatic venules (see eFig. 2-29B). Progression of the lesion is marked by scattered necrosis of a widening zone of centrilobular hepatocytes, disorganization, vacuolation because of fatty change, and accumulation of ceroid pigment in macrophages. Moderate centrilobular fibrosis is seen in later stages, as well as pronounced canalicular cholestasis. By this stage, affected animals begin to have icterus, inappetence, and depression. Bile ductular proliferation is not a marked feature. Death is attended by the usual signs of hepatoencephalopathy and tendency to bleed spontaneously. There is no evidence of direct neurologic damage as is seen in horses.

This intoxication is remarkable by virtue of its unpredictability. Experimental intoxication by pure indospicine has validly been shown to reproduce the naturally occurring intoxication caused by horsemeat feeding; however, liver failure can be produced by either means in only a small proportion of dogs so exposed. On the contrary, milder degrees of liver damage are reliably produced by both methods. Thus, it seems an idiosyncratic response is superimposed upon a more consistent effect of the toxin; the nature of the accompanying inflammatory response suggests that the former may be immunologically mediated. This has yet to be established, as has the proposal that the mechanism of the intoxication is the result of competitive inhibition of arginine.

Senna (Cassia) occidentalis

Ingestion of substantial amounts of seeds from *Senna (Cassia) occidentalis* in the family *Leguminosae* can produce acute hepatic necrosis in cattle, pigs, goats, and horses. Hepatic lesions range from vacuolation to scattered apoptosis and centrilobular necrosis. In all species, except for horses, significant cardiac and skeletal muscle injury and myoglobinuria are the predominant lesions, rather than hepatic injury. The toxic agent is not known currently.

Trifolium hybridum *(alsike clover)*

Two disorders result from alsike clover poisoning in herbivores. The first is primary photosensitization that occurs in cattle, sheep, swine, and horses. The second is hepatogenous photosensitization that is only reported in horses. *The toxic principle has not been isolated*, but it likely is in highest concentrations in the flowering stage used for hay. Although alsike clover is widespread in cultivation, *toxicity is rare*, which suggests that unknown contributing factors are involved. Toxicity usually occurs when alsike clover is a major component of pastures or hay, but some horses are believed to graze it selectively in a mixed pasture.

Clinical signs of poisoning initially include mild colic, ill-thrift, and anorexia, with increasing occurrence of signs of hepatotoxicity with cholestasis. In some, there can be icterus and photodynamic dermatitis. Exposure to the plant can occur for a year or more before signs of hepatic insufficiency develop, but cholestatic liver disease can be detected biochemically before horses become ill. More severely affected horses display neurologic disturbances, either excitement or mania in irregular episodes, or extended periods of extreme dullness, anorexia, apparent blindness, forced wandering, head pushing, and yawning. Clinical problems related to hypoproteinemia, such as coagulopathy or ascites, are not a feature of this disease, probably because most of the hepatocytes are not directly affected.

The lesions of alsike clover poisoning are those of *diffuse subacute-to-chronic ductular reaction (biliary hyperplasia) and fibrosis*, with the major lesions within and adjacent to all intrahepatic biliary tracts (Fig. 2-98). The liver may be enlarged, sometimes greatly so, or shrunken, pale, and tough or rubbery in consistency. The surface is smooth, but its appearance is mottled. The mottling is clear on the cut surface and is caused by bands of gray fibrous tissue, distinctly visible to the naked eye, surrounding and compressing each lobule. Near the margins of the liver and in some other areas, scar tissue may completely replace the parenchyma. Areas of parenchymal atrophy may occur upstream of some occluded ducts. Microscopically, there is pronounced proliferation of fibrous tissue in and around the portal tracts associated with hyperplasia of well-formed bile ducts (*ductular reaction*). Inflammation is rare and consists of mononuclear cells in portal tracts. In the initial stages, the proliferation of bile ducts is often greater than the proliferation of the fibrous tissue, but later the proportions are reversed. The proliferating tissue extends slowly to connect adjacent portal tracts, circumscribing areas that correspond to conventional lobules. The fibrous tissue does not permeate along the sinusoids, and there is gradual and uniform constriction of the parenchyma.

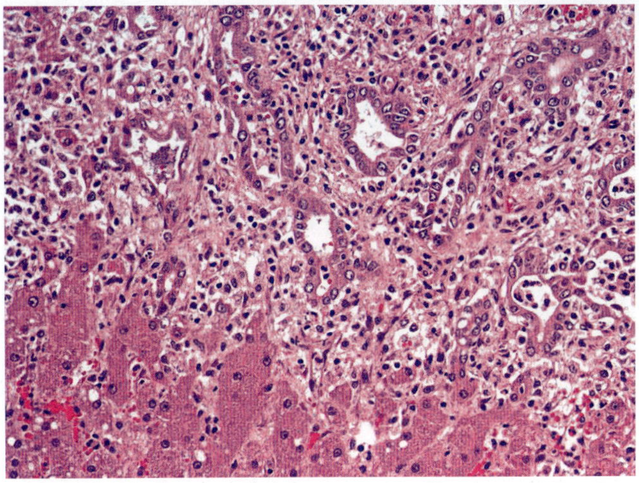

Figure 2-98 Chronic cholangiohepatitis caused by **alsike clover poisoning** in a horse.

The distribution of liver lesions suggests that the harmful factor in alsike clover is excreted into the bile in a form that damages the ducts. However, the biliary proliferation and fibrosis is like that observed in areas of the liver that are drained by chronically obstructed bile ducts, so it seems likely that some of the later changes are secondary to cholestasis. Agents that interfere with bile excretion have the potential to interfere with the elimination of various potentially injurious substances. Thus, it is possible that alsike clover ingestion might increase toxicity of other factors in the forage.

Tephrosia cinerea

Tephrosia cinerea is a member of the *Leguminosae* family and is found in Brazil. Prolonged ingestion causes chronic liver disease characterized clinically by wasting, and dramatic ascites in affected sheep. Hydrothorax and hydropericardium can also be present. Livers are pale with numerous ~1-mm nodules. The livers are firm, and the gallbladder is edematous. Histologically, there is portal fibrosis and ductular reaction that is typically more severe in the subcapsular region. Most hepatocytes are enlarged because of vacuolation. Scattered individual necrotic cells are present, and focally, there is evidence of bile stasis. Inflammation is modest.

Brassica rapa

Turnip *(Brassica rapa)* or other *Brassica* family forage ingestion by cattle on the North Island of New Zealand is incriminated as a cause of hepatogenous photosensitization and biliary injury. The injury can mimic sporidesmin toxicity clinically with elevated GGT and phytoporphyrin plasma levels. Histologically, bile ducts of smaller caliber than those injured by sporidesmin may be affected following turnip forage ingestion.

Copper

There is significant variation in species susceptibility to copper toxicosis. Sheep as a species are most prone to copper poisoning because of reduced biliary excretion of copper. Some sheep breeds are more susceptible than others, reflecting differences in the efficiency of intestinal absorption of copper, rather than differences in efficiency of biliary excretion. Altered biliary excretion of copper in sheep does not appear to be associated with alteration in the structure or expression of the gene for ATP7B, the copper transporting P-type ATPase that is defective in Wilson disease, the human autosomal recessive disorder of hepatic copper metabolism.

Excessive hepatic copper accumulation is important in chronic hepatitis in dogs and is discussed in further detail in the Chronic Hepatitis in Dogs section.

In cases of chronic hepatitis caused by copper accumulation, the liver is usually small, often with an accentuated lobular pattern; severely affected livers have architectural distortion, which ranges from a coarsely nodular texture to an end-stage liver. Depending on the duration of inflammation and injury, portal and periportal mononuclear cell inflammation and fibrosis of portal areas may extend into adjacent periportal areas of the lobule, leading to the prominent lobular pattern. *Small aggregates of pigmented macrophages*, containing copper and lipofuscin, surrounded by mononuclear inflammatory cells are a reliable feature of copper excess. With progression, hyperplastic nodules and bridging fibrosis develop.

In dogs and sheep, toxic amounts of copper can accumulate in the liver, although dietary copper levels are not excessive by standards for other species. Copper poisoning does occur in cattle, goats, and pigs, but in these species, it is because of abnormally high intake of the element. Acute copper poisoning can occur following either the ingestion or injection of excess copper, and *animals deficient in vitamin E or molybdenum appear especially susceptible to acute copper poisoning*.

Chronic copper toxicosis in sheep occurs because of 3 environmental factors acting alone or in concert. First, *excessive copper intake* may occur as a result of contamination of water (naturally occurring or through the use of copper piping or fixtures), pasture, or prepared feed; the latter is difficult to avoid when feed mills are preparing rations for different species and is probably partly responsible for the observation that housed sheep are more prone to copper poisoning than animals at pasture. Second, increased copper accumulation occurs because of increased availability of dietary copper; this happens when *dietary levels of molybdenum are unusually low*. Molybdenum, with sufficient sulfate, forms insoluble complexes with copper in the gut and liver, making the copper biologically inert. Subterranean clover growing on calcareous soils in southern Australia may be relatively deficient in molybdenum, and in these areas, British breeds of sheep are known to be more susceptible than Merinos to chronic copper poisoning. *Other hepatotoxins* constitute the third environmental factor that predisposes sheep to outbreaks of chronic copper poisoning. Examples include DHPAs (from *Heliotropium* or *Echium*) in eastern Australia, and phomopsin from lupins in western Australia and, possibly, South Africa.

The basis for chronic copper poisoning in sheep is the peculiar avidity of the liver for copper, coupled with the very limited rate at which sheep can excrete copper in the bile. After intraportal injection of a copper isotope, practically all of the radioactivity is removed during the first passage through the liver. Most of the copper is sequestered in hepatocellular lysosomes, where it does little damage at concentrations of up to 200-300 µg/g DW. As the concentration rises, there is presumably more interaction between other cell components and the copper. Lysosomal membranes may lose integrity and allow copper and lysosomal hydrolases to damage the rest of the cytoplasm. By the time the liver copper concentration has reached 300 µg/g or more, there is a histologically apparent increase in hepatocellular turnover, with single hepatocytes undergoing apoptosis within a dense knot of neutrophils. At still higher copper levels, the apoptotic rate increases, while all cells become swollen and their nuclei vesicular. The mitotic rate increases, presumably to keep pace with the accelerated loss of hepatocytes, and large macrophages appear in the sinusoids and stromal spaces about the vessels. These cells contain eosinophilic or somewhat brown, granular debris, which consists of *copper-containing lipofuscins*.

Sheep with liver copper concentrations >1,000 µg/g may be clinically and hematologically normal, as long as the increasing mitotic rate produces enough new hepatocytes to take up the copper released by dying cells. At this stage, however, activities of liver-specific enzymes will be elevated in the plasma. If the rate of hepatocellular loss exceeds the capacity of the liver to phagocytose and sequester cell debris quickly, the plasma copper levels can rise to levels that are high enough to damage circulating erythrocytes, and intravascular hemolysis ensues. *The effect of hemolysis and anemia on the liver is to accelerate the rate of hepatocellular necrosis; thus, copper enters the circulation at an increasing rate and acute copper toxic crisis is manifest*. The lethal clinical syndrome is then one of *paroxysmal intravascular hemolysis and liver failure*, in which a sheep may pass from apparent good health to death within ~6 hours. Stresses, such as brief starvation, may also precipitate the crisis in susceptible sheep, but the mechanisms involved are unknown. During the hemolytic crisis, some of the copper is lost from the disintegrating liver; some passes into the urine, and kidney copper concentration rises to 1,000 µg/g or more. *Blood or kidney copper levels* therefore give a truer indication of a prior hemolytic crisis caused by chronic copper poisoning than does elevation of liver copper alone.

The *gross lesions* of fatal chronic copper poisoning are those of acute copper toxicity. The carcass is discolored by marked icterus, superimposed on which is the red color imparted by free hemoglobin. Often, there is a brown hue as well because a proportion of the hemoglobin is oxidized to methemoglobin. The spleen is engorged, dark, and soft. The kidneys are deep red-brown to black and the urine deep-red, because of hemoglobinuria with oxidation to methemoglobin, and concurrent icterus (eFig. 2-30). The liver is often slightly soft and swollen, and deep orange, but if the condition arises after long-term liver injury, atrophy and fibrosis may be evident. The spectrum of liver lesions can be complicated by other causes of liver necrosis, including hypoxia caused by anemia, heart failure, and shock.

A breed of sheep from the Hebridean island of North Ronaldsay has apparently adapted to a seaweed diet low in both copper and molybdenum but rich in zinc. *Zinc is also capable of interfering with copper uptake*, and these sheep, although avoiding copper deficiency, are exquisitely susceptible to chronic copper poisoning when transferred to normal pasture. Hepatic disease associated with copper toxicity in this breed appears to differ morphologically from other domesticated sheep breeds. Experimentally, copper accumulation begins in centrilobular hepatocytes and progresses to panlobular. Scattered apoptosis and a few small aggregates of inflammatory cells scattered in hepatic lobules are observed after 4 months of copper supplementation. In chronic natural disease, panlobular copper accumulation, portal fibrosis progressing to panlobular pericellular fibrosis, admixed with a mild inflammatory infiltrate, and ductular proliferation are reported. North Ronaldsay sheep have been proposed as a possible animal model for human non-Wilsonian hepatic copper toxicosis and cirrhosis of infancy and for investigation of copper-associated hepatic fibrogenesis.

The events described in sheep also occur in **chronic copper poisoning in goats, pigs, and cattle**, and acute intravascular hemolysis may be seen, especially in calves. Usually, however, there is less of the acute terminal chain reaction in these species, and there is more evidence of chronic liver damage with extensive portal fibrosis and ductular reaction (biliary hyperplasia) within the portal tracts.

Acute copper poisoning *is most often seen in ruminants after accidental administration of single large doses of copper*, by either the oral or parenteral routes. Iatrogenic copper toxicosis has been induced by administering copper oxide boluses to neonatal calves, and by injection with copper disodium edetate in weanling calves. Doses of 20-100 mg/kg can produce acute poisoning in sheep. Copper toxicosis has also been reported in veal calves fed milk replacer supplemented with various copper-containing hematinics. Affected animals develop severe gastroenteritis, abdominal pain, diarrhea, and dehydration. The liver lesion varies with chronicity of exposure, from nonspecific acute centrilobular necrosis, to cholangiohepatitis with periportal fibrosis. Intravascular hemolysis may occur if plasma copper levels are sufficiently elevated.

Acute bovine liver disease

Acute bovine liver disease is a poorly understood entity that occurs sporadically in southern Australia. Outbreaks occur primarily in the spring and the autumn, and all ages of cattle can be affected. Sudden death or photosensitization may occur. There is an association with ingestion of *Cynosurus echinatus* (rough dog's tail). Gross lesions include serosal petechiae, gastrointestinal hemorrhage, and hepatomegaly with a pronounced hepatic reticular pattern. The characteristic histologic lesion involves periportal progressing to panlobular hepatocellular necrosis with ductular reaction. Necrosis is coagulative at first, and hydropic degeneration is frequent in remaining hepatocytes. Mycotoxin(s) produced by the fungus *Pyrenophora* (*Drechlera*) *biseptata* growing in some plants has been suggested to be the principal toxicant or cofactor in the syndrome.

HYPERPLASTIC AND NEOPLASTIC LESIONS OF THE LIVER, GALLBLADDER, AND BILE DUCTS

Remarkably, *the occurrence of fatal liver malignancies is rather uncommon in aged dogs and cats;* this suggests that they are either less exposed or they are more resistant to the etiologic agents responsible for liver neoplasia in humans. Dogs are not subject to significant chronic oncogenic viral infections, such as the hepatitis B and hepatitis C viruses that account for most human hepatocellular carcinomas. However, a hepadnavirus, related to human hepatitis B virus, termed domestic cat hepadnavirus, has been reported in cats. Chronic hepatitis and, possibly, hepatocellular carcinoma can develop in infected cats.

Ectopic, metaplastic, and hyperplastic lesions

Ectopic and metaplastic lesions in the gallbladder have been reported. Ectopic tissue includes hepatocyte nodules attached to or within the wall, and pancreatic islands, which may include islets of Langerhans. Gastric ectopia, readily distinguishable by the presence of chief and parietal cells, may form plaques or large polyps. Ectopia of gastric cardiac or pyloric mucosa is mimicked by metaplastic changes.

Nodular hyperplasia of hepatocytes is common in old dogs, but rare in other species. The lesions in dogs do not have a breed or sex predisposition, but their incidence increases sharply with age. Hyperplastic nodules typically develop in livers of normal mass; **regenerative nodules** arise because of compensatory hyperplasia of surviving hepatocytes in a background of hepatic injury, atrophy, and fibrosis (see the Responses of the Liver to Injury section).

Nodular hyperplasia often occurs as randomly distributed masses throughout the lobes. The grossly visible nodules are spherical, well circumscribed, varying in size from 2 mm to 3 cm or more, and may bulge from the capsular surface or be entirely hidden within the parenchyma (Fig. 2-99). They may be sharply distinct from the surrounding parenchyma because of color differences, either lighter than the surrounding liver because of increased lipid or glycogen content within hepatocytes comprising the nodule, or darker because of blood distending the sinusoids. Some nodules are the same color as the surrounding tissue and can only be identified by examination of a washed or blotted slice under a strong light.

The larger hyperplastic nodules grow expansively; they do not induce a fibrous capsule, but they can compress the surrounding parenchyma. The hepatocytes comprising nodular hyperplasia are often phenotypically different from those in adjacent parenchyma (Fig. 2-100). Old canine livers often have microscopic focal hyperplasia of similarly altered hepatocytes that can be distinguished from the surrounding parenchyma, but they evidently grow more slowly and do not compress their boundaries. These can be regarded as examples of the

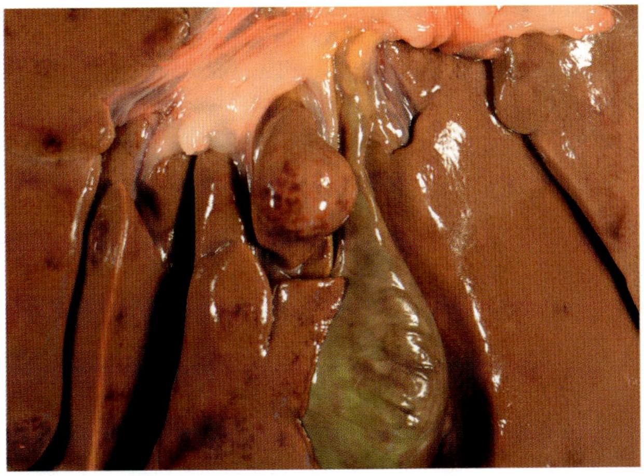

Figure 2-99 Nodular hyperplasia in the liver of a dog.

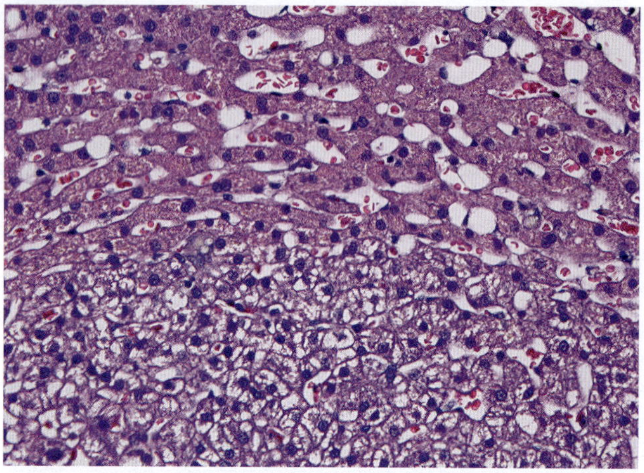

Figure 2-100 Nodular hyperplasia in the liver of a dog. These nodules have a discrete border with adjacent parenchyma and often are vacuolated.

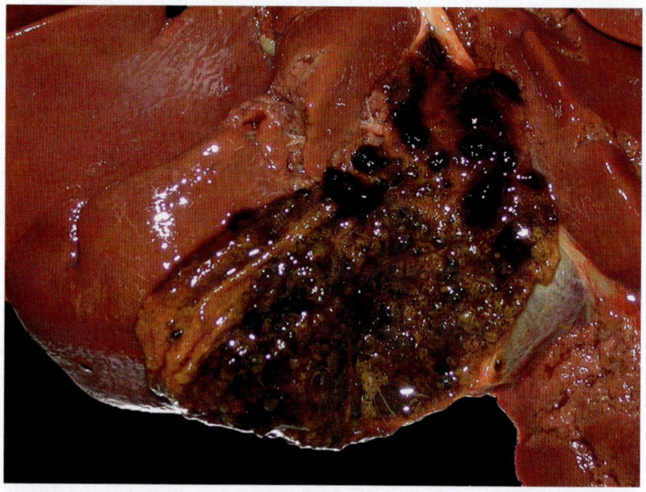

Figure 2-101 Cystic mucinous hyperplasia of the mucosa of the gallbladder in a dog.

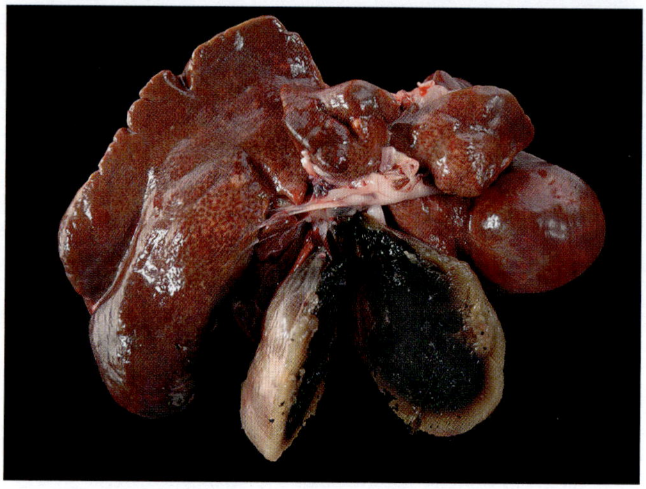

Figure 2-102 Gallbladder mucocele in a dog.

numerous atypical focal hyperplasias that arise as altered foci, nodules, plaques, or polyps in various tissues of old dogs. Mitotic figures are rare. Foci of extramedullary hematopoiesis are occasionally seen. Necrosis and hemorrhage in hyperplastic nodules are rare. *The significance of hyperplastic nodules in old dogs is usually negligible.*

Although hyperplastic nodules rarely progress to lesions with detrimental impact, they are often found during liver imaging, laparotomy, or biopsy and need to be differentiated from other focal lesions of more significance. Because they are atypically differentiated, they are the potential source of secreted products of clinical or diagnostic significance, but their potential in this regard is unexplored. *The hallmark of nodular hyperplasia, in contrast to the hepatic adenoma and hepatocellular carcinoma, is that it largely retains normal liver architecture, including a modified lobular structure with recognizable central veins and portal tracts.* However, this feature may be difficult to appreciate in small biopsies.

Regenerative nodules arise in a background of liver injury. They are typically multiple and often confluent. Histologically, the nodules typically lack portal tracts and mild pleomorphism is possible. The biologic distinction between atypical hyperplasia and neoplasia is sometimes equivocal. In small biopsy samples, it is challenging to separate regenerative nodules from hepatocellular adenomas.

Cystic mucinous hyperplasia *of the mucus-producing glands in the mucosa of the gallbladder* has been reported as an incidental lesion in dogs and sheep. The entire mucosa may be affected or nodular lesions may occur. These cystic hyperplastic nodules are often numerous, may be sessile or polypoid, and contain mucin (Fig. 2-101).

Gallbladder mucocele is recognized frequently in dogs; the gallbladder is dilated with accumulated mucoid secretion and mucosal hyperplasia. Histologically, fronds of epithelium extend into the clefts in the mucus, and mucus-filled cysts form. The gallbladder content is abnormally adherent laminated accumulations of pale basophilic mucus. Gallbladder infarction leading to ischemic necrosis and rupture can occur along with mucocele formation or independently (Fig. 2-102). Bile-laden mucus may also extend into the cystic, hepatic, and common bile ducts, resulting in variable degrees of extrahepatic biliary obstruction. The etiology of this condition is unknown, but metabolic abnormalities such as hyperadrenocorticism and hypothyroidism carry an increased risk.

There are also breed associations, with Cocker Spaniels, Shetland Sheepdogs, Chihuahuas, Border Terriers, and Miniature Schnauzers affected more often than other breeds, although any dog can be affected. Treatment with imidacloprid is also associated with an increased risk of gallbladder mucocele.

Mucosal hyperplasia in the large bile ducts is frequently observed in the long-standing mild cholangiohepatitis of fluke infection. The hyperplasia is of microscopic dimensions, but in some instances, it appears histologically to be atypical. Localized, polypoid foci of cystic hyperplasia are specific changes in cattle poisoned by highly chlorinated naphthalene.

Hepatocellular tumors

Primary epithelial neoplasms of the liver include tumors of hepatocellular, cholangiocellular, or neuroendocrine origin, and they are uncommon in most species, representing <1% of all neoplasms in cats and dogs. Pot-bellied pigs are a possible exception. *Proportionately, hepatocellular neoplasms are more common in dogs; cholangiocellular tumors predominate in cats in most studies.* Unlike the situation in humans, there are no clear associations in domestic animals between hepatocellular tumors, chemical carcinogens, mycotoxins, or drugs, such as synthetic steroids. There are no known virally induced hepatocellular neoplasms in most domestic species except in cats in which liver tumor development may be associated with infection with domestic cat hepadnavirus. *Hepatobiliary tumors in domestic animals are not obvious successors to recognized antecedent liver diseases*.

Histologic criteria have been established to diagnose hepatocellular tumors as either malignant or benign. However, there is not a great deal of clinical significance to this histologic distinction. In most species, morbidity or mortality is very uncommon because of metastatic disease. Morbidity or mortality arises most often from necrosis, and subsequent hemorrhage into the peritoneal cavity and hemoabdomen is reported to be roughly equal for diagnosed hepatocellular adenomas or hepatocellular carcinomas. Consequently, *the use of the general term hepatocellular tumor may be more appropriate* until studies with a robust number of cases can confirm the biologic behavior of neoplastic hepatocytes.

Hepatocellular adenomas, which are benign neoplasms of hepatocytes, are reported in dogs, cats, cattle, sheep, and pigs, but likely occur in all species. They are rarely of any clinical significance of themselves, but intratumoral necrosis can lead to increased morbidity or mortality if hemorrhage develops. Hepatocellular adenomas are typically solitary, but they can be multiple. They range from 2 to 12 cm in diameter and are roughly spherical masses. Typically, they are well demarcated from the adjacent parenchyma because of the compression caused by their expanding growth, but are not typically encapsulated. Hepatocellular adenomas often bulge from the capsular surface, or they can be pedunculated; in some instances, they may be found entirely within the hepatic parenchyma. The color of hepatocellular adenomas varies from yellow-brown to dark mahogany-red. Paler adenomas contain lipid or glycogen, and these lesions are often softer and more friable than normal liver (Fig. 2-103).

Histologically, the hepatocytes in hepatic adenomas may exhibit mild pleomorphism, do generally not differ markedly from normal hepatocytes or those in hyperplastic nodules, and often contain lipid, glycogen, or occasionally protein secretory vacuoles. Minimal anisocytosis and increased basophilia of the cytoplasm and prominence of nucleoli can be seen, but mitotic figures are uncommon. *Cells are arranged in cords or trabeculae that may be several cells thick, but the width tends to be consistent. There is a discrete well-defined border with adjacent parenchyma* (Fig. 2-104). *Adenomas lack normal lobular architecture*. Essentially, all the blood supplying adenomas come from the hepatic artery. Consequently, rather than portal tracts, isolated and various combinations of arteries, bile ducts, and hepatic veins can be found coursing through the mass. *Usually, no more than a single portal tract may be present, likely entrapped by the expanding hepatocyte population*. Extramedullary hematopoietic foci may sometimes be found in the adenomas, as well as ectatic vascular spaces. Focal necrosis and hemorrhage may occur.

Hepatocellular carcinomas are uncommon but occur in all veterinary species; they may be single and massive, nodular or diffuse. Several gross and histologic features suggest a malignant nature, including lack of pedunculation and lack of clear demarcation from the adjacent parenchyma. Because extrahepatic metastasis is quite uncommon, with one exception in dogs discussed below, the histologic appearance of hepatocellular tumors has little predictive value regarding biologic behaviors and *it may be preferable to use term hepatocellular tumor*. Varied coloration of the cut surface produced by hemorrhage and necrosis may be present in tumors diagnosed as benign or malignant (eFig. 2-31). *Venous invasion is typical of hepatocellular tumors*, and intravascular spread may extend to hepatic veins and vena cava leading to intrahepatic metastases. Hepatocellular carcinomas occasionally penetrate the capsule to implant on the peritoneum. *Metastasis is uncommon in all domestic species* but, when present, may be most common in the hepatic lymph node in dogs. Hematogenous metastases occur first in the lungs. Spontaneous rupture of any hepatocellular tumor may cause fatal blood loss, is the probable cause of morbidity and mortality in affected patients, and is a much more frequent cause of morbidity and mortality than metastatic disease.

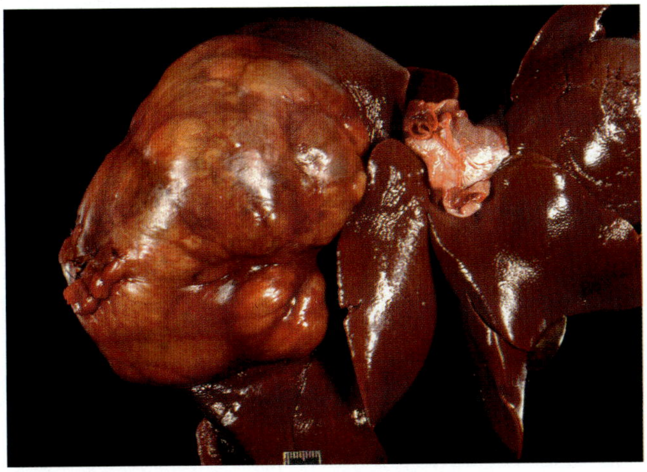

Figure 2-103 **Hepatocellular adenoma** in a dog.

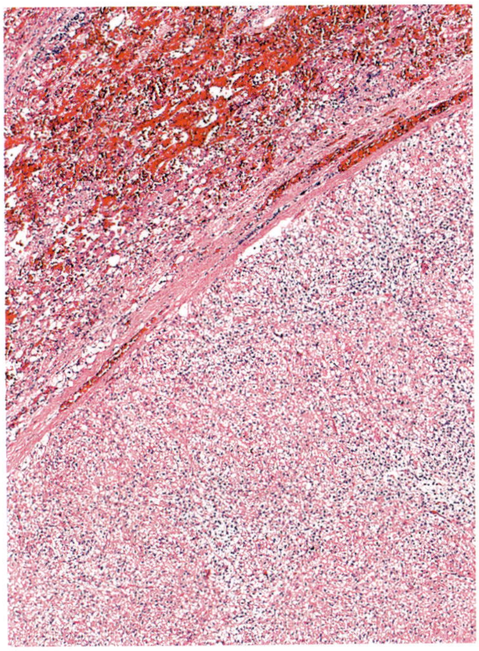

Figure 2-104 Histologic appearance of a canine **hepatocellular adenoma**. Compression of the adjacent parenchyma is apparent, and a capsule is evident at this site.

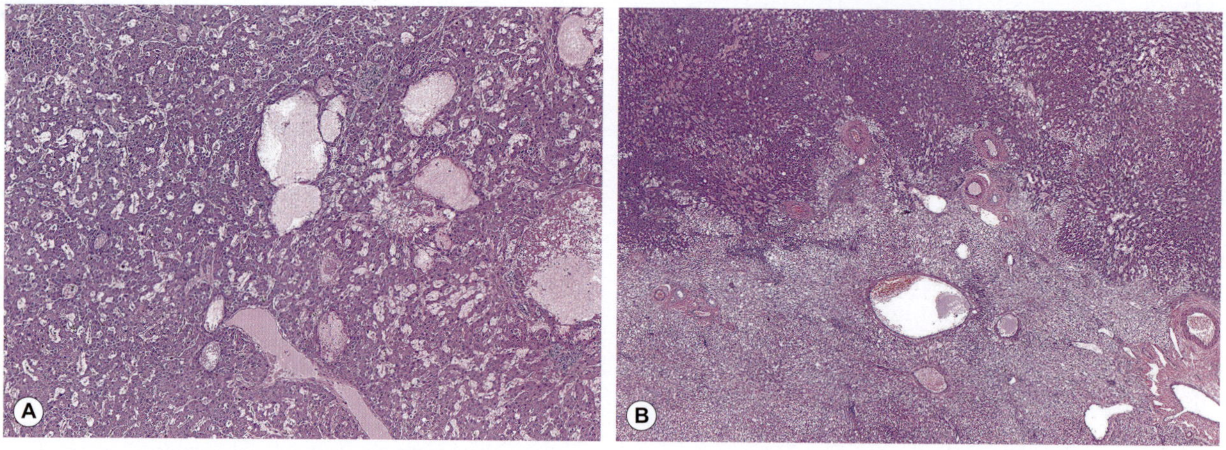

Figure 2-105 A. **Hepatocellular carcinoma** from a dog. B. Invasion at the margin of a hepatocellular carcinoma in the liver of a dog.

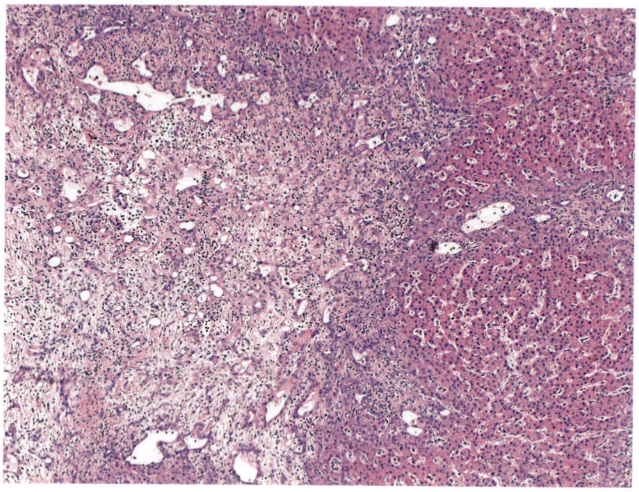

Figure 2-106 The **scirrhous variant of hepatocellular tumor** has areas of ductular proliferation and abundant connective tissue within areas of neoplastic hepatocytes. (Courtesy P. Pesavento.)

Hepatocellular carcinomas may be quite variable in histologic appearance, and various patterns may occur within a single neoplasm. ***Trabecular carcinomas** are the most common histologic pattern.* Neoplastic cells resemble normal liver and grow in irregularly thick plates or trabeculae that vary from few to many cells thick. Necrosis may be present, sinusoids may be dilated, and there may be large ectatic blood-filled spaces. Other patterns include ***pseudoglandular (adenoid) carcinomas***, characterized by tumor with frequent acini formation, and ***solid carcinomas***, characterized by solid sheets of poorly differentiated, often pleomorphic cells that do not form sinusoids (Fig. 2-105A and B). A **scirrhous variant**, which may be benign, has been described in dogs, characterized by multiple foci of CK19-positive ductular structures embedded in abundant fibrous stroma (Fig. 2-106). Giant cells are a feature of some hepatocellular tumors and are quite conspicuous by virtue of a large nucleus, multilobed nuclei, or multiple nuclei. Mitotic figures are more frequent in carcinomas than adenomas but may not be a prominent feature of well-differentiated carcinomas. Immunohistochemical staining using antibodies that bind a hepatocyte-specific antigen, HepPar1, identifies a large proportion of canine and all feline hepatocellular carcinomas. Some gastrointestinal tumors may also express HepPar1 complicating the identification of some metastatic lesions. Some canine hepatocellular carcinomas may not stain with HepPar1, but instead >5% of the cells can be stained with antibodies that recognize CK19, a marker of HPCs, immature hepatocytes, and biliary epithelial cells supporting less differentiated neoplastic cells and possibly a more aggressive behavior. These canine hepatocellular carcinomas have an aggressive growth pattern, including an increased incidence of intrahepatic and extrahepatic metastasis.

Some hepatocellular carcinomas in cattle are scirrhous, hard, and white. Paraneoplastic hypoglycemia may occur in animals with hepatocellular carcinoma.

Hepatoblastomas, rare benign tumors putatively originating from primitive hepatic precursor cells, have been reported most often in young horses, but also in sheep, dogs, cats, and a llama. Hepatoblastomas in humans are neoplasms of infancy and childhood. Cases in domestic species have been reported in both young and adult animals but are most often reported in *foals*. Hepatoblastomas are typically single, firm, lobulated masses with areas of necrosis and hemorrhage. Compression of adjacent parenchyma is evident, and, on occasion, invasion can be seen. The histologic patterns of hepatoblastomas can be epithelial, either fetal or embryonal, or mixed epithelial and mesenchymal. **Fetal hepatoblastomas** are composed of large, polygonal cells, approximately the size of adult hepatocytes, with round-to-oval nuclei and granular-to-vacuolated, eosinophilic-to-amphophilic cytoplasm (Fig. 2-107A). **Embryonal hepatoblastomas** form ribbons or rosettes of smaller basophilic cells with scant cytoplasm (see Fig. 2-107B). **Mixed epithelial-mesenchymal hepatoblastomas** contain variable amounts of fibrous connective tissue or other mesenchymal tissues, including cartilage or bone, in addition to epithelial cells. Combinations of these patterns are common. Portal tracts are absent. Immunohistochemical staining for α-fetoprotein is typically positive, and HepPar-1 staining is usually absent, supporting the view that they arise from precursor cells.

Cholangiocellular tumors

Cholangiocellular adenomas are rare benign neoplasms of biliary epithelium that are usually solitary, pale-gray to white, and well-circumscribed roughly spherical masses that tend to grow by expansion. They may distend the normal outline of the liver, although they can occur as intrahepatic masses.

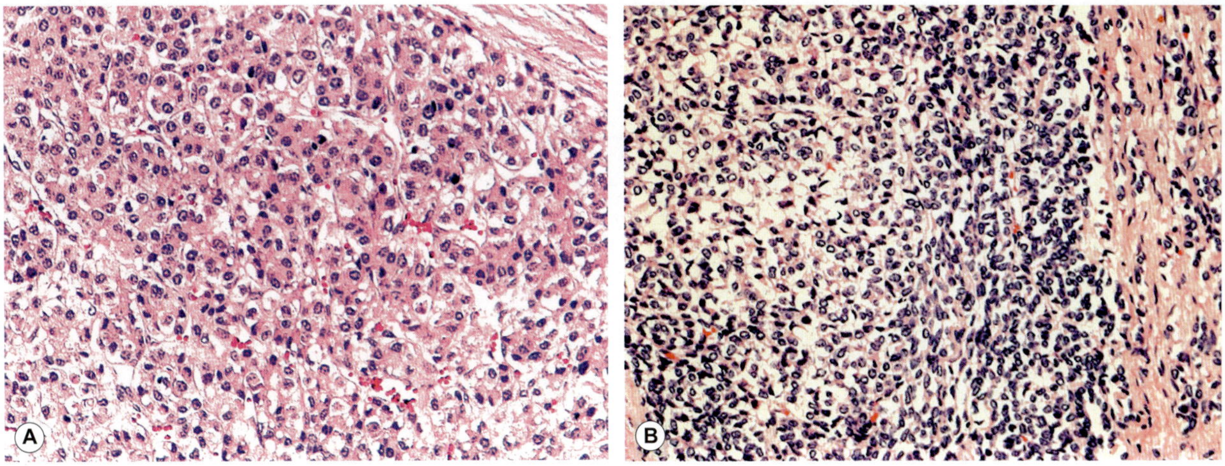

Figure 2-107 **Hepatoblastoma. A.** A **fetal pattern** from a foal. **B.** An **embryonal pattern** from a foal.

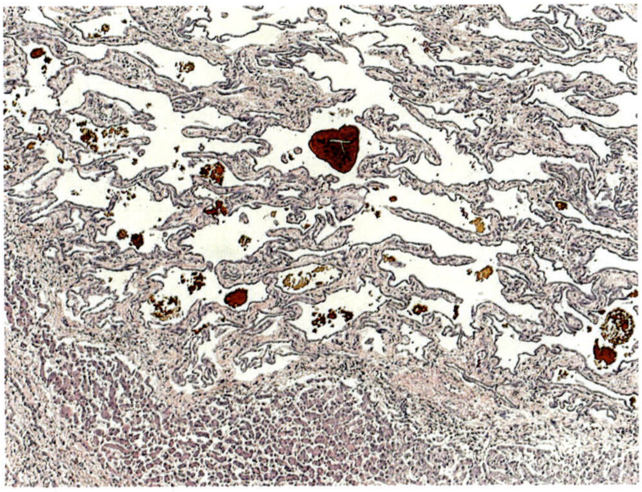

Figure 2-108 **Biliary adenoma** with uniform array of well-differentiated biliary epithelium forming uniform small tubules.

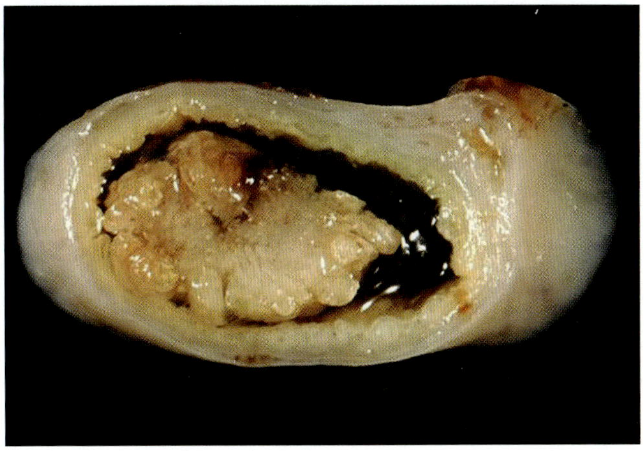

Figure 2-109 **Gallbladder adenoma** in a dog. (Courtesy J. Tobias.)

Cholangiocellular adenomas are composed of *tubules lined with a single layer of well-differentiated biliary epithelium and a moderate amount of intervening stroma*. The tubules may have narrow lumens, and there can be variable amounts of stroma within the mass (Fig. 2-108). Adjacent hepatocytes are usually compressed at the margins but are not found between tubules. The tubules contain clear watery-to-viscous fluid. Cuboidal or flattened neoplastic biliary epithelial cells have a moderate amount of pale eosinophilic cytoplasm. Nuclei are round-to-oval, vesicular, and oriented centrally. Nucleoli are small or inapparent. There are typically no mitotic figures.

Extrahepatic cholangiocellular adenomas are rare, except for gallbladder adenomas reported in abattoir surveys of cattle and rarely in domestic carnivores (Fig. 2-109). The smaller specimens may be solid on cut surface and white, but the large specimens, and many of the small ones, are cystic.

Lesions termed **biliary cystadenomas**, a subtype commonly seen in cats and occasionally in dogs, are most likely developmental anomalies of the embryonal biliary tree, termed **ductal plate anomalies;** however, there are no definitive criteria to distinguish the 2 lesions. The origin via ductal plate malformation is more clearly appreciated when biliary cysts are coincident with cystic renal developmental lesions, although either lesion may occur independently. The ductal plate anomalies can be multilocular and lined by bile duct epithelia that may be flattened by pressure or in some areas papillary. Entrapped hepatocytes are common and support ductal plate anomaly versus a biliary adenoma. The septal stroma is collagenous. Their recognition later in life may be the result of progressive secretion by the lining epithelial cells, creating cysts only when sufficient fluid has been produced.

Cholangiocarcinomas (cholangiocellular carcinomas) are reported in dogs, cats, sheep, cattle, horses, and goats. Affected livers are usually otherwise normal, with no suggestion as to an underlying cause, although there are associations with chronic fluke infections in humans and rarely in carnivores.

Cholangiocellular tumors can usually be distinguished from the hepatocellular variety by their multiplicity, firmness, pale-beige color produced by abundant stroma, and the typical umbilicate appearance of those that involve the capsule (Fig. 2-110). The central depressed area can be the result of necrosis or cavitation-associated collapse of tumor vessels in the central parts of the tumor nodules. Even several nodules may not cause much enlargement of the liver. In dogs and cats, the tumors are almost always multiple or diffuse. The several nodules of tumor might represent intrahepatic lymphogenous metastases, but the possibility of multicentric origin must be entertained. Hematogenous metastases are unusual, but metastases to the regional nodes are common. In cats especially, there is a tendency to invade the hepatic capsule and implant on the

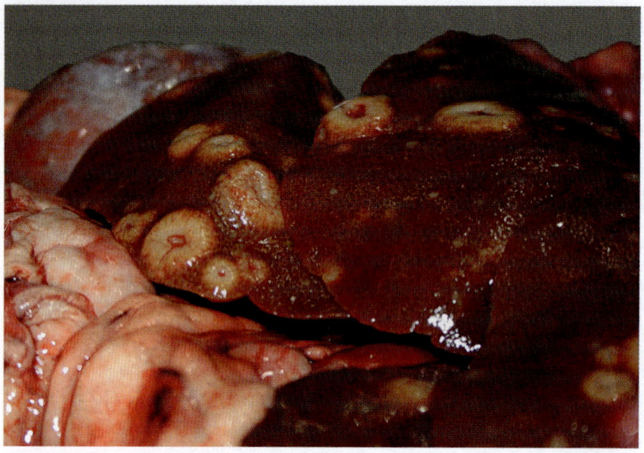

Figure 2-110 **Cholangiocarcinoma** in the liver of a dog; **umbilication** is prominent. (Courtesy J.L. Caswell.)

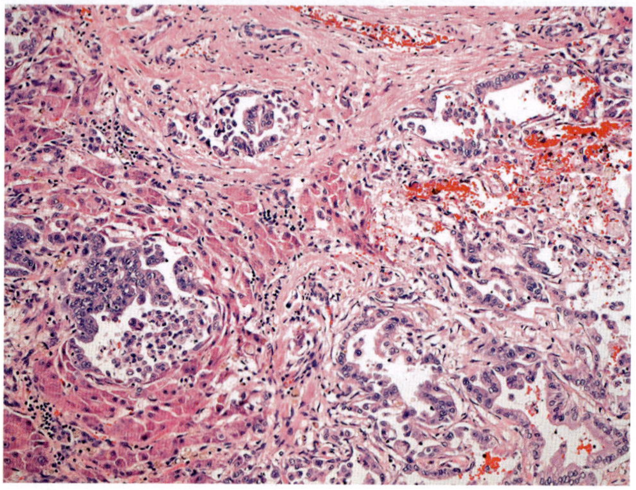

Figure 2-111 **Cholangiocarcinoma** from a cat with characteristic crude acini and tubules separated by abundant connective tissue.

peritoneum; the diffuse variety may cause great enlargement, although with retention of shape.

Microscopically, *cholangiocellular carcinomas form ductules and acini*, and sometimes papillary formations within the lumen of the neoplastic ducts (Fig. 2-111). The cells are cuboidal or columnar, with a small amount of clear or slightly granular cytoplasm. The nuclei are small and uniform, and nucleoli are not prominent. Mitotic figures are often abundant. The tubules do not contain bile, but in well-differentiated specimens they may contain mucins. The epithelial components are separated by fibrous connective tissue stroma, which may have pronounced collagen deposition, the so-called *scirrhous response* that gives the tumor a firm texture. In poorly differentiated cholangiocarcinomas, pleomorphic-to-anaplastic cells can be seen. It is not uncommon to encounter areas of poorly differentiated cells within a mass that is predominantly well differentiated. Foci of necrosis are common. *Cholangiocellular carcinomas have a highly invasive growth pattern*, and often metastasize to hepatic lymph nodes, lungs, and the peritoneal cavity.

Primary intrahepatic cholangiocellular carcinoma can be difficult, and often impossible, to distinguish from metastatic

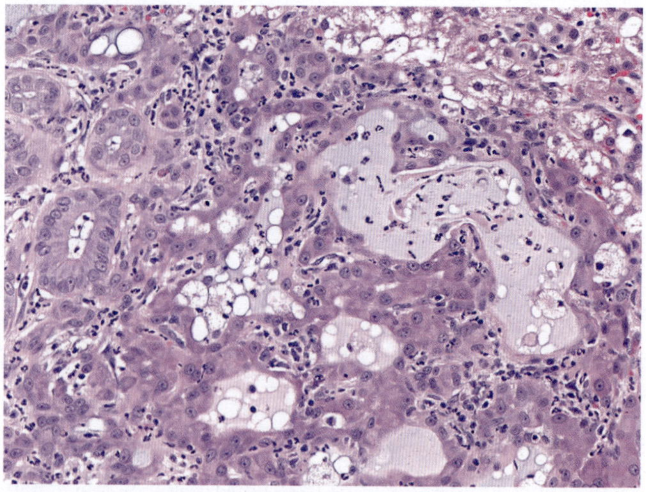

Figure 2-112 **Mixed hepatocellular and biliary carcinoma;** neoplastic cell populations have both biliary and hepatocellular phenotypes. H&E.

adenocarcinomas, especially those of pancreatic or mammary epithelial origin. Mucus secretion and intrasinusoidal permeation are more typical of biliary origin. Distinction from hepatocellular carcinoma of adenoid pattern may be assisted by demonstration of mucin, abundant mitotic figures, and a prominent connective tissue stroma, and immunohistochemically by diffuse staining with antibodies that recognize CK7 and CK19, as well as claudin-7.

Extrahepatic cholangiocellular carcinoma (or biliary cholangiocarcinoma) of the gallbladder or extrahepatic bile ducts is much less frequent than the intrahepatic form but has been reported in dogs, cats, cattle, and swine.

Mixed hepatocellular and cholangiocellular carcinomas

Rare hepatic carcinomas have the histologic and cytologic characteristics of both hepatocellular carcinoma and cholangiocellular carcinoma. These tumors likely arise from bipotential HPCs. The hepatocytic nature of some tumor cells can be confirmed with the monoclonal antibody HepPar-1, and cells of biliary phenotype can be stained by immunohistochemistry using antibodies that bind to CK7, a typical intermediate filament of biliary epithelium (Fig. 2-112).

Hepatic neuroendocrine carcinoma (carcinoid)

Hepatic carcinoids, presumably arising from the diffuse neuroendocrine cell population found among the biliary epithelium and possibly within the hepatic parenchyma, have been reported in dogs, cats, and cattle. They may arise within the liver, in the extrahepatic bile ducts, or within the gallbladder. The gross appearance of carcinoids is typically that of disseminated pale-gray to tan small masses within the liver, but on some occasions, only a single mass is formed (eFig. 2-32). Like other neuroendocrine tumors, *hepatic carcinoids typically form nests of cells separated by a fine fibrovascular stroma*. The cells are oval-to-fusiform and may form a rosette or pseudolobular pattern (Fig. 2-113). Mitotic figures are usually frequent. Argyrophilic cytoplasmic granules may be detected by silver impregnation stains; more precise identification of carcinoids may require immunohistochemical stains for neurosecretory products, such as neuron-specific

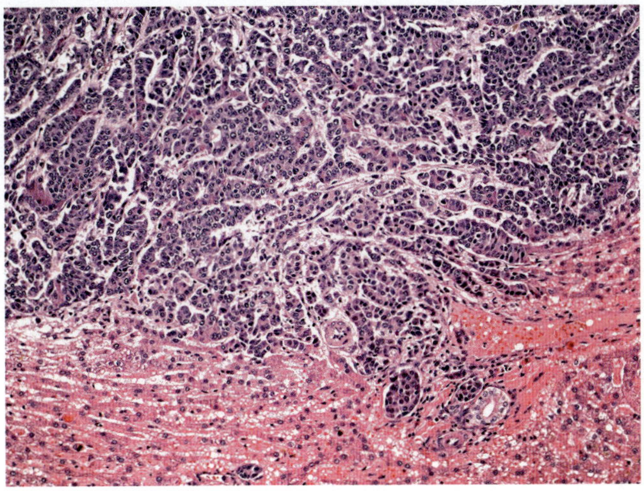

Figure 2-113 **Hepatic carcinoid** from a cat with characteristic islands and rosettes separated by fine fibrovascular stroma and with invasive behavior.

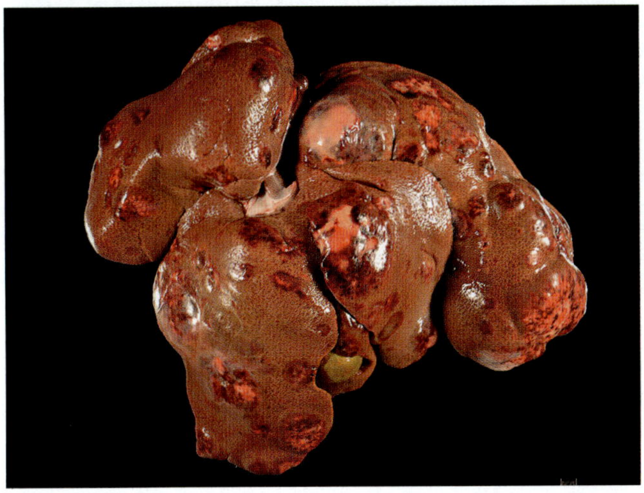

Figure 2-114 Hepatic **hemangiosarcoma** in a dog. Careful examination is required to distinguish primary from metastatic disease.

enolase or serotonin. These are aggressive neoplasms, with frequent intrahepatic spread, and metastasis to local lymph nodes, peritoneum, and lung. A thorough review of the entire body is necessary to confirm the identity of a primary carcinoid versus a metastatic lesion.

Mesodermal tumors

Primary mesenchymal tumors of the liver are quite uncommon. Of the mesenchymal tumors, primary **hemangiosarcomas** are likely the most frequent. Primary hepatic hemangiosarcomas occur in dogs, cats, cattle, and sheep. Hemangiosarcoma of the liver should always be considered metastatic until proven otherwise by diligent search. Some of these tumors are solitary, large, and gray-white, with scattered hemorrhagic areas; others are ill defined and cavernous (Fig. 2-114). The latter may rupture into the peritoneal cavity to produce severe hemorrhage. Microscopically, hepatic hemangiosarcomas resemble those found in other sites; however, it may be impossible to find malignant cells in or lining cavernous areas. At the margins of the tumor, there is a distinctive pattern or growth in which

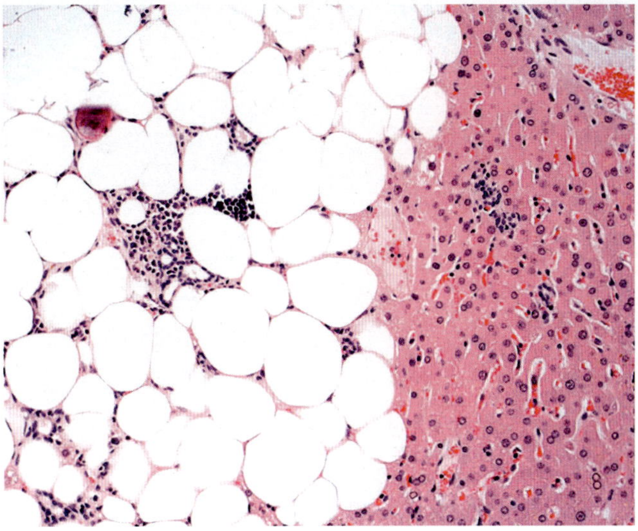

Figure 2-115 **Myelolipoma** of the liver of a dog.

small, solid nodules of malignant cells may be found, or these cells can be found forming capillary structures or invading along pre-existing sinusoids. The latter phenomenon is particularly characteristic. As the cells invade along the sinusoids, perhaps in single file, they initially produce little distortion of the hepatic cords. Behind them, the sinusoids are spread widely apart, and individual hepatocytes or portions of cords are isolated and appear to be floating freely, surrounded by a thin layer of connective tissue and neoplastic cells. Differential diagnoses other than metastatic lesions include the syndrome of telangiectasia in Pembroke Welsh Corgi dogs, telangiectatic lesions in older animals, and vascular hamartomas in cattle.

Hepatic **hemangiomas** have been reported in dogs and a pig.

Leiomyomas and **fibromas** are occasionally observed in the gallbladder of dogs and cattle. **Leiomyosarcomas** and **fibrosarcomas** have been reported in the liver of cats and dogs, *hemangiopericytoma* and *fibrosarcoma* in cattle, and a sole case of *botryoid embryonal rhabdomyosarcoma* in a cat. Other rare mesenchymal tumors reported in either dogs or cats include lymphangioma, plasmacytoma, osteosarcoma, nerve sheath tumor, liposarcoma, and chondrosarcoma.

The **myelolipoma** is an unusual tumor that develops most often in the livers of domestic cats and wild felids. The tumor develops as various growths, 0.5-5 cm diameter, in one or more lobes; if they project above the surface of the liver, they are irregularly nodular. Myelolipomas are friable, and yellow-to-orange because of their high fat content. The neoplasm is composed of normal-appearing, mature adipocytes with a variable admixture of myeloid cells, including both mature and immature cells of the granulocytic, erythrocytic, and megakaryocytic series (Fig. 2-115). In captive wild cats, similar lesions have been seen in the spleen. These were judged to be separate developments of the same process. Metastasis to other organs has not been reported.

Metastatic neoplasms

The liver is particularly "fertile soil"; *metastatic lesions markedly outnumber primary hepatic neoplasms.* Metastatic solid neoplasms may be multiple but are usually not numerous and usually do not elicit clinical or biochemical evidence of hepatic injury or dysfunction. Malignancies arriving via the portal vein, such as pancreatic or gastric carcinoma or hemangiosarcomas,

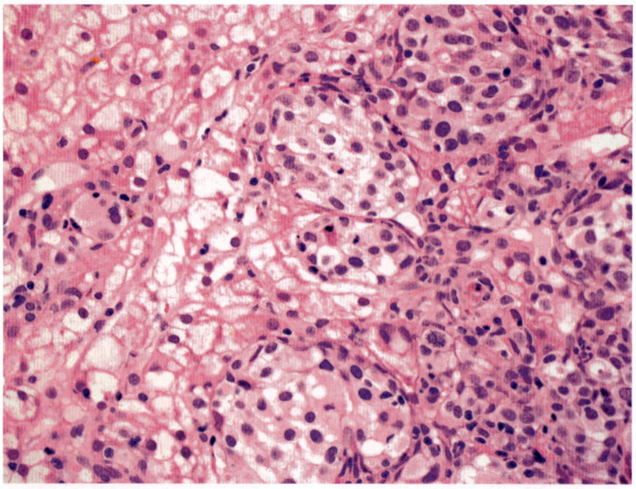

Figure 2-116 Histiocytic sarcoma in the liver of a dog.

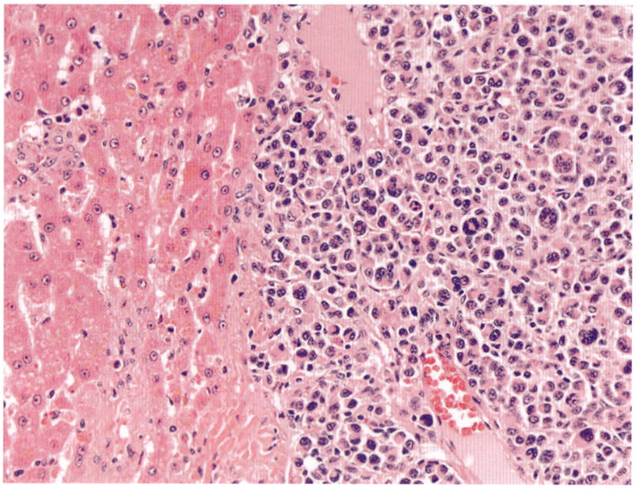

Figure 2-117 Primary hepatic plasmacytoma in the liver of a dog.

may practically replace the liver before producing clinical signs, one of which may be icterus caused either by extrahepatic bile duct obstruction, or by intrahepatic cholestasis, or both. In dogs, the most common metastatic hematopoietic, mesenchymal, and epithelial neoplasms are **lymphoma, hemangiosarcoma,** and **pancreatic carcinoma**, respectively. Some of the carcinomas (e.g., thyroid, mammary), melanoma, and sarcomas from more remote sites also metastasize to the liver via the lungs and hepatic artery, and some (e.g., ovarian carcinoma, mesothelioma) implant on the capsular surface from within the peritoneal cavity. Identification of metastatic lesions from carcinomas of the GI tract may be complicated by the fact that some of these tumors are stained by antibodies to HepaPar1, which are usually associated with hepatocytes.

The hepatic perisinusoidal and periportal compartments are hospitable to various hematopoietic neoplastic cell types. Accordingly, malignant histiocytosis, myeloid and erythroid leukemias, and mast cell tumors often localize in the liver along hepatic sinusoids. Some lymphomas, histiocytic sarcomas (Fig. 2-116), plasmacytomas (Fig. 2-117), and mast cell tumors also produce solid sarcoma masses in the liver as

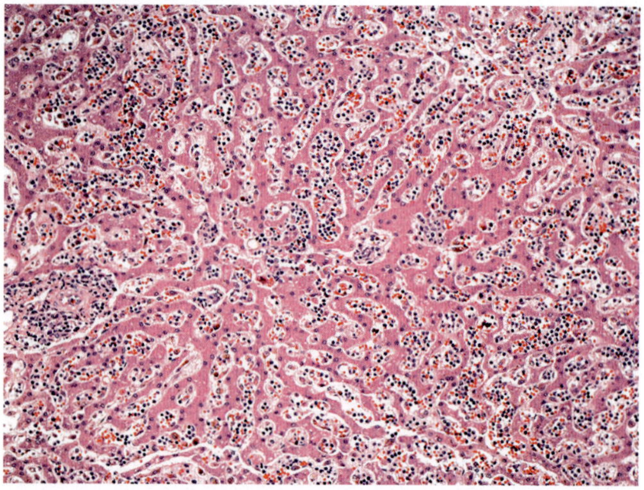

Figure 2-118 Monomyelocytic leukemia in a dog, with typical array of tumor cells along hepatic sinusoids.

primary or metastatic lesions. ***Lymphoma** in the liver is common*, especially when the spleen is involved, and occasionally, the liver appears to be the major or primary site affected. Typically, lymphoma is most apparent in the portal tracts, and the connective tissue surrounding the central veins can also be infiltrated, but late in the course of disease, the sinusoids are affected (eFig. 2-33). There are occasional exceptions to this pattern. Hepatosplenic γδ T-cell lymphomas (also CD3+ and CD11d+) in dogs preferentially involve the liver and spleen, and neoplastic lymphocytes are most common within the sinusoids. Hepatocytotropic lymphoma is typically a T-cell lymphoma variant (CD3+, CD11d–) that invades hepatic cords. Diffuse infiltration of the liver in myeloproliferative disorders and mast cell leukemia may also cause extreme enlargement of the organ; the infiltrates localize preferentially in and around the sinusoids (Fig. 2-118). Hepatic infiltration may be in discrete nodules 2 cm or more in size, particularly lymphoma in horses, but it is usually diffuse in the connective tissues of the portal tracts.

Melanomas and hemangiosarcomas have characteristic gross features in the liver, but most metastatic tumors cannot be distinguished by their gross appearance. Sarcomas do tend to form a few large, smooth-surfaced nodules, and carcinomas do tend to form more nodules and to be umbilicate when in contact with the hepatic capsule. Hemangiosarcomas come from the spleen, usually, and may virtually replace the liver with small, blood-filled caverns. Their microscopic appearance is the same as that of the primary tumors.

A non-neoplastic condition, **hepatic splenosis**, a rare condition in which normal splenic tissue becomes implanted into the liver, can be confused with metastatic disease. Normal spleen enters the liver via the portal vein after surgery or trauma to the spleen and soft red masses up to ~4 cm in diameter can develop. Histologically, the masses resemble splenic tissue.

Visit Elsevier eBooks+ (eBooks.Health.Elsevier.com) for eFigures and further readings.

CHAPTER 3

Pancreas

Andrew W. Stent

ACKNOWLEDGMENTS

This update of the Pancreas chapter is based on previous editions by Drs. Ken Jubb, Peter Kennedy, Nigel Palmer, and Jennifer Charles, and we gratefully acknowledge their contributions.

GENERAL CONSIDERATIONS

The pancreas has a reputation as an irascible organ, readily aggrieved by even minor insult. This notion is not entirely unfounded but has led to a certain trepidation in sampling the tissue for histologic examination. Biopsies are seldom performed and only under considerable duress, lest the manipulation further aggravate the organ. Consequently, early stages of pancreatic disease are not well examined, and minor lesions are often unnoticed given the sizeable functional reserve and regenerative capacity of the pancreatic parenchyma. However, improvements in imaging and biochemical markers of damage are easing constraints on the detection of early pancreatic lesions, leading to increased appreciation of the high prevalence of subclinical and clinical disease in dogs and other species.

As an amalgamation of exocrine and endocrine components within a single tissue, the pancreas illustrates the intimate relationship between the neurohormonal and digestive systems. Although often considered as distinct entities for the sake of simplicity—including within this chapter—*the significant interdependence between the endocrine and exocrine elements* of the organ is frequently underestimated. Hormones produced by the islets are important for regulating the structure and function of the surrounding exocrine tissue, with insulin and somatostatin being particularly influential. *Both insulin and pancreatic polypeptide are trophic for acinar tissue; somatostatin and glucagon are inhibitory*. The paracrine effects of these and other molecules are facilitated by intricate bidirectional circulation between islets and acinar parenchyma, which allows close discourse between the exocrine and endocrine tissues.

In addition to intraorgan stimulus, homeostatic maintenance of the pancreas is heavily reliant on trophic signaling from the broader gastrointestinal tract and beyond. Enteroendocrine hormones from the gastrointestinal mucosa exert considerable control of pancreatic function, with cholecystokinin providing critical stimulus for release of exocrine pancreatic enzymes; control of endocrine function is exemplified by the remarkable efficacy of gut-derived incretins such as glucagon-like peptide–1 in curbing hyperglycemia through regulation of islet hormone secretion. Both sympathetic and parasympathetic innervation are essential, with loss of either pathway triggering degeneration and atrophy of the exocrine and endocrine components of the pancreas. The enteric nervous system also assists in synchronizing the pancreatic response to ingesta, and regular nutritional stimulus is critical for maintenance of optimal parenchymal function and mass. This dependence on external inputs means that the pancreas is susceptible to secondary impairment stemming from a wide variety of gastrointestinal and extraintestinal vicissitudes.

The pancreas has long been a focus of research attention, largely reflecting the importance of diabetes mellitus in both human and veterinary medicine. However, it is important to note that the current understanding of pancreatic pathophysiology is based on in vivo and ex vivo investigations with a limited range of species, predominantly rodents and chick embryos, along with large-scale clinical investigations performed in humans. These studies often fail to acknowledge the immense interspecies variability in prenatal and postnatal development and maturation of the pancreas, and the relevance of published research data to domestic animals may be questionable, particularly as findings are often inconsistent among species and even individuals.

EXOCRINE PANCREAS

Early pancreatic **organogenesis** is best described in the mouse, but it is a reasonable assumption that, except for timing of events, the process is similar in other mammals. The incipient pancreas first emerges as a bud from the dorsal gut endoderm, shortly followed by ventral buds that form both pancreatic and bile ducts. Coiling of the gut tube brings the buds into proximity. As progenitor ducts project into the mesenchyme under the influence of epidermal growth factor (EGF), remodeling distinguishes future duct and acinar regions (Fig. 3-1A). Proliferation of the buds and formation of ducts may, in part, result from progressive branching, but the ductular architecture is more interlinked than this model implies, with anastomoses between ducts ultimately forming an interconnected plexiform system. In species suitably examined, the ductal systems of the 2 pancreatic anlagen form a fused network, with the dorsal bud giving rise to the left lobe and the accessory pancreatic duct; the ventral bud produces the pancreatic duct and the right lobe. Acinar cells arise from the tips of the ductular branches, and rapid growth is achieved through proliferation of these acinar progenitors (Fig. 3-1B).

There are **differences within and between species** as to which of the major ducts—the pancreatic or the accessory pancreatic duct—serves as the main conduit in the developed pancreas. The pancreatic duct develops from the dorsal anlage and opens into the duodenum at the major papilla, with or immediately adjacent to the bile duct. It is the only duct in small ruminants and in most cats; it is the main duct in horses, and in dogs it is the lesser duct and is occasionally absent. The accessory pancreatic duct, derived from the ventral anlage and entering the duodenum at the minor duodenal papilla, is the only duct in the pig and ox, the major duct in the dog, and a minor branch in the horse.

Innervation of the pancreas is important for regulating exocrine secretion. Parasympathetic autonomic stimulation derived from the vagus nerve prompts secretion of pancreatic juice, mediated by ganglion cells within the interstitial tissue.

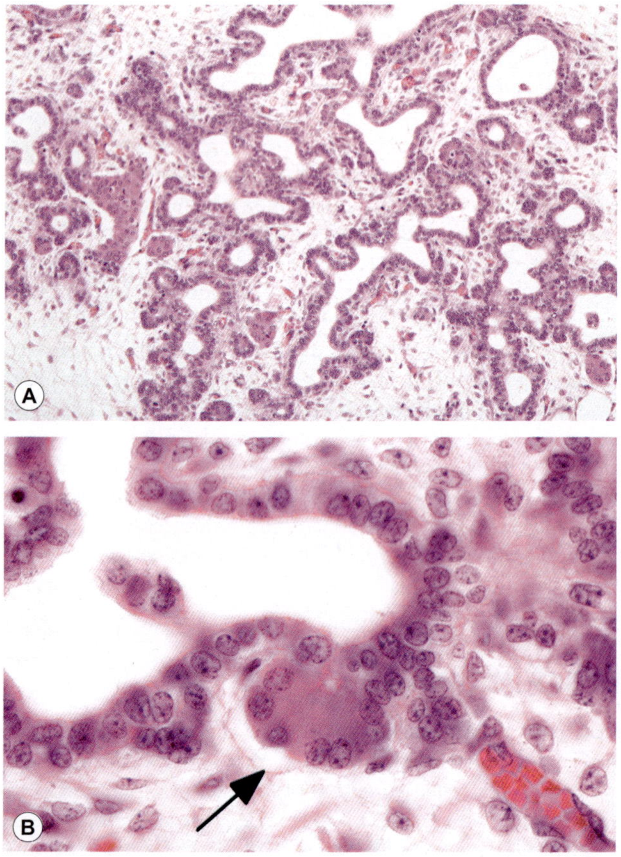

Figure 3-1 A. **Pancreatic organogenesis** in a lamb at day 48. Ductal epithelium invades through the mesenchyme, with scattered colonies of islet-like tissue distributed throughout. **B.** Details of (A). **Incipient acinar tissue** budding from embryonic ductular epithelium (arrow).

The ganglion cells are also innervated by the enteric nervous system, acting independently of central systems to coordinate secretory control by gastrointestinal hormones. *Lamellar (Pacinian) corpuscles* are normally prominent in the interlobular connective tissues of the pancreas of the cat and may be grossly visible as discrete 1-3-mm nodules.

By weight and volume, the pancreas is predominantly composed of acinar tissue. The organ lacks a conventional capsule but is organized into lobules separated by septa and enveloped in a thin condensation of connective tissue that also invests the ductal system. The lobules are composed of glandular acini that are distributed along the smaller ducts. Each acinus forms around an evagination of the ductal system that is called the *intercalated duct*. The intercalated duct is lined by cuboidal centroacinar cells, distinguishable in histologic sections by the clear unstained cytoplasm. Ductular epithelium progressively becomes more columnar along intralobular and interlobular ducts, and there is a corresponding alteration in epithelial secretory profile, with decreased bicarbonate secretion and increased production of mucins. Both enteric and pancreatic endocrine cell populations are also present within the ductular epithelium, but their functional importance remains unclear.

*The major **function of the exocrine pancreas** is the synthesis and secretion of digestive enzymes*. Acinar cells secrete trypsin, chymotrypsin, collagenase, phospholipase, elastases, and carboxypeptidases as inactive proenzymes; amylase and lipase are secreted in their active forms. The proenzymes and enzymes are packaged into membrane-bound zymogen granules within the cytoplasm of acinar cells. The entry of gastric acid and fatty acids into the duodenum causes local release of secretin, which in turn stimulates secretion of water and bicarbonate by pancreatic ductal epithelium, particularly by the centroacinar cells. The bicarbonate contributes to neutralization of gastric acid in the duodenum. However, this is not essential for maintaining a neutral pH, suitable for optimal activity of the digestive enzymes, given that the duodenal mucosa itself has an enormous capacity to secrete bicarbonate and absorb hydrogen ions. The presence of undigested lipid and amino acid peptides in the duodenal lumen promotes the release of cholecystokinin by mucosal endocrine cells; this secretagogue triggers rapid discharge of digestive enzymes from zymogen granules into the ducts and also has a direct, rapid, and substantial trophic effect on acinar cells.

Within the duodenum, exocrine secretions also inhibit bacterial proliferation, exert a trophic effect on the mucosa, and contribute to the normal degradation of exposed mucosal brush border enzymes. The exocrine pancreas also produces *intrinsic factor*, which is essential for the absorption of cobalamin (vitamin B12) in the ileum. In addition, the organ plays an important role in zinc homeostasis, accumulating zinc absorbed from the intestines and secreting excess into pancreatic juice. This function is partly mediated by the zinc-binding protein, metallothionein, which is present in acinar cells and exocrine secretions.

The exocrine pancreas is a labile organ. It synthesizes much more protein on a weight-for-weight basis than does any other tissue and consumes a correspondingly large amount of precursor substrate, but the mechanisms responsible for homeostatic regulation of pancreatic tissue remain incompletely understood. A degree of zonal variability and peri-islet hypertrophy is often observed in acinar tissue, reflecting exposure to trophic hormones secreted by the islets.

The response of the exocrine pancreas to changes in nutrient intake is rapid, and adaptation to new diets can produce dramatic alterations in the composition of pancreatic juice. Secretion of proteases is a reflection, in part, of dietary protein levels; amylase secretion is influenced by the level of dietary carbohydrate and by plasma levels of cortisol and insulin. The dietary influence on lipase secretion is less clear, but secretion is to some extent dependent on dietary protein levels. Acinar cell hypertrophy and hyperplasia leading to organ enlargement occurs in response to diets rich in protein and calories. When these substrates are withdrawn, the organ reverts to normal mass via autophagy and apoptosis. If dietary protein and energy become suboptimal, acinar cells and the exocrine organ are in general atrophy.

Maternal malnutrition during gestation and lactation may retard maturation of the exocrine pancreas of the offspring. Paradoxically, the enzyme content of the pancreas may increase in the offspring; whether this increase enhances the ability of the offspring to resist malnutrition remains unclear. The exocrine pancreas is normally functionally immature at birth, and the synthesis of some digestive enzymes may not commence postnatally for several weeks. Enzymatic activity of milk and proximal intestinal secretions compensate for this insufficiency in suckling animals. The weight of the pancreas increases rapidly during the immediate postnatal period, chiefly because of an increase in the number rather than size of acinar cells. Colostrum, which contains growth-promoting factors such as EGF and insulin-like growth factors (IGFs), plays a role in this early organ growth. Release of endogenous gut hormones such as gastrin that have trophic effects on the pancreas may contribute to this early development, and glucocorticoids also promote maturation of the acinar cells. At weaning, dietary and hormonal changes combine to cause abrupt increases in pancreatic enzyme synthesis and secretion. In animals weaned early, the surge in circulating glucocorticoids is considered to be more important than the dietary changes in triggering the alterations to enzyme output.

Acinar, ductal, and islet cells are all capable of **regeneration**, and restoration of the exocrine parenchyma typically proceeds rapidly following acinar destruction. Regeneration of exocrine components proceeds via the facultative progenitor potential of ductular epithelium, as well as proliferation of mature acinar cells through the formation of metaplastic ductular intermediates. The ductular progenitor cells display broad multipotency, and hepatocellular differentiation occasionally may be observed in regenerating pancreas. β-Cell regeneration appears to occur largely via mitotic division of the mature β-cell population, together with expansion of redifferentiated α-cells and ductular tissue. Adult stem cells are not currently thought to play a major role in the regenerative process, although this remains an area of active debate.

The regenerative capacity of the exocrine tissue is exemplified in cerulein toxicosis. Cerulein, an analogue of cholecystokinin, causes dose-dependent dissolution of the acinar cells in rodents that, even if total, can be fully repaired in a week or so. Slower regeneration of both exocrine and endocrine elements follows partial surgical ablation. Complete restitution of exocrine parenchyma by mitotic division and hypertrophy of viable acinar cells may follow minor cell loss. Extensive or persistent parenchymal injury may provoke proliferation of ductular epithelium and connective tissues.

Stellate cells akin to those of the liver have been identified in the normal pancreas in a periacinar location and appear to be the major mediators of pancreatic fibrogenesis. In the quiescent state, pancreatic stellate cells express desmin but not α–smooth muscle actin. Following activation by injury, these cells acquire a myofibroblastic phenotype and synthesize extracellular matrix, in particular type I collagen. Stellate cells also appear to have stem cell capabilities under some circumstances, although the extent and importance of this characteristic in vivo is still debated.

Developmental anomalies of the exocrine pancreas

The complex movements among embryonic tissues during pancreatic development provide abundant opportunities for malformations to arise.

Agenesis or **aplasia** (complete absence) of the pancreas may be associated with more generalized and severe malformations incompatible with survival.

Pancreatic hypoplasia occurs sporadically in calves. The defect is in the exocrine tissue; the islets are normal in number and morphology. The hypoplastic organ is small, pale, and loosely textured. Its margins are poorly defined, but the parenchyma is centered on a normal duct system. Microscopically, acinar tissue is present as small, scattered clusters of cells in glandular array. Some of the cells may appear well differentiated and contain zymogen granules, but most are small, basophilic, and of indifferent type.

Variations in the disposition of the ducts are common in dogs. Most dogs have 2 separate ducts opening into the duodenum, with interductal anastomoses within the pancreas, and with the accessory pancreatic duct the major conduit. A small percentage of dogs may have only an accessory duct entering the duodenum, and some may have 3 functional openings into the intestine.

An **annular pancreas**, characterized by a thin flat ring of normal pancreatic tissue completely encircling the duodenum, has been observed in dogs and piglets; the annulus may cause duodenal stenosis. This anomaly probably reflects the failure of normal embryonic rotation of the duodenal anlagen; the anomaly occurs sporadically, but can be induced experimentally in mice through inhibition of the Indian hedgehog signaling pathway.

Congenital stenosis or **cystic dilation of a pancreatic duct** is occasionally reported in domestic animals, and congenital intrapancreatic cysts lined by squamous or low cuboidal epithelium are occasionally seen in lambs. Cystic dilation of intralobular and interlobular pancreatic ducts accompanied by polycystic kidneys and cystic intrahepatic bile ducts is reported in cats, piglets, and goat kids (eFig. 3-1). Isolated pancreatic cysts lined by simple columnar epithelium are also rarely reported in dogs and cats. Saccular ductal distension to form a structure resembling a gallbladder and termed a **pancreatic bladder** has been described in cats and may be congenital or acquired. Such structures are usually subclinical, but large cysts may compress the bile duct to cause jaundice. True congenital **duplication of the gallbladder** with the accessory organ arising from the ventral pancreatic bud has also been observed in cats.

Ectopic or **accessory pancreatic tissue** forming small pancreatic nodules may be found in the submucosa, muscularis, or serosa of the stomach or intestine (especially in the duodenum), the mesentery, gallbladder, spleen, lymph node, or liver (eFig. 3-2). The ectopic rests are of normal morphology, although islets are not always present. Ectopia may result from dislocation of portions of the duodenal buds during development, from persistence of an anlage that would normally regress, or from activation of pancreatic transcription factors within pluripotential endodermal epithelium.

Splenic organogenesis occurs in close proximity to the developing pancreas within the dorsal splanchnic mesenchyme, and the organs continue to be connected in some reptiles and fish. In domestic species, they may be linked by a mesenteric band or, occasionally in dogs and cats, ectopic acinar tissue or islets may be found in the substance of the spleen. Conversely, **intrapancreatic accessory splenic tissue** is also identified in a range of domestic species, with a reported prevalence of 1.5% in pigs at slaughter. The foci can be large enough to be visible macroscopically, but are otherwise incidental findings.

Intrapancreatic hepatocytes are occasionally observed as an incidental finding, especially in neonates. Hepatocytes may also appear in the adult pancreas during attempted regeneration after massive lobular injury, reflecting pluripotency of regenerating ductular epithelium.

Regressive changes of the exocrine pancreas

Nonspecific degenerative changes are frequently observed within the exocrine tissue and should not be confused with **autolysis**, which occurs rapidly within the pancreas because of postmortem release and activation of digestive enzymes. Autolyzed pancreata are often discolored dark-red to brown, and there may be hemorrhage within the pancreatic interstitium and peripancreatic tissue after death, particularly in dogs and horses (Fig. 3-2). Histologically, the distribution of autolytic change is patchy. The cells separate and may be rounded, acinar tissue becomes smudged, and affected areas are poorly stained and display slate-gray coloration with H&E.

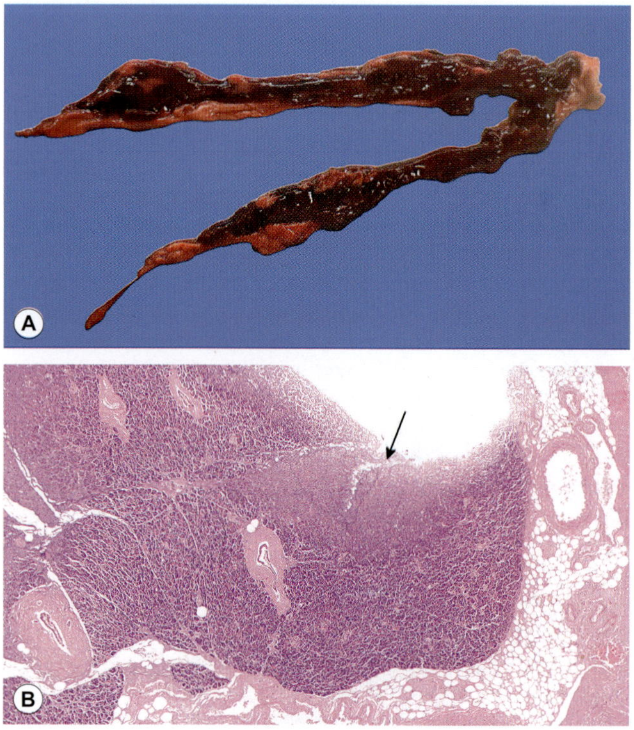

Figure 3-2 **A. Autolyzed pancreas** of a dog, uniformly discolored dark red with a gelatinous texture. **B. Histologic image of autolyzed pancreas**, with smudging and loss of cellular detail (arrow).

Insult to either the acinar or ductular epithelium frequently induces vacuolar hydropic change, reflecting membrane injury or failure of ion pumps with resulting accumulation of intracellular fluid. Autophagic vacuoles can also develop in acinar cells following toxic insult, as well as in atrophic or catabolic states. Microvesicular steatosis occasionally is observed in the cytoplasm of the acinar epithelium as early nonspecific pathologic degeneration. Cytoplasmic substrate accumulation occurs in lysosomal storage disorders, such as α- and β-mannosidosis and galactosialidosis. Vacuolation of ductal epithelium because of glycogen accumulation is a feature of diabetes mellitus.

Pancreatic lipofuscinosis is occasionally seen in dogs deficient in vitamin E. Accumulation of lipofuscin causes khaki-to-brown discoloration of the pancreas and of intestinal smooth muscle grossly; the urinary bladder and mesenteric lymph nodes may also be affected. The golden-brown pigment granules in the basal cytoplasm of pancreatic acinar cells and intestinal myocytes are periodic acid-Schiff (PAS) positive, sudanophilic, and weakly acid fast. Microscopic pigment accumulation may occur in other tissues, including the pigmented epithelium of the retina.

Lipomatosis of the pancreas occurs occasionally in dogs, cats, pigs, and cattle, usually as part of generalized obesity but sometimes restricted to the pancreas. Adipose tissue accumulates in the interstitium and dissects the parenchyma (eFig. 3-3). In most cases, the exocrine tissue is merely separated by the infiltrating adipocytes and organ function is spared, although examples of genuine pancreatic effacement by fat occur in dogs and cats. These animals had polyphagia, intermittent vomiting, and weight loss suggestive of exocrine insufficiency, and histologically, the exocrine tissue is mostly absent with variable depletion of endocrine tissue, although clinical endocrine dysfunction has not been described with this condition.

Exocrine degeneration and necrosis

Necrosis of individual acinar cells or local groups occurs in various local and systemic disorders, including febrile states, viral infections (most commonly those displaying epitheliotropism, including canine distemper, foot-and-mouth disease, and a number of adenoviral diseases), intoxications, and in hypovolemic or septic shock. Associated inflammation is often minimal. In most cases, the lesions are incidental to the course of the systemic disease.

Multifocal degeneration and necrosis also may be seen in many **intoxications**, including trichothecene mycotoxicosis of pigs resulting from consumption of T-2 toxin, deoxynivalenol (vomitoxin), or diacetoxyscirpenol (anguidine) produced by *Fusarium* species. These mycotoxins may also cause pancreatic interstitial edema, hyperplasia of ductular epithelium, and necrosis of islet cells. Cyclopiazonic acid synthesized by *Aspergillus* and *Penicillium* fungi can also damage the pancreas, in addition to broad toxic effects on the nervous, enteric, hepatic, renal, and lymphoid systems. Selenium excess may cause degenerative change in the exocrine pancreas, with experimental toxicosis in pigs producing acute pancreatic edema, hemorrhage, and acinar necrosis. Ingestion of *Cassia occidentalis* also has been reported to cause pancreatic necrosis in pigs.

Acute intoxication by **anticholinesterases** is recognized to cause exocrine degeneration in both humans and domestic species, manifesting as ballooning necrosis of acinar cells, together with interstitial edema and vasculitis. These lesions are theorized to reflect the inhibition of pancreatic pseudocholinesterase, resulting in excessive secretory stimulation of exocrine tissue as well as increased intraductal pressures. Cats appear relatively resistant to this form of toxicity because they possess low levels of pancreatic pseudocholinesterase, but clinical cases have still been reported. Although reports of pancreatic damage following anticholinesterase intoxication are rare in the literature, extensive use of these chemicals as pesticides within the veterinary field suggests that this phenomenon may be under-recognized.

Zinc toxicity causes striking pancreatic lesions in several species, including domestic animals and humans. There are numerous opportunities for exposure to zinc and narrow margins between safe and unsafe levels of exposure. Metallic zinc is available in alloys and galvanized products, zinc compounds are widely available in pesticides and herbicides, and zinc salts are occasionally used in the treatment of dermatologic conditions and for protection against facial eczema in cattle and sheep.

Zinc is an essential element for a multitude of biochemical processes in plants and animals, but the biologic and physiologic roles and homeostatic mechanisms remain incompletely understood. The most consistent expressions of zinc toxicity in animals are in the pancreas, liver, kidney, and blood, the latter manifesting as Heinz body hemolytic anemia. The pancreas is the major route of zinc excretion, and this is likely to explain the sensitivity of this organ to toxicity. The relative susceptibility of the pancreatic structures to zinc toxicity varies among domestic species, with the ductular elements affected first in sheep and other ruminants; acinar tissue is most vulnerable in pigs. Generally, *microvesicular degeneration and necrosis of acinar elements dominate early and are followed by acinar atrophy and fibrosis*. The islets are usually unaffected. There are associated changes in tissue concentrations of copper, iron, and manganese that raise the possibility that the hemolytic anemia and the hepatic necrosis, which is sometimes massive, may be caused by impaired capture of free radicals by various dismutases, rather than by the direct effects of zinc itself.

In acute zinc intoxication, the pancreas is enlarged and pale with prominent lobulation. The interlobular connective tissues are widened by slightly viscous edema fluid that may be stained by free hemoglobin. The liver may be reduced in size with a surface mosaic of prominent fatty degeneration and dark sunken areas of necrosis and collapse. Renal lesions such as tubular dilation and necrosis may not be present in acute intoxications. Histologically, the acinar cells are enlarged with vacuolated cytoplasm, and zymogen granulation may be prominent as an early change (Fig. 3-3). There is no or minimal inflammatory cell presence.

Progression of pancreatic toxicity is marked by shrinkage and nodularity of the organ, with some lobules appearing normal and others shrunken, although damaged lobules are generally uniformly affected. The interstitial edema is replaced by prominent fibrosis (Fig. 3-4). Acinar cells may become necrotic and exfoliate, and dilation of acinar lumina accompanied by attenuation of the lining cells often produces a pseudoacinar or tubular arrangement. Late in the disease progression, the liver may show postnecrotic scarring and there may be renal tubular degeneration affecting especially the straight ascending and descending limbs of the loops of Henle.

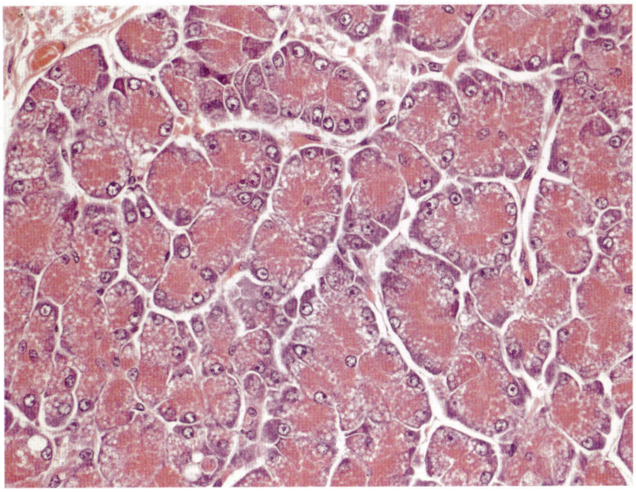

Figure 3-3 **Zinc toxicity** in a dog. In the acute phase, there is basilar vacuolar degeneration within the acinar cells.

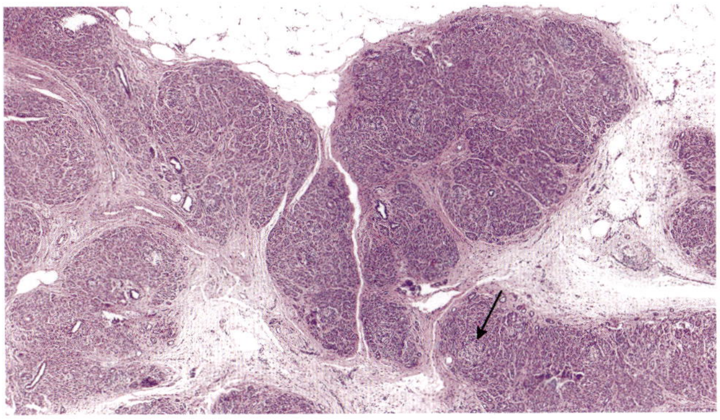

Figure 3-4 **Zinc toxicity** in a cow. With chronicity, the pancreas becomes markedly fibrotic with minimal associated inflammation and sparing of islets (arrow).

Although toxins may exert deleterious effects directly on exocrine tissue, *many chemicals, including ethanol, largely act via production of free radicals or other redox-reactive molecules*. The exocrine pancreas already generates a large free radical load during normal metabolic processes, and an additional burden produced by exogenous sources may overwhelm regulatory antioxidant pathways. Moreover, the exocrine acinar cells possess latent cytochrome P450 activity, and the oxidative damage of some pancreatic toxins may be amplified following biotransformation within the exocrine tissue. Agents that induce the cytochrome P450 pathway, including corticosteroids and even feeds rich in C18:2 fatty acids, such as corn oil, may potentiate pancreatic toxicity. Cytochrome P450 is also induced by chronic pancreatitis, thereby increasing the susceptibility of an already damaged organ to toxic insult.

Pancreatitis

Pancreatic inflammatory disease is common in a range of species but may not always be clinically significant. Histologic evidence of pancreatitis was identified in 66% of cats at autopsy; inflammatory pancreatic lesions were observed in 34-90% of dogs, but only a small minority of these animals had clinical signs of pancreatic disease. Conventionally, pancreatitis is defined as acute or chronic based on histologic characteristics, but in practice this distinction is often unclear. Both forms can have sudden onset of clinical signs, so rapid development of disease does not necessarily establish that the condition is acute. Moreover, lingering acute inflammation or periodic relapse can eventually impart features indistinguishable from the chronic form of disease. *Given the considerable clinical overlap between the specific types of pancreatic inflammation, clinicians tend to use the general term* pancreatitis *to describe any inflammatory disease of the pancreas*. However, more precise classification of pancreatic inflammation is useful whenever possible, as the different forms have distinct causes, pathogeneses, and clinical consequences.

Acute pancreatitis. ***Acute necrotizing pancreatitis****, also known as acute pancreatic necrosis, is the most common exocrine pancreatic disease in dogs and is recognized with increasing frequency in cats*. It most commonly manifests as a fulminant and potentially life-threatening condition, but mild or even subclinical episodes can occur, particularly if the disease only affects a small region of the pancreas. *Acute necrotizing pancreatitis begins with necrosis and saponification of fat in the peripancreatic mesentery*. This is followed by parenchymal damage that is concentrated at the periphery of the lobules, reflecting autodigestion of pancreatic tissue by activated enzymes. The duct system and centrilobular parenchyma are unaffected in the early stages of the disease, but parenchymal destruction and inflammation progress over time, accompanied by more-or-less extensive involvement of adjacent fat and other connective tissues.

Premature intracellular activation of zymogen-bound proenzymes is a key step in the **pathogenesis** of acute necrotizing pancreatitis. Normal enzyme secretion is triggered by rapid spiking of cytoplasmic calcium concentrations, but when the calcium increase is sustained—as occurs with hypoxia, hypercalcemia, hyperlipidemia, oxidative stress, and other cellular insults—ATP production is blunted, and the energy-intensive process of zymogen secretion is suppressed. Calcium then stimulates the fusion of the zymogen granules with lysosomes, resulting in intracellular activation of trypsinogen, and this, in turn, activates other proenzymes such as proelastase and prophospholipase. Diffusion of these activated digestive enzymes is considered to be responsible for the early fat necrosis. Amylase and lipase, normally stored in an active form, are liberated by autodigestion and are major contributors to adipocyte breakdown. Activated elastase and phospholipase A appear to be particularly important in expanding the area of pancreatic necrosis. Trypsin, phospholipase A, elastase, lipase, and colipase damage the walls of local blood vessels, inducing vasoactive amine release, increased vascular permeability, edema, hemorrhage, and thrombosis; enzymatic tissue necrosis may therefore be compounded by *superimposed ischemic necrosis*.

Exocrine cell injury in acute necrotizing pancreatitis is accompanied by upregulation of the NF-κB signaling pathway, which promotes the release of proinflammatory cytokines such as tumor necrosis factor (TNF), interleukin (IL) 1, IL6, IL8, and platelet-activating factor. Damaged acinar cells further augment the inflammatory response through the production of TNF. Some of these molecules stimulate chemotaxis of leukocytes, and the influx of inflammatory cells amplifies pancreatic damage via the generation of oxygen-derived free radicals and additional cytokines. Local activation of the complement cascade produces further deleterious effects, exacerbating inflammation, damaging cell membranes, and promoting thrombosis.

Under normal circumstances, the exocrine pancreas possesses robust **defenses against autodigestion**. Acinar cells possess intracellular hydrolases that are capable of degrading retained zymogen granules, and protease inhibitors such as pancreatic secretory trypsin inhibitor and α1-antitrypsin are packaged and cosecreted along with digestive enzymes to prevent premature activation. In acute necrotizing pancreatitis, these defense mechanisms appear to be overwhelmed, and experimental supplementation of these enzymes has been shown to ameliorate disease progression.

In many cases, the **inciting cause** of the disease is obscure. Because the periphery of the pancreatic lobule is also the periphery of the circulatory field, *hypoperfusion and possibly reperfusion may be important in the development of necrosis* and could account for its occasional onset after prolonged hypotension, following abdominal surgeries such as splenectomy and adrenalectomy, or in conjunction with gastric dilation-volvulus. Abdominal trauma may be the trigger in some animals, and the condition has been associated with infectious diseases, particularly blood-borne infections such as babesiosis, schistosomosis, and ehrlichiosis. Nutritional factors, especially diets high in fat and hyperlipidemia, appear to be important factors in the pathogenesis of necrotizing pancreatitis. This may partially reflect damage from lipid peroxidation, but hypertriglyceridemia can also lower the threshold for premature zymogen activation by increasing cytosolic calcium. High-fat diets may also promote hyperstimulation of the exocrine pancreas through excessive release of cholecystokinin. Pancreatic parenchyma also has drug-metabolizing activity and a capacity to produce toxic free radicals, which may subsequently induce oxidative tissue damage. Drugs reported as potential triggers of acute necrotizing pancreatitis include azathioprine, L-asparaginase, and anticonvulsants such as phenobarbital and potassium bromide. Various studies have demonstrated that corticosteroid administration does not directly induce acute necrotizing pancreatitis, at least in the short term, and may actually provide some therapeutic benefit in disease management. However, broader prospective studies of long-term treatment are required to exclude corticosteroid usage as a possible contributory risk factor, particularly because dogs with hyperadrenocorticism are recognized to be at increased risk of disease. Hypothyroidism, hypercalcemia, and uremia are additional factors that can predispose to acute necrotizing pancreatitis.

Middle-aged to older ***dogs*** *that are overweight or obese are at increased risk of acute pancreatic necrosis*. Miniature Schnauzers, Miniature Poodles, Yorkshire and Silky Terriers, and other terrier breeds are predisposed, and female dogs are more likely to be affected than male dogs. The prevalence of idiopathic hyperlipidemia in Miniature Schnauzers may in part explain their susceptibility, but many Schnauzers also carry a mutation in the gene encoding pancreatic secretory trypsin inhibitor (*SPINK1*), and these dogs may be more prone to premature activation of trypsin.

Grossly, in fatal cases of acute necrotizing pancreatitis, a small volume of turbid serous fluid containing free lipid droplets is usually present in the peritoneal cavity. Petechial and ecchymotic hemorrhages may be present in the pancreas and adjacent omentum and mesenteries, but extensive hemorrhage is not usually a feature. Numerous small white chalky areas of fat necrosis, each with an intensely hyperemic border, are present adjacent to the pancreas and in the mesentery

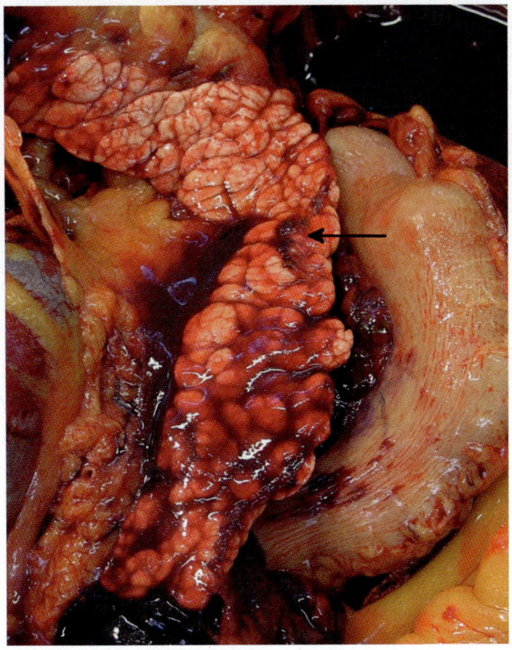

Figure 3-5 Acute necrotizing pancreatitis in a dog with peripancreatic hemorrhage, edema, and a focus of fat necrosis (arrow).

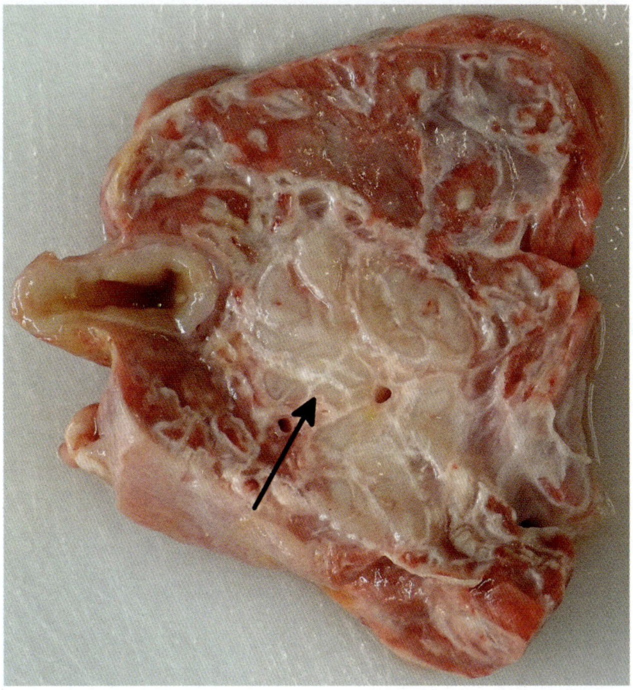

Figure 3-6 Cross-sectional view of the pancreas from a dog with recurrent necrotizing pancreatitis. Note the variegated appearance of the peripancreatic fat caused by hemorrhage, necrosis, dystrophic mineralization, and fibrosis. Remnant pancreatic tissue is indicated by the arrow; the duodenum is at the left of the tissue.

(eFig. 3-4). In some cases, foci of necrotic fat are widely distributed throughout the peritoneal cavity and may be detectable as far away as the ventral mediastinum, reflecting lymphatic dissemination of liberated digestive enzymes. The entire pancreas may be edematous, swollen, and soft (Fig. 3-5), or edema may be confined to localized areas. The necrotizing process may be confined to the central pancreas or one wing. Fibrin strands may overlie the surface of the affected pancreas and the omentum, mesenteries, and the visceral surface of the liver. The cut surface of the pancreas has a variegated appearance caused by merging of white areas of fat necrosis and gray-yellow areas of parenchymal necrosis; one or other appearance may predominate (Fig. 3-6). The texture is unusually greasy. Areas of parenchymal necrosis are soft and may liquefy.

Histologically, there is necrosis of peripancreatic adipose tissue and pancreatic parenchyma, accompanied by edematous separation of the interstitium and reactive inflammation (Fig. 3-7). Infiltrating leukocytes, chiefly neutrophils and macrophages, congregate at the boundary of necrotic and viable tissue. The necrotic fat saponifies and may undergo mild dystrophic mineralization. The initial parenchymal lesions at the periphery of the lobules are composed of small foci of coagulative necrosis in which the acinar cells become shrunken and acidophilic. These foci rapidly expand and liquefy, with smudging of the acinar cell detail and formation of large lakes of necrotic debris. The collagenous stroma resists digestion for some time. Phlebothrombosis, which may be associated with phlebitis or mural necrosis, may be apparent both adjacent to and distant from the parenchymal lesions; similar changes may occur in the small arteries, but these vessels are less susceptible to injury. Fibrin precipitates in the interstitium as a result of vascular injury and leakage, and circulatory compromise may contribute to the tissue necrosis. With the development of disseminated intravascular coagulation (DIC), microvascular thrombosis may be apparent in various organs.

Infrequently, inflammatory masses such as abscesses, pseudocysts, or phlegmon may develop in the pancreas in the aftermath of acute necrosis; these lesions are discussed later.

The intensity of inflammation associated with acute pancreatic necrosis may produce devastating **systemic consequences**. Recruitment of large numbers of leukocytes results in systemic release of proinflammatory mediators such as TNF, IL1, and chemokines such as IL8, and *this cytokine storm induces the systemic inflammatory response syndrome (SIRS) and multiple organ dysfunction*. Animals with acute pancreatic necrosis are highly susceptible to DIC because of activation of clotting factors combined with widespread endothelial damage. Mortality rates of 27-58% are reported in dogs with acute pancreatic necrosis, although most dogs with mild disease clinically recover within a few days. Although the extent of necrosis may well influence the outcome in dogs, secondary infection of the organ occurs rarely in this species. Other factors that have been associated with mortality in affected dogs have included obesity, concurrent diabetes mellitus, hyperadrenocorticism, hypothyroidism, epilepsy, and prior gastrointestinal disease.

A minority of dogs with pancreatic necrosis may develop **pancreatic panniculitis**, manifesting as painful nodules of fat necrosis along the flanks that often ulcerate. Comparable subcutaneous lesions have been experimentally induced in cats by ligation of the pancreatic ducts. Release of activated enzymes—particularly phospholipase A, lipase, amylase, and trypsin—into the systemic circulation has been incriminated in the pathogenesis of this condition.

Although most dogs survive an episode of acute pancreatic necrosis, in many cases *it is doubtful whether the pathologic process completely resolves*. Rather, the necrotizing process

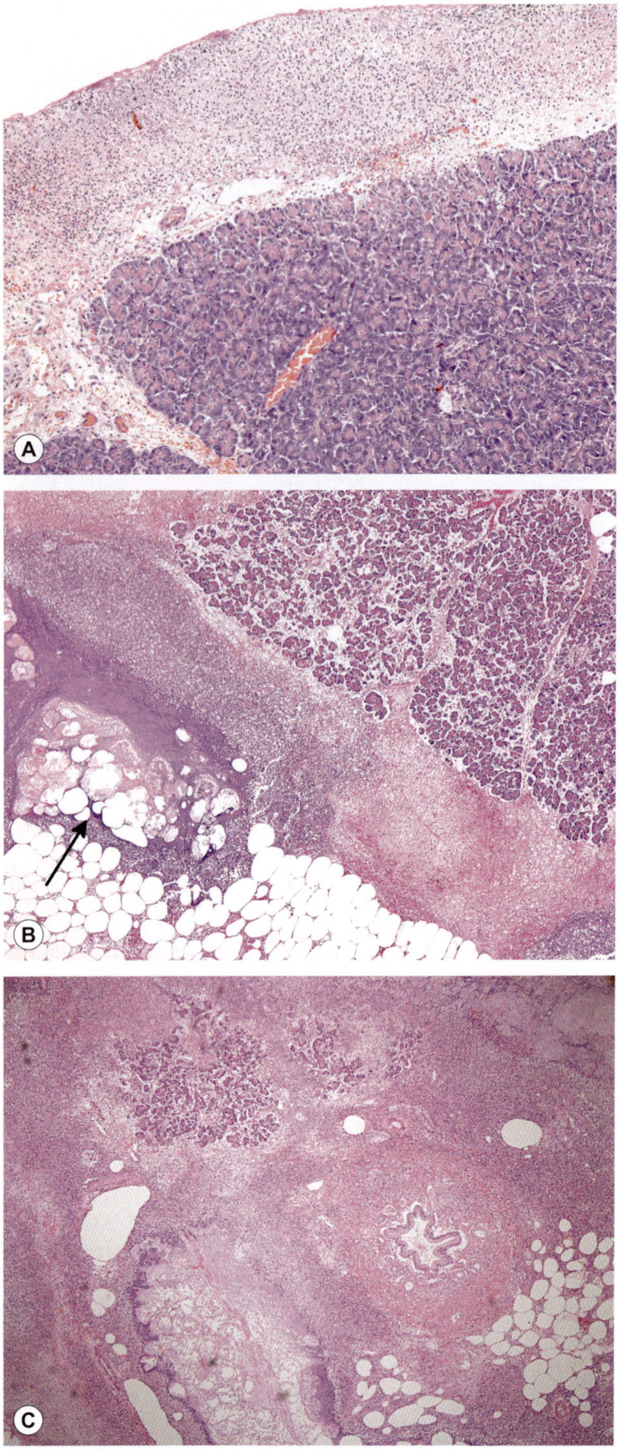

Figure 3-7 Progression of histologic changes in acute necrotizing pancreatitis. **A.** Peripancreatic hemorrhage, edema, and leukocyte infiltration with sparing of pancreatic parenchyma in early stages of the disease. **B.** Progression of disease with regions of fat necrosis and saponification (arrow). Note extension of the reaction into the adjacent pancreas. **C.** Advanced disease with widespread inflammation, fat necrosis, and destruction of pancreatic tissue.

smolders continuously and often subclinically until there is almost complete destruction of the pancreas. There is seldom any difficulty in finding microscopic areas of acute necrosis in chronically affected organs. Whether the apparently relentless course is the result of the persistence of the primary

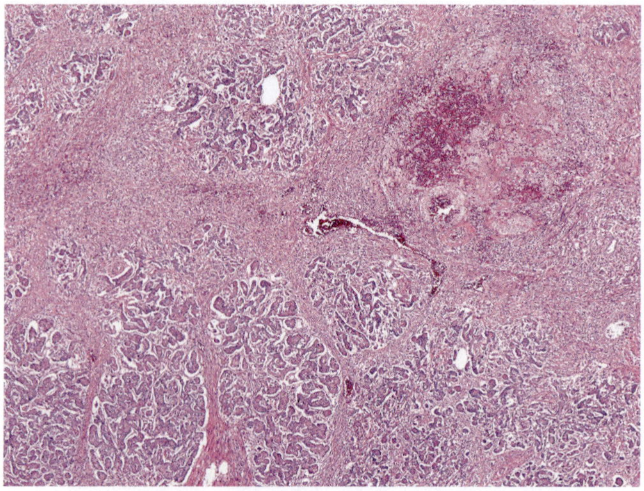

Fig 3-8 Chronic stages of necrotizing pancreatitis with fibrosis dissecting through remnant exocrine pancreatic lobules, accompanied by persistent inflammation.

pathogenetic mechanism or a self-perpetuating property of the lesion is not known. With chronicity, the organ may be irregular in conformation and knobby or reduced to a few distorted lobules adjacent to where the ducts enter the duodenum. In some cases, the remnants of the organ are too small to be visibly appreciated, but they may still be palpable in areas indicated by a slight puckering of the mesentery. Scar tissue is usually not extensive, and adhesions are absent or minor. Microscopically, a few small, rounded lobules remain, and these are compressed and atrophic (Fig. 3-8). Interstitial tissue is increased, but this is probably as much the result of condensation of stroma as by fibrosis. Blood vessels and nerves are also condensed into the small area of the pancreatic remnant. Islets often cannot be identified. Diabetes mellitus and exocrine pancreatic insufficiency (EPI) are common sequelae in chronic cases.

Acute necrotizing pancreatitis in **cats** is not readily distinguished clinically from chronic interstitial pancreatitis, and distinction relies on the gross and histologic appearance of the organ. The necrotizing form usually produces lesions similar to those described in dogs. However, in some cats, neutrophilic inflammation dominates the process, with relatively minor necrosis; it is not known whether this variation reflects a qualitative spectrum or divergent disease processes. Older domestic shorthair cats are most commonly affected by acute necrotizing pancreatitis, and there is no sex predisposition. The condition has been reported after abdominal trauma (including that associated with falling from a great height) and in cats with lipodystrophy, acute hypercalcemia, ductal reflux of duodenal contents, and organophosphate poisoning. Serious complications of acute necrotizing pancreatitis in cats are as described in dogs, but hepatic lipidosis, often severe, also may develop in affected cats.

Primary acute necrotizing pancreatitis is rare in **horses**, and the condition is more commonly associated with other gastrointestinal or hepatic diseases, particularly intestinal accidents, gastric dilation or rupture, and hepatitis. Strychnine intoxication can predispose to pancreatitis in horses. Occasionally, acute bacterial enteritis may extend to the pancreatic ducts and trigger pancreatitis, and cholangitis is often also present in these horses.

Other forms of acute pancreatitis. Multifocal necrosis of the exocrine pancreas with minimal response from inflammatory cells is common in systemic infections with epitheliotropic viruses but is incidental to the course of the systemic disease. Bacterial embolism to the pancreas is not uncommon in cats and dogs with septic peritonitis.

A form of acute pancreatitis with ductal or centrilobular distribution, sometimes referred to as **acute hemorrhagic pancreatitis**, is occasionally observed in cats, horses, and dogs. The inciting insult in this condition is believed to be reflux of activated digestive enzymes and bile salts into the main pancreatic duct. Reflux may be encouraged by increased luminal pressures during severe vomiting. In the initial stages, the organ is edematous and hyperemic, and the parenchyma becomes friable and hemorrhagic. Ductal necrosis resulting from autodigestion rapidly extends through periductal tissue and the broader parenchyma and may become confluent throughout most of the pancreas. Extensive hemorrhage may obscure the parenchyma and necrotic foci in adjacent adipose tissue. Apart from the intensity of accompanying hemorrhage, this stage may show some histologic overlap with the more common pattern of acute necrotizing pancreatitis that commences at the periphery of the organ.

Chronic pancreatitis. Aside from the dog, **chronic interstitial pancreatitis** is the usual pattern of inflammation seen in domestic animals. Lesions of chronic pancreatitis are frequently identified at autopsy of mature cats, and the condition is occasionally also observed in horses and dogs.

Ductal epithelial injury is a key step in the pathogenesis of chronic interstitial pancreatitis, and concordant with this, most cases of chronic interstitial pancreatitis arise as an extension from ductal inflammation. Ascending infection by intestinal bacterial flora or fluke migration are common triggers, and some cases also represent progression and persistence of acute pancreatitis. There is some evidence that chronic interstitial pancreatitis may develop as a manifestation of autoimmune disease, particularly in English Cocker Spaniels. This breed is susceptible to a specific form of chronic pancreatitis with prominent interlobular and periductal fibrosis accompanied by duct effacement and large interstitial aggregates of lymphocytes; these features closely resemble autoimmune pancreatitis type 1 in humans, an IgG4-related autoimmune disease.

In chronic interstitial pancreatitis, the organ may be enlarged or reduced in size. In horses, the tendency is for enlargement and the parenchyma may be replaced by a tough mass of scar tissue with adhesions to adjacent structures. Flattened remnants of pancreatic tissue may be visible near the surface of the mass. Incision reveals tortuous and eccentrically dilated ducts that may contain purulent exudate or a large volume of slightly viscid mucus.

In **horses**, chronic interstitial pancreatitis may be provoked by the larvae of *Strongylus equinus* or, less commonly, *Strongylus edentatus* that pass part of their developmental cycle in and about the pancreas. Hepatobiliary diseases, such as hepatitis, cholangitis, and cholelithiasis, may also predispose to development of chronic pancreatitis in horses.

Although most cases of feline chronic interstitial pancreatitis are idiopathic, the condition is sporadically associated with pathogens such as *Toxoplasma gondii*, feline infectious peritonitis virus, or the trematode *Eurytrema procyonis*. In **cats**, the pancreas is usually reduced in size and is firm, gray, and multinodular (Fig. 3-9). Clear retention cysts are often visible through the capsule and particularly on the cut surface. Fibrosis may not be recognizable on gross inspection but is typically extensive throughout the interlobular and intralobular

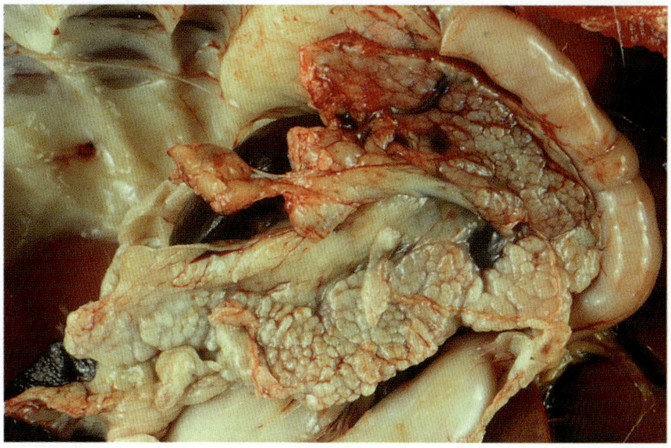

Figure 3-9 **Chronic interstitial pancreatitis** in a cat. The pancreas is pale with prominent nodularity.

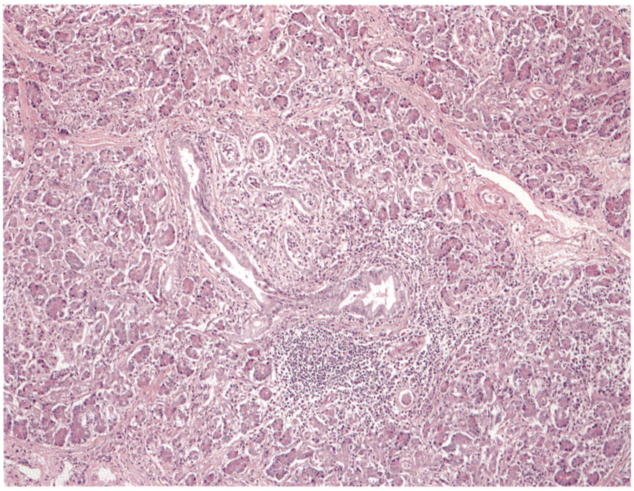

Figure 3-10 Histologic appearance of **chronic interstitial pancreatitis** in a cat. There is extensive interstitial and periductal fibrosis, and aggregates of lymphocytes that infiltrate through the acinar tissue.

septa. In exceptional cases, the whole organ may be converted into a shrunken, distorted, fibrous remnant. Histologically, the ducts may contain catarrhal exudate and are often enveloped by dense fibrous tissue (Fig. 3-10). Localized ductal stenoses and cystic dilations may occur. The epithelium of the ducts is hyperplastic, and there may be squamous metaplasia. Fibrous tissue extends from around the ducts to the interlobular stroma and subdivides many of the lobules. The interstitial tissues are permeated by leukocytes, chiefly lymphocytes and plasma cells. Acinar parenchyma atrophies as a consequence of fibrosis and ductal obstruction, but the islets are usually well preserved.

Chronic interstitial pancreatitis in cats often occurs in combination with cholangitis and inflammatory bowel disease in the syndrome of **triaditis**. This condition is thought to be a consequence of the unified outflow of the biliary and pancreatic ducts in this species, an anatomic feature that allows extension of inflammation and/or infection between organs. Inflammatory bowel disease may predispose to ascending bacterial infection, potentially through dysfunction of the sphincter of Oddi, although some evidence suggests that direct mucosal translocation of bacteria also occurs.

Inflammatory masses involving the pancreas and peripancreatic tissues are potential sequelae of chronic pancreatitis. A **pancreatic phlegmon** is a solid mass of indurated pancreas and adjacent tissues that results from inflammation, edema, and necrosis. A phlegmon may develop within a few days of onset of necrosis and typically resolves spontaneously within 2-3 weeks, after the necrotizing process subsides. Necrosis may cause some cavitation of a phlegmon.

Pseudocysts are intrapancreatic or peripancreatic, fluctuant pockets of pancreatic enzyme secretions, necrotic debris, inflammatory exudates, and blood. They are more common than abscesses as sequelae of acute or chronic pancreatic necrosis. Pseudocysts may develop within days to weeks of onset of pancreatic necrosis. Disruption of pancreatic ducts by inflammation (or necrosis) and duct occlusion contribute to their development. Pseudocysts are usually solitary and unilocular and may reach 10 cm in diameter, the wall formed by granulation tissue that matures to fibrous scar tissue. Unlike true cysts, there is no epithelial lining.

Pancreatic abscesses are pockets of purulent exudate and necrotic debris within the pancreas or adjacent tissues. Sterile abscesses may form within areas of intense liquefactive necrosis of parenchyma. Larvae of *Stephanurus dentatus*, migrating from the liver across the peritoneum to the perirenal area in pigs, may encyst in the pancreas and provoke abscessation. Septic abscesses may result from secondary infection of necrotic parenchyma or, less often, a pseudocyst. They can also arise by direct extension from a neighboring focus of infection, as they occasionally do from septic peritonitis and from perforated esophagogastric ulcers in pigs. Some may contain chyle as a result of lymphatic leakage, and gas bubbles occasionally may be present in abscesses.

Systemic **granulomatous infections** may involve the pancreas, but lesions are usually microscopic and less important than those in other viscera. Chronic sclerosing and granulomatous pancreatitis caused by zygomycotic fungi has been reported in dogs, and pyogranulomatous pancreatitis occurs in feline infectious peritonitis. Disseminated cryptococcosis may occasionally involve the pancreas of cats but is usually only associated with mild pyogranulomatous inflammation. Destructive granulomatous and eosinophilic pancreatitis can be a feature of multisystemic eosinophilic epitheliotropic syndrome of horses; a proportion of these cases may be associated with or precede the development of enteropathy-associated lymphoma.

In **pancreatolithiasis**, concretions form within the pancreatic duct system. The calculi are occasionally detected in cattle at slaughter, being slightly more common in cattle >4-years-old, but are rare in other species. The calculi are usually hard, white, numerous, and small, often resembling sand grains, and are chiefly composed of carbonates and phosphates of calcium and magnesium (Fig. 3-11). The calculi are associated with and may be a consequence of ductal inflammation, including that provoked by flukes, but are typically incidental findings, and rarely cause complete duct obstruction.

Exocrine atrophy

Although exocrine pancreatic atrophy may be secondary to other disorders of the pancreas or its ducts, primary pancreatic atrophy is also a common and significant consequence of nutrient deprivation, especially in those species genetically selected for rapid growth, and in populations subjected to intermittent or seasonal nutritional availability. Acinar atrophy occurs in starvation, prolonged anorexia, cachexia, protein-calorie deficiency, and maldigestive and malabsorptive syndromes. In protracted anorexia or starvation, the pancreas may be reduced to <10% of its normal mass; other tissues, particularly the liver, will also be reduced in mass in these conditions.

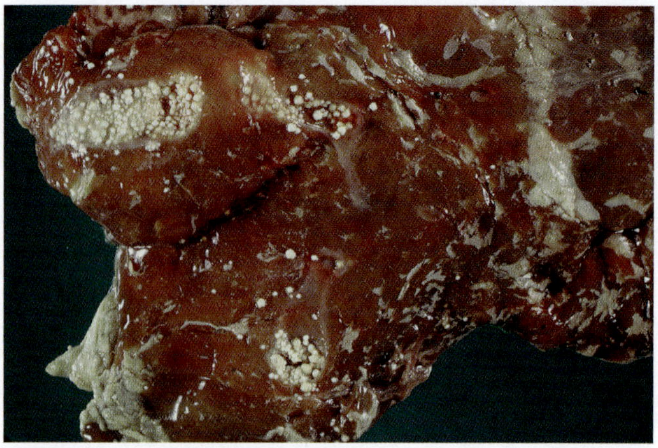

Figure 3-11 Ductal pancreatolithiasis in a cow.

The susceptibility of the exocrine pancreas to anatomic and functional atrophy is attributable to 2 characteristics. First, the pancreas utilizes large amounts of protein during normal activity, and protein stores in acinar cells are readily catabolized to compensate for nutritional shortfall, similar to the intestine, skin, and liver. Second, the pancreas is heavily dependent on neuroendocrine stimulus from the gastrointestinal and central nervous systems to maintain functional mass and is therefore prone to regression when stimulatory digestive signaling is suppressed.

Protein deficiency is a critical factor in nutritional atrophy of the exocrine pancreas and can induce rapid and profound regression of exocrine pancreatic tissue, regardless of overall caloric intake. Synthesis and secretion of digestive enzymes are reduced sequentially, with lipase depleted first, followed by trypsin; amylase is suppressed but not lost entirely. The morphologic effects can be profound, and in murine experimental models of protein deficiency, pancreatic mass has been shown to decrease by >75% in as little as 4 days, reflecting marked catabolism of nonessential cellular components without cell death. There is gradual disappearance of zymogen granules and reduced size of acinar cells, although early change may be subtle, with sparing of acini adjacent to islets as a result of trophic paracrine stimulation. Virtually all cellular organelles are altered; endoplasmic reticulum is reduced, mitochondrial size and shape varies widely, and the number of lysosomes is increased. With progression, there is loss and disorganization of acinar architecture, and dissociation of acinar cells into loose arrangement (Fig. 3-12). At this stage, nutritional correction can still restore acinar architecture and function, and this regeneration is mediated by the mammalian target of the rapamycin complex 1 signaling pathway, which suppresses autophagy and activates protein synthetic mechanisms when stimulated by branched-chain amino acids, in particular leucine. However, with chronicity the exocrine pancreas eventually loses this plasticity, and continued autophagy ultimately results in acinar cell apoptosis and tissue dissolution with attendant fibrosis, indicating irreversible change.

Aside from generalized protein malnutrition, **selective nutritional deficiency** may also cause significant atrophy of

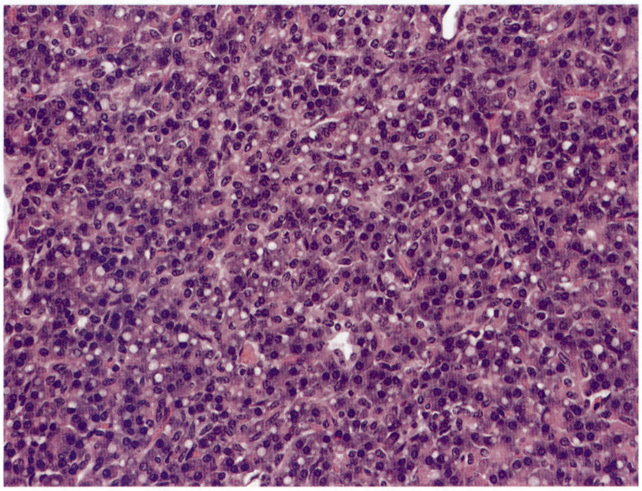

Figure 3-12 Exocrine pancreatic atrophy caused by starvation in a pig. Acinar cells are small and poorly granulated, and there is widespread dissociation of acinar architecture.

the exocrine pancreas. Selenium deficiency with or without concurrent vitamin E deficiency causes atrophic pancreatic lesions in chicks and mice in as little as 2 weeks, presumably reflecting oxidative stress caused by depletion of glutathione peroxidase. Histologically, there is acinar cell shrinkage and luminal dilation, together with abundant interstitial and periductal fibrosis. Inadequate intake of zinc, copper, vitamin A, and essential amino acids may also cause various degrees of exocrine atrophy.

Rapid atrophy also results from **obstruction of ductal drainage**, whether resulting from compression by adjacent inflammation or neoplasia, or from luminal occlusion by parasites, inflammatory exudate, or pancreatoliths. Atrophy in these cases is typically coupled with retrograde ductal ectasia, as well as proliferation and hyperplasia of new ductules.

Canine juvenile pancreatic atrophy. Pancreatic acinar atrophy of juvenile onset is a distinct subclass of exocrine insufficiency, which has in the past been designated erroneously as *pancreatic hypoplasia*. It was initially described in German Shepherd dogs and an association with particular alleles of the dog leukocyte antigen gene *DLA-DQB1* is recognized in this breed, as well as in Welsh Corgis. Familial predisposition has also been noted in Rough-Coated Collies, Chow Chows, and English Setters. The condition is reported sporadically in other breeds, including Beagles and Greyhounds. Clinical onset varies among breeds, with onset in English Setters in the neonatal period, whereas Beagles have more delayed onset with no signs of disease until animals are several months of age. Most cases do not develop EPI until 6-12 months of age. This variability in the age of onset suggests that juvenile pancreatic atrophy is a genetically diverse condition in different breeds. In a significant proportion of dogs, the clinical onset is precipitated by intercurrent gastrointestinal illness or a change in the normal household environment or diet.

Atrophy of the exocrine parenchyma is attended by intense but patchy infiltration by T lymphocytes, and the early stages of this process are sometimes referred to as *atrophic lymphocytic pancreatitis*. Cytotoxic CD8+ cells predominate over CD4+ cells in the pancreas as the disease progresses. The lymphocytes may be found both between and within acinar cells, and intraepithelial lymphocytes also may be observed within

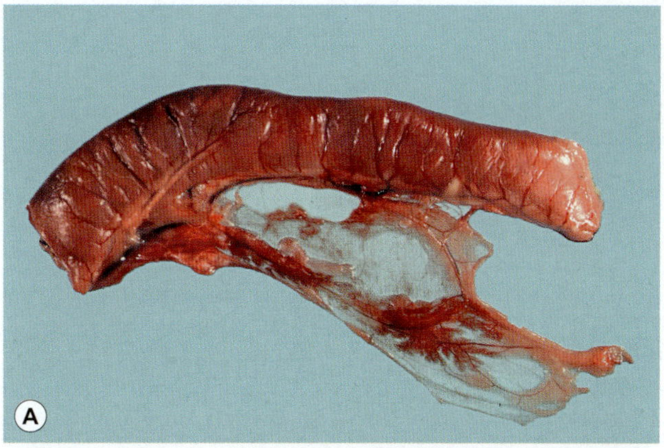

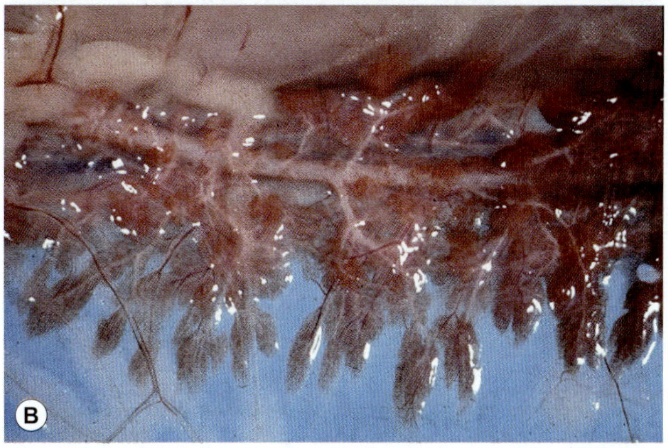

Figure 3-13 Juvenile pancreatic atrophy in a dog. **A.** Pancreatic volume is markedly reduced with only small remnants of tissue present in the duodenal mesentery. **B.** Detail of atrophic pancreas highlighting the prominent ductal architecture within the atrophic lobules.

the ductal epithelium. Lymphoid follicles may form in the parenchyma, and plasma cells, macrophages, and eosinophils may also infiltrate. Plasma cells are more commonly observed in areas of advanced parenchymal destruction. Reactive fibroplasia is not a significant feature of the process. *The nature of the lesion suggests that the condition may be an autoimmune cell-mediated process directed against acinar cells*, but there is currently no evidence to incriminate autoantibodies in the pathogenesis, and no inciting antigen has been identified.

By the time clinical signs emerge, exocrine atrophy is advanced and there is usually little remaining evidence of the preceding degenerative and inflammatory events. At autopsy of clinically affected dogs, the intestines are distended by bulky ingesta, reflecting maldigestion. The peritoneal cavity is devoid of fat, and transparency of the mesenteries allows the flimsy tissue of the atrophic pancreas to be recognized (Fig. 3-13A). The main ducts and their larger tributaries can be seen easily, and many of the smaller ducts are recognizable grossly with the aid of transillumination. The ducts are of normal size, length, and configuration. Surrounding them is a thin pink veil of residual acinar parenchyma (Fig. 3-13B). Microscopically, any remnant pancreatic lobules are small and composed of small acinar cells that stain darkly and do not assume a glandular arrangement. Tubular complexes—ductule-like structures lined by agranular, atrophic acinar cells—may be identifiable within the residual lobules. Occasional isolated lobules

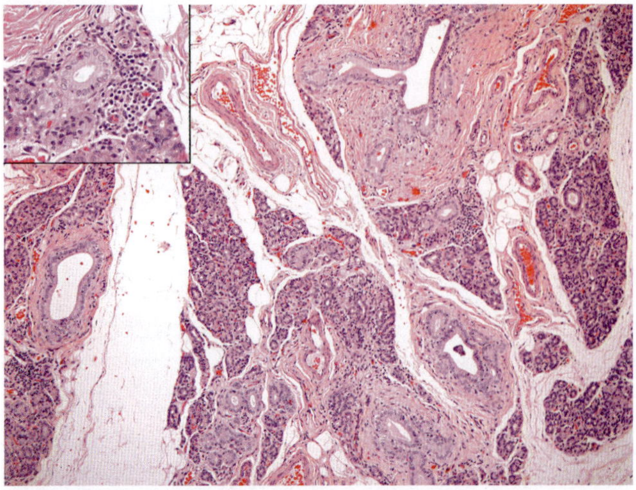

Figure 3-14 Histologic appearance of **juvenile pancreatic atrophy**. Pancreatic ducts are prominent among scant, atrophic exocrine tissue. Focal lymphocytic infiltrates are present within the interstitium (inset).

of normal appearance may be present. There is increased prominence of the connective tissues, ducts, islets, blood vessels, and nerves of the pancreas owing to condensation (Fig. 3-14). Mild interstitial and periductal fibrosis may be present, but fatty replacement of the organ is more common.

The islets are usually histologically normal, but dual loss of both exocrine and endocrine components has been reported in Greyhounds, several of which had insulin-dependent diabetes mellitus (IDDM). Diabetes mellitus has also been reported in a German Shepherd with juvenile pancreatic atrophy, and sporadically in other breeds. Haphazard distribution of various islet cell types, hyperplasia of pancreatic polypeptide and delta islet cells, and emergence of a profusion of nerve fibers immunoreactive for enkephalins and vasoactive intestinal peptide within islets have been noted in dogs with pancreatic acinar atrophy. The significance of these observations is uncertain.

Exocrine pancreatic insufficiency

Although the normal pancreas possesses abundant tissue reserve, significant impairment of exocrine function results in maldigestion and malabsorption of nutrients caused by reduced availability of pancreatic enzymes in the intestinal lumen. Exocrine pancreatic insufficiency (EPI) may occur as a consequence of congenital or acquired depletion of acinar tissue. The acquired form most commonly develops as a sequela to destruction of the exocrine pancreas and may be induced by almost any pancreatic disease of sufficient severity, including pancreatitis, toxic injury, localized and systemic infections, ductal disease (particularly in cases of obstruction), and neoplasia. Acquired EPI also may result from alterations in nutrient and neuroendocrine influences, reflecting the exocrine pancreas' heavy reliance on extrinsic signals for maintenance of functional mass. Physiologic activity of acinar tissue is dependent on a diverse range of stimuli—including vagal innervation, neuro-enteral signals from the gastrointestinal tract, and hormonal secretions from the pancreatic islets and the diffuse endocrine system of the gut—and withdrawal of these signals can lead to rapid decline in pancreatic function. Starvation or severe imbalances in protein, carbohydrate, and lipid intake may cause derangement of neurohormonal influences, as may structural or inflammatory disease of the gastrointestinal wall, to the detriment of pancreatic homeostasis.

Progression to insufficiency may be slow or rapid, but clinical disease only manifests when ~90% of secretory power is lost. Deficiency may be compensated in part by salivary and other alimentary secretions, delaying the onset of clinical disease.

EPI is observed commonly in dogs and is being recognized with increasing frequency in cats. Juvenile pancreatic atrophy is the most common cause of exocrine insufficiency in dogs. Excluding this syndrome, reports of EPI in dogs generally involve older age ranges, and both females and household pets are overrepresented. These risk factors are likely to reflect the higher incidence of acute necrotizing pancreatitis in such animals. For cats, although EPI is traditionally associated with chronic pancreatitis in older animals, the age range of affected cats is broad, with a number of cases detected at <6 months of age. Measurement of serum trypsin-like immunoreactivity is useful for clinical screening in dogs and cats; values <2.5 µg/L in dogs and <8 µg/L in cats are considered diagnostic, although there are occasional anomalous results. Isolated cases of EPI in horses are usually a result of chronic pancreatitis.

The most common clinical signs of EPI are loose feces and chronic weight loss despite a normal-to-voracious appetite. The haircoat may be of poor quality and marked muscle atrophy may be apparent in some animals. The feces are commonly pale, soft, voluminous, and malodorous, but may occasionally be watery or even of normal appearance. Steatorrhea is not invariably present, but can lead to greasy soiling of hair of the tail and perineum, especially in cats. There may be a pot-bellied appearance caused by bulky intestinal contents, and affected dogs are at increased risk of intestinal accidents, especially mesenteric torsion. Hepatic steatosis also may develop in dogs and cats with exocrine pancreatic atrophy.

Malassimilation of nutrients is not simply caused by failure of intraluminal digestion by pancreatic enzymes. Pancreatic proteases normally cleave proenzyme forms of small intestinal microvillar membrane enzymes and also inactivate or degrade exposed brush border enzymes. In several species, EPI is associated with increased activity of the jejunal brush border enzymes, sucrase and maltase, and an increase in high molecular weight microvillar membrane proteins, which are thought to be intestinal proenzymes. These alterations may impair the intestinal phase of digestion and absorption. Concurrent intestinal syndromes causing mucosal villus atrophy may compound the malabsorptive effects, and this phenomenon is often observed in neonates because of immaturity of the exocrine tissue. Increased activity of enterocyte lysosomal degradative enzymes also occurs in EPI, possibly to compensate for these changes. Protein synthesis by the jejunal mucosa is also reduced in affected dogs. The mechanism is unclear, but malnutrition and decreases in luminal trophic factors (e.g., pancreatic secretions and products of digestion) and humoral trophic factors (e.g., insulin, glucagon, gastrin) may be implicated. Intestinal transport mechanisms for monosaccharides, disaccharides, fatty acids, and amino acids are also disturbed, contributing to malabsorption. These functional changes in the intestinal mucosa are not usually associated with histologic lesions. However, dietary sensitivity leading to inflammatory bowel disease is also a potential consequence of EPI because there is increased intestinal mucosal exposure to antigenic macromolecules as a result of the deficiency of pancreatic proteases.

Small intestinal dysbiosis (also termed small intestinal bacterial overgrowth [SIBO]) frequently occurs with EPI, reflecting both the increased volume of undigested nutrients within the alimentary tract and the loss of the antimicrobial influence of pancreatic juice. Changes in intestinal flora are both quantitative and qualitative, and alterations in populations of *Bifidobacteriaceae*, *Enterococcaceae*, *Lactobacillaceae*, *Lachnospiraceae*, and *Ruminococcaceae* have been reported in dogs with EPI. The osmotic effect of excessive bacterial carbohydrate fermentation within the small intestine causes chronic or recurrent diarrhea, and this is often compounded by direct degradation of brush border enzymes, such as lactase, by bacterial proteases. Deconjugation of bile salts by aberrant intestinal flora impairs lipid processing, and the dysbiosis can damage the intestinal mucosa through induction of a mucosal immune response, as well as through direct effects of bacterial enzymes on enterocyte integrity. Enteric microorganisms also produce short-chain fatty acids and other nutrients that are important for gut health and function, and changes in intestinal bacterial populations can inhibit the synthesis of these factors. Dysbiosis alters normal production of cobalamin and folate by enteric flora, and both hypocobalaminemia and increased serum folate are common; cobalamin deficits are further exacerbated by impaired production of pancreas-derived intrinsic factor in cases of EPI. Intestinal flora alterations are recognized to be an important component in the development of inflammatory bowel disease in humans and domestic species, as well as having a wider influence on systemic immunity.

Diagnosis of small intestinal dysbiosis is problematic because histologic lesions are typically absent and there is considerable overlap between the flora in health and disease. Bacterial counts $>10^5$/mL in duodenal juice are historically deemed suggestive of bacterial overgrowth, although some investigators also consider anaerobe counts $>10^4$/mL as an additional diagnostic criterion. Quantitative PCR has shown promise for identifying specific alterations in intestinal flora that indicate dysbiosis, and panels that characterize the populations of important bacterial species have begun to supplant microbial culture as the quantification test of choice.

Parasitic diseases of the pancreas

The *pancreatic parenchyma* may be inadvertently affected by visceral migration of a variety of nematode parasites, although it is not specifically targeted in this process. As noted in previous sections, heavy burdens of *Strongylus equinus*, *S. edentatus*, and *Stephanurus dentatus* can cause a degree of pancreatitis, and abscesses can develop around migrating *S. dentatus*. Ascarid larvae may also journey through the pancreas occasionally, particularly in aberrant host species.

Various metazoan parasites may be found within the *pancreatic ducts* of domestic animals. Their significance depends on the extent to which they occlude the ducts, either by direct physical obstruction or by provoking inflammation and periductal fibrosis. Ascarids may invade the ducts from the intestine in pigs, horses, and dogs. *Thysanosoma actinioides*, the fringed tapeworm, may spill from the bile ducts of ruminants into the pancreatic ducts and small intestine. In heavy infestations in herbivores and carnivores, trematodes, such as *Dicrocoelium dendriticum*, *Opisthorchis tenuicollis*, *Opisthorchis felineus*, *Opisthorchis viverrini*, *Clonorchis sinensis*, *Platynosomum fastosum*, *Metorchis conjunctus*, and *Amphimerus pseudofelineus*, may be found in both the pancreatic and bile ducts.

Dicrocoelid flukes of the genus ***Eurytrema*** may inhabit both the pancreatic and biliary ducts but prefer the former. *Eurytrema pancreaticum* is the most important species and is a common parasite of the pancreatic and bile ducts of ruminants and other herbivores throughout Asia and South America, and is also reported in Russia and several African countries. *Eurytrema coelomaticum* is common in Brazilian cattle, where nearly 50% of the population are infected, and has been documented in ruminants in Asia. A third species, *Eurytrema cladorchis*, also occurs in cattle in southeast Asia. Snails and grasshoppers are the first and second intermediate hosts, respectively. The flukes are presumed to gain access to the pancreatic ducts directly from the duodenum following ingestion of an intermediate host.

Other species of *Eurytrema* are found in carnivores, wild herbivores, and birds. Pigs may harbor *Eurytrema* flukes of either herbivore or carnivore origin. *E. procyonis* is a common parasite of the pancreatic ducts of raccoons in many parts of the United States and has also been detected in red and gray foxes and domestic cats. In areas in which the fluke occurs, up to 14% of cats may be infected. The common garden snail, *Mesodon thyroidus*, and grasshoppers act as intermediate hosts. *E. procyonis* is infrequently reported in the bile ducts and gallbladder of cats.

Intraductal flukes may provoke only mild luminal and periductal inflammation, hyperplasia of the ductal epithelium, and periductal fibrosis. In some animals, however, there may be pronounced cording and dilation of the ducts and chronic interstitial pancreatitis, leading to near total loss of exocrine parenchyma and severe replacement fibrosis. Duct obstruction is largely thought to mediate the periductal fibrosis and the progressive atrophy of exocrine elements. Irritation of the ductal mucosa by the flukes and their ova and inflammation in response to dead flukes contribute to the progressive scarring.

E. pancreaticum preferentially targets the left pancreatic lobe in ruminants. Infestation of cattle with *E. pancreaticum* or *E. coelomaticum* may cause progressive wasting and emaciation, and death can occur with severe burdens. Although islets are preserved in most cases, progressive destruction culminating in diabetes mellitus has been reported in sheep. Glycosuria has also been noted in raccoons harboring *E. procyonis*. In cats, *E. procyonis* is found in the small- and medium-sized ducts of both pancreatic lobes, but the tail of the pancreas is usually more severely affected than the head. Duct obstruction causes substantial reduction in the volume of pancreatic secretions and in the content of digestive enzymes and bicarbonate. With heavy infestations, the major pancreatic duct may be greatly dilated and much of the organ is shrunken, pale, and fibrotic. However, infections in most cats are subclinical, and detection is by identification of typical dicrocoelid eggs with a single operculum in the feces.

Hyperplastic and neoplastic lesions of the exocrine pancreas

Unsurprisingly in an organ undergoing constant morphologic adaptation to nutritional influences, *hyperplasia is commonly encountered in the exocrine pancreas*, particularly in older dogs, cats, and cattle.

Exocrine hyperplasia typically occurs as small flecks or variably sized discrete nodules throughout the pancreatic parenchyma (Fig. 3-15). Their gray-white color and firm consistency contrast grossly with the color and texture of the

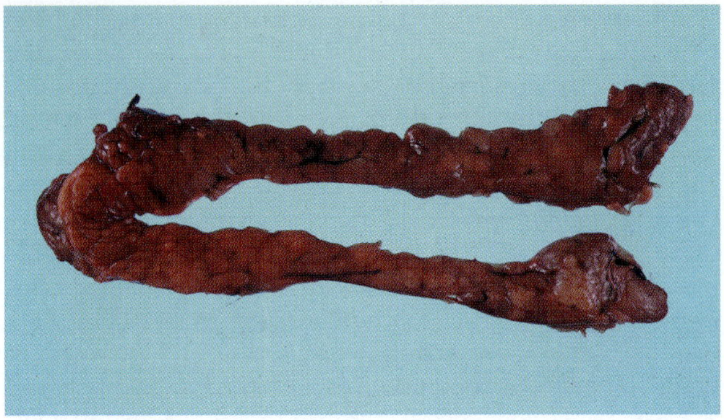

Figure 3-15 **Nodular pancreatic hyperplasia** in a dog.

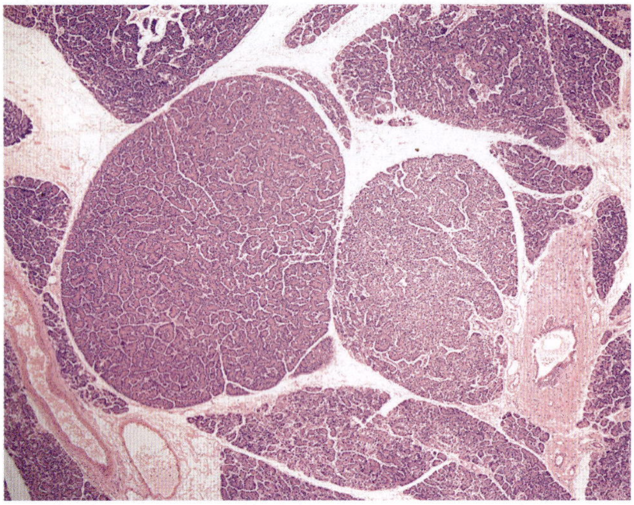

Figure 3-16 **Nodular pancreatic hyperplasia** in a cat. Acinar cells within the nodules are less intensely stained than the surrounding tissue and are diffusely enlarged with increased zymogen granulation.

normal pancreas. The lesions are incidental findings, and in most cases there is no identifiable preceding pancreatic insult. *Histologically, the hyperplastic tissue is nonencapsulated and does not compress surrounding parenchyma, differentiating it from an adenoma.* There may be a mosaic of normal and hyperplastic tissue within affected lobules. The hyperplastic cells may vary considerably in morphology and degree of zymogen granulation, but they are typically uniform within a single nodule (Fig. 3-16). Cells may be large and stain more intensely acidophilic than their normal counterparts, or alternatively may be small and poorly staining. The cells are often vacuolated, and there may be apparent loss of acinar architecture. Islet tissue is not affected, although exocrine hyperplasia may be particularly prominent in areas adjacent to islets, indicating a role for local trophic factors.

Hyperplasia of ductular epithelium is occasionally seen, often in an environment of chronic pancreatitis, exocrine parenchymal atrophy, and interstitial fibrosis, or within foci of nodular hyperplasia of the exocrine parenchyma. It is also reported as an aging phenomenon. The hyperplastic epithelium may protrude as papillae into the duct lumina, and the affected ducts may be dilated. Profound ductular hyperplasia often follows pancreatic outflow obstruction, with proliferation of small ductular branches amid abundant fibrous stroma similar to changes seen in the liver with biliary occlusion.

Exocrine pancreatic adenomas are rare, and some of those reported in older dogs, cats, and cattle may have been hyperplastic nodules. Adenomas are incidental findings at autopsy, and their rarity suggests that they do not give rise to pancreatic adenocarcinoma. Adenomas may protrude from the surface of the pancreas, and grossly, they more closely resemble normal parenchyma than do hyperplastic nodules. Tumors are usually encapsulated by fibrous tissue, and expansile growth causes compression of adjacent parenchyma. The histologic pattern of an adenoma may be predominantly tubular or rarely acinar. In the tubular type (which is thought to be derived from ductal epithelium), small or large cystic spaces are lined by cuboidal or columnar epithelial cells and may contain mucin. Mitoses are rare. Numerous recurrent pancreatic cysts suggestive of cystadenomas have been described in a cat with associated exocrine atrophy and eventual development of diabetes mellitus, presumably the result of compression atrophy of the adjacent parenchyma.

Exocrine pancreatic adenocarcinoma *is uncommon in all domestic animals*, but has predominantly been observed in dogs and cats. This malignancy generally occurs in older age but dogs as young as 3 years of age have been afflicted; a similar broad age range is reported in cats. Female dogs may be at slightly greater risk than male dogs.

Several factors have been implicated in the pathogenesis of pancreatic adenocarcinoma, although there is little work specific for domestic animals. Nitrosamines are found in a variety of foodstuffs, particularly processed meat containing nitrite preservatives, and their carcinogenic potential with regard to the pancreas is well established in humans and a range of animal models. Concurrent disease processes may also be associated with pancreatic carcinogenesis. There is a weak link between chronic pancreatitis and pancreatic malignancy, and an association with diabetes mellitus is well recognized in humans, but is yet to be proved unequivocally in veterinary species.

The most common clinical signs in dogs and cats with this neoplasm are nonspecific: anorexia, weight loss, depression, lethargy, and vomiting. As a result, diagnosis typically occurs late in the disease course. There is a tendency for these tumors to arise centrally within the gland or in the duodenal wing; and this may provoke early clinical signs of biliary obstruction and jaundice. Pancreatic panniculitis, a multifocal necrotizing steatitis affecting subcutaneous adipose tissue, has been observed in dogs with adenocarcinoma, although the syndrome may be seen with other pancreatic disease processes. In some cases, the foci of fat necrosis and inflammation are widely distributed throughout the body. A rare syndrome of paraneoplastic alopecia affecting the ventrum, legs, and often the face also has been observed in cats with pancreatic adenocarcinoma. The corneal layer of the affected skin is markedly atrophic and hypokeratotic, and there is attenuation of the follicular bulbs, resulting in a distinctive shiny appearance on gross examination. This condition is not pathognomonic for pancreatic adenocarcinoma, however, as it may also develop with intestinal and biliary malignancies. Pseudohyperparathyroidism leading to hypercalcemia has been reported in a dog with pancreatic adenocarcinoma, and progressive destruction of normal pancreatic tissue may eventually result in the development of diabetes mellitus or EPI. Episodes of hypoglycemia may occasionally occur, and in some instances this may reflect endocrine transdifferentiation within the neoplasm.

Pancreatic adenocarcinoma may occur as solitary or multiple masses, and although most are discrete, they may sometimes display poorly demarcated infiltration through the pancreatic parenchyma. The neoplasm is usually firmer than the adjacent pancreas. Some carcinomas are highly scirrhous and cannot be distinguished grossly from postinflammatory scarring. The cut surface of the neoplasm is typically heterogeneous and yellow to gray-white; areas of necrosis, hemorrhage, and mineralization may be obvious. Necrotic foci are often found in adipose tissue within and adjacent to primary and metastatic nodules, and there may be adhesions from the pancreas to adjacent tissues. Some tumors may contain mucin-filled cysts.

Four main histologic patterns of pancreatic adenocarcinoma are recognized: **acinar** (*the most common form*), **ductal/tubular**, **hyalinizing,** and **undifferentiated** (Fig. 3-17A-C). Well-differentiated *acinar* tumors are composed of small cells arranged into acini mimicking normal parenchyma, but poorly differentiated forms may be difficult to categorize, displaying scarce zymogen granulation, solid architecture with little acinus formation, and sometimes clear cell morphology. In the *ductal* forms, tubular or cystic structures resembling pancreatic ducts are formed by mucus-secreting cuboidal or columnar cells. Some tumors may contain localized ductular arrangements of well-differentiated cells that may be difficult to distinguish from the ductular response to incomplete obstruction. The *hyalinizing* form has been identified in the dog and is characterized histologically by large aggregates of PAS-negative hyaline material amid variable tumor architecture. *Undifferentiated* carcinomas do not form acinar or ductular structures. Some of these may be composed entirely of sheets of small anaplastic cells. These tumors usually have a higher mitotic count and a more pronounced fibrous stroma.

The *histogenesis* of pancreatic adenocarcinoma has not been elucidated in domestic animals. Traditionally, the tubular forms have been considered to be derived from ductal epithelium; tumor cells containing brightly eosinophilic zymogen granules have been interpreted to be of acinar origin. In practice, the histologic pattern often varies considerably within a single tumor, and this phenotypic variation can obscure the tumor origins. Based on limited cases, dual expression of cytokeratin-7 and cytokeratin-20 shows promise as an indicator of ductal origin, at least in cats.

The tendency of pancreatic adenocarcinomas to form tubules or acini usually permits their distinction from islet cell tumors, but cases of mixed acinar-endocrine cell neoplasia have been described in cats and dogs. Detection of eosinophilic granules in tumor cells permits distinction of pancreatic adenocarcinoma from invasive or metastatic adenocarcinoma of gastrointestinal or biliary origin. Electron microscopy or immunohistochemical analysis for secretory products may be needed to clarify the origin of poorly differentiated tumors, with most exocrine neoplasms in dogs displaying reactivity for amylase and carboxypeptidase. The normal acinar expression of claudin-5 junctional protein is lost in canine exocrine adenocarcinoma, and this observation may be useful as a marker of malignant transformation in equivocal cases.

The prognosis with pancreatic adenocarcinoma is grave; tumors metastasize widely and readily. The most common sites of metastasis are the liver, lungs, and regional lymph nodes, but other organs are often afflicted, including the spleen, kidneys, heart, pleura, ovaries, gastrointestinal tract, and brain. The tumors may also invade the wall of the adjacent duodenum or obstruct the pancreatic or bile ducts, and frequently disseminate through peritoneal implantation (Fig. 3-18). Neoplastic invasion of blood vessels and lymphatics may be

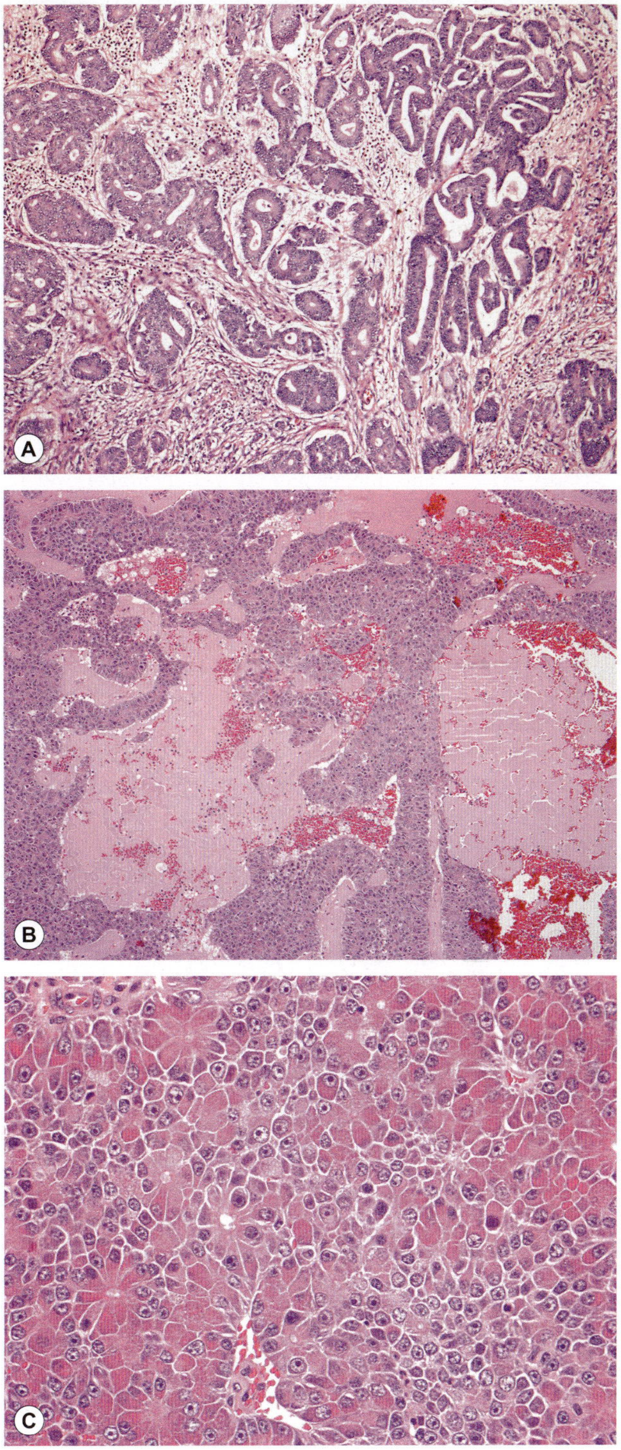

Figure 3-17 **A. Tubular form** of exocrine pancreatic adenocarcinoma accompanied by prominent scirrhous architecture. **B. Hyaline form** of exocrine pancreatic adenocarcinoma, with prominent interstitial aggregates of hyaline material. **C. Acinar form** of exocrine pancreatic adenocarcinoma, with the formation of atypical acinar structures.

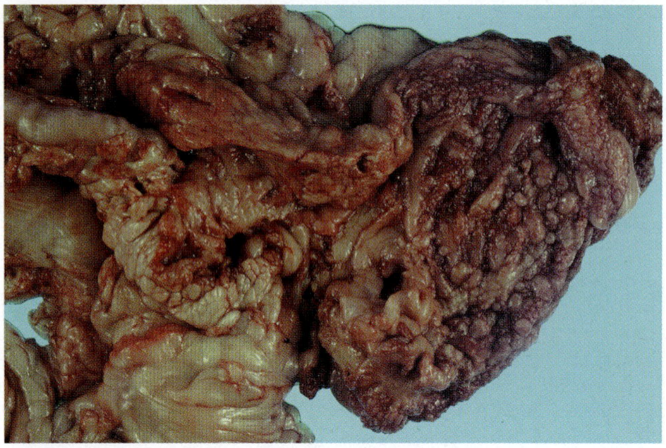

Figure 3-18 Exocrine pancreatic adenocarcinoma with peritoneal dissemination and implantation of metastatic foci over the attached mesentery and omentum.

obvious histologically in the pancreas (eFig. 3-5), with tumor cells often tracking in the perineural lymphatics, and they display a propensity to extend along visceral nerves to the dorsal ganglia. Prediction of metastatic behavior from histologic appearance is problematic, given that well-differentiated tumors can metastasize widely. A subset of cats survived for an extended period (>1 year), particularly if the neoplasm was excised prior to the onset of metastasis, but there was no correlation between survival and the histologic appearance of the tumor. However, based on limited numbers of reported cases, the hyalinizing form of adenocarcinoma may display less aggressive behavior.

Hepatopancreatic ampullary carcinoma has been reported in a single cat, as well as within many rhesus macaques from a single colony. Such tumors may cause obstruction of either or both ducts. In the cat, the tumor arose from the junction of the common bile duct and main pancreatic duct within the wall of the duodenum. The tumors affecting the macaques were typically aggressive, with duodenal invasion and metastasis to the lungs, lymph node, liver, and colon.

Nonepithelial neoplasms rarely arise in the pancreas. Those reported include fibrosarcoma, hemangiosarcoma, liposarcoma, neurofibroma, and neurofibrosarcoma.

Metastasis to the pancreas from malignancies arising elsewhere appears to be rare, but the paucity of reports may reflect lack of systematic examination and sampling of the organ at autopsy. The organ may become involved in hematopoietic malignancies and disseminated lymphoma. Neoplasms arising in the bile ducts, stomach, or duodenum, including intestinal lymphoma, may directly invade the pancreas.

ENDOCRINE PANCREAS

In pancreatic phylogeny, the development of the endocrine pancreas precedes that of the exocrine pancreas, commencing with establishment of the insulin-secreting β-cell population. In insects, concentrations of trehalose (a glucose homolog) in hemolymph are regulated by insulin-like and glucagon-like reactivities located exclusively within the brain. In more evolutionarily complex organisms, such as the protochordate lancelets, the cells that produce insulin-like peptide depart from the brain for the embryonic gut, accompanied by dispersed populations of other hormone-producing cell types. In the most primitive vertebrates—exemplified by hagfish—β-cells have separated completely from the gut tube to form islet-like structures in the lateral plate mesoderm supporting the gut tube, leaving behind the distributed population of other endocrine cell types. These dispersed cells in the gastrointestinal epithelium form the diffuse neuroendocrine system and are of physiologic significance and occasional clinical significance in domestic animals when neoplastic. Of particular relevance to the pancreas are the incretins: glucagon-like peptides (GLPs) produced by enteroendocrine K and L cells within the intestinal mucosa. These peptides, in particular GLP1, are released in response to nutrient passage, providing trophic stimulation for β-cells and transiently stimulating the release of insulin to maintain euglycemia. It is likely that these effects are mediated by the enteric nervous system.

In higher vertebrates, the distribution of islet-like colonies within the embryonic mesentery coincides with the regions of the gut tube involved in the budding of the biliary and pancreatic anlagen. Residual small clusters of islet cells may be seen in the gut and bile ducts in some mature animals as a reflection of this embryogenesis.

There is general consensus that growth and maturation of the pancreas in higher vertebrates, including ductular, acinar, and endocrine tissues, results from the differentiation of a common PDX1-positive endodermal stem cell, refuting the evolutionary evidence of a neural crest origin for pancreatic endocrine cells. The neural crest promotes differentiation of adjacent endoderm into insulin-secreting β-cells, but is otherwise not directly involved in the founding of islet cell populations. Neurogenin-3 is the key regulatory signal that initiates differentiation of endodermal precursors into endocrine cells.

As a broad definition for vertebrates, *an islet is a discrete glomerular organ composed of a variety of immunophenotypically distinct cells that produce specific endocrine, paracrine, and intracrine hormones*. The distribution of islets in the pancreas is not uniform in relation to the lobes or lobules or interstitial tissue. Islets have long been thought to have closed portal circulation, with blood flowing through the islets before perfusing the adjacent acinar tissue. However, in vivo studies have demonstrated that the vasculature is much more integrated, with extensive bidirectional flow of circulation between the islets and the adjacent exocrine parenchyma. This unified vascular architecture provides an environment for rich paracrine communication and enables a coordinated response to digestive and metabolic stimuli. Islet hormones directly regulate exocrine tissue, and this can often be appreciated histologically through the increased size and zymogen granulation of acinar cells adjacent to islets. Insulin provides the predominant exocrine trophic stimulus, with pancreatic polypeptide providing lesser influence; glucagon and somatostatin are inhibitory. Fenestration of the islet capillaries facilitates the permeation of hormones into the blood. With the exception of amyloidosis, pathologic changes related to the intra-islet vessels are not routinely sought, but specific responses to disease have been observed in the islet vasculature, such as the upregulation of endothelial cell adhesion molecules during type 1 diabetes mellitus.

There are 5 main **cell types** in the pancreatic islets identified by the hormones they produce. The **β-cells** that produce insulin and amylin (islet amyloid polypeptide) are the only ones present in all islets and comprise 60-70% of the islet cell population. The other types include **α-cells** that produce glucagon, **δ-cells** that produce somatostatin, **PP cells** that produce pancreatic polypeptide, and **ε-cells** that produce ghrelin. A range of other minor hormones, such as vasoactive intestinal peptide and urocortin-3, are also variably produced in the islets of domestic species.

The effects and interactions of the pancreatic hormones are complex (Table 3-1). **Insulin** is the major regulator of serum glucose and is released primarily in response to hyperglycemia. The hormone stimulates glucose uptake and glycogenesis by target cells, in particular hepatocytes, striated myocytes, fibroblasts, and adipocytes. Insulin has potent anabolic effects, promoting DNA, RNA, triglyceride, and protein synthesis, as well as suppressing proteolysis. Insulin also promotes cellular growth and differentiation in common with the insulin-related growth factors. The hypoglycemic effects of insulin are countered by **glucagon**, which promotes hepatocellular glycogenolysis and gluconeogenesis in response to low blood glucose, as well as stimulating lipolysis. Glucagon release is suppressed by **amylin**, which is cosecreted with insulin and also inhibits gastric secretory function and motility, as well as acting as a satiation signal. In contrast, **somatostatin** inhibits the release of glucagon, insulin, and pancreatic polypeptide and is thought to play a role in dampening the overall hormonal response to neuronal and nutritional stimuli. **Pancreatic polypeptide** and **ghrelin** exert opposing effects on the gastrointestinal tract: pancreatic polypeptide promotes satiety and delays gastric emptying as well as suppressing both gallbladder contraction and exocrine pancreatic function; ghrelin is orexigenic and stimulates gastrointestinal motility and secretory activity. Ghrelin is also produced by P/D1 cells in the gastric fundus, and secretion from this site may be responsible for most of the stimulatory gastrointestinal effects. Both pancreatic polypeptide and ghrelin also have minor paracrine influence over other islet cells, mediated in part through regulation of somatostatin secretion.

Synchronous islet response to secretory stimuli is largely achieved through a well-developed system of intercellular gap junctions that allows co-ordination of electrical signaling. This response is modified both qualitatively and quantitatively by a wide range of endocrine influences, including cholecystokinin, gastrin, and glucagon-like peptide 1, as well as the local paracrine effects of islet hormones as described previously. In addition to hormonal regulation, islet activity also may be modified by neuronal input. The islets are richly innervated by both

Table • 3-1

The effects and factors influencing secretion of the major islet hormones

HORMONE	PROMOTERS	INHIBITORS	MAJOR METABOLIC ACTIONS
Insulin	Glucose Amino acids Fatty acids Glucagon Incretins Parasympathetic stimulus	Somatostatin Leptin Ghrelin Sympathetic stimulus	↑ Glucose uptake ↑ Glycogenesis ↑ Protein anabolism ↑ Lipogenesis ↓ Glycogenolysis ↓ Gluconeogenesis ↓ Lipolysis
Glucagon	Amino acids Sympathetic stimulus	Glucose Insulin Amylin Somatostatin	↑ Glycogenolysis ↑ Gluconeogenesis ↑ Lipolysis ↑ Protein anabolism
Somatostatin	Glucose Fatty acids Amino acids Insulin Glucagon Ghrelin Urocortin-3 Incretins	Fatty acids Parasympathetic stimulus Pancreatic polypeptide	↓ Gastrointestinal motility and secretion ↓ Exocrine pancreatic secretion ↓ Gallbladder contraction
Pancreatic polypeptide	Ingesta Parasympathetic stimulus	Glucose Somatostatin	↑ Gastric acid secretion ↑ Gallbladder contraction ↓ Gastric motility ↓ Exocrine pancreatic secretion ↓ Appetite
Ghrelin	Fasting	Amylin Obesity	↑ Appetite ↑ Gastrointestinal motility and secretion ↑ Growth hormone secretion
Amylin (cosecreted with insulin)	Glucose Amino acids Fatty acids Glucagon Incretins Parasympathetic stimulus	Somatostatin	↓ Appetite ↓ Gastrointestinal motility and secretion

adrenergic and cholinergic autonomic systems, with dominant influence from the vagus nerve. Autonomic ganglia are distributed in the interstitial tissue and may contain islet tissue in a common capsule. Insulin secretion is stimulated by parasympathetic neurotransmitters and inhibited by sympathetic signals. In addition, the enteric nervous system, which may act autonomously from the central nervous system input, is important in enteropancreatic reflexes and exocrine secretion.

The arrangement of cells and their relative numbers are described for many vertebrate species, but there are inconsistencies in the descriptions between individuals and species that may reflect in part cellular plasticity, validity of immune reactants, or physiologic variability. Developmentally, islet cell distribution appears to reflect differential expression of cell adhesion molecules, in particular E-cadherin expression on β-cells and neural cell adhesion molecule expression on non–β-cells. However, it is likely that a degree of architectural plasticity persists in adult life, and alterations in cellular composition may occur as adaptations to changing physiologic and pathologic demands. The proliferative capacity of islet cells declines rapidly once cell populations are established in neonates, but a degree of regenerative ability persists in adulthood. Replication of β-cells can be experimentally stimulated by exposure to glucose, D-mannose, essential amino acids, glucocorticoids, gastrin, cholescystokinin, growth hormone, prolactin, insulin-like growth factors (IGF1 and IGF2), platelet-derived growth factor, epidermal growth factor, and indeed by insulin itself via stimulation of the IGF1 receptor. New islet cells may also arise from ductular hyperplasia and transdifferentiation. Despite this, proliferation is generally limited following pancreatic injury and is often insufficient to restore endocrine homeostasis following widespread islet destruction.

The peculiarities of endocrine tissue distribution in different domestic species warrant discussion. In **dogs**, there are fewer islets in the left lobe and larger compact islets in the tail of the organ. Most β-cells are in islets, but ~25% are interstitial in acinar tissue, probably mixed with other uncharacterized endocrine cells. The interstitial cells occur singly or in small clusters and may be sparse or abundant; their numbers and distribution may be correlated with systemic physiologic circumstances, but the distribution does not appear to be linked with abnormal insulin function.

In **cats**, the islets are large, of irregular shape and composed mainly of β-cells. Encapsulated interlobular islets can be seen in connective tissues and in and adjacent to ganglia. Mixed cell types, solitary or in small clusters, may be seen in ductal lining epithelium, in ganglia and nerves, or abundantly in the interstitium of acinar tissue.

In **ruminants**, including cattle, sheep, goats, deer, and buffalo, there are 2 populations of islets, large and small, throughout fetal development and extending into mature life. The cellular composition of fetal islets has been reported for sheep and cattle, with features that suggest that islet ontogeny may differ among species. The large islets are of round or irregular shape, measuring 200-1600 µm in fetal calves, and enmeshed in interlobular and periductal connective tissue without direct contact with acinar tissue (Fig. 3-19). They develop more or less concurrently with more regular small islets, but unlike their smaller counterparts, they do not continue postnatal proliferation and they are rarely encountered in adult pancreata. They are composed almost entirely of β-cells and are reminiscent of the initial β-cell organ of the embryonic gut tube in early vertebrates.

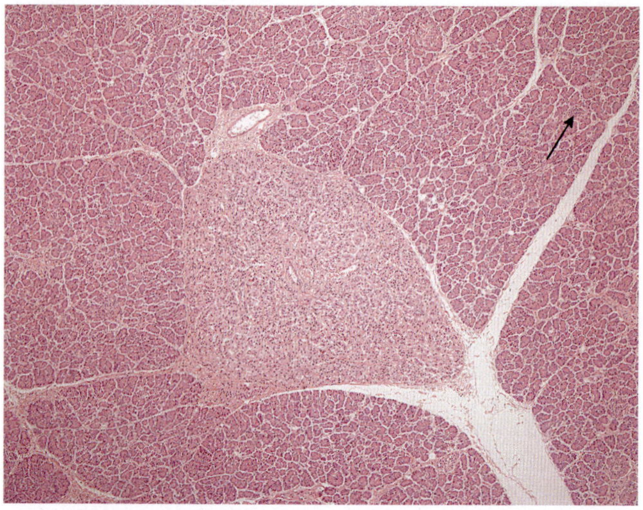

Figure 3-19 **Large islet** within the interlobular septa of the pancreas of a calf. A small islet is present within the adjacent exocrine tissue (arrow).

The small islets, which are usually <200 µm in size and are developmentally embedded in acinar tissue, contain β-cells with variable populations of α-cells, δ-cells, and PP cells. The β-cells display secretory granules at about the end of the first trimester, but remarkably they degranulate in late gestation and remain so for 2-6 weeks thereafter, when granulation is re-established. For several weeks postnatally, the small islets are difficult to distinguish from acinar tissue except by dense cellularity and indifferent cell character.

Many of the peculiarities of the ruminant endocrine pancreas are likely to reflect adaptation to different energy sources during fetal and postnatal life. Fructose is the most abundant hexose sugar in the fetal fluids of ungulate animals, including ruminants and pigs, but is negligible in humans and other species. Intravital exposure of the ovine fetus to either glucose or fructose in late gestation provokes minimal increase in plasma insulin, but postnatally, the fructogenic energy substrate of the ovine fetus is quickly replaced by glucose resulting in altered activity of islet hormones, with an increase in insulin responsiveness to glucose and—at least initially—short-chain fatty acids.

Like other endocrine glands, dysfunction of pancreatic hormones typically reflects excessive or insufficient secretion. In the case of the endocrine pancreas, excess is usually the result of unregulated neoplastic disease; insufficiency is almost exclusively restricted to insulin and is the important syndrome of diabetes mellitus. It is now established that, for some forms of diabetes mellitus, the thread of causation may stretch back to the pregnant uterus and that the intrauterine environment impacts the development of the endocrine pancreas and the β-cells. Influences such as maternal obesity and increased glucocorticoid exposure affect fetal islet development at different stages, with the common outcome of reduced islet size, reduced cell number, and altered responsiveness to higher glycemic levels during gestation and postnatally. Furthermore, intrauterine growth retardation resulting from a number of causes has been linked to epigenetic alterations that predispose to both β-cell dysfunction and insulin resistance in peripheral tissues.

Diabetes mellitus

Diabetes mellitus is a metabolic syndrome of sustained hyperglycemia, weight loss, polyphagia, and polyuria. Hyperglycemia may result from failure to synthesize or release adequate insulin in response to glucose or from resistance of tissues to insulin stimulation, especially the liver, striated muscle (including cardiac myocytes), and adipose tissue. Reduced end-organ sensitivity to insulin secretion suppresses cellular extraction of glucose from blood, consequentially leading to persistent elevation of blood glucose concentrations. In addition to impaired glucose entry into cells, hyperglycemia also reflects diminished glucose oxidation, enhanced glycogenolysis, and increased gluconeogenesis from amino acid sources. Diabetes mellitus is typically preceded by a period of impaired glucose tolerance, in which return to euglycemia after administration of glucose is slowed or incomplete. This prediabetic state is rarely detected in domestic animals, and most animals are only diagnosed after progression to clinical diabetes mellitus, by which time chronic hyperglycemia may induce significant degenerative changes in other organs.

Diabetes mellitus in veterinary medicine is broadly classified into 2 main categories—insulin-deficient diabetes mellitus (type 1) and insulin-resistant diabetes mellitus (type 2). Classification systems continue to evolve in recognition of the complexity of diabetic syndromes, and direct comparisons between veterinary and human disease (including nonobese mouse models) may not be entirely appropriate. In particular, longitudinal studies investigating the clinically silent phase of the disease in domestic animals are lacking, and so causal factors and early pathogenesis are poorly defined. The classification system for diabetes mellitus in dogs and cats devised by the European Society of Veterinary Endocrinology Project ALIVE (Agreeing Language in Veterinary Endocrinology) provides a comprehensive overview of potential etiological factors (Table 3-2). *It is important to note that more than one factor may contribute to the pathogenesis of diabetes mellitus*.

Type 1 diabetes mellitus is defined as hyperglycemia resulting from insulin deficiency, because of β-cell dysfunction, islet hypoplasia, or—more typically—death or destruction of β-cells. Clinically, this category is labeled as **IDDM**. Loss of β-cells can result from a wide range of insults, including viral infection, neoplasia, toxicity, and immune-mediated disease, but in many cases the depletion is idiopathic. Pancreatitis is often associated with the development of type 1 diabetes mellitus, but although this has long been supposed to reflect extension of inflammation from the exocrine tissue and islet bystander damage, the islet cell loss in such cases appears to be selective for β-cells and is not accompanied by insulitis, and hence, this β-cell depletion may involve other mechanisms or even represent a distinct pathologic process.

Type 2 diabetes mellitus is a complex multifactorial disease but is primarily seen as resistance to insulin stimulus in the face of a normal glycemic load. *Glycemic dysregulation in type 2 diabetes mellitus typically reflects both insensitivity of peripheral tissues to insulin signaling and diminished insulin secretion; there is thus some overlap in the pathogenesis of type 1 and 2 disease, although the interrelationship and relative importance of these factors remain uncertain*. Impaired insulin responsiveness suppresses glucose uptake by tissues—in particular skeletal muscle—following eating, resulting in sustained hyperglycemia. Insulin resistance also unshackles the normal insulinic restraint of gluconeogenesis within the liver, and this continued production of glucose exacerbates hyperglycemia. Lipolysis of adipose tissue proceeds unchecked without insulin regulation, and elevated circulating fatty acids may contribute to insulin resistance and also cause

Table • 3-2

Etiologic classification of diabetes mellitus in dogs and cats

TYPE	SUBCATEGORY

Insulin-deficient diabetes mellitus (β-cell–related disorders)	• Reduced insulin secretion
	  • β-Cell dysfunction
	  • β-Cell destruction
	    • Immune mediated
	    • β-Cell loss due to exocrine pancreatic disease
	      • Pancreatitis
	      • Neoplasia
	      • Idiopathic
	    • Toxicity (diazoxide)
	    • Infection
	    • Idiopathic
	  • β-Cell death (apoptosis)
	    • Glucotoxicity
	    • Lipotoxicty
	    • Idiopathic
	  • β-Cell aplasia/abiotrophy/hypoplasia
	• Production of defective insulin

Insulin-resistant diabetes mellitus (target organ–related disorders)	• Endocrine antagonism
	  • Growth hormone
	    • Endogenous hypersecretion
	      • Pituitary origin
	      • Mammary origin
	    • Exogenous growth hormone
	  • Steroid hormones
	    • Glucocorticoids
	      • Endogenous hypersecretion
	      • Exogenous glucocorticoids
	    • Progestagens
	      • Luteal phase secretion
	        – Pregnancy
	        – Diestrus (dog)
	      • Exogenous progestins
	    • Other
	  • Catecholamines
	  • Thyroid hormone
	    • Hyperthyroidism
	• Obesity
	• Drugs
	  • Thiazide diuretics
	  • β-Adrenergic agonists
	• Inflammatory mediators
	• Disorders of receptor and intracellular signaling

From European Society of Veterinary Endocrinology. Project ALIVE: Etiologic classification of diabetes mellitus. https://www.esve.org/alive/search.aspx.

β-cell lipotoxicity through oxidative injury and generation of ceramides.

The β-cells initially attempt to compensate for peripheral resistance by boosting insulin secretion, but eventually, they become refractory to hyperglycemic stimuli. The glucotoxic effects of persistent hyperglycemia can damage β-cells by increasing oxidative stress, altering gene transcription and secretory signaling, and inducing inflammatory and apoptotic pathways. Ultimately, these processes result in impaired glucose-induced insulin secretion and reduced β-cell functional mass, further promoting a persistent hyperglycemic state.

Although genetic factors participate in development of type 2 diabetes mellitus, many veterinary cases are further promoted by comorbidities, such as obesity, pancreatic disease, or other endocrine imbalances. Excess glucocorticoids, growth hormone, progesterone, and, to a lesser degree, thyroid hormone can all antagonize the effects of insulin on peripheral tissues. The influence of obesity on insulin resistance varies between species: cats are highly susceptible to obesity-related dysregulation of glycemic control; dogs are relatively unaffected.

Lesions within the islets can be subtle in diabetes mellitus. In most cases, the islets are small with a reduced or absent β-cell population, but other endocrine cells are often spared. The islets may become fibrotic, but frank insulitis is relatively uncommon, and is generally limited to a mild lymphocytic infiltrate when present.

Metabolic derangement caused by diabetes mellitus induces pathologic changes in many organs throughout the body, reflecting the ubiquity of glucose dependence. Muscle wastage occurs because of catabolism of proteins for glucogenic substrates, and insulin deficits also stimulate lipolysis and fatty acid mobilization from adipose tissue. Under normal circumstances, these lipids are processed into lipoproteins within the liver, but in diabetic animals this energy-intensive pathway is impaired by the inability to use glucose effectively. Hepatic lipidosis and hypertriglyceridemia result, and steatosis also develops within the proximal renal tubular epithelium. Metabolic dysfunction causes intracellular glycogen accumulation and vacuolation in many organs, particularly in rapidly progressing cases. Tissues affected include islet cells, renal tubules (especially the loops of Henle and distal convoluted tubules), and the pancreatic and biliary ductal epithelium (Figs. 3-20 and 3-21). In the dog, hepatocytes may also display intranuclear glycogen vacuolation, and islets may become fibrotic. Cataracts develop rapidly in the dog and also sporadically in cats, reflecting osmotic stress within the lens caused by accumulation of the glucose metabolite sorbitol. Osmotic diuresis and dehydration develop once the renal threshold for glucose resorption is exceeded, and loss of caloric stores through the urine contributes to the wasting effects of diabetes. Electrolyte disturbances, particularly hypokalemia, may occur because of solute loss in the urine.

In addition to the effects of metabolic dysregulation, chronic hyperglycemia itself can also induce a range of deleterious effects on tissues. Hyperosmotic cytoplasmic swelling occurs because of intracellular accumulation of polyols such as sorbitol derived from excessive glucose metabolism. Hyperglycemia promotes glycation of tissue proteins, especially within myelin sheaths and blood vessels, resulting in demyelination and loss of vascular compliance. Advanced glycation end products may also induce expression of proinflammatory cytokines by endothelial cells and macrophages, promoting inflammation. Oxidative stress within tissues is increased with diabetes mellitus, and excess glucose also stimulates the proinflammatory protein kinase C signaling pathway. These effects of hyperglycemia appear to be particularly important in the pathogenesis of *diabetic neuropathy*. Up to 8% of diabetic cats display evidence of this disorder, typically manifesting as a symmetric plantigrade hindlimb stance that is reversible in mild cases, although if unchecked this may progress to permanent paraparesis,

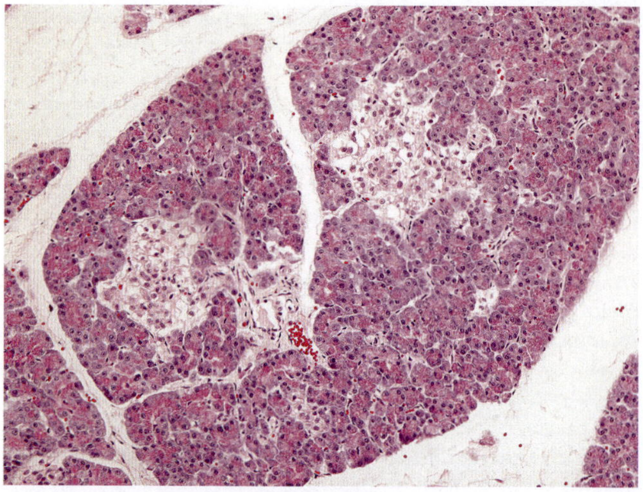

Figure 3-20 Pancreas from a cat with diabetes mellitus with **glycogen vacuolation** within islets.

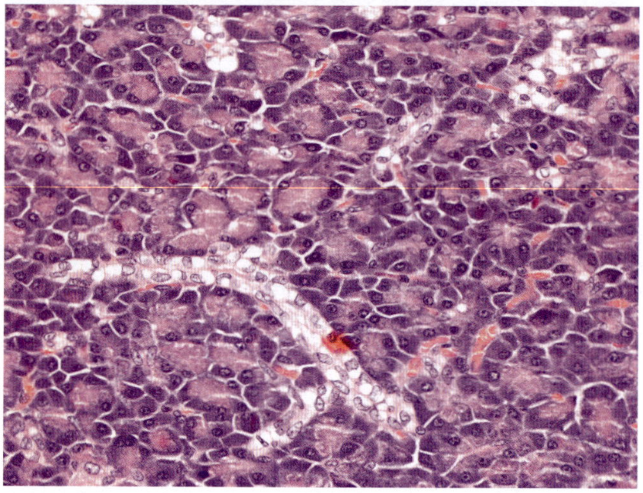

Figure 3-21 **Vacuolation** of pancreatic ductular epithelium in a dog with diabetes.

hyporeflexia, and proprioceptive deficits. *Diabetic nephropathy*, characterized by glomerulosclerosis, mesangial proliferation, and hyaline thickening of vascular basement membranes, may also develop as a response to hyperfiltration and derangement of local hemodynamic regulators, such as nitric oxide and the renin-angiotensin-aldosterone pathway. *Diabetic retinopathy* is diagnosed infrequently in dogs and only manifests 5 years or more after the onset of diabetes. The retinal vascular changes comprise venous dilation and tortuosity, saccular capillary microaneurysms, and focal hemorrhages that are most severe at the posterior pole. These lesions resemble the early nonproliferative stages of human diabetic retinopathy.

Significant morbidity and mortality accompany the metabolic dysfunction of diabetes mellitus, and death may result from *ketoacidosis*, wherein ketones such as β-hydroxybutyric acid and acetone are generated by the liver as it attempts to provide an alternative lipid-derived energy source as a replacement for glucose. Insulin deficiency suppresses the use of ketones by peripheral tissues while also stimulating lipolysis and ketogenesis within the liver, resulting in the accumulation of ketones within the circulation. This ketosis compounds the hyperosmolality and osmotic diuresis of diabetes, exacerbating dehydration, as well as causing marked acidosis and hypokalemia. If untreated, these physiologic derangements are frequently fatal, and disease progression is often exacerbated by renal failure, as well as thromboembolism caused by circulatory stasis and activation of clotting factors. In situations in which a low level of insulin efficacy persists, animals may become moribund in the absence of ketosis (nonketotic hyperosmolar diabetes), reflecting the hyperosmolar effects of marked hyperglycemia.

Early-onset diabetes mellitus has been reported in **dogs** that is consistent with the type 1 classification. Onset at birth is described in the Keeshond as a probable autosomal recessive defect. Juvenile onset is also described in a family of Samoyeds and in a single Chow Chow; these are classified as islet cell hypoplasia with diminished α- and β-cells. Diabetes mellitus with islet atrophy also occurs in some Greyhounds with juvenile pancreatic atrophy, discussed earlier. More typically, insulin-dependent diabetes develops in older dogs, and a breed predisposition is present in Cairn and Tibetan Terriers, Miniature Poodles, Miniature Schnauzers, and Rottweilers among others, indicating that there is a genetic component to spontaneous cases. Specific allelic variants in major histocompatibility complex genes have been shown to increase susceptibility in affected breeds. Although it has long been presumed that immune-mediated destruction is responsible for loss of β-cells in canine diabetes mellitus, the evidence for this is surprisingly tenuous. Autoantibodies against insulin and β-cell antigens have been reported in a minority of diabetic dogs, but can also be detected in some nondiabetic animals. Moreover, leukocytes are rarely identified in islets of diabetic dogs, despite ongoing β-cell loss. It therefore remains uncertain how much of a role autoimmunity plays in the pathogenesis of canine type 1 diabetes mellitus.

Many cases of canine diabetes mellitus are associated with concurrent or previous episodes of pancreatitis. Insulin resistance caused by glucose counter-regulatory hormones—such as glucocorticoids and progestagens derived from endogenous or exogenous sources—is also well documented in dogs, and these effects can precipitate the onset of type 2 diabetes mellitus. *Diestrus- and gestation-associated diabetes occurs in the female dog in the latter half of pregnancy*; it may be exacerbated by diets high in fat content. Progesterone released during pregnancy and pseudopregnancy stimulates the mammary gland to produce growth hormone, which is largely responsible for insulin resistance in this form of diabetes mellitus. Hormone profiles during diestrus, pseudopregnancy, and pregnancy are identical, but insulin insensitivity is more pronounced during pregnancy, suggesting that other factors may be involved beyond pure hormonal antagonism. Spontaneous remission can occur following completion of pregnancy or diestrus, but these female dogs frequently develop persistent diabetes mellitus during subsequent cycles.

Diabetes mellitus is relatively common in the **cat** and is most prevalent in older males, particularly Burmese. Obesity is recognized as a major risk factor, with obese cats 2-4× more likely to develop diabetes mellitus. The decline in function and number of β-cells characteristic of type 2 disease can often be ameliorated by modifying the diet to high protein and low carbohydrate content. Hormonal insulin antagonism is involved in many cases of type 2 disease in cats, especially hypersomatotropism, which is reported to be present in 15-32% of diabetic cats. Hypercortisolism, hyperprogesteronism, and hyperthyroidism are also sometimes associated with diabetes mellitus. Type 1 diabetes mellitus as a consequence of pancreatitis or pancreatic neoplasia appears to be rare in cats but may be under-recognized, particularly given that pancreatitis is more common in this species than historically assumed.

Amyloid deposits are commonly observed in feline islets (Fig. 3-22) and represent accumulation of insoluble aggregates of *amylin* (islet amyloid polypeptide), a digestive regulatory hormone that is cosecreted with insulin. The significance of islet amyloid in the pathogenesis of diabetes mellitus is uncertain, but the prevalence of amyloid is similar in diabetic and nondiabetic animals; therefore, *the finding of islet amyloidosis is not a useful criterion for confirmation of feline diabetes mellitus*. Diabetic cats have selective β-cell depletion and occasionally a degree of lymphocytic insulitis, and these features are more significant indicators of disease.

Diabetes mellitus has long been recognized in **cattle** persistently infected by foot-and-mouth disease virus. Reports also implicate bovine viral diarrhea virus in the pathogenesis of diabetes mellitus, and in view of the wide distribution and frequent persistence of BVDV infection, under-reporting of diabetic sequelae seems likely. Regardless, these observations support a role for immunoparticipant factors in the pathogenesis of many cases of bovine diabetes mellitus. Under the current classification system, the disease in cattle corresponds to type 1 diabetes, displaying immunodestruction of β-cells and retention of insulin responsiveness in tissues. Affected cattle have progressive emaciation, polydipsia, polyuria, and persistent hyperglycemia, reduced glucose tolerance, and glycosuria. Histologically, the cellularity of islets is reduced, with hydropic change and decreased granularity particularly affecting the β-cells. Lymphocytes infiltrate both small and large islets in all lobes in early stages, along with a small population of macrophages and plasma cells. Mild interlobular and interacinar fibrosis accompanies atrophy of acinar cells and reduction of zymogen granulation. In more chronic cases, endocrine cells including β-cells appear to be increased in periductal tissue, perhaps as a compensatory response.

Diabetes mellitus is rare in the **horse**. IDDM has been associated with a presumed autoimmune polyendocrine syndrome involving the pancreas, adrenal cortex, adrenal medulla, and thyroid gland. Chronic pancreatitis may reduce the islet-cell mass sufficiently to cause diabetes mellitus, and the condition

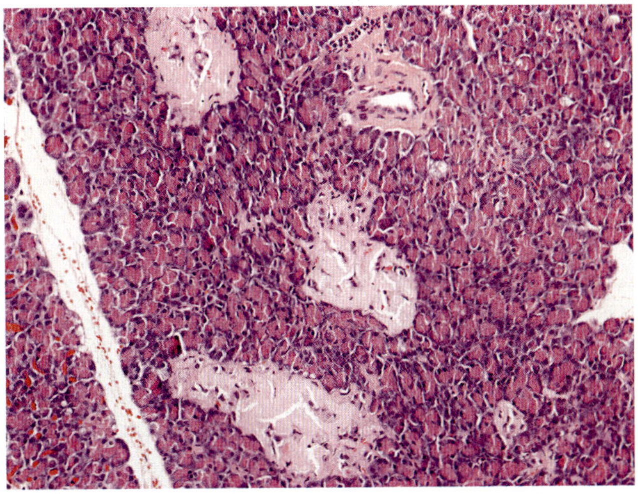

Figure 3-22 Islet amyloid deposition in a cat with diabetes mellitus.

has also been described in association with granulosa-cell tumors of the ovary and pheochromocytomas.

Insulin dysregulation and resistance are key features of **equine metabolic syndrome**, a common disorder in equids. Affected animals have elevated resting and postprandial insulin levels and may display impaired glucose regulation, but do not develop the marked and persistent hyperglycemia characteristic of overt diabetes mellitus. Obese or inactive animals are at increased risk of developing equine metabolic syndrome, potentially reflecting altered activity of adipokines, such as leptin and adiponectin, but it can also occur in non-obese equids. Genetic and epigenetic predispositions also contribute to the disease, with increased susceptibility reported in ponies, miniature horses, Morgans, Tennessee Walking Horses, and Arabians. Pituitary pars intermedia dysfunction may exacerbate insulin dysregulation and often occurs concurrently with equine metabolic syndrome. Laminitis is the most significant clinical consequence of equine metabolic syndrome and is thought to reflect the stimulatory effects of hyperinsulinemia on IGF receptors in the hoof lamellae.

Hyperplastic and neoplastic diseases of the endocrine pancreas

Islet hyperplasia and nesidioblastosis

Islet hyperplasia in domestic animals is often subtle and difficult to distinguish from normal islet variability, but has been reported in humans and other primates, mice, rats, hamsters, and horses. Histologically, the islets are enlarged—in some cases comprising up to 40% of the pancreatic tissue—and may compress the surrounding exocrine parenchyma (eFig. 3-6). The change is thought to represent a compensatory phenomenon, and in humans it may be observed in infants born of diabetic mothers, as well as those with hyperinsulinemic hypoglycemia, chronic pancreatitis, Zollinger-Ellison syndrome, and multiple endocrine neoplasia (MEN). In animals, the associations are less clear, although hyperplastic islets have been reported with pancreatic atrophy and fibrosis, potentially reflecting a nonspecific regenerative stimulus. Hyperplasia is also documented in aged rats and horses, sedentary obese rats, and hamsters treated with corticosteroids.

Nesidioblastosis (Fig. 3-23) *is described as a non-neoplastic proliferation of islet and ductular tissue* and has been reported sporadically in domestic animals, particularly the dog. Newly formed islet cells appear to bud from proliferating epithelium of small intralobular ductules and thence migrate and organize into discrete islets. Occasionally, the islet structures coalesce to form large aggregates, and these may appear similar to large islets observed in young ruminants. The majority of cells in the nesidioblastic foci are β-cells, but the other major cell types are also represented to a variable degree. The condition generally occurs as an aberrant regenerative response and may be induced by a range of pancreatic insults, including partial pancreatectomy, ectopic autotransplantation of pancreatic tissue, and ductular occlusion. It may also be observed in animals without other apparent pancreatic disease. Overexpression of *islet neogenesis-associated protein* appears to be important in the pathogenesis of nesidioblastosis; this protein is strongly expressed in nesidioblastic lesions and has been shown experimentally to induce islet differentiation in ductular epithelial cells. Hyperinsulinemic hypoglycemia is a common consequence of nesidioblastosis in humans, and although *most cases in animals are typically endocrinologically inactive*, there are reports of hypoglycemia in dogs and cats that resolve following lesion resection.

Pancreatic endocrine neoplasia

Pancreatic endocrine neoplasms are sporadically identified in domestic animals, particularly dogs, which may occasionally develop numerous independent tumors. They also occur as a component of the rare syndrome of **MEN** in several species. In these cases, there may be concurrent neoplasia or hyperplasia of the pituitary and parathyroid, in a presentation that is analogous to MEN type 1 in humans, but adrenal neoplasia can also accompany the islet tumors. Although many pancreatic endocrine neoplasms are functional and produce clinical signs of inappropriate hormone secretion, they may also be nonfunctional, typically occurring as an abdominal mass or metastatic disease. The true incidence of nonfunctional tumors remains unknown, however, as many remain clinically silent. Insulinoma is the most commonly identified neoplasm in the endocrine pancreas, but in truth *functional pancreatic endocrine tumors often produce various hormones*, and fewer than 10% of tumors in dogs purely express a single hormone.

The tumors typically occur as small (<2 cm), solitary, well-circumscribed, homogeneous nodular masses with the pancreas and may be missed on cursory examination (Fig. 3-24). In accordance with the cooperative relationships between islets, many islets may be larger than the average in

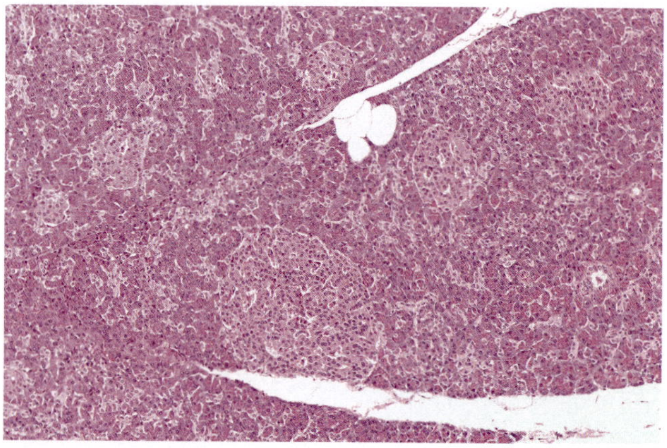

Figure 3-23 Nesidioblastosis in a dog displaying proliferation of ductuloinsular structures throughout the exocrine tissue.

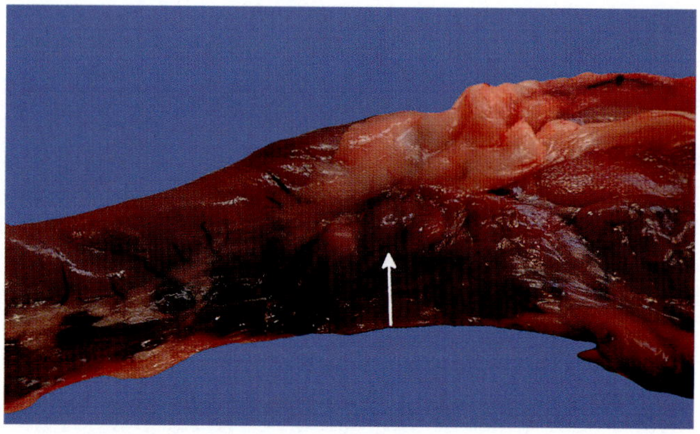

Figure 3-24 Insulinoma in a canine pancreas, with a small discrete nodule (arrow) within the parenchyma.

the organ and contain more nuclei, often clustered. Larger pancreatic endocrine neoplasms are unlikely to be functional. They are often lobular as a result of an expansive pattern of growth and may appear to be attached to adjacent structures. The main masses on cut surface are fibrotic or silky, firm, white and may have yellow foci of necrosis. In cases of carcinoma, metastases may not be grossly apparent on inspection of the liver, but, microscopically, they are expected to be widely distributed in the portal areas. Invasion of veins and lymphatics is best seen in marginal tissues. The tumors may spread from the local lymph node along perineural lymphatics to the sublumbar region.

The diagnosis of pancreatic endocrine neoplasm usually can be made on ordinary histologic examination, but identification of the cellular phenotype requires additional histochemistry. Immunohistochemistry may identify hormones normally produced within islets as well as others of ectopic origin. More than one hormone is often identified in a tumor, but it is possible that not all hormones detected are expressed functionally. In instances in which immunohistochemical assessment is not readily available, stains used to identify normal islet cell types such as Mallory-Azan may be beneficial, but staining is inconsistent in neoplastic tissue. Most pancreatic endocrine tumors in dogs are well differentiated, with sparse mitoses and relatively uniform nuclei containing a fine dusting of chromatin, although sporadic karyomegaly may be seen. Architecturally, there is a varied but characteristic organoid or pseudoalveolar pattern that, depending on orientation, may appear trabecular (Fig. 3-25A and B). Ductules may be present within the tumors, as well as aggregates of birefringent and congophilic islet amyloid polypeptide. Pancreatic endocrine tumors typically stain positively for chromogranin A and/or B, synaptophysin, and neuron-specific enolase. Distinguishing benign and malignant tumors may be difficult, and the classification is typically based on peripheral invasion and evidence of vascular or lymphatic metastasis. When present, large areas of necrosis, frequent mitoses, and marked cellular atypia are also useful indicators of malignancy. The following section describes the syndromic characteristics of pancreatic endocrine tumors expressing a single hormone, but it is important to note that the clinical presentation is determined by the specific balance of hormones produced.

Insulinomas are most prevalent in the dog, cat, and ferret. They also have been reported sporadically in horses and cattle, with concurrent pheochromocytomas often found in bovine cases. Clinical disease largely reflects neuronal glucose deficiency (neuroglycopenia), with depression, weakness, seizures (typically brief, reflecting transitory hypoglycemia), and muscle fasciculation commonly reported. Polyphagia may occur as an adaptive response, and drooling is a frequent finding in ferrets. In dogs, weakness may be exacerbated by the development of paraneoplastic polyneuropathy, characterized by demyelination and axonal degeneration. This is presumed to reflect the effects of hypoglycemia on energy supply, axonal transport, and myelin sheath integrity, and some dogs may show clinical improvement if euglycemia is restored. In severe cases, hypoglycemia caused by insulinoma can lead to neuronal necrosis within the superficial layers of the cerebral cortex.

Except for the ferret, in which the tumors are generally benign, insulinomas in domestic species are typically malignant and readily metastasize to the regional lymph nodes or the liver. Prognosis largely depends on the clinical stage, with the overall mean survival time for dogs of 12-18 months in different studies. Tumor characteristics associated with improved survival time include smaller tumor size, the presence of stromal fibrosis within the tumor, and a Ki67 index ≤2.5% in tumor cells.

Pancreatic neuroendocrine tumors that secrete IGF2 have been reported as a rare cause of hypoglycemia in dogs and should be considered as a potential diagnosis in hypoglycemic animals with a pancreatic mass but low serum insulin. These tumors may be less aggressive than insulinomas, and cases documented in the literature were not invasive, although metastases were present in the mesentery in a minority of cases. Prolonged survival followed complete excision of primary and secondary tumors.

Functional **glucagonomas** cause mild persistent hyperglycemia through stimulation of hepatic gluconeogenesis and glycogenolysis, and eventually, this can progress to diabetes mellitus. In dogs, glucagonomas are also associated frequently with the development of *superficial necrolytic dermatitis*. Affected animals have erythema, hyperkeratosis, and superficial erosions of the footpads, mucocutaneous junctions, and pressure points such as the elbow and hock. The skin lesions are identical to those present in *hepatocutaneous syndrome*, and it is likely that they share a common pathogenesis, but glucagonoma-associated cases lack the vacuolar hepatopathy

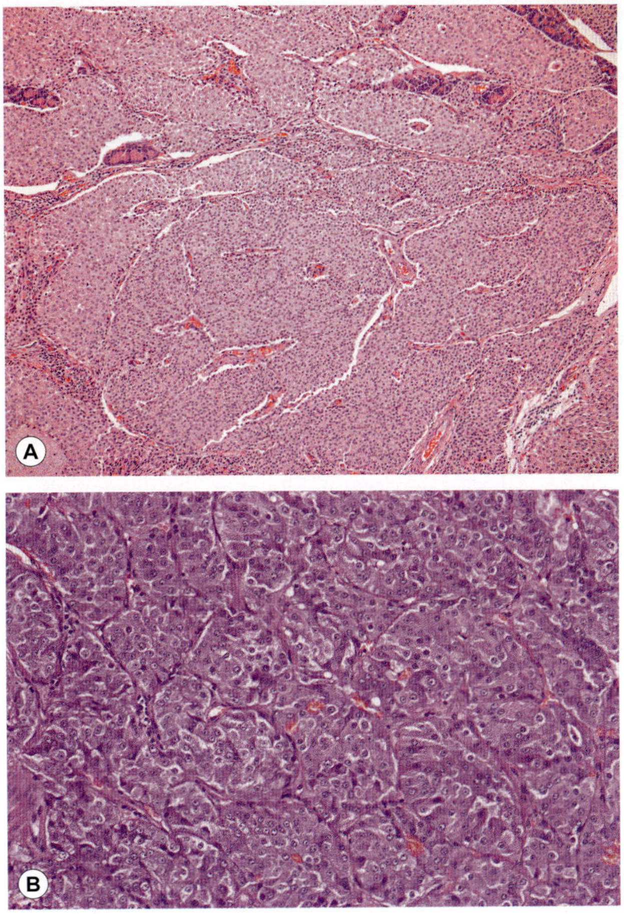

Figure 3-25 **A.** **Pancreatic endocrine neoplasia** in a dog. The tumor is composed of lobules of relatively uniform cells with pale acidophilic cytoplasm separated by fine fibrous septa. **B.** Higher magnification of a pancreatic endocrine neoplasm, composed of nests of relatively uniform endocrine cells.

seen with hepatocutaneous syndrome. Hypoaminoacidemia is a consistent finding in animals with superficial necrolytic dermatitis, with deficits in glutamine, glycine, alanine, hydroxyl-L-proline, proline, and threonine. Presumably, this amino acid depletion reflects dysregulated glucagon secretion, but as plasma glucagon levels are reduced rather than increased in dogs with hepatocutaneous syndrome, the pathogenesis of superficial necrolytic dermatitis may be more complex than simple hormonal excess.

Gastrinomas are infrequently reported in the dog and cat, and although often located within the pancreas, the lineage of these tumors is controversial, as the pancreas is generally considered an ectopic location for gastrin production. However, the detection of progastrin within pancreatic tissue of various species (including cats and dogs) suggests that the gastrin gene is, in fact, expressed by low numbers of endocrine cells throughout the pancreas. Moreover, the immunophenotypic characteristics of pancreatic gastrinomas—in humans, at least—are distinct from those of enteral gastrinomas, with pancreatic tumors displaying positivity for pancreatic polypeptide and the pancreatic differentiation marker PDX1, whereas those of duodenal origin express the sonic hedgehog marker. These observations suggest that the tumors are derived from intrinsic pancreatic endocrine tissue, rather than ectopic gastrointestinal G cells.

The primary presentation of gastrinoma is Zollinger-Ellison syndrome, wherein excess gastrin results in gastric acid hypersecretion, which induces antral mucosal hypertrophy and mucous metaplasia as well as gastroduodenal ulceration. Inactivation of pancreatic lipase and precipitation of bile salts at low pH in the duodenum may cause the development of steatorrhea. Gastrinomas typically metastasize early, but in contrast to other islet tumors are often highly invasive histologically.

There are rare reports of **pancreatic polypeptide-secreting islet neoplasia (PPoma)** in dogs with vague gastrointestinal signs, including vomiting, inappetence, watery diarrhea, weight loss, and upper gastrointestinal ulceration. The clinical signs are thought to reflect appetite suppression and decreased gastric motility caused by excess pancreatic polypeptide, with ulceration resulting from mild acid hypersecretion. Cases reported in the literature have been uniformly malignant, with metastases identified in the lymph nodes and liver.

Somatostatinoma has been documented in dogs with MEN, but the presence of concurrent endocrine tumors in these animals means that the isolated clinical effect of excessive somatostatin is poorly characterized. However, dogs with these tumors have variably had diabetes mellitus, cholelithiasis, weight loss, diarrhea, and anemia.

Visit Elsevier eBooks+ (eBooks.Health.Elsevier.com) for eFigures and further readings.

CHAPTER 4

Urinary System

Rachel E. Cianciolo • Shannon M. McLeland

ACKNOWLEDGMENTS

This update of the Urinary System chapter is based on previous editions by Drs. Ken Jubb, Peter Kennedy, Nigel Palmer, Grant Maxie, Shelley Newman, and John Prescott, and their contributions are gratefully acknowledged.

KIDNEY

GENERAL CONSIDERATIONS

The kidney is the central organ involved in the maintenance of a constant extracellular environment in the body. The vital homeostatic functions performed by the kidney include excretion of waste products, maintenance of normal concentrations of salt and water in the body, regulation of acid-base balance, production of a variety of hormones (e.g., erythropoietin, renin, prostaglandins), and metabolism of vitamin D to its active form, 1,25 dihydroxycholecalciferol ($1{,}25(OH)_2D_3$). *The essential requirements for normal renal function are adequate perfusion with blood (pressure >60 mm Hg), adequate amounts of functional renal tissue, and normal elimination of urine from the urinary tract.* Urinary tract disease is detected if any of these requirements are not met, and the outcome is always approximately the same; there is imbalance of salt and water, and of acids and bases, and there is retention of wastes. If urinary functions are sufficiently disturbed, retention of these wastes will result in the clinical condition of **azotemia**. If they are severely disturbed, the syndrome of **uremia** will occur.

Excretion of wastes and conservation of water in mammals require concentrating mechanisms capable of raising the osmolality of urine above that of plasma. In fact, the entire plasma volume of the body is dialyzed through the kidney many times a day, producing copious amounts of filtrate, of which almost all is resorbed. Although this system effectively rids the body of wastes, it requires a large expenditure of energy and a dependable renal blood supply. *Renal blood flow is normally high, up to 25% of the cardiac output.* Blood flow to the kidneys increases mildly after a high-protein meal and in certain systemic disease states, for example, fever. However, decreased blood flow causes injury more commonly than hyperperfusion. Whereas peripheral and splanchnic blood flow may be sacrificed in hypovolemia, renal blood flow is maintained and only decreases when perfusion of the brain and heart is impaired. Renal oxygen consumption equals ~10% of whole-body consumption. It is relatively small in relation to renal blood flow, but high compared with that of other tissues.

A unique feature of renal blood flow is that it varies little over a wide range of arterial pressures, thus ensuring a stable *glomerular filtration rate (GFR)*. The kidneys possess intrinsic mechanisms by which vascular resistance is varied to maintain constant glomerular filtration. Renal blood flow is normally directed predominantly toward the outer *cortical nephrons* rather than to the inner *cortical (juxtamedullary) nephrons*, but can be redistributed between the 2 areas. When reduction in renal perfusion occurs, it primarily affects the cortex. Depending on the severity and duration of the ischemic episode, it may lead to attenuation or atrophy of tubular epithelium, to necrosis of individual tubules (acute tubular epithelial cell injury), or to extensive necrosis of the renal cortex (infarct). Juxtamedullary nephrons are better at conserving water and concentrating urine. Therefore, redirection of blood flow toward these nephrons helps maintain circulating blood volume and elimination of wastes during periods of poor perfusion.

The **glomerulus** produces ultrafiltrate as the net result of the difference between high capillary hydrostatic pressure and low hydrostatic pressure in the urinary (Bowman) space as well as the difference between osmotic pressures in these 2 compartments. The glomerular basement membrane (GBM) is semipermeable, and dissolved substances (e.g., proteins, electrolytes) move across the glomerular capillary walls at rates determined by size, shape, and electrical charge. Malfunction of the glomerulus may result from inadequate glomerular blood flow and/or structural alterations that change its permeability.

After crossing the GBM, the ultrafiltrate exits the urinary space into the tubular lumens and is, in a strict sense, outside the body. Most of the filtered substances are retrieved by selective resorption, which requires special machinery and energy. If this function is defective, essential substances are lost in the urine, which occurs when enzymes are inhibited by toxins or drugs or are genetically deficient, tubular epithelial cells are injured, plasma levels of filterable substances are elevated, or the glomerulus has increased permeability. Myriad tubular functions are carried out sequentially, and the structure of the tubule varies along its length corresponding to the function to be performed.

The principal function of the kidney is the regulation of salt and water balance; this requires a system of monitors and feedbacks to achieve fine regulation. The hypothalamus and antidiuretic hormone (ADH, or vasopressin) control osmotic and volume regulation. The renin-angiotensin-aldosterone system (RAAS) is also involved in salt and water homeostasis and is described in more detail later.

According to the **"intact nephron"** hypothesis, nephron function is an all-or-none phenomenon. In progressive renal disease, the remaining nephrons respond by hypertrophy because new nephrons cannot be formed in a mature kidney. Glomerular filtration and tubular function of the remaining nephrons increase concomitantly to maintain homeostasis. *All of the renal components are interdependent, and if one component is irreversibly damaged, function of the other components will be impaired.* For example, glomerular disease can cause decreased peritubular capillary perfusion and tubular atrophy; tubulointerstitial disease can cause glomerular obsolescence. Interstitial inflammation and fibrosis may be primary events, but they also can be secondary to diseases of the glomeruli and tubules. *There is a tendency for chronic renal disease to affect various components of the kidney, resulting in chronic kidney disease (CKD) and shrunken, scarred* **end-stage kidneys;** at this stage, identification of the initiating cause may be impossible.

Anatomy

The *renal collecting system* is derived from the ureteric bud (metanephric duct), a diverticulum of the mesonephric (Wolffian) duct, and consists of *the ureter, pelvis, calyces, and collecting ducts*. Nephrons develop from the metanephric blastema and attach to the growing ends of the collecting system. The *uriniferous tubule* consists of the nephron and the collecting duct. Renal *calyces* are the cup-shaped recesses of the pelvis that enclose conical masses of medullary *pyramids*. The apex of a pyramid is referred to as a *papilla*, and its tip is fenestrated by collecting ducts (area cribrosa). The *fornix* is the uppermost blind end of a calyx or pelvis.

Kidneys of domestic animals are classified as **unipyramidal** (unilobar) or **multipyramidal** (multilobar). *Cats, dogs, small ruminants, and horses have unipyramidal kidneys.* In cats, one lobe is present, and papillary ducts open into a calyx through a single renal papilla. In dogs, small ruminants, and horses, there is complete or partial fusion of several lobes and a single crest-like papilla *(renal crest)*. *Pigs have multipyramidal kidneys* in which there are several distinct renal lobes, pyramids, and their respective papillae. Extensions of renal cortex between the pyramids are known as the *renal columns*. Simple papillae occur in central pyramids, and compound papillae occur in pyramids at the renal poles; this is of pathogenetic significance because compound papillae are more susceptible to ascending infection. The *kidneys of cattle are also multipyramidal*, but have distinct external lobation, with each lobe having one pyramid. The renal calyces of cattle join directly to form the ureter without forming a pelvis. Note the difference between a renal lobe and a renal lobule. A *renal lobe* consists of a pyramid and the overlying cortex. A *renal lobule* consists of a medullary ray and its associated nephrons. *Medullary rays* are seen histologically as lighter staining linear areas in the cortex and consist of collecting tubules, thick ascending limbs, and the straight portions of the proximal tubules. Histologically, the medullary rays have straight tubules running parallel to one another. On sagittal section of a kidney, *subdivisions of cortex and medulla* may be distinguished, particularly in dogs and sheep. The *cortex* has a darker outer zone, and a paler inner zone, which in mature dogs often has prominent pale streaks because of the fat in collecting duct epithelial cells. Depending on where the kidney is sectioned, outer and inner zones may be seen in the *medulla* of canine kidneys, and the outer zone may be further subdivided into outer and inner bands (stripes), owing to the thick segments of the descending and ascending limbs of the loop of Henle in the outer zone and only the thick ascending limbs in the inner stripe, respectively. The inner zone of the medulla contains the thin segments of the loop of Henle (Fig. 4-1). Mucous glands are large and prominent in the medulla of equine kidneys, and mucus and crystals are normally present in the equine renal pelvis.

Nephrons consist of the *renal corpuscle, proximal tubule, loop of Henle, distal tubule, connecting tubule, and collecting tubule.* The glomerulus and glomerular (Bowman) capsule comprise the **renal corpuscle**. The following approximate numbers of nephrons are present in each kidney—human, 200,000-1,800,000; cattle, 4,000,000; sheep, 650,000; pig, 1,250,000; dog, 400,000; cat, 200,000. The number of nephrons is fixed at birth in most mammals, although nephrogenesis may continue for several weeks after birth in animals with a short gestation period, such as dogs, cats, and pigs.

There are 4 main components of the kidney: blood vessels, glomeruli, tubules, and interstitium.

Vascular supply

Although the kidneys constitute only ~0.5% of body weight, *they receive 20-25% of cardiac output*. In multilobed kidneys, the *renal artery* divides in the pelvic region to form *interlobar arteries* that run in the renal columns, between lobes, up to the corticomedullary junction, where they branch to form *arcuate arteries*. These arteries run along the corticomedullary junction parallel to the renal capsule and terminate by becoming the radiating *interlobular arteries* in the cortex. Interlobular arteries give rise to prearterioles, which have a lumen diameter of <70 µm. The glomerular *afferent arterioles* (which are derived from the prearterioles) give rise to several glomerular capillary loops. The capillaries later rejoin to form the glomerular *efferent arteriole* and then divide again to form a peritubular capillary plexus. The juxtamedullary nephrons differ somewhat. Their efferent arterioles branch to form *descending vasa recta* (straight vessels), which enter the medulla. The ascending vasa recta form the medullary capillary plexus and are a *countercurrent exchange system* with their closely associated descending vasa recta. The glomerular capillary tufts are perfused at a high pressure that favors filtration; the peritubular capillary bed has low pressure, favoring resorption.

Because the renal artery and its branches are *end arteries*, occlusion of any branch leads to infarction. Furthermore, interference with glomerular capillary flow markedly alters peritubular blood flow, especially in the medulla. The medulla is particularly sensitive to ischemia because of its relative avascularity and the low hematocrit in medullary capillaries.

Intrarenal blood flow and GFR are controlled by complex mechanisms. The best understood regulatory mechanism is **tubuloglomerular feedback**, which is a negative feedback loop. It is mediated by the **juxtaglomerular apparatus (JGA)**, which consists of the *macula densa* of the distal convoluted tubule, extraglomerular mesangial cells at the glomerular hilus between the arterioles, and the renin-containing juxtaglomerular cells in the wall of the afferent arteriole. The architecture of the JGA is important because it allows communication between cells of the distal tubule and the glomerular hilus. Briefly, low GFR results in decreased NaCl delivery to the distal tubule. This is detected by the macula densa cells (via a Na-K-2Cl cotransporter at the apical membrane). The net result is contraction of the efferent arteriole with simultaneous dilation of the afferent arteriole, increasing the filtration pressure to deliver more NaCl to the macula densa. Increased GFR (or high NaCl) induces the opposite response. The molecular pathway is as follows: when macula densa cells detect low NaCl, they synthesize and secrete prostaglandin E2 (PGE2), which induces the release of renin from the afferent arteriolar juxtaglomerular cells. Renin cleaves angiotensinogen (made by the liver and released in plasma) to generate angiotensin I in the kidney, which is then cleaved by angiotensin-converting enzyme into angiotensin II. This latter molecule is a potent vasoconstrictor, and it has a greater effect on efferent than afferent arterioles. Angiotensin II also initiates adrenocortical synthesis of *aldosterone*, which, over the long term, increases resorption of sodium from the distal convoluted tubules and collecting ducts, resulting in water retention and expansion of the extracellular fluid volume. Angiotensin II also stimulates the secretion of ADH by the posterior pituitary, which helps raise the GFR by increasing water resorption through insertion of aquaporin-2 channels in the collecting duct. Other key mediators of tubuloglomerular balance include adenosine triphosphate (ATP), adenosine, nitric oxide (NO), myogenic control of afferent arteriolar tone, as well as other derivatives of angiotensin (angiotensin III, angiotensin IV, and angiotensin 1-7). Most of these additional mechanisms are involved in titrating the system so that GFR is kept within a narrow range. Interestingly, many angiotensin derivatives are vasodilatory (e.g., angiotensin 1-7) counteracting the vasoconstriction induced by angiotensin II, which underscores the complexity of this system.

The *renal venous system* begins with the formation of venules from the peritubular capillaries and vasa recta, and then closely parallels the arterial system. Veins in the outer cortex drain into stellate veins, which in cats are prominently visible on the capsular surface, and then into interlobular

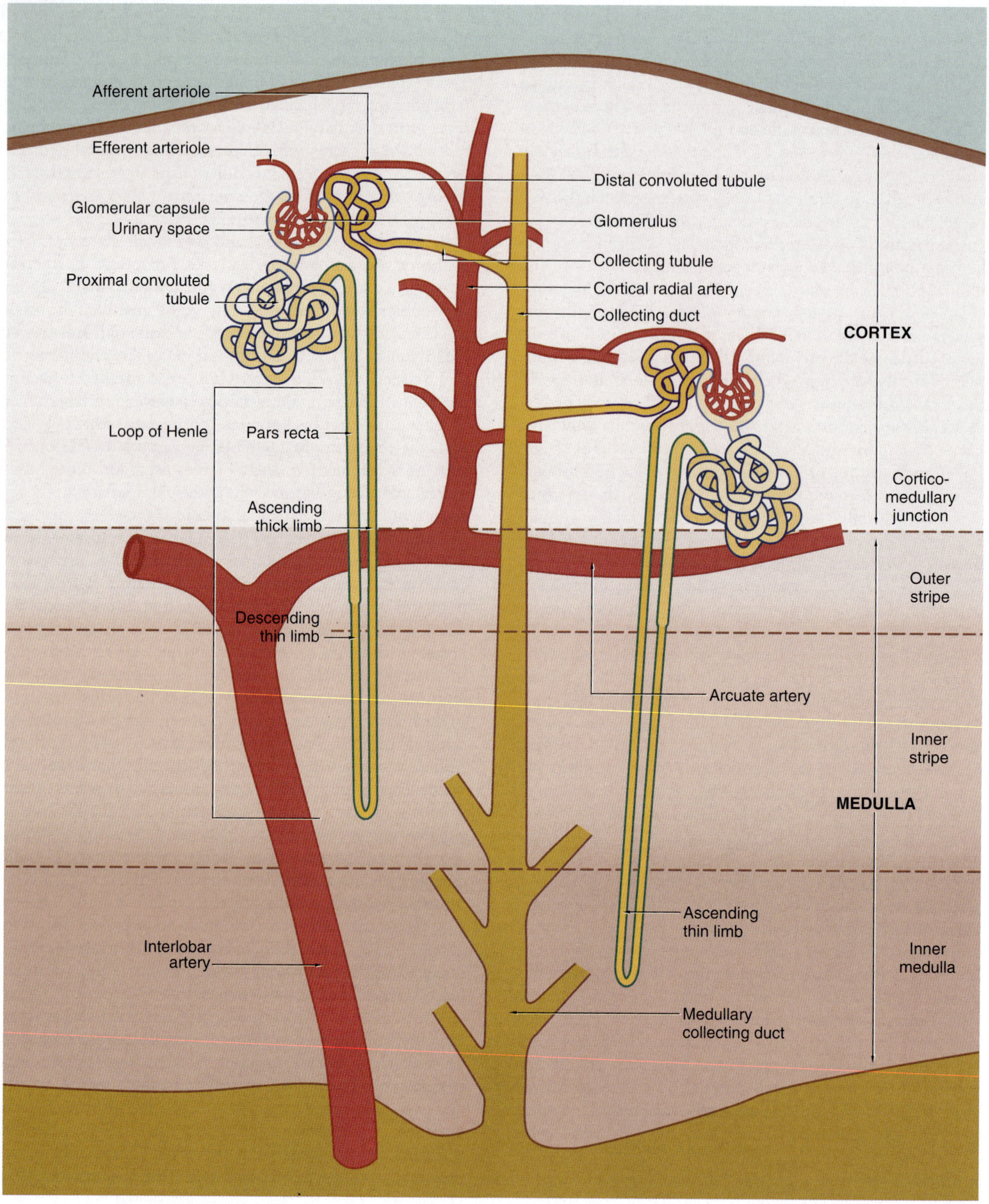

Figure 4-1 Basic organization of the nephron, collecting system, and renal vasculature. (Modified from Young B, et al. Urinary system. In: Wheater's Functional Histology. 6th ed. Elsevier, 2014: 292–317.)

veins. Veins within the kidney have very thin walls and are susceptible to compression.

Lymphatics are present in the renal cortex and medulla. One set of lymphatics drains the cortical and medullary interstitium and follows the pattern of the vascular system; another set of lymphatics drains the capsular area. Lymphatic flow increases after urinary obstruction and in interstitial disease.

Glomerulus

The glomerulus is a vascular-epithelial structure designed for the ultrafiltration of plasma (Fig. 4-2). It develops embryologically by the invagination of a capillary-rich meshwork into an epithelium-lined sac, which connects to the proximal tubule. The visceral epithelium (podocytes) covers the abluminal surface of glomerular capillaries; the parietal epithelium lines the

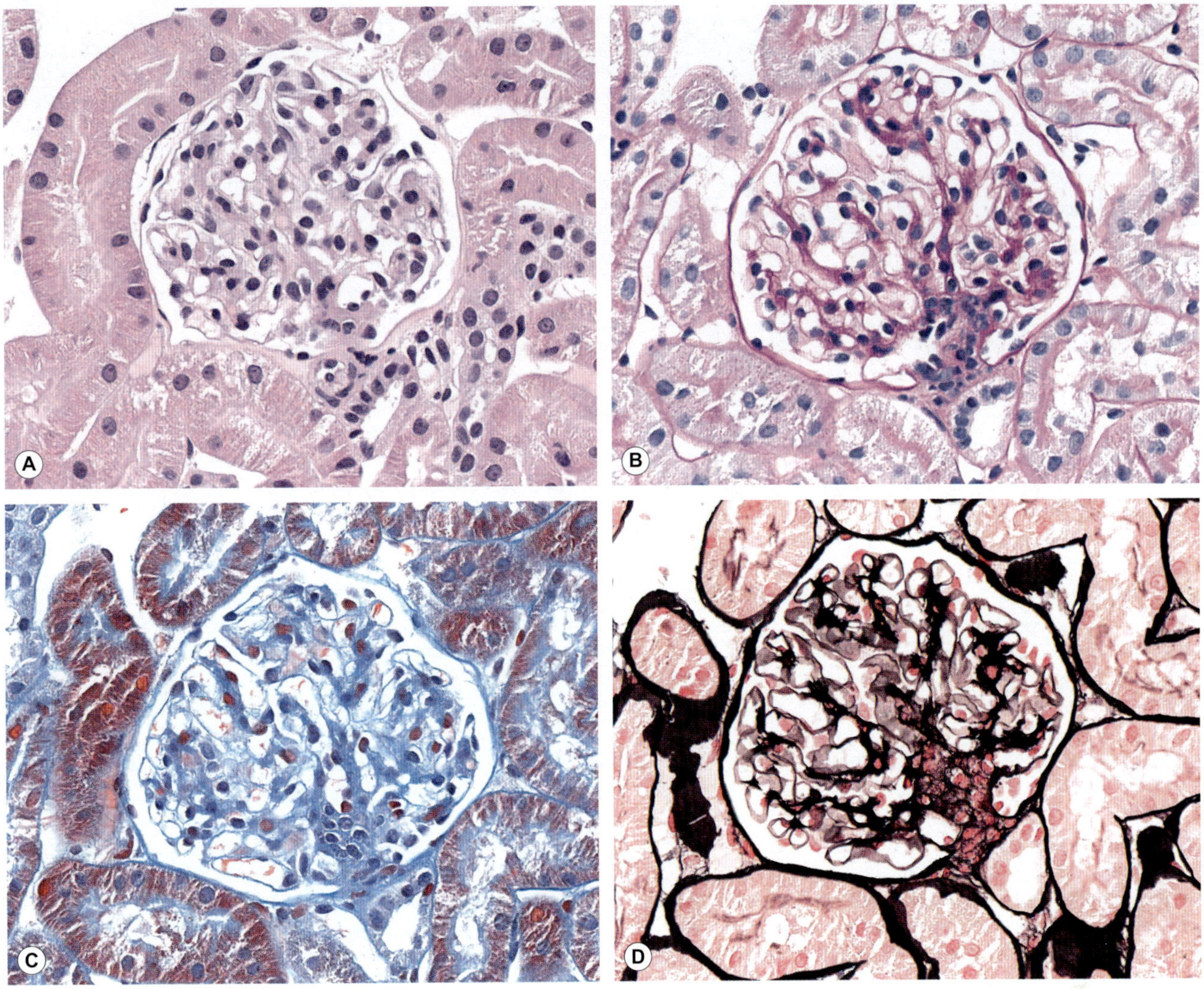

Figure 4-2 Normal canine glomerulus and macula densa, sectioned at 3 μm thickness. **A**. H&E. **B**. Podocytes can be clearly distinguished on the abluminal side of the delicate glomerular basement membrane, and mesangial zones contain <3 nuclei. PAS stain. **C**. Mesangium at vascular pole may contain >3 nuclei. Masson trichrome stain. **D**. Note the smooth outer contour of the glomerular basement membrane. Jones methenamine silver stain.

basement membrane of the glomerular capsule. This capsule encircles the urinary space that receives glomerular ultrafiltrate. The arterioles enter and leave the glomerulus at the *vascular pole*, and urine enters the proximal tubule at the *urinary pole* of the glomerulus. The *glomerular filtration membrane* (Fig. 4-3) consists of 3 layers: 1) capillary *endothelium* with 50-100-nm fenestrae and coated by a thick glycocalyx on the luminal side; 2) the *GBM*, which is 100-300 nm thick and consists of a central electron-dense lamina densa and peripheral electron-lucent layers, the lamina rara interna and externa; and 3) *podocytes*. The podocytes have complex interdigitating trabeculae whose *foot processes (pedicels)* are embedded in the lamina rara externa of the GBM. The foot processes are separated by 25-50-nm–wide *filtration slits*, which are bridged by thin *slit diaphragms* with 6-9 nm pores. The GBM is produced continuously by the podocytes and endothelium, but it does not completely encircle the glomerular capillaries. At the base of the capillary loop, the endothelial cells are in direct contact with mesangium. The GBM is a complex porous meshwork composed of collagen (primarily type IV in mature glomeruli), laminin, polyanionic proteoglycans (mainly heparan sulfate), fibronectin, entactin, and other glycoproteins.

A large volume of glomerular ultrafiltrate is formed as a product of the high hydrostatic pressure of arteriolar blood, and the selective permeability of the filtration membrane. The entire plasma volume is filtered about 100 times per day. The GBM is a *size-dependent barrier* to filtration, prohibiting passage of particles with radius >3.5 nm. It is highly permeable to water and small solutes, but virtually excludes high–molecular-weight (HMW) plasma proteins from the filtrate. It had been assumed that the GBM also prohibited the filtration of medium–molecular-weight (MMW) proteins, such as albumin, because micropuncture studies did not identify it in the filtrate of the proximal tubules; however, it is now known that albumin can pass through the GBM relatively easily, but is reabsorbed immediately by the cells adjacent to the urinary pole as soon as it enters the proximal tubule. Therefore, the cells nearest the junction with the glomerular capsule play a special role in albumin retrieval, and damage to this segment can impact the amount of albumin detected in the urine. The

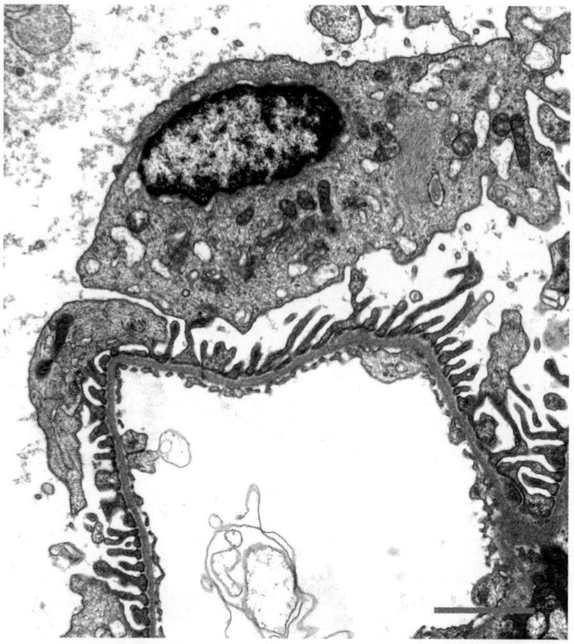

Figure 4-3 Transmission electron micrograph of a **normal canine glomerular filtration barrier**, consisting of the internal fenestrated endothelium, glomerular basement membrane (GBM), podocyte foot processes that are perpendicular to the GBM, and the podocyte cell body. Bar = 2 μm. (From Cianciolo R, et al. Atlas of Renal Lesions in Proteinuric Dogs. The Ohio State University, 2018.)

filtration barrier also excludes particles from filtration on the basis of *charge*. Thus, anionic molecules are repelled by virtue of the negatively charged sialoglycoproteins in the lamina rara interna and externa and the negatively charged glycocalyx of the endothelial cells. *Changes in porosity or charge of the filtration membrane alter glomerular permeability and can lead to proteinuria, a hallmark of glomerular damage.*

The **mesangium** is the central region of the glomerulus that forms a supporting framework about which the glomerular capillaries arborize. *The mesangial matrix is basement membrane–like periodic acid-Schiff (PAS)–positive glycoprotein, and the mesangial cells are phagocytic, contractile cells, which are derived from vascular smooth muscle cells.* These cells function in phagocytic removal of deposited macromolecules, removal of GBM, and may modulate intraglomerular blood flow. Mesangial cells both respond to and produce a variety of cytokines. Mesangial cell hyperplasia and increased mesangial matrix are common in glomerular disease.

Tubules

The kidney functions by producing a large volume of glomerular filtrate from which the body resorbs the constituents it needs and rids the body of wastes. Thus, about 99% of the filtered sodium chloride and water are resorbed. The tubules are the main resorptive mechanism. The *structure of a tubule segment is correlated with its function.* Cells of the proximal convoluted tubule have a well-developed brush border to increase surface area with myriad transporters and numerous mitochondria. Energy for the sodium pump in this actively resorptive area is provided by mitochondrial oxidative phosphorylation; this area is especially vulnerable to hypoxia. Also, if toxins are resorbed by or created by the proximal tubule, there can be chemical-induced cell injury.

The proximal tubule actively resorbs large quantities of sodium and chloride, and water passively follows. *Tubules and peritubular capillaries are in close apposition to allow rapid removal of resorbed sodium chloride and water from the tubular epithelial cells.* In addition to salt and water, proximal tubules resorb glucose, amino acids, calcium, phosphate, uric acid, proteins, and potassium; hence, 60-80% of the glomerular ultrafiltrate that enters the proximal tubule is reabsorbed. Transport of these molecules is often interconnected. For example, movement of sodium ions down its concentration gradient into the proximal convoluted tubule cell provides energy to resorb glucose and amino acids via a cotransporter mechanism. The sodium concentration gradient is maintained by Na^+/K^+ ATPases located at the basal surface of the proximal tubular epithelial cells.

Many substances, such as glucose, amino acids, and water-soluble vitamins, are almost completely resorbed, unless there is an abnormally high level filtered by the glomerulus. Above these threshold concentrations, the tubular transport maximum is exceeded, and the substance will appear in the urine. For example, hyperglycemia of diabetes mellitus exceeds what can be reabsorbed by the proximal tubule, leading to glucosuria and osmotic diuresis. Proximal tubules are also involved in the trafficking of hydrogen ions, and ~90% of the hydrogen ion excretion by the kidney occurs in the proximal tubule. Last, proximal tubules are involved in the movement (reabsorption or excretion) of organic acids, p-aminohippurate, penicillin, aminoglycosides, and some iodinated radiopaque materials.

After exiting the proximal tubule, the filtrate enters the loop of Henle. Interestingly, juxtamedullary nephrons have long loops of Henle, extending into the deep medulla; cortical nephrons have variable lengths of their loops of Henle. The length of the loop of Henle (nephron loop) is based on the presence and length of the ascending thin limb. In short loops of Henle, the ascending thin limb is either absent or very short, such that the descending limb connects almost directly into the ascending thick limb (see Fig. 4-1). *Urine concentrating ability of a nephron is directly proportional to the length of its loop of Henle.* Environment and evolution have impacted the ratio of short to long loops in a species. For example, species that evolved in biomes with easy access to water (e.g., beavers, hippopotamuses) have predominantly short-loop cortical nephrons. Species that evolved in desert environments (e.g., cats, dogs, chinchillas) have mostly or all long loops of Henle. Notably, humans and pigs have a high proportion of short loops of Henle.

The loops of Henle serve as *countercurrent multipliers* and the capillaries as simple *countercurrent exchangers*, with the flow in each occurring in opposite directions. The countercurrent multiplier uses energy to produce a solute gradient that becomes greater toward the tip of the papilla and therefore is an active process. The gradient is passively preserved by vasa recta countercurrent exchange. Sodium chloride is actively pumped from the ascending limb of the loop of Henle into the interstitium, in turn drawing water from the descending limb, and progressively increasing the solute concentration in the lumen of the descending limb. The ascending limb is impermeable to water. Thus, as sodium chloride leaves the lumen and the filtrate returns to the cortex, the degree of hypertonicity of luminal fluid lessens. More salt may be resorbed by the collecting ducts, further changing the tonicity of the fluid.

Water diuresis occurs during a state of water excess or when ADH is not released from the neurohypophysis. If water preservation is required, ADH is released and makes the epithelium of the collecting duct highly permeable to water, producing concentrated urine, up to 3-4 times the blood osmolality (280 mOsm/L). The water resorbed in the medulla is passively transported into the ascending vasa recta to be delivered back to the systemic circulation. The solute concentration of the medulla consists mostly of sodium and urea, the latter of which is produced in the liver as a byproduct of ammonia breakdown. During antidiuresis, ADH renders the *cortical portions* of the collecting ducts permeable to water but not to urea, thus increasing the urea concentration of the luminal fluid. ADH also increases the permeability of the *medullary portions* of the collecting ducts to urea and water; urea then diffuses from collecting duct to interstitium, and water follows. Neonatal nephrons have immature functional capacity and a relative inability to conserve sodium and water. Specifically, immature neonatal tubules in most species cannot produce a medullary solute gradient to concentrate urine. Neonatal pigs, in particular, are thus very susceptible to dehydration. In contrast, renal functional capacity of calves approaches that of adult cattle within 2-3 days of birth.

Either osmotic diuresis or water diuresis may result in **medullary solute washout** because of increased tubular flow rates and hence decreased efficiency of the countercurrent multiplier in the loop of Henle. The quantities of urea and sodium chloride resorbed are decreased because tubular fluid transit time quickens. Hence, the medullary solute gradient decreases, as does urine concentrating ability. The same mechanism is operative in CKD, in which there are higher tubular flow rates in the small number of remaining hypertrophic tubules.

Although plasma buffers and pulmonary control of carbon dioxide excretion are the first lines of defense in protecting the pH of the extracellular fluids, *it is the action of the kidneys that ultimately corrects acid-base balance*. For example, the kidneys can correct metabolic alkalosis by excreting alkaline urine containing the excess bicarbonate. Furthermore, the kidneys can correct metabolic acidosis by increasing resorption of filtered bicarbonate, excreting titratable acids (hydrogen ions), and producing ammonia.

Interstitium

The interstitium normally contains peritubular capillaries, pericytes, dendritic cells, and a few fibroblasts. Interstitial tissue is usually only obvious around interlobar, arcuate, and interlobular arteries. *Expansion of the cortical interstitium is abnormal* and may occur because of edema, cellular infiltration, or fibrosis. Interstitial fibrosis can result in loss of the peritubular capillaries, promoting tubular hypoxia and atrophy. This has been observed in humans, rodents, and cats with CKD. The glycosaminoglycan content of the medullary interstitium increases with age and ischemia. Specialized interstitial cells produce prostaglandins, particularly PGE2 and PGF2α.

Examination of the kidney

Gross examination

The systematic gross inspection of a kidney entails observation of its *size, shape, color, and consistency*. The kidneys are usually equal in size and ~3 vertebrae long. Mild renal enlargement may occur because of the addition of blood, edema, fat, or swollen or hypertrophic nephrons. Mild-to-severe renomegaly can occur with urine accumulation in the renal pelvis or renal cysts. Acute inflammation causes renal enlargement from both interstitial edema and leukocyte infiltration; chronic inflammation causes scarring and atrophy of parenchyma. The kidneys are usually bean or horseshoe shaped, although the bovine kidney is lobated externally. Focal lesions, such as those caused by infarction or pyelonephritis, may markedly distort the capsular surface, whereas more generalized diseases, such as glomerulonephritis (GN), do not. The normal renal color is brown-red, except in mature cats, in which the cortices are yellow because of their high lipid content. The fat content in cats is apparently hormonally determined; pregnant females and sexually inactive old males have the most fat, pseudopregnant females and castrated males have somewhat less, estrous females and sexually active males have moderate amounts, and anestrous females have little or no renal fat. Kidneys autolyze fairly rapidly after death, particularly in obese animals in a warm environment.

The urinary system may be kept intact during examination, or the kidneys may be removed from the carcass. In small animals, the kidney should not be severed from the ureter until the absence of hydronephrosis has been established. Each kidney is cut in the sagittal plane, and the cut surface is examined. The *normal cortex-to-medulla ratio* in this plane is about 1:2 or 1:3. *The cortex normally accounts for 80% of the renal mass*, a fact that is better appreciated in a coronal section than in a sagittal section. Diffuse diseases of the kidney usually respect the integrity of the medulla; however, pyelonephritis and papillary necrosis center on the pelvis and papilla/medulla. Pallor of the cut surface suggests the deposition of fat, acute tubular necrosis (ATN), or possibly glomerular disease. If the surface bulges slightly when sectioned, diffuse tubular injury and interstitial edema are likely. Focal glomerular lesions do not cause glomerular prominence, but diffuse lesions, such as amyloidosis or diffuse GN, might be seen as red pinpoint foci throughout the cortex. *Removal of the renal capsule is essential for examination of the outer surface of the cortex*. The capsule should strip easily and leave a smooth surface underneath. Tearing of the cortex may indicate scarring, except in the horse, which normally has trabeculae attached to the capsule. In cattle, the left kidney is often shorter and wider than the right kidney. The size of bovine kidneys is also influenced by age and breed. Specifically, kidneys from cows >6-years-old are significantly smaller than those <6-years-old. Holsteins have significantly larger kidneys than Limousin-cross cattle. It is unknown if this breed-associated size difference can be generalized to all dairy versus beef cattle. Additionally, there is a wide variation in the number of lobes within bovine kidneys, ranging from 13 to 35 (mean of 20) within a single study cohort. Most of the lobes are present in the midsection of the kidney (at the level of the hilus), whereas the fewest lobes are at the cranial pole.

Histologic examination

The kidney must be trimmed so that a section from the capsule to papilla is available. The section should first be examined subgrossly for evidence of localized lesions, for example, infarcts, abscesses, granulomas, pyelitis, mineralization, neoplasia, scars, and medullary loss. The section is then scanned at low power. Glomeruli are normally distributed randomly throughout the cortex, with ~1 or 2 present per 40X field (0.24 mm^2). Tubules should be tightly packed, with little intervening connective tissue (Fig. 4-4). In dogs, the diameter but not the number of glomeruli is significantly correlated with the body

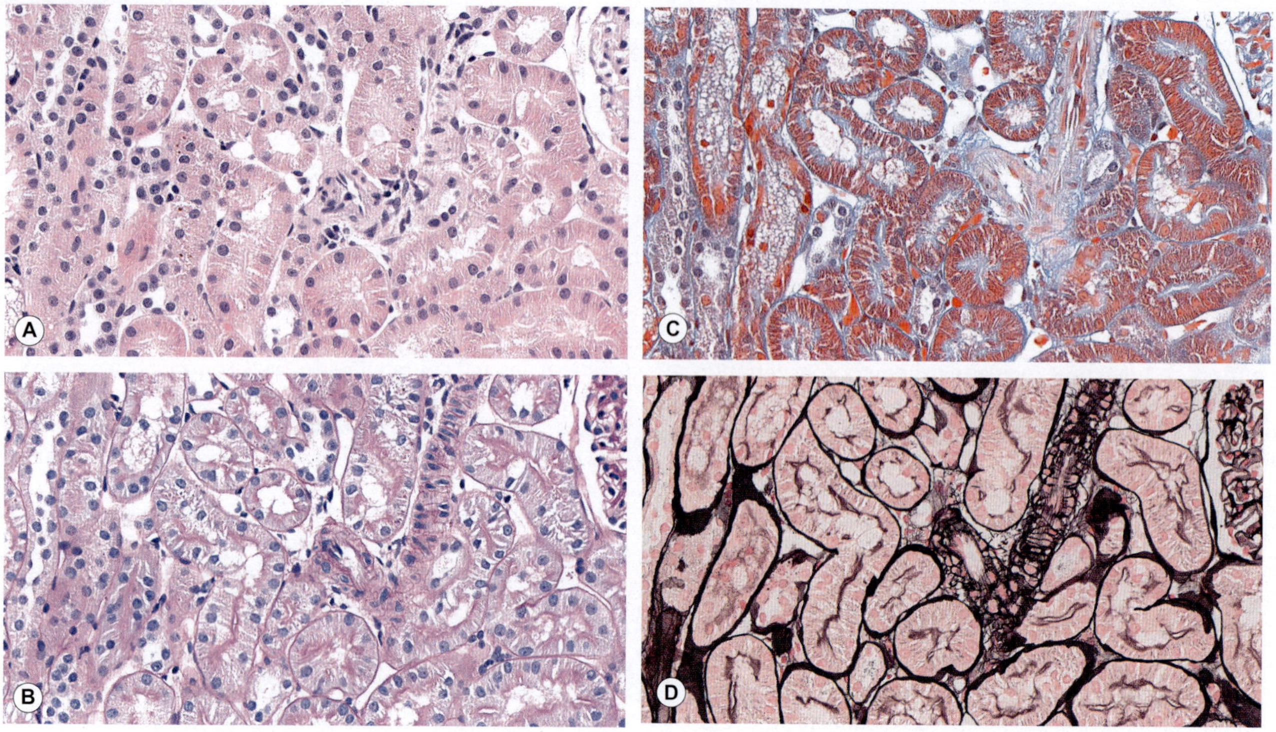

Figure 4-4 Normal canine tubulointerstitium, sectioned at 3 μm thickness. **A.** H&E. **B.** Apical brush border of proximal convoluted tubules is intact and stained pink, and peritubular capillaries are immediately adjacent to tubular basement membranes. PAS stain. **C.** Apical brush border of proximal convoluted tubules is blue, and interstitial fibrosis is not present. Masson trichrome stain. **D.** Jones methenamine silver stain.

surface area. This suggests that large-breed dogs have larger nephrons than small-breed dogs, as opposed to having more nephrons. Goat and sheep glomeruli are more cellular than those of most other species. Horses have the largest glomeruli of domestic animals (up to 200 μm diameter). Glomeruli in neonatal kidneys are small and hyperchromatic, particularly in the outer cortex (Fig. 4-5). Nephrons may be seen in the "S" stage of development in the outer cortex of fetuses and also in neonates with ongoing renal development, such as dogs, cats, and pigs (eFig. 4-1).

After scanning the section, the 4 basic elements of the kidney should be systematically examined, namely, glomeruli, tubules, interstitium, and blood vessels, to determine which structure is primarily injured.

Reactions of **glomeruli** to injury consist basically of combinations of cellular proliferation, mesangial expansion, leukocyte recruitment, remodeling of the GBM, and sclerosis. Epithelium of the proximal tubule might be present in the glomerular urinary space in acute tubular injury (ATI) or, more commonly, due to squeezing the kidney during gross examination, especially if the kidney is autolytic. This autolytic change is termed *tubular regurgitation* or *infraglomerular herniation or reflux*. Comparison of autolyzed feline kidneys to contralateral kidneys harvested immediately after euthanasia revealed that autolyzed kidneys weighed more and had increased glomerular diameters. However, the thickness of the GBM, the intact foot processes, and the number of cells per glomerulus did not change after a 24-hour postmortem interval.

Tubules, especially proximal convoluted tubules, are the portions of the nephron that are most susceptible to ischemia and many toxins. Degenerative changes are nonspecific in character and usually not diagnostic of the causative condition. The proximal convoluted tubule is the longest cortical part of the nephron, and hence, proximal tubules comprise the bulk of the cortex. Proximal tubules are more eosinophilic than the other tubules and have a brush border that is visible in nonautolyzed specimens. The brush border can be easily seen as bright pink with the PAS stain (see Fig. 4-4B) and blue with the Masson trichrome stain (see Fig. 4-4C). Long delays

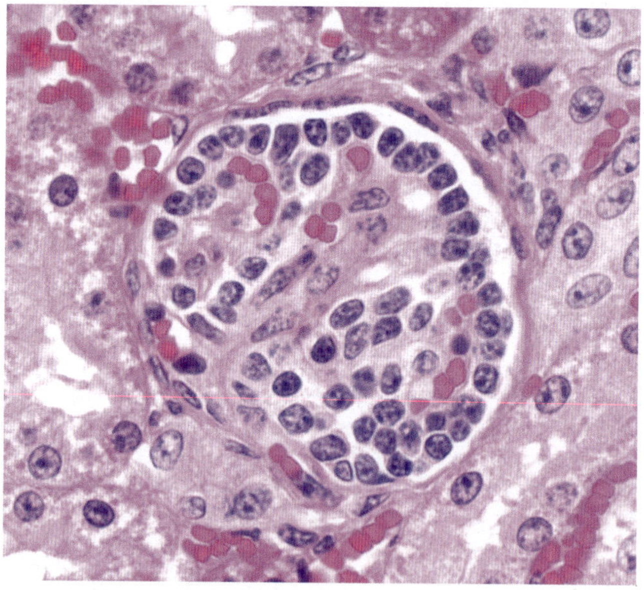

Figure 4-5 Normal fetal glomerulus in a neonatal piglet.

in fixation lead to sloughing of the apical cytoplasm into tubular lumina. Because cells of the distal tubule do not have a brush border and are flatter, the tubular lumina appear larger. Interstitial fibrosis, particularly in areas of the **interstitium** lacking large blood vessels, is abnormal and indicates that tubular-peritubular capillary interactions are disrupted, which can result in tubular hypoxia by increasing the distance between the peritubular capillaries and tubules and can also impede transport of reabsorbed important molecules. Complete loss of the peritubular capillary bed might eventually develop. Interstitial fibrosis might cause tubular obstruction and create *retention cysts* proximally.

Vascular changes may occur in various systemic diseases, for example, arterio- and arteriolosclerosis in hypertension, arteritis in malignant catarrhal fever, and phlebitis in renal feline infectious peritonitis.

The **renal medulla** should be examined closely because this is the site of urine concentration and the accumulation of protein casts. Tubules and ducts in the medulla are normally separated by more connective tissue and ground substance than those in the cortex. Tubulointerstitial mineralization is common in renal disease and may be seen along with cortical mineralization in cases of hypercalcemic nephropathy. The papilla should be carefully examined for evidence of papillitis (an early lesion in pyelonephritis), for interstitial amyloid, and for papillary necrosis. Inclusion bodies can be prominent in pelvic urothelium of dogs; they may be nonspecific protein droplets or could be canine distemper viral inclusions.

Renal biopsy

Renal biopsy is useful in evaluating renal disease in domestic animals and *may be of particular use in cases of acute GN, nephrotic syndrome, asymptomatic proteinuria, and acute kidney injury* (AKI). Biopsy techniques vary and include ultrasound-guided percutaneous, laparoscopic, surgical core, or surgical wedge procedures. In small animals, 16-gauge needles are preferred. The use of 14-gauge needle has been shown to include unwanted medullary tissue, and 18-gauge needles capture significantly fewer entire glomeruli than 16-gauge needles. Importantly, renal biopsy cores and wedges must be evaluated grossly to ensure that glomeruli are present in the sample. To do this, the tissue can be placed in a small Petri dish of physiologic saline and examined with a dissecting microscope or a magnifying glass. Small red dots are perfused glomeruli and should be easily visible in fresh biopsy tissue (Fig. 4-6). Once an adequate sample has been obtained, a small piece (1-2 mm^3)

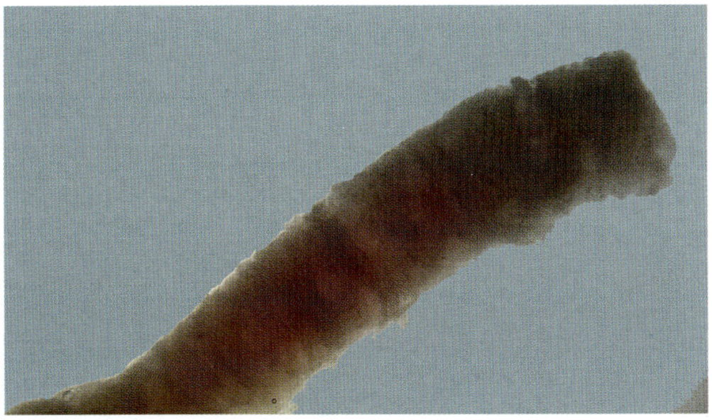

Figure 4-6 Biopsy core of renal cortex with small pale foci, which are glomeruli. (Courtesy S. Linn-Peirano.)

can be removed and placed in glutaraldehyde for possible ultrastructural evaluation. Alternatively, formalin-fixed tissue can be postfixed in glutaraldehyde and used for transmission electron microscopy (TEM). If immunofluorescence (IF) evaluation is desired, an unfixed core can either be immediately embedded in optimal cutting temperature compound and quickly frozen or a core can be placed in Michel buffer for transfer to a service that has IF capabilities.

Although most renal biopsies are performed in small animals, one study reported that the procedure has low morbidity in horses and can provide diagnostic tissue in >90% of cases. It is usually possible to obtain 10-20 glomeruli from an adult dog by using an automated spring-loaded biopsy instrument, such as the EZ core or Monopty biopsy needle. Of note, at least 20 glomeruli might be necessary to detect a focal glomerular disease process. The main risk of renal biopsy is vascular puncture and hemorrhage, which, on rare occasions, can be fatal.

In addition to the usual H&E staining of paraffin sections of the kidney, several other techniques are useful. The special stains and techniques are listed below together with the features they can highlight. Thin sections (3 µm) must be used. Photomicrograph examples of these various features are presented together with their associated disease processes.

1. *PAS* stain highlights glomerular and tubular basement membranes, mesangial matrix, glomerular capsule basement membrane, and apical brush border of proximal tubules. This stain can also help differentiate the podocyte cytoplasm from the underlying capillary walls. When there are increased numbers of cells within glomeruli, this stain is useful in discerning their location (e.g., within mesangium vs. within capillary lumens vs. both). Last, this stain shows differential staining intensity for protein casts; Tamm-Horsfall (uromodulin) casts stain bright pink, whereas other protein casts do not stain as intensely. The PAS-methenamine silver technique is an improvement of the PAS stain.
2. *Jones methenamine silver* (JMS) method, a methenamine silver-periodic acid stain, enables visualization of all basement membranes and mesangium. This stain is mostly used to assess the smoothness, thickness, and contour of the GBM. If the mesangium does not stain dark gray or black, there is either additional material within the mesangium (e.g., amyloid) or lysis of the mesangial matrix (mesangiolysis).
3. *Masson trichrome stain* facilitates evaluation of interstitial and glomerular scarring, and in some cases, immune complexes (ICs) can be identified as red nodular material along the GBM. The various proteinaceous substances in capillary walls or mesangium will result in the orange-to-peach-to-red coloration of the glomerular tufts (e.g., hyalinosis or amyloidosis). Interstitial fibrosis is best assessed with this stain.
4. *Other special stains for fibrin, amyloid, and lipids.* Microscopic resolution of glomerular lesions can be improved by the use of 1-µm-thick methacrylate-embedded sections.
5. *Immunofluorescence* studies for localization of immunoglobulins, complement, and foreign antigens, especially in glomeruli.
6. *Immunoperoxidase* techniques for localization of a wide variety of antigens.
7. *Transmission electron microscopy* particularly for identification and localization of electron-dense deposits or fibrillar material (e.g., amyloid). Abnormalities in podocytes, GBM, and endothelial cells mesangium can also be assessed.

Renal disease (AKI and CKD) and uremia

Renal disease, which encompasses **any deviation from normal renal structure or function**, is often subclinical. *Clinical renal disease* is typically divided into acute, chronic, and "acute-on-chronic" forms. Creatinine is a waste product generated from creatine in muscle. It is filtered freely through the glomerulus and is not reabsorbed by the tubules. In many types of renal disease, the ability of the kidney to eliminate creatinine is hampered, so it accumulates in the serum. Notably, urea is another waste product that is often retained in the serum with renal disease. Increases in serum creatinine above the reference interval is called "azotemia." For many reasons, urea is a less reliable biomarker of disease, and the diagnosis of azotemic kidney disease should not be based on elevated blood urea levels alone.

Acute kidney injury (AKI) usually results in a rapid increase in serum creatinine and/or proteinuria; it may result from acute glomerular or interstitial injury or from ATI, and it is often reversible. **Chronic kidney disease (CKD)** is characterized by prolonged azotemia and/or proteinuria, often with isosthenuria. The clinical signs might improve and even normalize, but there is almost always irreversible damage to the renal parenchyma. Last, acute clinical disease can be superimposed on CKD or subacute disease. One example of this scenario could be an abrupt worsening of azotemia in a patient that previously had stable CKD. Alternatively, patients that had been diagnosed with CKD based solely on the basis of proteinuria, persistent isosthenuria, or abnormal renal shape (e.g., maldevelopment) might eventually lose enough nephrons to progress to azotemic kidney disease. In this latter scenario, the clinical progression might appear rapid, but the histology could show significant renal scarring. Clarification of terminology is in order:

Uremia literally means urine in the blood. It is a *clinical syndrome of the inability of the kidneys to excrete toxins and/or toxic metabolites*, with biochemical disturbances, and often also with extrarenal lesions. Although uremia often carries a poor prognosis, it can be reversible. Some patients might even experience various uremic crises with intervening periods of improved renal function. Dogs and cats being managed with chronic hemodialysis are examples of patients that can fluctuate between uremic states and nonuremic CKD.

Azotemia can be of renal or of extrarenal origin.

- **Prerenal azotemia** results from renal hypoperfusion, the result of conditions such as congestive heart failure, shock, moderate-to-severe hemorrhage, or dehydration.
- **Renal azotemia** results from intrinsic renal disease.
- **Postrenal azotemia** occurs due to obstruction of the lower urinary tract. Notably, the blockage is often in the urinary bladder or urethra but could also occur if both ureters are obstructed.

The evolution from normal renal function to uremia over the course of progressive renal disease occurs through *4 overlapping stages:*

1. In the stage of **diminished renal reserve**, the GFR can be decreased to ~50% of normal. The animal is subclinical but has an increased susceptibility to additional renal insults.
2. At the stage of **renal insufficiency**, GFR is 25-50% of normal; the animal is azotemic.
3. As GFR further decreases (estimated at GFR of 5-25%), the kidneys cannot maintain homeostasis, and uremia ensues, with its attendant gastrointestinal, cardiovascular, respiratory, and skeletal complications.
4. When GFR falls below 5% of normal, the uremic patient is often diagnosed with "end-stage kidney disease" **(ESKD)**. Importantly, however, the diagnosis of ESKD needs to be based on evidence of significant irreversible renal scarring either with advanced diagnostic imaging or histology. The pathologist's and radiologist's interpretations of renal biopsies and imaging, respectively, can influence the outcome of patients. If terminology such as ESKD is misused (e.g., in a patient with severe but reversible AKI), euthanasia might be elected even though the patient would have recovered from the episode if given appropriate treatment. *With the increasing availability of veterinary hemodialysis and the change in owners' perceptions of veterinary intensive critical care, pathologists need to be cognizant of the wording used in their biopsy reports.*

Staging systems for CKD in small animals have been created by the International Renal Interest Society (IRIS); there are IRIS grading systems for AKI as well. Notably, patients with Stage 1 CKD and Grade 1 AKI are not azotemic, underscoring the fact that creatinine is not the sole biomarker of renal disease. Veterinarians use these clinical guidelines for prognosis and treatment or management of their patients. As such, pathologists should familiarize themselves with the relevant IRIS literature, especially if they are interpreting renal biopsies or if they are examining kidney samples for prospective or retrospective case series research.

The biochemical disturbances of uremia reflect impairment in the kidney's maintenance of fluid volume, regulation of electrolyte and acid-base balance, excretion of waste products, and synthesis and/or metabolism of hormones. The clinical signs may be related to the renal disease itself, as with pyuria or renal pain; to the effects of reduced renal function, as with metabolic acidosis or dehydration; or to the compensatory responses to renal dysfunction, as with hyperparathyroidism.

Dysregulation of **fluid volume** may result in either dehydration or anasarca. *Dehydration* resulting from reduced renal concentrating ability may be related to lesions of the renal medulla and juxtamedullary nephrons. Vomition and/or diarrhea can exacerbate the dehydration. Dehydration due to decreased access to water has an inherently different pathogenesis and must be differentiated from dehydration secondary to renal disease. *Anasarca* occurs infrequently. It usually occurs with a marked reduction in GFR and/or inappropriate activation of the RAAS. There might also be a superimposed component of iatrogenic overhydration. Edema and/or cavitary effusions can also be due to hypoproteinemia resulting from the loss of protein through injured glomeruli; if severe, the patient can develop anasarca. Disturbances in **electrolyte balance** include excesses and deficits of plasma sodium, potassium, calcium, and phosphate. The handling of these substances by the kidney is complex, even in health; in disease, it is often paradoxical and involves disordered tubular function, compensatory mechanisms, and endocrine imbalances. Excesses of plasma sodium, potassium, and calcium/phosphate contribute to anasarca, cardiotoxicity, and mineralization, respectively; deficits may cause dehydration, muscle weakness, tetany, and osteodystrophy.

Several aspects of the uremic syndrome contribute to **acid-base imbalance** and metabolic acidosis. Compensatory hyperventilation may occur. The main factors leading to acidosis in uremia are reduced capacity of distal and collecting tubules to produce ammonia, increased retention of acidic hydrogen ions, and impaired resorption of bicarbonate ions at a time of increased utilization. The term **uremic acidosis** encompasses simultaneous azotemia, anion retention, and acidosis; **renal tubular acidosis (RTA)** is a more limited term and is discussed later in the Specific Tubular Dysfunctions section. **Failure to excrete metabolic wastes** is the basis for tests of renal function; *elevated blood concentrations of urea and creatinine are often used as biomarkers to indicate reduced glomerular filtration*. Postmortem collection of vitreous humor to measure creatinine and blood urea can provide evidence of AKI or CKD in animals that did not have clinical evaluation prior to death. As stated above, a diagnosis of azotemia should not be based solely on urea levels.

Some animals can *reversibly* or *irreversibly* lose the function of ~75% of their nephrons before becoming azotemic. Because of the disconnect between the proportion of nonfunctional nephrons and elevations in serum creatinine and urea, they are considered to be insensitive indicators of renal disease. Changes in the excretion patterns of other metabolic wastes might be more sensitive and specific, and this is an area of intense research in humans and animals. Symmetric dimethyl arginine (SDMA) has been identified as an earlier indicator of decreased GFR, although its specificity has been called into question as well. Breed-related variations in serum creatinine and SDMA have been reported in the dog (Greyhounds) and cat (Birman). Therefore, even this promising biomarker has caveats in interpretation.

With the advent of "-omics" analyses, metabolites, mRNAs, micro-RNAs, and lipids can be efficiently screened to identify specific and sensitive biomarkers of renal disease. For example, a metabolomic study was performed using samples from adult colony cats (maintained by a pet food company) wherein serial plasma samples were collected and autopsies were performed. Cats diagnosed with azotemic renal disease, cats with calcium oxalate nephrolithiasis, and normal cats were compared. There were metabolomic profiles unique to each cohort, with renal disease impacting serum levels of many amino acids, fatty acids, and their derivatives, such as ketones. Through these types of analyses, we might eventually be able to better hone our diagnoses to identify the region of the urinary tract affected and perhaps even the specific segment(s) of the nephron that are injured or abnormal. Ultimately, however, diagnosis of renal disease should be based on various lines of evidence, as opposed to a single clinical parameter.

Disturbances in endocrine function are important causes of signs and lesions in uremic animals. Retention of phosphate, resulting from reduced glomerular filtration, causes increased synthesis and secretion of parathyroid hormone (PTH), and development of secondary hyperparathyroidism (see Fibrous osteodystrophy in Vol. 1, Bones and Joints). Reduced renal catabolism of PTH, and end organ resistance to PTH, may contribute to hyperparathyroidism. Most uremic animals have hyperphosphatemia, hypercalcemia, and hyperparathyroidism. The PTH release will increase reabsorption of calcium from bone and renal tubular lumens, as well as increasing enteric calcium absorption. Fibroblast growth factor (FGF) 23, which is released from bone in response to elevated serum phosphate levels, and PTH promote phosphate loss in the urine (phosphaturia), but hyperphosphatemia is often a losing battle at this stage. Hyperparathyroidism promotes the activation of $1,25(OH)_2D_3$, whereas FGF23 has the opposite effect. To add even more complexity to the situation, FGF23 requires Klotho as a cofactor to bind its receptor. Klotho is mostly synthesized by the kidney itself (as well as choroid plexus). Therefore, if there is significant renal scarring, FGF23 loses its important cofactor, impacting the effectiveness of this pathway. FGF23 is considered a prognostic biomarker of CKD in cats and dogs, and Klotho shows promise as well. The balance of calcium and phosphate is intricate and can vary across patients. Even though most dogs with moderate-to-severe renal disease are hypercalcemic and hyperphosphatemic, sometimes hypercalcemia and hypophosphatemia occur, possibly because of lack of feedback inhibition of PTH release. Similar changes occur in some uremic horses and may be related to decreased renal excretion of calcium. However, cats with moderate-to-severe CKD are almost always hyperphosphatemic, unless treated.

Nonregenerative **anemia** in CKD is of multifactorial pathogenesis, including decreased renal production of erythropoietin and hepcidin-mediated iron deficiency. Hepcidin is increased in CKD due to inflammation and impaired renal clearance. Thus, hepcidin increases in circulation and sequesters iron, further contributing to anemia of CKD. Other mediators of anemia in CKD include PTH and FGF23 (see Vol. 3, Hematolymphoid System).

In uremia, "**uremic toxins**" accumulate in the body. The list of uremic toxins is lengthy, and there is variability across species. Various toxins are thought to be responsible for the profound malaise that characterizes the uremic syndrome. Uremic toxins include low–molecular-weight (LMW), MMW, and HMW molecules. LMW molecules (500 Da) include guanidines (e.g., creatine, creatinine), oxalates, indoxyl sulfate, methylamines, phenylacetylglutamine, phosphate, polyamines, pseudouridine, purines (e.g., uric acid), pyrimidines (e.g., thymine, uridine), and urea. "Middle molecules" (500-5,000 Da) include α- and β-chains of fibrinogen, immunoglobulin light chains, retinol-binding protein, endothelin 1, and adipokines. HMW molecules (>5,000 Da) include various peptides and cytokines, such as **PTH**, β2 microglobulin, and proteins that have roles in the immune system. Some uremic toxins have both HMW and LMW forms, and imbalance of the sizes can indicate uremia. For example, LMW hyaluronic acid promotes renal injury, whereas HMW forms dominate in uremia. The *cause of death in uremia* varies from case to case. Metabolic acidosis, hyperkalemia, and hypo- or hypercalcemia may be severe enough to be fatal. Most companion animals, however, are euthanized due to declining quality of life.

Prerenal azotemia due to reduced renal blood flow and glomerular filtration is unlikely to progress to uremia. When ischemia is severe or prolonged, intrarenal mechanisms that divert blood flow away from cortical nephrons to juxtamedullary nephrons may produce patchy or diffuse cortical ischemia and necrosis. In such cases, prerenal azotemia may be followed by renal azotemia and potentially uremia. *Postrenal azotemia is always the result of obstruction to the outflow of urine, and hence the patient is oliguric or anuric*. These patients often become uremic.

A form of neonatal uremia, distinct from those mentioned, occurs in *newborn animals*, especially pigs, with very high levels of blood urea. The kidneys of newborn pigs, dogs, and cats are functionally "immature" and incapable of producing hypertonic urine. Normally, this is of no consequence, because milk provides enough fluid to excrete the small amount of waste produced in their hypotonic urine. However, when these newborn animals are anorectic, they lack both nutrients and fluid, so they catabolize tissue proteins and purines. Being unable to excrete the excess solute from protein and purine breakdown, their blood urea and uric acid reach very high levels. Because anorexia is usually associated with fever, vomition, or diarrhea, fluid loss is rapid. In pigs, the excess solute is deposited in the inner medulla as streaks of light-yellow urate precipitates (Fig. 4-7), which disappear during histologic processing. Pigs are apparently unique among mammals in that their tubules do not resorb urates from the glomerular filtrate, which accounts for their concentration in the medulla.

The **nonrenal lesions of uremia** occur inconstantly and unpredictably, although they tend to be seen most often in dogs and cats, especially those with severe CKD rather than AKI. Many animals dying with uremia are cachectic. This is probably caused by anorexia, vomition, and diarrhea, as well as by body tissue catabolism to supply energy. Besides this general lack of body condition, several distinctive lesions may develop in the gastrointestinal, cardiovascular, respiratory, and skeletal systems.

Ulcerative, necrotic stomatitis occurs in dogs and cats, and there might be a foul-smelling brown film coating the tongue and buccal mucosa (Fig. 4-8). Oral lesions are more common in chronic than in acute uremia. The pathogenesis of the ulcers is not always clear, but some are associated with fibrinoid necrosis of small vessels, and some are related to bacterial production of ammonia from urea in the saliva. In dogs, large areas of the *gastric mucosa* are often swollen, suffused with red-black blood. Regions may be mineralized and partly ulcerated (Fig. 4-9). This lesion, often called "gastritis," is initially noninflammatory, although opportunist bacteria may infect the ulcerated mucosa, attracting inflammatory cells. Mucosal infarction occurs secondary to vascular necrosis. *Mineralization of the middle and deep zones of the gastric mucosa is common* (Fig. 4-10). Necrosis and mineralization of the muscular tunics are sometimes present. Intestinal lesions resemble those in the stomach, but they are less frequent, less severe, and without mineralization. Gastrointestinal lesions probably account for much of the vomition, diarrhea, and melena of uremic dogs. Intestinal intussusceptions sometimes develop in dogs with gastrointestinal lesions. Cats might have mineralization, but they rarely develop ulcers or gastritis. In uremic cattle, colitis is more common, and the stomach and proximal intestine are merely edematous. Hyperamylasemia and hyperlipasemia occur in some uremic dogs and may be the result of concurrent pancreatitis rather than the result of reduced renal clearance of the enzymes.

Systemic *arterial lesions* found in animals with AKI or CKD are discussed elsewhere (see Vol. 3, Cardiovascular System). Lesions of various organs, such as uremic gastric infarction in dogs, may result from arterial injury and thrombosis. Arterial lesions in the myocardium sometimes cause ischemia and necrosis. In moderate-to-severe CKD, the left ventricle might be hypertrophied. *Hypertension* is common in canine and feline kidney disease, and left ventricular hypertrophy may be caused by or amplified by the hypertension. Lesions in the circulatory system are occasionally identified but might be

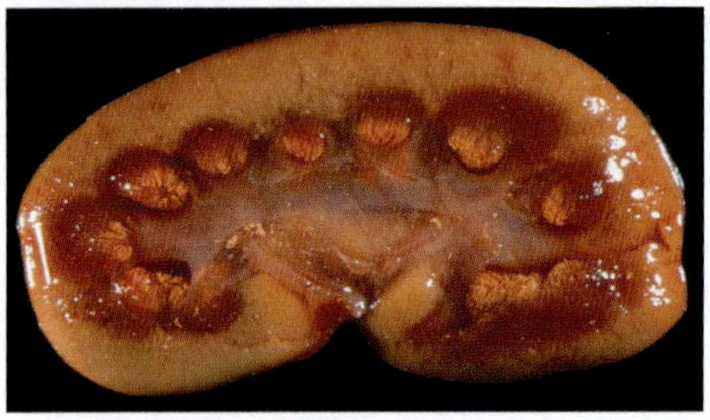

Figure 4-7 **Urate calculi** in renal medulla of a neonatal dehydrated piglet. (Courtesy K.G. Thompson.)

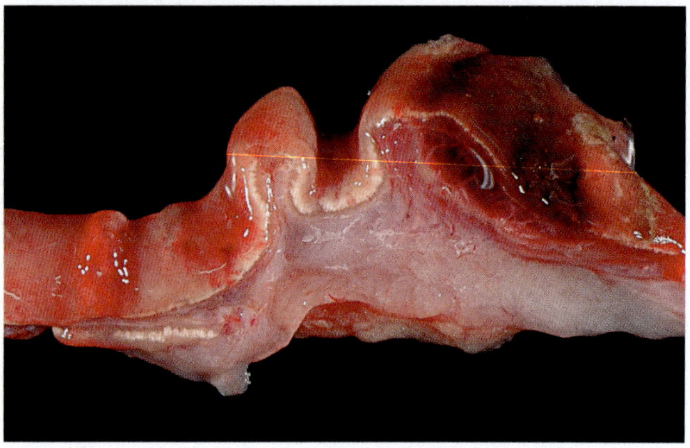

Figure 4-9 **Uremic gastritis** with hemorrhage and mineralization of the mucosa in a dog. (Courtesy M.K. Keating.)

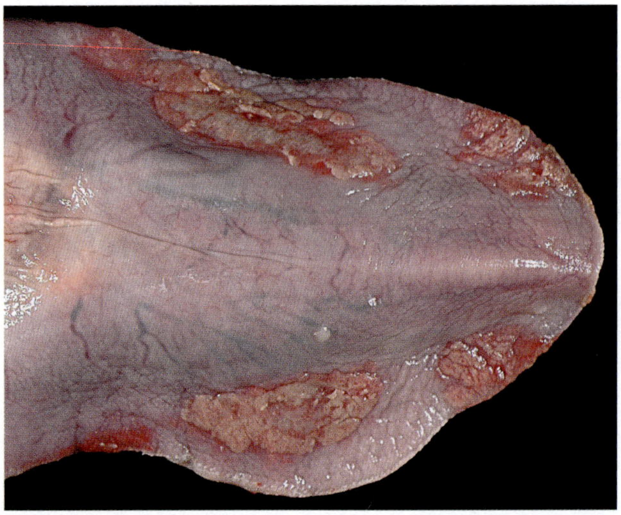

Figure 4-8 **Ulcers** on lateral margin and ventral surface of the tongue of a dog with **uremia**. (Courtesy M.K. Keating.)

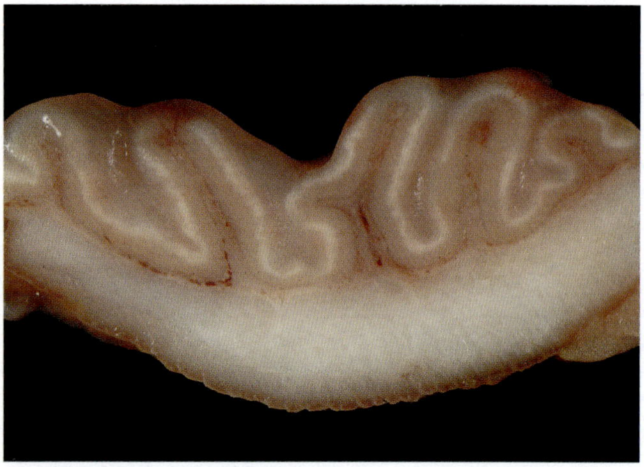

Figure 4-10 Marked **gastric mucosal mineralization** in a uremic dog. (Courtesy S. Jennings.)

overlooked. Arterial injury may occur in the intestines in cattle with ATI and contribute to the colonic lesions of acute uremic syndromes in this species. Some causes of ATI (e.g., oak toxicity in cattle) are mediated by endothelial cell damage, which can explain the vascular lesions. In cattle with urethral calculi, there is often anasarca and pericardial effusion. Edematous distension of retroperitoneal tissue, expressed particularly as *perirenal edema*, occurs in pigs and cattle; the underlying renal lesion is usually ATI caused by ochratoxin or *Amaranthus retroflexus* in pigs, and oak poisoning in cattle (see the Iatrogenic Nephrotoxicity section).

Most animals dying with uremia develop *terminal pulmonary edema*. The mechanism is unknown, but increased permeability of alveolar capillaries is the suspected pathogenesis. In a few animals, acute pneumonia develops terminally. It may be associated with aspiration of gastric content, and its fulminant nature is possibly related to the immunosuppression that develops in uremia. Pulmonary mineralization occurs in chronically uremic dogs and cats. Mineral is deposited in the walls of the alveoli and pulmonary arterioles. Dull granulations of the visceral pleura may be present over the cranial lobes. Occasionally, in uremia, spectacular pulmonary lesions develop. They may be visible in radiographs as lines of increased density spreading out from the hilus due to interstitial edema and mineralization. At autopsy, the lung is edematous and resilient, and the alveolar spaces contain fibrin in the fluid. Leukocytes are present but may be a response to superimposed infection. Mineralization is extensive, with deposition particularly on reticulin of the widened alveolar walls (eFig. 4-2). The lesion is referred to as uremic lung or *uremic pneumonitis;* it is not common, and when it occurs, it may be patchy.

Perhaps the most "classic" lesion in the dog is *mineralization beneath the parietal pleura* in the intercostal spaces (Fig. 4-11). It is preceded by necrosis of the subpleural connective tissue with extension to intercostal muscle and overlying pleura. Once mineralization has occurred and the pleura repaired, the lesion appears as gray-yellow thickenings, perpendicular to the ribs, and somewhat wrinkled. The cranial intercostal spaces are involved first; when deposition is extensive, many more spaces may be affected. To our knowledge, this lesion only occurs in uremic states.

The *pathogenesis* of diffuse tissue mineralization in uremia is not clear. There are at least 2 types of mineral deposits, and serum concentrations of calcium, magnesium, phosphate, and carbonate probably determine the type of calcium phosphate compound that is formed. When calcium is higher than magnesium, apatites are formed; the opposite relationship favors deposition of amorphous calcium phosphate. The regularity with which certain tissues and organs are mineralized is no doubt related to local characteristics, such as tissue glycosaminoglycans, local pH, and cellular factors.

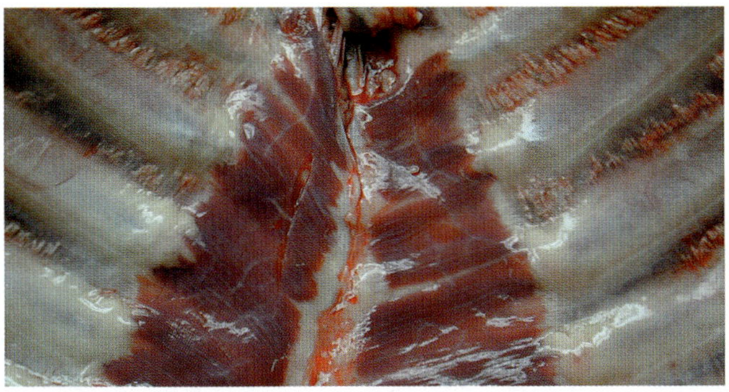

Figure 4-11 Necrosis and mineralization beneath the intercostal pleura in a uremic dog.

The effects of chronic uremia on the *skeleton* are discussed in Fibrous osteodystrophy, Vol. 1, Bones and Joints. *Enlarged parathyroids* are common in dogs and cats with CKD; osseous lesions are less so.

Uremic encephalopathy is an uncommon complication of uremia in domestic animals. It has been reported in dogs, ruminants, and horses and is expressed as white matter spongiform degeneration that may be accompanied by reactive astrogliosis.

The *immune system* is also impacted with CKD and uremia. This is often manifested as a proinflammatory state that is less effective at responding to infectious agents. For example, azotemic CKD cats have a decreased lymphocyte count at the end of life and a higher neutrophil count compared with their baseline levels and to healthy cats. In dogs, the uremic toxin, methylguanidine, promotes neutrophil apoptosis.

The **renal lesions of uremia** are varied, but if the syndrome is chronic, certain common changes tend to occur. *The end result is a fibrosed, mineralized kidney with globally sclerotic glomeruli, and a mixture of atrophic and hypertrophic tubules*. Often, this can only be diagnosed as **"end-stage kidney."** Severe mineralization may diffusely involve glomerular capsules and tubular basement membranes. Less commonly, arterial walls and the glomerular tufts themselves will mineralize. According to the "precipitation-mineralization hypothesis," phosphorus absorbed from the intestines in excess of the excretory capacity of nephrons will induce precipitation of calcium phosphate microcrystals in tubular lumina, the interstitium, and renal capillaries. Dietary phosphate restriction may slow renal mineralization and its attendant inflammation, scarring, and loss of nephrons.

Interstitial fibrosis and glomerulosclerosis (GS) are slowly progressive lesions that are common in the end stages of many renal diseases. *Progressive interstitial fibrosis is thought to be the final common pathway of CKD*. Hypertrophy of remaining nephrons is an inconstant compensatory change. Adaptive changes in the remaining intact nephrons can help maintain renal function at an adequate level. The glomerulus is probably the limiting factor in this compensatory mechanism because it has a relatively limited ability to increase its size. However, if renal injury occurs in young dogs or horses, the glomeruli can hypertrophy to degrees not seen in adults. It seems unlikely that uremia provides a suitable environment to permit or encourage compensatory hypertrophy, and it is likely that enlargement of nephrons is an early response to a reduction in nephron number, rather than a late adaptation to uremia.

Regardless of the initiating cause, **CKD tends to be progressive**, due to persistence of the primary insult and/or the addition of other complications, such as urinary tract infection (UTI), systemic hypertension, and intrarenal deposition of mineral. Additionally, compensatory mechanisms may contribute to CKD progression. These compensatory factors include glomerular capillary hypertension, hyperfiltration, and podocyte hypertrophy. Chronic glomerular hyperperfusion and podocyte hypertrophy can lead to segmental GS with proteinuria (see the Glomerulosclerosis and Focal Segmental Glomerulosclerosis section). Additionally, there is increased renal oxygen demand by the remaining hypertrophied tubular epithelial cells (often in the setting of anemia) as well as increased renal ammoniagenesis. High dietary protein intake increases renal blood flow and GFR, so restricting protein intake minimizes renal hemodynamic changes and slows the progression of CKD.

Normal aging changes accumulate in any aged animal and occur in the absence of a specific renal insult; these "background" senescence changes lead to decreased renal reserve, but they are usually subclinical. In aged dogs, for example, *renal weight is reduced* by 20-30% because of nephron senescence. Microscopic features of renal aging in cats include an increase in GS, tubular atrophy, interstitial inflammation, fibrosis, and tubular and interstitial lipid with age. Additionally, p16-mediated renal senescence, measured by p16 IHC staining in cortical and corticomedullary tubules, is positively correlated with age in cats. However, no significant differences in telomere length or percentage of short telomeres have been reported in aging healthy cat kidneys. This is in contrast to cats with CKD, which have telomere shortening as well as increased renal senescence and nitrosative stress. In geriatric humans, there are intrarenal vascular changes, such as arteriosclerosis, glomerular obsolescence, and tubular atrophy. In general, glomerular mesangial volume increases with age, proximal tubule volume and length decrease, and interstitial connective tissue increases. Changes in the ground substance of medullary connective tissue can reduce medullary hyperosmolality and hence renal concentrating ability. Aged animals with purely senescent renal changes have *decreased compensatory abilities* and are hence more susceptible to renal insults.

Renal transplantation is available in a number of centers as a therapeutic option for cats with ESKD. Various immunosuppressive protocols are used to prevent postoperative rejection of the transplanted kidney, particularly necessary when the donor is unrelated to the recipient. Cats have limited major histocompatibility complex (MHC) variability, so graft rejection is milder than in dogs. Surgical complications may be noted at autopsy, for example, avulsion of the renal vein, torsion of the vascular pedicle, and retroperitoneal fibrosis. The various stages of rejection of renal allografts have been extensively categorized in human pathology (Banff criteria); however, small animals do not seem to fit into the same diagnostic categories. Histologic evaluation of >70 allograft feline kidneys revealed evidence of cyclosporine toxicity, necrotizing glomerulitis and vasculitis (suggestive of acute antibody-mediated rejection), and subcapsular and intralobular phlebitis. The latter feature is not described in the Banff scoring system, and its significance is unknown. Although a feline renal transplant recipient may enjoy long-term (months to years) success, the pre-existing condition, for example, systemic hypertension, might persist and lead to failure of the transplanted kidney. Complications of immunosuppressive therapy in allograft recipients include a spectrum of infections, including a wide range of bacterial (*Mycobacterium*, *Actinobacillus*), yeast/fungal (*Candida*, *Penicillium*, *Encephalitozoon*), and protozoal (*Toxoplasma*, *Pneumocystis*, *Giardia*) diseases. In general, the uninephrectomized kidney donor survives well, and its remaining kidney hypertrophies to meet the body's needs. As alluded to earlier, renal transplantation has been performed in dogs with limited success because of the high rate of rejection.

Terminology for renal disease in young animals

Many terms are used to describe renal diseases that are hereditary and/or developmental. In the literature, **juvenile nephropathy** and **renal dysplasia** are used interchangeably as diagnoses of renal lesions in young dogs. Unfortunately, these terms are vague and often used (sometimes inappropriately) to diagnose kidney disease of any etiology in young dogs. Because of the confusion that these terms can create, veterinary nephropathologists recommend usage of the terms "juvenile-onset chronic kidney disease (**JOCKD**)" and "renal maldevelopment." The first term, JOCKD, should be used for any young animal with azotemia, proteinuria, isosthenuria, misshapen kidneys, and/or histologic evidence or renal disease. Young dogs are those <3-years-old. *Importantly, JOCKD does not imply a genetic basis of the CKD.*

The term **renal maldevelopment** describes lesions that are indicative of abnormal formation or maturation of the kidney parenchyma. Notably, renal maldevelopment is a well-described (but poorly understood) entity in dogs but is rarely reported in other domestic species. This is likely because optimal evaluation of renal parenchymal function and morphology in young animals of other species is uncommonly performed. It is our opinion that renal maldevelopment in cats is exceedingly rare, given that renal samples from kittens are frequently examined and do not have histologic lesions of abnormal development or maturation. **Familial nephropathy** and **breed nephropathy** are terms applied to renal disease observed in *families or breeds of animals*, particularly dogs. Of note, familial nephropathy can include genetic diseases as well as lesions in litters exposed to the same infectious agent or environmental stresses. **Hereditary nephropathy** *is the definitive term used once the inheritance of the nephropathy has been determined, through pedigree analysis, test matings, and eventually identification of underlying genetic abnormality.* A list of reported familial and breed nephropathies, many of which are suspected or proven to be hereditary, is provided in Table 4-1. This list will continue to change as inheritance of disease entities is defined; classifications will also be further refined as the pathogeneses of somewhat obscure familial and juvenile diseases are more fully characterized. Given greater knowledge of heritability, breed societies are able to undertake control programs.

Examples of specific familial and/or hereditary renal diseases abound and will be discussed later under their respective sections of developmental defects, glomerular disease, tubular disease, and renal neoplasia. *In general, the canine familial renal diseases are seen clinically as CKD in a group of related immature or young-adult dogs.* For most breed nephropathies, only terminal clinical signs and end-stage lesions are described; inheritance, pathogenesis, and early morphologic changes are not reported. The age of onset of CKD varies from a few weeks to several years but, in most cases, is 4-18 months. This wide age range and the lack of renal biopsies before end-stage disease hinder the diagnosis and investigation of pathogenesis. Therefore, there is a danger that azotemia in a young purebred dog (secondary to nephrotoxicity or infection) will be misdiagnosed as maldevelopment or breed-related nephropathy. It is also possible that some of the chronic interstitial nephritides assumed to be secondary to infection are indicative of breed nephropathies and/or renal maldevelopment. These diagnostic dilemmas underscore the importance of histopathology and the risks of making a diagnosis based solely on clinicopathologic and signalment data.

Table • 4-1

Suspected or proven familial and/or breed-related nephropathies in domestic species

BREED	LESION	GENE/INHERITANCE
Abyssinian cat	Amyloidosis (medullary and glomerular)	Autosomal dominant with incomplete penetrance, suspected
Alaskan Malamute	Immature glomeruli and tubules; glomerular hypertrophy; glomerulocystic atrophy; glomerulosclerosis; adenomatoid tubular epithelia; mineralization of tubular basement membranes; severe interstitial inflammation in 2 of 3 dogs	Not identified
Basenji	Fanconi syndrome; histologic lesions are minimal and include tubular epithelial cell hypertrophy and karyomegaly	Not identified
Beagle	Glomerular and medullary AA amyloidosis affecting various dogs of a single litter	Not identified
	Primitive mesenchyme; persistence of metanephric ducts; asynchronous differentiation of nephrons and atypical tubular epithelium in related laboratory Beagles	Not identified
	Unilateral renal agenesis	Not identified
Bedlington Terrier	Increased interstitial connective tissue without inflammation; consolidated glomeruli and dilated, thickened glomerular capsules; occasional cystic tubules	Not identified; only reported in 3 offspring of 2 litters from a single sire
Bernese Mountain Dog	Immune complex–mediated membranoproliferative glomerulonephritis with IgM and C3 deposition in glomeruli	Autosomal recessive, with an epigenetic influence by a sex-influenced genetic determinance
Boxer	Immature glomeruli and/or tubules; primitive mesenchyme	Not identified
	Small kidneys with cortical scars; nephron atrophy; paucity of glomeruli; glomerulocystic lesions; tortuous arteries with intimal thickening; immature glomeruli and/or metanephric tubules	Not identified
Bracco Italiano	Renal amyloidosis	Not identified
Brittany Spaniel	Membranoproliferative glomerulonephritis with IgG deposition, lacking C3, in glomeruli; part of hereditary canine C3 deficiency syndrome; dogs with recurrent systemic infections also have a predisposition to develop renal AA amyloidosis	Autosomal recessive caused by a deletion of a cytosine at position 2136, resulting in a frameshift mutation that generates a premature stop codon
Bullmastiff	Uncharacterized glomerulonephropathy (segmental mesangial expansion and hypercellularity); small glomeruli, thickened glomerular capsule, glomerulocystic atrophy; tubular atrophy: interstitial inflammation and fibrosis	Autosomal recessive (suspected)
Bull Terrier	Polycystic kidney disease	Autosomal dominant caused by a missense mutation (G to A) in exon 29 of the *Pkd1* gene, which replaces glutamic acid with lysine in polycystin 1
	Basket weaving of the GBM, suggestive of Alport syndrome; however, both α3(IV) and α5(IV) collagens are present; sometimes concurrent polycystic kidney disease	Autosomal dominant
Cairn Terrier	Polycystic kidney disease	Autosomal recessive (suspected)
Chow Chow	Immature glomeruli and glomerulocystic atrophy in radiating bands of interstitial fibrosis; compensatory glomerular hypertrophy in adjacent renal parenchyma	Not identified
Cocker Spaniel	Glomerulocystic atrophy; segmental accumulation of fibrocellular material in urinary space (suggestive of fibrous crescents); some glomerular capsules contained an amorphous protein coagulum that variably stained positive for fibrinogen/fibrin in urinary space	Not identified; of note the lack of EM evaluation of the GBM precludes comparison of this familial nephropathy to that of English Cocker Spaniels

Continued

Table • 4-1

Suspected or proven familial and/or breed-related nephropathies in domestic species—cont'd

BREED	LESION	GENE/INHERITANCE
Dalmatian	Basket weaving of the GBM, suggestive of Alport syndrome; however, both α3(IV) and α5(IV) collagens are present	Autosomal dominant
	Urate calculi resulting from a transport defect in uric acid, which is generated during normal purine metabolism. This leads to hyperuricosuria and hyperuricemia	Autosomal recessive caused by a mutation in *SLC2A9*, a putative renal and hepatic urate transporter
Doberman Pinscher	Glomerulosclerosis; glomerulocystic atrophy; mesangial hypercellularity; EM of some dogs reveals lamination of the lamina densa rarely with intramembranous electron-dense material; other dogs had material resembling fibrillar collagens within the GBM; IF studies revealed IgM staining in only 1 of 10 dogs	Not identified; affected females may have concomitant unilateral renal agenesis
Dutch Kooiker	Asynchronous differentiation of nephrons; persistent mesenchyme; persistent metanephric ducts; adenomatoid proliferation of the tubular epithelium	Not identified
English Cocker Spaniel	Proliferative and sclerosing glomerulopathy; basket weaving of the GBM	Single nucleotide substitution at 115 in *COL4A4*
Finnish Landrace sheep	Membranoproliferative glomerulonephritis with crescents; C3-dominant IF staining with variable IgM, IgA, and IgG IF staining	Autosomal recessive deficiency of complement factor C3
French Mastiff	Glomerulocystic atrophy; hypercellular glomeruli; thickened capillary walls without immune complexes	Possibly autosomal recessive
Gelbvieh cattle	Mesangial expansion and hypercellularity with glomerulosclerosis; affected calves also had a peripheral neuropathy	Unknown
German Shepherd dog	Renal cystadenocarcinomas; part of the renal cystadenocarcinoma/nodular dermatofibroma disease complex; female dogs may also have uterine leiomyomas	Autosomal dominant
German Shorthaired Pointers	Membranous glomerulonephritis in proteinuric dogs that are also diagnosed with exfoliative cutaneous lupus erythematosus	Single base pair variant in *UNC93B1*
Golden Retriever	Radiating bands of interstitial fibrosis; glomerulocystic atrophy with or without primitive metanephric ducts and persistent mesenchyme	Not identified; not confirmed to be familial
Irish Terrier	Cystinuria and cystine calculi	X-linked
Japanese black (Wagyu) cattle	Chronic interstitial nephritis with zonal fibrosis; kidneys often have cystically dilated tubules and glomerular capsules, resembling multicystic renal dysplasia	Autosomal recessive null mutation in *claudin-16*; 2 separate mutations have been identified
Keeshond	Cystic collecting ducts; glomerulocystic atrophy	Not identified
Lhasa Apso	Radiating streaks containing immature and fetal glomeruli and tubules with paucity of collecting ducts and normal adjacent cortical parenchyma	Not identified
Miniature Schnauzer	Radiating bands of immature glomeruli; sclerotic glomeruli; glomerulocystic atrophy; reduced number of glomeruli; mesangial cell hyperplasia; interstitial fibrosis and tubular atrophy	Not identified
Newfoundland	Glomerulosclerosis and glomerulofibrosis; EM revealed fibrillar collagen deposition in the mesangium and subendothelial space	Not identified
	Cystinuria and cystine calculi	Nonsense mutation in exon 2 of the *SLC3A1* gene
Norwegian Elkhound	Interstitial and periglomerular fibrosis; sacculations in distal tubules and collecting ducts	Likely autosomal dominant; mutations in *COL4A3* and *4A4* have been excluded as causes
Old English Sheepdog	Radiating bands of interstitial fibrosis; cystic tubules; glomerulocystic atrophy	Not identified; not confirmed to be familial

Table • 4-1

Suspected or proven familial and/or breed-related nephropathies in domestic species—cont'd

BREED	LESION	GENE/INHERITANCE
Pembroke Welsh Corgi	Telangiectasia	Not identified
	Glomerulosclerosis; glomerulocystic atrophy; interstitial fibrosis and tubular atrophy; interstitial inflammation; hyperplasia of collecting duct epithelium	Not identified
Persian cat	Polycystic kidney disease	Autosomal dominant inheritance; missense mutation (C to A) in exon 29 of *Pkd1* that results in a premature stop codon (at what would be position 3284 of the human polycystin 1 protein)
Rottweiler	Glomerulocystic atrophy; mesangial hypercellularity; glomerulo-sclerosis; lamination of the lamina densa	Not identified
Samoyed	Proliferative and sclerosing glomerulopathy; basket weaving of the GBM	X-linked; nonsense mutation in codon 127 of *COL4A5* that changes a glycine to a stop codon
Scottish Terrier	Cystine urolithiasis	Likely X-linked
Chinese Shar-Pei	Amyloidosis	Likely autosomal recessive inheritance; gene not identified
Shih Tzu	Incomplete lobulation (gross); immature glomeruli and tubules; adenomatoid proliferation of tubular epithelium; metanephric tubules; cortical cysts; persistent mesenchyme and interstitial fibrosis	Likely autosomal recessive inheritance
Soft Coated Wheaten Terrier	Podocytopathy and segmental glomerulosclerosis	Podocytopathy is linked to mutations in *NPHS1* and *KIRREL2*
	Radiating bands of dense interstitial collagen; cystic tubules; sclerotic and immature glomeruli; affected dogs may also have podocytopathy with segmental sclerosis in bands of more normal parenchyma	Not identified
Standard Poodle	Immature glomeruli; glomerulocystic atrophy; interstitial fibrosis and tubular atrophy; interstitial inflammation	Not identified
West Highland White Terrier	Polycystic kidney disease; cysts also present in the liver	Autosomal recessive

EM = electron microscopy; GBM = glomerular basement membrane; IF = immunofluorescence; IgA, IgG, and IgM = immunoglobulins A, G, and M, respectively.

ANOMALIES OF DEVELOPMENT

The embryology of mammalian kidneys involves the sequential development of 3 successive but overlapping structures: the *pronephros, mesonephros*, and *metanephros*. The first 2 become vestigial, but act as inducers of the definitive kidney, the metanephros. Pronephric tubules, arising in the intermediate mesoderm of the cervical region, form the pronephric duct by fusion and extension of their caudal ends. This duct opens into the cloaca, but the pronephric tubules are not functional in mammalian embryos. However, the pronephric duct is used by the mesonephric tubules, hence the pronephros has potential significance as a source of renal anomalies. Mesonephric tubules develop from thoracic mesoderm caudal to the pronephros. The mesonephros is functional in mammalian embryos, but degenerates before birth. In males, some of the caudal tubules persist as efferent ducts of the epididymis, and the duct itself is used as the vas deferens. In females, cystic remnants of mesonephric tubules in the mesovarium may form the epoophoron and paroophoron, and remnants of the duct are known as the Gartner duct.

The formation of the **metanephros**, *the definitive kidney*, begins with the development of a *ureteral bud* from the mesonephric duct immediately cranial to its junction with the cloaca. The bud, accompanied by vessels and nerves, grows into a mass of mesenchymal cells, the *metanephric blastema*. Normal renal and ureteral development depends on the interaction of these 2 structures. As the bud grows into the blastema, it makes a specific number of successive, dichotomous divisions. The tubes formed by early divisions of the ureteral bud dilate and become the pelvis and calyces of the kidney. Tubes formed by later divisions develop into collecting ducts, and the last divisions give rise to collecting tubules. As the blind end of each collecting tubule, the *ampulla*, grows into the metanephric blastema, it induces compact masses of cells to form about it (so-called "cap mesenchyme"). These masses soon cavitate, become S shaped, and unite with the side of the ampulla. The cavitated cell masses develop into nephrons. Connection of the lumens of the nephron and the collecting tubule occurs very soon after the cell mass cavitates. Glomerular development involves the formation of a lateral invagination in the S-shaped mass by mesenchymal cells that differentiate into endothelial and mesangial cells and become linked with the renal vasculature.

The complicated formation of the kidney provides many patterns of malformation. The interaction of ureteral bud and metanephric blastema involves mutual inductions, and malformations of renal tissue are often accompanied by ureteral anomalies. *Ectopic budding of the ureter from the mesonephric duct* appears to be a primary event that precedes many congenital anomalies of the kidney and urinary tract (CAKUT). Ectopia results in hypoplastic kidney, ectopia of the ureterovesical orifice, urinary outflow obstruction, and/or reflux. The genes involved in navigating ureteric budding to the correct site often also regulate later developmental events of the kidney and urinary tract. Candidate genes have been proposed for a wide range of urinary developmental defects in humans and laboratory rodents, but specific genetic defects have not yet been associated with maldeveloped kidneys in domestic animals.

The prevalence of urinary tract anomalies is not known for most species. Survey results from large numbers of lambs suggest that anomalies occur more often than commonly believed.

Abnormalities in the amount of renal tissue

Lack of renal tissue may be complete *(agenesis)* or partial *(hypoplasia)*. Renal agenesis may be caused by developmental failure of the pronephros, mesonephros, or ureteral bud; by absence or unresponsiveness of the metanephric blastema; or by complete degeneration of the metanephric blastema. Partial degeneration or partial responsiveness of the blastema to the inductive influences of the ureteral bud probably leads to renal maldevelopment. Even a fragment of recognizable metanephric tissue necessitates the diagnosis of maldevelopment or dysplasia instead of agenesis.

Agenesis may be unilateral or bilateral. Bilateral agenesis is inconsistent with postnatal life. As is the case with all renal anomalies, agenesis may be associated with other urogenital deformities. Unilateral renal agenesis is compatible with normal life if the other kidney is normal; however, contralateral maldevelopment, or even hypoplasia, may be present, in which case CKD ultimately develops. The ureter may be absent or malformed with a blind end that terminates in connective tissue at the renal site. Renal agenesis occurs infrequently in all species, except when there is a *familial incidence*, as in some Beagles, Shetland Sheepdogs, and Doberman Pinschers, and in Large White pigs. Bilateral agenesis may account for some stillbirths, but this can only be assessed by careful examination of fetuses.

The small size of **hypoplastic kidneys** is the result of *a reduced number of histologically normal nephrons, lobules, and calyces.* Renal hypoplasia is a quantitative defect caused by reduced mass of metanephric blastema or by incomplete induction of nephron formation by the ureteral bud. When the amount of blastema is normal, but there is malfunction of the ureteral bud, maldevelopment probably develops. *Most of the small kidneys diagnosed as hypoplastic are actually probably abnormally developed or scarred.* The term "cortical hypoplasia" should be avoided because it is inconsistent with established concepts of renal embryology and anatomy. *Renal hypoplasia is rare.* It may be unilateral or bilateral. When unilateral, contralateral hypertrophy is expected.

Bilateral hypoplasia will likely lead to CKD, and this often complicates the diagnosis because of the secondary changes that develop. Several forms of renal hypoplasia occur in humans, but, because of the confusion of terminology, the variations and incidence of the condition in animals is not well described. Kidneys suspected of being hypoplastic should be weighed along with the contralateral organ and examined for evidence of maldevelopment. In humans, in the absence of acquired disease, a decrease in size of one kidney by >50% or reduction of total renal mass by more than one-third is taken as evidence of hypoplasia. Similar guidelines are not established in domestic species.

Details regarding **excess renal tissue** are not well documented. *Duplication of ureters and kidneys* occurs in cattle, pigs, and dogs, but it is not clear whether total renal mass is increased.

Anomalies of renal position, form, and orientation

The kidneys develop in the pelvis and migrate to their sublumbar location, meanwhile rotating so that the ureters attain their normal orientation. During this movement, the blood supply shifts from the iliac arteries to the aorta. Various disruptions of this procedure may occur. Vitamin A deficiency in sows may cause anomalies such as those described later.

Malposition of the kidneys *(renal ectopia)* is observed more frequently in swine than in dogs or cats. Malpositioned kidneys are usually in the pelvic or inguinal location. One or both kidneys may be displaced. The kidneys may be normal or abnormally small. The renal arteries arise close to the bifurcation of the aorta or from the iliacs. The ureter is short, but it may be kinked and thereby predisposed to hydronephrosis and pyelonephritis, or may empty into the genital tract, causing urinary incontinence. *Crossed renal ectopia* refers to malposition of a kidney that has crossed the midline; it may fuse with its contralateral partner.

Fusion of the kidneys may occur in utero. *Horseshoe kidney*, or *ren arcuatus*, seen in all species, results from fusion of the cranial or caudal poles of the kidneys (Fig. 4-12). The fusion

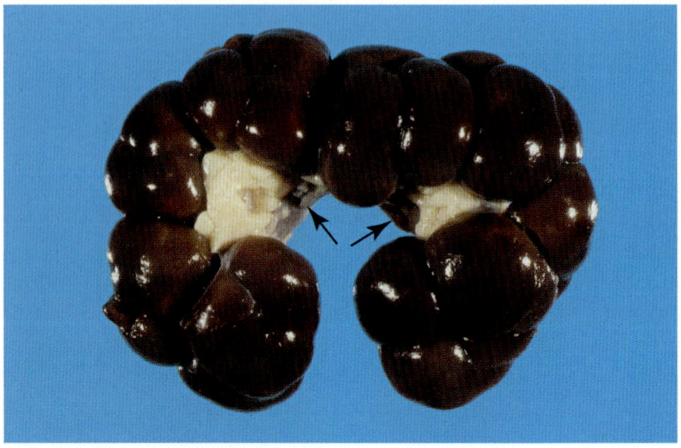

Figure 4-12 Horseshoe kidney in a calf. Ureters have been severed (arrows). (Courtesy University of Guelph.)

may involve only a small portion of the capsule or parenchyma or be sufficient to produce a common pelvis. The ureters are not involved, and their location depends on whether the cranial or caudal poles are fused. Such kidneys function normally.

Fetal lobations, which are normal in embryos and cattle, may persist (eFig. 4-3) in other species if there is failure of fusion of individual renal segments. They are not of pathologic significance.

Renal maldevelopment

Renal maldevelopment (also referred to as "renal dysplasia") is disorganized development of renal parenchyma because of anomalous differentiation. If normal development of the collecting duct system ("renal branching morphogenesis") is disrupted, then renal maldevelopment can result. Transcription factors, growth factors, and cell surface signaling peptides are critical in regulation of renal branching morphogenesis. Renal lesions may be gross or microscopic. Renal maldevelopment is *usually congenital*. But in cats, dogs, and pigs, which have an active subcapsular nephrogenic zone at birth, maldevelopment could be caused by disease in the early neonatal period until differentiation of the nephrogenic tissue is completed. Developmental lesions may be obscured by secondary compensatory, degenerative, and inflammatory changes.

The **causes** of renal maldevelopment are ill-defined, but some may be *hereditary*. Cases of familial renal disease in several *dog* breeds often have evidence of interrupted development or maturation (see Table 4-1). An autosomal dominant form of cystic renal dysplasia has been reported in *Suffolk sheep*. Many *human* cases of renal maldevelopment/dysplasia are associated with intrauterine *ureteral obstruction*, and some animals probably have the same cause. The term congenital anomaly of kidney and urinary tract (CAKUT) emphasizes the frequency with which renal maldevelopment and lower urinary tract abnormalities occur concomitantly. Of note, rapid growth and the increased activity of the intrarenal RAAS in the fetus may cause greater susceptibility to permanent renal injury if the fetus (or newborn, depending on the normal rate of maturation for that species) is exposed to a virus, toxin, or teratogen. Renal dysplasia in pigs has been attributed to *hypovitaminosis A;* formation of the trigonal wedge and proper insertion of the ureteral buds into the bladder, and hence proper renal development, are mediated by vitamin A and proto-oncogene *Ret* signaling pathways.

There is considerable variation in the appearance of abnormally developed kidneys. Most are *small*, which accounts for their frequent misdiagnosis as hypoplastic. They are usually *misshapen and fibrotic* with thick-walled cysts and dilated tortuous ureters. One or both kidneys may be affected, and accessory vessels are occasionally identified (Fig. 4-13). If the lesion is unilateral, the ipsilateral ureter should be examined for anomalous valves, diverticula, or atresia. When both kidneys are involved, scrutiny of the bladder and lower urinary tract is indicated. If the diagnosis rests on ultrasonographic and/or renal biopsy findings, then examination of the entire urinary tract via contrast imaging studies could help characterize the lesions. Some maldeveloped kidneys may be only slightly irregular in contour or may appear normal, in which case microscopic examination is required for diagnosis. Considerable emphasis has been placed on the size of renal arteries in renal maldevelopment, but changes should be interpreted with caution because degenerative lesions in the renal parenchyma may be accompanied by vascular remodeling.

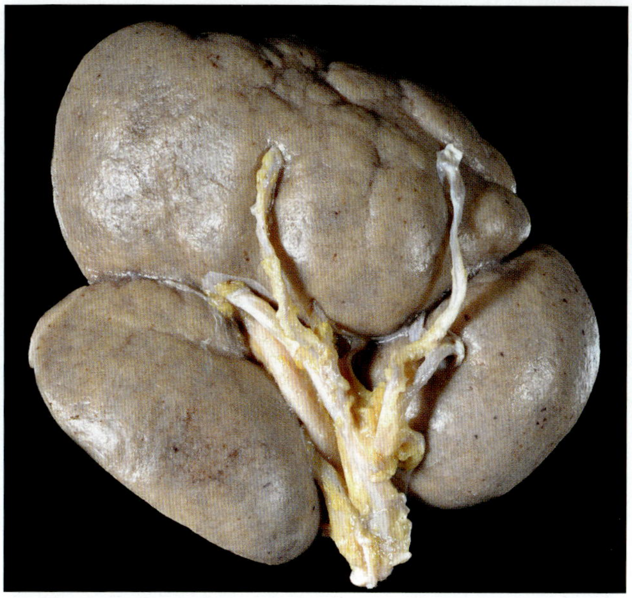

Figure 4-13 Malformed kidney with **accessory vessels** in a young horse. (Courtesy E. Clark, P. Stromberg.)

Previously, the **microscopic criteria** of human renal maldevelopment/dysplasia were applied to kidneys from young dogs. Specifically, *areas of undifferentiated mesenchyme, groups of immature glomeruli* (small glomeruli with peripheral nuclei and inapparent capillaries) (Fig. 4-14A), *primitive (metanephric) ducts* lined by cuboidal or columnar epithelium (Fig. 4-14B), sometimes surrounded by concentric layers of mesenchyme, and *dysontogenic (cartilaginous or osseous) metaplasia* were all assessed. Notably, cartilaginous or osseous metaplasia, which occurs in many dysplastic human kidneys, were rarely present in domestic animals. The other features could be identified in many of the maldeveloped kidneys, but many dogs did not have all of the features in one region. Other lesions have also been proposed as evidence of abnormal development. For example, bands or regions of collagen with a paucity of tubules with no or few leukocytes indicate a failure of the ureteric bud to branch in that region (Fig. 4-14C; eFig. 4-4). Few leukocytes in that region suggest that the collagen is not secondary to previous infection or inflammation. Importantly, the proportion of renal parenchyma that is abnormally developed impacts whether the patient will develop clinical signs of CKD. For example, due to the large renal reserve, if only 5% of the renal parenchyma has lesions of maldevelopment, then it is likely that the animal will not be azotemic.

Because *ureteral anomalies* are often concomitant, dysplastic kidneys are abnormally susceptible to pyelonephritis.

Renal cysts (pre- and post-natal)

Cystic diseases of the kidney include various conditions with one or more grossly visible cystic cavities in the renal parenchyma. No satisfactory classification of renal cysts exists, but location of cysts, mode of inheritance (or lack thereof), lesions in other organs, and the clinical course in affected animals are important aspects to consider.

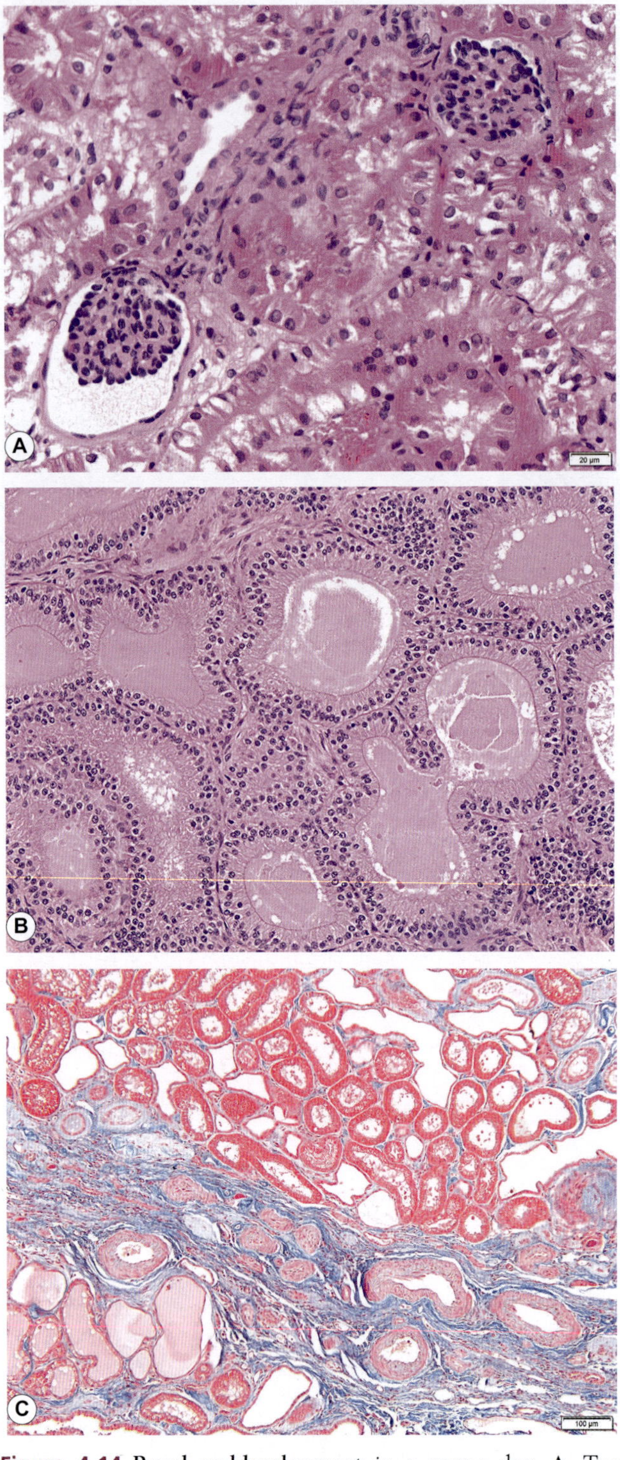

Figure 4-14 Renal maldevelopment in a young dog. **A**. Two **immature glomeruli**, one of which has a mildly dilated glomerular capsule. **B**. Persistent medullary metanephric ducts. **C**. Fibrotic area lacks tubular profiles and inflammation.

Cysts can arise during organogenesis and may be associated with histologic criteria of renal maldevelopment. Cysts can also develop in nephrons and collecting ducts after the end of nephrogenesis. Cysts can occur in any part of the nephron, including the urinary space, or in the collecting system. Analyses of their content indicate that they are part of functional nephrons.

Three **mechanisms**, which are not mutually exclusive, can lead to the formation of renal cysts:

1. Renal cysts may be caused by *obstructive lesions;* examples are the acquired retention cysts of chronic renal disease, some dysplastic cysts, and possibly those of glomerulocystic disease.
2. A fundamental change, of unknown origin, may occur in the *tubular basement membrane* and result in formation of saccular dilations of the tubules. Some dilated segments may detach from the tubule and form spherical cystic structures. Likewise, detachment of the proximal tubule from the urinary pole will result in dilated glomerular capsules and so-called "atubular glomeruli."
3. Disordered growth of tubular epithelial cells may lead to *focal hyperplastic lesions* and cyst formation.

Mutation of polycystic kidney disease (PKD) genes in humans may alter production of *polycystin* proteins, which are important in cell-cell and cell-matrix interactions; altered tubular epithelial growth and differentiation may lead to cyst formation. Renal cysts are seen in humans with primary aldosteronism or primary renal potassium wasting, perhaps as a consequence of chronic hypokalemia and tubular obstruction by proliferating tubular epithelial cells. Renal cysts are dynamic structures, and their growth may be modified by pharmacologic means.

Many *chemicals*, such as long-acting corticosteroids, diphenylamine, polychlorinated biphenyls, 5,6,7,8-tetrahydrocarbazole-3-acetic acid, alloxan, diphenylthiazole, and nordihydroguaiaretic acid, cause renal cysts in experimental animals. Corticosteroids induce hypokalemia, and cyst formation can be prevented by injections of some potassium salts, but in general, the mechanisms of cyst development are not known. It seems possible that some of the therapeutic, prophylactic, and pollutant chemicals to which animals are exposed could be responsible for sporadic cases of renal cysts.

Renal cysts vary in size from the barely visible to structures that exceed that of the organ itself. Cysts are often more numerous in the cortex than in the medulla, this may simply reflect the relative volumes of the 2 regions. The content is watery, and cysts are lined by flattened or cuboidal epithelium. Some cysts are subdivided by thin trabeculae, but most are unilocular and roughly spherical, ovoid, or fusiform.

Simple renal cysts occur in all species but are most common in pigs and calves. There are different patterns of occurrence in pigs, but it is not clear whether similar patterns exist in other animals. The usual finding in pigs is one or a few unilocular ~1-2 cm cortical cysts that bulge from the renal surface or are exposed when the kidney is sliced. They are usually bilateral and are incidental findings in young pigs. Affected kidneys are discarded in abattoirs. Although usually regarded as sporadic occurrences, these lesions may be examples of a cystic renal disease that is inherited as an autosomal dominant trait. Polygenic inheritance may determine the number of cysts in animals with the dominant gene. In this condition, a few cysts are present at birth, but they gradually increase in number, and there may be 80-90 by 1-year-old. Azotemia is not seen, but the condition has similarities to a human cystic disease in which CKD develops in adults; a similar course in mature swine is conceivable.

Occasionally, areas containing many small cysts occur in one lobe of a bovine kidney or one pole of an equine kidney. They are not significant clinically.

Polycystic kidney disease (PKD) occurs in 2 major forms:

1. **Autosomal dominant polycystic kidney disease** (ADPKD), in Bull Terriers and Persian cats (Fig. 4-15A), is similar to

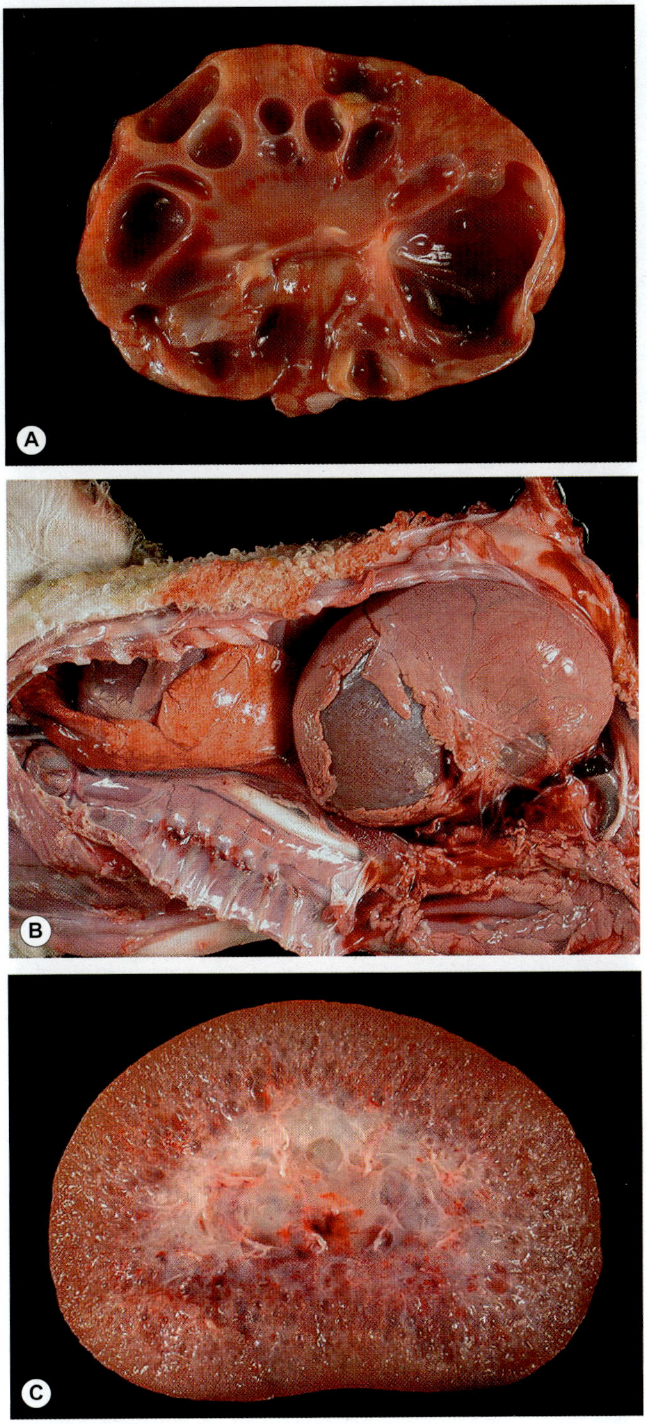

Figure 4-15 **A. Polycystic kidney disease** in a Persian cat. **B, C. Congenital polycystic disease** in a Perendale lamb. Kidneys are grossly enlarged by numerous parenchymal cysts. **C.** Sagittal section of B. (Courtesy K.G. Thompson.)

the *adult-onset* form of PKD in humans, which is linked to defects in genes *PKD1* and *PKD2*. Polycystin 1 and 2 are encoded by *PKD1* and *2*, respectively, and localize to the primary cilia present on the apical surface of the tubular epithelial cells. There is one primary cilium per epithelial cell, and its purpose is to translate a physical event (fluid movement through the tubular lumen) into an intracellular calcium signal. The basal body of the primary cilium also plays a role in cell division, wherein the cilium is reabsorbed and serves as the centriole during mitosis, thereby linking the cilium to cell proliferation. Renal cysts develop bilaterally, are of proximal or distal tubular origin, grow progressively over time, and lead to chronic tubulointerstitial nephritis and azotemia in adult life. ADPKD in Persian cats (see Fig. 4-15A), linked to a *PKD1* gene defect, is commonly accompanied by hepatic cysts and/or hepatic fibrosis, and pancreatic cysts. Genetic sequencing of *PKD1* identified a substitution of cytosine for adenine in exon 29 (position 3284). The substitution leads to a shortened mRNA due to a premature stop codon; ~25% of the C-terminus portion of *PKD1* is missing, and this genetic variant has a reported prevalence of ~30% in the Persian breed. It is also documented in other feline breeds (e.g., Scottish fold, American shorthair). Bull Terriers with ADPKD also have a mutation in *PKD1*, and some of the affected dogs may also have abnormal GBMs, as discussed later.

2. **Autosomal recessive polycystic kidney disease** (ARPKD), described in West Highland White and Cairn Terriers, and Perendale sheep, is similar to the *childhood* form of PKD in humans and may be accompanied by hepatic biliary cysts. In sheep, cysts are congenital and lambs die in utero or shortly after birth (see Fig. 4-15B and C). In humans, ARPKD has been linked to a mutation in the *PKHD1* gene, which encodes fibrocystin, another component of the primary cilia. A genetic cause for the disease in domesticated species has not been identified.

Congenital PKD, of unknown inheritance, occurs in piglets, lambs, calves, goat kids, puppies, kittens, and foals. In humans, this variant is often diagnosed as *multicystic dysplasia*. There may be concurrent cystic bile ducts, bile duct proliferation, and sometimes pancreatic cysts. This form of PKD in domestic animals is manifested by stillbirths or death in renal failure during the first few weeks of life. Grossly, the kidneys are large and pale, and contain numerous 1-5 mm cysts that involve both cortex and medulla. Bile duct cysts range from barely visible up to 3 cm across, and the gallbladder and biliary system are often distended with bile that discolors the liver.

Glomerulocystic disease is the term used when cysts involve glomerular capsules, and they may be the result of periglomerular fibrosis and stenosis of the glomerulotubular junction (Fig. 4-16). Although a few scattered dilated glomerular capsules may not be clinically significant, renal insufficiency can be seen when many glomeruli are affected.

Acquired cysts of the kidney develop when tubules are obstructed by scar tissue. They are multiple and small, rarely exceeding 1.0 cm in diameter (eFig. 4-5). Most are located in convoluted tubules and urinary spaces. Hyperplastic collecting ducts are sometimes grossly visible as elongated cysts in the medulla of dogs with renal failure. These acquired cysts are distinguishable from primary cysts because they occur in kidneys with extensive scarring.

Perinephric pseudocysts occasionally develop unilaterally or bilaterally as a collection of fluid, which may be urine, blood, lymph, or transudate, in the space between the renal capsule and the renal reflection of the peritoneum (Fig. 4-17A and B). It can be seen in any species but is most commonly observed in cats. *The space is not lined by epithelium* and is thus a pseudocyst. Potential causes include trauma, ureteral or lymphatic obstruction, venous congestion, and hypertension. Affected cats often have concomitant chronic renal disease.

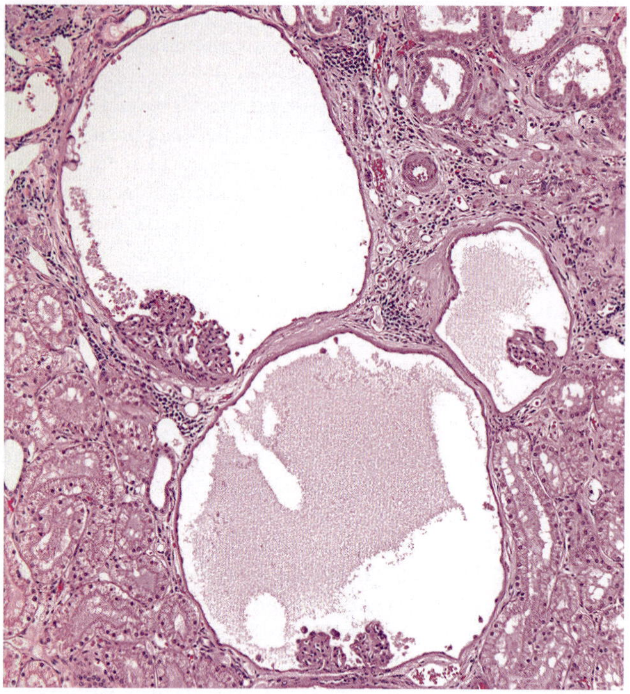

Figure 4-16 Glomerulocystic disease. Several severely dilated glomerular capsules in a dog. Glomerular tufts are compressed and atrophic.

CIRCULATORY DISTURBANCES AND DISEASES OF THE BLOOD VESSELS

Renal hyperemia

Active hyperemia is seen in acute nephritis but especially in acute septicemia and endotoxemia. Kidneys are swollen and uniformly dark, although in some cases, the hyperemia may be largely restricted to the medulla. Microscopically, all vessels, especially capillaries, are filled with blood. *Passive hyperemia (congestion)* follows the usual principles. Affected kidneys are enlarged and dark, and the capsular vessels are injected. On cut section, the corticomedullary junctional zone is dark and prominent, with engorgement of visible tributaries. Acute congestion with intertubular hemorrhages occurs in clostridial enterotoxemia of lambs and calves.

Renal hemorrhages

Hemorrhages are especially common in the renal cortex in a variety of bacteremias and viremias and sometimes in healthy slaughtered animals. Petechiae are very common in piglets dead of any cause. Many or few pinpoint hemorrhages occur beneath the capsule in classical swine fever (hog cholera), African swine fever, and porcine salmonellosis. In porcine erysipelas, the hemorrhages tend to be larger and more irregular in size and shape (Fig. 4-18). Severe hemorrhage in the wall of the renal pelvis and the medulla sometimes occurs in classical swine fever, in other acute infections of swine, and in the hemorrhagic diatheses; hemorrhage occurs from rupture of congested medullary vessels. Extensive subcapsular hemorrhage is common in clostridial enterotoxemia of calves; it produces a black cast molded to the shape of the cortex.

Renal infarction

Infarcts of the kidney are common lesions of localized coagulative necrosis produced by embolic or thrombotic occlusion of the renal artery or of one of its branches (Fig. 4-19). The sequelae depend on whether the obstructing material is septic or sterile and on the size and number of the vessels obstructed. Thrombi produce typical infarcts; septic thrombi produce abscesses that

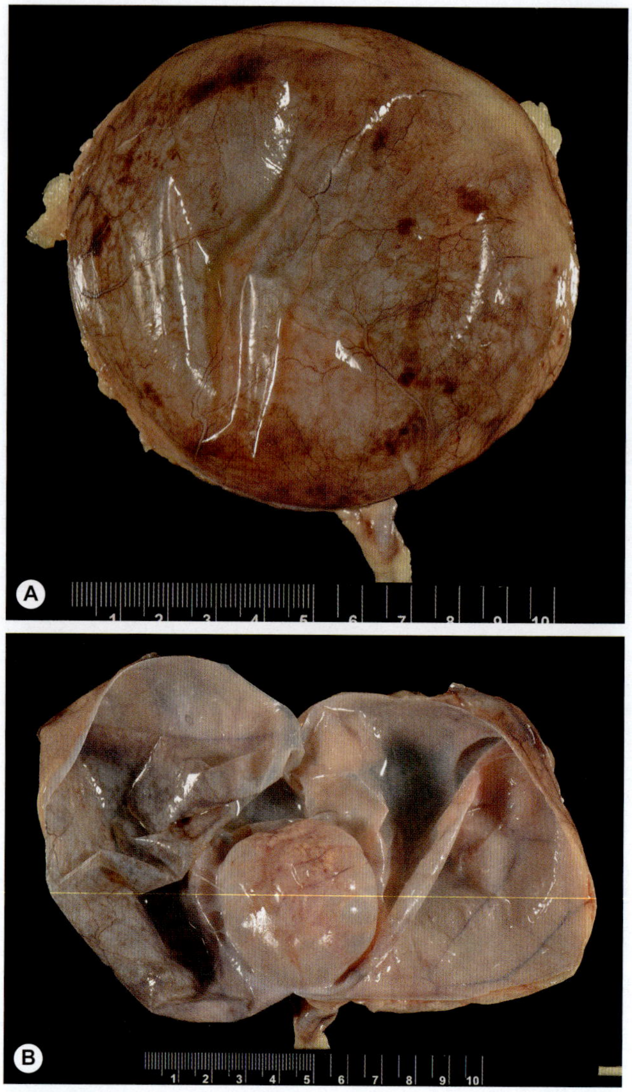

Figure 4-17 Large **perinephric pseudocyst** from a cat. **A**. Intact. **B**. Opened. (Courtesy R. Kohnken.)

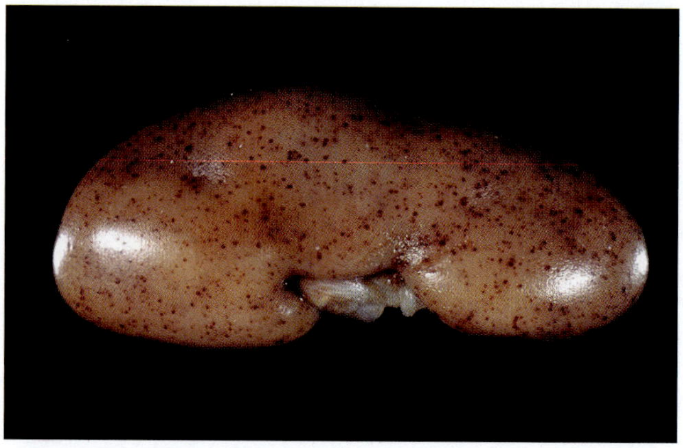

Figure 4-18 Renal cortical petechiae in a pig with erysipelas. (Courtesy P. Stromberg.)

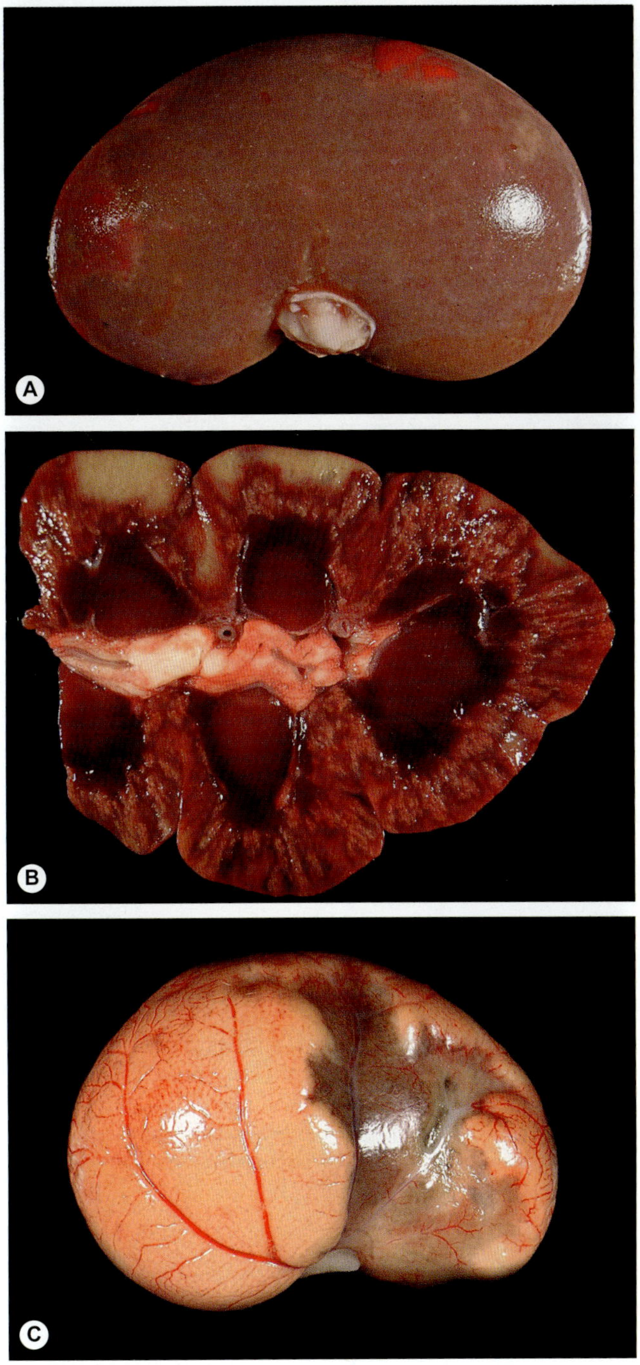

Figure 4-19 **Renal infarction. A. Acute renal infarcts** in a dog are raised and red as the result of hemorrhage and edema. (Courtesy B. Harrington, P. Stromberg.) **B. Renal infarcts** in a cow associated with ascending pyelonephritis caused by nonhemolytic *Escherichia coli* and *Trueperella pyogenes*. (Courtesy M. Gramer.) **C. Chronic infarcts** and scarring in a cat. (Courtesy S. Chaney, P. Stromberg.)

may heal, sequester, or discharge into the pelvis. Thrombosis of a trunk of a renal artery will produce total or subtotal necrosis of the kidney, the extent of the latter depending on the presence and efficiency of parahilar and capsular collaterals. If an arcuate artery is obstructed, then there is necrosis of a wedge of both the cortex and medulla. If an interlobular vessel is involved, infarction is limited to the cortex. The ease and frequency with which the kidneys are infarcted result from their vascular architecture being of the "end-artery" type and the large volume of blood that continually traverses them. In cats, renal infarcts (see Fig. 4-19C) may serve as an indicator of underlying hypertrophic cardiomyopathy and distal aortic thromboembolism.

Soon after total obstruction of a vessel, the related wedge of tissue is swollen, intensely cyanotic, and congested by the blood that oozes into the vessels from collateral vessels. There is no sharp line between the infarcted zone and the adjacent normal tissue; instead, there is a transition zone in which blood continues to ooze slowly toward the central region of the infarct. In the outer part of the marginal zone, the red cells survive and circulation may be re-established. This zone persists for the first 2-3 days; it has been referred to, erroneously, as the zone of reactive hyperemia (see Fig. 4-19B). The extent of useful diffusion determines the actual limit of the infarct, and it is here that dehemoglobinization begins, neutrophils accumulate, and cells undergo necrosis. The dehemoglobinization begins at about 24 hours and may be complete by 2-3 days when the infarcted area then becomes white. Before decoloration begins, the affected area is outlined by a thin but distinct white line of leukocytes.

The *sequence of degenerative changes* in the infarcted tissue reflects the specialization and sensitivity of the various structures. At the outer margins, only a few proximal tubules have epithelial necrosis. More centrally, every proximal tubule is dead, and inside the zone of diffusion everything is dead. In the central dead zone, there may be some revascularization within 1-2 weeks. The zone is progressively replaced by fibrous tissue, and healed infarcts persist as pale gray-white scars, wedge shaped, and depressed. The scars may be difficult or impossible to distinguish grossly from focal healed pyelonephritis.

Minute emboli that lodge in the glomerular or peritubular capillaries may produce small infarcts that are not detectable macroscopically. Because of the small size of such infarcts, there may be adequate diffusion across the infarcted zone so that leukocytes do not accumulate, epithelial necrosis is minimal and soon repaired, and circulation is re-established. Commonly, infarcts of various ages in a kidney indicate recurrent embolic episodes.

Primary vascular disease includes various processes, such as renal arteriosclerosis, arteriolosclerosis, arteriolar hyalinosis, and arteritis (eFig. 4-6), with "polyarteritis nodosa" and systemic diseases such as malignant catarrhal fever being examples of the latter category. A variety of degenerative proliferative arterial changes occur in chronic diffuse inflammatory diseases. Although they are probably secondary, they may be magnified by the *hypertension* that is expected to develop. Hypertension is common in moderate-to-severe canine and feline renal disease (both AKI and CKD) and can lead to further deterioration in renal function by causing additional glomerular and tubular damage. *Renal telangiectasia, aneurysms*, or *pseudoaneurysms* are rarely reported to cause hematuria. Renal telangiectasia has been documented in related Pembroke Welsh Corgis and Labrador Retrievers.

Renal cortical necrosis and acute tubular necrosis

Acute tubular necrosis (ATN) and renal cortical necrosis are grouped together here for purposes of discussion; ATN is also discussed in more detail later. These lesions occur infrequently in animals, but if severe, may cause AKI and death. *Either variety of renal necrosis is usually a manifestation of hypoperfusion, or "shock,"* which may be classified as cardiogenic, hypovolemic, septic, or neurogenic. Renal cortical necrosis and ATN occur in cattle in a variety of endotoxemic conditions, such as mastitis or metritis, and in gastrointestinal diseases, such as severe enteritis and grain overload. Bilateral cortical necrosis is a rare complication of esophagogastric ulceration in swine and apparently results from hemorrhagic shock.

ATN, sometimes referred to as **ATI**, is demonstrated by patchy necrosis of segments of both proximal and distal tubules; necrotic tubular epithelial cells become casts, which cause tubular blockage and oliguria. Other contributors to oliguria are tubular backleak through disrupted tubular basement membranes, compression of medullary tubules by edema and inflammation, reflex constriction of afferent arterioles, and decreased glomerular membrane permeability. In **renal cortical necrosis**, there is destruction of both tubules and glomeruli, and this can result from patchy or complete renal ischemia.

The usual balance between the RAAS and the eicosanoid systems that maintain fine regulation of intrarenal blood flow is disrupted during ischemia. During hypotension, perfusion of outer cortical nephrons is reduced, while perfusion of inner cortical nephrons is maintained; *intrarenal blood flow is redistributed toward the inner cortex and medulla*. This occurs because the vasoconstrictive effects of angiotensin II and adrenergic stimulation are unopposed in the outer cortex, whereas in the inner cortex, prostaglandins modulate vasoconstriction; PGE2 is produced in the medulla in response to ischemia, travels in tubular fluid to the area of the JGA, and causes vasodilation of afferent arterioles of juxtamedullary nephrons.

The duration of ischemia is of obvious importance for the pathogenesis of necrosis. Complete ischemia of <2 hours duration can be expected to be followed by *good reflow* if cardiac output and blood pressure are restored to normal, whereas total ischemia of longer duration may be followed by patchy reflow or complete failure of reflow in the cortex, medulla, or both. Reflow is inhibited primarily because of vascular congestion by red cells swollen by plasma water uptake, and perhaps also by ischemia-induced swelling of endothelial cells of glomeruli, vasa recta, and peritubular capillaries. This *"no-reflow" phenomenon* contributes to further renal ischemia and AKI. It is mediated by the pericytes surrounding vasa recta and the peritubular capillaries; glomerular perfusion is not affected in a similar manner. Severe ischemic injury can permanently alter peritubular capillary density, resulting in decreased urinary concentrating ability and predisposing to interstitial fibrosis. This capillary loss might be mediated through local synthesis of *angiostatin*, a proteolytic cleavage product of plasminogen that inhibits angiogenesis, promotes endothelial cell apoptosis, and disrupts the integrity of capillaries.

Renal cortical necrosis can also occur in *disseminated intravascular coagulation*, which is often the result of gram-negative endotoxemia. Endothelial injury in glomerular and peritubular capillaries leads to microthrombosis and hemorrhagic renal cortical necrosis. This severe degree of renal damage is usually rapidly fatal, but milder lesions can be seen in a number of bacteremic diseases as petechiae or cortical hemorrhages.

The cellular destruction that occurs in ischemic renal injury begins with a decreased ability to produce ATP and hence an increase in membrane permeability that allows influx of calcium into the cell. Excess free cytosolic calcium activates phospholipases that further increase membrane permeability and lead to membrane disruption and generation of toxic lipid byproducts. Increased intracellular calcium also interferes with mitochondrial respiration and causes increased production of free radicals that further injure cell membranes and mitochondria. Unfortunately, reperfusion can be deleterious because reoxygenation increases the production of free radicals.

The **gross appearance** of the kidneys, other than those with hemorrhagic renal necrosis, varies considerably from case to case; it is determined by the severity, distribution, and duration of the ischemia and the quality of the reflow. In ATN, the cortices are finely mottled or flecked by small yellow foci of necrosis. Renal cortical necrosis can be diffuse, or the injury may be patchy; pigs tend to develop a "turkey egg" pattern marked by hemorrhagic glomeruli, but most die before more extensive necrosis is evident (see Fig. 4-18), whereas cattle sometimes develop a distinctive patchy cortical necrosis (see Fig. 4-19B). The reaction is the same as for infarction given previously. A narrow subcapsular rim of viable tissue may remain. The affected areas of cortex are pale, almost white, slightly swollen, and stop sharply at the corticomedullary junction. The irregular areas of cortical infarction may be outlined by hemorrhage. The medulla may be normal, but in some cases, there is severe congestion of the inner stripe of the outer medulla or the whole medulla, so that it is swollen and resembles a blood clot.

The **histologic appearance** of a kidney with ATN includes irregular necrosis of the proximal tubules, with or without disruption of the tubular basement membranes. Hyaline and granular casts are present, particularly in distal tubules and collecting ducts. There can be interstitial edema as a result of tubular leakage. Preferential damage occurs to the pars recta and thick ascending limb because of their location in the poorly perfused outer medulla and because of their higher oxygen requirement. Microthrombi may be seen in capillaries, interlobular and stellate veins. If the animal survives the ischemic episode, evidence of regeneration may be seen in ~1 week. Tubules are lined by flattened epithelial cells with karyomegaly and occasional mitoses.

Renal medullary necrosis

Under certain circumstances, medullary necrosis is the primary manifestation of renal injury. As noted previously, renal hypotension usually results in cortical necrosis because of redistribution of blood flow to juxtamedullary nephrons. However, medullary vessels are damaged when ischemia lasts longer than 2 hours. In the case of venous occlusion, the elevated intrarenal blood pressure maintains the patency of lower resistance cortical vessels but not of higher-resistance medullary vessels, and hence medullary infarction predominates.

Toxic and hypoxic insults to the kidney are synergistic, and several protective mechanisms must be incapacitated to produce medullary injury. Prostaglandins are important autoregulators of renal perfusion. *Nonsteroidal anti-inflammatory drugs* (NSAIDs)—such as aspirin, phenacetin, phenylbutazone, flunixin meglumine, ibuprofen, and meloxicam—inhibit cyclooxygenase, resulting in decreased production of PGE2 and loss of its vasodilatory effect on arterioles of juxtamedullary nephrons. Additionally, NSAIDs cause constriction of the pericytes of vasa recta, impeding perfusion of the medulla and papilla. Dehydration likely contributes to the pathogenesis. In toxicity studies, there is evidence of papillary interstitial cell degeneration and necrosis when laboratory Beagles are dosed daily with 50 mg/kg of ibuprofen for 5 weeks.

Papillary necrosis is characteristic of **"analgesic nephropathy,"** such as renal crest necrosis in dehydrated horses treated with phenylbutazone (Fig. 4-20A and B; eFig. 4-7). *Dehydration* is involved in the pathogenesis of papillary necrosis in racing Greyhounds. Accidental ingestion of a combination of monensin and roxarsone has caused renal medullary necrosis in normally hydrated dogs. Papillary necrosis occurs in dehydrated lambs and calves when treated with phenothiazine, and the necrosis is due to a combination of dehydration and ischemia.

Urinary obstruction, pyelonephritis, and amyloidosis can cause papillary necrosis in animals. Compression of thin-walled interstitial vessels is probably the mechanism by which all of these processes cause papillary necrosis. Specifically, outflow obstruction will cause collecting ducts to dilate, pyelonephritis will lead to significant interstitial inflammation and edema, and amyloid may be deposited directly in the medullary interstitium.

The *gross lesions* of medullary necrosis vary greatly in their extent and stage of development. Acute papillary infarction may be an incidental finding in an animal dead of other causes, such as dehydration and electrolyte imbalances in neonatal diarrhea. Massive medullary infarction will cause AKI, possibly leading to death. In an animal that survives an episode of medullary necrosis, medullary scarring occurs, the papilla may slough, and secondary cortical scarring is seen. The sloughed papilla may remain in the pelvis and may become mineralized. *Microscopic lesions* cover the usual range of necrosis and scarring. *Sequelae* to medullary necrosis include inability to concentrate urine, CKD, and uremia.

Hydronephrosis

Hydronephrosis is dilation of the renal pelvis and calyces associated with progressive atrophy and enlargement of the kidney (see Fig. 4-21). The cause is *urinary obstruction*, which may be complete or incomplete, existing at any level from the urethra to the renal pelvis. The obstruction may be caused by anomalous development of the lower urinary tract, or it may be acquired. *Acquired causes* include urinary calculi in any location; prostatic enlargement in the dog; cystitis, especially if it is hemorrhagic; compression of the ureters by surrounding inflammatory or neoplastic tissue; displacement of the bladder in perineal hernias; and acquired urethral strictures. Depending on the site of obstruction, hydronephrosis may be unilateral or bilateral, and there may be some degree of hydroureter and dilation of the bladder.

The pathogenesis of hydronephrosis is based on the persistence of glomerular filtration in the presence of urinary obstruction. Even with sudden complete obstruction, glomerular filtration continues because filtrate diffuses into the interstitium and perirenal spaces, where it is drained by lymphatics and veins. However, continued filtration creates increased pressure throughout the nephrons, collecting ducts, calyces, and pelvis. Pressure atrophy and apoptosis of tubular epithelium occur, diminishing tubular function and concentrating ability. Blood vessels are compressed, particularly hilar veins and inner medullary vessels, leading to *papillary ischemia and necrosis*.

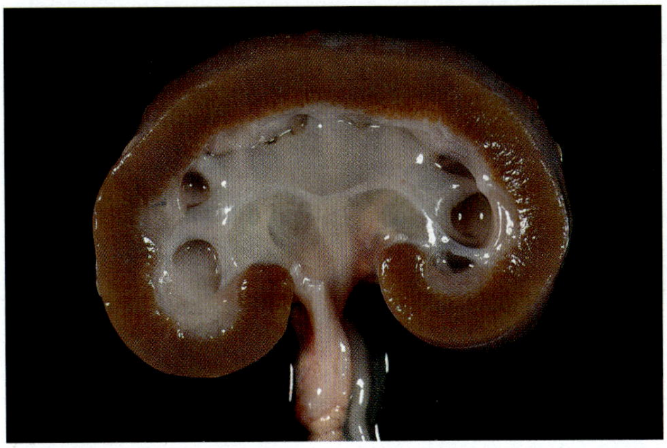

Figure 4-21 Hydronephrosis in a sheep. (Courtesy L. Himmel, C. Premanandan.)

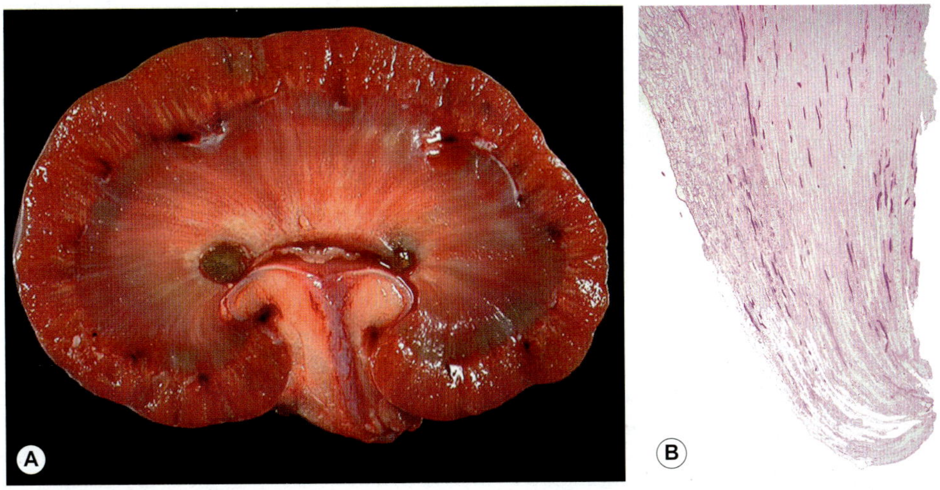

Figure 4-20 A. **Renal crest necrosis** in a dog caused by nonsteroidal anti-inflammatory drug (NSAID) toxicity. (Courtesy K.G. Thompson.) B. Histology reveals **coagulative necrosis with minimal inflammation** of the renal papilla of a cat with NSAID (meloxicam) toxicity.

Interstitial inflammation is triggered by activated tubular epithelial cells and leukocytes releasing vasoactive factors, growth factors, and cytokines. Glomerular filtration eventually decreases because of intrarenal vasoconstriction. Nephrons atrophy and are replaced by progressive interstitial fibrosis.

Complete bilateral obstruction results in early death from uremia. Unilateral obstruction produces the greatest degree of hydronephrosis, especially if the obstruction is incomplete or intermittent, because glomerular filtration can continue. If an obstruction is removed within about 1-week, renal function returns. After about 3 weeks of complete obstruction, or several months of incomplete obstruction, irreversible renal damage occurs. In unilateral hydronephrosis, the contralateral kidney can compensate if it is normal. Urinary stasis predisposes to infection; hence, pyelonephritis might be superimposed on hydronephrosis.

Early *gross changes* consist of progressive dilation of the pelvis and calyces with blunting of the apices of the pyramids. Eventually, these may become excavated to form multilocular cysts communicating with the pelvis and separated by intricate ridges that represent original septa. In advanced cases, the kidney is transformed into a thin-walled sac with only a thin shell of atrophic cortical parenchyma.

Microscopically, there is dilation of the proximal convoluted tubules, followed shortly thereafter by dilation of distal and straight segments. The latter persists, with atrophy of the epithelium, but dilation of proximal tubules subsides. Instead, cortical tubules atrophy and are separated or replaced by fibrosis. Much of the tubular atrophy may be through apoptosis. The glomeruli can persist for a long time. Various degrees of ischemia or infarction may develop in the cortex if the obstruction is sudden and complete; the infarcts are venous in origin. There is progressive destruction of the pyramids that spares the pelvic epithelium. Necrotic tissue is removed, and pyramids are gradually destroyed. Inflammatory response is often minimal to mild.

GLOMERULAR DISEASE (GENERAL TERMINOLOGY)

Glomerular disease is of central importance in the kidney because interference with glomerular blood flow alters filtration and impairs peritubular capillary perfusion, which can lead to loss of the entire nephron.

- The term **glomerulonephritis (GN)** implies *cellular or molecular inflammation* that is predominantly focused on glomeruli. In some diseases [e.g., immune-complex-mediated membranous glomerulonephritis (MGN)], inflammatory cells are uncommon, which is analogous to certain dermatitis lesions that are "cell-poor."
- The term **glomerulitis** is sometimes used when inflammation is restricted to glomeruli, as may occur in acute septicemias.
- **Glomerulopathy** refers to glomerular disease with uncertain etiology or pathogenesis.
- Glomeruli may also be significantly affected in a variety of systemic diseases, such as **amyloidosis**, which is discussed later, bacterial endocarditis, and in various vasculitides.

Clinical presentations can be nonspecific and include proteinuria, hematuria, oliguria, hyposthenuria, and azotemia. Some dogs develop vascular thrombosis (i.e., pulmonary arteries or renal veins) because they are in a *hypercoagulable state* resulting from stimulation of production of acute-phase proteins, such as fibrinogen, while simultaneously losing LMW anticoagulants, such as antithrombin III, into urine.

Proteinuria, occurring in the absence of urinary tract inflammation, is suggestive of glomerular damage, namely, as the result of increased glomerular permeability. Proteinuria is usually measured by calculating the ratio of urine protein to urine creatinine (UPC). This technique is preferable to only measuring urine protein because it accounts for differences in urine concentration. A small amount of protein in a dilute urine sample is clinically more significant than the same amount of protein in a concentrated sample. Mild proteinuria (usually UPC 0.5-3) could be the result of tubular and/or glomerular injury. However, if the UPC is >3, then protein loss is presumed to be at least partly glomerular in origin and might lead to development of the **nephrotic syndrome** in which proteinuria, hypoalbuminemia, generalized edema, and hyperlipidemia and/or hypercholesterolemia occur. Edema in the nephrotic syndrome is less common in dogs than in humans - results from decreased plasma colloid osmotic pressure, stimulation of the RAAS, and release of ADH in response to hypovolemia. The hepatic response to hypoproteinemia is a generalized increase in production of proteins, including lipoproteins, leading to hyperlipoproteinemia and hypercholesterolemia. In dogs, the nephrotic syndrome connotes a worse prognosis compared with patients with only proteinuria (based on matched UPC values). The term "nephritic syndrome" refers to patients with proteinuria and an active urine sediment; they are often also azotemic. In proteinuric patients, evaluation of the lower urinary tract must be performed to rule out the possibility of its contribution to proteinuria.

Depending on the type or severity of the glomerular disease, there may be an increase in MMW and/or HMW proteins in the urine. Additional biomarkers of glomerular disease include urinary albumin and urinary immunoglobulin G (IgG). Albumin is thought to indicate early kidney disease (and is sometimes referred to as microalbuminuria when it is mildly elevated); the presence of large molecules, such as immunoglobulins, suggests a marked increase in glomerular permeability. Urinary protein electrophoresis can reveal "glomerular" or "tubular" patterns of injury, based on the size of the proteins in the urine. However, most small animals undergoing renal biopsy and serum protein electrophoresis fall into a "mixed glomerular and tubular" pattern because of the interaction of the 2 compartments.

The following terms are generally accepted for the description of glomerular disease:

- **Diffuse:** involves >50% of glomeruli
- **Focal:** involves <50% of glomeruli
- **Global:** involves the whole glomerular tuft
- **Segmental:** involves only part of the glomerulus
- **Mesangial:** affects primarily the mesangial area

Classification of GN in humans is relatively complex, based on extensive clinicopathologic correlations and responses to therapy. The following terms are currently used for the histologic description of GN in domestic animals.

- **Membranous GN (MGN):** GBM remodeling that is secondary to immune complex (IC) deposition on the abluminal (subepithelial) surface of the GBM with normocellularity to mild hypercellularity (Fig. 4-22). The deposits stain red with Masson trichrome (see Fig. 4-22B). Over time, the subepithelial ICs are separated by projections *(spikes)* of basement membrane material synthesized by podocytes. Eventually, they become encircled by and incorporated within the GBM, which can be visualized with PAS or JMS as *holes* in the GBM (see Fig. 4-22C). IF shows positive granular staining for immunoglobulins (see Fig. 4-22D), and electron-dense deposits are seen with TEM (see Fig. 4-22E).

- **Proliferative GN:** increased cellularity without significant alterations to the GBM; ICs may or may not be identified (Fig. 4-23; eFig. 4-8).
- **Mesangioproliferative GN:** increased cellularity limited to the mesangium with evidence of IC deposition within the mesangium (Fig. 4-24; eFig. 4-9).
- **Membranoproliferative glomerulonephritis (MPGN)**, also called "mesangiocapillary GN": proliferation (endocapillary and mesangial) with remodeling of the capillary loop resulting from IC deposition (usually between the endothelial cell and the GBM; Fig. 4-25; eFig. 4-10). In MPGN, thickening of the glomerular capillary walls results from subendothelial IC deposition as well as from mesangial cell interpositioning. This can be seen with JMS as a characteristic *double-contoured GBM* or *"tram-tracks"* (see Fig. 4-25C).
- **Segmental glomerulosclerosis (GS):** segmental effacement of peripheral capillary loops by extracellular matrix; notably, GS can be superimposed on the above patterns or can occur as the sole pathologic process (Fig. 4-26; eFig. 4-11). **Hyalinosis** is often seen concurrently with GS as glassy PAS-positive material in the capillary wall. Hyalinosis indicates plasma insudation into the wall of the capillary loop.
- **Global glomerulosclerosis (glomerular obsolescence):** tuft is shrunken, eosinophilic, and hypocellular (Fig. 4-27; eFig. 4-12).

Lesions in the glomerular capsule and urinary space may occur because of various combinations of hyperplasia of parietal epithelial cells, crescents, invasion by monocytes, thickening of the basement membrane, and periglomerular fibrosis. Importantly, thickening and splitting of the glomerular capsule basement membranes can be a nonspecific lesion in older dogs and cats (eFig. 4-14).

Secondary histologic changes in GN include *tubular protein casts* (Fig. 4-30). Proteinuria can damage and activate tubular epithelial cells, releasing proinflammatory cytokines resulting in acute and chronic inflammation. Tubular epithelial cells also release growth factors that induce *interstitial fibrosis*. Indeed, the amount of tubulointerstitial fibrosis is often closely correlated with the degree of azotemia in glomerulopathies. Histologic changes may also be of *ischemic origin* because of decreased glomerular and peritubular blood flow. Advanced glomerular lesions are often concurrent with interstitial fibrosis and tubular atrophy, eventually producing the nonspecific histologic picture of *end-stage kidney*.

Glomerular cystic atrophy (Fig. 4-28 may occur subsequent to tubulointerstitial scarring, which constricts tubules, inhibits or stops tubular fluid flow, and dilates glomerular capsules. In humans and experimental animal models, this lesion is often referred to as "atubular glomeruli"; however, technically, this latter term requires serial sections of entire glomeruli to demonstrate the lack of a connection between the glomerular capsule and the proximal tubule. If glomerulocystic atrophy is diffuse and severe, small cysts can be seen grossly in the cortex and it is called **glomerulocystic disease** (see Fig. 4-16).

There is an important distinction between the *patterns* of glomerular lesions and the *diagnostic terms*. For example, a diagnosis of MGN requires identification of IC on the abluminal surface of the GBM via IF, TEM, and/or special stains. In the early stages of the disease, the GBM may not be thickened at all, and deposits are only seen with TEM and IF. Furthermore, there are other diseases that result in thickened GBM that should not be diagnosed as MGN. This is because MGN does not simply refer to a histologic pattern of thickened capillary walls, but instead is a diagnosis of a specific type of **IC-mediated glomerulonephritis (ICGN)**. Similarly, some glomerular diseases may have an "MPGN pattern" on histology because there is hypercellularity and thickening of the GBM, but the lack of definitive ICs indicates that they are not ICGN. Examples of "MPGN pattern" in dogs and humans include Alport syndrome and thrombotic microangiopathies, both of which are discussed in detail later.

A few veterinary nephropathology services offer routine TEM and IF evaluations. In autopsy specimens or cases with financial restrictions, one will almost always forego these advanced diagnostic modalities. In these situations, the pathologist can equivocate and merely provide a diagnosis of GBM thickening with or without hypercellularity. However, it is necessary to differentiate between ICGN and non-ICGN when examining renal biopsy tissue. This helps the nephrologist make appropriate therapeutic decisions. Notably, epidemiologic studies based solely on histologic pattern (without the use of advanced modalities to detect IC) will skew impressions about common pathogeneses and prognoses of glomerular diseases.

Glomerulonephritis

Lesion development may be at different stages in glomeruli of the same kidney, and the type of glomerular reaction may not be uniform among glomeruli. Glomeruli commonly exhibit a spectrum of histologic changes. Glomeruli may be nonspecifically involved in renal diseases such as renal cortical necrosis, or they may be secondarily impacted by tubulointerstitial diseases such as pyelonephritis. Septic emboli frequently lodge in the glomerular and peritubular capillary beds, causing focal glomerulitis and focal interstitial nephritis in diseases such as porcine erysipelas and in actinobacillosis of foals. Diffuse glomerulitis (also referred to as "diffuse proliferative glomerulonephritis") can be seen in acute septicemia and is characterized by increased endocapillary cellularity.

Cellularity of the glomerular tuft may be increased by any combination of:

1. recruitment of leukocytes
2. proliferation of endothelial cells or mesangial cells
3. hypertrophy of endothelial cells, mesangial cells, or podocytes

The term "endocapillary hypercellularity" is often used as a generic descriptor of increased numbers of nucleated cells within glomerular capillary lumens. This assessment is usually subjective. There should only be a single endothelial nucleus in a glomerular capillary lumen in small animals; 2 or more nuclei indicates hypercellularity. That being said, the lesion should be present in many glomeruli. In other words, a small proportion of glomeruli with a few circulating leukocytes does not warrant the diagnosis of "endocapillary hypercellularity." Hence, the subjective nature of the lesion. Likewise, mesangial cells in glomeruli of dogs usually occur singly or in pairs, and more than 3 mesangial cells in close proximity warrants the diagnosis of **mesangial cell hyperplasia**. Mesangial cell number in other species may vary. Proliferation of endothelial versus mesangial cells may be difficult to distinguish in standard H&E sections. Hypercellularity that is limited to the mesangium can often be easily distinguished using PAS or trichrome stains on thin (3 μm) sections. If there is difficulty discerning the location of the increased cellularity, it is often assumed that at least some of the cells are inside capillary loops, distorting the architecture and precluding identification of the proliferating population.

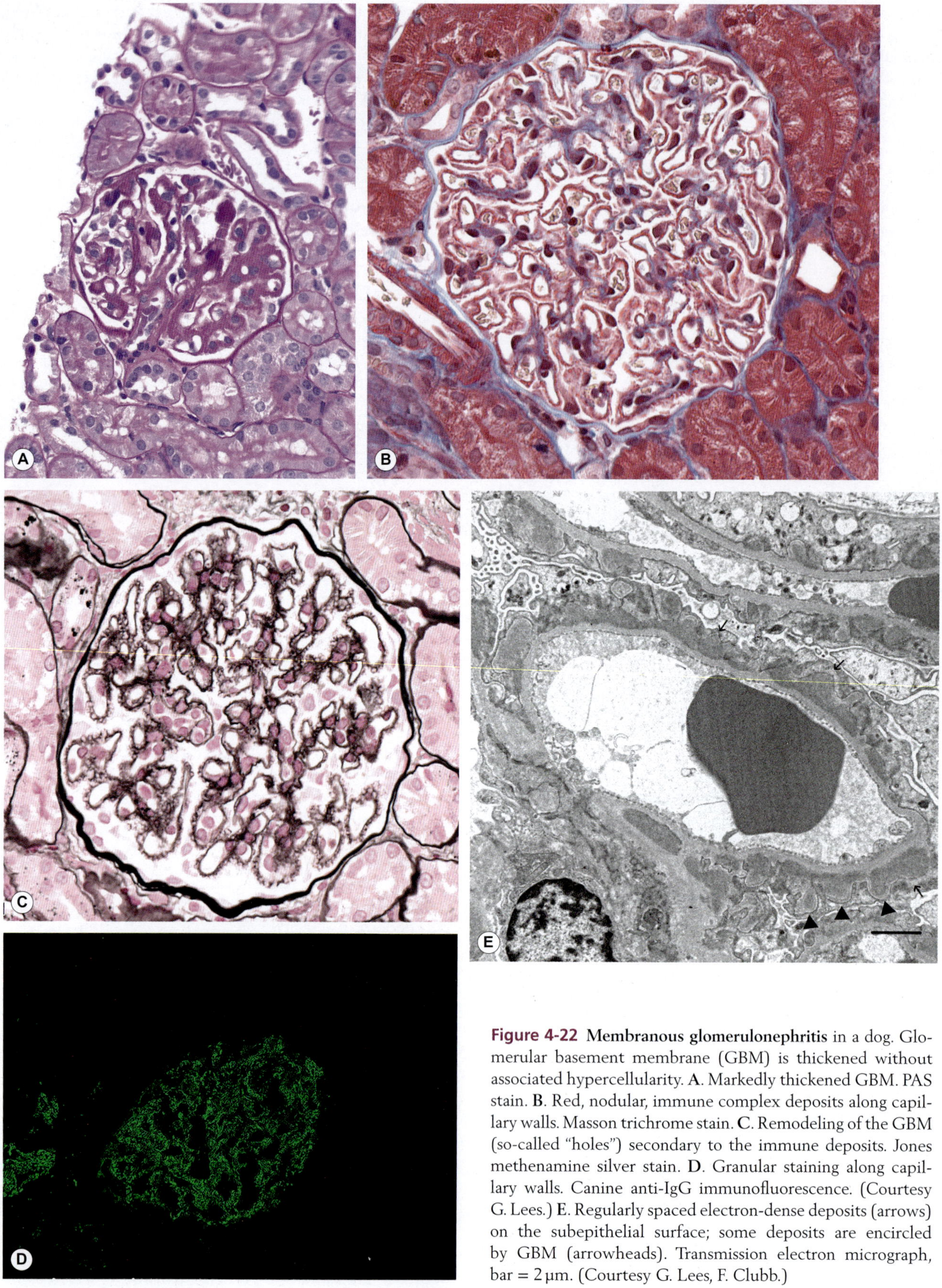

Figure 4-22 Membranous glomerulonephritis in a dog. Glomerular basement membrane (GBM) is thickened without associated hypercellularity. **A**. Markedly thickened GBM. PAS stain. **B**. Red, nodular, immune complex deposits along capillary walls. Masson trichrome stain. **C**. Remodeling of the GBM (so-called "holes") secondary to the immune deposits. Jones methenamine silver stain. **D**. Granular staining along capillary walls. Canine anti-IgG immunofluorescence. (Courtesy G. Lees.) **E**. Regularly spaced electron-dense deposits (arrows) on the subepithelial surface; some deposits are encircled by GBM (arrowheads). Transmission electron micrograph, bar = 2 μm. (Courtesy G. Lees, F. Clubb.)

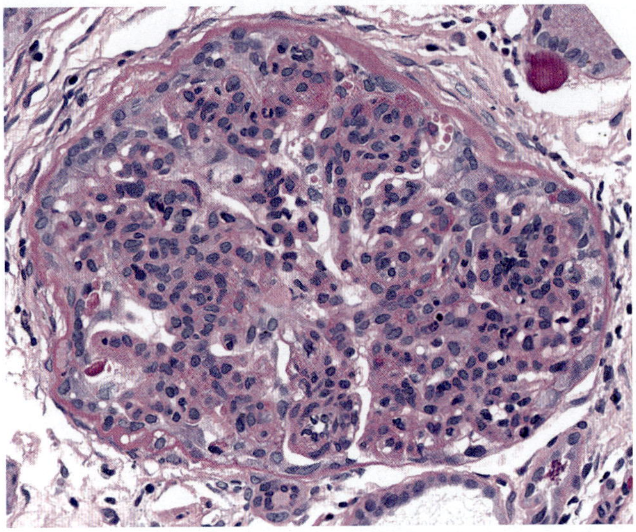

Figure 4-23 **Proliferative glomerulonephropathy** in a young dog. Note marked mesangial and endocapillary hypercellularity. PAS stain. (Courtesy G. Lees, F. Clubb.)

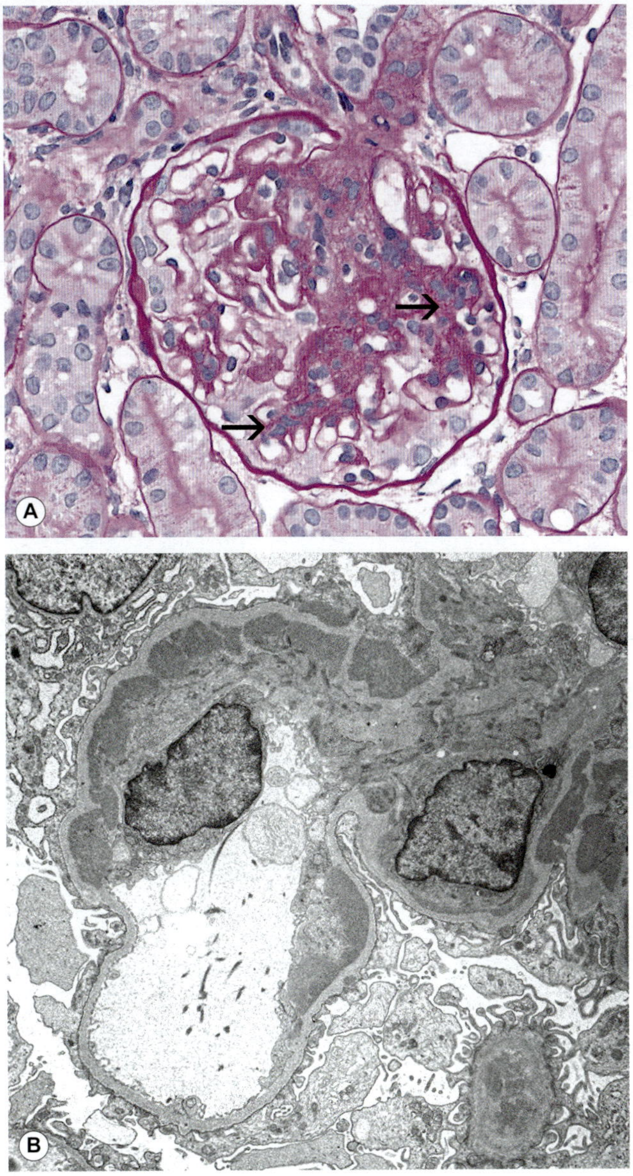

Figure 4-24 **Mesangioproliferative glomerulonephropathy** in a dog. **A.** Note increased mesangial cellularity (arrows). PAS stain. **B.** Large electron-dense deposits in the mesangium and extending into the base of the capillary loops. Transmission electron micrograph. (Courtesy G. Lees, F. Clubb.)

In addition to cell proliferation and leukocyte recruitment, a glomerulus can appear hypercellular if endothelial cells, mesangial cells, or podocytes undergo hypertrophy. This cellular and nuclear enlargement will make it more likely that the nucleus appears in the tissue section. Additionally, hypertrophied mesangial cells can migrate out into the capillary wall (mesangial cell interpositioning), which will also contribute to the appearance of hypercellularity within a capillary loop. It is important to remember that mesangial hypercellularity and endocapillary hypercellularity can occur alone or together and that the use of proper stains on appropriate sections can help the pathologist localize the source of the increased cellularity. If both are present, then both should be included in the histologic description. If, however, only mesangial cells are increased, then the correct morphologic diagnostic term is "mesangioproliferative."

Fibrin exudation into the urinary space, which occurs in severely damaged glomeruli with rupture of the GBM or glomerular capsule, leads to the proliferation of both visceral and parietal epithelial cells, and often the infiltration of macrophages and neutrophils (Fig. 4-29; eFig. 4-13). These represent an uncommon but important form of glomerular hypercellularity, called a **glomerular crescent**. Some of the cells produce collagen, and fibroblasts from the interstitium can also invade the glomerular capsule. Experimental evidence implicates transforming growth factor–β as being integral in the transition from a "cellular" to a "fibrocellular" to a "fibrous" crescent. In humans, crescents are most commonly seen in cases of rapidly progressive GN; however, they are only indicative of severe glomerular damage and not pathognomonic of any one disease. Crescents are rare in cats and dogs, but may occur with some frequency in certain types of porcine and ovine GN.

Ultrastructural evaluation is the optimal way to assess podocytes. The **swelling of foot processes** and their subsequent retraction is a reversible lesion in podocytes and is associated with protein leakage. Although it is often stated that podocytes do not replicate postnatally, various lines of evidence in humans and experimental glomerular diseases have questioned this concept. It is safe to say that podocytes replicate slowly or infrequently. Severe injury can cause loss of podocytes and exposure of "bare" GBM, which can adhere to the glomerular capsule (**synechiae**; see Fig. 4-26). If the adhesion is extensive, the glomerular filtrate can diffuse into the interstitium surrounding the glomerulus.

Glomerular capillary walls may appear thickened in H&E-stained sections because of endothelial or podocyte swelling and/or **thickening and/or remodeling of the GBM**. The GBM is easier to visualize when special techniques, such as PAS or JMS, are used on thin (1-3 µm) sections. TEM is required to characterize the morphology of the thickened GBM, which may be regular with a smooth outer contour or irregular because of deposition of electron-dense material in *subendothelial, intramembranous,* or *subepithelial* locations. *These electron-dense deposits are usually ICs.*

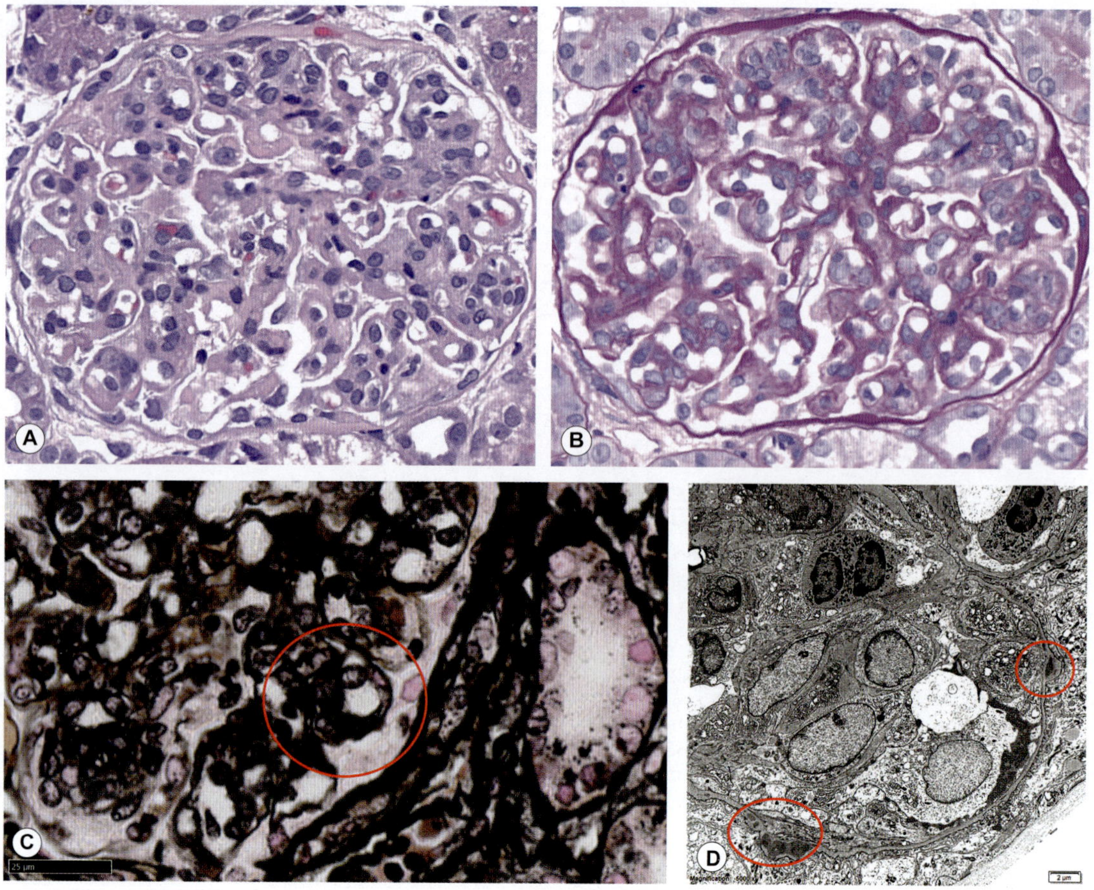

Figure 4-25 **Membranoproliferative glomerulonephritis** in a dog. **A.** H&E. **B.** Endocapillary and mesangial hypercellularity. PAS stain. **C.** Double contours (circled; also referred to as glomerular basement membrane remodeling) of the capillary wall. Jones methenamine silver stain. **D.** Small subendothelial electron-dense deposits (circled), endothelial cell swelling, and numerous circulating red and white blood cells. Transmission electron micrograph. (Courtesy G. Lees, F. Clubb.)

Thickened peripheral capillary walls are particularly prominent in cases of MGN and MPGN (described later). As stated above, **GS** is the accumulation of extracellular matrix that effaces the lumens of peripheral capillary loops and eventually results in consolidation of the tuft. Both GS and hyalinosis are possible sequelae to ICGN. It is important to realize, however, that not all cases with GS have an underlying IC-mediated pathogenesis. Therefore, TEM and IF are needed to correctly classify these cases. Primary GS is described in more detail later.

Pathogenesis of immune-complex-mediated glomerulonephritis

GN often results from the deposition in glomeruli of circulating ICs, which is referred to as immune-complex-mediated glomerulonephritis (**ICGN**). GN can also be caused by formation in situ of antibodies against the GBM, or from activation of the alternative pathway of complement. Many types of GN are of unknown pathogenesis.

In **ICGN**, circulating antigen-antibody complexes of nonglomerular origin localize in glomeruli and are visible by IF or TEM. The classic experimental model of ICGN is intravenous injection of foreign protein resulting in IC deposition in glomeruli. This condition (referred to as "chronic serum sickness") models the continued antigenemia that occurs during various bacterial, viral, and parasitic infections, such as feline leukemia virus (FeLV; *Retroviridae, Gammaretrovirus felleu*) infection and canine dirofilariosis. In addition to exogenous antigenemia, endogenous antigens are also important. Examples of endogenous antigens are nucleoprotein in human systemic lupus erythematosus, or tumor-associated antigens. Importantly, although some infections and inflammatory conditions are associated with ICGN in domestic species, the specific antigens have only been definitively identified in IC in research settings. *There are no routinely available tests to label the antigens within the IC in biopsy or autopsy samples*. Comprehensive analysis of ICGN cases shows a *characteristic granular staining pattern, as seen by IF*. With TEM, the complexes are seen as electron-dense deposits in a subendothelial, subepithelial, or intramembranous location, or within the mesangium. ICs usually contain complement proteins as well as antigens and antibodies. In general, it is thought that IC deposition occurs during the period of equivalence of antigen and antibody concentrations or during slight antigen excess. It is also possible that some antigens are capable of penetrating the GBM, where they bind antibody of low avidity. For example, dirofilarial antigens circulate in ICs and also may be deposited directly in the GBM, inducing formation of in situ ICs. The relative

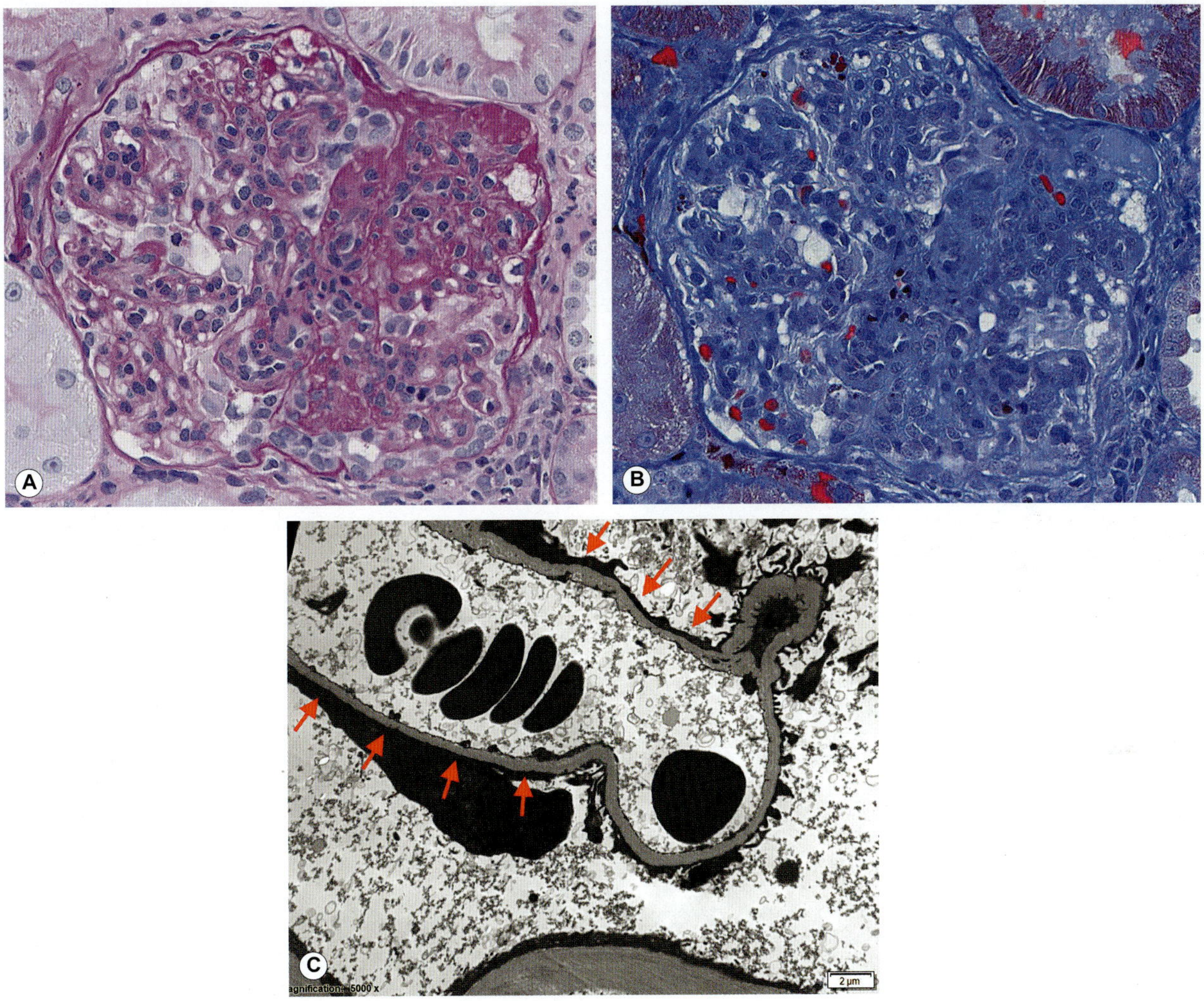

Figure 4-26 Focal segmental glomerulosclerosis in a dog; <50% of glomeruli in the biopsy were affected by this process. **A.** Segmental effacement of the peripheral capillary lumens by extracellular matrix. This segment is adherent to the glomerular capsule (synechia). Degree of cellularity can vary in this lesion. PAS stain. **B.** The additional matrix has staining properties similar to mesangial and glomerular basement membrane material. Masson trichrome stain. **C.** Segmental podocyte foot process effacement (arrows) and the absence of electron-dense deposits. Transmission electron micrograph.

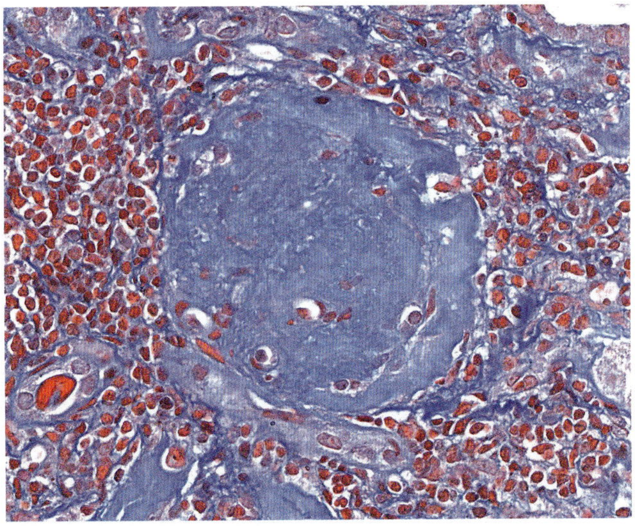

Figure 4-27 Global glomerulosclerosis (obsolescence) in a dog. The glomerulus is a meshwork of collagenous material and has very few nuclei. Masson trichrome stain.

importance of circulating soluble ICs versus in situ formation of complexes in causing ICGN is not resolved.

The reasons for *localization of ICs* in various glomerular sites, namely, subendothelial, intramembranous, subepithelial, or mesangial, are complex. Localization may be affected by the size, shape, charge, and chemical composition of the complexes. Penetration of the GBM by the complexes may be aided by products of inflammation. The location of deposits may also change with time due to remodeling of the GBM. *Modification of glomerular ICs occurs;* they may be removed or they may enlarge. Complexes may be eliminated by solubilization, phagocytosis by neutrophils, macrophages, or mesangial cells, passage through the mesangium and egress at the vascular pole, degradation within the mesangial matrix, or by extracellular degradation by proteases. Thus, for example, removal of the source of persistent antigenemia in pyometra of dogs by hysterectomy results in resolution of GN and cessation of proteinuria. Conversely, complexes may enlarge through combination with various blood-borne reactants, such as small amounts of antigen, free antibody, ICs of the same or different specificity, complement components,

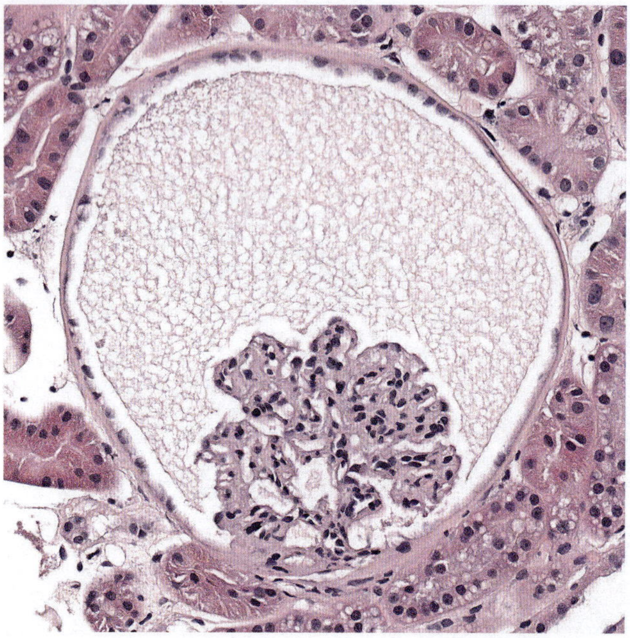

Figure 4-28 **Glomerulocystic atrophy** in a dog. Although this lesion can be a nonspecific finding in older dogs, these glomeruli are nonfunctional. Therefore, if they are common within a specimen, there may be renal insufficiency. PAS stain.

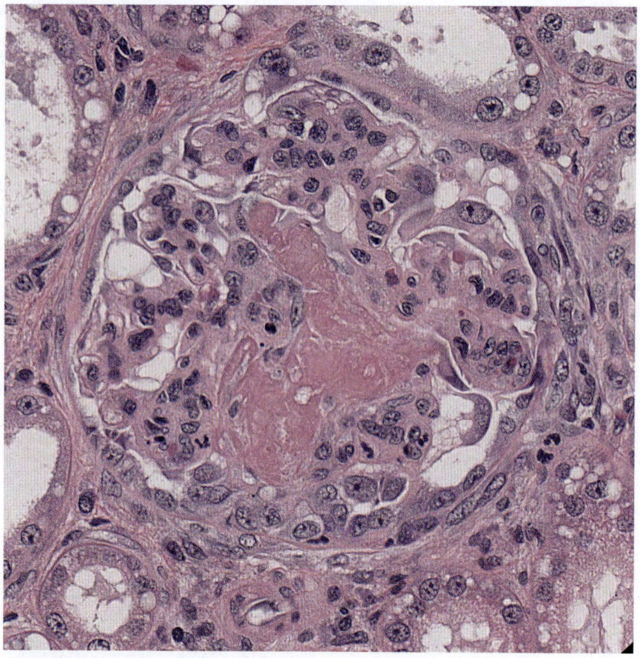

Figure 4-29 **Cellular crescent** in a dog. Cells have accumulated in the urinary space due to rupture of the capillary walls. This dog had immune-complex–mediated glomerulonephritis, consistent with membranoproliferative glomerulonephritis. PAS stain.

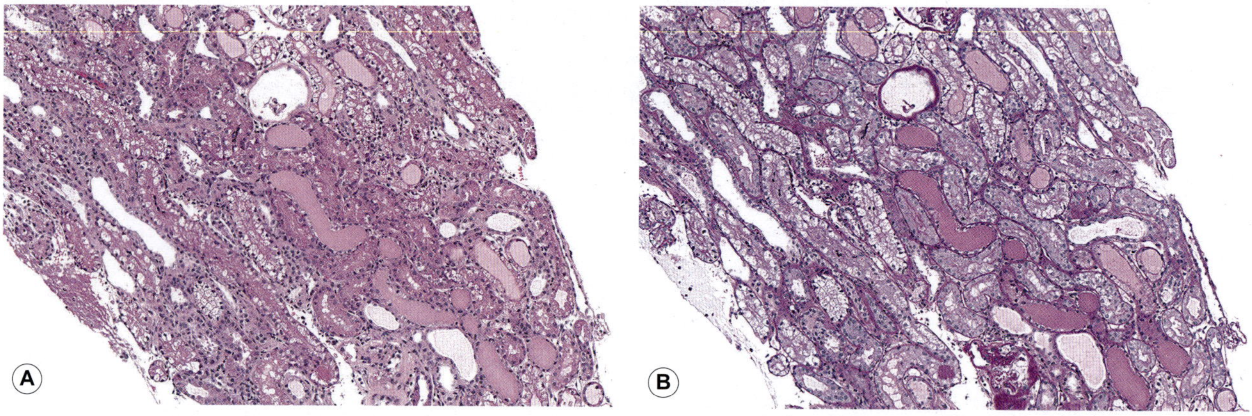

Figure 4-30 A. Tubulointerstitium from a proteinuric dog diagnosed with **focal segmental glomerulosclerosis**. Additionally, there is vacuolar degeneration of tubular epithelial cells. H&E. B. Same region. There are bright-pink intratubular casts of Tamm-Horsfall mucoprotein. PAS stain.

or antibodies against immunoglobulins or complement components.

Several mechanisms result in glomerular injury once ICs are formed in situ or are deposited in glomeruli. The best-established mechanism is that of complement fixation with resultant chemotaxis of neutrophils. Notably, in MGN there is minimal endocapillary hypercellularity because the activation of the complement system occurs on the opposite side of the GBM. This is in contrast to MPGN, in which the IC are predominantly subendothelial, resulting in complement activation near the capillary lumen. Complement components C3a, C5a, and C567 attract neutrophils, which, in the process of ingesting IC, release lysosomal enzymes, arachidonic acid metabolites, and oxygen-derived free radicals, causing GBM damage. The terminal membrane-attack complex of complement, C5b-9, can injure glomeruli by releasing oxidants, cytokines, and other mediators that damage podocytes, endothelial, and mesangial cells. Complement fragments cause release of histamine from mast cells, and hence increased capillary permeability, which may allow deposition of more ICs in the capillary wall.

Chemokines (chemotactic *cytokines*) produced by glomerular, mesangial, tubular, and interstitial cells activate circulating leukocytes bearing the respective surface receptors. Local attachment of leukocytes occurs through interaction of leukocyte integrins with adhesion molecules, such as intercellular adhesion molecule 1 and vascular cell adhesion molecule 1, on endothelial, mesangial, and interstitial cells. Activated leukocytes initiate their effector functions, such as respiratory burst, phagocytosis of IC, release of hydrolases, and removal of matrix, cell debris, and apoptotic cells. Activated leukocytes also release additional mediators, chemokines, and cytokines in an amplification loop to recruit more leukocytes. It is paradoxical that, although complement participates in glomerular injury, it is also capable of solubilizing ICs to facilitate their removal. Hence, hereditary hypocomplementemia, as occurs in Finnish Landrace lambs, leads to persistence of ICs and glomerular injury. Interaction of complement fragments with platelets leads to coagulation, thrombosis, and fibrinolysis. Hageman factor links the complement, coagulation, and kinin-forming pathways. Fibrin and its degradation products are often present in inflamed glomeruli, and fibrinogen that leaks into the urinary space is a stimulus for monocyte infiltration, proliferation of parietal epithelial cells, and crescent formation.

There also can be electron-dense deposits composed solely of components from the complement system, but they are not ICs. In humans, the MPGN-pattern of injury is subdivided into 2 main categories (*IC-mediated GN* and *C3 GN*). This division is important because it has etiologic, prognostic, and therapeutic implications; a similar division of GN may be useful in veterinary species. Specifically, there are examples of breed-related/familial abnormalities in the complement system that can result in GN. However, in many veterinary cases, this type of classification system is purely academic.

In **anti-GBM GN**, *antibodies are formed against intrinsic GBM antigens*, resulting in a *linear pattern of IF* reflecting the uniform distribution of immunoglobulins and complement proteins along the GBM. There is a notable lack of electron-dense deposits on TEM examination. In humans, this causes severe crescentic GN without significant hypercellularity. Anti-GBM GN occurs as a component of Goodpasture syndrome in humans, which is the combination of anti-GBM antibodies together with antibodies against pulmonary capillaries, which can lead to acute pulmonary hemorrhage and death. Aside from humans, anti-GBM antibodies have only been documented in a single horse. The lack of histologic lesions in that horse and the linear IF staining in other horses without detectable anti-GBM antibodies suggest that spontaneous *anti-GBM disease* is limited to humans. It can be modeled in rats by injection of anti–rat kidney antibodies obtained from rabbits or ducks immunized with rat kidney tissue; this experimental model is also referred to as *nephrotoxic nephritis*. The animal model only acutely mimics the human anti-GBM disease, because with time, the typical linear IF pattern is gradually converted to the granular pattern typical of ICGN. Ultrastructural evaluation reveals ICs in subepithelial and subendothelial locations.

The role of **mesangial cells** in the development of glomerular injury is increasingly recognized. Mesangial cells may initiate inflammation in the absence of leukocytes because they can produce inflammatory mediators, including oxygen free radicals, interleukin 1 (IL1), arachidonic acid metabolites, and a variety of growth factors. Likewise, mesangial cells can be stimulated to proliferate when macrophages and other immune cells release IL1, β-endorphin, tumor necrosis factor, and platelet-derived growth factor (PDGF). In these scenarios, there is also an increase in mesangial matrix. Proliferating mesangial cells release autacoids, such as IL1 and PDGF, producing an amplifying loop of inflammation. Transforming growth factor–β induces synthesis of mesangial matrix. Immunomodulatory peptides released by proliferating mesangial cells stimulate replication and activation of macrophages, which both amplify the inflammatory lesion and ameliorate it by the phagocytosis of ICs.

In addition to the immunologic causes of GN discussed previously, there are a number of *nonimmunologic causes of glomerular injury*. These include increased glomerular capillary pressure, coagulation in response to endothelial injury, serum lipid abnormalities, and glomerular hypertrophy, and they are discussed later.

Morphology of glomerulonephritis

Acute GN may not significantly alter the gross appearance of the kidney, or it may be slightly or markedly enlarged, pale, soft, and edematous. Petechiae may be visible (Fig. 4-31A). In **subacute GN**, the kidney is often enlarged and pale-tan with a smooth surface and nonadherent capsule. The capsule is tense, and the cut surface bulges. The pale-tan cortex is well demarcated from a normal-colored medulla. This subacute phase is anatomically and developmentally arbitrary and progresses to the **chronic** phase, in which the kidney is shrunken and contracted with generalized fine granularity of the capsular surface (see Fig. 4-31B). When contraction is severe, it is grossly indistinguishable from diffuse chronic interstitial nephritis. The capsule may be adherent. On cut surface, the cortex is often uniformly narrowed. Small cysts, which are obstructed tubules, are often present.

Histology reveals strikingly different lesions depending on the location of the ICs. In the **acute phase of proliferative GN or MPGN**, there is hypercellularity, usually because of influx of inflammatory cells. Neutrophils and/or monocytes marginate in the capillaries and, together with the swollen proliferating endothelial and mesangial cells, give a distinct impression of hypercellularity (see Fig. 4-25). Occasionally, fibrin thrombi form in the capillaries, or there is fibrinoid necrosis of the tuft. This form of GN with the formation of fibrin thrombi is the usual picture seen in swine with petechiae. In **acute MGN**, glomeruli appear completely normal, in which case TEM and IF are needed to identify ICs. The tubulointerstitial compartment can be normal (most commonly in MGN), or there may be edema, inflammation, or tubular epithelial injury (usually in acute proliferative or MPGN).

Although clinical signs can vary greatly, some can be anticipated. The swelling of the kidney can result in oliguria. There is proteinuria, and there may be hyaline, granular, and/or red blood cell casts. In fact, RBC casts in urine are highly specific for active GN in humans. Although hematuria can be observed in many types of renal and lower urinary tract disease, the cast shape indicates an intrarenal source of the RBCs. RBC casts are occasionally seen in dogs and cats with severe acute GN (eFig. 4-15).

In the **subacute** phase, there is often mesangial hypercellularity and/or remodeling of the GBM. Subendothelial deposits will result in double contours of the GBM, whereas subepithelial deposits will induce spike formation between deposits. Repeat biopsies of the same patient might even reveal a change in the distribution of the deposits over time. Segmental

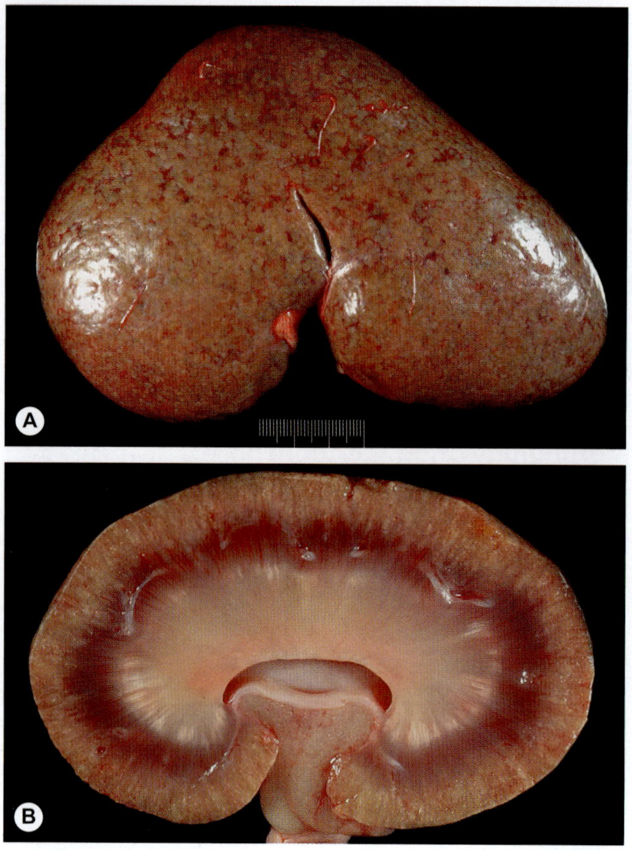

Figure 4-31 **Glomerulonephritis.** **A**. In a horse, the cortical surface is pale-tan and with widespread petechiae. (Courtesy L. Himmel, P. Stromberg.) **B**. In a dog, the cortex is pale-tan and slightly irregular. (Courtesy D. Russell, P. Stromberg.)

GS and synechiae may be present. There is often increased tubulointerstitial scarring.

In the **chronic** phase, scarring of glomeruli occurs. There may be a reduction in the apparent number of glomeruli as obsolescent glomeruli blend with surrounding scar tissue. Although all glomeruli usually have IC, the development of GS varies. The interstitial reaction initiated during the acute phase progresses with fibrosis and lymphocytic infiltration. Large numbers of tubules undergo atrophy and are replaced by scar tissue. The fibrosis becomes slowly self-perpetuating. Tubules that remain connected to functioning glomeruli may become dilated and develop epithelial hypertrophy and hyperplasia. Azotemia can occur, with an increased volume of urine of low specific gravity. Proteinuria can vary and casts may be absent. The frequency with which GN leads to CKD is not known. Therefore, prospective studies in many species would help pathologists draw conclusions regarding prognosis. Furthermore, the anecdotal evidence about the success of immunosuppressive therapy in small animals with IC-mediated GN has led to the development of guidelines for immunosuppression in these patients.

Once the GFR has decreased to 30-50% of normal, progression to end-stage renal disease tends to be inevitable. This occurs partly because of continuation of the primary glomerular disease, partly because of the addition of complicating factors such as hypertension, and partly because of adaptive changes in glomeruli in a failing kidney. These *adaptive changes* include hypertrophy and increased workload of the remaining nephrons, with resulting epithelial and endothelial injury and proteinuria.

Prevalence of glomerulonephritis

The frequency of diagnosis of GN in domestic animals has increased dramatically, mostly because of increased awareness and understanding of GN by clinicians and pathologists. ICs commonly circulate throughout life, but few individuals develop significant lesions, so various factors such as genetic susceptibility, defective immune systems, or other mechanisms may be operative in affected animals. Many associations of infectious and other diseases with GN have been identified. In essence, *any infection that can produce persistent antigenemia has the potential to cause IC disease*. The morphology of the glomerular lesion is of little assistance in identifying its cause because many agents can cause the same type of lesion, and conversely, one agent can produce a spectrum of glomerular changes. Diseases known or suspected to induce ICGN are listed in Box 4-1. Most cases in animals are *idiopathic*; those occurring in association with other diseases or in which glomerular lesions contain known antigens are referred to as *secondary*.

Dogs

One large study of 89 dogs diagnosed with glomerular disease via comprehensive biopsy analysis used unbiased hierarchical cluster analysis to group cases based on lesion scores (but not based on clinical data or outcome). The presence (or absence) of IC deposits was the first branch point between groups, indicating that it was an important feature in lesion phenotype. Interestingly, when the algorithm used the same scores but only considered values from histologic evaluation, ~25% of the cases were misclassified. More importantly, the incorrect categorization would have impacted treatment. In other words, there was a ~25% chance that a case with definitive ICs (verified by TEM and IF) would be diagnosed as non-ICGN, and vice versa. This underscores the need for advanced diagnostic techniques in the evaluation of proteinuric kidney disease. An additional study showed that IF is currently superior to IHC in labeling canine ICs. A study compared lambda light-chain IHC and IF to TEM (gold standard) in dogs. It showed complete agreement between the TEM and IF results and frequent disagreement between IHC and TEM. The IHC had both false-positive and false-negative results. The authors noted that additional optimization of the IHC techniques might improve specificity and sensitivity; however, the ease of direct IF will likely support its use in routine renal biopsy evaluation by veterinary nephropathology centers.

Almost half (48%) of the North American dogs that underwent biopsy for the clinical indication of proteinuria had ICGN, with GS and amyloidosis also being common glomerular diseases. Data from the International Veterinary Renal Pathology Service show a similar proportion of ICGN versus non-ICGN cases (data not published). Interestingly, ICGN has geographic variability, based on commonality of infectious diseases. Proteinuric dogs from the United Kingdom, undergoing comprehensive renal biopsy evaluation, were less likely to have ICGN. Specifically, 17 of 62 (27%) dogs had demonstrable ICs. This lower prevalence in the United Kingdom is posited to be associated with the low level of tick-borne infections (*Borrelia* and *Leishmania*, both discussed later). Although the UK study was retrospective and case-control comparisons could be performed, there was a noticeable difference in outcome between

Box • 4-1

Causes of immune-complex–mediated glomerulonephritis in domestic animals

Viral
African swine fever virus
Aleutian mink disease virus
Bovine viral diarrhea virus
Canine adenovirus 1 (infectious canine hepatitis)
Classical swine fever virus
Equine infectious anemia virus
Feline leukemia virus

Bacterial/fungal
Borreliella (Borrelia) burgdorferi
Canine pyometra
Campylobacter fetus
Encephalitozoon cuniculi
Septic valvular endocarditis

Protozoal
African trypanosomosis
Babesia gibsoni
Leishmania infantum
Coccidiosis

Helminths
Dirofilaria immitis

Neoplasms
Various

Autoimmune
Various autoimmune diseases suspected

Hereditary
Abnormal complement system of Bernese Mountain Dogs
Dense-deposit disease of pigs
Hypocomplementemia in Brittany Spaniels
Hypocomplementemia in Finnish Landrace lambs

ICGN dogs that were immunosuppressed versus ICGN dogs that were not. Specifically, 6 dogs received some form of non-steroid-based immunosuppression, and all were alive at the time at the end of the study (up to 3.5 years after diagnosis). Only 1 of 6 ICGN dogs that were not immunosuppressed was alive (median survival time 300 days).

Canine adenovirus 1 (CAdV1; *Adenoviridae, Mastadenovirus canidae*), *Dirofilaria immitis*, *Borreliella (Borrelia) burgdorferi*, and *Leishmania infantum* (either singly or as coinfections) have all been associated with the development of ICGN. Exudative GN has been associated with acute leptospirosis in dogs in Europe.

Experimental infections with **CAdV1** have shown that the virus is present in glomerular endothelial cells within 4 days (as demonstrated by IF for anti-CAdV antigen and viral inclusions on TEM). Histologically, endothelial cells are swollen and vacuolated. Within 7 days, viral antigen, IgG, C3 staining, and electron-dense deposits can be detected in the mesangium but not at the periphery of capillary loops. At this stage, there are increased numbers of mesangial cells and infiltration of the tufts by neutrophils. Some glomeruli contain thrombi, and there may be segmental necrosis of the tuft.

Experimental chronic **dirofilariosis** was reported to cause either a strong immune response and clearance of microfilariae or a weaker response that cannot clear the microfilariae. In the strong response scenario, there was a strong granular pattern of IgG deposition in the mesangium, mesangial electron-dense deposits, and various degrees of mesangial hypercellularity. In the weaker response scenario, there were small electron-dense particles (<25 nm) distributed continuously along the GBM and in the mesangium. This was correlated with a linear or pseudolinear staining pattern of IgG along capillary walls, whereas C3 had a granular pattern. Hypercellularity was mild and limited to the mesangium. Taken together, the authors suggested that uniform localization of filarial antigens along the GBM elicited an antibody response resulting in a linear (or "pseudolinear") appearance of the IgG. In addition to these phenotypes, MGN with subepithelial IC, mesangioproliferative GN with scattered mesangial and subendothelial IC, and focal segmental glomerulosclerosis (FSGS) without IC have all been reported in chronic experimental or spontaneous dirofilarial infections. Microfilariae may be observed in glomerular or peritubular capillaries (Fig. 4-32). Patients with dirofilariasis might also have changes in the distribution and number of negatively charged macromolecules of the GBM, many of which are assumed to be proteoglycans, specifically heparan sulfate. This process might lead to proteinuria via a pathway that is not IC mediated. Importantly, spontaneous infections might not result in histologic glomerular lesions or only equivocal evidence of ICs.

A unique form of rapidly progressive MPGN (eFig. 4-16) is putatively associated with infection by ***Borreliella (Borrelia) burgdorferi***, a spirochete transmitted by *Ixodes* ticks. Golden Retrievers and Labradors are predisposed, but it has been seen in many other breeds. Serologic tests for antibodies against the bacterial outer surface proteins (Osp) C and F or the recombinant protein C6 (which mimics the bacterial protein called variable major protein–like sequence, expressed) are often used as evidence of infection. Lyme nephritis has been reported to occur in <2% of serologically positive dogs, and <30% of the nephritic patients had concurrent or prior lameness. Definitive diagnosis of Lyme nephritis is difficult because *B. burgdorferi* organisms are not frequently found in the kidney, and disease is thought to be driven by ICs containing a variety of antigens, including OspA, OspB, and/or flagellin. A validated consistent immunohistochemical test for these bacterial antigens is not commercially available, and elution of ICs from kidney tissue is not feasible as a routine test. It has been reported that dogs with signs of Lyme disease have significantly more *B. burgdorferi*–specific IC in circulation compared with subclinical Lyme-positive dogs; however, there are subclinical dogs that also have very high levels of circulating ICs.

Renal biopsies of proteinuric dogs naturally infected with ***Leishmania*** spp. have demonstrated mesangioproliferative GN (with IC limited to the mesangium), MPGN (with subendothelial and mesangial IC), and GS without definitive IC deposition. Notably, biopsies 60 days after the initial biopsy rarely demonstrated a change in the severity of the glomerular lesion, suggesting that both progression and resolution are slow processes. Elution studies were performed to assess the composition of glomerular ICs, and they revealed antibodies directed against parasite membrane antigens. Although there were small variations in antibody characteristics, such as isoelectric points, they were not correlated with clinical signs

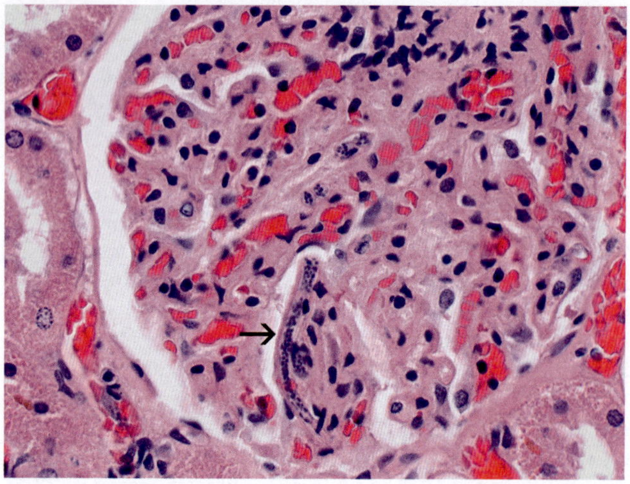

Figure 4-32 ***Dirofilaria immitis*** **microfilaria** (arrow) in a glomerular capillary of a dog.

or whether the deposits were located in the mesangium or capillary wall. Similar to borreliosis, many dogs are serologically positive and do not have clinical signs. However, dogs with medium-to-high antibody and low IFN-γ levels as well as having *Leishmania* DNA (as evidenced by positive PCR) were more likely to have clinicopathologic abnormalities compared with dogs that were infected but clinically healthy. Specifically, the clinicopathologic abnormalities included hypoalbuminemia, hyperglobulinemia, proteinuria, and lymphopenia. Therefore, host immune factors play a critical role in the development of renal disease in dogs with leishmaniosis.

In canine **pyometra**, ICGN can occur but may be less significant than tubulointerstitial lesions, the latter of which may be an age-related change as opposed to being secondary to the pyometra.

Deposition of **IgA** was reported 47 of 100 autopsied dogs in Japan with or without clinical renal disease, and IF labeling was considered moderate to marked in 22 dogs. The most common histologic lesion was mesangial expansion and hypercellularity with segmental sclerosis. Immunogold TEM demonstrated IgA deposits in mesangial locations. Although these lesions are similar to IgA nephropathy in humans, there are likely some differences in lesion pathogenesis. IgA in humans is the result of aberrant glycosylation patterns (often hypoglycosylation) of the IgA1 isoform. Only primates are known to synthesize IgA1; they also synthesize IgA2. Nonprimate species only make the IgA2 isoform. Therefore, the pathogenesis of human IgA nephropathy is quite different from IgA deposition observed in dogs.

Proteinuria and azotemia together with MPGN (diagnosed via renal biopsy) were observed in a dog infected with ***Babesia gibsoni***. Resolution of infection and restoration of renal function followed appropriate antibiotic therapy and a short course of immunosuppressive therapy. A 7-month-old dog that had been vaccinated once per month for 7 months with the distemper-hepatitis-leptospirosis-parainfluenza-parvovirus vaccine (without veterinary supervision) developed MPGN, and antigen from the vaccine was also detected in the glomeruli.

Canine breed-associated immune-mediated glomerulonephritides. Breed-associated glomerulonephritides associated with electron-dense deposits have been reported rarely. Immune-complex–mediated MGN occurs in German Shorthaired Pointers with concurrent exfoliative cutaneous lupus erythematosus. The cutaneous lesion is due to a mutation in *UNC93B1*, which is a chaperone protein for Toll-like receptor (TLR) 7 that helps the TLR traffic from the endoplasmic reticulum to endosomes. Although the pathogenesis is not yet completely understood, the disrupted trafficking pattern is posited to lead to autoimmunity. These dogs will have ulcerative dermatitis, polyarthralgia, lymphadenopathy, and infertility. Some of the dogs will be proteinuric and have IgG deposits along the subepithelial surfaces of capillary walls (in a membranous pattern).

In humans, electron-dense deposits can be indicative of IC deposition or abnormalities in the complement system. Notably, complement system defects can have a genetic basis, which means that there is often a familial basis to complement-mediated GN. Likewise, there are 2 known breed-associated GNs, with electron-dense deposits that are likely to have complement-based pathogeneses. In young-adult **Bernese Mountain dogs**, MPGN with proteinuria and azotemia occurred in an autosomal recessive inheritance pattern. There was concurrent tubulointerstitial nephritis. GBMs were remodeled, and there was mesangial interpositioning in GBMs, and subendothelial deposits of IgM and C3. Inherited deficiency of the third component of complement in **Brittany Spaniel dogs** led to the development of MPGN. Affected dogs also had increased susceptibility to infections. Interestingly, treatment of dogs with exogenous C3 resulted in increased proteinuria and more severe glomerular lesions. Both these diseases have likely been removed from the breeding population, as they are no longer commonly observed in these breeds. The lack of a commercial serologic assay for C3 means that many of these types of diseases are likely missed or incorrectly attributed to more commonly seen GN such as ICGN.

Cats

Although most feline glomerulonephritides have been diagnosed as MGN, many have not been verified with TEM and/or IF. It is easy to mistake primary segmental GS for MGN with secondary sclerosis via histology. Therefore, caution should be used when interpreting the histologic lesion without TEM or IF. Even so, TEM- and IF-proven MGN and MPGN do occur in cats. In a study of 57 proteinuric cats (that underwent renal biopsy and comprehensive tissue evaluation), more than half of them had ICGN. Interestingly, cats diagnosed with ICGN had lower UPC and were older than cats with non-ICGN diagnoses. The main negative prognostic factor of survival (in both ICGN and non-ICGN cats) was development of effusion. Cats that were definitively diagnosed with ICGN and received immunosuppressive therapy survived longer than those that did not, underscoring the importance of a correct diagnosis in the selection of therapeutic plans. Both FeLV and feline immunodeficiency virus (FIV; *Retroviridae, Lentivirus felimdef*) in proteinuric cats have been associated with an increased risk of ICGN compared to cats with renal disease not attributable to IC. Notably, the non-ICGN group in that study included cats with primary tubulointerstitial lesions, so the cohorts were not entirely comparable.

Case reports of hematopoietic tumors and plasmacytic pododermatitis have documented glomerular disease (both ICGN and amyloidosis) as a comorbidity.

Horses

GN is observed in horses, but end-stage kidney disease is rare. MPGN often occurs in horses with equine infectious anemia. *Streptococcus equi* and herpesviral infections are also suggested as causes of GN in horses. TEM in horses with proliferative GN may reveal atypical ICs, which can vary from fibrillar to crystalline and rhomboid. In one horse, the ICs had a distinct fibrillar substructure. The outer diameters of the fibrils were 35-40 nm, and they contained a central pore. This appearance is similar to that of humans with immunotactoid GN and may imply a specific etiopathogenesis. Diagnosis of ICGN in horses via renal biopsy could guide therapy; however, immunosuppression in horses is less common compared with small animals because of cost and inherent risks.

Swine

Acute fatal GN occurs sporadically in swine, but is of little economic importance. Deposition of ICs containing IgG and C3 is common in the mesangium of normal slaughter swine, but the mesangioproliferative GN is not of clinical significance. The *porcine dermatitis and nephropathy syndrome* (PDNS) in feeder pigs is associated with systemic necrotizing vasculitis. It appears to be immune mediated, and it results in proliferative GN, fibrin exudation in the tuft, cellular crescent formation, and interstitial nephritis. The lesions are associated with porcine circovirus 2 (PCV2; *Circoviridae, Circovirus porcine2*) infection with a coinfection of porcine parvovirus (PPV; *Parvoviridae, Protoparvovirus ungulate1*) or porcine reproductive and respiratory syndrome virus (Fig. 4-33). PDNS lesions have been induced experimentally by porcine circovirus 3 (PCV3; *Circoviridae, Circovirus porcine3*) alone; immunohistochemistry demonstrated positive staining for the virus in renal tubular epithelial cells.

An autosomal recessive *hereditary deficiency of factor H*, a complement inhibitory protein, caused lethal dense-deposit disease (also called MPGN type II) in Norwegian Yorkshire pigs; factor H deficiency led to massive glomerular deposition of complement, large sausage-shaped intramembranous dense deposits, and mesangial hypercellularity. This genetic deficiency has been eradicated from the porcine population.

Experimental infections with classical swine fever virus (hog cholera virus, CSFV; *Flaviviridae, Pestivirus suis*) led to proliferative ICGN with mesangial IgG deposits and intraglomerular viral antigen. Mesangial IC deposits, with fewer subendothelial and subepithelial deposits, were verified ultrastructurally. GN of unknown pathogenesis was reported in 4 laboratory Göttingen minipigs. Because TEM and IF were not performed, the role of IC deposition is not known. Two pigs had protein in the urinary space, resembling the early crescent formation that occurs in other swine breeds.

Ruminants

Immunologic evidence of GN is common in ruminants, but clinical disease is not. Glomeruli of healthy sheep and goats are often hypercellular and have thick GBM, but the changes appear to have little clinical significance, suggesting that there are variabilities in the GBM of healthy small ruminants. An interesting exception is the *MPGN of* **Finnish Landrace sheep**, which is present at birth and is the result of recessive inheritance of a deficiency of the complement component C3; in affected lambs, blood levels of C3 are ~5% of normal. This congenital deficiency contributes to the development of MPGN, probably because of impaired complement-mediated solubilization of ICs in glomeruli. Affected lambs are clinically normal at birth but die at 1-3-months-old in renal failure. At autopsy, the kidneys are enlarged with pale cortices and glomeruli that are grossly visible as red spots. The glomerular lesion consists of mesangial cell proliferation, capillary wall thickening, and often the formation of glomerular crescents. Subendothelial electron-dense deposits are present and consist of C3, smaller amounts of IgM and IgA and, with prolonged survival, progressively larger amounts of IgG. Glomerular changes begin in the lambs in utero and develop progressively after birth. Choroid plexus lesions also result from IC deposition and lead to encephalopathy.

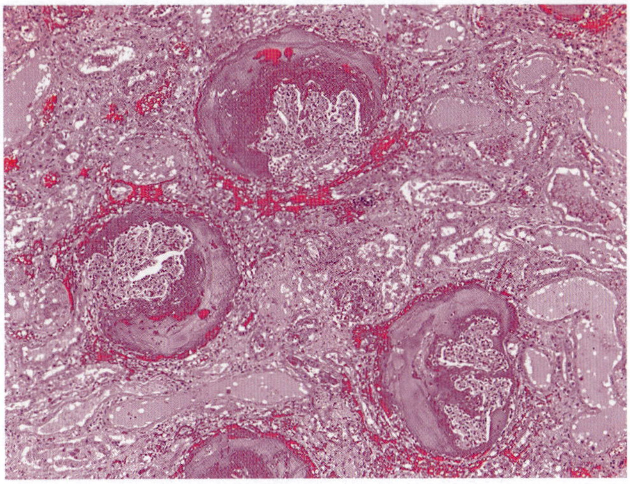

Figure 4-33 Crescentic proliferative glomerulonephritis in a pig with porcine dermatitis and nephropathy syndrome from porcine circovirus 2 infection. (Courtesy T. Clark.)

Visna/maedi viral infection has been associated with histologic evidence of MPGN in sheep, but investigations lacked TEM and IF. Immunohistochemistry revealed viral antigen in tubular epithelial cells and interstitial cells. Glomerular staining was not reported. *Bovine viral diarrhea viral antigen* can be detected along the GBM and in the mesangium of persistently infected cattle. Glomeruli have mesangial hypercellularity and slight thickening of the GBM. IF has demonstrated viral antigen, IgG, and complement components in the glomerulus, but similar histologic lesions with concomitant IgG and scattered C3 staining have been observed in bovine viral diarrhea virus (BVDV)–negative cattle. Unfortunately, TEM was not performed in those studies. Comprehensive evaluation of renal tissue from a calf infected with BVDV1 demonstrated MPGN, subendothelial electron-dense deposits along with a similar positive IF staining pattern as described above.

Glomerular diseases that are not immune-complex mediated

Amyloidosis

Amyloidosis is a group of disorders in which *amyloid—an eosinophilic, homogeneous, proteinaceous material*—is deposited in the walls of small blood vessels and extracellularly in a variety of sites, particularly in glomeruli. All amyloid fibrils have a β-pleated sheet structure. Deposition of amyloid causes pressure atrophy of adjacent cells, and, depending on the organs involved, can lead to CKD, nephrotic syndrome, thrombosis, hepatic failure, spontaneous hepatic hemorrhage and rupture, arthritis, or diabetes mellitus. Amyloidosis is seen in a number of presentations:

- **Reactive systemic amyloidosis** (secondary, or AA) is the most common form of amyloidosis in domestic animals (dogs, cattle, horses, cats; rare in swine and goats). **AA amyloid** is derived from *serum amyloid A* (SAA), an acute-phase apolipoprotein made predominantly by hepatocytes. SAA is produced in excess as a result of chronic antigenic stimulation, such as in persistent infectious, inflammatory, or neoplastic conditions. Of note, there are various *SAA* genes (some species have 4) that mainly differ in the N-terminal sequence, and this impacts the ability of each SAA protein to form an amyloid fibril. This genetic influence on "fibrillogenesis" can partially explain why certain species (or breeds) are more likely to develop amyloidosis when they have elevated SAA production.
- **Immunoglobulin-derived amyloidosis** (primary, or AL) is the most common form in humans, but it is uncommon in domestic animals (dog, horse, cat). **AL amyloid** is produced from *immunoglobulin light chains* in plasma cell dyscrasias as a product of monoclonal B-cell proliferation. Either λ or κ light chains may predominate in this dysproteinemia. Systemic κAL amyloidosis has been described in a Holstein cow with bovine leukocyte adhesion deficiency.
- **Familial** amyloidosis occurs in a number of species and breeds. Systemic AA amyloidosis occurs in Beagles, Chinese Shar-Peis (likely autosomal recessive), Bracco Italiano, gray Collies, English Foxhounds, Abyssinian cats (likely autosomal dominant with incomplete penetrance), and Siamese and Oriental cats.
- **Apolipoprotein A-I** (apoA-I)–derived amyloidosis affects the pulmonary vessels of old dogs.
- **Islet amyloid polypeptide**–derived amyloidosis is common in the pancreatic islets of cats with non–insulin-dependent diabetes mellitus.

Both AA and AL amyloidosis can occur in either systemic or localized forms. The *cause* of amyloid fibril formation and deposition is obscure, but the *nidus theory* postulates that amyloid fibrils serve as templates for further fibril growth and as scaffolding for fibril polymerization; this is similar to how prions induce transformation of their own precursor proteins. Macrophages appear to be important in the conversion of precursor proteins to amyloid fibrils. Other extracellular matrix components, including serum amyloid P component (a glycoprotein of the pentraxin family), glycosaminoglycans, and proteoglycans, are always associated with amyloid. The associated proteins comprise a variable but significant amount of the mass of the amyloid deposits. Serum amyloid P component is a plasma protein that can bind bacteria, fungi, and even viruses. It can either promote a stronger inflammatory response to the infectious agent (e.g., *Aspergillus fumigatus*) or it can protect the organism from phagocytosis (e.g., some types of *Escherichia coli* and *Candida albicans*). When serum amyloid P component binds to amyloid fibrils, it can impede their proteolysis, thereby stabilizing them. Notably, the variability of the types and amounts of associated proteins can impact the histologic appearance of amyloidosis, especially in glomeruli. Most cases of amyloidosis in domestic animals are of the reactive systemic type. Deposits of AA amyloid may be found in many organs, but *the kidney is the organ most commonly involved*. Localization of amyloid is usually *glomerular* in most breeds of dogs, but *medullary* localization predominates often in Shar-Pei dogs, cats, and occasionally cattle.

Amyloidosis is most common in older **dogs** and is usually idiopathic, although some cases occur in association with chronic neutrophilic and granulomatous lesions in other tissues. Canine glomerular amyloidosis has been associated with *Hepatozoon americanum* and *Ehrlichia canis* infections. Dogs with glomerular amyloidosis develop progressive renal insufficiency and proteinuria that may cause the *nephrotic syndrome*. Dogs with medullary amyloidosis without glomerular involvement may have little or no proteinuria. This clinical presentation is most often seen in Shar-Pei dogs because amyloid tends to be medullary as opposed to glomerular in this breed. The literature reports a poor prognosis for dogs diagnosed with amyloidosis, but this is not our experience; we are aware of dogs that have survived >1 year after the diagnosis of moderate-to-severe glomerular amyloidosis on renal biopsy.

The prevalence of amyloidosis in **cats** is much increased on diets that provide excess vitamin A (see Vol. 1, Bones and Joints). Shelter cats have an increased risk of multiorgan (including the kidney) amyloidosis, and cats with longer stays in shelters have more severe disease. Amyloid fibrils have been identified in excreted bile, which could serve as a fecal-oral route of amyloid fibrils to spread throughout a shelter, serving as a nidus for amyloid development in co-housed cats as discussed above. Liquid chromatography-mass spectrometry of urine from Italian shelter cats with amyloidosis identified a potential urinary biomarker, apolipoprotein C-III, which was elevated compared with values from shelter cats that did not have amyloidosis. One case report documented glomerular amyloidosis with concurrent ICGN with a membranous pattern in a cat, demonstrating that more than one glomerular disease can occur in the same patient.

In **cattle**, glomerular amyloidosis can cause severe proteinuria; medullary amyloidosis is reported as a common subclinical disease. Renal amyloidosis is an uncommon comorbidity in cattle with mastitis, pododermatitis, and traumatic reticuloperitonitis. AA amyloidosis occurs systemically in **horses** used for antiserum production; AL amyloidosis occurs in the skin and the upper respiratory system. **Sheep and goats** can develop glomerular and medullary amyloidosis in the course of chronic inflammatory processes.

Grossly, with small deposits of amyloid, the kidney may be only mildly increased in size. Characteristic renal changes include pallor, enlargement, and a waxy consistency. The capsule strips smoothly, and the cortical surface has a finely stippled appearance because of numerous fine yellow spots (glomeruli) and gray translucent points (dilated tubules). *Affected glomeruli stain brown-red when exposed to an iodine solution, and subsequent exposure to acetic acid changes the color to purple* (Fig. 4-34). In animals with predominantly medullary and papillary amyloidosis, the kidneys might be indistinguishable from those with nonspecific chronic interstitial nephritis. The papillary amyloidosis can lead to papillary necrosis and even detachment and sloughing of the necrotic papilla.

Histologically, amyloid is first deposited in the mesangial area and in the subendothelial zones of glomerular capillaries. Nodules of amyloid gradually develop until the glomeruli are enlarged and converted to homogeneous foci lacking endothelial and mesangial nuclei. In a study of glomerular lesions in proteinuric dogs, there was also often podocyte loss and secondary synechiae. Similarly, amyloid can be deposited in tubular basement membranes, and eventually broad cuffs of amyloid appear around the tubules. The physical presence of amyloid causes ischemia and atrophy of nephrons, and resultant scarring. If medullary amyloidosis is present (Fig. 4-35), there may also be some degree of tubulointerstitial scarring.

Amyloid is eosinophilic in H&E sections, pale-pink in PAS, a mix of pale-blue to orange on trichrome, and does not take up silver in the JMS stain (Fig. 4-36; eFig. 4-17). *The histologic diagnosis must be confirmed with the Congo red (CR) stain*, with which it stains peach or orange-red, and exhibits apple-green birefringence in polarized light. Importantly, to enhance the sensitivity of the CR stain, slides should be cut at 8-10 μm thickness. Elimination of the CR staining affinity by oxidation of tissue sections in potassium permanganate suggests that it is AA amyloid. Retention of congophilia after pretreatment with potassium permanganate indicates the presence of AL amyloid; the potassium permanganate reaction may be unreliable in cats. Amyloid exhibits bright-yellow fluorescence after staining with *thioflavin-T*, which may be required in cats because of variable staining of amyloid with CR in this species. The above staining patterns of amyloid result from its characteristic β-pleated pattern, which also promotes insolubility and a resistance to proteolysis. Specific IHC stains can be useful in identifying amyloid and in distinguishing amyloid types. Subtyping of amyloid requires mass spectrometry to isolate the amyloid, followed by amino acid sequencing. Characteristic nonbranching 7-10 nm fibrils of amyloid may be seen by electron microscopy (see Fig. 4-36D and E).

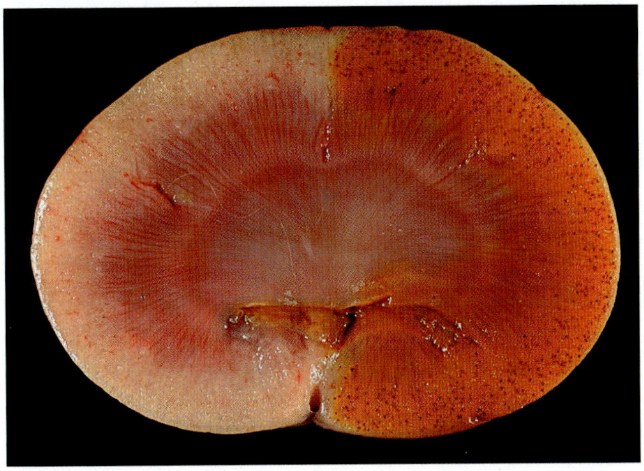

Figure 4-34 Renal amyloidosis in a cat. Right half of the kidney was treated with Lugol iodine to demonstrate the amyloidotic glomeruli, resulting in red discoloration of the cortex. (Courtesy M.K. Keating.)

In scenarios in which mass spectrometry and amino acid sequencing have been performed, the amino acid sequences of feline SAA and AA amyloid varied slightly between Abyssinian and Siamese cats. Genetic sequencing of *SAA* genes is also informative. Pigs have 4 *SAA* genes, all differing in the N-terminus sequence with differing fibrillogenesis capabilities. In this species, inflammatory states lead to synthesis of the SAA isoform that forms amyloid poorly. This explains why pigs rarely develop amyloid even with chronic inflammation. However, subtyping of the amyloid fibrils (via mass spectrometry and peptide sequencing) was performed in 2 pigs that did develop renal amyloidosis. These 2 studies demonstrated a specific amyloid peptide sequence that can form particularly rigid fibrils. In vitro, these rigid fibrils can change the amyloidogenic potential of other SAA fibrils, again providing evidence for the prion-like nature of amyloidosis in animals.

Of note, rare cases of nonamyloidotic fibrillary material have been observed in cats, dogs, and humans. Therefore, birefringence on the CR stain is required for a definitive diagnosis of amyloidosis. Ultrastructural analysis of nonamyloidotic fibrillary glomerulopathy reveals fibrils with a larger diameter than amyloid. In one such example in a cat, the material stained positively for IgM and IgG but negatively for C3. The significance of the IF staining pattern in that particular cat is unknown. In humans, fibrillary GN and immunotactoid GN result from *fibrillogenesis of portions of immunoglobulin molecules*. These immunoglobulins activate complement, and there is usually strong C3 staining on IF. Fibrils that have a larger diameter than amyloid are identified via TEM in human fibrillary GN. In immunotactoid GN, the fibrils have a microtubular structure with a central pore. We have observed definitive, well-characterized examples of both of these types of fibrils, but not yet reported in the peer-reviewed literature.

Glomerulosclerosis and focal segmental glomerulosclerosis

Glomerulosclerosis (**GS**) means "scarring of the glomerulus," and *global GS* is synonymous with glomerular obsolescence. *Focal*

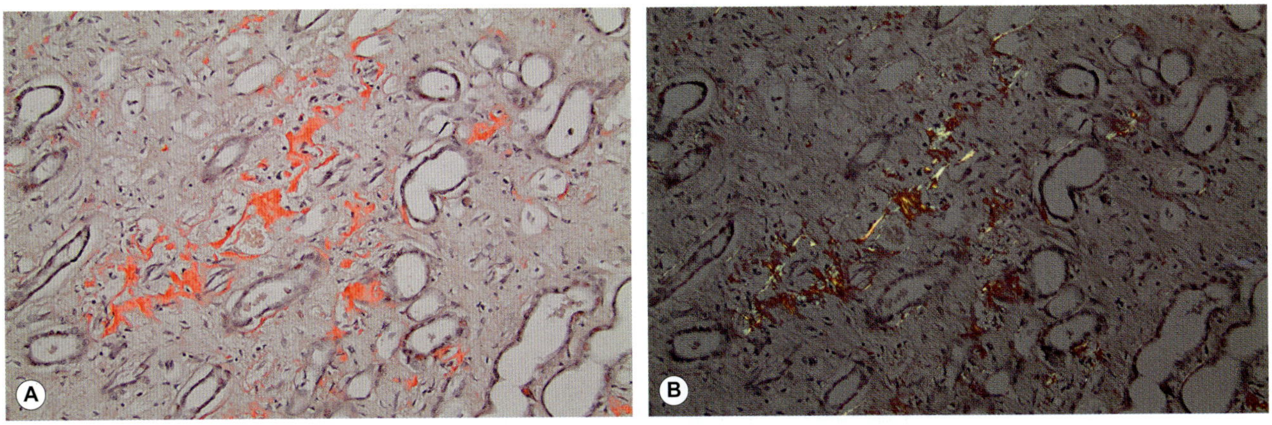

Figure 4-35 Medullary interstitial amyloidosis in a dog. **A.** Congo red staining of the medullary interstitium. **B.** Same field as **A**, polarized light reveals apple-green birefringence of a small portion of the orange material. Moving the polarizer will shift the apple-green birefringence to other regions of the interstitium.

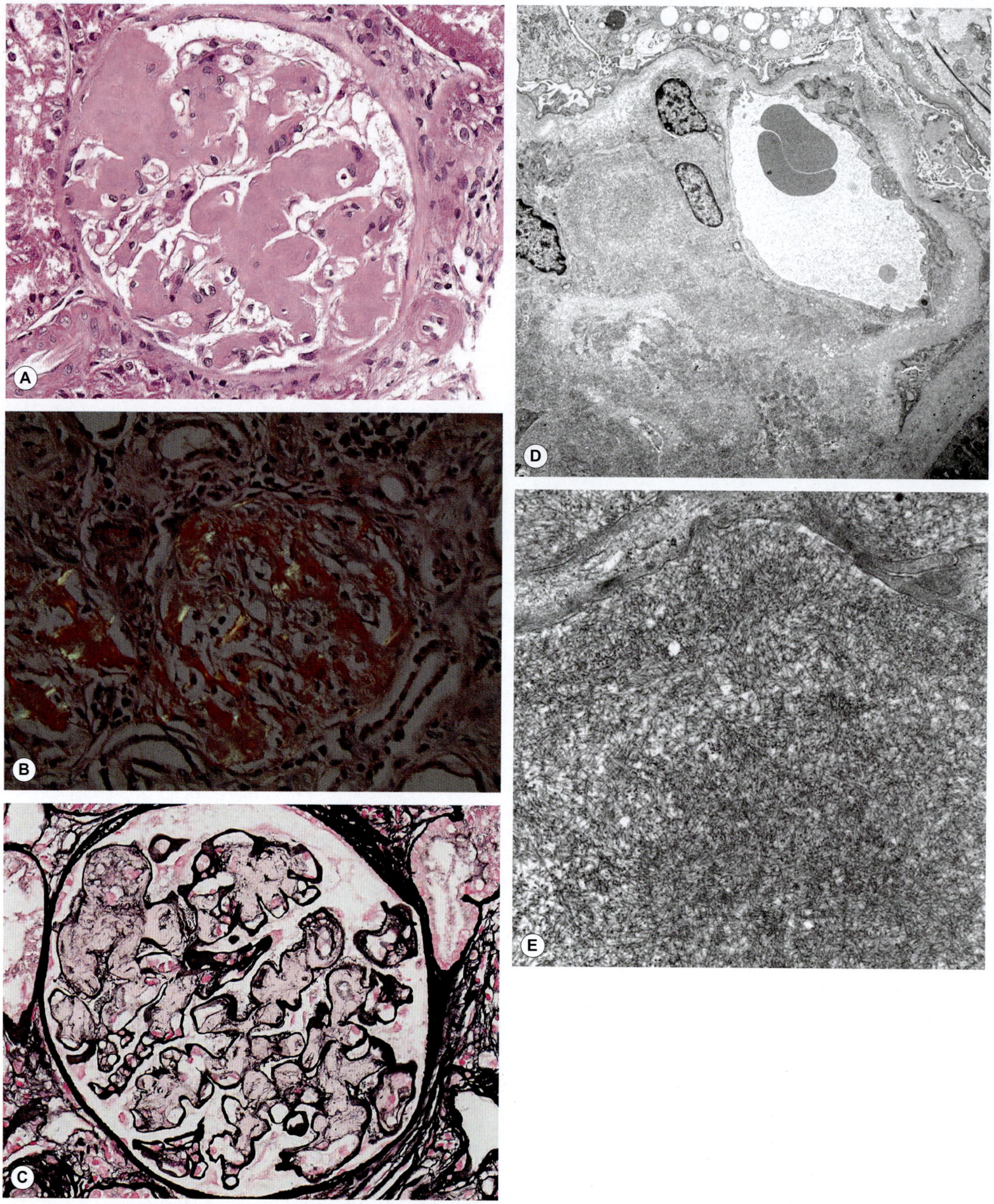

Figure 4-36 Glomerular amyloidosis in a dog. **A**. The material is pink and glassy-to-waxy. H&E. **B**. Polarized light, demonstrating apple-green birefringence. Congo red stain. **C**. Amyloid does not take up silver. Jones methenamine silver stain. **D**. Large accumulations of fibrillar material in the mesangium and smaller amounts in the glomerular basement membrane. Podocyte foot processes are globally effaced. Transmission electron micrograph (TEM). **E**. Higher magnification of **D** reveals haphazardly arranged nonbranching 7-10 nm fibrils. TEM. (D, E courtesy G. Lees, F. Clubb.)

*segmental glomerulosclerosis (**FSGS**) describes portions of glomerular capillary tufts effaced by extracellular matrix, and ICs are not identified*. Even though it is technically a histologic pattern, it has also become a diagnostic entity in human nephropathology. In humans, dogs, and cats, it is a common cause of moderate-to-severe proteinuria. There are widely variable causes of FSGS. Even though the causes might differ, a unifying step in the pathogenesis involves podocyte injury, detachment, and loss. Because podocytes cannot be replenished easily, the denuded GBM can be covered by cytoplasmic projections from neighboring podocytes. Alternatively, the GBM may adhere to the glomerular capsule (synechia). In the setting of minimal podocyte loss, the neighboring podocytes can handle the extra workload. However, if many podocytes are lost (either in a monophasic insult or repeated podocyte injury), the neighboring podocytes can no longer compensate, and they will detach too. After enough of the podocytes are lost, there is an increase in the amount of extracellular matrix produced in that segment of the glomerular tuft. The relationship between podocyte injury and increased synthesis of extracellular matrix is not entirely understood. Often, insudation of hyaline material (plasma) is also present in the glomeruli. On H&E, hyalinosis and sclerosis appear similar. Special stains show that hyalinosis is often a different hue of pink (with PAS) or blue (with Masson trichrome), compared with the adjacent GBM and mesangium. Sclerosis should have the same tinctorial properties as the GBM and mesangium.

Using a genetically modified rat model in which specific amounts of podocytes can be killed in a dose-dependent manner, loss of >40% of the podocytes (all at once) resulted in rapid progression of azotemia, proteinuria, and frequent segmental-to-global GS. Loss of 20-40% of podocytes caused mild proteinuria, FSGS, and synechiae, but not azotemia. When <20% of podocytes were killed, there was transient proteinuria, mild mesangial expansion, and normal serum creatinine. This indicates that there is a threshold of podocyte loss, which can be impacted by a wide variety of factors. Segmental sclerosis can be due to innate podocyte defects (e.g., a mutation in a podocyte or slit diaphragm protein) or secondary to direct podocyte injury (e.g., from a toxic insult, hypertension, obesity). Additionally, glomerular tuft enlargement in animals with a low nephron endowment (e.g., from renal maldevelopment or unilateral renal agenesis) can cause podocyte stretching and stress.

ICGN can damage glomeruli such that podocytes are also injured and lost. Therefore, chronic ICGN may have superimposed segmental sclerosis. This has led to the misconception in veterinary pathology that all cases with segmental GS have underlying IC disease. However, TEM and IF evaluations of canine renal biopsies have revealed that ICs are not present in a considerable proportion of patients with segmental GS (see Fig. 4-26; eFig. 4-11). These cases fall into the diagnostic category of FSGS. In fact, 20% of North American dogs that underwent a renal biopsy for the clinical indication of proteinuria had FSGS. Female dogs were over-represented in a case series of 76 dogs with FSGS. FSGS dogs were proteinuric and often mildly hypertensive but infrequently azotemic at the time of diagnosis.

In humans, the region of the kidney affected and the histomorphology of the sclerotic lesion within the glomerulus all have etiologic and prognostic implications; however, similar insights have been infrequently established in domestic species. For example, in aging laboratory Beagles, the glomeruli in proximity to arcuate vessels and medullary rays are predisposed to undergo segmental sclerosis, suggesting that these glomeruli (and podocytes) are exposed to injuries and stresses that do not affect other glomeruli.

There are 3 important points about segmental GS:

1. It should be rare-to-absent in normal kidneys and should not be considered as a step on the pathway to nephron senescence; when a nephron undergoes senescence, the entire glomerulus scars all at once.
2. Because the lesion is focal, an adequate number of glomeruli need to be sampled in a renal biopsy. In humans, a biopsy core with 10 glomeruli has a 65% chance of detecting FSGS, even when only one-tenth of the glomeruli are involved. The likelihood of detecting FSGS increases to 88% if the core contains 20 glomeruli. Although similar studies have not been done in veterinary species, it is assumed that a similar number of glomeruli should be evaluated to rule out FSGS in a biopsy core.
3. Segmental sclerosis can be secondary to any glomerular insult that damages podocytes, which means that it can be seen in the setting of underlying ICGN. If ICs are not identified with advanced modalities, then a diagnosis of FSGS should be considered. Notably, segmental sclerosis secondary to GN lesions should be mentioned in the morphologic diagnosis because it connotes irreversible glomerular scarring (e.g., membranous glomerulonephropathy with secondary segmental sclerosis).

In addition to its association with ICGN, some natural and experimental infections with *D. immitis* led to fraying and thickening of the GBM with associated segmental GS. ICs were not identified with TEM and IF studies. This suggests that some diseases can damage glomeruli through various pathways (both ICGN and non-ICGN). FSGS has been reported in a colony of Maltese Beagle dogs with *glucose-6-phosphatase deficiency* (glycogen storage disease Ia). Nephrotic syndrome secondary to FSGS has also been reported in a yearling Standardbred colt; TEM and IF studies did not reveal IC deposition.

The protein-losing nephropathy (PLN) in **Soft Coated Wheaten Terriers** is characterized by segmental sclerosis, and podocytes are often swollen with large cytoplasmic protein resorption droplets. Genome-wide association studies have revealed mutations in 2 podocyte genes, *NPHS1* and *KIRREL2*. Some of these dogs also have features of renal dysplasia. Food hypersensitivity was reported in a subset of dogs, suggesting abnormalities of the immune system in this breed. In the general pet population, PLN and FSGS in Soft Coated Wheaten Terriers often occur in the absence of IC deposits, as demonstrated by TEM and IF.

One specific subset of sclerosing glomerulopathies is **diabetic nodular GS of humans**. In this entity, sclerosis is limited to the mesangium, and it has a very characteristic histologic appearance, known as *Kimmelstiel-Wilson (KW) nodules*. This phenotype has only been demonstrated experimentally in diabetic rodents. Mesangial sclerosis without KW nodule formation was documented in uninephrectomized dogs that were made diabetic at 9-months-old. These dogs also had significant generalized thickening of the GBM compared with control dogs, which is another characteristic lesion of diabetic nephropathy in humans, noted on TEM. Glomerular lesions in spontaneously diabetic dogs are usually limited to mild mesangial expansion, occasionally associated with lipid in the mesangial matrix or cell cytoplasm. Histologic evaluation of diabetic cats with age-, sex-, breed- and body weight–matched controls revealed no difference in glomerular morphology between the 2 groups. However, cats that lived with diabetes for >1 year had more glomerular and vascular lesions than diabetic cats that died within 1 year of diagnosis. This suggests that diabetic kidney disease is a slowly progressive process.

Collagenofibrotic glomerulonephropathy can have a histologic appearance similar to GS, but the *primary lesion is deposition of collagen type III* in glomeruli; only *collagen type IV* should be present in normal adult glomeruli. This disease has been reported in humans, dogs, pigs, a monkey, and a cat (Fig. 4-37; eFig. 4-18). Proteinuria and **azotemia** result from sclerosis and obliteration of capillary lumina. Deposition of **fibronectin** in the mesangium has also been reported in a dog. GS resulting from fibrillar collagen deposition that was not subtyped was reported in Newfoundland dog littermates. *Collagenofibrotic glomerulonephropathy* and *fibronectin glomerulonephropathy*, both of which are well characterized although poorly understood glomerular disease in humans, are differential diagnoses for young animals with marked mesangial expansion and variable degrees of mesangial hypercellularity. The PAS stain (and sometimes the trichrome stain) is useful for the diagnosis of these rare diseases because there is a tinctorial change between the matrix and the capillary walls (see eFig 4-18B). In the more common condition of FSGS, the staining intensity of the 2 compartments is similar.

Minimal change disease (podocytopathy)

Histologic glomerular changes are slight, but clinical signs are marked, in **minimal change disease (MCD)**. It is also called **podocytopathy**. In this disease, reversible global effacement of podocyte foot processes is accompanied by significant proteinuria (Fig. 4-38; eFig. 4-19). MCD has been produced experimentally in dogs by infection with *Ehrlichia canis*. Global foot process effacement with severe proteinuria has also been documented secondary to treatment with tyrosine kinase inhibitors in a cat and 2 dogs. One dog with severe MCD later developed AKI, which is a well-known clinical scenario in humans. In MCD with AKI, azotemia follows an abrupt onset of severe proteinuria. MCD is a diagnosis that *requires* TEM and IF to verify that ICs are not present. Notably, early MGN can be histologically identical to MCD and the 2 diseases are often only differentiated by TEM and/or IF. Because treatment for the 2 diseases is different, it is important that the pathologist recommend these advanced diagnostic tests when evaluating biopsy material.

MCD (podocytopathy) and FSGS are 2 opposite ends of a spectrum of podocyte injury. MCD is due to reversible podocyte injury; however, if the insult is persistent, podocytes can become irreversibly damaged and FSGS ensues. Therefore, when MCD is diagnosed in a renal biopsy, a careful review of the history to identify any potential podocyte toxins is necessary to prevent continued podocyte injury.

Abnormalities of the glomerular basement membrane

There are several canine breed-related glomerulopathies that strongly resemble a hereditary glomerular disease in humans known as *Alport syndrome*. The basis of the disease is an abnormal, multilaminated GBM (seen on TEM) that results from various genetic mutations in type IV collagen α-subunits. Clinically, young dogs (<1-year-old) have proteinuria, hematuria, progressive azotemia, and JOCKD. Histology of late-stage disease shows mesangial hypercellularity, dilated glomerular capsules, numerous segmentally to globally sclerotic glomeruli,

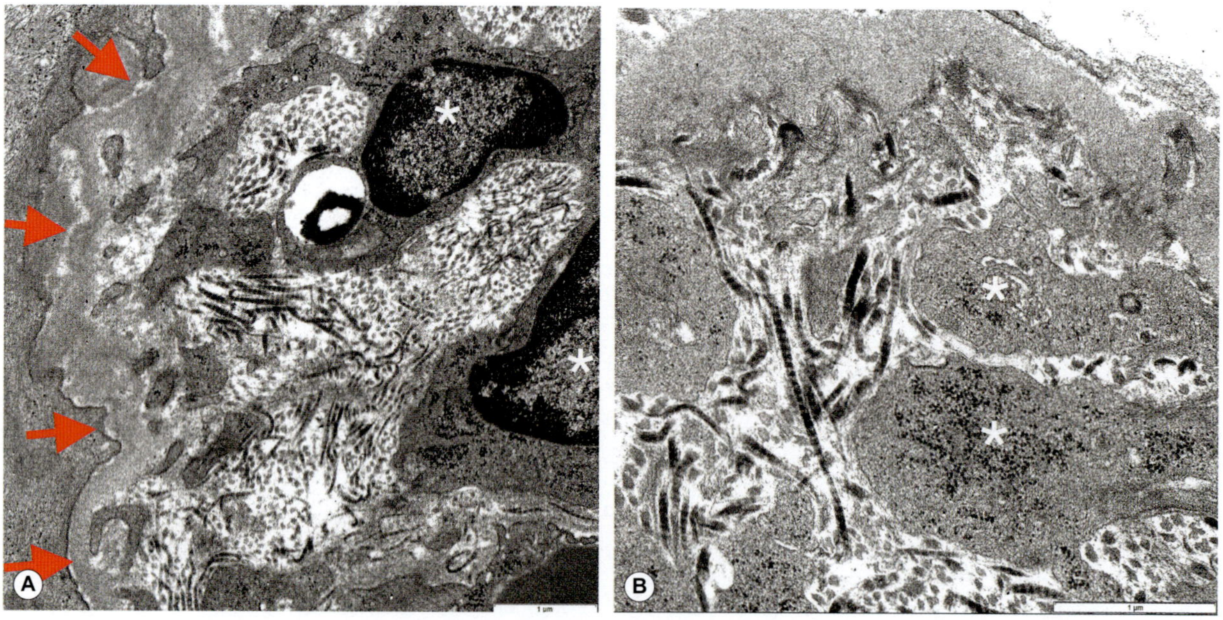

Figure 4-37 **Collagenofibrotic glomerulonephropathy** resulting from the deposition of fibrillar collagen in the glomerular basement membrane (GBM) in an azotemic, mildly proteinuric young cat. **A.** Haphazardly arranged collagen fibers within the GBM (delineated by the red arrows). Transmission electron micrograph (TEM). **B.** Note the periodicity of the fibers and the intermingled mesangial cell processes (asterisks). The fibrillar collagen is usually type III collagen, which may be caused by overproduction or failure of the fetal glomerular type III collagen to switch to the adult glomerular type IV collagen during maturation. TEM.

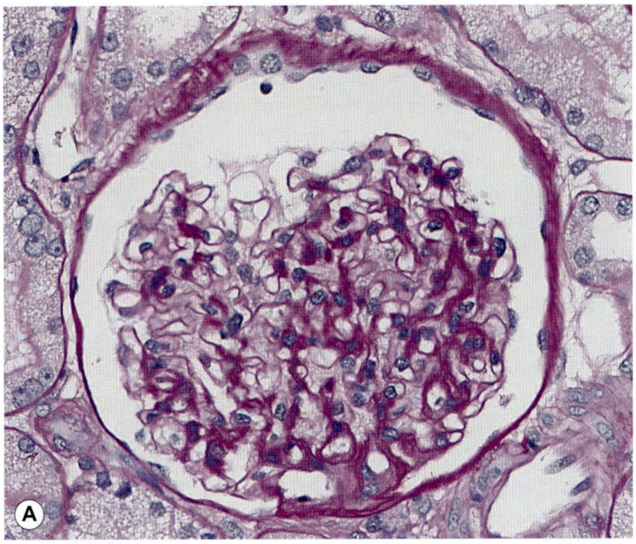
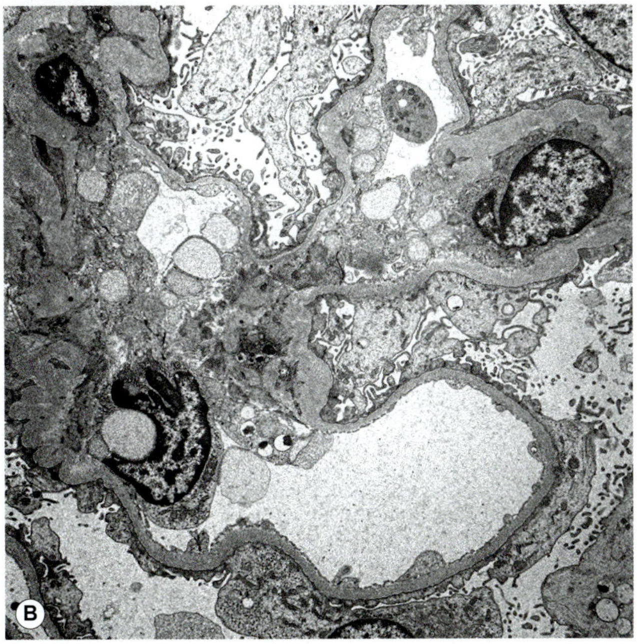

Figure 4-38 Minimal change disease in a severely proteinuric adult dog. **A**. Glomeruli are normocellular and the glomerular basement membrane (GBM) is within normal limits. PAS stain. (Courtesy G. Lees.) **B**. Global effacement of podocyte foot processes. Neither immune complexes nor GBM abnormalities are present. Transmission electron micrograph. (Courtesy G. Lees, F. Clubb.)

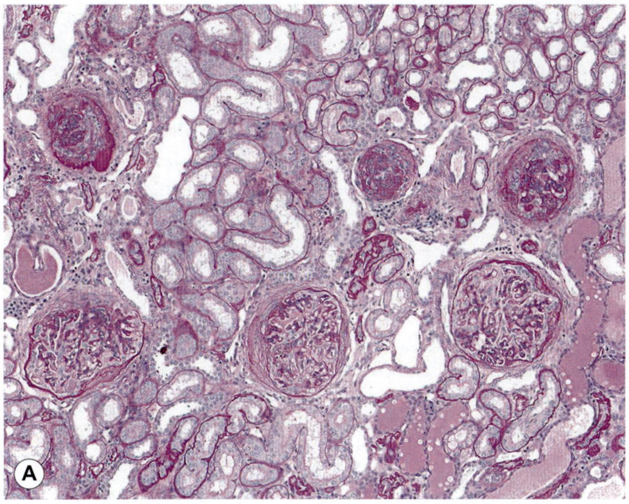
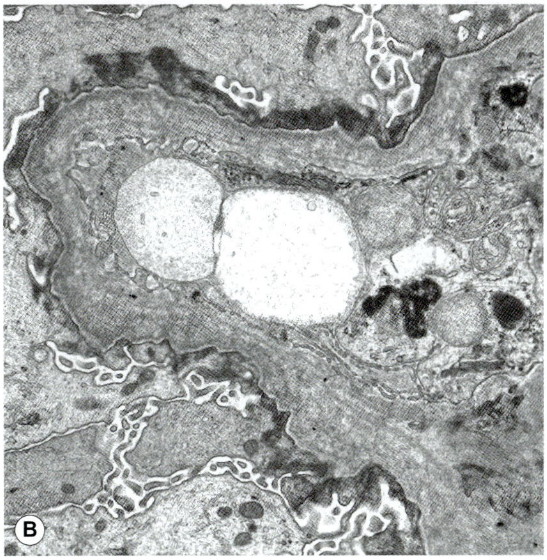

Figure 4-39 Canine Alport syndrome (hereditary nephritis) resulting from mutated type IV collagen in a severely azotemic and proteinuric 10-month-old dog. **A**. Glomerulosclerosis, mesangial hypercellularity, and glomerular basement membrane (GBM) thickening with accumulation of collagen and plasma in urinary spaces. Tubules are at various stages of degeneration and atrophy. PAS stain. **B**. Severe lamination of the GBM in a glomerular capillary loop. Electron-dense deposits are not present. Transmission electron micrograph.

and moderate-to-marked interstitial inflammation with fibrosis and tubular atrophy (Fig. 4-39A; eFig. 4-20). Depending on the stage of the disease, there is extensive multilamination of the GBM and podocyte foot process effacement on TEM (see Fig. 4-39B).

Type IV collagen is the main structural subunit of the GBM in adult dogs and humans. It is a heterotrimer, composed of 3 intertwined chains (α3-5) encoded by the genes *COL4A3-5*, respectively. *COL4A5* is located on the X chromosome in humans and dogs, and mutations in *COL4A5* can result in X-linked Alport syndrome in both species. Because of the extrarenal expression of *COL4A5*, human patients also have hearing deficits and ocular abnormalities. There are 2 canine models of X-linked Alport syndrome: **Samoyed hereditary glomerulopathy** (the result of a mutation in exon 35 of the *COL4A5* gene) and a colony of **mixed-breed dogs** (the result of a 10-base pair deletion in exon 9 that causes a frameshift and a premature stop codon in exon 10 in the *COL4A5* gene). Mutations in both canine models result in decreased collagen expression in the GBM. IF tests to detect the α-chains of type IV collagen have been used to verify decreased (or lack of) protein expression. Unfortunately, these IF antibodies are no longer available for routine diagnostic testing.

In both models of X-linked Alport syndrome, male dogs are more severely affected than female dogs and have an earlier onset of clinical signs. Dogs do not have hearing loss or ocular disease; therefore, the canine signs do not entirely mimic those of humans. The clinical progression of Samoyed hereditary nephropathy is as follows: affected males develop proteinuria and poor body condition at 2-3-months-old, azotemia after 5 months, uremia after 7 months, and death by 15-months-old.

In Samoyeds, there is a 90% reduction in the amount of α5 chain in GBMs, leading to inadequate cross-linking of collagen type IV. The mixed-breed dogs with this disease have also been well characterized. Labeling of α3-6 collagen chains was absent from GBMs in the affected mixed-breed dogs. As an aside, some normal adult dogs have expression of an α6 chain of type IV collagen in their GBM in addition to the α3-5 chains. Because IF staining of the GBM can no longer be used for the diagnosis of this disease, sequencing of the relevant genes is now the recommended diagnostic test.

Both *COL4A3* and *COL4A4* reside on canine chromosome 25 and human chromosome 2, therefore mutations in these genes will result in an autosomal recessive disease. The canine model for autosomal recessive Alport syndrome is **English Cocker Spaniel hereditary nephritis**, which is the result of a single nucleotide substitution that causes a premature stop codon in exon 3. In affected dogs, α1-α2(IV) are increased, α3(IV) and α4(IV) chains are absent, α5(IV) chains are markedly decreased, whereas α6(IV) chains are present.

Last, there is also an autosomal dominant form of Alport syndrome in humans, and **Bull Terriers** have been proposed as animal models for this subtype. Although mutations in *COL4A3* and *COL4A4* genes have been documented in humans, the specific mutations have not been identified in Bull Terriers. A group of related Dalmatian puppies in Australia were suspected to have autosomal dominant Alport syndrome, but the ultrastructural lesion has never been observed in additional relatives or in Dalmatians from other countries. Neither IF labeling to prove the absence of type IV collagen nor genetic testing was performed in that original cohort, so the cause of the abnormal GBM remains uncertain.

Other examples in which there is ultrastructural evidence of marked GBM lamination on TEM have been identified. These diseases and lesions are not yet well characterized, and more research into their pathogeneses is needed. There is a familial tendency in **Doberman Pinschers** to develop proteinuria and CKD; the precise mode of inheritance is unknown. Grossly, the kidneys are light brown, slightly small, and have diffuse, fine, subcapsular pits that appear as radial streaks on cut surface. Females may have concomitant unilateral renal agenesis. The histologic renal lesion is mesangial hypercellularity with irregularly thickened GBM and various degrees of tubulointerstitial disease. Ultrastructurally, GBMs display 2 distinct lesions: the lamina densa may be lamellated and contain intramembranous electron-dense material, or there may be diffuse attenuation of the lamina densa with thickening of the GBM by collagen fibers. Notably, the electron-dense material only stained positively for IgM in 1 of 9 dogs examined, and therefore this is not an example of familial ICGN. There is also a familial glomerulopathy of **Rottweilers** with multilaminated GBM; however, the disease phenotype and the pathogenesis are uncharacterized.

Familial glomerulopathies in other dog breeds

Familial renal diseases of uncertain inheritance occur in other breeds (see Table 4-1). Glomerular lesions (fetal and immature glomeruli, glomerulocystic atrophy) are prominent, but there are also significant tubulointerstitial lesions, making it difficult to definitively determine which compartment was primarily affected.

Familial renal disease in **Norwegian Elkhound** dogs is seen as rapidly progressive renal failure in juvenile dogs; the mode of inheritance is unknown. Glomerular changes begin as *periglomerular fibrosis* with hypertrophy and hyperplasia of parietal epithelium and progress to diffuse fibrosis of cortex and medulla and progressive loss of glomeruli. In contrast to the hereditary glomerulopathies discussed previously, the lesion in Norwegian Elkhounds may represent a primary tubular lesion with secondary prominent glomerular changes because microdissection of nephrons in early cases reveals saccular dilations of the distal segments. Genetic analysis has ruled out the possibility of an Alport-like syndrome.

Lipid-mediated glomerular lesions

Large *foam cells*, which contain sudanophilic (lipid) droplets, may be found in one or more lobules of glomerular tufts in adult dogs. This condition is rarely seen in other domesticated species. The cells are closely packed and finely vacuolated, and the cell boundaries are distinct (Fig. 4-40; eFig. 4-21). The source of these cells is unknown, but mesangial and endothelial cells have been proposed. Although **glomerular lipidosis** is thought to be an incidental finding, involvement of many glomeruli, and aneurysmal dilation of capillary loops with associated mesangiolysis suggests a more serious disease process. The original literature reported that most dogs with this lesion did not have renal dysfunction, based solely on lack

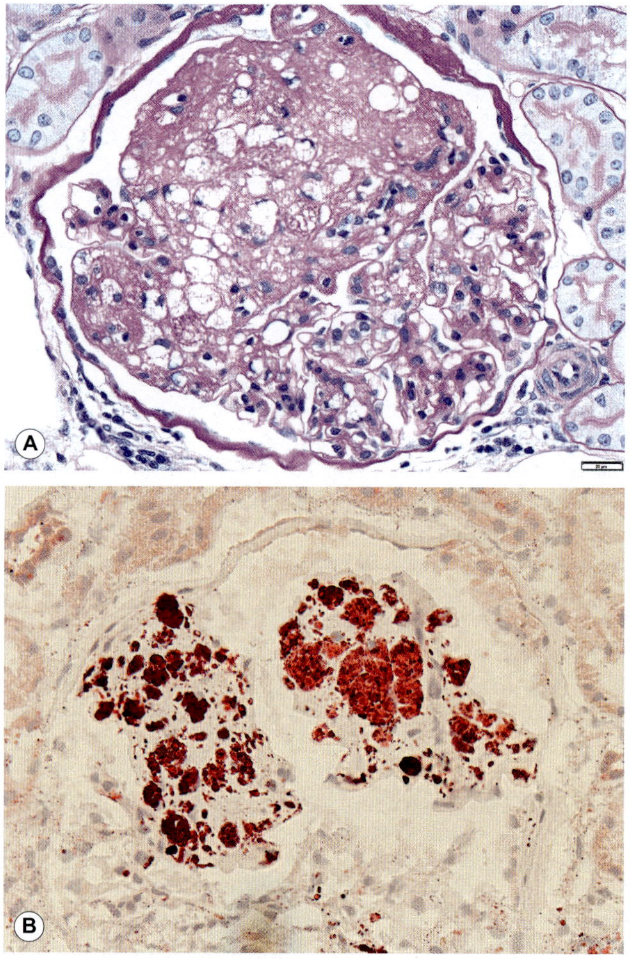

Figure 4-40 **Glomerular lipidosis** in a 1-year-old dog with marked proteinuria. **A.** PAS stain. **B.** Stain on unprocessed renal tissue reveals numerous lipid droplets expanding capillary lumens. Oil red O stain.

of azotemia; UPC and urinalysis results were not provided. Glomerular lipidosis in many glomeruli has been identified as the sole lesion in proteinuric dogs. Glomerular lipidosis has also been diagnosed in dogs with other (possibly unrelated) glomerular diseases (e.g., FSGS, ICGN). Furthermore, experimental models of vascular injury in dogs via intravenous injection of biologic toxins (i.e., snake venom and diphtheria toxin) resulted in glomerular lipidosis. Ultimately, glomerular lipidosis should be recognized as a degenerative lesion because the foam cells impair the filtration capacity of the glomerulus. Its clinical relevance depends partly on the proportion of the glomeruli affected and the severity of the lesions within each tuft. As with many *focal* glomerular lesions, describing and/or diagnosing glomerular lipidosis in a renal biopsy sample is necessary; however, a few glomeruli with lipidosis in a cross section from an autopsy sample might not be clinically significant.

Lipid embolization of renal arterioles and glomerular capillaries occurs occasionally in dogs with diabetes mellitus, dyslipidemia, or following trauma. The lipid emboli are intravascular rather than within foam cells (Fig. 4-41; eFig. 4-22). Miniature Schnauzers are predisposed to the development of this lesion, likely associated with the dyslipidemia commonly seen in that breed. Cholesterol clefts may also be observed in glomerular capillaries and interstitial vessels.

A syndrome of **idiopathic cutaneous and renal glomerular vasculopathy** has been documented in Greyhounds. Most dogs are diagnosed based on characteristic ulcers of the distal extremities, thrombocytopenia, and AKI. Histologically, there is frequent necrosis of glomerular afferent arterioles with coagulation and necrosis of the tufts. Pulmonary and cutaneous vessels are sometimes similarly affected. Acutely, the ultrastructural lesions consist of endothelial cell injury and necrosis with aggregated platelets and fibrin. Over time, there is thickening of the glomerular capillary walls and associated narrowing of the lumens by cellular interpositioning and electron-densities that, based on lack of IF staining, are not consistent with ICs. The clinical presentation and the glomerular ultrastructure are *suggestive of primary endothelial cell injury* [so-called thrombotic microangiopathy (TMA)], which is not mediated by ICs. TMA is well described in humans, but is only rarely documented in other species (Fig. 4-42; eFig. 4-23). Dogs of various breeds in the United Kingdom have been diagnosed with various manifestations of the cutaneous lesions and renal TMA. The cases are rare (~300 over the course of 10 years). Most cases occur in summer months, suggesting environmental exposure or infectious agent, although none has been identified.

Experimentally induced **pregnancy toxemia in sheep** led to significant proteinuria and azotemia. Glomerular abnormalities were characterized ultrastructurally by double contours of the GBM, occlusion of the capillary lumens by swollen endothelium, widespread fusion of podocyte foot processes, and absence of IC deposits. Affected sheep had significantly higher plasma levels of renin without a change in substrate concentration. Although comparisons to the glomerular TMA that can occur in human pre-eclampsia are understandable, the pathogenesis may be different. Specifically, the role of placental production of soluble vascular endothelial growth factor (VEGF) receptors in the pathogenesis of pre-eclampsia has been clearly demonstrated in humans, but similar research in sheep is lacking. Furthermore, hypertension is a key feature in human pre-eclampsia but was not reported in the sheep.

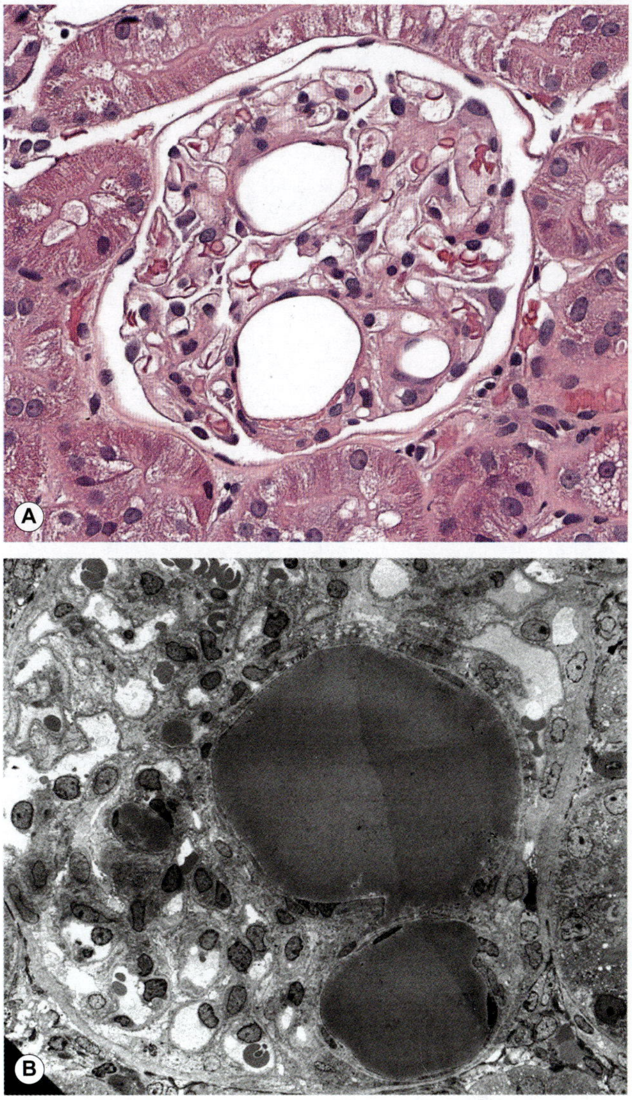

Figure 4-41 Glomerular lipid emboli in a severely proteinuric adult dog. **A**. PAS stain. **B**. Large osmiophilic lipid droplets distort glomerular capillary loops. Transmission electron micrograph. (Courtesy G. Lees, F. Clubb.)

Mesangial hyaline droplets, of unknown pathogenesis and significance, were reported in 3 pigs; 2 of the pigs had concurrent mastocytosis and the third had mesangial cell proliferation. Droplets were assumed to be plasma constituents because IF demonstrated that they contained albumin, IgG, and fibrinogen, similar to protein droplets present in proximal tubules.

DISEASES OF TUBULES

Tubular diseases are primarily reflected in morphologic changes in the epithelial cells; specific functional abnormalities that result from enzyme deletions may not be visible histologically. Patients are often azotemic or have abnormal urinary profiles. For example, glucosuria and amino aciduria in the setting of normal plasma levels can indicate proximal tubular defects, even when the serum creatinine and the histology are normal. Novel urinary biomarkers that have shown promise in identification of dogs with ATI before the development of azotemia include retinol binding protein, neutrophil

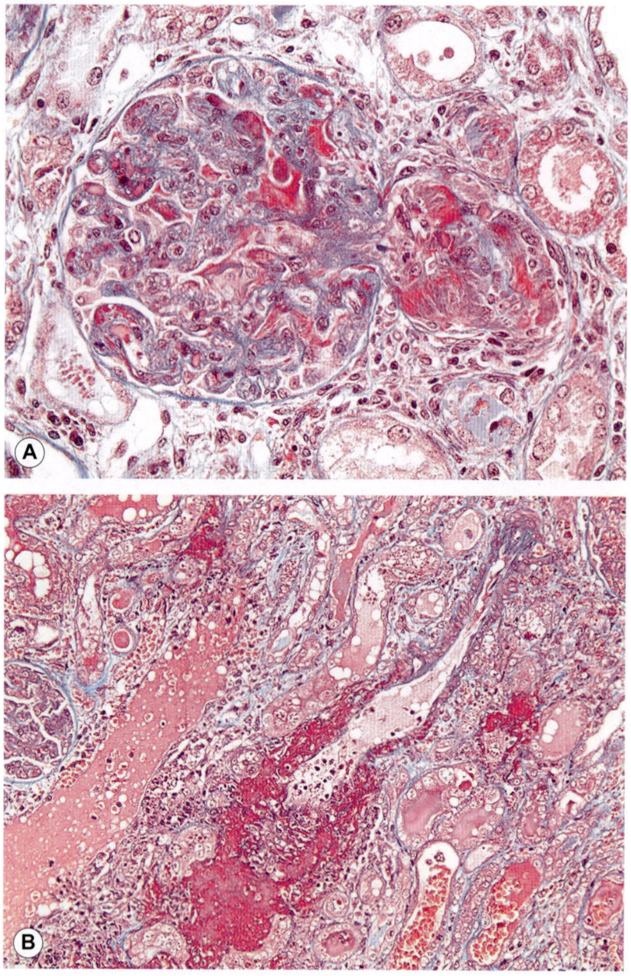

Figure 4-42 Thrombotic microangiopathy in a dog with acute renal failure and mild proteinuria. **A**. Fibrinoid necrosis of the afferent arteriole. **B**. Fibrinoid necrosis of an intralobular artery. Masson trichrome stain.

gelatinase-associated lipocalin, N-acetyl-β-D-glucosaminidase, β2-microglobulin, cystatin C, cystatin B, and kidney injury molecule 1. *The tubules and interstitium are intimately associated, and damage to one affects the other.* Diseases that involve both compartments are discussed later under the **Tubulointerstitial Diseases** section. Regeneration of tubular epithelium can occur, but postnatal development of entire nephrons is limited, depending on species. The response of the kidney to destruction of tubules is limited to *compensatory hypertrophy of remaining nephrons*. Thus, the tubules remaining in damaged kidneys are often large and dilated.

Degeneration and swelling of tubular cells cause the kidney to enlarge and bulge on cut surface. *Acute cellular swelling* results from damage to mitochondria and is visualized by the formation of clear spaces in the cytoplasm with some discrete vacuoles (Fig. 4-43A). It is potentially reversible. *Necrotic tubular cells* are eosinophilic, have pyknotic nuclei, and slough into the lumen, where they form cellular or coarsely granular casts (see Fig. 4-43B). In addition to tubular epithelial cell necrosis, the cells might undergo anoikis, which is detachment of viable epithelial cells into tubular lumens. When those viable cells exit via the urine, they can be recovered and grown in in vitro cultures.

Tubules filled with *proteinaceous fluid* usually indicate that there is increased glomerular permeability in that nephron. *Tamm-Horsfall mucoprotein*, which is produced in the distal segment of the nephron, is bright magenta with the PAS stain and pale-blue to pale-peach with the Masson trichrome stain. *Hyaline droplets*, which are pink homogeneous globules of protein, appear in the cytoplasm of proximal tubular cells in nephrons with increased glomerular permeability. The hyaline droplets are lysosomes swollen by resorbed protein that is undergoing proteolysis and will be returned to the circulation as amino acids. Proteinaceous hyaline droplets are normal in proximal tubular epithelial cells of neonatal piglets. Protein resorption by proximal tubules is a physiologic process; hyaline droplets indicate that this mechanism is saturated. *Tubular lipidosis* is seen in swine, dogs, and cats, which normally have considerable quantities of fat in the renal epithelium. The lipid is usually found in the cells of the convoluted tubules.

Thickening of the tubular basement membrane is seen in a variety of situations involving chronic damage and is usually associated with atrophic tubular epithelium. In renal *amyloidosis*, amyloid can be deposited on the tubular basement membrane, as well as in glomeruli. Disruption of the tubular basement membrane indicates severe or prolonged tubular injury and may allow herniation of tubular epithelial cells, with some of these cells persisting as interstitial foam cells.

Acute tubular injury

The terminology used to describe and diagnose tubular injury has evolved in response to our ever-increasing understanding of lesion pathogenesis. "**Nephrosis**" was the oldest term to describe an acute injury to the tubular portion of the nephron—it should no longer be used. Next, the term **acute tubular necrosis (ATN)** was put forth as being more accurate. Unfortunately, this term implies that the functional disturbances in the kidney are the result of tubular epithelial cell death. This term can lead inexperienced pathologists astray by suggesting that overt necrosis is needed to make the diagnosis, when in fact the lesion may be limited to swollen, degenerate epithelial cells. The dead cells might have already undergone detachment. Furthermore, severe functional deficits may result from cell degeneration, followed by sloughing of the apical portion of the cell into the lumen, and maintaining the basal portion attached to the tubular basement membrane (so-called "simplification"). Examination of renal tissue over the time course of AKI has revealed that these attenuated cells are present early in the disease before any reparative phase. Therefore, **acute tubular injury (ATI)** is now the preferred term because it connotes a *functional disturbance* that can result in *significant azotemia* without implying the presence of coagulative or liquefactive necrosis. Even so, "ATN" is still often used by nephrologists and nephropathologists because it has been such a prominent part of our parlance.

ATI is a reversible condition mediated by tubular degeneration and is an important cause of acute kidney injury (**AKI**). Affected animals might be *oliguric or anuric* and die within a few days unless given appropriate therapy. *The principal causes of ATI are ischemia and nephrotoxins*. The renal tubules, in particular the proximal straight tubule and the medullary thick ascending limb, are highly active metabolically and are the segments most susceptible to ischemia or nephrotoxins.

Ischemic or **tubulorrhectic ATI** follows a period of hypotension and/or marked renal ischemia. Tubulorrhexis means rupture of the tubule. *Prolonged renal ischemia causes renal*

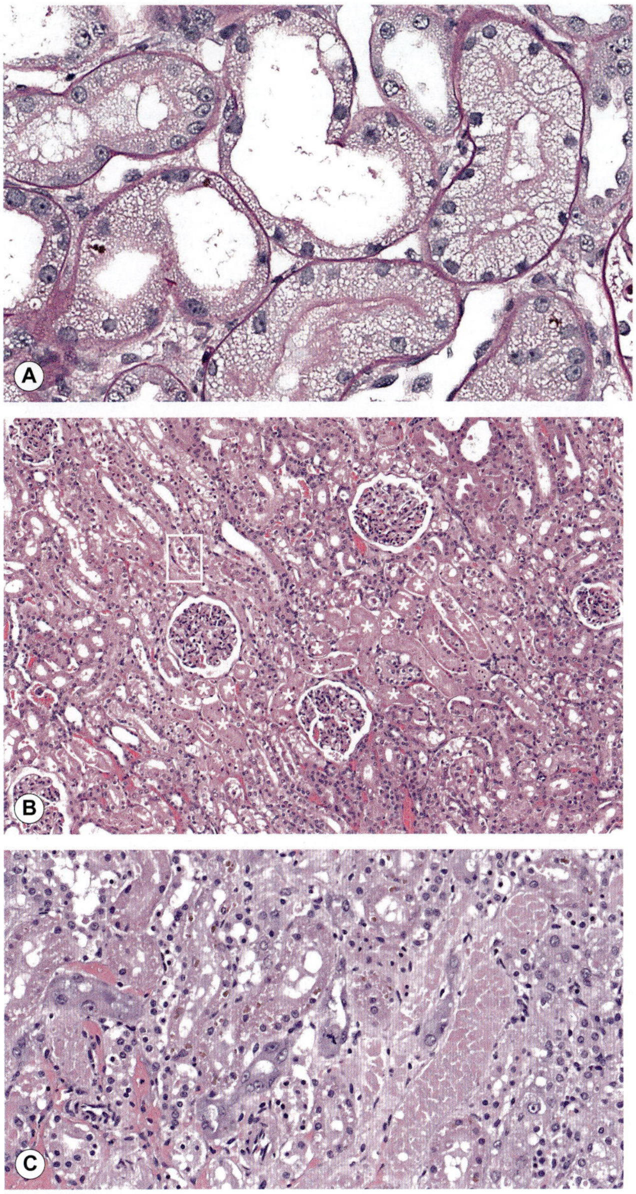

Figure 4-43 Various lesions of **acute tubular epithelial injury**. **A**. Tubulointerstitium from a dog with loss of the apical border (tubular simplification), attenuated epithelial cells, and marked isometric vesiculation. PAS stain. **B**. Segmental tubular necrosis affecting all of the tubules marked with asterisks. There are sloughed epithelial cells (boxed) as well. Interstitial inflammation is not a feature. H&E. **C**. Later stage of tubular necrosis with cells stretching to cover previously denuded tubular basement membranes, cytoplasmic basophilia, and scattered mitotic figures. Adjacent tubules have more recent necrosis and are filled with sloughed eosinophilic cellular debris. H&E.

cortical necrosis, that is, all cortical structures are affected. Ischemic ATI ranges in severity depending on length of the hypotensive episode. *Mild ischemic ATI* is characterized histologically by proximal tubular epithelial cell degeneration, and dilated, empty tubular lumens resulting from loss of the apical brush border. This apical portion is often rich in cytochrome pigments, and these cell portions can be identified as muddy brown casts in the urine if a specimen is collected

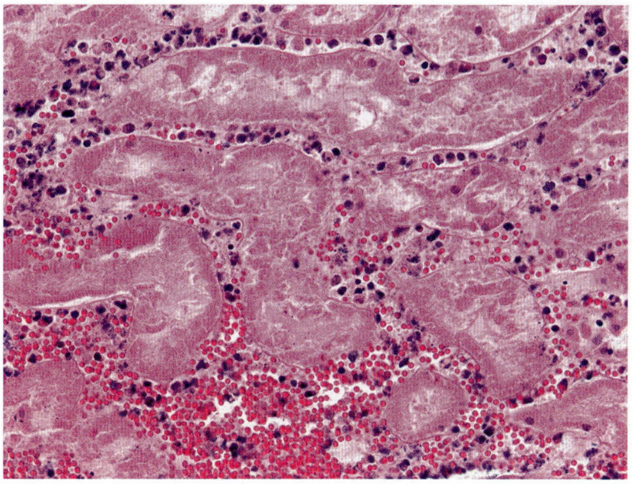

Figure 4-44 Ischemic tubular necrosis in a sheep with a **renal infarct**. Tubular outlines are preserved, and the interstitial acute inflammation provides evidence of reperfusion.

soon after the insult. *More severe cases of ischemia* can affect distal tubules to some extent and also cause generalized tubulorrhexis. Eosinophilic hyaline and granular casts commonly occur in the distal tubules and collecting ducts. They consist of Tamm-Horsfall mucoproteins, dead epithelial cells, and other plasma proteins. Interstitial edema and accumulation of leukocytes in dilated vasa recta are common findings, especially acutely (Fig. 4-44). Glomeruli vary from normal to slightly wrinkled due to poor perfusion. After about 1 week, *epithelial regeneration* may be seen as tubules lined by flattened, basophilic, karyomegalic epithelium, with mitotic figures (see Fig. 4-43C). If the initial injury is mild and/or supportive therapy is adequate, *recovery* of architecture may be complete within about 2-3 weeks.

Nephrotoxic ATI differs in pathogenesis but often can overlap with ischemic ATI morphologically. Renal tubules, especially proximal tubules, are particularly susceptible to a wide variety of toxic agents as a consequence of their high metabolic activity and their exposure to agents in the ultrafiltrate that they contact during urine formation. Cellular enzyme systems are inactivated by toxic agents such as heavy metals, which bind to sulfhydryl groups. *Preservation of tubular basement membranes provides the framework for epithelial regeneration and is an important prognostic feature to evaluate in renal biopsies*. Ischemia, however, often complicates toxic ATI because edema compresses peritubular capillaries and decreases blood flow. Another example of the interaction between ischemic and nephrotoxic ATI is seen with hemolytic anemia. Massive hemolysis causes ATI and produces a pattern known as *hemoglobinuria-associated ATI* (previously called hemoglobinuric or pigmentary nephrosis) (Fig. 4-45). The role of hemoglobin (and myoglobin) as a nephrotoxic agent is acknowledged, but the pathogenesis is unclear. Even so, the kidney is simultaneously exposed to nephrotoxic hemoglobin in a setting of anemia-induced renal ischemia. *It can be difficult to discern the etiology of ATI in diagnostic cases. Given the interaction of ischemic and nephrotoxic ATI, there are no pathognomonic lesions for either pathogenesis*.

The *pathogenesis* of AKI and oliguria in either ischemic or toxic ATI is multifactorial. Obstruction of tubular flow by cellular debris and casts and by interstitial edema appears to be

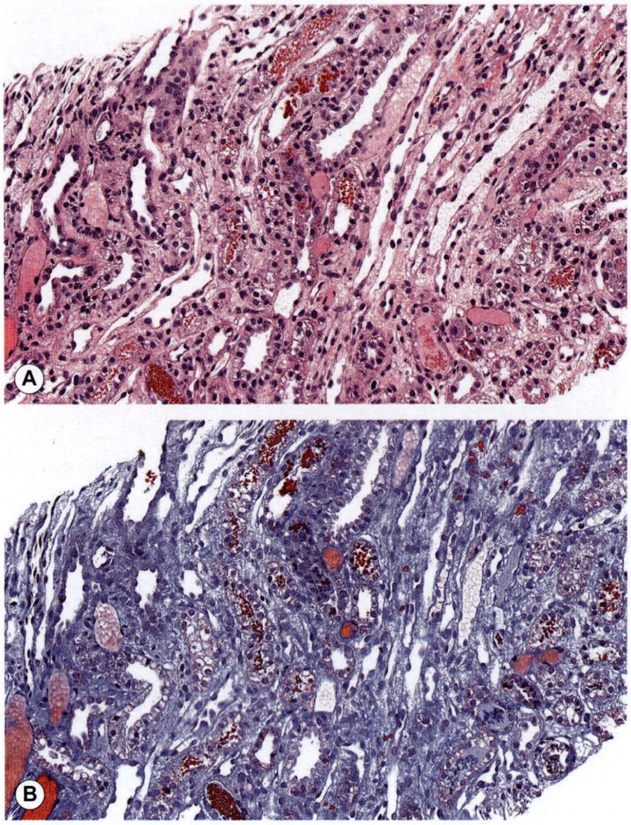

Figure 4-45 Myoglobin-induced acute tubular injury in an adult dog secondary to marked myonecrosis. **A.** H&E. **B.** Masson trichrome stain. Within the medulla, there are numerous intratubular granular-to-globular casts that are bright red-brown on both stains. There is associated vacuolar tubular degeneration. Of note, hemoglobin casts have a histologically identical appearance.

an important factor. Disruption of the actin cytoskeleton of proximal tubular cells and sloughing of apical brush border can impede tubular flow. One molecule—apoptosis inhibitor of macrophages (AIM)—is involved with clearance of debris. Interestingly, this molecule is in circulation with IgM. During AKI, AIM dissociates from the immunoglobulin and transfers into the tubular lumen, where it can participate in removal of necrotic cell debris. There is species-dependent variation in the affinity AIM for IgM. Feline AIM has a binding affinity that is 1,000× stronger than murine AIM. This means that cats have impaired ability to use AIM as a mechanism for clearance of cellular debris during an AKI event. Genetically modified mice (which express feline AIM) also show decreased tubular clearance and worse clinical outcomes, underscoring the importance of this molecule in recovery from AKI.

Other proposed mechanisms include preglomerular vasoconstriction, possibly because of activation of the RAAS; leakage of tubular fluid into the interstitium (tubular backleak); and impaired glomerular permeability or vascular reactivity. Redistribution of tubular cell membrane proteins causes loss of cell polarity, abnormal ion transport across tubular cells, and increased delivery of sodium to the distal tubule. The resulting tubuloglomerular feedback leads to vasoconstriction of afferent arterioles. *Oliguria* is the result of various combinations of these factors. At the oliguric stage of AKI, hyperkalemia can be life threatening. If the animal survives the oliguric phase, diuresis may occur, and electrolyte imbalances, such as

Box • 4-2

Agents that are nephrotoxic in domestic animals

Exogenous

Animal venoms
Antimicrobials
- Aminoglycosides (neomycin, kanamycin, gentamicin, streptomycin, tobramycin, amikacin)
- Amphotericin B
- Cephalosporins
- Polymyxins
- Sulfonamides (sulfapyridine, sulfathiazole, sulfadiazine)
- Tetracyclines

Antineoplastic agents (cisplatin, doxorubicin, methotrexate)
Cantharidin (blister beetle)
Chlorinated hydrocarbons
Contrast media
Ethylene glycol
Menadione (vitamin K_3)
Metals (arsenic, bismuth, cadmium, lead, mercury, thallium)
Methoxyflurane
Monensin
Mycotoxins (citrinin, ochratoxin A)
Paraquat
Plants
- *Amaranthus retroflexus* (pigweed)
- *Isotropis*
- *Lantana camara*
- Oxalates (various plants)
- *Quercus* spp. (oak; tannins)
- *Terminalia oblongata* (yellow-wood)

Sodium fluoride (superphosphate fertilizer)

Endogenous

Bile
Hemoglobin
Myoglobin

hypokalemia, may contribute to death. As tubular regeneration proceeds, azotemia resolves and tubular function slowly returns.

Numerous toxic substances can cause ATI in domestic animals (Box 4-2). Some of these agents are no longer important as nephrotoxins. For example, organomercurials were commonly used as fungicides on grains that were occasionally inadvertently fed to animals and humans with disastrous results. This use of mercury has been banned. Similarly, highly chlorinated naphthalenes, which cause hyperkeratosis and AKI in cattle, have been mostly excluded from the farm environment.

Heavy metals in the environment, such as lead, arsenic, and cadmium, can infrequently result in accidental exposure to livestock. **Lead** exposure is seen in farms adjacent to battery manufacturers and zinc-lead smelter factories; individual exposure can also occur from lead-acid batteries and lead-containing paint. Lead toxicity is multisystemic, affecting the gastrointestinal, central nervous, and musculoskeletal systems. In acute toxicity, cattle might die within 24 hours. With respect to the kidney, there can be acute and chronic toxicities. In acute nephrotoxicity, there might be intranuclear inclusions composed of lead and associated proteins. Chronic exposure will lead to hyperuricemia, hypertension, and nonspecific glomerular and tubular lesions. Lipid peroxidation and reactive oxygen species are important in both scenarios. Critical antioxidant enzyme systems that can be inhibited by lead include: glutathione synthase/transferase/peroxidases, catalases, glucose-6-phosphatase, and superoxide dismutase. Lead promotes tubular epithelial cell apoptosis. Interstitial nephritis is also commonly seen in these cases.

Arsenic exposure from the environment, feed, water and parasiticides will cause renal toxicity as well as gastrointestinal disease, central nervous system signs, mucosal and conjunctival lesions, and decreased milk production. Similar to lead, arsenic causes lipid peroxidation and inhibits antioxidant pathways. Additionally, there is evidence of DNA damage. Specifically, methylation of arsenic is an early step in detoxification of the metal. But it can lead to hypomethylation of DNA, changing gene expression. Histologic lesions of arsenic toxicity are nonspecific GS and tubular necrosis.

Cattle can ingest **cadmium** in a variety of forms, but most commonly in water. Cadmium accumulates in the S1 segment of the proximal tubule, disrupting cellular transport proteins and mitochondria. It also can impact gene expression. Cadmium toxicity might not show histologic lesions, even if it disturbs bicarbonate, phosphate, and amino acid reabsorption. Taken together, aside from intranuclear inclusions that can occasionally be seen with **lead toxicity**, *heavy metal intoxication causes nonspecific renal lesions*. Knowledge of the environment surrounding the farm and their feeding practices as well as assays of heavy metal concentrations from various tissue samples are more important in the diagnosis of nephrotoxicity than histology. In these cases, the histologic lesions serve a supportive role for the final diagnosis.

The toxicity of many of the exogenous agents is exacerbated by various systemic states, such as dehydration or shock, which concomitantly impair renal function in the affected animal.

Iatrogenic nephrotoxicity

Aminoglycosides

These antibiotics are widely used against gram-negative infections and include, in decreasing order of nephrotoxicity, **neomycin, kanamycin, gentamicin, streptomycin, tobramycin**, and **amikacin**. Aminoglycosides can be ototoxic as well as nephrotoxic. Foals are particularly prone to nephrotoxicosis. Aminoglycosides are not metabolized but instead are eliminated from the body primarily by glomerular filtration. They selectively accumulate in and damage proximal tubules. The tubulotoxic effects of aminoglycosides include loss of the brush border and formation of cytosegrosomes and myeloid bodies. Overloading of lysosomes with phospholipids (lysosomal phospholipidosis) results from aminoglycoside-induced inhibition of phospholipases. Lysosomal dysfunction and/or leakage may lead to tubular cell injury and death. Damage is dose related and is enhanced by pre-existing renal impairment and dehydration. Toxicity is manifested clinically by an inability to concentrate urine, polyuria, enzymuria, proteinuria, hematuria, and azotemia. Aminoglycoside nephrotoxicity is reversible, and recovery may occur in the face of continued therapy because the regenerating cells have increased resistance to aminoglycoside toxicity.

Tetracyclines

An overdose of oxytetracycline can produce ATI and renal failure in dogs. Tetracycline administration has been reported to cause ATI and death in calves because of tetracycline degradation products; high doses of oxytetracycline are nephrotoxic to cattle. *The use of tetracyclines is contraindicated in animals in azotemic CKD.* Tetracyclines are excreted from the body primarily by the kidneys; thus, renal dysfunction leads to increased serum drug concentrations and enhanced nephrotoxic potential. Doxycycline, a semisynthetic tetracycline, is not nephrotoxic.

Sulfonamides

Severe injury may follow ingestion of excessive doses of sulfonamides, especially in dehydrated patients. Toxicity was more common previously when formulations were relatively insoluble. *Crystalline nephropathy is now rare because newer shorter-acting sulfonamides have greater solubility*. Affected kidneys are slightly enlarged and congested, and the sulfonamide crystals are grossly visible in the medulla, pelvis, and in some cases even in the bladder. The deposits are yellow and form pale radial lines in the medulla. Crystals are not observed in histologic sections because they are dissolved during processing. Epithelial cells of the proximal convoluted tubules and of glomerular capsules undergo severe acute swelling. There is little evidence of necrosis in the distal and collecting tubules, but epithelial proliferation and swelling are prominent, and the tubules become densely populated with large basophilic cells. Some papillary projections into the lumen may result from the regenerative proliferation. It appears that the *renal lesions are the result of both local toxic and obstructive effects* and that hypersensitivity does not play a role in animals, as it apparently does in humans.

Amphotericin

Amphotericin B is an antifungal agent, a polyene antibiotic, whose most important toxic effect is renal dysfunction. It causes decreased renal blood flow and glomerular filtration because of *renal vasoconstriction* and is also *directly toxic* to renal tubular epithelial cells. Necrosis of proximal and distal tubules occurs, and there is mineralization of intratubular casts. Nephrotoxicity of amphotericin B has been reduced by complexing the drug with lipids or entrapping it in liposomes.

Environmental nephrotoxicity

Ethylene glycol

Dogs and cats are commonly poisoned by ingestion of ethylene glycol. The seasonal incidence of this poisoning coincides with the changing of engine antifreeze solutions in the spring and autumn. Cattle are also occasionally poisoned. Ethylene glycol, which is present in a 95% concentration in antifreeze solutions, has a sweet taste and is usually ingested voluntarily, especially by young dogs. Cats are more susceptible, but less commonly affected, than dogs; the minimum lethal dose is 1.5 mL/kg for cats and 6.6 mL/kg for dogs.

Ethylene glycol, which itself is of low toxicity, is rapidly absorbed from the gastrointestinal tract. Most is excreted unchanged in the urine. A small percentage is oxidized by alcohol dehydrogenase in the liver to glycolaldehyde, which is in turn oxidized to glycolic acid, glyoxylate, and finally oxalate. *Glycolaldehyde and glyoxylate, the primary nephrotoxic metabolites*, cause depletion of ATP and damage to membrane phospholipids and enzymes. Other end products of metabolism are lactic acid, hippuric acid, and carbon dioxide.

Depression, ataxia, and osmotic diuresis develop within a few hours after ingestion of ethylene glycol. Although oxalate crystals are deposited around cerebral vessels and in perivascular spaces (Fig. 4-46A and B), nervous signs are attributed to the aldehydes and the severe metabolic acidosis from accumulation of lactic acid, glycolate, and glyoxylate. Over the next 12 hours, pulmonary edema, tachypnea, and tachycardia occur. Any of these early effects could result in death. Therefore, renal lesions might not be present in cases in which the patient dies soon after ethylene glycol ingestion. If the animal survives for 1-3 days after ingestion, AKI develops, primarily as the result of nephrotoxicity. Severe renal edema impairs intrarenal blood flow and contributes to injury. Soluble calcium oxalates in the blood precipitate in the ultrafiltrate of the renal tubules as the pH of the fluid decreases. *Oxalate crystals may be found in tubular lumens, in tubular cells, and in the interstitium*; they are light yellow, arranged in sheaves, rosettes, or prisms, and are birefringent with polarized light (see Fig. 4-46C and D). Crystals with a purple tint have calcium in addition to the oxalate component. Tubular lesions, which are most severe in proximal tubules, range from acute cellular swelling to necrosis to regeneration.

In animals surviving the acute toxic insult, calcium oxalate crystals are thought to be of importance in causing renal failure. *Large numbers of crystals in tubules are virtually pathognomonic of ethylene glycol poisoning; rare scattered oxalate crystals can be seen in many types of CKD*. Occasional calcium oxalate crystals are normally seen in urine sediment of dogs; large numbers of these crystals are highly suggestive of poisoning. Hypocalcemia resulting from the formation of crystals is usually mild in dogs. Animals that survive acute exposure may develop tubulointerstitial scarring. Few crystals may be left in the tubules; they tend to be removed in the weeks following their deposition. The diagnosis may be confirmed by detection of ethylene glycol in stomach content or blood by gas chromatography early in the toxicosis, or by detection of glycolic acid

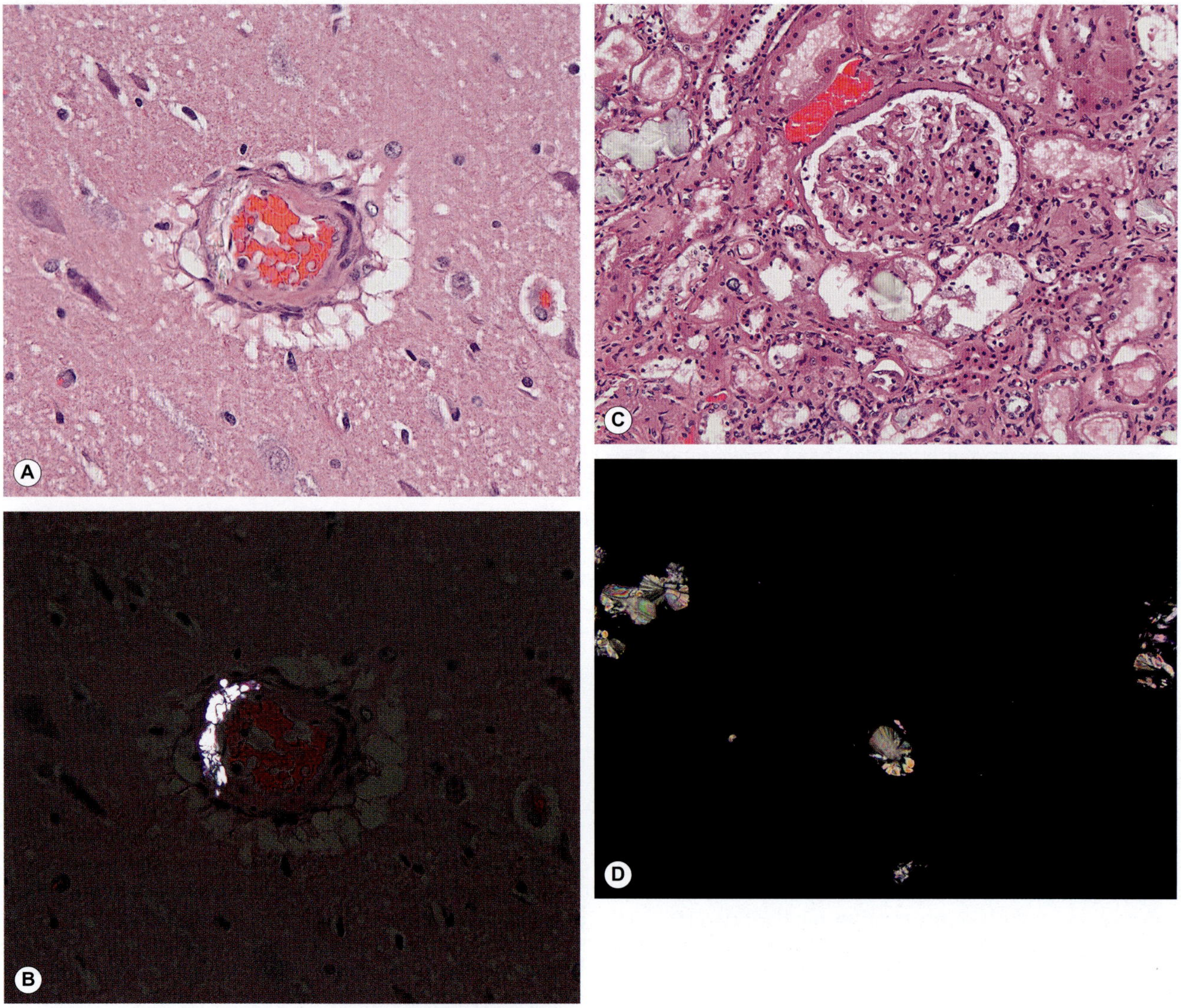

Figure 4-46 Ethylene glycol intoxication. A. Oxalate crystals in the wall of a vessel in the brain of a dog. **B.** As in **A**, with polarized light to demonstrate refractile calcium oxalate crystals. (**A, B** courtesy J. Davies.) **C.** Acute tubular necrosis in a cat, with oxalate crystals within tubular epithelial cells and tubular lumens. **D.** As in C, with polarizer, to demonstrate refractile oxalate crystals with the "sheaves of wheat" appearance.

in urine, serum, or ocular fluid by mass spectrometry later in the toxicosis. In dogs dying from ethylene glycol intoxication, the renal calcium-to-phosphorus ratio is often >2.5, whereas it is <0.1 in normal dogs.

Oxalate

Plants are the usual source of oxalate poisoning in sheep and cattle. Plants that can contain toxic amounts of oxalate are *Halogeton glomeratus*, halogeton; *Sarcobatus vermiculatus*, greasewood; *Rheum hybridum*, the common garden rhubarb; *Oxalis cernua*, soursob; and *Rumex* spp., sorrel, dock. Plants of lesser importance are *Portulaca oleracea*, *Trianthema portulacastrum*, and *Neobassia (Threlkeldia) proceriflora*, as well as some cultivated species, such as mangels and sugar beets. Young plants may contain ≥7% potassium oxalate; the amount decreases with maturity and drying of the plant. The above-listed plants are only eaten in unusual circumstances. Species of **grasses** in the genera *Cenchrus*, *Panicum*, and *Setaria*, which are widely cultivated in tropical and subtropical areas and accumulate large amounts of oxalate, have also been associated with renal oxalosis in cattle and sheep and with skeletal disease in horses; the latter is the result of calcium deficiency (see Vol. 1, Bones and Joints).

The **fungi** *Aspergillus niger* and *A. flavus* can produce large quantities of oxalates on feedstuffs. Large doses of **ascorbic acid** (vitamin C) have caused oxalate nephrotoxicosis in humans and in a goat; ascorbic acid is a metabolic precursor of oxalate. **Primary hyperoxaluria**, a rare inherited metabolic condition, occurs in humans, cats (inbred colony of domestic shorthairs), dogs (families of Tibetan Spaniels, and Shih Tzu), Beefmaster cattle (likely autosomal recessive), and Zwartbles sheep. **Pyridoxine (vitamin B_6)** deficiency and **methoxyflurane** anesthesia can also cause renal oxalosis.

Mortality rates of 10% may occur in sheep when they graze almost pure stands of halogeton or soursob. It is more usual, however, for fatalities to be sporadic. Under natural conditions, sheep may ingest up to 75 g of oxalate per day; *the rumen degrades the salt efficiently by metabolism of oxalate to bicarbonate and carbonates*. Depending on the microbial composition of the rumen, some variation is expected in the ability of ruminal microbiota to degrade the oxalate. Cattle are less commonly affected under range conditions than are sheep, but cattle and sheep are equally susceptible to experimental poisoning. Horses are resistant to oxalate-induced nephrotoxicity and succumb to acute gastroenteritis only after receiving unnaturally large amounts of the chemical; they may develop fibrous osteodystrophy with prolonged exposure.

Chelation of calcium by unmetabolized oxalate in the ingesta contributes to hypocalcemia. Following absorption, oxalates combine with calcium to form insoluble calcium oxalate; hypocalcemic tetany may result. Calcium oxalate may crystallize in vessel lumens or walls, causing vascular necrosis and hemorrhage, or in renal tubules, causing tubular obstruction and AKI. The nephrotoxicity of oxalates may also be partly due to intracellular chelation of calcium and magnesium and hence interference with oxidative phosphorylation. Clinically, weakness, prostration, and death may follow within 12 hours of ingestion of oxalate-containing plants.

Endogenous oxalates are produced by the degradation of glycine, an important constituent amino acid of collagen and elastin. Uptake of normal dietary oxalate may increase in a variety of enteric diseases (enteric oxalosis). *Oxalosis can be prominent in the kidneys of aborted bovine fetuses* and may reflect maternal intake of oxalate-containing plants or moldy feed. A few oxalate crystals can frequently be found in scarred tubules in any species; these crystals are usually without significance.

Melamine and cyanuric acid

Outbreaks of nephrotoxicity occurred in dogs, cats, pigs, aquatic animals, and human infants as the result of a combination of melamine and cyanuric acid in adulterated food, including pet food, pig feed, and baby formula. The lesion involves the distal nephron, which contains prominent green to gold-brown circular melamine cyanurate crystals with radiating spokes (Fig. 4-47). Scattered oxalate crystals were also present, secondary to renal failure as opposed to being the cause. Interestingly, prolonged formalin fixation (>6 weeks) led to dissolution of crystals. Although many pets likely ingested the contaminated pet food, only some developed renal failure. The difference in response likely depended on underlying renal disease and urine pH.

Mycotoxins

Aspergillus and *Penicillium* spp. produce a number of nephrotoxic mycotoxins, namely, **ochratoxins, citrinin, fumonisin, oxalate**, and **viridicatumtoxin**, which can contaminate feed grains. *Ochratoxin A (OTA)* is the most significant; OTA is produced by *Aspergillus ochraceus* and *Penicillium verrucosum*. In pigs, OTA and citrinin produce proximal tubular degeneration and atrophy with cortical interstitial fibrosis, but the renal insufficiency produced is usually subclinical. When AKI does occur, it is manifested by severe perirenal edema resembling that produced by redroot pigweed (*Amaranthus retroflexus*). Ochratoxicosis also increases the susceptibility of pigs to secondary bacterial infections. Ochratoxins are normally degraded in the rumen; thus, toxicity is unlikely to occur in ruminants.

Moldy feed also produces mycotoxic nephropathy in horses. **Fumonisins**, mycotoxins produced by *Fusarium* fungi, alter sphingolipid metabolism and cause leukoencephalomalacia in horses and pulmonary edema in pigs; they are hepatotoxic in all species. Fumonisins are nephrotoxic in sheep and cattle; renal lesions include vacuolar change, apoptosis, karyomegaly, and obstruction of proximal tubules.

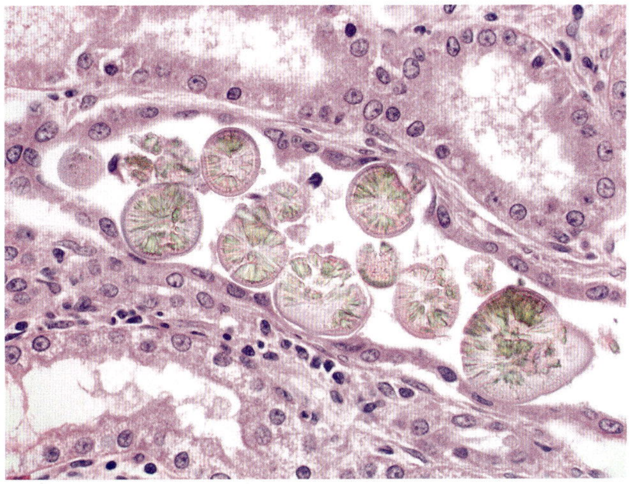

Figure 4-47 **Acute tubular injury** in a cat that consumed melamine and cyanuric acid in contaminated pet food. Melamine cyanurate crystals are often circular and gold-brown.

Amaranthus

Ingestion of redroot pigweed, *Amaranthus retroflexus*, causes *perirenal edema and AKI in swine and cattle*, and uncommonly in horses and lambs. The nephrotoxic principle of *A. retroflexus* has not been identified, but extracts of leaves were more toxic to in vitro cultures of murine fibroblasts compared with other plant parts. Overall, *Amaranthus* plants have abundant nitrogen-containing compounds, some of which are rarely seen in other vegetation. Because this genus survives in harsh environments and has high amino acid levels in its leaves, it can serve as a complete protein resource for livestock and humans. Amaranth components are used medicinally, as well as nutritionally. Phytotoxicity appears to be limited to the *A. retroflexus* spp. Experimentally, a small peptide was eluted from *A. retroflexus* leaf extracts, which was necessary to induce murine fibroblast toxicity. The peptide mimics one involved in cell signaling.

Lush growth of pigweed occurs in early summer, and this plant often dominates the weed growth in disused lots to which animals are moved when other pasture is depleted. Weakness, recumbency, and often death follow 5-10 days after grazing begins. Grossly, there is *marked perirenal edema*, which may be blood stained and may be accompanied by edema of the mesentery, intestinal wall, and ventral abdominal wall, with moderate ascites and hydrothorax (Fig. 4-48). The kidneys are pale-tan but not usually enlarged. Histologically, there is coagulative necrosis of both proximal and distal tubules and intratubular granular casts. There might also be mild glomerular epithelial injury and hypercellularity. The perirenal edema seen in acute cases is apparently the result of tubular backleak, with subsequent lymphatic drainage and leakage into perirenal connective tissue. The probable cause of death is heart failure resulting from *hyperkalemia*. Survivors may develop renal interstitial fibrosis and tubular atrophy.

Oak toxicity

Poisoning of ruminants and occasionally of horses by *blossoms, buds, leaves, stems, and acorns* of **oak shrubs and trees (*Quercus* spp.)** can occur. There are many species and varieties of oaks, but not all are palatable. They are all potentially poisonous by virtue of the *tannins* they contain, but toxicity is dose dependent. Ingestion of large amounts of the material can cause hydrothorax, ascites, perirenal edema, alimentary tract ulceration, ATI, microscopic hematuria, and death. The toxic substances are **gallotannins;** they are hydrolyzed to tannic acid, gallic acid, and pyrogallol, which appear to be the active toxic metabolites. Binding of tannins to endothelial cells results in *endothelial damage* and leads to perirenal edema, hydrothorax, and ascites. The alimentary lesions result from the binding of oak tannins to peptide bonds within endothelial cells, which precipitates protein. The gastrointestinal ulcers are also partly the result of disseminated intravascular coagulation.

In acute oak poisoning, there is marked perirenal edema and hemorrhage. The kidneys are swollen and pale-tan and, in cattle, have 2-3-mm cortical hemorrhages. Glomeruli are ischemic. After several days, dilation of glomerular capsules may be present. Necrosis of the epithelium of the proximal tubules can be complete, producing homogeneous casts within the basement membranes. In less severe injury, adjacent groups of tubules may vary considerably in the extent of injury and necrosis. Animals may recover with or without scarring of the renal parenchyma. *Frank necrosis in groups of tubules with intratubular hemorrhage distinguishes the nephrotoxicity of acute oak poisoning from that of most other causes.*

Other plant toxicoses

Poisoning by the **yellow-wood tree, *Terminalia oblongata***, in Australia is reputed to produce lesions similar to those of oak poisoning. Yellow-wood produces at least 2 toxic factors: punicalagin, a tannin that is hepatotoxic, and terminalin, a condensed tannin that is nephrotoxic. In acute yellow-wood poisoning of cattle and sheep, coagulative periacinar hepatic necrosis predominates over the nephrotoxic injury. Subacute and chronic intoxications result in renal fibrosis and atrophy.

Several species of the genus ***Isotropis*** are toxic to ruminants. In both cattle and sheep, there is abomasitis, enteritis, perirenal edema, and accumulation of fluid in the body cavities and subcutis. The renal lesion is necrosis of proximal tubular epithelium. In many acute poisonings, there is abundant proteinaceous fluid in urinary spaces.

Various members of the ***lily* family, *Liliaceae***, of plants are nephrotoxic in animal species, for example, *Narthecium ossifragum* (bog asphodel) in ruminants, and *Lilium* spp. in cats. Intoxicated cats are polyuric, polydipsic, glucosuric, proteinuric, isosthenuric, and azotemic. In addition to proximal tubular necrosis (Fig. 4-49), cats also have acute pancreatic

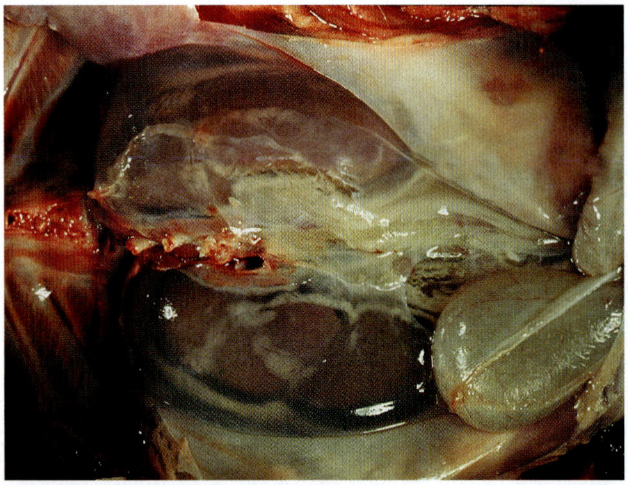

Figure 4-48 Perirenal edema caused by *Amaranthus retroflexus* toxicity in a pig. (Courtesy K. Potter.)

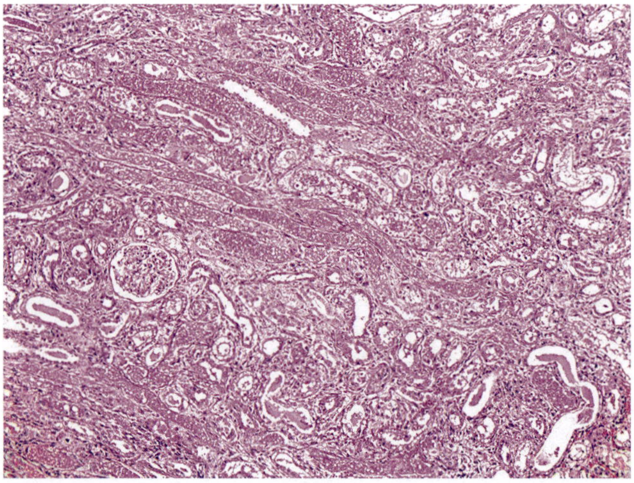

Figure 4-49 Acute tubular necrosis caused by **lily intoxication** in a cat. Entire nephron segments have coagulative necrosis and some have sloughed cellular debris.

necrosis and elevated creatine kinase. Ultrastructurally, renal tubules have swollen mitochondria, megamitochondria, and lipid accumulation.

Grapes, raisins, and currants (*Vitis vinifera* plants) occasionally causes proximal renal tubular degeneration and/or necrosis in dogs. Histology reveals the intracellular gold-brown globular pigment that variably stains positively for iron with the Prussian blue stain. Dysregulation of calcium homeostasis might be involved in the pathogenesis because high calcium and high calcium:phosphorus products at the time of presentation are poor prognostic indicators. AKI associated with ingestion is idiosyncratic; dogs are more likely to vomit after ingestion, and AKI is actually rare. It is possible that early intervention in dogs known to have ingested grapes and raisins has prevented AKI. Tartaric acid is purported to play a role in the pathogenesis because it is a documented toxin in dogs that ingest cream of tartar, the baking ingredient. It is present in variably high levels in grapes, raisins, and tamarinds. In vitro exposure of cultured Madin-Darby canine kidney (MDCK) cells to tartaric acid is cytotoxic, but human kidney (HK) 2 cells are resistant. This difference in susceptibility might be based on species variations in organic anion transport (OAT) 4 proteins. Blocking the OATs (with probenecid) prevents toxicity, and transfection of MDCK cells with human OAT4 also prevents toxicity.

Specific tubular dysfunctions

Renal tubular dysfunction may occur secondary to other systemic conditions. For example, glucosuria occurs when tubular transport for glucose is exceeded in diabetes mellitus, stress, and acute enterotoxemia; heavy metal toxicity causes glucosuria and aminoaciduria because of tubular injury. Primary tubular transport defects identified in domestic animals are *hyperuricosuria in Dalmatian dogs, essential cystinuria, a syndrome of resorptive defects in Basenji dogs, renal tubular acidosis (**RTA** types I-IV)*, and *primary renal glucosuria*. Hyperuricosuria and cystinuria predispose to urolithiasis and are discussed in that section.

Basenjis and several other breeds of dogs may develop a *proximal renal tubular disorder* similar to the **Fanconi syndrome** (also called "proximal tubulopathy") in humans; the condition is hereditary in Basenjis. The syndrome in dogs is one of polyuria, polydipsia, hyposthenuria, glucosuria with normoglycemia, hyperphosphaturia, proteinuria, and aminoaciduria. The aminoaciduria may be generalized or limited to cystinuria. Affected dogs have impaired renal tubular resorption of glucose, phosphate, sodium, potassium, uric acid, and amino acids. Research implicates abnormal fluidity of the proximal tubule brush border membrane resulting from significantly increased levels of cholesterol in affected Basenjis compared with normal dogs. This likely affects the resorptive capacity of the proximal tubule. Polyuria results from the glucosuria and natriuresis. The syndrome develops in adult dogs and is usually slowly progressive. Dehydration and acidosis might result in renal papillary necrosis, uremia, and death. Histologic renal lesions are nonspecific and include interstitial fibrosis and tubular atrophy. Affected dogs often have marked karyomegaly in scattered tubular cells. Ultrastructural abnormalities have not been noted in tubular cells. Acquired proximal tubulopathy has been reported in dogs in association with gentamicin nephrotoxicity, ethylene glycol nephrotoxicity, primary hypoparathyroidism, and copper storage hepatopathy (Fig. 4-50). This clinical syndrome has also been reported in small-breed dogs that were fed certain types of jerky treats.

Type II renal tubular acidosis (RTA) is a specific type of **proximal tubular** disease due to failure to resorb filtered bicarbonate. Proximal RTA is usually a self-limiting disease that is not evident clinically. **Distal, or type I, RTA** is caused by defective excretion of hydrogen ions by distal tubules and produces hyperchloremic metabolic acidosis that is more severe than that of type II RTA. It occurs in dogs, cats, and horses. Untreated distal RTA can result in osteomalacia, nephrocalcinosis, nephrolithiasis, and azotemia. A mixed pattern of RTA (proximal and distal) is diagnosed as **type III; type IV RTA** is due to low renin and aldosterone levels. There are case reports of both of these conditions in dogs and horses.

Primary renal glucosuria may occur as a singular transport abnormality without other defects. This defect is an inherited disorder in Norwegian Elkhounds.

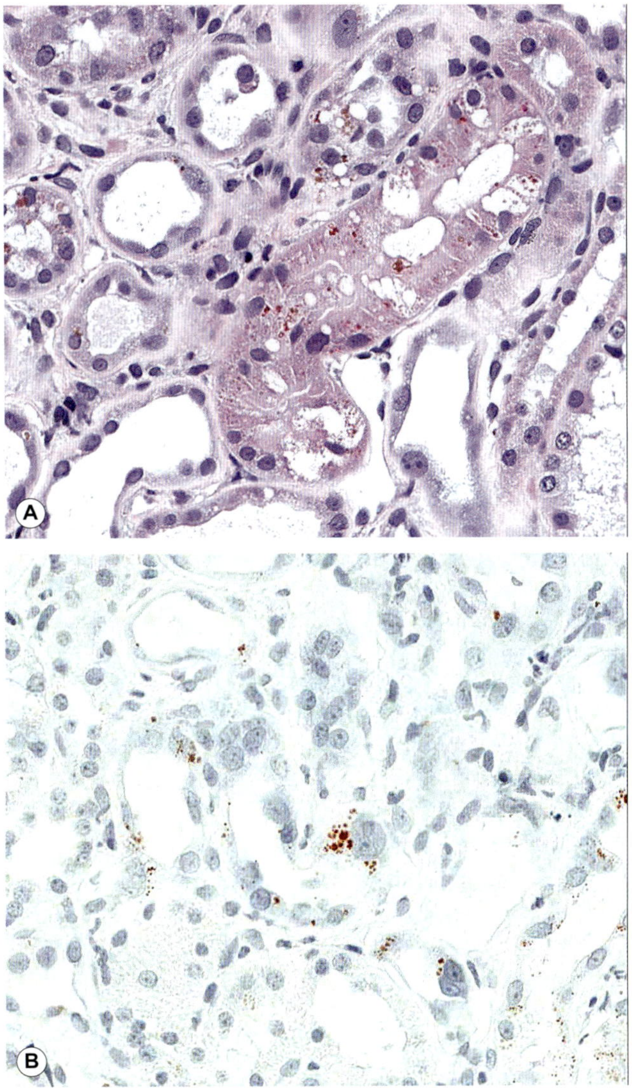

Figure 4-50 A. **Acute tubular injury** with karyomegaly in a dog with acquired **Fanconi syndrome**. H&E. **B**. This case was associated with hepatic copper storage disease, and the rhodanine stain demonstrates small intracytoplasmic red-brown granules.

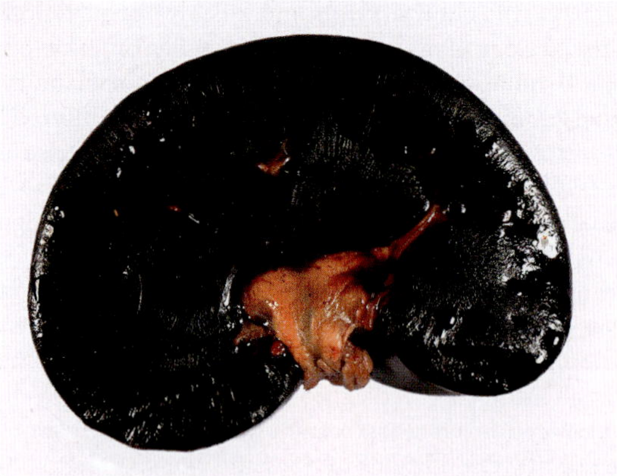

Figure 4-51 Marked discoloration (dark-brown to black) of the renal parenchyma in a goat following a **hemolytic crisis in chronic copper poisoning**. (Courtesy E. Clark, D. Russell.)

The mannosidoses, hereditary **lysosomal storage diseases**, can cause vacuolation of neurons, renal tubular epithelial, and other cells in humans, cattle, goats, and cats. Salers calves affected with autosomal dominant *β-mannosidosis* have a variety of neurologic deficits and greatly enlarged kidneys, with marked vacuolation of the cytoplasm of proximal tubular epithelial cells. Although the renal lesion is marked, azotemia is not reported (see Vol. 1, Nervous System). Importantly, similar tubular epithelial vacuolation can be caused by some plant intoxications, for example, *Swainsona, Astragalus, and Oxytropis*.

Pigmentary changes

Following acute hemolytic crises, *the kidneys may be very dark, almost black*, as a consequence of concentrated **hemoglobin** (Fig. 4-51). Initially, the discoloration is uniform, but the kidneys soon have small foci of brown discoloration as a result of retention of hemoglobin in scattered nephrons. The gross lesion is commonly observed in the hemolytic crisis of chronic copper poisoning in sheep. Microscopically, the hemoglobin appears as fine red granules in the epithelial cells of the tubules and as red granular casts in the lower nephron, especially the loop of Henle and collecting tubules (see Fig. 4-45). Myoglobin casts are histologically indistinguishable from hemoglobin casts. The same histologic picture occurs following incompatible blood transfusions. In horses, hemoglobinuria resulting from *Acer rubrum* intoxication or neonatal isoerythrolysis should be differentiated from myoglobinuria, which can be seen in trauma, exertional rhabdomyolysis, polysaccharide storage myopathy, or intoxication with drugs (monensin) or plants (e.g., white snakeroot, coffee senna). Hemoglobin and myoglobin pigments persist in tubules after they are no longer detectable in urine samples. Heme proteins (hemoglobin and myoglobin) can reduce renal blood flow and are also cytotoxic. Other factors, such as anemia and dehydration, likely also contribute to renal failure. Tubular obstruction by myoglobin exacerbates AKI in horses with severe rhabdomyolysis.

Hemosiderosis results from chronic hemolytic anemia and from acute hemoglobinuric episodes. The pigment is found in epithelial cells of proximal tubules, where it is produced by the degradation of resorbed hemoglobin. It may be sufficient to produce brown discoloration of the cortex.

Lipofuscinosis of the kidneys of adult cattle is the result of *deposition of brown iron-free pigments* with staining characteristics of lipofuscin. On cut surface, the kidney has radiating dark lines in the cortex, but the medulla is spared. Microscopically, the pigment is present as fine, brown granules in the epithelial cells of the convoluted tubules.

Cloisonné kidney is a nonclinical pigmentary condition in goats. The renal cortices are uniformly brown or black because of *thickening and brown pigmentation (ferritin and hemosiderin) of basement membranes* of proximal convoluted tubules, presumably as the result of repeated episodes of intravascular hemolysis.

In congenital **porphyria** of cattle, swine, and cats, the renal cortices are discolored brown. Histologically, the pigment is present in the tubular epithelium and interstitium, and the pigment is excreted in the urine. When exposed to light, the urine develops a port-wine color because of photic activation of porphyrins. Urine and tissues fluoresce blue-green in ultraviolet light.

Green-yellow pigmentation of swollen kidneys is common in **icterus** of hepatic origin and less notably in hemolytic icterus unless there is concomitant hepatic injury. It is described in the Hepatorenal Syndrome section. Olive-green coloration of the renal cortex is common in newborn lambs, calves, and foals. The pigment is bilirubin, and its presence is probably due to immaturity of hepatic conjugating mechanisms.

Light-green to green-yellow discoloration of renal and other abdominal lymph nodes is occasionally observed in cattle at slaughter. Histologically, numerous red-brown acicular crystals are present in the cytoplasm of renal tubular epithelial cells and hepatocytes. Crystals may be present in renal tubules, and renal calculi are rarely present. The crystals are **2,8-dihydroxyadenine (2,8-DHA)**, a metabolite of the purine adenine. The crystal deposition and pigmentation are of little significance, and the cause of this condition in cattle is unknown. In humans, these pigmented crystals are the result of adenine phosphoribosyltransferase deficiency and may result in urolithiasis. A case of 2,8-DHA urolithiasis has been reported in a dog; management for this disease is similar to that of urate urolithiasis.

Miscellaneous tubular conditions

Hepatorenal syndrome

The term **hepatorenal syndrome** is applied to *AKI that occurs in human patients with cirrhosis and ascites;* an exact parallel has not yet been identified as a spontaneous disease in domestic animals. Splanchnic vasodilation will result in underfilling of general circulation, mimicking hypovolemia. This can cause activation of renal feedback mechanisms to preserve volume. Cirrhosis also leads to an imbalance of vasodilators (e.g., nitric oxide) and vasoconstrictors (e.g., endothelin). Hypotension may result from the vasodepressors and the diuretic effects of cholemia; thus, the azotemia in icteric patients may be of prerenal origin. Concentrations of bilirubin and bile acids are greatly elevated in the blood, especially in obstructive jaundice. Bile pigment accumulates in tubular epithelial cells, which are frequently swollen. In severe liver dysfunction, bile casts may form in tubules, resulting in so-called *"bile cast nephropathy."* Therefore, the renal histology can range from normal, to ATI, to bile casts in tubules. In humans, resolution of liver disease or liver transplantation will allow the kidneys to regain normal function. Experimentally, hepatorenal syndrome has been induced in dogs by complete surgical ligation of the common bile duct at its entry point into the duodenum.

Pseudohepatorenal syndromes include conditions in which the liver and kidneys are both affected, but the renal disease is not *secondary* to hepatic disease; included are a wide variety of infectious, circulatory, genetic, toxic, and other systemic disorders.

Glycogen accumulation in tubules

In diabetes mellitus in dogs and cats, glycogen accumulates in tubular epithelium, producing marked cytoplasmic clear spaces in the epithelial cells in the outer medulla and inner cortex. Glycogen can be readily demonstrated by appropriate techniques. The deposition occurs in the ascending limb of the loop of Henle, disappears following insulin administration, and has no effect on renal function.

Nephrogenic diabetes insipidus

This condition has been reported in dogs and foals with polyuria, polydipsia, and hyposthenuria. Affected animals are unresponsive to water deprivation, to exogenous administration of ADH, and to infusion of hypertonic saline. The basis of the defect is a *lack of responsiveness of the cells of the distal tubules and collecting ducts to ADH*. The defect may be *congenital* (possible X-linked disorder in 2 foals) or *acquired* as the result of tubulointerstitial diseases, such as pyelonephritis or hypercalcemic nephropathy, or drugs such as tetracycline. If there is interference with production of ADH by the hypothalamus or ADH release from the posterior pituitary, the disease is referred to as *central or neurogenic diabetes insipidus*.

Hypokalemic nephropathy

Chronic potassium depletion can result in defects in urine concentration and polyuria. Hypokalemia may be caused by diarrhea, hyperaldosteronism, and some renal diseases. Chronic potassium depletion can lead to lymphoplasmacytic tubulointerstitial nephritis and interstitial fibrosis. Vacuolar change of proximal tubular cells is a prominent lesion seen in human renal biopsies. It might be more striking in humans because vacuoles are not expected in that species, whereas they are more commonly seen in dogs and cats. Similar tubular epithelial cell vacuolation was reported in ewes deliberately given 11-17 times the recommended dose of *thiabendazole*. Many of the ewes developed hypokalemia, hypoproteinemia, and uremia, and died; potassium loss was thought to occur through the kidneys. *Corticosteroids* produce hypokalemia and reversible vacuolar change of tubular cells. Hypokalemia may be related to the tubular dilation commonly seen in piglets with *diarrhea* and is related to experimentally induced renal cysts.

Miscellaneous

There are several miscellaneous histologic changes that may be found in renal epithelium. *Some of the* **pyrrolizidine alkaloids** *cause megalocytosis in the proximal tubules*. The lesion is similar in type to that in hepatocytes, but less conspicuous, and does not cause functional disturbance. Some pyrrolizidine alkaloid–containing plants, particularly *Crotalaria* spp., cause significant glomerular megalocytosis (see Vol. 2, Liver and Biliary System).

Occasional nuclei in tubules of old dogs may be **polyploid**. *In the proximal tubules, eosinophilic, crystalline, intranuclear inclusions* **("brick inclusions")** *are commonly encountered in old dogs*. Similar inclusions occur in the liver. Their source is unknown, and they do not cause clinical disease. Their significance is the result of their similarity to certain heavy metal inclusions. Subacute **lead poisoning** produces amorphous *acid-fast inclusion material* in proximal tubular epithelial nuclei that are large, pale, and vesicular (see the Iatrogenic Nephrotoxicity section).

Large, eosinophilic, intranuclear glycogen inclusions occur in hepatocytes and renal collecting duct epithelial cells in goats. The pathogenesis of this **nuclear glycogenosis** is unknown, and it does not appear to be of functional significance. Intranuclear glycogenosis is occasionally observed in humans with diabetes mellitus.

Eosinophilic intracytoplasmic inclusion bodies have been reported in the renal collecting duct epithelial cells of dogs. The inclusions consisted of **iridovirus** particles, and the infection was not clinically significant.

TUBULOINTERSTITIAL DISEASES

This term encompasses *diseases that involve primarily the interstitium and tubules*, and it acknowledges that inflammatory and degenerative interstitial diseases almost always impair tubular function. Hence, **interstitial nephritis** and **pyelonephritis** are classified as tubulointerstitial diseases. There is obviously overlap with the previous category of ATI because animals often develop secondary interstitial inflammation and fibrosis after ATI. *Tubulointerstitial nephritis can be caused by a vast array of agents*, including infections, toxins, chemicals, therapeutic drugs, and immunologic disorders. Immunologically mediated tubulointerstitial disease has been identified in humans, and rarely in domestic animals. Hypersensitivity reactions occur to a variety of drugs, for example, methicillin. Tubular immune-complex disease occurs in some humans with lupus nephritis and GN, indicating that autoantibodies might cross-react with glomerular and tubular basement membranes; antitubular basement membrane autoantibody has been identified in a dog.

Histologic features of tubulointerstitial diseases include interstitial inflammation, interstitial fibrosis, and tubular atrophy. Pyelonephritis is usually caused by infectious agents, although they may not be identified, especially in chronic cases. Interstitial nephritis is common in dogs and cats, can be a primary disease or secondary to glomerular disease, and can be the result of infectious or noninfectious inflammatory conditions. AKI, including GN, leads to release of a wide array of cytokines and growth factors from tubular epithelial cells and peritubular capillaries, resulting in interstitial inflammation and ongoing tubulointerstitial damage. Monocytes are recruited, interstitial fibroblasts are activated, interstitial myofibroblasts appear, and fibrosis ensues. Glomerular diseases can also incite the above sequence of events through the action of filtered proteins on tubular epithelial cells. However, injury to glomeruli may occur secondarily in tubulointerstitial disease because of the interdependence of renal structures. In any case, *destructive fibrosis and nephron loss underlie progressive renal disease*.

The hallmark of glomerular disease, clinically, is persistent proteinuria; tubulointerstitial diseases are more likely to demonstrate azotemia, defects of concentrating ability, or specific tubular defects of resorption or secretion. However, the end point of both types of renal disease is decompensated renal function with isosthenuria and azotemia, possibly progressing to uremia.

Mononuclear interstitial nephritis

Focal lymphohistiocytic inflammation with slight scarring is common in the kidneys. The causes are seldom known and probably not specific. Mononuclear interstitial nephritis may be acute or chronic, and multifocal or generalized, depending on the intensity of the insult and the efficiency of the host response. **Acute interstitial nephritis** *is characterized by acute clinical onset, and histologically by interstitial edema, leukocytic infiltration, and focal tubular necrosis*. In **chronic interstitial nephritis**, *there is mononuclear cell infiltration, interstitial fibrosis, and generalized tubular atrophy*. Many infectious agents are capable of causing mononuclear interstitial nephritis. Unfortunately, agents are often not identified, especially in chronic cases or when antibiotics were administered prior to tissue harvest.

Leptospira interrogans serovars Canicola and Icterohaemorrhagiae have been associated with acute generalized interstitial nephritis in dogs, although their importance has declined because of the efficacy of vaccination. In survivors of acute infections, there may be marked interstitial fibrosis and tubular atrophy. Diffuse interstitial nephritis is less common in large domestic animals than in dogs; the usual end result of leptospirosis in cattle and swine is multifocal interstitial nephritis. Leptospirosis is discussed in detail later.

Encephalitozoon cuniculi, an obligate intracellular microsporidian parasite, causes diffuse mononuclear-to-granulomatous interstitial nephritis and granulomatous encephalitis in immature dogs and rabbits. The renal lesion is a heavy, almost pure, interstitial infiltrate of plasma cells. The gram-positive organisms occur in tubular epithelial cells, tubular lumens, and vessel walls. Encephalitozoonosis is discussed in Vol. 1, Nervous System.

The best-known form of multifocal mononuclear interstitial nephritis is the *"white-spotted kidney"* of calves. It is common and is largely an incidental finding in young calves that can progress to scar tissue with advancing age. The cause is usually undetermined but is thought to be the result of neonatal bacteremia; *E. coli* can occasionally be recovered from the lesions. *Salmonella* and *Brucella* are other suggested causes. Affected kidneys contain up to 1-cm white nodules throughout the cortex (Fig. 4-52). Histologically, the initial lesion are microabscesses, which are soon replaced by numerous lymphocytes, plasma cells, and macrophages. Progressive fibrosis results in healing by scar tissue. The inflammation and scarring may cause tubular obstruction and/or atrophy.

Multifocal interstitial nephritis also occurs in cattle during the course of *malignant catarrhal fever, theileriosis, and lumpy skin disease*. It can also be seen in a fatal *autosomal recessive disorder* in Japanese Black cattle (Wagyu) resulting from a null mutation of *claudin-16* gene (analogous to *paracellin-1* in humans), which is a tight junction protein expressed between tubular epithelial cells. Affected cattle are azotemic and proteinuric and have increased urinary magnesium excretion but normal serum magnesium levels. Homozygous animals usually die before 6 months of age, and interstitial inflammation and zonal fibrosis are marked, with cystically dilated tubules and glomerular capsules. The relationship between the genetic mutation, abnormal magnesium dynamics, interstitial inflammation, and cystic tubules has not been clearly elucidated.

Interstitial nephritis is also seen in sheep infected with sheeppox virus (SPV; *Poxviridae, Capripoxvirus sheeppox*) and visna/maedi virus (VMV; *Retroviridae, Lentivirus ovivismae*); the latter infection can also cause MPGN. Goats with caprine arthritis encephalitis virus (CAEV; *Retroviridae, Lentivirus capartenc*) infections also have interstitial nephritis. The virus has been detected in tubular epithelial cells and renal arteries via IHC.

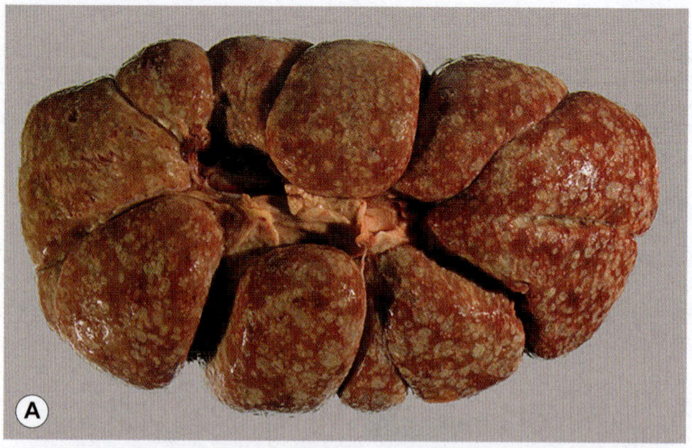

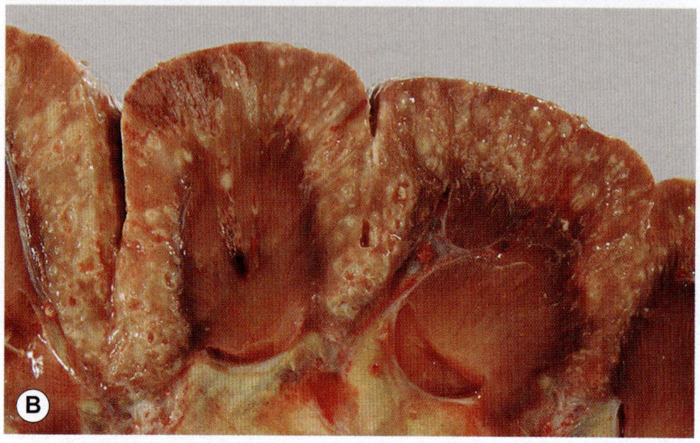

Figure 4-52 **A. "White-spotted kidney"** (multifocal mononuclear interstitial nephritis) from a calf. **B.** Cross section with white spots distributed throughout the cortex and rarely present in medulla. (A, B courtesy J.J. van der Lugt.)

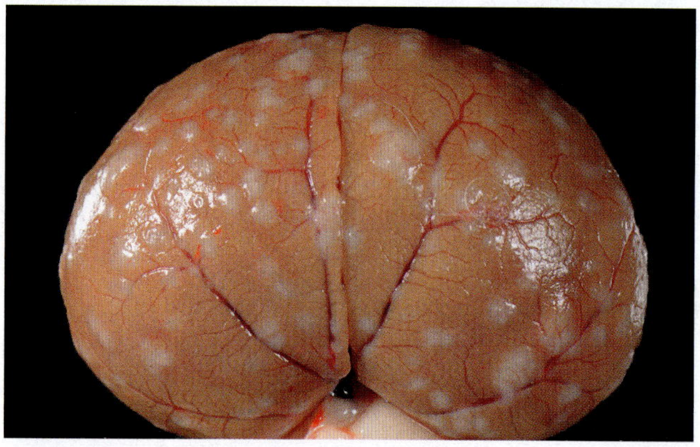

Figure 4-53 **Perivascular pyogranulomatous nephritis** in a cat with feline infectious peritonitis. (Courtesy R. Kohnken.)

There are also amplifiable proviral sequences in homogenized renal tissues of affected goats. In the horse, interstitial nephritis has been associated with equine infectious anemia. The renal lesions do not contribute significantly to the course of these diseases, but are diagnostically important. Their gross and histologic features are given elsewhere. Multifocal pyogranulomatous lesions are a rather consistent finding in the kidneys of cats with feline infectious peritonitis (Fig. 4-53). Canid alphaherpesvirus 1, canine herpesvirus (CaAHV1, CHV; *Orthoherpesviridae, Varicellovirus canidalpha1*) (Fig. 4-54) produces severe necrotizing nephritis as part of the systemic disease in puppies (see Vol. 3, Female Genital System). Other causes of mononuclear interstitial nephritis in dogs include *Leishmania* spp., *Borrelia burgdorferi*, *Hepatozoon canis*, and CAdV1.

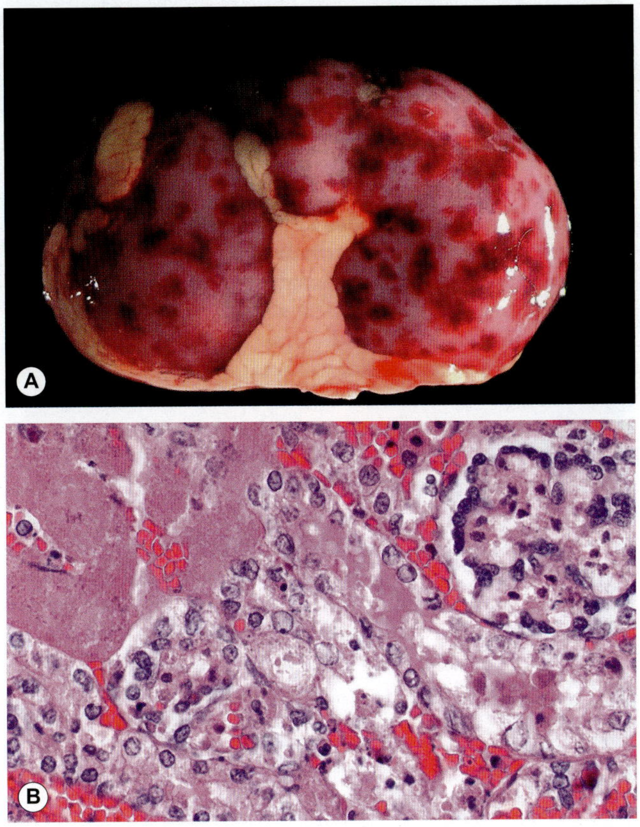

Figure 4-54 A. **Multifocal renal cortical hemorrhages** in a puppy infected with canid alphaherpesvirus 1. **B. Segmental tubular necrosis** and interstitial hemorrhage. H&E. (A, B courtesy L. Fry.)

Cattle and horses grazing *vetch* (*Vicia* spp.) can develop dermatitis, diarrhea, and ill-thrift. They develop lesions in the skin, kidney, and other internal organs, with multifocal eosinophilic granulomatous inflammation. Similar lymphocytic-to-granulomatous lesions are reported in cattle fed *citrus pulp*.

Neutrophilic interstitial nephritis

Bacterial infection of the kidneys may be either **hematogenous** or **ascend from the lower urinary tract**. The former causes embolic neutrophilic nephritis; the latter causes pyelonephritis, with inflammation in both the pelvis and renal parenchyma.

Adenoviral infection of sheep primarily causes pneumonia, but also can cause mild, multifocal, neutrophilic interstitial nephritis, with characteristic large, basophilic, intranuclear inclusion bodies in endothelial and/or interstitial cells. Two young horses from the same farm succumbed to equine polyomavirus (*EPyV; Polyomaviridae, Betapolyomavirus equi*) infection of the kidney. There was marked interstitial nephritis and tubulitis. Intranuclear inclusions were identified in tubular epithelial cells, with the distal nephron being primarily affected (eFig. 4-24). Immunohistochemistry revealed viral infection of most organs in one horse; infection was limited to the kidney and a few cells of the gastrointestinal tract in the other. Immunosuppression in human renal transplant recipients puts them at risk of developing polyomaviral and adenoviral infections of the allograft kidney.

Embolic nephritis

Embolic nephritis is analogous to abscess formation in any organ and occurs when bacteria are seeded in the kidneys in the course of bacteremia or septic thromboembolism. Bacteria alone or in

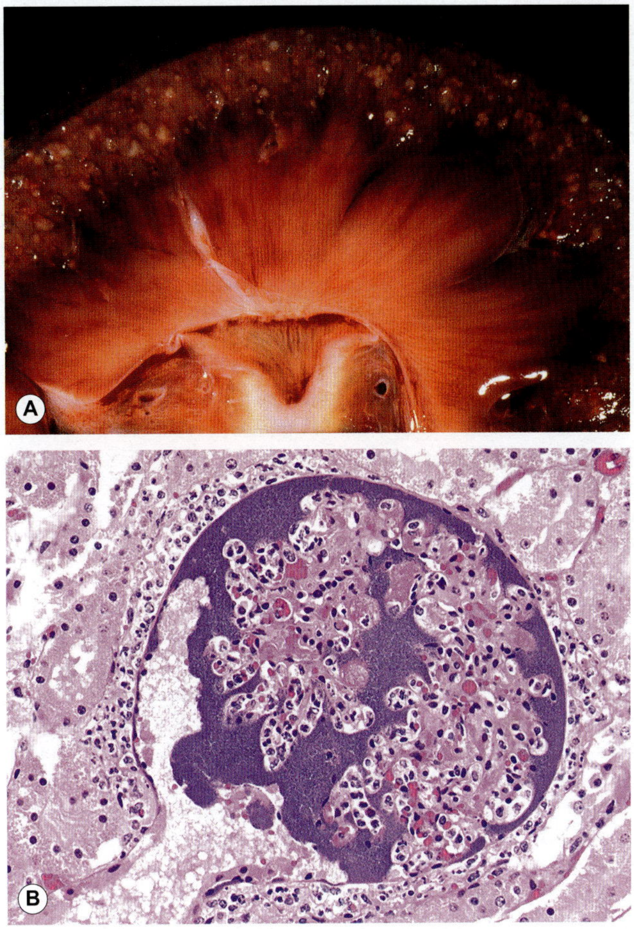

Figure 4-55 A. *Actinobacillus equuli* **embolic nephritis** in a foal. (Courtesy K. Potter.) **B.** Myriad cocci fill the urinary space of a glomerulus. H&E.

small septic emboli lodge mainly in glomerular and peritubular capillaries and may produce variably sized *abscesses*. Larger emboli lodge in arteries, producing unilateral or bilateral *septic infarcts*.

Many bacteria undoubtedly pass through the glomerular capillary walls into the tubules, where they are probably harmless unless there is stasis of urine. Abscesses are generally cortical rather than medullary; however, gram-negative enterobacteria can cause microscopic neutrophilic foci in the medulla. Healing of neutrophilic lesions occurs by scar formation.

In **horses**, the most common cause of embolic neutrophilic nephritis is *Actinobacillus equuli*, which is acquired in utero, during parturition, or shortly after birth as an umbilical infection. Death may occur because of fulminant septicemia. In foals that survive for several days, microabscesses are seen in the kidneys and other organs, and polyarthritis is present (Fig. 4-55; eFig. 4-25). The abscesses are usually green-yellow, up to 3-mm foci. The most common cause of embolic nephritis in **swine** is probably *Erysipelothrix rhusiopathiae*. Embolic GN may be seen grossly as glomerular hemorrhages. Microabscesses form in the interstitium. In adult **cattle**, most cases are caused by *Trueperella pyogenes* from valvular endocarditis. Septic emboli often produce large, randomly distributed abscesses and infarcts. In **sheep and goats**, renal abscesses caused by *Corynebacterium pseudotuberculosis* are common. In **dogs**, systemic protothecosis can involve the kidneys and is likely embolic; *Prototheca zopfii* organisms have been identified in glomerular capillaries, interstitial granulomas, and urine (eFig. 4-26).

Leptospirosis

Leptospirosis is a zoonotic disease caused by pathogenic spirochete bacteria of the genus *Leptospira*. The organisms are delicate, slender spirochetes (6-20 × 0.1 µm), with hooked ends like question marks, which led to the name *L. interrogans*. *Leptospirosis is particularly important as a cause of abortion and stillbirth in farm animals, but also causes acute disease (septicemia, hepatitis, nephritis, meningitis) in these and other species*. Many aspects of leptospirosis are poorly understood because of epidemiologic factors, difficulties in diagnosis, and the complexities of host-leptospiral relationships. Although generalizations are helpful, leptospirosis may best be understood in terms of the individual relationship between specific serovars and particular host species.

Several hundred serovars, based on outer lipopolysaccharide antigens, classified into ~20 antigenically related serogroups have been documented for *Leptospira* species. Unfortunately, neither serogroup nor serovar reliably predicts the species of *Leptospira*, because the same serogroup (i.e., shares some common antigenic determinants) or serovar (i.e., antigenically indistinguishable isolate) may occur within 2 or more species. Thus, some genetically unrelated leptospires can be antigenically identical. Serotyping is increasingly being replaced by restriction enzyme analysis of chromosomal DNA to identify *"genotypes."* Based on sequence composition, *Leptospira* species are grouped into 2 pathogenic subclades, P1 (pathogens 1, pathogenic species) and P2 (pathogens 2, intermediate pathogenicity), and 2 saprophytic subclades, S1 and S2. **P1 species**, which include *Leptospira interrogans*, *Leptospira borgpetersenii*, and *Leptospira kirschneri*, are most often implicated in canine leptospirosis. However, P2 species have also been associated with severe disease. The reader is referred to relevant microbiology textbooks and references for further detail on serotype and genotype classification of *Leptospira*. In addition, pathologists should refer to their regional diagnostic microbiology laboratory regarding common species and strains relevant for their cases.

Although many serovars are recognized globally, only a limited number are usually endemic to a particular region (Table 4-2). Geographic differences in the distribution of serovars are marked, but the true incidence and prevalence of leptospirosis are largely undetermined for most countries and regions. Serologic surveys tend to be flawed because antigens chosen may not represent serovars present in the country, because serologic prevalence does not necessarily indicate disease significance, because sampling is often done on the basis of convenience rather than in a carefully designed manner, and because titers designated as "significant" [usually ≥1:100 in the microscopic agglutination test (**MAT**)] may underestimate the true seroprevalence of some host-adapted serovars.

Each serovar is adapted to and may cause disease in particular *"maintenance" hosts*, although they may cause disease in other species, the *"incidental" hosts*. The general distinctions between these types of host are shown in Table 4-3. *The natural reservoir of pathogenic leptospires is the proximal convoluted tubules of the kidney and, in certain maintenance hosts, the genital tract.*

In maintenance hosts, transmission may be direct through contact with urine, postabortion discharges, milk, or through venereal or transplacental transmission. Infection of incidental hosts is often indirect, via environmental contamination with urine of carrier animals. Optimal conditions for survival of leptospires are moist, warm (optimal 28°C), and neutral or mildly alkalinized. Under ideal conditions, leptospires may survive weeks or months in waterlogged soil ("mud fever") or stagnant water. Under adverse conditions, survival is measured in minutes. *Leptospirosis thus occurs especially in the autumn in temperate climates ("fall fever") and in the winter in tropical climates.*

Leptospires penetrate exposed mucosal surfaces or water-softened skin and disseminate throughout the body. Leptospiremia lasts up to 7 days. Organisms multiply especially well in the liver, kidneys, lungs, placenta, udder, and cerebrospinal fluid. Development of agglutinating and opsonizing antibody ~6 days after infection clears the organisms from most organs except certain sites (e.g., proximal convoluted tubules of the kidney, cerebrospinal fluid, vitreous humor of the eye). Certain serovars can also survive in the genital tract of maintenance hosts.

Most leptospiral infections are supposedly subclinical, particularly in nonpregnant and nonlactating animals, and can only be detected by the presence of antibody or *minor lesions of interstitial nephritis at slaughter*. Infection may also cause *acute or subacute systemic disease* (i.e., nephritis, hepatitis, endotoxemia, hemoglobinuria) during the leptospiremic phase. After

Table • **4-2**

Common leptospiral serovars of disease significance in domestic animals

SEROVAR	MAINTENANCE HOST	DISTRIBUTION	SPECIES DISEASE SIGNIFICANCE
Autumnalis	Rodents	Asia, Americas	+ Possibly dogs
Bratislava	Pigs, horses (possibly dogs?)	Global Africa, Americas, Europe	+ + + + Pigs + + + Horses, dogs
Canicola	Dogs	Global Africa, Americas, Asia, Europe	+ + + Dogs + All species
Grippotyphosa	Raccoon, skunk, small rodents	Global	+ + Dogs + All species
Hardjo type Hardjo-bovis type Hardjoprajitno	Cattle, sheep Cattle	Global Global? (some exceptions)	+ + Cattle, sheep + + + Cattle, sheep
Icterohaemorrhagiae	Rats	Global? (some exceptions) Africa, Americas, Asia, Europe	+ + + Dogs, humans
Pomona type Kennewicki	Pigs	Global? (some exceptions)	+ + + + Pigs + + + Cattle, all species
Tarassovi	Wildlife, cattle, pigs	Europe, Australasia	+ + + Pigs

Table • 4-3

General distinctions between maintenance and incidental hosts in leptospiral infection

CHARACTERISTIC	MAINTENANCE HOST	INCIDENTAL HOST
Susceptibility to infection by the serovar	+ + + +[a]	+ +
Endemic transmission within host species	+ + + +	+
Pathogenicity for the host	+ +	+ + +
Type of disease caused	Chronic, reproductive loss especially, nephritis	Acute or chronic
Persistence in kidney	+ + + +	+
Persistence in genital tract	+ + + (Bratislava, Hardjo)	–
Microscopic agglutinating antibody response	Low titer, sometimes nil	High titer
Efficacy of vaccination in controlling losses	± to + + + +	+ + + +
Examples	Pig: Bratislava, Pomona; dog: Canicola	Pigs and cattle: Canicola, Grippotyphosa; cattle: Pomona

[a]Arbitrary scale for comparison.

leptospiremia has ceased, *chronic disease* can manifest as abortion, stillbirth, infertility, or recurrent uveitis.

Acute and severe disease can occur in the leptospiremic phase, particularly in young animals. Clinically, there may be fever, icterus, hemolytic anemia, hemoglobinuria, pulmonary congestion, or occasionally meningitis. Capillary injury is caused by inflammatory cytokine release. *Icterus* is a common manifestation of acute disease and might be the result of hemolysis from hemolysin production or because of toxic and/or ischemic hepatocellular injury. *Anemia* is initially the result of bacterial hemolysins but may later be the result of intravascular hemolysis caused by reaction of antibodies with leptospiral products coating erythrocytes. Localization of leptospires in the kidneys is associated with focal or diffuse *interstitial nephritis and acute, transient tubular injury*.

Progression of tubulointerstitial nephritis to tubular atrophy and fibrosis, as a consequence of chronic infection with Canicola and other serovars, can occur in dogs. This progression is not often described in other animals, even though active interstitial nephritis, especially in pigs, can be extensive. *Interstitial nephritis can be caused by all serovars*. Leptospires reach the kidney hematogenously and migrate randomly, persist briefly in the interstitium, and enter tubules at all levels of the nephron. Tissue invasion may be accomplished by corkscrew motion that may facilitate binding to vascular endothelial cadherin and weakening of endothelial cell barriers. Once antibodies develop, the leptospires localize to the proximal convoluted tubules, where they may multiply. The filtrate in the distal nephron damages leptospires; they are eliminated in that nephron segment. The *interstitial phase* is accompanied by marked vascular alterations that produce hyperemia, edema, and endothelial swelling. Tubular epithelial necrosis is likely the combined result of various factors, including hypoxia resulting from hypovolemia and hemolysis; bacterial toxins, including lipooligosaccharides and sphingomyelinases; free hemoglobin; and interstitial inflammation. Leptospiral antigen is demonstrable by IHC staining in tubular epithelial cell phagosomes. Minute, round, black spherical bodies can be seen with the Warthin-Starry stain. By 2 weeks, the tubular changes are accompanied by *interstitial infiltration of plasma cells and lymphocytes*. Leptospiral antigen is present in peritubular macrophages. The renal lesions may be clinically insignificant or might result in various degrees of CKD.

Alterations in expression of MHC class II may play a role in the development of interstitial nephritis in animals. In healthy dogs, the expression of MHC class II molecules is usually limited to interstitial dendritic cells. However, in dogs with chronic tubulointerstitial nephritis, tubular epithelial cells and peritubular capillary endothelial cells begin to express MHC class II molecules, attracting leukocytes. This spreading of MHC class II expression is not specific to cases of canine leptospirosis and can occur in other interstitial nephritides. Pigs seropositive for leptospirosis (with various patterns of nephritis) had MHC class II expression in interstitial histiocytes and lymphocytes as well as regenerating tubular epithelium. But colocalization of tubular MHC class II and leptospiral expression was not observed. This indicates that MHC class II contributes to renal inflammation and acts as a potential defense mechanism for renal tubular colonization. However, the lack of colocalization of MHC class II and leptospiral organisms suggests that the pathway for inciting inflammation remains ambiguous.

Abortion, stillbirth, or the birth of congenitally infected young may occur weeks to months after maternal leptospiremia and is the most important form of the disease in ruminants and pigs. Serovar Bratislava and serovar Hardjo may also cause infertility in swine and cattle, respectively. Horses are particularly likely to develop *recurrent uveitis* ("periodic ophthalmia") following serovar Pomona infection, but uveitis can develop in other species as well.

Leptospires do not stain with usual aniline bacterial dyes but may be stained by Giemsa or, in tissue, by silver impregnation techniques of Levaditi or Warthin-Starry. Dark-field microscopy of fluids is generally used in routine laboratory study. *Demonstration of leptospires by dark-field microscopy and silver staining of tissue sections are insensitive methods that give both false-negative and false-positive results*. IF of urine or of homogenates of tissues (e.g., fetal lung and kidney, or placenta) is an excellent detection technique, almost equivalent in sensitivity to isolation by experienced laboratorians. Difficulties may be experienced with serovar Bratislava because of the small size of these organisms. A number of PCR procedures are available, which generally are more reliable for urine than for tissues. Leptospires die readily in tissues or body fluids unless kept at 4°C. Results may be improved if tissues are submitted to laboratories in leptospiral transport medium.

Culture is expensive and often time consuming, and usually restricted to highly specialized laboratories. The *MAT*, which is serovar specific, and to some extent serogroup specific, has been a mainstay of diagnostic approaches and interpretation is often made by comparison of acute to convalescent titers. In the diagnosis of abortion, the MAT suffers sometimes from the low titers that may occur with host-adapted serovars in their maintenance host and also from difficulties in interpretation of titers. Titers may fail to rise between acute and convalescent phases because abortion may follow many weeks after infection in a maintenance host. In fetuses, MAT on fetal fluids is often a useful diagnostic approach, but dilutions should start at 1:10.

Cattle

The most severe (but uncommon) manifestation of acute leptospiral infection occurs in calves infected with incidental serovars, especially **Pomona**. Hemoglobinuria is usually the first clinical sign and may be transient. In fatal cases, the urine is a port-wine color. Hematuria from hemorrhage into renal tubules may lead to blood clots in the urinary tract. There is fever, anemia, icterus, dyspnea because of pulmonary congestion, and occasionally meningitis. Albuminuria and bilirubinuria can be severe. In cows, agalactia with small quantities of discolored, viscous milk is also typical. Abortion may occur during the acute phase or several weeks later during convalescence. The fetus is frequently decomposed, indicating death some time before abortion. Fetuses that are aborted in late stages of gestation might be icteric; stillborn fetuses might have petechiae in the thymus, heart, thyroid glands, lungs, mesentery, pleura, and peritoneum. In experimental leptospiral abortions, the only consistent lesion is that of renal tubular necrosis with lymphoplasmacytic and neutrophilic interstitial nephritis.

The most common form of the disease is a less severe, "subacute" form characterized in dairy cows by a 2-10-day drop in milk production with transient pyrexia. In this "milk drop syndrome," the milk has the consistency of colostrum, with thick clots and yellow discoloration, and the udder is soft. This form is commonly associated with serovar **Hardjo type Hardjoprajitno**, but may be caused by all serovars. Hemoglobinuria is uncommon in milder infections. The chronic form of the disease, most commonly associated with serovars **Hardjo** and **Pomona** in pregnant cows, is seen as abortion, stillbirth, or the birth of premature and weak infected calves as the result of fetal infection. The cow may have had an episode of illness up to 6 weeks (Pomona) or 12 weeks (Hardjo) earlier.

The postmortem appearance of an animal that dies of acute leptospirosis is one of mild icterus and severe anemia. Hemorrhages may be absent, or ecchymoses may be numerous on serous membranes and in the subcutis. The lungs are pale-pink and edematous, and the liver is enlarged, friable, pale tan-yellow, with or without hemorrhages and small zones of necrosis around central veins. Massive hepatocellular necrosis is not typical. Hemoglobinuria may or may not be present. The kidneys are swollen. Depending on the duration of clinical disease, their gross appearance ranges from diffusely dark red-brown (due to hemolysis in the early stages of disease), to pigment restricted to small groups of tubules resembling numerous small hemorrhages, to rather indistinct, small gray foci more numerous in the cortex than in the medulla.

It is doubtful that cattle die from chronic leptospiral interstitial nephritis. In animals that have recovered from the acute disease, foci of renal inflammation might be the only morphologic traces remaining. Although leptospiral infection has been implicated in the pathogenesis of "white-spotted kidneys" in neonatal calves, various studies have implicated other pathogens or excluded leptospires as an etiology.

The histologic changes in most cases of bovine leptospirosis may be mild and nonspecific. There may be mild multifocal pulmonary edema and periacinar hepatocellular necrosis (from anemia). Kupffer cells are increased in number and contain excessive amounts of hemosiderin. There is diffuse but mild cellular infiltration in the portal triads. In the uncommon infections caused by Icterohaemorrhagiae, necrosis in the liver and dissociation of hepatic cords may occur. Depending on the stage of the infection and degree of hemolysis, biliary canaliculi may contain bile plugs.

In acutely fatal disease, there are often marked degenerative changes in the epithelium of the cortical renal tubules. The changes vary in severity from acute cellular swelling to necrosis and desquamation. The detached epithelium forms granular and cellular casts, in addition to the protein, red blood cell, and pigment casts. There is also interstitial edema with mild diffuse infiltration of plasma cells and lymphocytes. *In acute disease, organisms can often be demonstrated by appropriate stains in the liver*, in which they are partly intracellular, *and in the kidneys*, in which they occur in the tubular epithelium and frequently as clusters in the tubular lumen.

After recovery from acute disease, and in subclinical illness, organisms localize in the kidneys and appear as *intratubular aggregates*; it is rare to find organisms in the interstitium. *There are widespread foci of interstitial nephritis*. The mononuclear inflammatory reaction is virtually confined to the cortex, and lymphocytes and plasma cells predominate. The reaction subsides slowly, and inflammatory cells decrease in number as the lesions scar. An odd feature of active lesions is an atypical regenerative pattern of tubular epithelium within the areas of inflammation wherein regenerating cells produce a few bizarre syncytia or a few giant cells.

Sheep, goats, and deer

Sheep, goats, and deer may be less susceptible than cattle to clinical leptospirosis. The major serovar in sheep is **Hardjo**, which has a maintenance cycle independent of cattle. Acute disease in lambs resembles that of calves and mainly causes renal discoloration at autopsy (Fig. 4-56A). Hardjo infection of ewes may cause late-term abortion, stillbirth, weak lambs, and agalactia. Leptospirosis in goats is not often described, but clinical and pathologic changes are similar to those described for cattle. Fatal nephritis of farmed young red deer caused by serovar Pomona has been described in New Zealand. Kidneys were markedly enlarged because of severe chronic active cortical interstitial nephritis.

Dogs

Dogs are susceptible to infection with a number of serovars, but those best recognized to cause severe diseases are **Canicola** and **Icterohaemorrhagiae**. Canicola is host maintained in the dog, but widespread use of vaccination has dramatically reduced incidence of disease attributable to this serovar as well as to Icterohaemorrhagiae. Icterohaemorrhagiae is generally acquired from rats, and other serovars (**Autumnalis, Bratislava, Pomona**) from their respective hosts. Serologic evidence of infection with serovar Bratislava has been associated with nephritis and abortion in dogs. It has been suggested that this serovar is host adapted to the dog, pig, and horse. Leptospirosis has resurged in urban dogs in northeastern North America and elsewhere, associated with Grippotyphosa, Pomona,

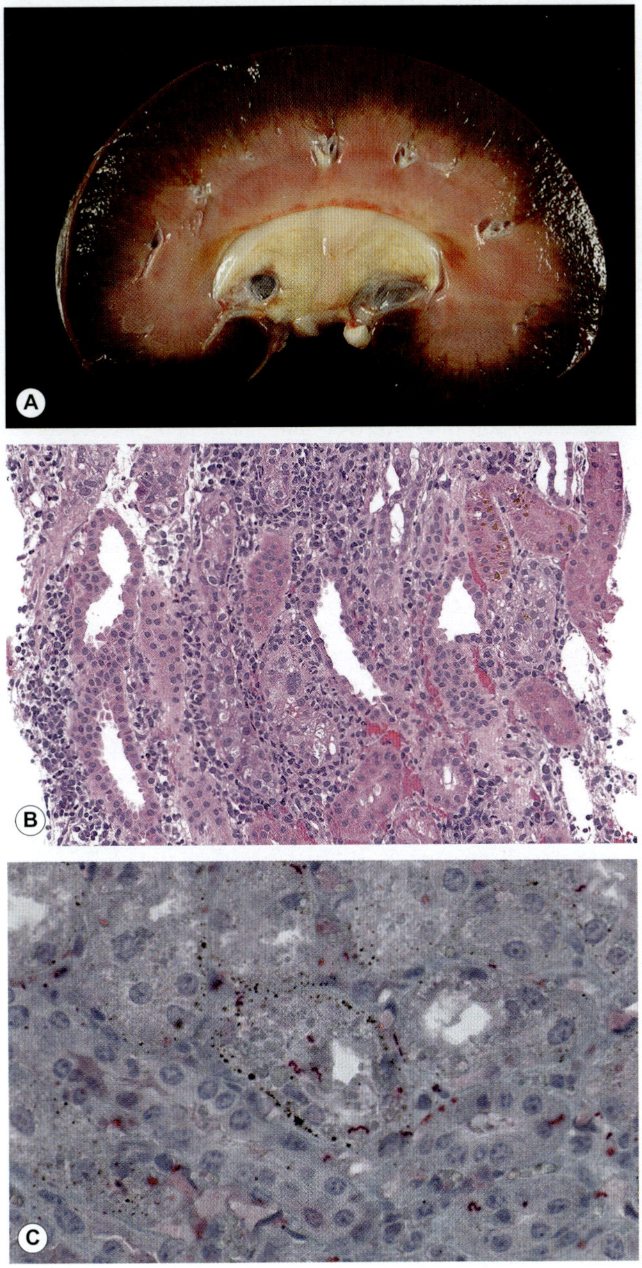

Figure 4-56 A. Kidney from a sheep with **leptospirosis**. (Courtesy K. G. Thompson.) B. Severe neutrophilic and histiocytic **tubulointerstitial nephritis** in a dog with acute leptospirosis. C. **Leptospires** in a bovine kidney. Immunohistochemistry. (Courtesy J. Ramsay.)

possibly Autumnalis, and rarely other serovars acquired from urban wildlife. Clinically normal dogs can shed pathogenic leptospires in urine, which may pose a zoonotic risk. Serologic testing is a poor predictor of urinary shedding. Current Canicola- and Icterohaemorrhagiae-based vaccines provide only serovar-specific protection.

As a generalization, Icterohaemorrhagiae exerts its effect predominantly on the liver, whereas Canicola damages the kidney, although there may be overlap in the clinical presentations. Other serovars can affect both organs, although disease is usually less severe.

Hyperacute infection, which is usually seen in puppies and caused by Icterohaemorrhagiae, causes fulminant septicemia; death occurs in a few hours to 2-3 days. There is fever, dehydration, hypersensitivity, hematemesis, melena, epistaxis, and petechiae on the mucous membranes. Icterus is usually absent in hyperacute infection; it is prominent in *acute disease* and may be the first abnormality observed. Fevers are usually mild.

Widespread hemorrhages characterize both the hyperacute and the acute disease. The most consistent gross lesions in acute cases consist of *subcapsular renal cortical hemorrhages*. With chronicity, these foci become pale-tan, and the capsule adheres to the cortex. Lesions in dogs given viable Canicola and killed 100 days later consisted of symmetrically enlarged kidneys with nodular and wedge-shaped 4-8-mm lesions at the corticomedullary junction. Lesions in the liver of dogs with spontaneous infections of Grippotyphosa vary from gross enlargement to fibrosis with nodular hyperplasia to atrophy.

In animals dying acutely, focal hepatocellular necrosis is often, but not always, present. *The characteristic change is dissociation of the cells of the hepatic cords, but this is not pathognomonic*. Dissociated cells are discrete and rounded with eosinophilic, coarsely granular cytoplasm, and pyknotic or karyorrhectic nuclear debris. Regeneration is sometimes prominent and evidenced by cytomegaly, binucleation, and mitoses. Kupffer cells contain excess hemosiderin, and many canaliculi contain bile plugs. Organisms can be demonstrated by appropriate techniques in sinusoids and in hepatic epithelial cells. Serovar Grippotyphosa may cause chronic active hepatitis, with peribiliary fibrosis, lobular disarray, and irregular fibrosis.

In dogs, there is usually concurrent renal and hepatic injury, but sometimes they are seen as solitary diseases. Clinical signs are those of *renal insufficiency* and vary in severity and progression. Death may occur rather rapidly from AKI. But some cases can apparently smolder over the course of years, eventually leading to CKD from interstitial nephritis, tubular atrophy, and fibrosis. In the acute phase, the renal changes are severe but are largely tubular injury rather than inflammation. The brunt of the injury is borne by the convoluted tubules, with epithelial changes ranging from acute cellular swelling to necrosis. The latter may be extensive enough to denude considerable areas of tubular basement membrane. In the course of a couple of days, regeneration begins and atypical syncytial giant cells may form (see Fig. 4-56B). This is accompanied by interstitial edema and a diffuse but sparse infiltration by lymphocytes and plasma cells. Leptospires are demonstrable in the tubular epithelium and in the lumens of tubules, frequently in clusters (see Fig. 4-56C). Early on, organisms may be found in any part of the cortex, but later they are restricted to superficial, subcapsular areas. Glomerular disease has been reported in Swiss dogs with acute severe disease. The glomerular lesion is diffuse, global exudation of fibrin, erythrocytes, and neutrophils, which obscures glomeruli. In addition to glomerular injury, there may be fibrinoid occlusion of afferent and efferent arterioles, interstitial hemorrhage, tubular necrosis, and interstitial nephritis. Comprehensive evaluation of the kidneys (with TEM and IF) was not performed in those cases, so the role of ICs is unknown.

With chronicity, the interstitial inflammation decreases and fibrosis increases. Glomerular capsules may be thickened, and there may be periglomerular fibrosis, although both lesions are nonspecific. Likewise, lesions in the renal medulla are nonspecific and include fibrosis with mild inflammation. Lymph nodes and spleen may be enlarged and edematous or hemorrhagic, and microscopically, there is depletion of lymphocytes and increase of sinusoidal reticular cells. Erythrophagocytosis is prominent.

Cats

Although clinical disease is rarely reported in **cats**, there is a wide range of seroprevalence, and cats can shed leptospires in their urine. Furthermore, there was a significant difference in seropositivity between cats with kidney disease (15%) and healthy cats (7%), suggesting a role of exposure in the pathogenesis of feline kidney disease. There was not a significant difference in PCR positivity, however. The most commonly detected serovars were **Pomona** and **Bratislava**. Additionally, liver lesions have been reported in association with feline leptospirosis and include chronic inflammation, fibrosis, and multifocal hepatic necrosis.

Swine

Although any leptospiral serovar may cause disease in pigs, the most important serovar recognized in North America is serovar **Pomona** (type **Kennewicki**), which is host adapted to swine. In Australia and some European countries, **Tarassovi** (formerly Hyos), another pig-adapted serovar, causes serious losses. The understanding of leptospirosis in swine has changed with the recognition of the widespread and dominant prevalence of antibodies to the Australis serogroup and the isolation of Bratislava and Muenchen from aborted and stillborn pigs. Only a small proportion of infected animals develop clinical illness, usually an unrecognized transient episode of mild fever, anorexia, and depression. Hemoglobinuria and icterus may occur rarely in piglets. The principal aspect of the disease in pigs, apart from transmissibility to other species, *is abortion and the birth of small litters of weak piglets*, which may reach outbreak proportions. This is particularly liable to occur if pregnant sows with no acquired immunity are exposed during the second month of pregnancy. Abortion is associated with heavy leptospiral infection of the fetus.

The usual pattern of leptospirosis in pregnant sows, caused by serovars other than those of the Australis serogroup, is for the litter to be delivered 1-3 weeks prematurely, with some of the fetuses dead and some born alive, only to die shortly afterward. Not all aborted fetuses in the litter will yield leptospires. The organism can usually be recovered from the fresher ones. Straw-colored pleural effusion, somewhat viscid, may be accompanied by effusion of lesser volumes in the other serous cavities. Petechial hemorrhages may be present in the pleura, epicardium, renal cortex, and peripelvic tissue, and occasionally elsewhere. The liver and spleen are swollen and dark, with tan 2-5-mm foci of necrosis, especially near the margins.

Histologic changes are also variable. Hepatitis is acute, consisting of neutrophils and lymphocytes in portal areas and surrounding the foci of coagulative necrosis. Focal mononuclear myocarditis with coagulative necrosis is less frequent than mild epicarditis and endocarditis. These latter mononuclear infiltrates can be quite diffuse. In addition to many minor foci of interstitial inflammation in the kidney, there may be large discrete infiltrates of mononuclear cells in the peripelvic parenchyma, sometimes involving the papilla and encroaching on the adjacent cortex. The medulla may contain myriad organisms. Infection with serovars belonging to the Australis serogroup produces subtler losses than those described for Pomona or other serovars, and lesions have not been described. In Northern Ireland and the United States, late-term abortion is uncharacteristic, but stillbirths occur, with the birth of live, dying, and dead piglets within a litter. Diagnosis is problematic because of the extreme difficulty of isolation of serovars Bratislava and Muenchen, but approaches include fetal and maternal serology, IF of fetal lung and kidney homogenates, and PCR-based detection.

A distinct *infertility ("repeat breeder") syndrome* is associated with Australis serogroup infection. Disease is most noticeable in sows bred to infected boars for the first time or when susceptible animals are introduced into infected herds. Serovars Bratislava and Muenchen are commonly isolated from the genital tracts of sows and boars in infected herds. Venereal transmission is thought to be common.

Most cases of chronic interstitial nephritis in pigs, which is often observed at slaughter, are thought to be leptospiral in origin, particularly associated with serovar Pomona.

Horses

There is widespread serologic evidence of leptospiral infection in horses, but acute disease is apparently rare. Clinical features include fever, anorexia, depression, and icterus (acutely) and abortion, premature foaling, and uveitis/periodic ophthalmia (chronically). Horses are maintenance hosts for **Bratislava**. In foals, leptospires are involved in fatal hepatic and renal disease. Acute respiratory distress and failure has been reported in foals and adults, wherein bronchoscopy reveals pulmonary hemorrhages.

Leptospires of a variety of serovars have been isolated or identified by IF in neonatal foals or adults with fatal icterus. Various serovars can also cause subacute disease, with fever, with or without icterus, in adults. Although of generally minor significance per se, these infections have important chronic sequelae in the form of abortion or chronic uveitis. In North America, serovars involved in *leptospiral equine abortion* are **Pomona, Grippotyphosa**, and **Bratislava**. Abortion tends to occur in late gestation. *Giant cell hepatitis in aborted fetuses* has been associated with leptospiral infection; the lesions included dissociation of hepatocytes, disruption of hepatic cords, and numerous large, multinucleate hepatocytes. The placenta is edematous with necrotic, mineralized villi, and cystic adenomatous hyperplasia of the allantoic epithelium. Leptospires can be demonstrated in the placental villi and stroma.

Recurrent uveitis may develop several months after leptospiral infection, particularly with serovar Pomona. There is a genetic predisposition for Appaloosas and German Warmbloods, with the MHC1 haplotype ELA-*A9* being at higher risk. Following an acute infection, there may be recurrent ocular disease with a thick hyaline membrane at the posterior iris, and the nonpigmented epithelial cells of the ciliary body can contain eosinophilic linear cytoplasmic inclusions. The inflammation can lead to cataracts, synechiae, lens luxation, and retinal detachment. Expression of the leptospiral proteins LruA and LruB in the eye, together with elevated antibodies against these proteins, has been demonstrated. Because the antibodies in the aqueous humor exceed serum antibody levels, local production is presumed. Furthermore, these antibodies can cross-react with normal ocular components. Specifically, LruA antibodies cross-react with α-crystalline B and vimentin, whereas LruB antibodies cross-react with β-crystalline B2.

Pyelonephritis

Pyelonephritis is inflammation of the pelvis and renal parenchyma (renal papilla or crest radiating toward the cortex), usually resulting from infection ascending from the lower urinary tract. Hematogenous pyelonephritis is extremely uncommon. Ascending pyelonephritis involves inflammation, necrosis, and eventually deformity of the calyces. The location distinguishes pyelonephritis from other forms of nephritis. It is usually accompanied by ureteritis and cystitis. In *acute pyelonephritis*, inflammation and necrosis predominate, with the pelvis and papilla or crest being more severely affected than the cortex. In *chronic pyelonephritis*, fibrosis replaces inflammation. In both cases, the disease can be asymmetrical within a kidney, and it can be unilateral or bilateral. Chronic pyelonephritis

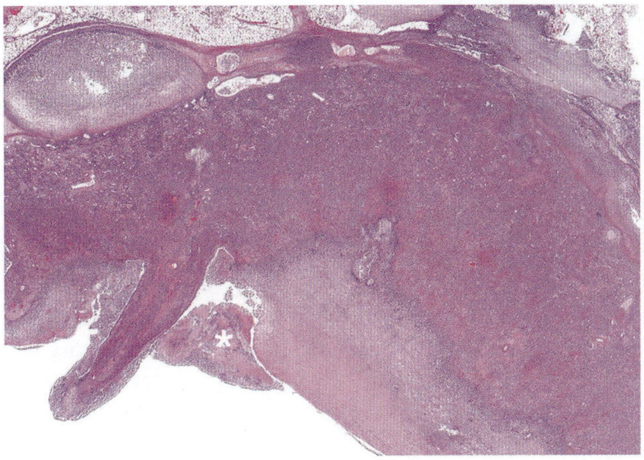

Figure 4-57 **Pyonephrosis** in a dog, which ruptured through the renal cortex to become a perinephric abscess. H&E.

produces irregular contracture of the kidneys with pelvic deformities. **Pyonephrosis** denotes severe suppuration of the kidney in the presence of complete or nearly complete ureteral obstruction; the infected hydronephrotic kidney is converted to a sac of pus. Suppuration may extend through the renal capsule during the course of pyelonephritis to produce a **perinephric abscess** (Fig. 4-57).

The pathogenesis of pyelonephritis begins with establishment of infection in the lower urinary tract. Organisms involved in UTI are usually endogenous bacteria of the bowel and skin, such as *Escherichia coli*, *Klebsiella*, staphylococci, streptococci, *Enterobacter*, *Proteus*, and *Pseudomonas*, and more specific urinary pathogens, such as *Corynebacterium renale*, *C. cystitidis*, and *C. pilosum* in cattle, and *Actinobaculum (Eubacterium) suis* in pigs. Mycoplasmas are rarely involved in cattle. Infections can be mixed. Fungal infections are rare causes of pyelonephritis in dogs.

Virulence of bacteria in the urinary tract is enhanced by the pili on their surface. For example, pili assist in adhesion of *C. renale* to urinary epithelium in a pH-dependent manner, and *C. renale* is an obligate parasite of urinary mucosae. The type of pili expressed by the bacteria can also be important later in the course of pyelonephritis. Regarding *E. coli*, uropathogenic varieties have the ability to survive in the urinary tract and are thus referred to as uropathogenic *E. coli* (UPEC). There is not a specific genetic marker of UPEC because there are many factors that can confer persistence in the urinary tract. One of these factors is cytotoxic necrotizing factor 1 (CNF1), which enables bacterial colonization of tissue. It stimulates cytokine production and enhances tissue invasion and injury. Hemolysin A is also an important virulence factor for UPEC; it can initiate apoptosis of host epithelial cells and macrophages. Type 1 fimbriate *E. coli* induce greater activation of neutrophils and hence more renal scarring than nonfimbriate or P-fimbriate *E. coli*.

One of the *urinary tract defenses* against bacterial infection and colonization is shedding of mature epithelial cells with attached bacteria. Normal voiding of urine helps maintain the sterility of the bladder. Once bacteria enter the bladder, they grow well in urine with low osmolality or alkaline pH. *Stasis of urine* is an important predisposing factor in the pathogenesis of cystitis and of pyelonephritis. Urinary obstruction (partial or complete) can be caused by ureteral anomalies in young animals, kinked ureters in pigs, pregnancy, urolithiasis, and prostatic hypertrophy. *Females are predisposed to UTI* because of their short urethras, more frequent urethral trauma, and possibly because of hormonal effects. Clinically, urinary infection is indicated by bloody or cloudy urine, pyuria, and/or bacteriuria.

Once infection is established in the bladder, probably the most significant mechanism in causing renal infection is **vesicoureteral reflux**. This retrograde flow of urine up the ureters and into the kidney *(intrarenal reflux)* during micturition may carry bacteria as far as the urinary space of glomeruli, especially if there is urinary obstruction. It can also occur during manual compression of the bladder in dogs and cats for collection of urine samples. Swine have a long intravesical ureter—5 mm at birth, 36 mm at maturity—that should prevent reflux in mature animals. Transient vesicoureteral reflux is common in puppies and is related to the immaturity of the ureterovesical junction, wherein pressure in the bladder overcomes the vesicoureteral valve. Reflux should decrease with age because the intravesical portion of the ureter lengthens and has a more oblique entry through the bladder wall. Vesicoureteral reflux of sterile urine does little renal damage, but the ureteral muscular layers may hypertrophy. Cystitis and mucosal edema may impede the valve function, leading to reflux in adult dogs. Importantly, vesicoureteral reflux is a clinical diagnosis based on contrast radiographs or advanced imaging. Positioning of the patient, especially dogs, may affect the clinician's ability to detect this phenomenon, wherein dogs in lateral recumbency may have reflux that is not repeatable when they are in a supine position. Movement of the urinary bladder with kinking of the ureters is the likely cause of this discrepancy.

Cystitis can alter normal ureteral peristalsis, perhaps causing reversed peristaltic waves. Hence, persistent pyelonephritis may result from vesicoureteral reflux, and possibly from reversed peristalsis in animals with cystitis. Progression of pyelonephritis probably depends on persistence of bacterial infection or bacterial antigens.

For a number of reasons, *the medulla is the part of the kidney most susceptible to infection*. It is relatively hypoxic because of the low hematocrit in vasa recta. Hypertonicity depresses the phagocytic activity of leukocytes, and ammonia may interfere with activation of the complement system. In pigs, the renal poles are more susceptible to intrarenal reflux and infection because the collecting ducts serving those lobes do not collapse as readily as do those of the central lobes when exposed to increased pelvic pressure. Bacterial invasion of the renal papilla progresses by way of the collecting ducts, as is suggested by lines of neutrophils along the straight tubules and the bacterial colonies within tubules. There can also be direct invasion across the eroded pelvic urothelium.

Pyelonephritis can be unilateral or bilateral; however, unilateral pyelonephritis will be clinically silent. A general description will be given of acute and chronic pyelonephritis before species differences are noted in more detail. **Acute disease** typically begins with necrosis and inflammation of the papilla or renal crest ("necrotizing papillitis") in an irregular pattern. Bacteria may be abundant in the collecting ducts. Associated wedge-shaped areas of parenchyma are swollen, dark-red, and firm. As hyperemia subsides, *neutrophilic tubulointerstitial nephritis and ATI* develop in radially distributed wedges. Tubules are obliterated by the inflammation, and neutrophils cross the tubular basement membrane to enter the tubular lumen (tubulitis; Fig. 4-58; eFig. 4-27). Leukocytic casts formed in the tubules may be found on urinalysis. Tubular dilation and obstruction are common.

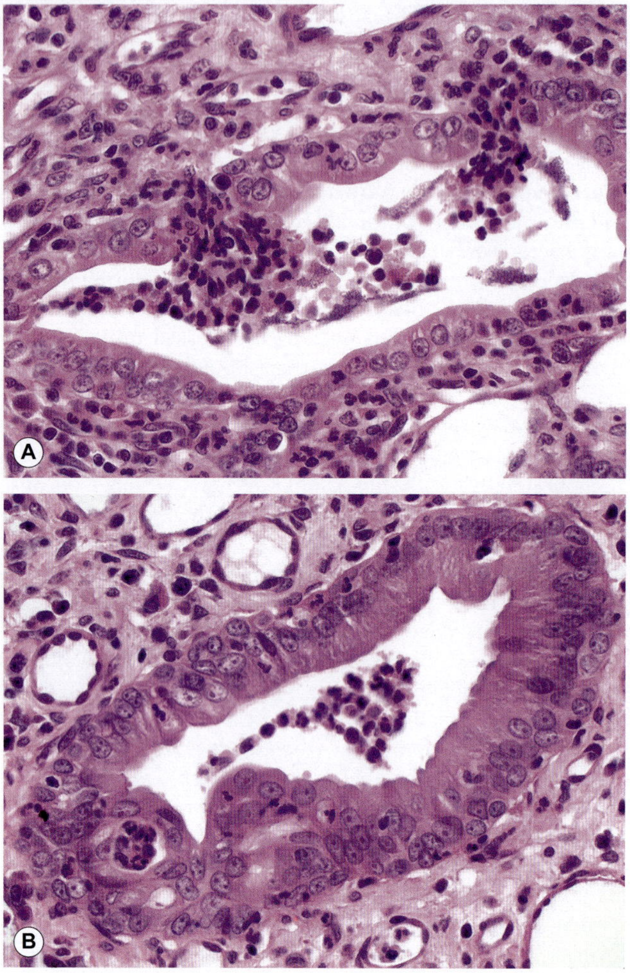

Figure 4-58 Acute pyelonephritis in a dog. **A**. Neutrophils cross the basement membrane of a collecting duct that contains cocci. **B**. Neutrophils might make microabscesses between tubular epithelial cells. H&E.

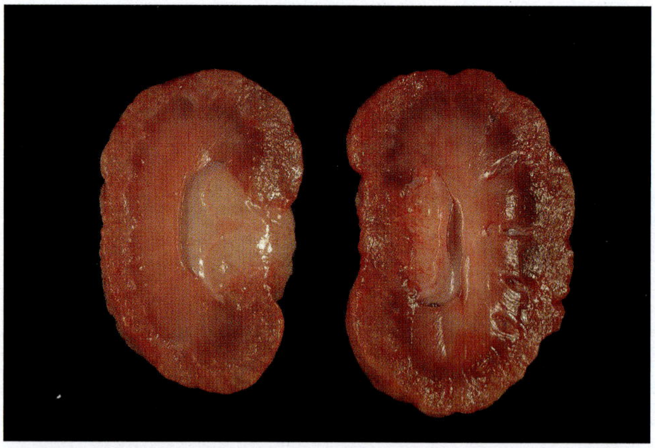

Figure 4-59 Chronic pyelonephritis in a dog. The renal parenchyma is scarred and atrophic. (Courtesy A. Koehne.)

Glomeruli, although initially uninvolved, may eventually be obliterated. As the process becomes **chronic**, mononuclear cells replace neutrophils, and fibrosis develops. Contraction of the scars results in deep, cortical depressions (Fig. 4-59). The *scars in pyelonephritis* extend from the pelvis to the capsule. They can be distinguished from those of other nephritides and infarcts by the fibrosis and deformation of the renal papilla. The calyces and pelves are dilated and often contain exudate and debris. Papillary defects may be subtle in mild cases. Generalized involvement of the kidney will produce a firm pale shrunken kidney with an irregular surface, and this will be difficult to differentiate from end-stage kidneys of other etiologies.

In **dogs** and **cats**, acute pyelonephritis can go undetected, but scars attributed to chronic pyelonephritis are common. In dogs, accumulation of colloid-like material in tubules and glomerular capsules dilated from scarring produces a thyroid-like histologic appearance, called "thyroidization." Calculi can form in the pelvis on the nidi provided by cellular debris. Neither thyroidization nor pelvic calculi are pathognomonic for pyelonephritis, however. In *emphysematous pyelonephritis*, an uncommon variant caused by gas-forming organisms in dogs and cats with diabetes, gas is present in the renal parenchyma, collecting system, or perinephric space.

In **swine**, acute pyelonephritis is seen occasionally, but chronic disease is rare. Shortening of the intravesical portion of the ureter and widening of the ureteric orifices occur in sows as a consequence of cystitis. This can facilitate vesicoureteral reflux and pyelonephritis. *Acute pyelonephritis occurs in sows postpartum or 3-4 weeks postbreeding.* Young males are occasionally affected, and some of these have urinary tract anomalies. Blood-stained urine or discharge can be seen, but it is not unusual for prostration and death to occur in 12 hours or so. Severe cystitis and ureteritis are usually present with yellow-brown or bloody mucoid exudate. The renal poles are preferentially involved, and the infection may be fulminant, erupting through the renal capsule to produce retroperitoneal hemorrhage and inflammation. Less severe disease is seen as pale-tan areas of leukocytic infiltration involving wedges or entire lobes. Swine kidneys have been documented to contain *E. coli* species that can colonize the human intestinal tract and eventually cause UTI in humans. In one study, kidneys were harvested at slaughter from 24 clinically healthy pigs: 12 had gross renal lesions and 12 did not. Histologically, all kidneys had evidence of pyelonephritis, and *E.coli* was cultured from all of them. They all expressed CNF1, which is one of the commonly expressed virulence factors of UPEC. This study suggests that pyelonephritis due to UPEC is likely common in swine, even in those that appear clinically healthy.

In **cattle**, pyelonephritis is a significant sporadic disease. Unilateral pyelonephritis is as common as bilateral disease, which means that many animals are not azotemic. Neutrophilic destructive papillitis may predominate; tubulointerstitial nephritis may be minimal. The medulla of each lobe might be destroyed. Eventually, the cortex remains as a narrow capsule surrounding large amounts of pus in the calyces. Alternatively, a pattern of radially distributed tubulointerstitial nephritis can be the main histologic pattern (eFig. 4-28). The kidney may have a granular surface because of interstitial inflammation and fibrosis. Rupture of the kidney occurs in males with bacterial-associated obstructive urolithiasis, but it is less common in cattle than in swine. Pyelonephritis is uncommon in **sheep**. Pyelonephritis is also uncommon in **horses**; but it can cause life-threatening hematuria that requires transfusion and may recur intermittently.

Hypercalcemic nephropathy

Hypercalcemia may be sufficiently severe to cause azotemia (hypercalcemic nephropathy) in dogs and cats.

- A common cause *is hypercalcemia of malignancy, or pseudo-hyperparathyroidism,* a paraneoplastic syndrome. Lymphoma and adenocarcinoma of the apocrine glands of the anal sac can stimulate bone resorption via production of parathyroid hormone–related protein (PTHrp), a peptide that resembles PTH (see Vol. 3, Endocrine Glands and Vol. 3, Hematolymphoid System). Hypercalcemia of malignancy is less commonly caused by osteolytic neoplasms.
- Poisoning by *rodenticides containing vitamin D* (0.075% cholecalciferol) is an important cause of hypervitaminosis D and hypercalcemia in dogs and cats. The same syndrome follows ingestion of *human antipsoriatic preparations* that contain synthetic vitamin D analogues, for example, calcipotriol and tacalcitol. Diagnosis of cholecalciferol rodenticide poisoning may be aided by determination of the renal 25-hydroxyvitamin D (25(OH)D_3) concentration. The renal calcium:phosphorus ratio is <0.1 in normal dogs, but 0.4-0.9 in cholecalciferol-poisoned dogs.
- Hypercalcemia can also be seen in primary hyperparathyroidism, CKD with secondary hyperparathyroidism, and hypoadrenocorticism.
- Hypercalcemia resulting in nephrocalcinosis and mineralization of other soft tissues is well known in grazing animals that ingest plants containing vitamin D_3 sterol (e.g., *Solanum glaucophyllum, Cestrum diurnum, Trisetum flavescens, Medicago sativa)*.

Hypercalcemia results in inactivation of adenylyl cyclase, and hence decreased cAMP formation. Sodium transport is impaired in the ascending limb of the loop of Henle, the distal tubule, and collecting ducts, resulting in natriuresis. Hypercalcemia also interferes with ADH receptors in the collecting ducts, leading to nephrogenic diabetes insipidus. The resultant polyuria and compensatory polydipsia are reversible if the primary cause of the hypercalcemia is removed. If hypercalcemia persists, *progressive renal mineralization* occurs, beginning with basement membranes of tubules and glomerular capsules, particularly in the outer zone of the medulla (Fig. 4-60) and eventually involving the interstitium, vessels, and glomeruli. Tubular epithelial mineralization and cast formation cause tubular obstruction and eventually loss of nephrons. These latter lesions are irreversible.

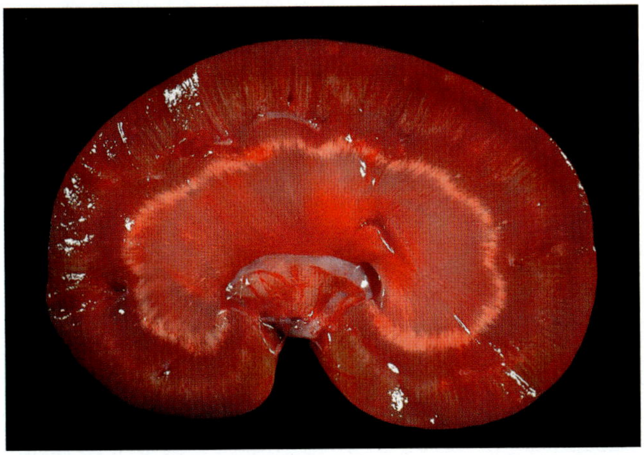

Figure 4-60 Hypercalcemic nephropathy in a dog. (Courtesy J. Grieves, P. Stromberg.)

Other less significant examples of renal mineralization also occur. The deposition of calcium salts in the form of clumps of granules in the lumen and basement membrane of collecting ducts and in the adjacent interstitium is rather common. They are associated with hypomagnesemia in some species and are not considered to be significant.

Mineralization is very common in dogs and cats, but unusual in other species. Cellular casts, injured epithelium, and basement membranes can mineralize quickly (eFig. 4-29). In uremia, glomeruli and small blood vessels may also be mineralized. Renal mineralization is a frequent result of *secondary hyperparathyroidism* induced by chronic renal insufficiency and coexists with similar deposits in the lungs, gastric mucosa, and other organs (discussed above). Dogs fed a high-phosphorus diet similarly develop diffuse renal mineralization.

Miscellaneous interstitial lesions

Extramedullary hematopoiesis occurs in the kidneys of dogs under a variety of circumstances, all of which probably have a common denominator of bone marrow suppression or increased peripheral demand for leukocytes. When the kidneys are sites of hematopoiesis, the liver, lymph nodes, spleen, adrenals, and lungs are usually also involved. Pronounced hematopoiesis can occur in canine pyometra.

Bone occasionally develops in the urinary tract, for example, following urinary tract surgery or in hydronephrotic kidneys. Urothelium stimulates transformation of mesenchymal cells to osteoblasts (eFig. 4-30).

Renal telangiectasia occurs in cattle, dogs, cats, mink, and ferrets; it is familial in Pembroke Welsh Corgis and Golden Retrievers (eFig. 4-31). It is a rare cause of hematuria in dogs.

Parasitic lesions in the kidneys

Toxocara canis

The most common parasitic lesion in the kidneys is a focal scar secondary to *Toxocara canis* larval migration in canine kidneys. These 2-3-mm granulomas are found in the cortical parenchyma. Early lesions are gray-yellow with soft centers; later, they become firm and white, and the superficial ones cause dimpling of the cortex. *Each granuloma surrounds an entrapped larva,* which may be hard to find in histologic sections (eFig. 4-32). Healing occurs after death and removal of the larvae. Residual scars typically consist of dense concentrically arranged fibrous tissue. Similar lesions are produced in calves by the migratory larvae of *T. cati* and *T. canis* acquired by fecal contamination of feed, and by *T. vitulorum*, especially in buffalo.

Stephanurus dentatus

Stephanurus dentatus is the kidney worm of swine. It is widely distributed in tropical and subtropical countries, and the prevalence in grazing swine can be very high. *The worms encyst in perirenal fat and adjacent tissues, and the cysts communicate with the renal pelvis.* The life cycle of *S. dentatus* can be direct or involve earthworms as transport hosts; the latter mechanism has not been shown to occur naturally. Eggs are passed in the urine of the pig, and the larvae hatch in 2-3 days. Infective stages are vulnerable to sunlight and drying. Infection may occur by penetration through the skin or by ingestion, and prenatal infections occur. Following oral infection, third-stage larvae migrate from the small and large intestine via the portal circulation and mesenteric lymphatics to the liver. A few migrate across the peritoneal cavity. After skin infection, most larvae migrate to the lungs and reach the intestines following

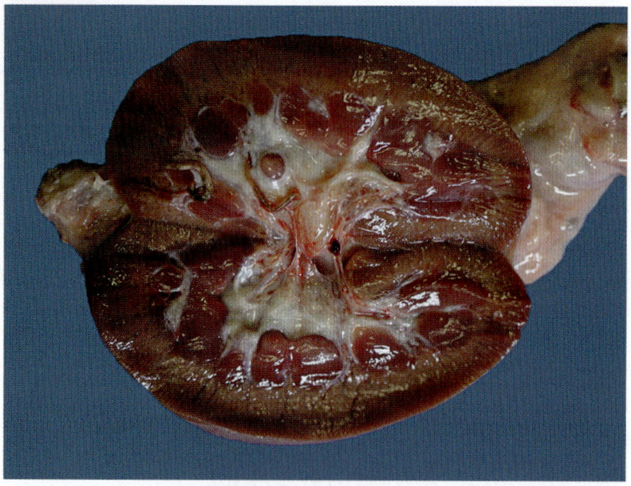

Figure 4-61 Encysted ***Stephanurus dentatus*** in the hilus of a porcine kidney. (Courtesy O. Illanes.)

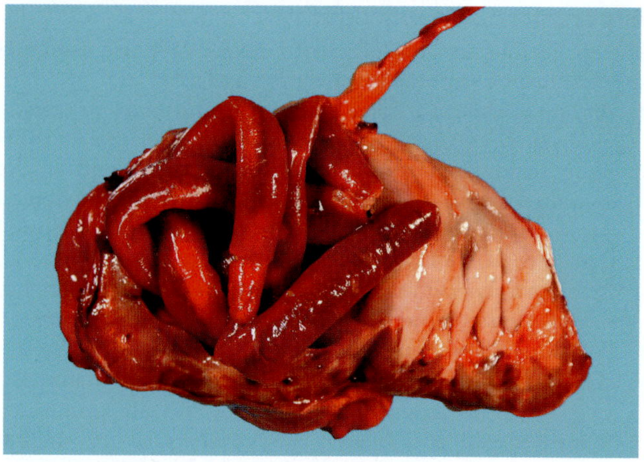

Figure 4-62 Adult ***Dioctophyme renale*** within the kidney of a dog. (Courtesy B. Lillie.)

tracheal migration. Deaths resulting from peritonitis and intestinal intussusception occur in some pigs 20-30 days after heavy infections. These are associated with larval migration from the mesenteric nodes to the liver. Infective larvae may migrate in the liver for several months. Hepatic migrations can cause severe hepatitis, with lesions similar to, but often more severe than, those produced by *Ascaris suum* larvae. *S. dentatus* also produces portal phlebitis with thrombosis in some pigs (see Vol. 2, Liver and Biliary System). The liver is usually enlarged and may be very firm. The lobulation is enhanced by perilobular fibrosis. Lobules may be obliterated by contracting and proliferating scar tissue in the portal areas.

Many larvae are destroyed in the liver by encapsulation in small abscesses. *From the liver, the larvae migrate across the peritoneal cavity to the perirenal region.* Many become encysted in abscesses in adjacent tissue, especially the pancreas. It is not unusual for some to invade the vertebral canal causing paraplegia. The definitive site is the tissue around the renal pelvis and ureter, wherein the adults encyst (Fig. 4-61; eFig. 4-33). Occasionally, cysts may be found in the kidney itself. The cysts communicate with the lumen of the ureter, allowing escape of eggs. Developmental stages in the definitive host take a long time, and patent infections may not be established for 9 months or more. Mature females may lay eggs for 3 years or longer.

Dioctophyme renale

Dioctophyme renale is the *giant kidney worm*, the largest of parasitic nematodes. It has a worldwide distribution, but its incidence is unknown. The worm is red and cylindrical, and adult females are 20-100 cm long and 4-12 mm diameter. Males are 14-45 cm long and 4-6 mm diameter. *D. renale* is usually found in dogs, mink, cats, and other fish-eating mammals, but has been reported in the pig, ox, and horse. Definitive hosts are wild fish-eating carnivores, especially mink, in which the worms are smaller and usually located in the kidney.

The life cycle involves 2 aquatic intermediate hosts. Eggs passed in the urine are resistant to the external environment and may survive for 2-5 years. Embryonation requires 1-7 months, depending on the climate. Embryonated eggs are ingested by the intermediate hosts, which are aquatic oligochaetes ("mud worms"; *Lumbriculus variegatus*), and develop through first and second larval stages. Third- and fourth-stage larvae can either develop directly in the worm or within fish or frog intermediate hosts, for example, the northern black bullhead *[Ameiurus (Ictalurus) melas]* and green frog *[Lithobates (Rana) clamitans]*. Following ingestion by mammals, infective third- or fourth-stage larvae penetrate the gut wall and migrate across the peritoneal cavity to the kidney. The life cycle from egg to adult requires 3.5-6 months, but may take up to 2 years.

Adult worms live in the renal pelvis but may also encyst in a body cavity, the uterus, mammary gland, or bladder (Fig. 4-62; eFig. 4-34). Adults are very destructive in the kidney, causing hemorrhagic pyelitis that becomes neutrophilic. The renal parenchyma is then progressively destroyed until the renal capsule only contains the worm and exudate.

Dogs are regarded as abnormal hosts because only one or a very small number of worms is present, worms of both sexes are found in only about one-third of infections, and most infections are not patent. *Intrarenal parasites in dogs and mink are more common in the right kidney than in the left kidney.* In ~60% of infected dogs, parasites are only in the peritoneal cavity. *D. renale* may encircle a lobe of the liver, causing infarction or rupture with or without hemoperitoneum. Simultaneous renal and peritoneal infections occur in ~15% of dogs.

Pearsonema plica

Pearsonema (Capillaria) plica may be found in the lumen of the renal pelvis, ureter, or urinary bladder of dogs, foxes, and smaller carnivores. Although widely distributed, it is uncommon. The life cycle is not clearly known but is probably indirect, with earthworms as intermediate hosts. Ingestion of earthworms from infected premises causes patent infections in 61-68 days. Pathologic effects are not usually attributed to *P. plica* infection, but hematuria and dysuria are occasionally seen. Worms embedded in the bladder, ureter, or pelvis may invoke mild submucosal inflammation.

Other species of *Pearsonema* occur in the urinary bladder of other animals—*P. mucronata* in mink and *P. feliscati* in the cat; the latter may be the same as *P. plica*. Light infestations are common but harmless. At most, the rostral end of the worm embedded in the surface layer of epithelium may incite mild submucosal inflammation.

Klossiella equi

Klossiella equi is an *apicomplexan parasite of the kidney of the horse and its relatives*, including the zebra, donkey, and burro.

Infections are usually incidental. The life cycle is not fully known. It is thought that after infection with sporocysts from the environment, sporozoites are released and enter the circulation. One schizont generation develops in glomerular endothelium and another in proximal tubular epithelium. Sporogony occurs in the epithelium of the thick ascending limb of the loop of Henle (Fig. 4-63), and sporocysts may be passed in the urine. Heavy infections can result in rupture of tubules and lymphoplasmacytic interstitial nephritis.

Granulomas may be found in the renal pelvis in **schistosomosis** of cattle and sheep (see Vol. 3, Cardiovascular System) and larvae of ***Setaria digitata*** may produce granulomas in the bladder of cattle in Asia (see Vol. 2, Alimentary System).

Halicephalobus gingivalis

Halicephalobus gingivalis (formerly *Micronema deletrix)* is a saprophagous nematode that produces granulomatous masses in the nasal cavity of horses and is occasionally responsible for cerebral vasculitis and granulomatous nephritis. Granulomas contain numerous larval and adult female rhabditiform nematodes and embryonated eggs. Urine and semen of infected horses may also contain various life stages of the parasites (Fig. 4-64).

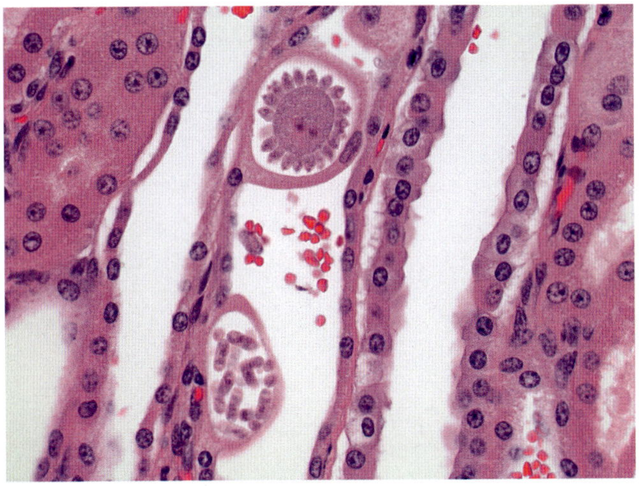

Figure 4-63 ***Klossiella equi*** in tubular epithelial cells of an equine kidney.

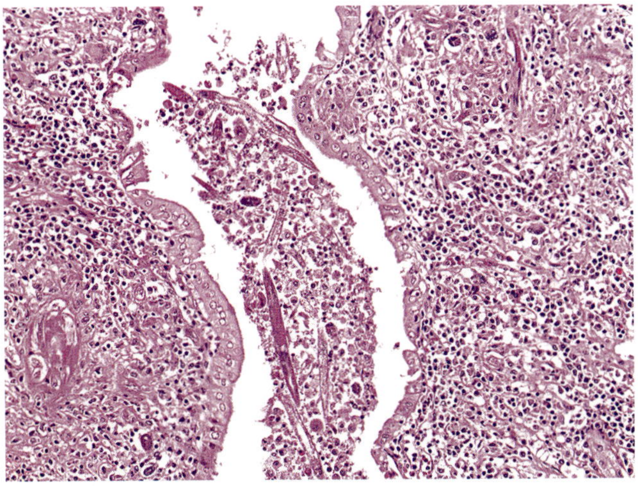

Figure 4-64 ***Halicephalobus gingivalis*** nematodes in a tubule of an equine kidney with associated marked pyogranulomatous inflammation.

RENAL NEOPLASIA

Primary renal tumors are uncommon. One abattoir survey in the United Kingdom found 8.5, 0.9, and 4.3 cases per million animals in cattle, sheep, and pigs, respectively. Renal tumors were found in ~0.15% of horses in 2 large surveys. Primary renal tumors comprise about 1% of all canine neoplasms and 1.5-2.5% of feline neoplasms. In one large retrospective study of primary canine renal neoplasms, most were of epithelial origin (85%), metastasized, and had an associated poor prognosis (mean survival 6.8 months). A separate study reported that of 82 dogs diagnosed with primary (nonlymphoma) neoplasia, 60% were carcinomas, 34% were sarcomas, and 6% were nephroblastomas. Notably, because the proximal tubules were initially metanephric mesenchymal tissue, they can sometimes have a spindle-cell phenotype. Some renal cell carcinomas (RCCs) therefore will have regions with a sarcomatoid morphology. These sarcomatoid RCCs have been observed in dogs, cats, and rodents. The literature discussing the incidence of renal neoplasia might be skewed if samples are small, and IHC is not performed.

The vast majority of renal neoplasia is metastatic to the kidney, by hematogenous or lymphatic spread or by direct extension. The following is an overview of primary renal neoplasia.

Renal adenoma

Renal adenomas are rare; they are said to occur more often in cattle and horses than in other species. In dogs, they comprise ~3% of primary renal epithelial tumors, based on compilations of various studies and review of the data from the Veterinary Medical Database. Adenomas are usually incidental autopsy findings. Renal adenomas arise from tubular epithelium. Grossly, they tend to be solitary nodules, <2 cm diameter but occasionally are larger (Fig. 4-65). Neoplastic cells are cuboidal with moderate-to-abundant eosinophilic cytoplasm. They form solid sheets, papilliform or tubular structures, and stromal tissue is scant. Tumors with mixed architectural patterns occur. Histologic differentiation of adenoma and renal carcinoma is sometimes impossible, requiring serial sections to look for evidence of invasion. Some adenomas might be histologically indistinguishable from well-differentiated carcinomas.

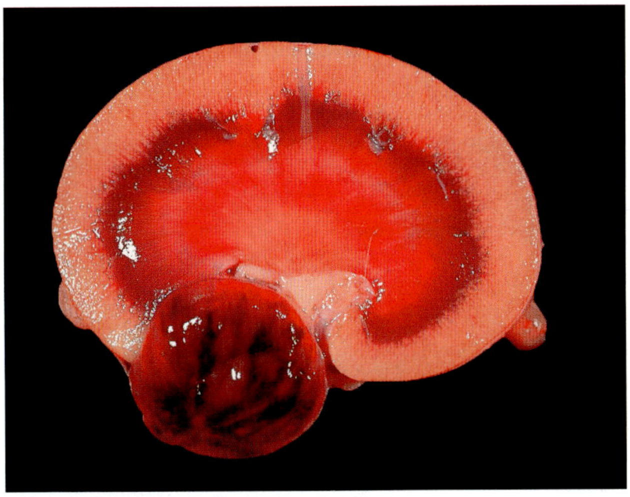

Figure 4-65 **Renal adenoma** in a cat. Incidental finding. (Courtesy N. Vapniarsky.)

Renal carcinoma

Renal cell carcinomas (RCCs) are the most common primary renal tumors of dogs, cats, cattle, and horses. There are only sporadic reports in sheep and pigs. These tumors occur in mature and old animals; thus, their incidence is relatively low in some species. The average age of affected dogs is ~8 years, although this tumor has been reported in dogs <2-years-old. Males are affected about twice as often as females. This is in contrast to the overwhelming higher occurrence in cows, likely because of a preponderance of females in the aged cattle population. Common presenting signs are hematuria, palpable abdominal mass, and weight loss. Polycythemia caused by excessive erythropoietin production is rarely seen in animals, although paraneoplastic erythrocytosis occurs in 1-5% of humans with RCC. Hypertrophic osteopathy may be seen in cases of RCC with pulmonary metastases. Disseminated intravascular coagulation, extreme neutrophilic leukocytosis, leukemoid blood response, and bone infarcts are additional rare paraneoplastic syndromes in dogs. Leukocytosis has been associated with synthesis of granulocyte-macrophage colony-stimulating factor by neoplastic cells.

Grossly, RCCs are spherical or ovoid masses, typically located in one pole of the kidney. Usually, they are well demarcated from the remainder of the kidney, which is atrophic and compressed. The tumor may be much larger than the original size of the kidney. The mass is usually gray or light yellow, often with darker areas of necrosis and hemorrhage (Fig. 4-66). Invasion of the renal pelvis, ureter, renal vein, and hilar lymphatics may be visible.

In humans, the types of RCC are recognized based on neoplastic cell morphology and organization and include clear cell and papillary RCCs, both arising from the proximal tubule, and chromophobe RCC and oncocytoma, both arising from the collecting duct, as well as other less common variants. Biallelic loss of the von Hippel-Lindau *(VHL)* gene has been documented in a majority of human clear cell RCCs, but sequence analysis of *VHL* exons in canine RCC has not revealed mutations.

Histologically, cell types and architectures vary, and there is often a mix of clear cells, poorly stained chromophobe cells, and eosinophilic cells. They may be arranged in sheets, papillary or tubular structures (Fig. 4-67; eFig. 4-35), and occasionally, they line small cystic spaces. As stated above, rare tumors in cats and dogs will have foci that have a sarcomatoid appearance intermixed with regions with a more typical RCC architecture. All of these patterns may occur in a single tumor, and the various patterns have not been associated with specific prognoses in veterinary species. A meta-analysis of 21 studies of canine RCC included 258 tumors. Papillary RCC and tubular RCC were the most common histologic phenotypes, each representing ~33% of cases. Solid RCC accounted for 24% of the tumors. RCCs with mixed patterns and cystic renal carcinomas were less common, all representing <6% of cases. Mitotic count was prognostically significant in a study of 70 canine RCCs, which reported a median survival time of 187 days if the mitotic count was >30 in 10 hpf (~2.4 mm^2). This was significantly shorter than dogs with a mitotic count <10 in 10 hpf (which was >1,100 days). The median survival time for dogs with an intermediate mitotic count (10-30) was ~450 days.

Immunohistochemistry and lectin staining can help distinguish cell of origin because there are segment-specific patterns within the various levels of the nephron. Normal canine proximal tubules stain positively for CD10 and pancytokeratins; normal distal convoluted tubules coexpress vimentin, cytokeratin, and uromodulin (i.e., Tamm-Horsfall protein). Additionally, IHC for cytokeratins AE1/AE3 labels normal distal convoluted tubules as well as collecting ducts. Although uncommonly used, lectin stains that can label the distal portion of the nephron include: *Dichloros biflorus* agglutinin, peanut agglutinin, and *Ulex europaeus* agglutinin I.

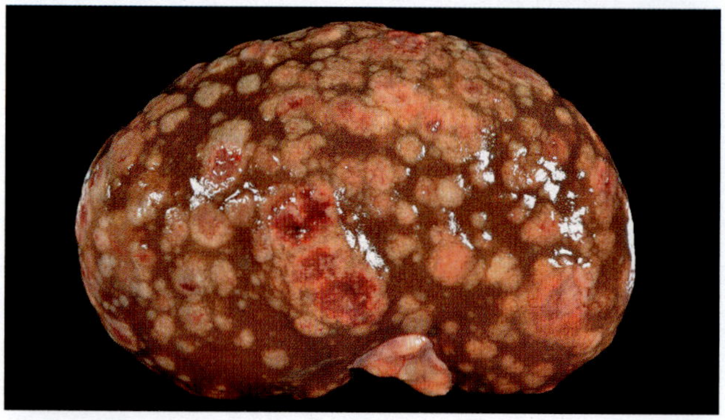

Figure 4-66 Renal carcinoma with intrarenal metastasis in a dog. (Courtesy E. Clark, P. Stromberg.)

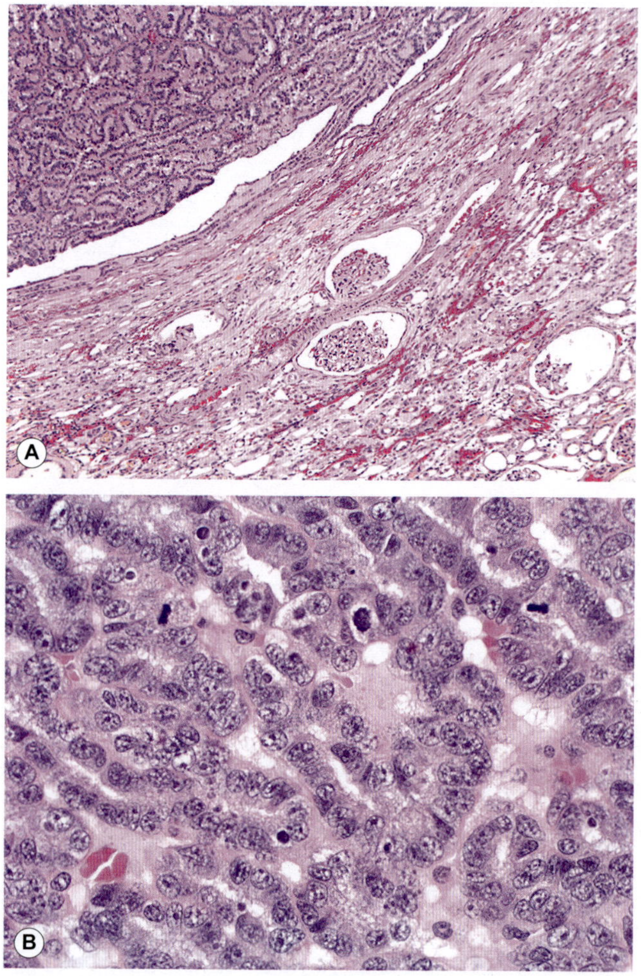

Figure 4-67 A, B. Renal cell carcinoma in a dog compressing adjacent parenchyma and consisting of tubules and ducts. H&E.

A study of 13 canine RCCs reported that all expressed uromodulin and thus arose from the distal segment of the nephron. Other studies have shown that canine RCCs often express vimentin and some coexpress vimentin and cytokeratins. This supports the theory that canine RCC is more commonly derived from the distal portion of the nephron, likely the distal convoluted tubule. Papillary, tubulopapillary, and cystic carcinomas frequently express cytokeratins; solid carcinomas (with sheetlike arrangements of neoplastic cells) are usually cytokeratin negative. Expression of CD10, a marker for proximal tubules, is sporadic in canine RCCs, but cKIT is expressed in most cases. This staining pattern is in contrast to that of human RCCs, with frequent CD10 and absent cKIT expression. Taken together, these data suggest that many canine RCCs arise from a different segment of the nephron than do human RCCs.

IHC can also be useful in confirming the epithelial origin of sarcomatoid RCC by showing cytokeratin expression in spindle cells. An additional IHC stain that can support the epithelial origin of some spindle cell tumors in the kidney is PAX8. This is a transcription factor expressed in the nuclei of canine RCCs of both proximal and distal tubular origins. In normal canine kidneys, PAX8 is expressed in tubular epithelial cell nuclei of canine cortical and medullary tubules (the literature does not state which specific segments) as well as in some parietal epithelial cells of glomerular capsules. In normal cat kidneys, PAX8 has strong expression in the loop of Henle, as well as expression in some cortical tubules. Therefore, positive IHC labeling of cytokeratins, vimentin, and PAX8 supports a diagnosis of RCC (eFig. 4-36), even if the cellular morphology resembles a mesenchymal neoplasm.

Last, IHC can provide prognostic information, although not used routinely in diagnostic cases (Table 4-4); the literature regarding these IHC markers is retrospective in nature. Positive IHC labeling of 14-3-3σ in canine RCCs was associated with a shorter survival time. This is an oncoprotein that has been identified in other canine cancers, but it is not expressed by normal tubular epithelial cells. Cox2 expression in RCCs is also associated with worse outcomes.

The stroma of RCCs is scant but highly vascularized, which predisposes to the extensive hemorrhage often seen grossly. Microvascular density (calculated as the mean number of vessels per mm^2 of tissue) was significantly higher in canine RCCs compared with normal renal parenchyma, and these cases demonstrated VEGF expression, whereas control dogs did not. Although IHC staining revealed the expression of VEGF in both tumor cells and cells surrounding the tumor, there was no colocalization of VEGF expression and increased microvascular density. Two other possible angiogenic mediators, TNF and HIF1α, were also evaluated in the same study, but neither showed a statistically significant association with microvasculature. Regarding metastatic disease, satellite nodules can develop in the kidney.

Table • 4.4

Immunohistochemical markers for normal kidneys and for neoplasms

	CANINE				
	NEOPLASM				
MARKER	RCC (n = 13)	NEPHROBLASTOMA	INTERSTITIAL CELL TUMOR	ONCOCYTOMA[a]	NON-NEOPLASTIC, NORMAL RENAL TISSUE
CD10	3/13 + variable exp				PT
KIT	12/13+				DCT
Vimentin[b]	11/13 VM+[c]; 7/13 VM+/CK+	+	+	–	DCT
Cytokeratin[b]	9/13CK+[d] 7/13 VM+/CK+	+ (glomeruloid and tubular epithelium)	–	+	PT (panCK); DCT, CD (AE1/AE3)
PAX8[b]	+nuclear				CT, MT, parietal epithelial cells (nuclear)
CEA	7/13+ [all 3 solid RCCs moderate CEA+)				
Uromodulin (Tamm-Horsfall protein)	13/13+				DCT
Lectin stains[e]					DN
14-3-3 σ oncoprotein	+=shorter survival				–

Continued

Table • 4-4

Immunohistochemical markers for normal kidneys and for neoplasms—cont'd

CANINE					
	NEOPLASM				NON-NEOPLASTIC, NORMAL RENAL TISSUE
MARKER	RCC ($n = 13$)	NEPHROBLASTOMA	INTERSTITIAL CELL TUMOR	ONCOCYTOMA[a]	
COX2	+=worse outcomes		+		
VEGF	+				
Wilms tumor 1		+			
GFAP		–		–	
Histochemical stain PAS			+	+ (mitochondria)	

FELINE						
	NEOPLASM			NON-NEOPLASTIC, NORMAL RENAL TISSUE		
MARKER	RCC	SARCOMATOID RCC[f]	ONCOCYTOMA[g]	NORMAL DCT	NORMAL PT	UROTHELIAL CELLS AND CD
Cytokeratin AE1/AE3	$n = 20$ + 11/11+	–	+	+		+
Vimentin	$n = 19/20$ +, 10/11	1/1+	–	+		
PAX8	$n = 19/20$+			Loop of Henle and some CTs (cat).		
KIT	12/20+	1/1–		+		+
CD10	15/20+	1/1+			+	
CK7	9/11	1/1–				+
CK20	10/11+	1/1–		+		+
AQP1	Solid anaplastic $n = 1$ +	$n = 1$+			+	
EMT-related markers						
E-cadherin	+	+				
B-catenin	+(cytoplasmic)	+ (nuclear)				
Twist	1/6+	+				
Twist w/beta-catenin in nuclei	–	+				
N-cadherin	3/6+	+				
SMA	–	+				
Desmin	–	–				

[a]IHC: desmin, vimentin, GFAP, S-100, lysozyme, alpha 1-antichymotrypsin negative. Oncocytoma in a Greyhound (Buergelt CD, 2000).
[b]Immunopositivity for cytokeratins, vimentin, and transcription factor PAX8 supports diagnosis of RCC.
[c]All (2 of 13) papillary-cystic RCCs were VM-.
[d]All (3 of 13) solid RCCs were CK-.
[e]Lectin stains (e.g., *Dichloros biflorus* agglutinin, peanut agglutinin, *Ulex europaeus* agglutinin I).
[f]Widespread metastasis and poor prognosis ($n = 12$ study).
[g]IHC: CK+; vimentin, chromogranin A, neuron-specific enolase –. Renal oncocytoma in a cat. (Lee S, 2017).
CD = collecting ducts; CT = cortical tubules; DCT = distal convoluted tubules; DN = distal nephron; MT = medullary tubules; PT = proximal tubules; RCC = renal cell carcinoma.

Lymphovascular invasion is concerning but does not always lead to metastases. Peritoneal implantation may occur. Usually by the time a dog is presented for examination, widespread metastases are present, especially in the lungs and liver, but also in the brain, heart, and skin. In cases without metastases, unilateral nephrectomy might be curative.

RCCs are rarely diagnosed in **cats**, but typically occur unilaterally, in older cats (mean 9 years), with no sex or breed

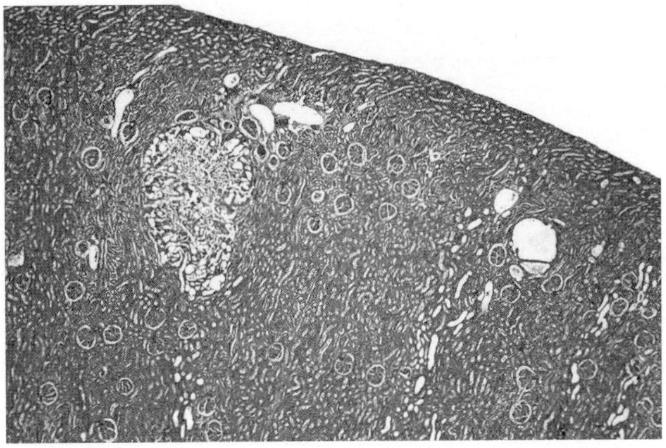

Figure 4-68 Renal cystadenocarcinoma from a German Shepherd dog. H&E.

predilection and only sporadic metastases. In a study of 20 feline RCCs, all samples stained positively for cytokeratins AE1/AE3 and 19 stained positively for vimentin (expressed by distal convoluted tubules) and PAX8. Fewer samples expressed cKIT and CD10 (marker of proximal tubules). In a study of 12 feline RCCs in nephrectomy samples that focused on outcome, the RCCs often expressed CK7, CK20 (both of which are usually expressed by urothelial cells and collecting ducts), CD10, and vimentin. This study included one case of sarcomatoid RCC, and it expressed aquaporin 1 (marker of proximal tubules). The sarcomatoid RCCs also expressed N-cadherin and Twist with an accumulation of β-catenin in nuclei. The sarcomatoid RCCs had widespread metastasis and a poor prognosis, but the other cats had favorable outcomes following nephrectomy. Notably, when a nephrectomized renal mass is examined, assessment of the non-neoplastic portions of the kidney is imperative. It can provide information about the status of the remaining kidney.

Bovine RCCs often contain corpora amylacea. One study reported that they all stain positively for uromodulin via IHC, indicating that they are derived from distal segments of the nephron, similar to dogs. Cattle have a low rate of systemic metastasis, but bilateral renal involvement is common. This might be explained by multiple de novo development as opposed to intrarenal metastasis. Reports of **equine** RCCs are rare in the literature, but they are considered to be locally invasive with potential for metastasis.

Middle-aged and older **German Shepherd dogs** with generalized *nodular dermatofibrosis* concurrently also have **renal cystadenocarcinomas** or cystadenomas, which are usually bilateral (Fig. 4-68; eFig. 4-37). The carcinomas will occasionally metastasize to regional lymph nodes, peritoneum, liver, spleen, lung, and bone. Affected females also often have uterine leiomyomas. The syndrome is *inherited in an autosomal dominant mode in German Shepherd dogs*, and genetic mapping has linked the disease to mutations in the Birt-Hogg-Dubé locus located on chromosome 5. Mutations in this gene have previously been associated with a similar phenotype in humans. Because nodular dermatofibrosis with various cystic renal diseases has been reported in a variety of dog breeds, some postulate that there is concurrent initiation of fibrosis in both the skin and the kidney. Renal fibrosis can result in outflow obstruction of renal tubules with expansion and eventual cyst formation. There can be progression through a continuum of lesions, including renal epithelial cysts, cystic adenomatous hyperplasia, renal cystadenoma, and cystadenocarcinoma, with purebred dogs perhaps being prone to more rapid transformation to malignancy. Thus, all dog breeds are potentially at risk.

Nephroblastoma

Nephroblastoma (embryonal nephroma, Wilms tumor) is the most common primary renal tumor of ***pigs*** *and* ***chickens***. Abattoir surveys of pigs in the United Kingdom found 3.5 per million swine slaughtered, and in the United States, 43.5 per million, with a frequency of 197 cases per million in one area. Nephroblastomas occur far less often in calves and in dogs, and are uncommon in sheep, horses, and cats. They are usually seen in young animals and sometimes in fetuses. They may be seen in mature sows, and they are more common in juvenile or adults dogs than in pups. Rarely, *polycythemia* is seen as an associated paraneoplastic syndrome in nephroblastoma.

In rats, various carcinogens, including dimethylnitrosamine, can induce formation of nephroblastomas. Additionally, nephroblastematosis is a spontaneous precursor lesion to nephroblastoma in Sprague-Dawley rats. These precursor lesions begin as foci of interstitial immature blastema cells in the inner cortex that can replace normal architecture with increasing size and neoplastic transformation.

Nephroblastomas are *true embryonal tumors* that arise in primitive nephrogenic blastema. These tumors establish the important principle that all component tissues of the kidney arise from a common blastema. This neoplasm may represent a form of arrested development. Finding nephrogenic rests of nodular renal blastema in dogs suggests that this species shares a similar pathogenesis and histogenesis to that seen in Wilms tumors in humans.

Grossly, nephroblastomas can be large enough to cause abdominal distension. They can be multiple in the affected kidney, growing expansively and compressing the adjacent parenchyma (Fig. 4-69). They are usually unilateral, but a few are bilateral, and these sometimes unite across the midline to form a single large mass. Widespread metastases to the lung and liver occur in more than half of the canine cases, but are rare in pigs and calves. The cut surface of a nephroblastoma is *lobulated with myxomatous soft, gray-white or tan spongy tissue*. Larger tumors have extensive hemorrhagic necrosis. Rarely, these tumors are seen as primary extramedullary and intradural *spinal canal masses* between T10 and L2 and are called *thoracolumbar spinal tumor* of young dogs. German Shepherd and male dogs seem to be over-represented with the spinal form, which may occur in the absence of renal involvement.

Histologically, the characteristic features are primitive glomeruli, abortive tubules, and a loose spindle cell stroma that may have some differentiation to a variety of mesenchymal tissues, including *striated muscle, collagen, cartilage, bone, and adipose tissue*. The mesenchymal components may predominate over epithelial elements in certain tumors, especially in ruminants. When all 3 components (blastemal, epithelial, and stromal) exist in equal proportions, these forms are referred to as *triphasic (mixed)*. Glomeruloid structures can be rare in some tumors. Commercially available antibody to the human Wilms tumor 1 successfully binds with canine nephroblastomas. These tumors are also typically glial fibrillary acidic protein negative and variably vimentin and cytokeratin positive. Tubular and glomerular differentiation indicates a good prognosis; anaplasia and sarcomatous stroma are associated with metastasis and poor prognosis. Please note that *a sarcomatoid RCC could be misdiagnosed as nephroblastoma because of the biphasic histologic pattern*. Again, this underscores the need for

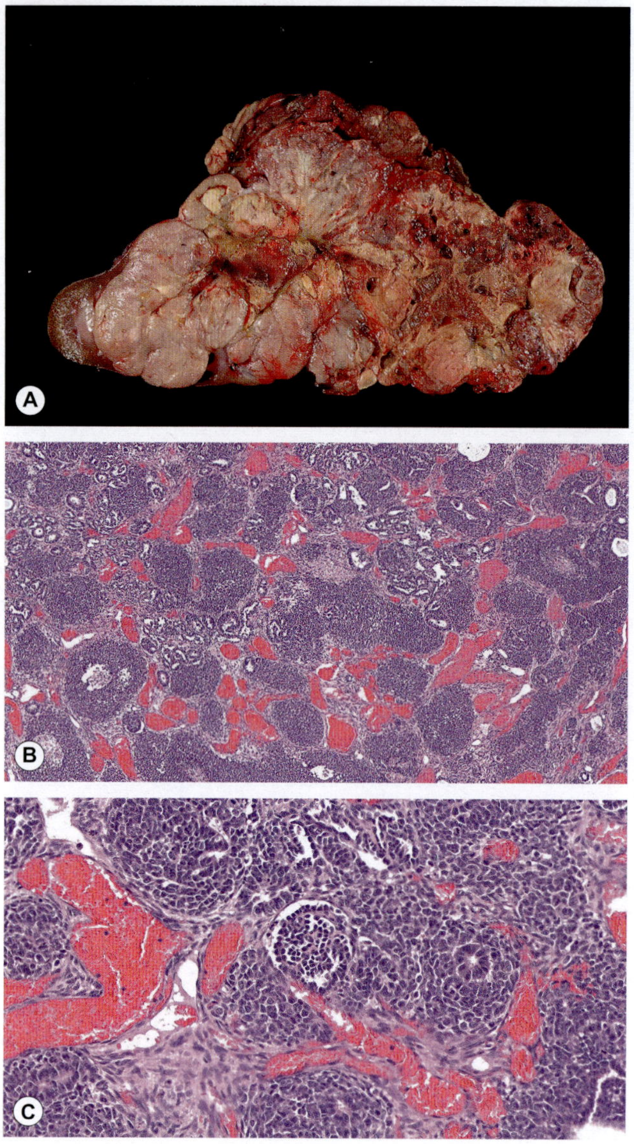

Figure 4-69 **Nephroblastoma** from a dog. **A**. The kidney is irregularly shaped, and the masses are of various sizes. (Courtesy J. Luff, P.A. Pesavento.) **B**. Biphasic pattern of tubular epithelial cells and abundant stromal mesenchymal cells. H&E. **C**. Occasional glomeruloid structures are identified among the epithelial and mesenchymal cells. This latter feature can be rare-to-absent, depending on the sample. The presence of glomeruloid structures is not required for the diagnosis of nephroblastoma. H&E.

IHC (PAX8 and Wilms tumor 1) when examining cases with these histologic patterns.

In pigs, the mesenchymal component of nephroblastomas can be immunolabeled with vimentin; all tubular structures are labeled with CK19. Embryologically, this particular cytokeratin is transiently expressed as the epithelial cells of tubules undergo differentiation and then CK19 becomes limited to the parietal epithelium and distal tubules. This widespread presence of a transiently expressed protein in porcine nephroblastomas supports the embryonic origin of the neoplasm. Interestingly, glomeruloid structures do not contain factor VIII–positive cells, demonstrating a lack of capillary invasion.

Other tumors

Urothelial papilloma and **carcinoma** of the renal pelvis are rare tumors, which occur in the dog, cat, cow, pig, and

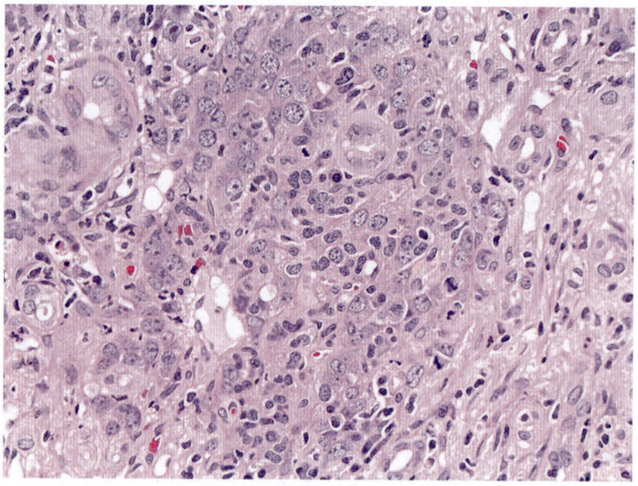

Figure 4-70 **Urothelial carcinoma** arose from the proximal ureter and invaded the renal parenchyma in a dog. H&E.

horse (Fig. 4-70). Squamous and glandular metaplasia can develop within carcinomas; however, neoplastic urothelium remains the predominant cell type. Primary pelvic **squamous cell carcinoma** is rare, but they have been noted in dogs in association with pelvic calculi. Cats with CKD of various etiologies frequently have hyperplasia of the collecting duct epithelium and renal pelvic urothelium. Dysplasia of these epithelial cells is occasionally observed, and some cats have concurrent hyperplasia and carcinomas. This suggests that the pelvic urothelial hyperplasia in cats might progress through a dysplastic phase and eventually to neoplasia.

Primary mesenchymal tumors of the kidney occur, but may be diagnosed only after very careful examination to exclude a primary focus in some other tissue. The prognosis associated with renal mesenchymal neoplasms is usually grave. Fibrosarcomas and vascular tumors are the most common types. **Hemangioma** is the most frequently encountered benign mesenchymal renal neoplasm in dogs; hematuria is the most consistent accompanying sign. Renal **interstitial cell tumors** occur near the corticomedullary junction, arising from cells distinct from interstitial fibroblasts. These tumors will have positive COX2 IHC labeling; renal interstitial cells in normal kidneys have labeling for that marker as well. **Benign cortical fibromas** also occur in older dogs. Other rare primary renal tumors include *spindle cell sarcomas* and *oncocytoma*. **Renal oncocytomas** are rare, usually unilateral, benign tumors composed of oncocytes, which are large polygonal cells with bright eosinophilic granular cytoplasm. PAS stain accentuates the cytoplasmic granules, which on electron microscopy are mitochondria. The cells are typically arranged as compact nests, cords, or tubules. The histogenesis is unclear, but it is thought that these tumors originate from intercalated cells of the collecting ducts; the cells express cytoplasmic keratin.

Metastatic tumors are common in the kidneys, and disseminated neoplasms of any type are likely to localize there, typically with bilateral involvement of the cortices. Many such metastases are microscopic (eFig. 4-38) and of hematogenous origin. Retrograde lymphatic invasion along the renal lymphatics may occur from carcinomas in adjacent organs.

In dogs, primary **pulmonary adenocarcinoma** with renal metastases may be difficult or impossible to distinguish from

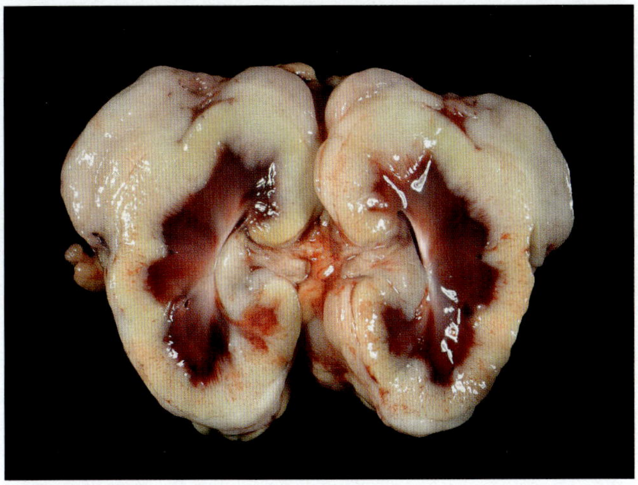

Figure 4-71 **Renal (cortical) and perirenal lymphoma** in a cat. (Courtesy E. Clark, D. Russell.)

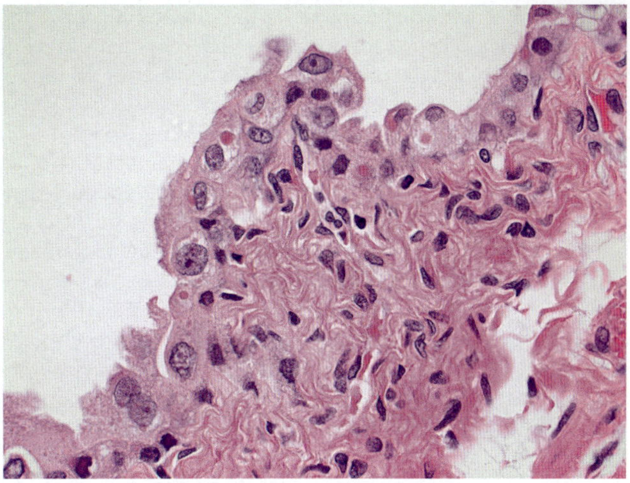

Figure 4-72 **Intracytoplasmic inclusion bodies** in the urothelium of a dog infected with canine distemper virus. H&E. (Courtesy E. Clark, P. Stromberg.)

primary renal carcinoma with pulmonary metastases because their microscopic appearance is quite similar. Positive PAX8 IHC can help support the renal origin of the neoplasm in these scenarios.

Renal involvement in **lymphoma** is common in those species in which the neoplasm is common. This is the most common renal neoplasm in cats, but is more often a metastatic rather than a primary lesion (Fig. 4-71; eFig. 4-39). The involvement may be diffuse or nodular and possibly bilateral. When the nodular lesions are grossly visible, they are numerous, poorly defined, fatty in appearance, and project above the surface. Diffuse lymphoma results in generalized enlargement with a uniform white fatty appearance. In cats, some types of lymphoma are limited to the cortex and stop abruptly at the corticomedullary junction. Metastases of other round-cell tumors have similar gross appearances (eFig. 4-40). Differentiation of metastatic lymphoma from interstitial nephritis may require microscopic examination. Peripelvic and periureteral lymphoma, which can cause hydronephrosis, is seen in cattle.

LOWER URINARY TRACT

GENERAL CONSIDERATIONS

The lower urinary tract consists of the **ureters, urinary bladder**, and **urethra**. The ureters and bladder, and also the renal pelvis, are lined by nonkeratinizing, stratified epithelium—the **urothelium**. The ureters are of uniform diameter throughout, and usually course directly to the bladder, although they may be tortuous. They are dilated distally in baby pigs. The ureters enter the bladder wall obliquely and are covered by a mucosal flap. Histologically, the ureteral mucosa is present in longitudinal folds; there are poorly defined internal and external longitudinal muscle layers, a prominent middle circular layer, and either adventitia or peritoneal serosa. Ureters and the renal pelves of horses have simple branched tubuloalveolar mucous glands that connect to the lumens. Histologically, the bladder is an expanded ureter, lined by stratified urothelium 3-14 cells thick, depending on the species and degree of distension. Superficial cells, which contain tubulovesicular compartments, supply additional membrane so the cells can stretch during bladder distension. The basolateral cell membrane of the superficial cells and the cell membrane of the intermediate layer of urothelium interdigitate and are attached by desmosomes that provide structural stability and elasticity during distension and relaxation. Lymphoid nodules are commonly found in the lamina propria of all domestic animals. Eosinophilic intracytoplasmic inclusion bodies of canine distemper seen in urinary bladder epithelial cells (Fig. 4-72) must be differentiated from similar nonspecific inclusions.

The function of the ureter is to propel urine from the kidney to the bladder by peristalsis. Ureteral peristalsis is complex and influenced by the rate of urine production as well as external pressures. For example, peritonitis can interfere with ureteric peristalsis. The ureters pass obliquely through the muscular wall of the bladder at the ureterovesical junction. *This intravesicular segment of a ureter forms the basis of the* **vesicoureteral valve**, *which prevents reflux of urine from bladder to ureter*. When the length of the intravesical ureter is short, as is often the case in puppies, reflux frequently occurs. Thus, the angle of the ureteral entry and the thickness of the bladder wall influence the competence of the valve. The urinary bladder stores urine and, in concert with the urethra, expels it. In general, the bladder is relatively flaccid, and the urethra acts as a valve. During micturition, contraction of the *detrusor muscle*—the urinary bladder musculature—pumps urine through the relaxed urethra. Sphincter mechanism incompetence or detrusor dysfunction can lead to incontinence, seen most commonly in female dogs.

Embryologically, the ureters are formed by buds from the mesonephric ducts, which develop craniad to their entrance into the cloaca. The cloaca is divided into a dorsal rectum and ventral urogenital sinus by the urorectal fold such that the urogenital sinus is continuous with the allantois. The allantois originates as an evagination of the hindgut. At this stage of development, the mesonephric duct and ureteral bud form a Y shape; one arm of the Y is the ureteral bud, and the other arm plus the stem of the Y are formed by the mesonephric duct. As the allantois and urogenital sinus develop, the stem of the Y is absorbed, and the mesonephric duct and ureteral bud enter the urogenital sinus independently. In females, the entire urethra, plus the vaginal vestibule, is derived from the urogenital sinus, but in males, only the prostatic urethra is derived in that manner. The penile urethra forms by closure of the urethral groove on the caudal face of the penis. The bladder, which is formed from the cranial part of the urogenital sinus and the caudal part of the allantoic diverticulum, communicates with the allantois via the urachus, a part of the intraembryonic allantoic diverticulum. The communication is severed at birth, and the urachus closes but remains as the umbilical ligament of the bladder.

Most ailments of the lower urinary tract are associated with obstruction and infection, which can be concomitant. Unlike the gastrointestinal tract, which has a normal microbial flora throughout its length, only the most distal part of the male urethra, and the female vagina, normally host microorganisms. The operation of sphincter-like mechanisms in the urethra and vesicoureteral valves, and the intermittent pulsatile flow of urine from the kidneys and bladder, normally prevents the movement of organisms higher up the tract. The susceptibility of the urinary bladder of the female to infections is undoubtedly related to its short distensible urethra and its proximity to the external environment and rectal flora. On the contrary, the anatomy of male urethras, with their flexures, ossa, and appendages, make them prone to obstruction, particularly by calculi. Specific factors concerned in the establishment and maintenance of infections in the urinary bladder and their spread to the kidney are discussed in the sections General cystitis and Pyelonephritis. The causes and effects of obstruction are considered in the sections Urolithiasis and Hydronephrosis.

The **urothelium** of the renal pelvis, ureter, and perhaps the trigone of the bladder originates from mesoderm; in the rest of the bladder, it has an endodermal origin. The urothelium responds to chronic irritation from infections, calculi, and excreted chemicals by proliferation and/or metaplasia, both of which are regarded as premalignant changes. Proliferation of urothelium, a common reactive change, results in groups of proliferating cells isolated in the submucosa, known as **Brunn nests**. If the center of the nest undergoes liquefactive necrosis, *cystitis cystica*, *ureteritis cystica*, or *pyelitis cystica* results. *Cystitis glandularis* develops if the epithelium lining the cyst undergoes mucous metaplasia. Squamous and/or mucous metaplasia is often superimposed on predominantly proliferative lesions. The male urethra has a thin lining of urothelium; that of the female is similar but has stratified squamous epithelium at its termination. Urothelium can also undergo metaplasia to an intestinal-type epithelium; this most commonly occurs in cystic urachal remnants.

Dog and cat bladders can appear thickened at autopsy, due to peri- or postmortem muscle contraction. If the bladder can be dilated by pulling it between the fingers, the thickening is not pathologic. Horse urine normally contains mucus and crystals.

ANOMALIES OF THE LOWER URINARY TRACT

As stated above, developmental anomalies of the urinary tract often are associated with renal maldevelopment, and these anomalies should be diagnosed as CAKUT. Previously, diagnosis of these conditions often occurred at autopsy; however, with advanced diagnostic imaging, the diagnoses can be established so that they can be surgically corrected. As such, communication among pathologist, radiologist, and clinician is imperative so the anomalies can be described correctly.

Ureters

Agenesis of the ureters is the result of failure of the ureteral bud to form and may be unilateral or bilateral. In dogs, it is often accompanied by renal agenesis (see the Anomalies of Development section). **Duplication** of a ureter is caused by the formation of 2 ureteral diverticula from the mesonephric duct. In these scenarios, the caudal ureter, which drains the caudal part of the kidney, empties normally. The cranial ureter is usually ectopic, draining the cranial part of the kidney. Duplication is rare but occurs in dogs and pigs. **Ureteral dysplasia** often occurs in association with renal maldevelopment. **Ureteral valves** are occasionally seen in dogs and can impede urinary flow. **Retrocaval ureter** (also called "circumcaval") is a condition in which one ureter (often the right) traverses dorsal to the vena cava and then wraps around to run ventral to it (Fig. 4-73). Although it can be seen incidentally in cats, it might predispose to unilateral obstruction secondary to either ureterolithiasis or ureteral stricture.

Ectopic ureter *is the most important ureteral anomaly*. Rather than terminating at the trigone of the bladder, the affected ureter may empty into the vas deferens, vesicular gland, or urethra of the male, or the bladder neck, urethra, or vagina of the female (Fig. 4-74). In female dogs, the ectopic ureter usually terminates in the vagina or urethra; in cats, urethral termination is most common. There are 2 possible causes: either the ureteral bud arises too far craniad to be incorporated into the urogenital sinus or the differential growth of the sinus is abnormal and the ureter fails to migrate to its usual location. Ectopic ureters occasionally empty into the rectum because of anomalous cloacal division by the urorectal fold. Very rarely, they empty into the cervix, uterus, or uterine tube, possibly as a result of aberrant origin from the paramesonephric (Müllerian) duct. Even more rarely, an ectopic ureter may be blind-ended cranially in cases with accompanying renal agenesis.

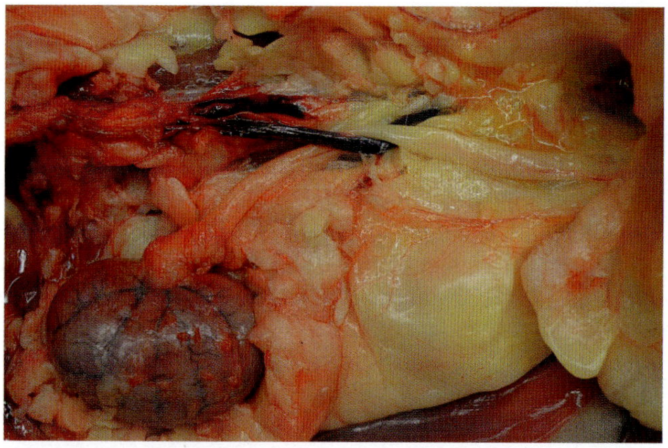

Figure 4-73 **Retrocaval ureter** in a cat. Incidental finding.

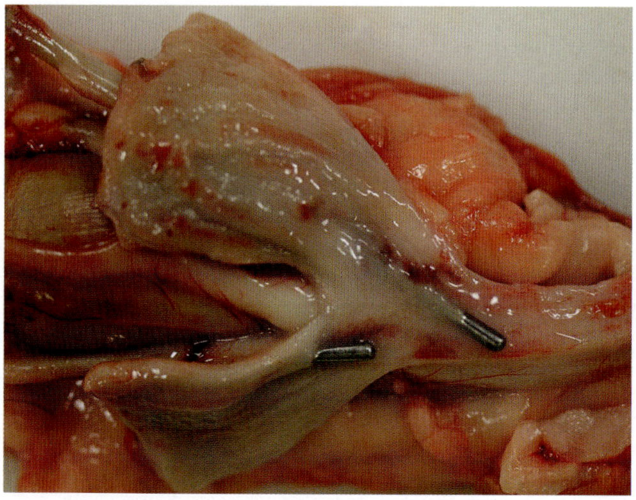

Figure 4-74 **Ectopic ureter** in a dog, demonstrated by insertion of probes through the ureters. (Courtesy J. Davies.)

Ectopic ureter is most common in dogs and is diagnosed up to 20 times more frequently in females than in males. However, this sex difference may be exaggerated because affected females are usually incontinent from birth, whereas affected males may not be. Termination of the ectopic ureter proximal to the external urethral sphincter in males leads to retrograde filling of the bladder rather than to incontinence. Ectopia can be unilateral or bilateral and is often associated with other urinary tract abnormalities, including bladder agenesis or hypoplasia, renal agenesis or hypoplasia, ureteral or bladder duplication, and branching of the terminal ureter. Ectopic ureter also occurs in White Shorthorn bulls and tends to involve the region of the seminal vesicles. It is rare in horses.

A **ureterocele** is a congenital abnormality that is *a focal submucosal dilation of the distal ureter*, especially involving that portion that lies within the urinary bladder wall. It may be associated with normal anatomic emptying or it can be ectopic. *Ureteral anomalies often predispose to hydronephrosis/hydroureter and UTI that may culminate in pyelonephritis*. **Ureteral diverticula** result from urothelial hyperplasia, mucous metaplasia, and submucosal urothelial proliferation with the formation of small cysts. Neoplastic transformation may occur more readily in such sites. **Congenital hydroureter** and hydronephrosis often occur in piglets in association with epitheliogenesis imperfecta.

Urinary bladder

Duplication of the urinary bladder occurs rarely in dogs and causes dysuria, incontinence, and, less frequently, abdominal distension and cryptorchidism. The extra bladder originates dorsally between the urinary tract and the uterus or rectum. Cystic remnants of the urorectal fold may be responsible for this defect.

Patent urachus is the *most common malformation of the urinary bladder* and is seen more often in foals than in other animals. Animals with this defect dribble urine from the umbilicus because the urachal lumen fails to close and is a channel between the apex of the bladder and the umbilicus. A patent urachus is susceptible to infection. **Rupture of the urachus** causes uroperitoneum. The condition must be differentiated from perinatal rupture of the bladder. Occasionally, urachal closure is partial, and **urachal cysts** remain between the umbilicus and the bladder. Although these cysts may become quite large, they are usually small, multiple, and attached to the midline of the bladder. Occasionally, they adhere to the intestinal serosa. The urachus is normally lined by urothelium, but metaplasia to squamous or mucus-secreting columnar epithelium is common in urachal cysts. Urachal remnants in the bladder wall can be a nidus for cystitis (infectious or sterile) and may give rise to neoplasms.

Diverticula of the bladder may be primary or acquired secondary to partial obstruction to urine outflow, or as the result of pressure changes exerted during normal contractions. Diverticula are usually seen at the apex, where they represent incomplete closure of the urachus (vesicourachal diverticulum) with an area of discontinuity in the muscle. They can also occur in the trigone region in association with a malformation of the bladder muscle wall. Similar to urachal remnants, stasis of urine in the diverticulum can lead to persistent infection and inflammation. Calculi may form in the diverticulum. If the distal urachus remains patent to the exterior through the umbilical opening, it is called a **urachal sinus**.

Urethra

Urethral **agenesis, duplicated** urethra, **ectopic** urethra, and **imperforate** urethra occur rarely in dogs. Hypospadias occurs with male genitalia. *The most common urethral anomaly is* **urethrorectal** or **rectovaginal fistula**, which is caused by incomplete division of the cloaca into the rectum and urogenital sinus by the urorectal fold. In males, the communication involves the pelvic urethra, and affected dogs urinate from the rectum. In females, the opening is in the vagina and may be associated with imperforate anus. These defects are reported in dogs, cats, pigs, rabbits, alpacas, and foals, often as one of several congenital anomalies. These changes usually predispose to urogenital tract infections, but sometimes are incidental autopsy findings.

In male ruminants and swine, a **urethral recess** is normally present near the ischial arch and is an impediment to catheterization. Dilation of the urethral recess can cause midline perineal swelling in ruminants.

Urethral atresia and **urethral hypoplasia** have been noted in newborn freemartin intersex calves with uroperitoneum following rupture of the urethra or urinary bladder. **Urethral strictures** have been documented in intersex ruminants, a llama, and a Nubian goat.

Acquired anatomic variations

Displacements of ureters and urethra can be caused by local inflammation and neoplasia. Their significance is related to obstruction of urine flow. Ureteral and urethral displacements may also occur with variations of position of the bladder.

Torsion of the bladder is uncommon; it may be partial or complete about the long axis of the organ. The presence of part of the bladder within the pelvis, so-called *"pelvic bladder,"* is a clinical diagnosis made via contrast urethrocystography; its clinical significance as a cause of UTI or incontinence is controversial in dogs. **Retroflexion** of the bladder can occur from vaginal prolapse in cows, sows, and female dogs, and occasionally in perineal hernia of older male dogs. In these cases, the retroflexed bladder may be present in the hernial sac with obstructive kinking of the neck of the bladder and sometimes of the urethra and ureters. If the ureters are patent, the accumulation of urine in the bladder contributes to the size of the hernia. Hydronephrosis or rupture of the bladder may occur if the condition is not corrected.

Eversion of the bladder *(invagination into and through the urethra)* occurs in females because the female urethra is short and wide. The bladder may evert to the level of the vagina. This is an issue in large animals, especially mares. Eversion occurs in circumstances in which increased intra-abdominal pressure or straining occurs, often after parturition. Hypocalcemia in periparturient dairy cows may contribute by resulting in decreased bladder tone before eversion. The everted bladder may allow for herniation of the intestine. Rarely, *umbilical eversion* of the bladder can occur in foals that experience traumatic tearing of the umbilical cord and urachus during birthing. Eversion of the bladder should be distinguished from **prolapse** of the bladder. In eversion, the mucosal surface protrudes from the vulva; *in prolapse the bladder is displaced through a rent in the vagina, and the serosal surface appears*.

Hydroureter, or *dilation of a ureter* (eFig. 4-41), may be caused by obstruction by calculi, neoplasms, inflammation, scar tissue, or the result of accidental ligation during surgery (e.g., ovariohysterectomy). It will lead to hydronephrosis. Dilation without physical obstruction can occur with peritonitis and may be because of loss of muscle tone. Dilation of ureters is often present in neonatal pigs with enteric infections. Ureters may **rupture** as a consequence of blunt physical trauma or rarely in association with parturition. Foals can have bilateral involvement after nonpenetrating, blunt trauma, which suggests a possible congenital predisposition. Ureters may also be accidentally **transected** during surgery (e.g., ovariohysterectomy). Leakage of urine from a traumatized ureter is the most common cause of a **paraureteral or uriniferous pseudocyst**, which is basically a fibrous wall without an epithelial lining. Urethral obstruction and urine leakage from a rent in the renal capsule are also documented causes. **Perinephric pseudocysts** are similar but surround the kidney and are seen most commonly in cats.

Dilation of the bladder may be the result of obstruction or neuromuscular disease. Severe or prolonged distension may result in loss of tone and a thin wall. It can be complicated by bacterial infection. *Causes of obstruction* include calculi, prostatic enlargement, inflammatory debris or blood clots in the urethra, urethral strictures, and tumors of the neck of the bladder or urethra. Detrusor atony of the bladder may follow prolonged dystocia in the dog. *Neurogenic disorders of micturition* can arise from abnormalities of the sphincter or bladder, and also from failure to store and/or void urine. Neurogenic distension follows spinal injury, with loss of tonic parasympathetic outflow from the sacral plexus. In the dog, it most commonly follows herniation of intervertebral discs. Spinal myelitis can also cause paralysis of the bladder. Cystitis and ischemic necrosis, secondary to compression of vessels within the distended urinary bladder wall, are possible complications. In horses, bladder paralysis and distension may lead to sabulous urolithiasis, resembling sand (Fig. 4-75). Descriptions of *detrusor-urethral dyssynergia* in dogs have been rarely documented in young and middle-aged large-breed dogs. This condition is a functional disorder of the voiding phase of micturition because of involuntary contraction of the external urethral sphincter in the postprostatic urethra, the smooth muscle of the neck of the bladder, or the prostatic urethra (internal sphincter). Typically, these animals have dysuria with interrupted spurting of urine and a large residual urine volume.

Sphincter mechanism incompetence *is the most common cause of urinary incontinence in middle-aged, spayed female dogs*, but the prevalence is also higher in those with body weights >30 kg, and docked breeds (Doberman Pinschers, Old English Sheepdogs, Rottweilers, Weimaraners, and Setters). In females, an intrapelvic bladder neck, a short urethra, reduced urethral tone, and neutering before first estrus predispose to this condition. Restoration of normal anatomic location of urethra/urinary bladder by surgical procedures is often curative. Bladder neck position (i.e., intrapelvic), breed, prostate size, and castration status are significant risk factors for incontinence in male dogs. Congenital urethral sphincter mechanism incompetence in cats has been associated with genitourinary dysplasia (urethral hypoplasia and vaginal and/or uterine hypoplasia/aplasia).

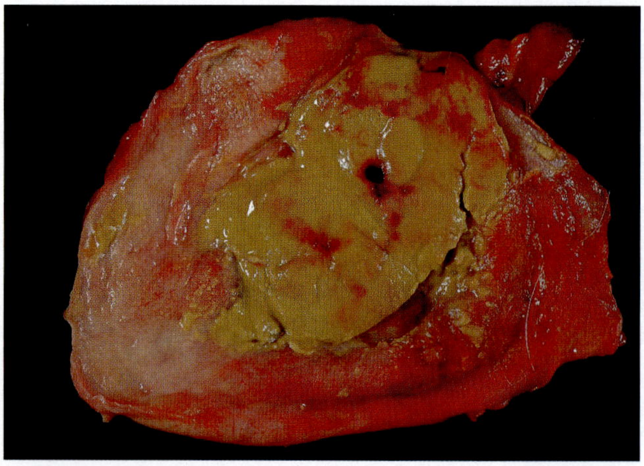

Figure 4-75 Sabulous cystitis in a horse. (Courtesy S. Siso, B.G. Murphy.)

Hypertrophy of the bladder wall is fairly common in dogs and less so in other species. It is a response to long-standing partial obstruction to the outflow of urine.

Rupture of the bladder (cystorrhexis) often occurs following urethral obstruction, such as in urolithiasis. Rarely, it is secondary to pelvic trauma or dystocia. The interval between obstruction and rupture depends somewhat on the competence of the vesicoureteral valve and whether hydronephrosis develops. Rupture of the bladder occurs in newborn foals, with an incidence of 0.2-2.5%, affecting either the dorsal or ventral aspect of the organ. Males are most often affected. Some ruptures are congenital and are probably caused by birth trauma. Twists in the amniotic portion of the umbilical cord may compress the urachus, causing distension of both bladder and urachus and predisposing to rupture. Only rarely is the urinary bladder rupture secondary to atrophy of circular smooth muscle fibers in the dorsal bladder wall.

Urine in the peritoneal cavity, or **uroperitoneum**, follows leakage from the kidneys, ureter, bladder, or urethra. Diagnosis of uroperitoneum is supported by the finding of peritoneal-to-serum ratios for potassium, phosphate, and creatinine >2:1. Calcium carbonate crystals are occasionally seen in the peritoneal fluid. In foals, uroperitoneum is associated with positive sepsis scores and a negative prognosis. *Escherichia coli*, *Actinobacillus equuli*, and, less commonly, *Clostridium perfringens* are implicated in urosepsis or urachal infections. Abdominal trauma is a common cause of urine leakage from the bladder in dogs and cats. Catheterization and bladder expression are the most common causes of urethral leakage in cats. Urinary calculi and obstruction by urothelial carcinoma (UC) are also causes.

Although uncommon in domestic swine, **urethral polyps** have been reported in Vietnamese pot-bellied pigs. It seems most likely that these lesions arise secondary to trauma to the mucosal folds of the urethral recess associated with repeated catheterization. **Urethral caruncles** have been described in humans and dogs, and form as a result of chronic inflammation of the urethral mucosa. In this lesion, urothelial hyperplasia overlies an inflamed stromal expansion, often with glandular structures, and can produce an obstructive mass.

CIRCULATORY DISTURBANCES

In the ureters and urethra, **hemorrhages** are associated with obstructive calculi or acute ascending infections. Urethral hematomas following pelvic trauma may predispose to urinary bladder rupture. In the bladder, hemorrhages are typically located in the lamina propria and may occur in any inflammatory condition. Small hemorrhages or hematomas are common and considered diagnostically significant in classical swine fever, African swine fever, porcine salmonellosis, and equine purpura hemorrhagica. Larger hemorrhages are seen in bracken fern poisoning of cattle. Hemorrhage occurs with acute cystitis and neoplasia and following rupture of the bladder. In our experience, intramural fibrinoid vascular necrosis has been observed in small animals with obstruction and bladder rupture.

UROLITHIASIS

Urolithiasis is the presence of calculi (uroliths or stones) in the urinary passages. Calculi are grossly visible aggregates of precipitated urinary solutes, urinary proteins, and proteinaceous debris. Minerals predominate in **calculi;** matrix usually predominates in **urethral plugs**. *Calculi typically have a central nidus, surrounded by concentric laminae, an outer shell, and surface crystals*. Many calculi are hard spherical or ovoid structures with a small amount of organic matrix impregnated with inorganic salts. *Urethral plugs are masses of sandy sludge with a much higher organic component* whose form is largely determined by the shape of the cavity they fill. Even densely mineralized calculi of the same type may have quite a different appearance, depending on whether they are located in renal pelvis or urinary bladder. Many calculi contain significant quantities of "contaminants," such as calcium oxalates in "silica" calculi. A few calculi are relatively pure.

The diseases caused by uroliths are among the most important urinary tract problems of domesticated animals. Calculogenic material must occur in urine in quantities sufficient to be precipitated. Sometimes this concentration is achieved because a substance is metabolized in an unusual way, as is uric acid in Dalmatian dogs. Also, a substance may be processed abnormally by the kidney, as is cystine in cystine stone formers, or may be in abnormally high levels of a substance in the diet, such as silicic acid in native pastures. Regardless of the type of calculus, certain factors are important: **urinary pH** and **reduced water intake**, in relation to the degree of urine concentration. Other predisposing conditions include **infection** (see the Struvite Calculi section), obstruction, structural abnormalities, foreign bodies, and drug-induced changes in urine composition, for example, by sulfonamides. A foreign body, such as a suture, grass awn, catheter, or needle, can act as a nidus for urolith formation. Deficiency of vitamin A is frequently suggested as a factor predisposing to urolithiasis, but the evidence is equivocal; it may contribute in exceptional circumstances by producing metaplastic changes in the urinary epithelium.

Urine **supersaturation** is the essential precursor to initiation of urolith formation (nucleation). Supersaturation may be in the **unstable** region in which spontaneous precipitation occurs (homogeneous nucleation), or in the **metastable** range, in which precipitation occurs by heterogeneous nucleation (one type of crystal grows on the surface of another type). When proteins are admixed in the urolith, there could be coprecipitation of proteins and minerals, or the proteins could be adsorbed onto formed crystals. It is also possible that crystals of one salt, for which urine is supersaturated in the unstable range, induces precipitation of crystals of another salt, for which supersaturation is metastable. Crystals are much more common in urine than are calculi. Even though equine urine, for example, is normally supersaturated with calcium carbonate and crystalluria is normal, horses experience a low prevalence of calculi.

The factors that promote crystal growth and crystal aggregation or, more importantly, prevent them in some animals, are poorly understood. Experimentally, high levels of urinary inorganic pyrophosphate and magnesium are important inhibitors of calcium phosphate and calcium oxalate crystallization, and pyrophosphate also inhibits aggregation of calcium phosphate crystals. Certain urinary macromolecules, probably glycosaminoglycans, are also strong inhibitors of crystal aggregation in experimental systems. Deficiency of inhibitors of crystallization might be important in calcium oxalate and calcium phosphate calculogenesis. The important types of urinary calculi are listed according to species in Table 4-5. Although one mineral may predominate in a urolith, *many uroliths are of mixed composition*. Overlap in the gross appearance of uroliths usually precludes specific gross diagnosis of mineral type. *In general, calculi are important in cattle, sheep, dogs, and cats, less important in horses, and unimportant in pigs*. In *pigs*, uroliths are occasionally found in the renal pelvis of old animals and, more often, in the pelvis of dehydrated piglets [see the Renal Disease (AKI and CKD) and Uremia sections]. In *horses*, they occur sometimes as single or several, spherical or faceted carbonate stones in the bladder; urethral obstructions are rare. In *dogs*, several breeds are predisposed to formation of calculi.

Table • **4-5**

Composition and importance of urinary calculi

SPECIES	COMMON TYPES	UNCOMMON TYPES
Dog	Struvite Oxalate Purines (urate, uric acid, xanthine)	Silica Cystine Calcium phosphate
Cat	Struvite Oxalate	Urate Cystine
Ox	Silica Struvite Carbonate	Xanthine
Sheep	Silica Struvite Oxalate "Clover stones" Carbonate	Xanthine
Horse	Carbonate	
Pig		Urate

Calculi may form in any part of the urinary duct system, from the renal pelvis to the urethra. Some uroliths clearly originate in the lower urinary tract, but the point for development of most is not known (Fig. 4-76, eFig. 4-42). Obstructive nephroliths and ureteroliths occasionally develop in horses and cats can be associated with chronic tubulointerstitial nephritis. Sometimes, there is renal medullary crest necrosis resulting from the use of NSAIDs in dehydrated horses and cats, with subsequent mineralization of the sloughed necrotic renal crest material. Nephroliths are uncommon forms of uroliths in most species, representing only 1-4% of canine uroliths (Fig. 4-77).

Small calculi may be voided in the urine, but *obstruction in the urethra is common in males*. The common sites of urethral impaction are the ischial arch, the sigmoid flexure of ruminants (Fig. 4-78), the vermiform appendage of rams, the proximal end of the os penis in dogs, and anywhere along the urethra of male cats. At the point of obstruction, there is pressure necrosis with ulceration of the mucosa. Because urinary stasis favors bacterial growth, acute infectious urethritis can develop and ascend to the bladder and kidney. Hydronephrosis is not common with completely obstructive urethral calculi because the urethra or bladder typically ruptures prior to dilation of the renal pelvis.

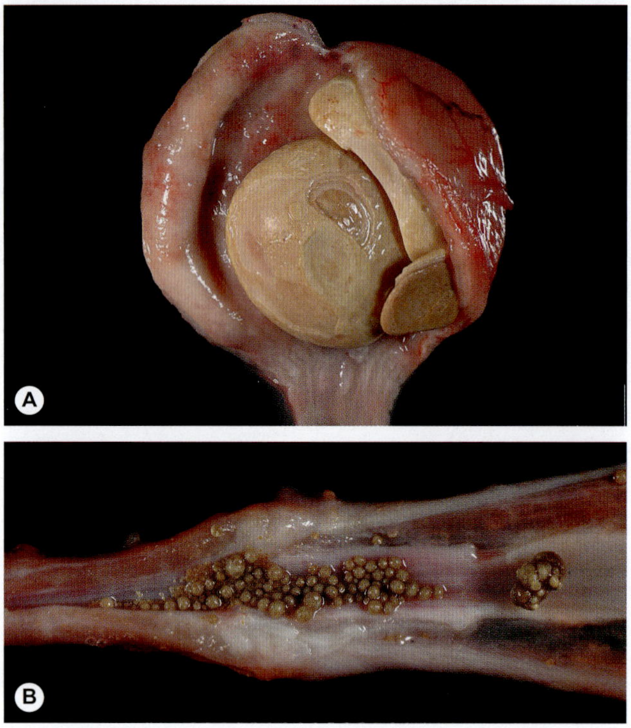

Figure 4-76 A. **Urolithiasis** in the urinary bladder of a dog. (Courtesy L. Himmel, C. Premanandan.) **B.** Numerous small uroliths in the urethra of a cat. (Courtesy C. Martin, C. Premanandan.)

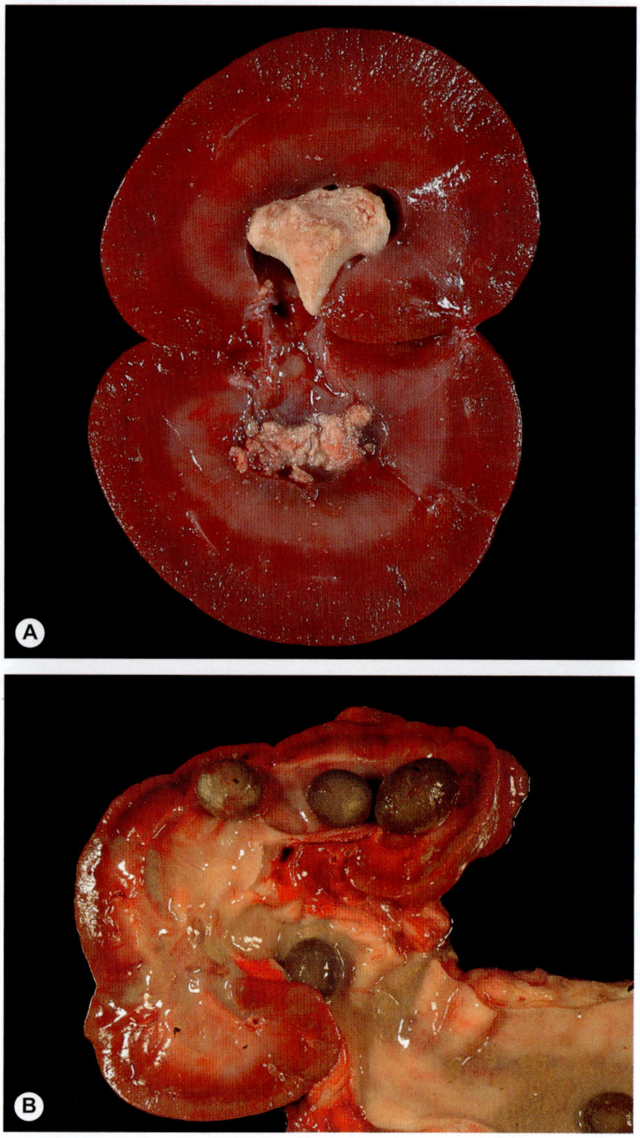

Figure 4-77 A. **Staghorn calculus** in the renal pelvis of a dog. (Courtesy L. Himmel, C. Premanandan.) **B. Uroliths** in a hydronephrotic equine kidney. (Courtesy S. Jennings.)

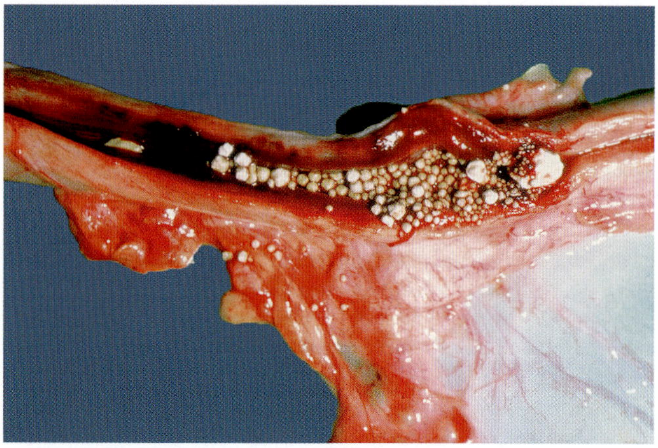

Figure 4-78 **Obstructive urolithiasis** and hemorrhagic urethritis resulting from impaction of numerous calculi at the sigmoid flexure of the penis in a steer. (Courtesy University of Guelph.)

Large numbers of companion animal uroliths have been studied, and knowledge is expanding on the prevalence of mineral composition, breed predilections, geographic region prevalence, and the association with UTIs.

Silica calculi

In **ruminants**, these calculi are hard, white to dark-brown, radiopaque, often laminated, and up to 1 cm across. They are spherical, ovoid, or mulberry shaped, and have smooth surfaces in the bladder of ruminants, but in the kidney, they are angular and irregular, having the shape of the minor calyces, where they are located almost exclusively.

"Pure silica" stones contain ~75% silica as silica dioxide. Mixed calculi contain some calcium oxalate or carbonate. Silica calculi often contain ~20% organic matter. Most have a friable core, which is high in amorphous silica and low in organic matter. The core is surrounded by a layer of organic matter, which separates it from the outer concentric laminations that are rich in silica.

Silica calculi are very common in pastured ruminants and are a major cause of urinary tract obstruction. They occur with increasing prevalence in dogs and rarely in horses. Silica calculi are present in >50% of steers on native ranges in western Canada; <5% develop urethral obstruction. The singularity of adjacent laminae in the calculi is consistent with intermittent deposition as urine composition changes. Certain grasses contain 4-5% or more of silica; the level increases through the growing season. Most of it is relatively insoluble, but some is soluble, unpolymerized silicic acid. Rumen fluid becomes saturated with silicic acid. After absorption, some is returned to the gut in digestive secretions; <1% of dietary silica is excreted in urine, and up to 60% is resorbed from the filtrate. However, when urine production is very low, because of dehydration, the concentration of silicic acid in urine may reach 5 times the saturation level. Even so, precipitation from solution requires other substances, probably proteins of renal or serum origin, in the urine. Calculus formation is reduced to subclinical levels by adding salt to the ration, thereby increasing water consumption. Reduction in the dietary calcium:phosphorus ratio and feeding an acidic diet can also reduce silica urolith formation.

In **dogs**, silica calculi are detected primarily in males, are located in the bladder and urethra, and often cause urinary obstruction. Male German Shepherd dogs and Old English Sheepdogs are at increased risk for formation of these calculi. Unlike cystic silica calculi in ruminants, bladder stones in dogs have very irregular shapes with surface protrusions. Silica uroliths in dogs may be multilayered or single layered and may contain calcium oxalate and struvite. Silica uroliths are likely less soluble in acid than in alkaline urine. Large quantities of plant-derived ingredients, particularly corn gluten feed, rice hulls, and soybean hulls, in dry dog food are implicated as risk factors for development of silica uroliths. Some geographic regions of Mexico have a higher incidence of silica uroliths; a proposed association with higher silica levels of tap water might partially explain this increased incidence. Some canine cases are associated with lower UTIs, often with *Staphylococcus* species.

Struvite calculi (magnesium ammonium phosphate calculi)

Struvite is *magnesium ammonium phosphate hexahydrate* ($MgNH_4PO_4 \bullet 6H_2O$) and is also called a MAP urolith. Struvite stones are white or gray, radiopaque, chalky, usually smooth, and easily broken. They may be pure struvite but usually contain other compounds, such as calcium phosphate (which may form a shell around a struvite calculus), ammonium urate, oxalate, or carbonate. They may be single and large, or numerous and sand-like. Single struvite calculi can form masses that mold to the shape of the cavity they occupy. They have also been referred to as "triple phosphate," a misnomer, and as "infection calculi" in recognition of their common association with infection.

Urolith analysis centers have reported trends of stones analyzed and epidemiologic data on patients. Even with some fluctuations over the past 40 years, struvites and calcium oxalates remain the 2 most common calculi in small animals, usually representing >80% of all stones analyzed. In **dogs**, struvites occur more commonly in females, perhaps because they develop bladder infections more often than males. Ureases from *Staphylococcus* and *Proteus* spp. induce supersaturation of urine with struvite by increasing urine pH and ammonium ions. Bacteria can be cultured from struvite uroliths, with *Staphylococcus pseudintermedius* being the most commonly cultured organism. Alkaline urine decreases struvite solubility and increases ionization of trivalent phosphate, both of which favor calculus formation. Primary pores in struvite calculi are an important feature and may allow dietary and medicinal manipulations to dissolve these uroliths. The occasional refractory response of struvite calculi to medical or dietary manipulations in dogs is suggested to be due to hydroxyl apatite and concentric laminations, which have low porosity. Pugs and some families of Beagles are predisposed to developing both struvite uroliths and struvite urethral plugs, without evidence of underlying UTI.

In **cats**, most cases of the heterogeneous group of disorders referred to as **feline lower urinary tract disease** (FLUTD) are idiopathic and are discussed in the General Cystitis section. One manifestation of FLUTD is urolithiasis, in which discrete calculi develop in the urinary bladder of young to middle-aged cats (increased risk for cats 4-10-years-old). Additional risk factors are associated with Russian Blue, Himalayan, or Persian breed, and castrated male or spayed female status. Intact females had a reduced risk. Struvite crystalluria is often seen in cats with and without calculi; the reasons for aggregation of crystals into sterile calculi are obscure. The prevalence of struvite uroliths and struvite urethral plugs has declined since the mid-1980s when cat foods were reformulated; there has been a concomitant increase in calcium oxalate urolithiasis in cats. Formation of struvite uroliths can be induced in previously normal cats fed calculogenic diets containing 0.15-1.0% dry weight magnesium. Coagulase-positive staphylococci and other bacteria may be cultured from the urine or calculi of some affected cats. Formation of infection-induced struvite calculi is similar to that seen in dogs, but these calculi are less common than sterile struvite uroliths.

Of considerably more importance than discrete calculi are the amorphous accumulations of protein, cellular debris, and struvite crystals that form *sabulous (matrix-crystalline)* ***urethral plugs*** *in male cats*, with castrated males being at a higher risk and spayed females at the lowest risk. Animals 2-7-years-old are predisposed. FLUTD was previously known as *feline urologic syndrome*, and it results from concomitant occurrence of urinary tract inflammation and various types of urine crystals. Clinically, dysuria, hematuria, and urethral obstruction occur. If unrelieved, the obstruction can lead to bladder distension, hemorrhagic cystitis, azotemia, and death. *The obstructive material, which becomes molded to the shape of the urethra in male cats, may be either struvite "sand" or rubber-like protein matrix, or a mixture of the two;* the matrix contains Tamm-Horsfall mucoprotein, albumin, globulins, cells, and cellular debris. The inflammatory component of plugs may be influenced by concurrent infections. The addition of magnesium and phosphate to the diet causes urethral plugs in some cats, and, conversely, the reduction of dietary magnesium reduces the incidence. Alkaline urine pH is likely of more significance in the formation of struvite crystals than is magnesium intake. The increased incidence during cold winter months may be the result of decreased fluid consumption or increased intervals between urinations. The incidence of urethral plugs has decreased as more cats have been fed magnesium-restricted/pH-controlling diets.

In **ruminants**, struvite calculi usually occur in feedlot cattle or sheep on high grain rations, and obstruction may develop in up to 10% of steers. As in cats, *calculi usually form a gritty sludge with a high proportion of matrix.* Inhibition of urethral growth by early castration predisposes to obstruction, and increased water consumption tends to prevent obstruction. Animals with crystalluria often have crystals adhering to preputial hairs. Diets high in phosphate are associated with a high incidence of calculi in sheep, wherein a calcium:phosphorus ratio of 1:2 or greater appears to be the critical cutoff. The balance of other constituents, such as magnesium, sodium, and potassium, is probably also important. Additional potassium tends to promote phosphate urolithiasis. There may also be a genetic effect on urolithiasis in sheep because it is more likely to develop in sheep that excrete phosphorus mainly in urine as opposed to fecal excretion.

Oxalate calculi

Oxalate calculi are hard, heavy, white or yellow, and typically covered with jagged spines, although some are smooth. They tend to be large and solitary in the bladder.

Oxalate calculi occur as calcium oxalates, *either calcium oxalate monohydrate* or *calcium oxalate dihydrate*. Their development is not well understood, but *hypercalciuria and hyperoxaluria are involved*. There are several causes of hypercalciuria (see the Hypercalcemic Nephropathy section). Oxalic acid is synthesized from glyoxylic and ascorbic acid and may be ingested in certain foods. Hyperuricosuria may be involved in oxalate precipitation because sodium hydrogen urate may act as a heterogeneous nucleator. Dietary magnesium and citrate inhibit the formation of calcium oxalate uroliths by forming soluble complexes with oxalate and calcium, respectively.

Oxalate (and silica) calculi may be important in **sheep** grazing grain stubble, but the source of the oxalate is not known. Oxalate-containing plants are not apparently a source because oxalate is metabolized in the rumen; nonetheless, occasional exceptions to this general rule do occur. Feeding a low-calcium diet (0.3% Ca) has produced oxalate urolithiasis in steers, possibly because of increased bone resorption resulting in increased plasma concentrations of hydroxyproline, an oxalate precursor. High magnesium intake inhibits the formation of oxalate calculi; low levels induce formation in some species.

In **dogs**, oxalate calculi are second to struvite calculi in prevalence and are of increasing importance, but little is known of their origins. Calcium oxalate and calcium phosphate (hydroxyapatite or calcium apatite) calculi occur in dogs with primary hyperparathyroidism, hypercalcemia, hyperadrenocorticism, or following exogenous steroid administration. Canine dietary factors, such as high protein, fat, Ca, P, Mg, Na, K, Cl, and use of canned foods, are thought to decrease the risk of development of these stones. Males are more frequently affected than females, and these calculi are seen more commonly in older animals. Breeds at increased risk include the Miniature Schnauzer, Bichon Frise, Lhasa Apso, Yorkshire Terrier, Shih Tzu, and Miniature Poodle. In predisposed Miniature Schnauzers, idiopathic hypercalciuria, decreased urinary oxalate, normal urinary citrate, increased brushite (calcium hydrogen phosphate dihydrate), urinary relative supersaturation, lower urine volume, and elevated excreted uric acid levels have been reported. Idiopathic hypercalciuria also appears to play a role in oxalate urolithiasis in Shih Tzu and Bichon Frise breeds, and it is theorized to result from any of the following: intestinal hyperabsorption, decreased renal resorption, or increased bone resorption of calcium. Genetic variations and different urinary proteomic profiles have been identified in oxalate stone formers versus healthy dogs. Specifically, metabolism of vitamin D might play a role in stone development because single nucleotide polymorphisms in the vitamin D receptor are associated with increased risk of developing stones and higher urinary calcium:creatinine ratios. The proteome of oxalate stone formers showed higher levels of urinary thrombomodulin compared with healthy dogs.

The prevalence of oxalate uroliths in **cats** temporarily increased from the early 1980s through the 1990s. This increase was accompanied by a marked decline in the prevalence of struvite uroliths. However, these trends have since reversed such that oxalates are once again less common in cats. The underlying cause for oxalate uroliths in cats is multifactorial and likely related to diet. Several dietary factors can contribute to calciuria, including high animal-source protein, low magnesium, high sodium chloride, and diets formulated to acidify urine. Risk factors also include feeding a single brand of cat food, and keeping cats in an indoor environment. Persian and Himalayan breeds are at increased risk; cats with calcium oxalate uroliths tend to be older than cats with struvite uroliths. In addition, male and neutered cats are at higher risk for the development of oxalate calculi. Oxalate uroliths in cats have been associated with parathyroid neoplasia, as in dogs.

Uric acid and urate calculi

These *purine-based calculi* are usually multiple, hard, concentrically laminated, and brown-green. In the bladder, they are frequently spherical and <5 mm across. At physiologic pH, urate is more common than uric acid; the terms are used interchangeably. Most urate calculi contain ammonium urate with some uric acid and phosphate; in others, sodium urate is the predominant salt.

Urate stones are most common in dogs, especially Dalmatians, but also occur in pigs and rarely in cats. Most species, except humans and great apes and some dogs, excrete purine catabolites as allantoin, which is a highly soluble product of purine catabolism. However, humans, great apes, Dalmatians, and spontaneous cases of other dog breeds excrete uric acid as their purine breakdown product. In Dalmatians, this is due to an inherited autosomal recessive trait. It is linked to a mutation in *SLC2A9*, a glucose and urate transporter in the liver and renal proximal tubule. Early research showed that hepatic uricase levels are normal, and Dalmatian hepatocytes could catabolize uric acid to allantoin. However, the defective transporter cannot take up urate into hepatocytes, and proximal tubules cannot reabsorb any urate from the urinary filtrate. (In most species and non-Dalmatians, abundant urate is filtered through the glomerulus, but there is net reabsorption along the proximal convoluted tubule.) This means that in affected dogs, all the filtered urate will be excreted into the urinary bladder, promoting stone formation. Predisposing factors for urolith formation include male sex, hyperuricemia, hyperammonemia, hyperuricosuria, hyperammonuria, and aciduria. Other dog breeds with a higher incidence of urate urolithiasis include English Bulldogs and Black Russian Terriers. Affected dogs of those breeds also have the similar *SLC2A9* genotype. Interestingly, the gene is in close proximity to one of the 3 spotting genes, which is likely why the trait has become fixed in the Dalmatian breed.

Dogs and cats with *portosystemic shunts* have ammonium biurate crystals in their urine and may have urate-containing calculi in the kidneys and bladder. Surgical shunt correction will prevent further urate stone formation; however, recurrence of the shunts has been associated with additional episodes of urate urolithiasis. Although **cats** with portosystemic shunts develop urate stones, this pathogenesis only explains a minority of the cases. In general, feline urate urolithiasis remains poorly characterized. Over-represented breeds in the population of cats with urate urolithiasis include Siamese, Egyptian Mau, and Birmans. Associated genetic mutations have not been reported in cats. Neonatal **piglets** in a negative energy balance produce increased purine catabolites, thus predisposing to urate urolithiasis. Urea-splitting organisms might also be important in the development of urate calculi because production of ammonium ion favors calculus formation.

Xanthine calculi

Xanthine stones are yellow to brown-red, often concentrically laminated, friable, and irregularly shaped. They are radiolucent. *Xanthine is a metabolite of purines*, which seldom appears in urine because it is normally degraded by xanthine oxidase to uric acid.

Xanthine calculi occur occasionally in dogs and are reported in sheep, calves, and cats. A high incidence in sheep was circumstantially related to deficiency of molybdenum in unimproved pasture because molybdenum is a component of xanthine oxidase. Several cases in calves in Japan were also associated with deficiency of xanthine oxidase. Xanthine precipitates in acid urine. Calculi usually form in the collecting ducts and calyces of the kidney and may cause hydronephrosis.

Two forms of xanthinuria exist in **dogs**. The *primary form* is inherited as an autosomal recessive and is caused by mutations in either of 2 genes. The first gene (*XDH*) codes for xanthine dehydrogenase, which catalyzes 2 sequential steps in degradation of purines, namely, conversion of hypoxanthine to xanthine, and then xanthine to uric acid. Notably, xanthine oxidase and xanthine dehydrogenase are different enzymes, but they both use the same substrates (hypoxanthine and xanthine) to produce uric acid. However, xanthine dehydrogenase uses NAD as a cofactor, generating NADH during the conversion, whereas xanthine oxidase generates a superoxide anion during uric acid production. The other genetic defect in canine xanthinuria is in the molybdenum cofactor sulfurase gene (*MOCOS*), which is needed for *XDH* activity, and again highlights the role of molybdenum in the function of xanthine dehydrogenase. Primary xanthinuria has been noted most often in Dachshunds and in a family of Cavalier King Charles Spaniels; examination of unrelated Cavaliers did not reveal abnormal excretion or metabolism of uric acids and xanthines. The *secondary form of xanthinuria* (iatrogenic) is more common in dogs, especially Dalmatians, and is usually the result of previous treatment with allopurinol, which binds to and inhibits the action of xanthine oxidase.

Cystine calculi

Cystine calculi are small and irregular, soft and friable, waxy, and light-yellow to red-brown, turning to green on exposure to daylight. Many cystine calculi consist of pure cystine; others may also contain calcium oxalate, struvite, and complex urates.

*Cystine stones occur in **dogs**, ferrets, and rarely in cats*. They comprise <1% of canine calculi in North America, but 20-30% in some European countries, being second to struvite calculi in prevalence. Cystinuria occurs in both males and females, but cystine calculi and urinary obstruction occur almost exclusively in males. They are primarily found in the urinary bladder, but nephroliths are common in Irish Terriers, Scottish Terriers, and Newfoundlands. Other predisposed breeds include Dachshunds, Bulldogs, Mastiffs, Basset Hounds, and Tibetan Spaniels. Although blood cystine levels are normal, urinary cystine levels are high because of defective proximal tubular resorption from glomerular filtrate. The renal tubular transporter system for basic amino acids in dogs, cats, and humans is a tetramer composed of 2 heterodimers of the $b^{0,+}$AT protein (encoded by *SLC7A9*) and rBAT (encoded by *SLC3A1*). Many dogs with cystinuria also have high levels of other amino acids (ornithine, lysine, and arginine) in their urine, but these are more soluble than cystine. Cystine precipitates in acid urine, but factors other than urinary pH are probably important in the genesis of cystine stones because dogs with crystalluria do not always form stones. The incidence of recurrent urolithiasis is enhanced in those dogs with higher excretions of urinary cystine. In some dogs, the severity of cystinuria may decrease with age. Mutations in *SLC3A1* cause **type I-A** and **type II-A cystinuria** in dogs, and these types are autosomal recessive and autosomal dominant, respectively. Type I-A cystinuria is documented in Newfoundlands and Labrador Retrievers; type II-A is reported in Australian Cattle Dogs. Mutations in *SLC7A9* cause autosomal dominant type II-B cystinuria. Last, there is androgen-dependent cystinuria, which is only reported in mature intact male dogs and is referred to as **type III cystinuria**. Castration is considered curative in those animals.

Clover stones

***Sheep** grazing estrogenic pastures*, particularly subterranean clover, or sheep *injected or implanted with estrogens*, may have an incidence of fatal urinary obstruction as high as 10%. There are probably 3 *separate developmental patterns*, and in each, the obstructing material is soft or pulpy and scantily mineralized. Probably, the most common pattern is urethral obstruction by desquamated cells and secretions of accessory glands originating in the pelvic urethra under the influence of estrogen. The second type, the so-called "clover stone," is usually found in the renal pelvis as yellow, soft material, which eventually leads to scarring of the kidney. It affects both sexes equally. These calculi contain *benzocoumarins*, which may be metabolites of phytoestrogens. Finally, sudden and serious mortalities may occur in male sheep grazing subterranean clover *(Trifolium subterraneum)* during its period of rapid maturation. The urethral process becomes impacted with soft white paste consisting mainly of calcium carbonate and an unidentified organic material probably related to *isoflavones*.

Other types of calculi

Several other types of calculi develop in animals. They may be important locally, or iatrogenic and rare, such as **tetracycline, sulfonamide**, and **barium** stones. Dried solidified **blood calculi** are identified in cats and rarely dogs. In some cases, the mineralization might be limited (and therefore the term "calculus" might be a misnomer). Even so, they can block the renal pelvis or ureter, resulting in similar obstructive nephropathy. The source of the hemorrhage might be from tubular red blood cell casts or from vascular damage; both lesions have been seen histologically in the kidneys of cats where blood calculi are present at autopsy.

Cats treated with the antiviral compound, **remdesivir** or its metabolite GS 441524, for feline infectious peritonitis rarely form a new type of urolith. Spectrographic analysis of the metabolite and the stones have been identical, and the metabolite has limited solubility in water. After this discovery, veterinarians have been encouraged to closely monitor cats treated with this medication for clinical signs of dysuria or stranguria.

Stones with high **carbonate** content are associated with very alkaline urines and are seen in ruminants consuming high-oxalate plants or clover-dominated pastures.

In horses, **calcium carbonate** crystals are seen commonly in normal urine. Calculi are much less frequent, but are most commonly composed of calcium carbonate, usually in the crystalline form of calcite, and similar compounds where the Ca of $CaCO_3$ is replaced in various amounts by Mg, K, and Mn. Calcium oxalate dihydrate may also be present. Alkaline pH and dietary factors are implicated in their formation.

Uncommonly, canine uroliths are composed of **calcium phosphate**. Factors that decrease calcium phosphate solubility, predisposing to urolith formation include alkaline urine, hypercalcemia and hypercalciuria (due to hyperparathyroidism), reduced concentrations of crystallization inhibitors (inorganic pyrophosphates, citrate, magnesium ions, nephrocalcin), or increased concentrations of crystallization promoters (calcium oxalate and urate crystals).

INFLAMMATION OF THE LOWER URINARY TRACT

Inflammation of the lower urinary tract centers on involvement of the urinary bladder, that is, **cystitis. Ureteritis** is rare in the absence of cystitis, and clinical **urethritis** in animals is usually associated with obstruction by a calculus from the bladder. Under normal circumstances, the bladder is resistant to infection, and bacteria are quickly eliminated by the normal flow of normal urine. *Predisposition to UTI* occurs when there is stagnation of urine because of obstruction, incomplete bladder emptying (because of upper or lower motor neuron disease or dysautonomia), or urothelial trauma. *Other risk factors for UTI* include catheterization, vaginoscopy, urinary incontinence, vaginitis, or administration of antibiotics or corticosteroids. Of itself, normal voiding is not sufficient to prevent or eliminate bladder infection. *Defense mechanisms* in the bladder and urethra, which prevent bacterial adhesion to mucosal surfaces, are essential if bacteria are to be removed by urine flow. *Uromodulin* (also called Tamm-Horsfall mucoprotein), produced in the kidneys, may bind to bacterial adhesins and prevent adherence. Local production of IgA and a surface glycosaminoglycan layer is probably important in preventing attachment of organisms to the normal urothelium, and IgG may have similar activity in specific UTIs. Urinary oligosaccharides may be able to detach adherent bacteria. Voiding of sloughed urothelial cells with attached bacteria aids their clearance. Incomplete voiding at micturition may be a result of diverticula of the urinary bladder or vesicoureteral reflux. Residual urine can maintain a bladder infection, allowing organisms to take advantage of any opportunity to invade the urothelium.

Unlike human urine, which tends to be a good medium for bacterial growth, animal urine usually has antibacterial activity. This activity is related to urine pH and particularly to urine osmolality. In general, the further the pH is from the optimum range of 6-7, the less likely it is to support bacterial growth. The antibacterial effect of acidic urine is related to the concentration of undissociated organic acids. High urine osmolality also contributes to bacteriostasis.

To infect the urinary tract, uropathogens must compete with the normal bacterial flora of the distal urethra, vulva, or prepuce. *The usual causes of cystitis are* ***bacteria*** *from the urethra, the origin of which is almost always the rectal flora.* Cystitis is common in young animals with patent urachus, and the bacterial flora is mixed. When bacteria breach the surface defenses of the urothelium and attach to the epithelial cells, the cells are desquamated through a rapid apoptosis-like mechanism. If the urothelium is penetrated, clearance is prevented and neutrophils and macrophages in the submucosa respond.

Various **bacteria** may be involved in bladder infections and these include in all hosts: uropathogenic *Escherichia coli (UPEC)*, *Proteus vulgaris*, streptococci, staphylococci, and enterococci. Other uropathogens include *Klebsiella*, *Pasteurella*, *Mycoplasma*, *Enterobacter*, and *Pseudomonas* spp. Coinfections with more than one bacterium are common. The *Corynebacterium renale* group (*C. renale*, *C. pilosum*, *C. cystitidis*) is important in cows, and less so in other species, where it is usually part of a mixed infection. *C. urealyticum* can cause "encrusting cystitis" in dogs and cats with deposition of struvite (magnesium ammonium phosphate) and calcium phosphate along the bladder mucosa secondary to ammonia release by these urease-producing bacteria. Likewise, *Staphylococcus felis* and *Proteus mirabilis* have been associated with pseudomembranous cystitis that has foci of mineralization. *Actinobaculum (Eubacterium) suis* is the primary cause of cystitis and pyelonephritis in swine and is an important cause of death in sows; *A. suis* infections typically produce gross hematuria and alkaline urine.

Mycoplasmas are uncommon causes of UTI in dogs and cattle. In the latter species, *Mycoplasmopsis (Mycoplasma) bovirhinis* (a typical isolate from the respiratory tract) can also be isolated from semen and then may travel retrograde through the female reproductive tract to the bladder in recently bred cows and bulls with urethral obstruction. Urogenital infections causing prostatitis, orchitis, nephritis, and cystitis may occur in canine **blastomycosis**. *Aspergillus*, *Candida*, and *Nocardia* are unusual causes of cystitis in dogs and cats. *Candida* infections can be seen more commonly with predisposing factors, such as diabetes mellitus, prolonged antibiotic or glucocorticoid usage, aciduria, indwelling catheters, or an immunocompromised state.

Bacterial pathogens of the urinary tract, such as *Escherichia coli*, can express a formidable array of *virulence factors*. The most urovirulent strains often express various virulence factors simultaneously, producing a synergistic or additive effect and are classified as UPEC. As discussed previously (in Pyelonephritis), there is not a single genetic marker of UPEC. These organisms are defined based on their ability to survive in the urinary environment. These factors include fimbriae or pili adhesins (*P fimbriae, type 1 fimbriae*), nonfimbrial adhesins, CNF1, aerobactin (an iron chelator), hemolysin A, capsular polysaccharide, and anticomplementary serum resistance. Certain virulence factors, such as *adhesins*, specifically favor the development of pyelonephritis; others favor cystitis. In human UPEC, P fimbriae bind to renal pelvic urothelium and are thought to be responsible for pyelonephritis. *Type 1 fimbriae (pili)* are more important in bladder colonization. Type 1 pili tips interact with membrane glycoproteins of urothelial cells, known as *uroplakins*. In contrast, gram-positive bacteria use extracellular polysaccharides for adhesion.

Once attached, UPEC can invade the urothelial cell and replicate to create small intracellular bacterial colonies. Interestingly, UPEC can replicate rapidly without increasing in length and change from a coliform morphology to a more coccoid shape. The clusters of bacteria have *biofilm properties* and will eventually distort the apical membrane of the superficial urothelial cell. Later, UPEC become motile and detach from the clusters to exit the cell. At this time, the bacteria attain a filamentous morphology, which helps them survive attacks by neutrophils. These bacterial morphologic changes occur in human UTI and experimentally in some rodent models. Their relevance to UTI in animals is unknown. Urothelial cells will exfoliate as part of an innate host defense system.

Last, subclinical bacteriuria is occasionally seen in small animals. These patients have bacterial colonization of their bladder (often with UPEC, but other organisms as well). If there are no clinical signs, such as difficulty urinating or ascending pyelonephritis, treatment might not be warranted.

In fact, newer antimicrobial stewardship policies state that these animals should not be treated because it risks development of antimicrobial-resistant bacteria.

General cystitis and specific variants

Cystitis is a clinically significant disease in many species. There is a higher incidence in females, which is probably associated with their shorter urethra. Hormone-induced changes, such as hyperestrogenism, can also affect the functional integrity of the urethral and vesicular epithelium. The role of hormones in the production of glycosaminoglycans in the urogenital tract might also change the susceptibility to UTIs. During estrus in sows, estrogen causes the urine pH to rise, producing an alkaline environment suitable for the growth of *Actinobaculum suis*.

Animals with diabetes mellitus, hyperadrenocorticism, or pyometra are at increased risk of developing UTIs with *E. coli*. Glucosuria in diabetes mellitus promotes bacterial growth, but other factors (e.g., decreased leukocyte efficiency) might also be significant in this condition. **Emphysematous cystitis** develops rarely in dogs and cats with diabetes mellitus and is thought to be a result of fermentation by glucose-fermenting bacteria. Emphysematous cystitis is less commonly detected in nondiabetic animals (Fig. 4-79).

Malakoplakia is a rare but classic lesion in which defective macrophages cannot digest phagocytosed *E. coli*. It has been reported in puppies (Pugs and Bulldogs) with histories of chronic recurrent UTI. Histologically, the lamina propria is expanded by sheets of macrophages that contain granular-to-globular debris in the cytoplasm (Fig. 4-80). The material stains positively with PAS (see Fig. 4-80B). Occasionally, myriad intracellular bacteria can be demonstrated with Giemsa; however, other stains for infectious agents (traditional Gram stain, Ziehl-Neelsen, and GMS) are negative. This severe cystitis is untreatable and might have a pathogenesis akin to histiocytic ulcerative colitis, especially given the similarity in breeds affected.

In addition to UTIs, *other types of diseases* also induce urinary tract inflammation with or without hemorrhage of the lower urinary tract. Hemorrhagic cystitis sometimes occurs in *malignant catarrhal fever* in cattle and deer, and occasionally is the dominant gross lesion. In horses eating alfalfa hay, hematuria should raise the clinical suspicion of *cantharidin* intoxication. In *Schistosoma mattheei* infections in cattle, linear granulomas occur in the renal pelvis, ureter, and bladder. UTI has been associated with recent calving, inadequate sanitation, and omphalitis in dairy cattle, but azotemia is uncommon. Cystitis in horses and cattle (but not sheep) grazing *Sorghum* sp. is associated with ataxia caused by degenerative encephalomyelopathy; the bladder lesions are almost certainly neurogenic in origin.

Feline lower urinary tract disease (FLUTD) may result from UTI, uroliths, urethral plugs, congenital or acquired anatomic defects of the bladder or urethra, or iatrogenic causes. Even when discrete uroliths cannot be identified, crystals can be embedded along the urothelial mucosa (Fig. 4-81), suggesting previous urolithiasis, urinary sludge, or abrasion by the crystals. Abyssinian cats, cats >10-years-old, and spayed females are predisposed to bacterial UTI. Although some studies report the absence of

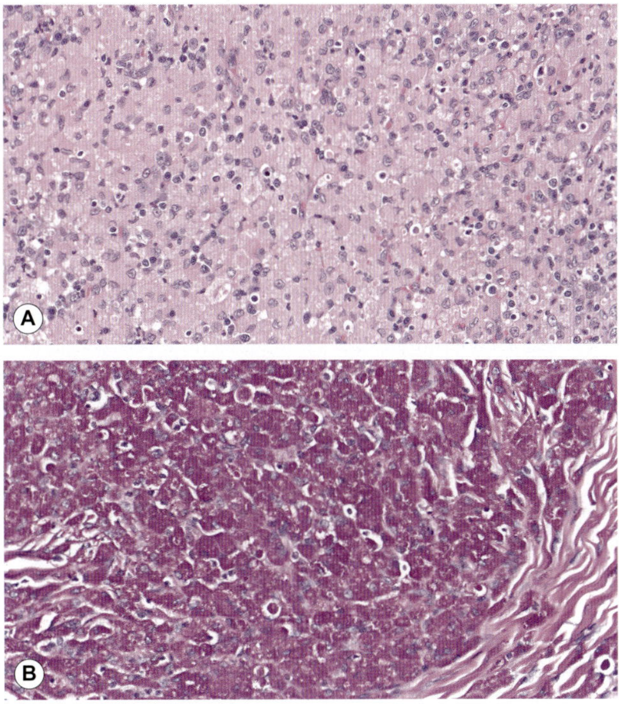

Figure 4-80 Malakoplakia in a dog. **A**. The urinary bladder wall is effaced by macrophages that contain eosinophilic granular material. H&E. **B**. The granules stain bright pink and are phagocytized *Escherichia coli* that cannot be digested. PAS stain.

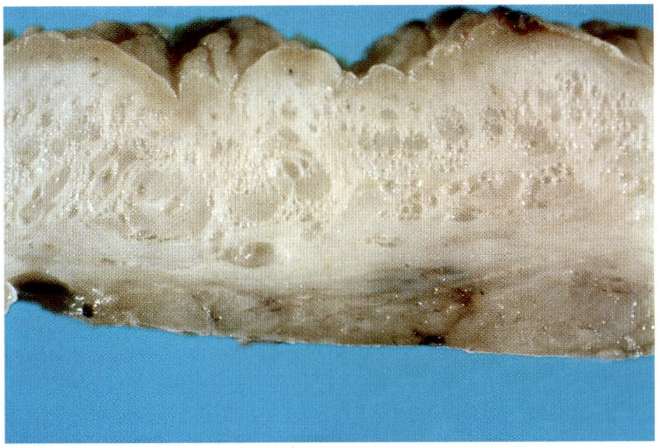

Figure 4-79 Emphysematous cystitis in a dog; not associated with diabetes mellitus. (Courtesy University of Guelph.)

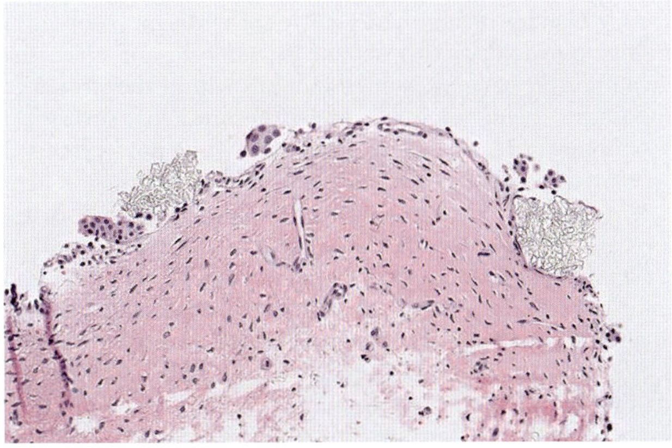

Figure 4-81 Erosive cystitis with embedded oxalate crystals in the urinary bladder of a cat with clinical signs of feline lower urinary tract disease.

infection in most cases of FLUTD, other studies have demonstrated bacteriuria in up to one-third of cats with these clinical signs. Differences in prevalence may be the result of patient population, geographic location, and primary practice versus tertiary referral care centers. Various viruses, including feline syncytia-forming virus and novel feline caliciviruses, have been implicated as potential urinary pathogens in FLUTD cats. *Mycoplasma* or *Ureaplasma* have also been suggested to play a role. There is no concrete evidence that any of these infectious agents are involved. Cats with antibodies to feline morbillivirus 1 (FeMV; *Paramyxoviridae, Morbillivirus felis*) had a higher risk of FLUTD in comparison to those that do not. Interestingly, antibodies to feline morbillivirus 2 were more commonly seen in cats with azotemic CKD but not FLUTD.

Many cases of FLUTD are idiopathic and bear considerable resemblance to the somewhat obscure condition in humans called "interstitial cystitis." The **feline version of interstitial cystitis** results in chronic irritative voiding signs (dysuria, hematuria, pollakiuria, and/or inappropriate urination), sterile and cytologically inactive urine, and cystoscopically visible submucosal petechiae. This common feline condition may result from decreased urinary excretion of glycosaminoglycans, increased bladder permeability, and neurogenic inflammation. Increased sympathetic activity is confirmed in feline interstitial cystitis cases, and this affects bladder function locally. Nonspecific histologic changes in the bladders of affected cats include submucosal edema, dilated submucosal vessels with margination of neutrophils, and submucosal hemorrhage; numbers of submucosal mast cells may also be increased. Cats 4-10-years-old are predisposed.

Sterile hemorrhagic cystitis may occur in dogs and cats treated for neoplastic or immunologic diseases with *cyclophosphamide*. Activated metabolites of the drug cause mucosal ulceration, hemorrhage, and edema. Signs of cystitis occasionally follow an 8-week course of therapy, but have also been noted within 24 hours of administration of the first therapeutic dose. Concurrent treatment with other drugs, degree of diuresis, and pre-existing cystitis may influence the prevalence of cyclophosphamide-induced lesions. Fibrosis and mineralization of the bladder may result in persistent hematuria and incontinence. UC may develop in the bladder of dogs in association with prolonged cyclophosphamide therapy.

Eosinophilic polypoid cystitis is an uncommon form of cystitis in older dogs with a history of urolithiasis and with a predominance of eosinophils in a proliferative fibroblastic mass (Fig. 4-82). Surgical excision is considered curative. In our experience, eosinophils are frequently identified in many urinary bladder inflammatory polyps. The diagnosis of eosinophilic polypoid cystitis should be reserved for cases that have multiple aggregates of eosinophils within the stroma (as opposed to being targeted toward the urothelial surface). If eosinophils are lacking, the diagnosis of "polypoid cystitis" is warranted.

Cystitis is differentiated into acute and chronic forms, but there is considerable overlap in both the lesions and the causes. In simple **acute** catarrhal inflammation, there is moderate hyperemia and submucosal edema, and the surface is covered with a layer of tenacious catarrhal exudate. The urine is cloudy. Histologically, there is necrosis and desquamation of the epithelium and prominent leukocytic infiltration. Submucosal vessels are dilated and cuffed by leukocytes. In more severe inflammation, leukocytes may infiltrate all layers of the bladder wall, the mucosa may ulcerate, and hemorrhage from the submucosal vessels may be severe enough to produce blood clots in the bladder lumen. These hemorrhagic complications are common in cystitis following urethral obstruction, especially in cats and cattle. When the inflammation is severe, the cystitis may be erosive to ulcerative (Fig. 4-83). There might be superficial fibrinous or a deeper diphtheritic covering of the denuded regions. In both, there is a thick, dirty-yellow friable surface encrustation, which may peel with difficulty. Ulcerations may penetrate the wall to the serosa or predispose to rupture.

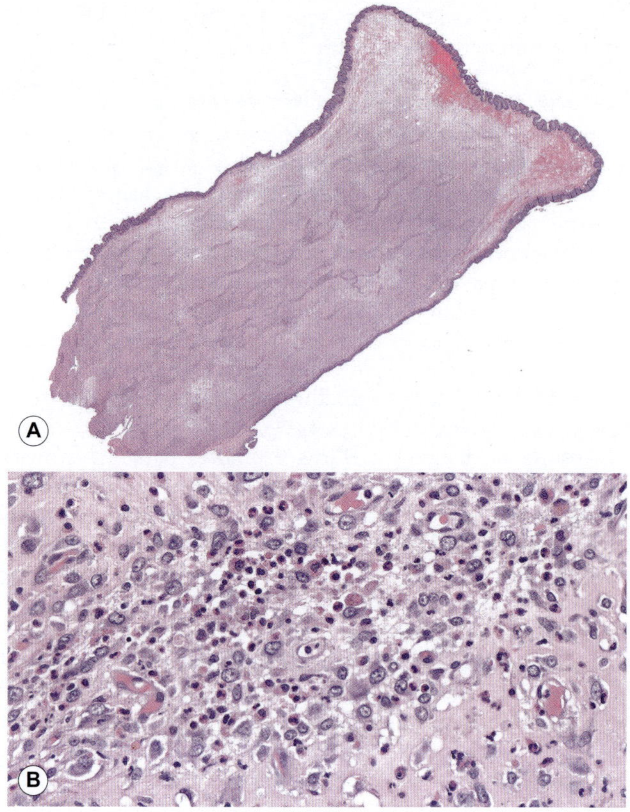

Figure 4-82 Fibrurothelial polyp in the urinary bladder of a dog. **A**. The lesion has hyperplastic urothelium and a stromal core. Invasion of the urothelium is not present. **B**. Some polyps have a prominent population of eosinophils in the stroma. In those scenarios, the diagnosis of "eosinophilic stromal polyp" is often used. H&E.

Chronic cystitis may also have different patterns. The simplest occurs in association with calculi. The mucosa is irregularly reddened and usually thickened. There is some urothelial desquamation, and the submucosa is infiltrated by mononuclear inflammatory cells; there are few neutrophils (eFig. 4-43). In addition, there is often submucosal fibrosis and hypertrophy of the muscularis. In **follicular cystitis**, which is common in dogs, the mucosa is studded with gray-white ~1-mm nodules, which may be confluent or surrounded by a zone of hyperemia (Fig. 4-84). Histologically, the nodules are aggregates of proliferating lymphocytes. These are immediately beneath the epithelium, which may be normal or ulcerated. **Chronic polypoid cystitis** is common in any species. The mucosa is thrown into many folds or villus-like or sessile projections. The polyps are covered by epithelium over a core of proliferated connective tissue densely infiltrated with mononuclear leukocytes. The polyps can undergo mucoid degeneration, or the epithelium might undergo metaplasia to a mucus-secreting, glandular type, resembling colonic epithelium. Polyps can break down, causing intermittent hematuria or outflow obstruction. With the increasing number of cystoscopic biopsy sample submissions, it can sometimes be difficult to differentiate polyps with Brunn nests or cystitis glandularis from fragments of malignant tumors that have true invasion. Identification of basement membrane around the Brunn nests or glands can support the diagnosis of a benign hyperplastic process, but this feature might not always be visible. Immunohistochemistry should show that the nests or glands will express basal cell IHC markers (AE1/AE3) but will not express CK7, which should label mature, superficial urothelial cells (see Table 4-4).

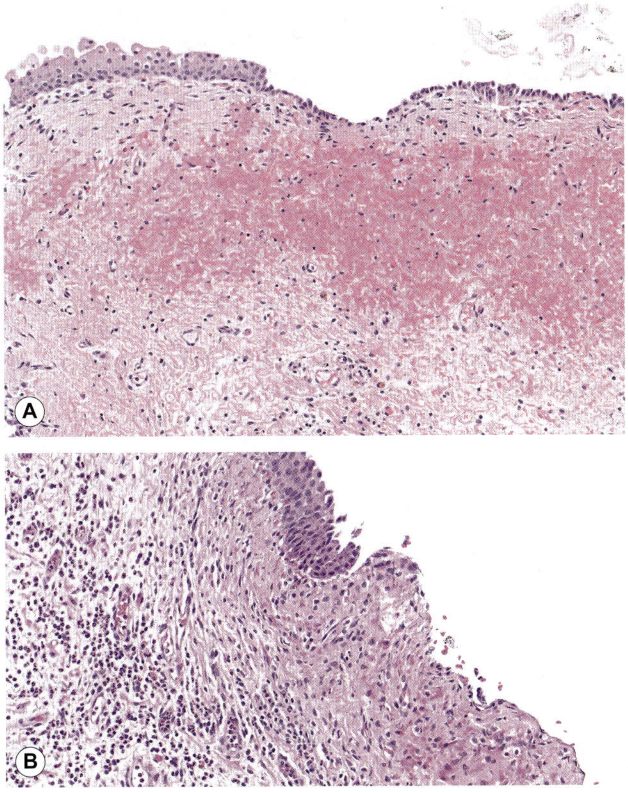

Figure 4-83 **Cystitis** in dogs. **A**. Focal erosion of the urothelium with acute lamina proprial hemorrhage. **B**. Ulcerative cystitis in a different dog with many neutrophils in the lamina propria.

Enzootic hematuria

Enzootic hematuria is a syndrome in mature **cattle** seen as *persistent hematuria* and anemia, and is associated with *hemorrhages or neoplasms in the lower urinary tract*. In >90% of cases, the hematuria originates from **tumors of the urinary bladder**. Outbreaks of the disease are also reported in sheep.

Enzootic hematuria occurs on all continents, but is restricted to particular locations. In endemic areas, up to 90% of adult cattle may be affected. *The syndrome is attributed to chronic ingestion of* **bracken fern** and is reproducible experimentally. The extent and persistence with which toxic ferns are grazed probably influences the incidence of bladder lesions. There are 2 subspecies of bracken fern: *Pteridium aquilinum* subsp. *aquilinum* and *P. aquilinum* subsp. *caudatum*. It is not known whether all varieties are toxic. *P. revolutum*, a species of bracken fern common in South Asia, and *P. esculentum*, a bracken fern of Australia, also produce enzootic hematuria. In areas where bracken does not grow, other ferns, such as *Cheilanthes sieberi* (mulga or rock fern from Australia), are capable of producing enzootic hematuria.

Bracken fern is very common and may be the only plant that causes naturally occurring tumors in animals. *It contains several toxic substances*, including a thiaminase, a variety of carcinogens (quercetin, shikimic acid, prunasin, ptaquiloside, ptaquiloside Z, aquilide A, and others), and a "bleeding factor" of unknown structure. Following administration of ptaquiloside to guinea pigs, hemorrhagic cystitis results, suggesting that this is one of the toxic principles in bracken fern hematuria. There is a strong link between bracken fern and bovine papillomavirus 2 (BPV2) in the development of bladder neoplasms in animals with enzootic hematuria; the relationship of oncogenic viruses to bracken is discussed in Vol. 2, Alimentary System.

Cattle fed low levels of bracken fern develop microscopic, followed by macroscopic, hematuria. Microhematuria is usually associated with petechiae, ecchymoses, or suffusive hemorrhages in the urothelium of the renal calyces, pelvis, ureter, and bladder (Fig. 4-85). These lesions appear to be a manifestation of the hemorrhagic syndrome characteristic of acute bracken fern poisoning. In some cases, microscopic hematuria occurs before gross lesions are visible. Diffuse or patchy areas of pink discoloration develop in the bladder mucosa, and microscopically, ectatic and engorged capillaries are present. These altered vessels are prone to hemorrhage into the

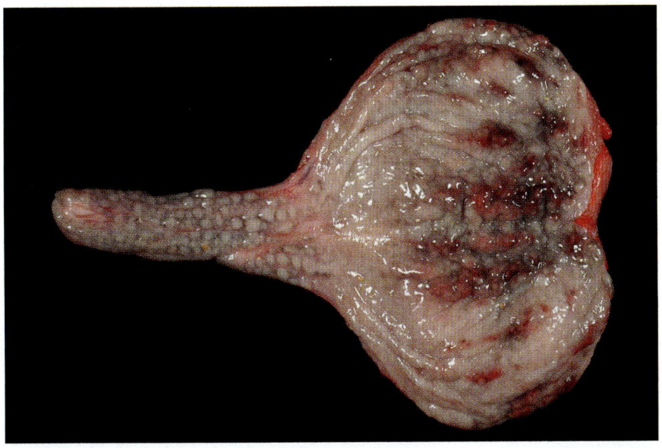

Figure 4-84 **Follicular cystitis** in a dog. (Courtesy D. Russell.)

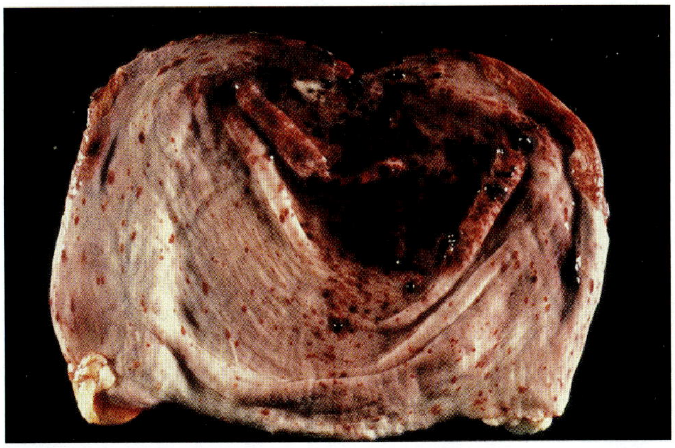

Figure 4-85 Hemorrhagic urinary bladder mucosa in **enzootic hematuria** in a cow. (Courtesy K. Potter.)

bladder wall or lumen, and nodular vascular lesions develop in affected areas. Macroscopic hematuria is usually, but not always, indicative of tumors, which ulcerate and bleed into the lumen. Occasionally, tumors also develop in the renal pelvis and ureter, and hepatic hemangiomas accompany bladder tumors in a few animals. Most neoplasms are located on the ventral and lateral walls of the bladder, where constant contact with urine occurs.

Several types of epithelial and mesenchymal neoplasms may develop, including UC, SCC, papilloma, adenoma, hemangioma, hemangiosarcoma, leiomyosarcoma, fibroma, and fibrosarcoma. Various tumors of more than one type may be present, and in >50% of affected cattle mixed epithelial-mesenchymal neoplasms develop. *Papillomas, fibromas, and hemangiomas with carcinomas are the most common types*. Malignant types may invade locally, and ~10% of epithelial malignancies metastasize to iliac nodes or lungs. Chronic cystitis usually accompanies the neoplastic changes. Brunn nests may develop in the mucosa. Epithelial neoplasms appear to develop from the hyperplastic and metaplastic (squamous and mucous) changes in the urothelium that often accompany the vascular lesions. A pagetoid variant of urothelial carcinoma in situ has been reported in a cow that also had enzootic hematuria and concurrent BPV2 infection; fragile histidine triad (Fhit) protein, expressed by the tumor suppressor gene *FHIT*, was found to be absent in some of the pagetoid cells, correlating with late-stage neoplastic progression. Uroplakins are urothelial cell differentiation products that are more consistently expressed in the superficial urothelium. In high-grade urothelial carcinomas that invade muscle, the immunohistochemical uroplakin III staining of the neoplastic cells decreases; cytokeratin-7 expression is maintained. Research indicates that cyclin D1 may be dysregulated in all tumors (benign and malignant) from cattle with enzootic hematuria; malignancies often have p53 mutations. Although it is not necessarily of use prognostically, staining for uroplakins may help identify metastatic urothelial cell clusters.

NEOPLASMS OF THE LOWER URINARY TRACT

Neoplasia of the lower urinary tract is uncommon, but occurs most often in dogs, cats, and cattle (see the Enzootic Hematuria section, which is associated with almost all bovine bladder neoplasia). Equine bladder neoplasia is rare, but SCC of the bladder has been reported in this species. There are few data for other animals; thus, the following discussion concerns mainly small animals. Because of the overwhelming proportion of UC among urinary bladder cancers, almost all epidemiologic trends concern this subtype. Therefore, signalment trends are discussed below in that subtopic. Most tumors of the urinary bladder are malignant and will metastasize, and most bladder neoplasms in small animals are epithelial in origin. With the exception of rhabdomyosarcoma, neoplasia of the lower urinary tract usually occurs in old animals. Clinical signs are often related to the urinary system with hematuria, stranguria, pollakiuria, and urinary incontinence. UTIs are occasional comorbidities. In those cases, the bladder mass might not be identified until after recurrence of clinical signs post-treatment.

Bladder neoplasia may be caused by a variety of industrial chemicals, chronic irritation, foreign bodies (sutures), viruses, bracken fern, and cyclophosphamide. *Staging of urinary tract neoplasms according to tumor invasiveness, lymph node involvement, and metastases [the tumor-node-metastasis (TNM) system]* can assist with prognostication and selection of therapeutic plans. The clinician is responsible for determining the stage, often requiring diagnostic imaging. Obviously, input from the pathologist is required for staging.

Notably, the various tumor types discussed below can occur anywhere in the lower urinary tract. Because of the relatively large surface area of the urinary bladder, most descriptive studies report characteristics of tumors in this location. However, urethral neoplasia can be more clinically significant, resulting in obstruction even when the tumor is fairly small. In contrast, ureteral neoplasia might be clinically silent because only one kidney is obstructed. With the advent of less invasive biopsy techniques and advancements in urologic surgery techniques, more samples from the urethra or ureters will be submitted for evaluation. As such, it is likely that trends in tumor types and associated signalment data might shift when sufficient numbers of those types of samples are amassed.

It is rare for malignancies in other organs to metastasize to the bladder. These rare metastases usually originate from other levels of the urinary tract (renal, ureteral, urethral, prostatic), or as peritoneal implants of local pelvic neoplasia.

A literature review collated data from various studies reporting numbers and types of urinary bladder neoplasia (from the 1960s to the 1990s) for dogs, cats, and cattle and also added cases from the Veterinary Medical Database (previously unpublished data). The prevalence data below are based on this review. For perspective, there were 2,421 canine bladder neoplasms, 2,131 bovine bladder neoplasms (all associated with enzootic hematuria), and 119 feline bladder neoplasms.

Epithelial tumors

Urothelial carcinomas (UCs), formerly called *transitional cell carcinomas* (TCCs), account for 2% of all canine malignancies, and are less prevalent in cats. In dogs, spayed females are over-represented. The sex bias is less pronounced in the predisposed breeds: Scottish Terriers, Shetland Sheepdogs, Wirehaired Fox Terriers, and West Highland White Terriers. Epithelial tumors (papillomas, adenomas, carcinomas) comprise 75-90% of canine and feline lower urinary tract neoplasms, and most of them develop in the bladder of old animals.

Papillomas are uncommon in small animals, comprising 2% of all canine and feline bladder neoplasms. They represent 22% of bovine bladder neoplasms. A papilloma is a focal (singular) projection of urothelium covering a narrow stalk of stromal tissue. The urothelium is well differentiated, <8 cell layers thick, does not have cellular or nuclear atypia, and mitoses are not observed. Sometimes a basement membrane between the urothelium and the supporting stroma can be identified. The urothelium does not invade the supporting stroma. Additionally, the stromal connective tissue should not be inflamed. Notably, there are histologic similarities among papillomas, polyps, and polypoid cystitis, so it is possible that some papillomas are placed into non-neoplastic diagnostic categories (and vice versa). Polyps will also be single (focal); polypoid cystitis will be multifocal. Both polyps and polypoid cystitis will have inflammation, neovascularization, and frequently granulation tissue within their stromal cores. The urothelium of polyps and polypoid cystitis can be >7 cell layers thick, and it might be eroded or undergoing squamous metaplasia. The urothelium often extends into the stroma (e.g., forming Brunn nests and cystitis glandularis lesions). Last, bladders with polyps and polypoid cystitis will have evidence of inflammation in other regions of the organ. In cattle, where the samples are obtained at slaughter or autopsy, the pathologist can be certain that the lesions are singular and that they are harvested such that the underlying bladder wall can be assessed for evidence of invasion or inflammation. This can facilitate accurate diagnoses of papillomas. Obtaining ideal samples to enable differentiation of these lesions can be more difficult in small animals, especially if the masses are harvested via cystoscopy. Experimentally, papillomas have been documented to undergo malignant transformation to UC. This presumably occurs in spontaneous tumors as well; however, documentation of this process via partial or incisional biopsy of a papilloma with long-term follow-up to show tumor progression has not been reported in cats or dogs.

Adenomas are rare in all species; they originate from areas of mucous metaplasia of the urothelium and may have a papillary or pedunculated appearance. In fact, distinguishing an adenoma from a papilloma is based solely on histologic architecture. Microscopically, they form glandular structures, some of which contain mucin. The glandular structures can extend into the lamina propria but do not invade the smooth muscle.

Carcinomas may be solitary or multiple and usually do not reach a large size before they cause hematuria or death from urinary complications. *Grossly*, UCs can be papillary, polypoid, or sessile (Fig. 4-86). They may be difficult to distinguish from inflamed, thickened mucosa, even though the bladder wall is infiltrated diffusely. UC may be present in any part of the bladder, but are often in the bladder neck or trigone. Tumors originating in the prostatic urethra are easily overlooked at autopsy. *Histologically*, UC is divided into papillary versus nonpapillary and infiltrating versus non-infiltrating. Both features are usually included in the UC diagnosis. In dogs, the most common histologic phenotype is *papillary and infiltrative UC* (Fig. 4-87), which extends toward the bladder lumen as well as through the lamina propria and into the detrusor wall. In contrast, *nonpapillary and infiltrative UC*, which is the second most common canine histologic phenotype, forms a plaque-like or sessile mass of sheets of neoplastic urothelial cells. Islands of neoplastic cells invade the wall, providing evidence of malignancy. *Papillary and non-infiltrative UCs* grow toward the lumen but do not invade past the lamina propria or do not invade the stalk of the polypoid mass. The least common type is *nonpapillary and non-infiltrative UC*. It has flat or slightly raised urothelium with cellular atypia and frequent mitoses, lacking deeper invasion. It is comparable to a diagnosis of *carcinoma in situ* of other organs.

There have been many grading and classification systems of canine UC since the 1990s. However, the systems have rarely been used in routine diagnostic pathology. The prognostic value of these systems has been called into question, and the lack of clearcut criteria has resulted in significant interobserver variability. Grading systems with 5 and 3 grades have been proposed, ranging from urothelial papilloma through low-grade and high-grade carcinomas of typical anaplastic characteristics. Consistent application of these grading systems and collection of outcome data are needed for validation.

The proposed grading system with 5 categories is as follows. Urothelial papillomas should have ≤7 layers of cells, lack cellular and nuclear atypia, have no mitoses, and have thin, uninflamed stroma. Grade 1-4 UCs can all be papillary or nonpapillary. Grade 1 UCs have cellular characteristics similar to papillomas, but will be >7 cell layers thick. They have rare-to-no mitoses, and they do not invade. Grade 2 UCs will have mild atypia, enlarged nucleoli and visible nucleoli, rare-to-no mitoses, and lack invasion. Grade 3 UCs have loss of cellular polarity with moderate atypia, visible nucleoli, common

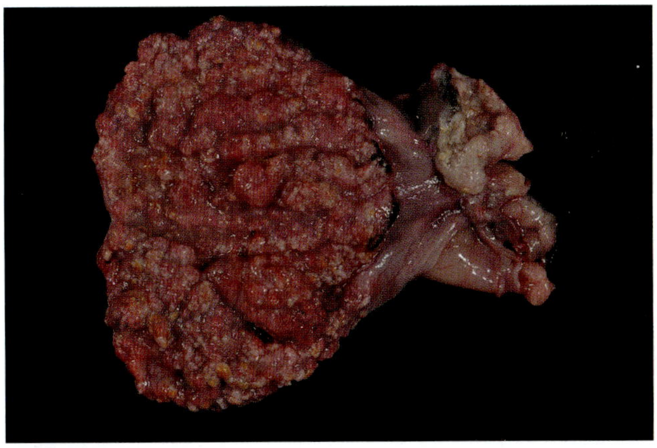

Figure 4-86 Urothelial carcinoma in the urinary bladder of a dog. (Courtesy E.E.B. LaDouceur.)

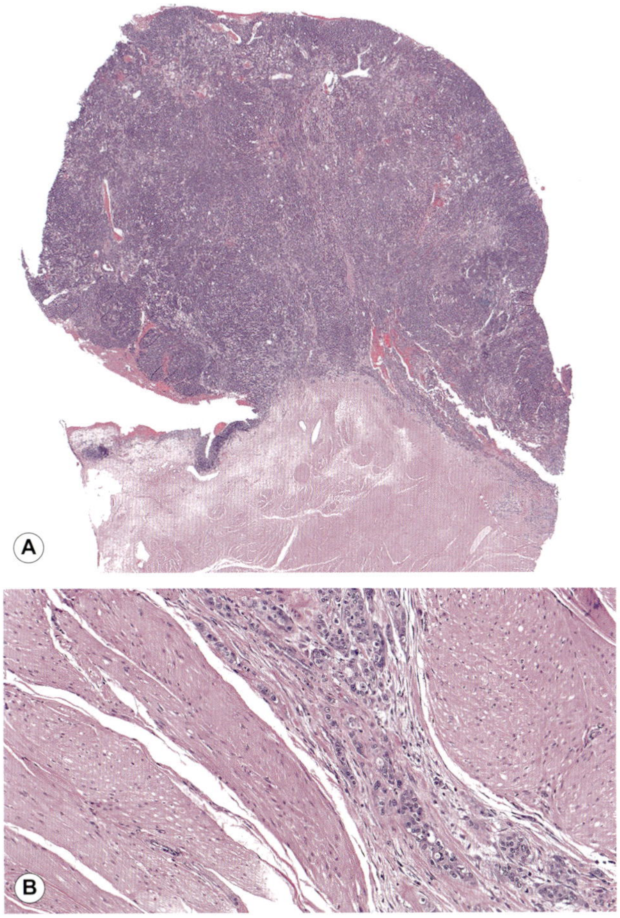

Figure 4-87 Papillary and infiltrative urothelial carcinoma in the urinary bladder of a dog. **A**. The mass has papillary projections toward the lumen. **B**. The tumor infiltrated the detrusor muscle. H&E.

mitoses, and often invade the lamina propria. Grade 4 UCs have disorganized growth, marked cellular atypia, clumped chromatin, many mitoses, and invade past the lamina propria. The proposed grading system with 3 categories merely combines grades 1 and 2 UCs (both considered low grade). Grades 3 and 4 UCs are combined as high-grade carcinomas. Urothelial papilloma is the third category.

Urothelial cell proliferation and invasion often promotes a desmoplastic response. Rarely, the desmoplastic areas contain foci of heterotopic bone. A few UCs contain areas of squamous metaplasia or glandular structures (eFig. 4-44A). There is often distant evidence of inflammation and hyperplasia with Brunn nests and cystitis glandularis lesions (see eFig. 4-44B). Careful evaluation of the lamina propria and smooth muscle is required to identify areas of potential lymphovascular invasion. Metastatic disease is identified in 50-90% of UC cases at autopsy and is often widespread, and UC is considered to be one of the "most malignant" tumors in veterinary medicine; <20% of dogs treated for UC (grade not specified) will survive longer than 1 year.

The usual pattern for metastasis is to regional lymph nodes and lungs, but peritoneal metastasis or retrograde lymphatic spread to the soft tissue and bones of the hindlimbs or vertebrae also occur. Occasionally, there is solitary metastasis to bone. Pulmonary metastasis is present at the time of UC diagnosis in ~20% of cases. Likewise, at the time of UC diagnosis, metastasis to regional lymph nodes and regional pelvic tissue or bones can be identified in 15% and 6% of cases, respectively. In dogs, *eosinophilic cytoplasmic inclusions*, called "Melamed-Wolinska bodies," in a metastatic lesion can suggest a urothelial lineage (Fig. 4-88). The droplets are easier to visualize with cytologic evaluation but can often be seen histologically as well; the bodies are often seen in neoplastic urothelial cells, but they are nonspecific and can be identified in other neoplasms. If these droplets are found in an epithelial cell population in a lymph node aspirate, and the dog has a mass in the urinary bladder, it is very likely to be UC with metastasis. Melamed-Wolinksa bodies are also seen in human UC. They are less common in feline UC and have not been reported in bovine UC.

Canine and bovine UC have been evaluated with IHC (Table 4-6). The information regarding urothelial markers of bovine tumors is discussed in the Enzootic Hematuria section. In dogs, IHC is performed either to verify that the cells are urothelial in origin or to provide evidence of potential aggressive biologic behavior. Mature urothelial cells express CK7, CK20, uroplakin III (UPIII), and GATA3 (nuclear staining); basal urothelial cells express p63 and 34βE12. *UPIII is reported to be a specific and sensitive marker for canine UC*. The presence of UPIII was not noted to be correlated with tumor grade (using a previous grading system). Because

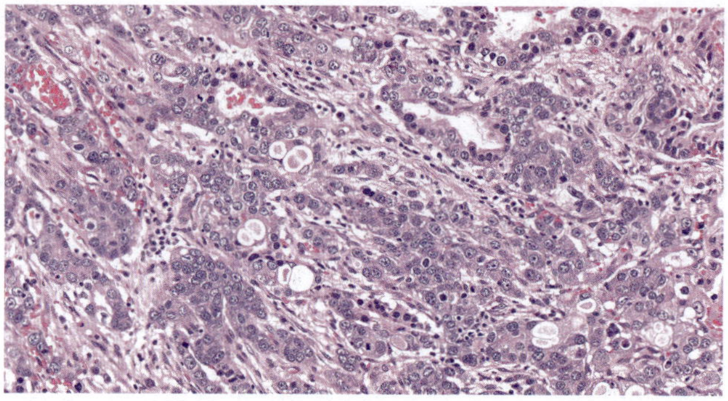

Figure 4-88 Melamed Wolinska bodies in the cytoplasm of neoplastic urothelial cells in a dog. They are variably sized eosinophilic droplets, sometimes encircled by vacuoles. H&E.

Table • 4-6

Immunohistochemical staining patterns of lower urinary tract neoplasms

MARKER	UROTHELIAL CELL CARCINOMA (UC)	NON-NEOPLASTIC URINARY BLADDER TISSUE
CK7	Labeled 53 of 54 UC, and 5 of 5 metastatic sites; can help identify areas of invasion into bladder wall	Diffuse cytoplasmic staining of mature urothelial cells +++
CK20	Labeled 37 of 54 UC, and 1 of 5 metastatic sites; can help identify areas of invasion into bladder wall	Diffuse cytoplasmic staining of mature urothelial cells ++
Uroplakin (UP) III*	Labeled 50 of 55 UC, and 4 of 5 metastatic sites; can help identify areas of invasion into lamina propria and also metastatic sites	Umbrella urothelial cells and some intermediate cells +++; typical stain cell membrane but occasionally label the cytoplasm
GATA3	Can help identify areas of invasion; but might represent metastasis from another organ	Mature urothelial cells ++, nuclear labeling
p63	Decreased staining seen in UC and was significantly associated with vascular invasion and metastasis	Nuclear labeling; more prominently expressed by basal layer of urothelial cells
34βE12	Not reported	Cytoplasmic labeling of basal layer of urothelial cells
β-catenin	Decreased staining seen in UC	Cytoplasmic labeling; more prominently expressed by basal layer of urothelial cells
HER2 (also called EGFR2/ ERBBN2/NEU)	Expressed in neoplastic urothelial cells in 60% of dogs with high-grade UC	Not expressed
COX2	Expressed in neoplastic urothelial cells	Not expressed

UPIII should only be seen on the bladder surface, this IHC marker can highlight foci of invasion. If that IHC marker is not available, then CK7, CK20, and GATA3 can help identify islands of invasion. Since these proteins are expressed by other cell types in the body, the argument could be made that the positively labeled cells might represent metastasis from elsewhere. However, it is rare for malignancies of other organs to metastasize to the luminal aspect of the bladder. Therefore, these stains are often considered sufficient evidence for diagnosis of UC, especially infiltrative UC. Expression of COX2 can occur in neoplastic urothelium, but not in normal urothelium, suggesting that it may be a useful marker for neoplastic transformation and growth and can be targeted for therapeutic effects. Likewise, HER2 (also called EGFR2/ERBB2/NEU) is expressed by neoplastic urothelium but not non-neoplastic urothelial cells; 2 studies have shown expression of this marker in ~60% of canine high-grade (invasive) UC.

In addition to IHC, other tools can assist in the diagnosis of canine UC. A widely used test, likely because of its noninvasive nature and commercial availability, is a PCR assay of the *BRAF* gene. The PCR test can identify a mutation of this gene (valine is substituted by glutamic acid at position 595, $BRAF^{V595E}$), which has been associated with UC in dogs. This amino acid substitution mimics the phosphorylation of its nearby amino acids. The result is constitutive activation of the MAPK pathway with increased expression of ERK1/2, and uncontrolled cell proliferation. The reported relative proportion of BRAF+ versus BRAF− tumors varies in the literature, with some sources indicating that the Cadet-BRAF test identifies 80-95% of UC, and other literature reporting that 46% of 79 canine UC did not have the mutation. Moreover, BRAF mutation status was not an independent predictor of patient outcome in the latter study.

Other canine UC diagnostic tests (which have often been reported in retrospective research) include urinary levels of basic fibroblastic growth factor, urinary bladder tumor antigen (V-BTA), urothelial cell telomerase activity, urinary survivin levels, urinary calgranulins (S100A8, A9, and A12), and fluorescence in situ hybridization for detection of chromosomal aberrations in urothelial cells. All of these have variable sensitivities and specificities. For example, the V-BTA has low specificity, and the antigen can be detected in dogs with cystitis or polyps. However, because of its high sensitivity, when the V-BTA test is negative, it is extremely unlikely that the patient has UC. Taken together, these additional diagnostic tests can be part of a portfolio to provide evidence of UC, especially when biopsy samples are small or fragmented. Transcriptomics and micro-RNA analysis of UC compared with normal tissue have identified future potential biomarkers and therapeutic targets. Currently, however, these "-omics" approaches have been limited to small numbers of cases and controls. Promising markers need to be further validated before being considered as diagnostic tools. Even if more diagnostic tests are developed and become commercially available, they should not replace the pathologist's diagnosis or tumor grade. For example, many UC do not carry the BRAF mutation; while it is helpful to know the BRAF status, a negative BRAF test should not preclude a diagnosis of UC.

SCCs and **adenocarcinomas** are usually nonpapillary infiltrative growths, which grossly are nodular or sessile and often ulcerated. They develop in areas of squamous or mucous metaplasia. Histologically, they are "pure," without urothelial cell areas. SCCs and adenocarcinomas occur in dogs, cattle, and cats. SCCs are the most common urinary bladder neoplasm in horses; they occur most often in female dogs in the urethra, the distal two-thirds of which is lined by stratified squamous epithelium. Apparently, SCCs are less likely to metastasize than UCs. Adenocarcinomas can develop in regions of previous glandular metaplasia or cystitis glandularis. Some might develop in regions of urachal remnants, so knowing the location of the mass can be helpful in making this diagnosis.

Undifferentiated carcinomas are rare primary neoplasms that do not conform to one of the histologic types mentioned previously. Because some UCs have foci of marked cellular atypia and variations in cellular arrangement, the diagnosis of undifferentiated carcinoma should not be confused with high-grade UC that has marked anaplasia.

Mesenchymal tumors

Mesenchymal tumors comprise ~10% of tumors of the canine lower urinary tract. Neoplasms associated with enzootic hematuria in cattle are ~10% mesenchymal and 55% mixed, with most of the nonepithelial tumors in these mixtures being hemangiomas. A few vascular tumors also occur in the bladder and the urethra of dogs, but most mesenchymal tumors in dogs are leiomyomas or fibromas. **Leiomyomas** originate in the smooth muscle of the urinary bladder and form well-defined projecting spherical white nodules. The nodules may be multiple and seem to have a predilection for the neck of the bladder, where they may interfere with urine outflow. **Leiomyosarcomas** are rare and generally do not metastasize; IHC staining for smooth muscle actin and desmin are expected. One study reported that leiomyomas should have mitotic counts of <5 in 10 hpf, whereas leiomyosarcomas will often have 10-20 mitoses in 10 hpf.

Fibromas probably arise from suburothelial connective tissue, are usually solitary, and have a typical gross and microscopic appearance. **Fibrosarcomas** are rare. Because of the overlap between fibroma/fibrosarcoma and fibrous polyps, it has been suggested that the diagnosis of neoplasia should be limited to tumors developing within the smooth muscle tunic or completely confined within the lamina propria. If masses grow toward the lumen, then they are more likely to represent a polyp as described tab above. This distinction is supported by the fact that polyps and polypoid cystitis are often inflamed and will have concurrent urothelial cell proliferation. The literature regarding follow-up for biopsies of inflammatory polyps (especially those containing eosinophils) have a favorable outcome, following tumor resection. Reserving the term fibroma/fibrosarcoma for neoplasms that consist only of spindle cell proliferations should prevent this potential misclassification.

Botryoid (shaped like a bunch of grapes) **rhabdomyosarcoma** occurs in the urinary bladder and occasionally the urethra of young dogs (Fig. 4-89). Large breeds, particularly the Saint Bernard, seem to be over-represented. Basset Hounds also are over-represented. The young age of the affected animals (<2-years-old in most cases) raises the possibility that these tumors arise in rests of embryonic myoblasts. Grossly, the tumors usually occur at the trigone and project into the bladder as botryoid masses. They may metastasize but are usually identified because of urinary obstruction before this

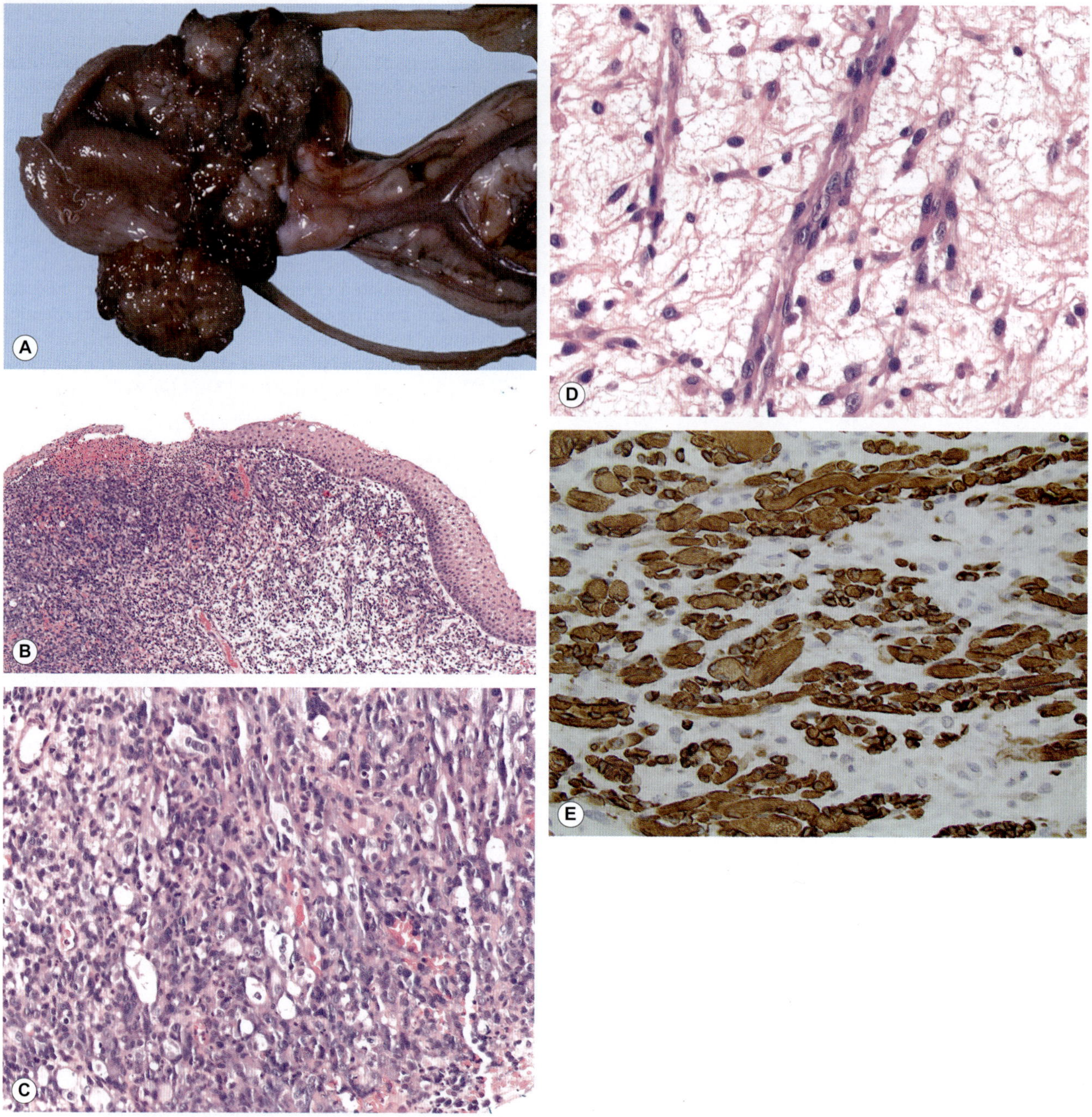

Figure 4-89 Botryoid rhabdomyosarcoma in the urinary bladder of a young dog. **A.** The bladder has many confluent masses. (Courtesy K. Potter.) **B.** From a different dog; inflamed mesenchymal proliferation beneath a focally ulcerated urothelium. H&E. **C, D.** Multinucleate round and spindle cells with occasional strap cells that have cytoplasmic striations. H&E. **E.** Diffuse cytoplasmic desmin positivity in neoplastic cells. Immunohistochemistry.

occurs. This tumor has been rarely associated with hypertrophic osteopathy in dogs. Microscopically, there is usually a mixture of fusiform and pleomorphic cells, with some strap cells and multinucleate cells. Cytoplasmic cross-striations are sometimes present. PTAH staining and IHC for desmin (see Fig. 4-89E), smooth muscle actin, and MyoD1 can assist in difficult cases.

Involvement of the urinary bladder in primary **lymphoma** has been reported only rarely in domestic animals; primary canine epitheliotropic T-cell lymphoma involving the urinary bladder is even more rare.

Visit Elsevier eBooks+ (eBooks.Health.Elsevier.com) for eFigures and further readings.

CHAPTER 5

Respiratory System

Jeff L. Caswell • Kurt J. Williams

ACKNOWLEDGMENTS

We gratefully acknowledge the contributions to prior editions of this chapter by Drs. Ken Jubb, Peter Kennedy, Nigel Palmer, and Donald Dungworth.

GENERAL CONSIDERATIONS

Of all of the organ systems, *the respiratory tract may be unique in its vulnerability to injurious* agents. The involuntary nature of ventilation, necessitated by aerobic respiration and the need for oxygen, actively pulls large volumes of air into the lungs (estimated at 5400 L/day in dogs and 11,400 L/day in horses). Along with this air come a variety of potentially injurious materials. In addition, the entire cardiac output of blood passing through the extensive and delicate vascular bed of the gas exchange region of the lungs provides a separate avenue for the delivery of potentially harmful substances to the respiratory tract. The dual exposure routes are particularly important in determining the expression of disease in the lung, with *distinct patterns of lesions depending on whether the route of entry is airborne (aerogenous) or vascular (hematogenous)*. The array of potentially injurious agents includes airborne microorganisms, particulates, and toxic gases in ambient air, and a wide variety of infectious agents and extrinsic or intrinsic toxins delivered via the pulmonary circulation. Together, the injury, inflammation, and reparative responses to these insults compromise the gas exchange functions of the respiratory system.

The upper airway

The nasal cavity comprises the nares, vestibule, and maxilloturbinate, nasomaxillary, and ethmoidal regions. The ventral, middle, and dorsal *meatuses* are demarcated by the osseous and cartilaginous dorsal and ventral *conchae* (turbinates). Air flows past the *ethmoid conchae* in the caudal nasal cavity, through the *choanae* and into the nasopharynx. Respiratory turbinates are restricted to mammals and birds and are assumed to be important in the evolution of endothermy and the high levels of oxygen consumption associated with metabolism in these species; similar structures are not present within ectothermic animals.

Functionally, the *respiratory turbinates warm and humidify the inspired air* to prevent desiccation of the lower respiratory tract and reclaim moisture and heat from the saturated vapor leaving the lungs. The nasal submucosa is richly supplied with a complex vascular plexus, nerves, and mucosal glands. In addition to the air-warming functions, most species have vascular shunts between the respiratory turbinates and the brain vasculature, suggesting a role in *cooling the brain* during periods of intense activity in mammals and birds. Stimulation of the parasympathetic innervation in the nasal cavity leads to increased vascular permeability and mucosal gland secretion, which may occlude the nasal airways and increase resistance to airflow. This is countered by the sympathetic nerve fibers, which favor vasoconstriction and decreased vascular permeability.

The mucosa of the nasal cavity has distinct epithelial types: 1) *stratified squamous*, 2) *transitional*, 3) *ciliated respiratory, and* 4) *olfactory*. The relative distribution and extent of each of these cell types vary among species. Stratified squamous epithelium is confined to the nasal vestibule at the entrance to the nasal cavity. Separating the squamous epithelium from the more caudal respiratory epithelium is a zone of nonciliated cuboidal-to-columnar cells, the transitional epithelium. Most of the nasal mucosa is lined by *pseudostratified respiratory epithelium*. This is a complex epithelium that includes ciliated, mucous, nonciliated, and basal cells (Fig. 5-1). *Olfactory epithelium is located in the caudal and caudodorsal nasal cavity*, covering the ethmoid conchae. The epithelium is composed of olfactory sensory neurons—bipolar neurons that have nonmotile apical cilia forming dendritic knobs bearing the olfactory receptors—as well as sustentacular cells and basal cells. Olfactory mucosa is readily recognized by a line of sustentacular cell nuclei at the midlevel of the epithelium, basal cells adjacent to the basal lamina, and olfactory neuron nuclei scattered between these 2 layers; as well as the olfactory (Bowman) glands and prominent olfactory nerves in the lamina propria (see Fig. 5-1). *Olfactory epithelium is rich in cytochrome P450 monooxygenases*. These enzymes are essential for olfaction, and their biotransformation activity confers susceptibility to inhaled or ingested toxins, such as 3-methylindole in horses.

The **nasopharynx** is lined by ciliated pseudostratified epithelium with zones of stratified squamous epithelium. *Lymphoid nodules* are abundant throughout the submucosa and are one of the components of the pharyngeal lymphoid (Waldeyer) ring, a collection of lymphoid tissues that encircle the oropharynx and nasopharynx. *The auditory (Eustachian) tubes* extend from the nasopharynx to the middle ears. In horses, diverticula of each auditory tube form the *guttural pouches*, which are located caudodorsal to the caudal pharynx. The guttural pouches function to cool blood destined for the brain during periods of intense activity. This respiratory-based cooling mechanism is facilitated by the anatomy of the internal carotid artery as it courses in a crease along the caudal wall up to the dorsal surface of the pouches. As with the pharynx and auditory tube, the mucosa of the guttural pouches is lined by pseudostratified ciliated epithelium.

The **larynx** forms a complex of cartilage plates lined by stratified squamous epithelium as well as pseudostratified ciliated respiratory epithelium. The larynx is at the boundary between the respiratory system and the pharynx and communicates directly with the laryngopharynx. The cartilage of the larynx is important in vocalization in animals and also resists deformation and obstruction from ingesta, external pressure, and the negative internal pressures experienced during inhalation.

The **trachea** extends from the terminus of the larynx to the *carina*, the branch point for the principal bronchi leading into the right and left lungs. With its relatively simple gross anatomy, and seemingly simple function serving as the conduit for

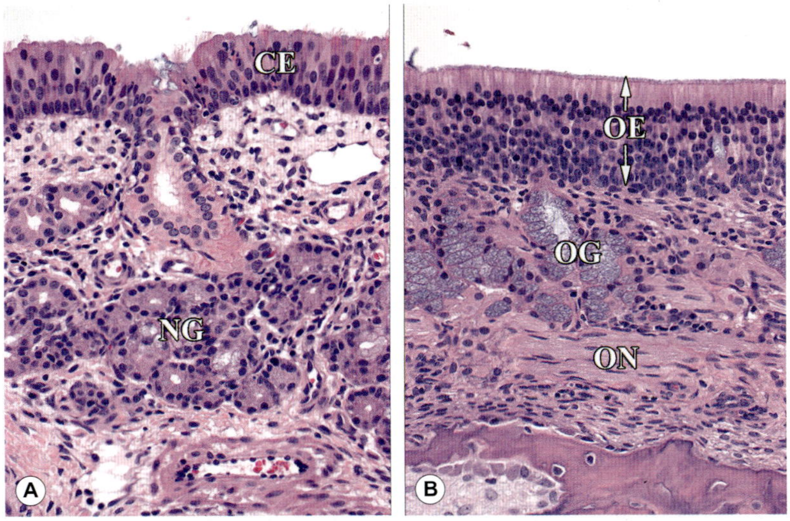

Figure 5-1 Microscopic anatomy of nasal epithelium in a pig. **A**. Respiratory epithelium is pseudostratified and contains ciliated epithelial cells (CE), with nasal glands (NG) in the lamina propria. **B**. Olfactory epithelium (OE) has dendritic knobs at the surface, apical cytoplasm, a mid-level layer of sustentacular cell nuclei, and nuclei of basal cells and bipolar neurons in the basal half of the epithelium. The lamina propria contains olfactory glands (OG) and prominent olfactory nerves (ON).

air traveling to and from the lungs, the trachea is often overlooked in routine pathology examinations. The upper third of the trachea is arbitrarily considered to be the most distal part of the upper respiratory tract.

Organization of the lung

The organization and subdivision of the lower respiratory tract arise as a function of the development of the organ and vary considerably by species (lung development is reviewed later in the chapter). Many of these gross features are important in the pathogenesis of disease and susceptibility of individual species to infectious agents, inhaled toxins, and particulate matter. In addition, knowing the names of these anatomic structures is the foundation for observing and precisely describing gross lung lesions at the time of autopsy.

The divisions of the lungs, from largest to smallest, include lobe, bronchopulmonary segment, and terminal acinus. All domestic species have a right and left lung, each of which is served by a single **principal bronchus** (primary bronchi) arising at the tracheal bifurcation. Each of the 2 lungs is further subdivided into individual lobes. *A* ***lung lobe*** *is defined as the gas exchange region ventilated through a* **lobar (secondary) bronchus**. The numbers and distribution of lung lobes vary by species. All domestic species except the horse have 2 lobes in the left lung (cranial and caudal lobes) and 4 lobes in the right lung (cranial, middle, caudal, and accessory); the horse lacks a right middle lung lobe. The cranial lobe of the left lung is subdivided into a cranial and caudal part in all species, except the horse, and the right cranial lobe of domestic ruminants is similarly divided into a cranial and caudal part. The lobar bronchus **(tracheal bronchus)** of the right cranial lung lobe of ruminants and pigs arises from the trachea, proximal to the tracheal bifurcation.

Depending on the species, further subdivisions into individual **lobules** by connective tissue septa may or may not be grossly visible; when present, these interlobular septa are contiguous with the pleura. *In humans, pigs, and cattle, lobulation is highly developed, with individual lobules readily seen on the pleural surface of the lung. Equine, ovine, and caprine lungs are intermediate in lobulation; canine and feline lung are essentially devoid of septation and lobule formation.* A **bronchopulmonary segment** is the area served by a tertiary bronchus that arises from the lobar (secondary) bronchi. Well-developed interlobular septa that nearly completely surround individual bronchopulmonary segments, as in the pig and cow, limit collateral ventilation as well as the movement of cells and molecules between adjacent segments. Functionally, this is important in these species because it limits spread of inflammation between lobules. Well-developed connective tissue septa can effectively sequester inflammation in affected lobules, leading to the characteristic gross lesions especially common in bacterial bronchopneumonia, with severely affected lobules adjacent to those less affected.

The **terminal acinus** *is composed of one terminal bronchiole and its associated gas exchange region*. The anatomy of the terminal acinus varies among domestic species, especially the segment between the terminal bronchiole and the alveoli. This junction is composed of respiratory bronchioles and/or alveolar ducts, depending on the species. **Respiratory bronchioles** (prominent in dogs, cats, ferrets, and humans, but not in horses, cattle, sheep, or pigs) are lined by cuboidal epithelium that is interrupted by periodic alveolar outpocketings before transitioning into the gas exchange region. **Alveolar ducts** are cylindrical airways lined by a membranous epithelium and have numerous circumferential communications with alveoli; they may have smooth muscle in their wall.

Vascular supply to the lung

The vascular supply to the lung is dual, arriving through both the pulmonary and bronchial circulation. This unique system of perfusing the lung with blood has implications in the pathogenesis of pulmonary disease. The **pulmonary arterial circulation** receives the entire output of the right ventricle and is a high-flow, low-pressure system. In contrast, the **bronchial arterial circulation**, being a part of the systemic arterial blood vasculature, is a low-flow, high-pressure system. The bronchial circulation can arise from a variety of sites, including the aorta, intercostal arteries, and subclavian arteries. It delivers nutrition to the bronchi and bronchioles, and in some species also to the blood vessels, pleura, and much of the interstitium. Species vary in their vascular supply: the bronchial artery supplies the airways of dogs and its obstruction causes bronchiolar necrosis; this does not occur in rabbits because of contributions by the pulmonary artery. In cattle, sheep, pigs, and horses, the bronchial circulation also supplies the pleura; in species with thin pleurae (dogs, cats, rodents), the pulmonary circulation serves this function. The pulmonary circulation nourishes the alveolar parenchyma and delivers blood to the site of alveolar gas exchange.

Thus, species vary in anatomic details of their terminal airways, interlobular septa, and vasculature. Dogs and cats have thin pleura supplied by the pulmonary artery, inapparent interlobular septa, well-developed respiratory bronchioles, and pulmonary veins that are nonmuscular and present in the interlobular septa. Cattle, sheep, pigs, and horses have thick pleura and interlobular septa supplied by the bronchial artery, lack respiratory bronchioles, and have pulmonary arteries that are more muscular and become more hypertensive in hypoxia; in cattle and pigs, the pulmonary veins are muscular and contained in the bronchopulmonary sheath. The pulmonary and bronchial arteries supply the alveoli of horses; alveoli are supplied by only the pulmonary artery in other species.

The morphology of the 2 vascular systems in most species can be discerned histologically, at least in their normal state (Fig. 5-2). Pulmonary and bronchial arteries are adjacent to bronchi and bronchioles, but the pulmonary artery is much larger (at least half the diameter of the airway) than the bronchial artery. Furthermore, large muscular pulmonary arteries have an internal and external elastic lamina of similar thickness; the muscular bronchial arteries have an internal elastic lamina, but the external lamina is indistinct or absent. At the pulmonary trunk, the arteries of most species have considerable numbers of elastic fibers interspersed with smooth muscle; the more distal arteries and arterioles do not have elastic fibers. The smaller branches of pulmonary arteries vary considerably between species in their morphology, especially in the thickness of the tunica media. *Cats, pigs, and cattle have the thickest pulmonary arteries of the domestic species*. Because of the presence of smooth muscle in the small pulmonary arterioles of many domestic species, care needs to be taken in diagnosing pulmonary arterial hypertension based simply on arteriolar morphology.

Pulmonary veins drain the entire lung except the proximal trachea and lymph nodes. Cardiac muscle is present in the large proximal veins of rodents but not domestic species. The pulmonary veins follow the bronchial tree in most domestic

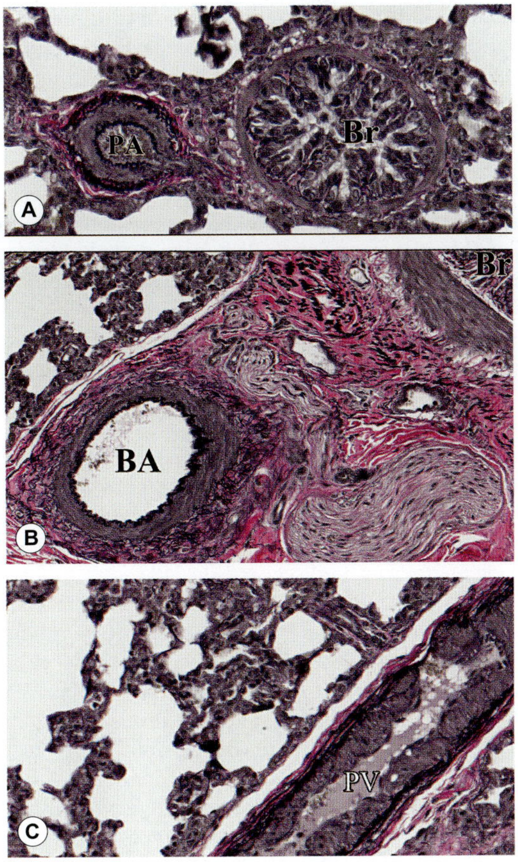

Figure 5-2 Microscopic anatomy of pulmonary vessels in a calf. Verhoeff-van Gieson elastic stain. **A.** The pulmonary artery (PA), located in the connective tissue ensheathing the bronchiole (Br), has both internal and external elastic laminae and is about half the diameter of the bronchiole (Br). **B.** The bronchial artery (BA) also follows the bronchiole (Br) but is smaller than the pulmonary artery and has an internal but not an external elastic lamina. **C.** The pulmonary veins (PV) are most easily seen in the lung parenchyma and may have an external but no internal elastic lamina. Pulmonary veins of cattle, shown here, have thick beaded smooth muscle in the tunica media.

species (in contrast to humans) and have a thin fibrous wall in all species except for cattle, small ruminants, and pigs, in which smooth muscle is prominent. Cattle >3-months-old have thick muscular veins next to airways and in the interstitium that can resemble arteries (see Fig. 5-2), but the veins have muscular sphincters that protrude into the lumen and give a beaded appearance. In all species, the larger pulmonary veins are recognized by an external elastic lamina between the tunica media and the adventitia, but no internal elastic lamina.

The **lymphatic system** is the least well understood of the vascular systems in the lung. Lymphatic vessels are present within the visceral pleura and surround airways and blood vessels, but do not extend into the alveolar septa. The morphology of the pulmonary lymphatics varies by their location. Within the pleura and just below it, the interstitial space leading into proper lymphatics can be considered as prelymphatic space. This is a site of fluid accumulation during pulmonary edema and also, given that it collects fluids bathing the entirety of the surrounding tissue, is important in delivering antigens to regional lymph nodes. The prelymphatics in the pleura blend into reservoir lymphatics, which eventually connect with conduit lymphatics. Within the lung, saccular and tubulosaccular lymphatics surround all airways and noncapillary blood vessels (arteries and veins). These lymphatics are large (some >100 µm) and thin walled. Although they are histologically indistinct and are often overlooked, the lymphatics sometimes distend with fluid in cases of pulmonary edema or pneumonia. Metastatic emboli filling lymphatics sometimes reveal the distribution of the pulmonary lymphatic system, and aggregates of inflammatory cells may accumulate around terminal airways and blood vessels in association with the local lymphatics. Thus, the lung lymphatic system is important in fluid movement, regulating alveolar hydration, and acting as a conduit for the movement of antigens, leukocytes, and metastasizing neoplasms.

Architecture and cell biology of the lung

The cellular constituents of the respiratory system are functionally interdependent in relation to organ development, homeostasis, and response to injury. This interdependence is first evident in the close interactions between endodermal and mesodermal components in lung development (see the Lung Development and Growth section). In the adult lung, this anatomic and functional relationship has been termed the *epithelial-mesenchymal trophic unit* and includes the interactions among respiratory epithelial cells, smooth muscle cells, endothelial cells, extracellular matrix proteins, and leukocytes during development, health, and disease.

In all domestic species, the **trachea and bronchi** *are surrounded by rings of hyaline cartilage*. These rings help maintain the patency of the upper airways, which would otherwise collapse from the negative intraluminal pressures needed to draw in air. Despite their greater diameter, relative to the bronchioles, ~80% of the resistance to pulmonary airflow resides within the first 4-7 generations of the conducting airways. Partly because of this, any process that results in significant narrowing of the bronchi can result in clinically detectable changes at an earlier stage than a similar process involving the bronchioles.

Bronchioles, in contrast to bronchi, *have no cartilage in their walls to prevent airway collapse*. Bronchiolar airway patency is dependent on the connective tissue that attaches the alveolar septa to the bronchiolar wall. An exception is marine mammals, both cetaceans and pinnipeds, which possess well-developed cartilage rings around even the smallest bronchioles that prevent airway collapse from the supra-atmospheric pressures of the ocean depths. In terrestrial mammals, the radially arranged alveolar septa are tethered to and pull on the bronchiolar wall to maximize the luminal diameter during inspiration. During expiration, as the forces from the alveolar septa decrease, the bronchiolar lumen decreases in diameter. Because of their smaller diameter, collapsibility, and thin-walled structure, bronchioles are much more susceptible to disease processes occurring in the surrounding alveolar parenchyma than are bronchi, and they individually have a higher resistance to airflow than individual bronchi. Despite this, there is less resistance to airflow in the distal airways because of the higher number of bronchioles. Therefore, a large percentage of bronchioles must be affected before clinical evidence of disease is detected.

Histologically, there is great cellular diversity within the epithelium of the conducting airways, the cell populations changing depending on the species and airway generation.

The trachea, bronchi, and proximal bronchioles are lined by pseudostratified epithelium composed of a mix of ciliated, mucous, club, serous, and chemosensory/brush cells. In general, the numbers of ciliated and mucous cells decrease within the distal airways, with a greater proportion of nonciliated cells present within the bronchioles (see Figs. 5-1 and 5-76). This affects the species- and region-specific susceptibility of the airway epithelium to infectious agents, particulate matter, and especially inhaled or systemic toxins.

The **ciliated cells** function mainly in clearance of airway-lining fluid and also have secretory functions. The **secretory cells** include mucous cells, serous cells, and club cells; single-cell mRNA sequencing suggests functional subsets of each of these and differences between proximal and distal airways. The morphologic and functional differences between these secretory cells are not considered immutable, and microenvironmental conditions induce metaplasia from one type to the other. The contribution of these cells to the airway surface liquid includes not only mucus but also innate defense molecules (see the Lung Defenses section), immunoregulatory proteins such as club cell secretory protein and annexin A1, and cellular defense molecules including antioxidants and trefoil factor. **Mucous cells** (goblet cells) are a source of mucins that form the mucus layer of the epithelial lining fluid. **Club cells** are nonciliated non–mucus-secreting cells that predominate in the distal airway of many species. The club cell functions as a *progenitor cell* for epithelial repair within the airway mucosa, given that it has the capacity to divide and differentiate into other secretory cells or ciliated cells. Club cells of many species have abundant smooth endoplasmic reticulum that has high concentrations of cytochrome P450 monooxygenase enzymes. Indeed, on a per-cell basis, club cells of some species have greater metabolic capacity than even hepatocytes. Therefore, *club cells are extremely sensitive to a variety of xenobiotics;* metabolism of these toxins can generate intermediate metabolites that form adducts with macromolecules and lead to cellular injury. Finally, club cell secretory protein, secreted in response to adrenergic stimuli, may dampen the inflammatory response by inhibition of phospholipase A2. **Chemosensory or brush cells** are infrequent neuroendocrine cells that are thought to detect irritants in the inhaled air. Additional epithelial cell types include basal cells and ionocytes. In addition to these cells lining the airway surface, **tracheobronchial glands** in the lamina propria are the major source of mucus in these large airways.

Smooth muscle cells are located around the circumference of the bronchi and bronchioles, and extend to the ostia of alveolar outpocketings in the respiratory bronchioles, and into the alveolar ducts of some species. Historically, the *airway smooth muscle cell* was primarily seen as the transducer of bronchoconstriction and bronchodilation. However, smooth muscle cells can undergo hyperplasia in response to paracrine signals arising from the airway epithelium in inflammatory diseases, and this doubtless contributes to the accentuation of smooth muscle found histologically in chronic bronchitis and asthma. Furthermore, smooth muscle cells *produce a wide array of cytokines, chemokines, growth factors, and extracellular matrix metalloproteases*, allowing them to modify the interstitial matrix directly around smooth muscle bundles. These cells also *secrete matrix proteins*, including fibronectin, elastin, and a variety of laminins and collagens, which then modulate the proliferation, migration, and apoptosis of the smooth muscle cells. For example, plasmin can stimulate release of active transforming growth factor–β from these cells, which in turn promotes collagen synthesis by the smooth muscle cells. This paradigm may partly explain the increased extracellular matrix found around smooth muscle bundles in chronically inflamed airways.

The **alveoli** are the site of the most essential function of the lung, that being *gas exchange to support cellular aerobic respiration*. Regardless of the media for gas exchange (water or air), the essential design of the gas exchange membrane in animals is remarkably similar, consisting of an epithelial layer exposed to the exchange medium, in close apposition to blood-filled capillaries. This relatively simple arrangement belies the complexity of the biology of the region. In mammals, there are 5 major cell types associated with the alveolar parenchyma: *type I and type II pneumocytes, capillary endothelial cells, interstitial fibroblasts*, and *alveolar macrophages*.

Type I pneumocytes *are large, flat, membranous epithelial cells that line ~93% of the alveolar surface*. They are considered the broadest cell in the body, each cell covering an ~80-μm-diameter meshwork of capillaries. But at ~0.1 μm thickness, only their nuclei can be discerned on H&E-stained histologic sections, and thus loss of these cells can only be visualized with other methods. Type I pneumocytes are terminally differentiated and nonmitotic. They are particularly vulnerable to injury because of their large membrane surface area, paucity of cytoplasmic organelles, and low levels of antioxidants, especially reduced glutathione. Irreversible injury to type I cells is quickly followed by sloughing of the cells from the alveolar basement membrane, which triggers a rapid regenerative response orchestrated by the type II pneumocytes. This description of type I cells suggests a passive role in the lung, facilitating gas exchange across the plasma membrane, and poised for injury and loss following any number of insults. Although this is true, they also play a critical part in maintaining normal lung fluid composition, forming the main barrier to movement of fluid into the alveolus, and clearing fluid and protein from the alveolus during pulmonary edema.

Type II pneumocytes *are the main cuboidal cell lining the alveolus*; the brush cell or type III pneumocyte is also cuboidal, but much less numerous. Type II pneumocytes are found most commonly at the intersection of alveolar septa, the so-called "corners" of the polygonal alveoli. Ultrastructurally, the type II pneumocyte has apical microvilli and characteristic cytoplasmic osmiophilic lamellar bodies, which are the site of surfactant storage. The primary functions of type II pneumocytes are to *synthesize pulmonary surfactant*, to serve as *progenitor cells* for replacement and turnover of alveolar epithelium, and to *metabolize xenobiotics*.

Pulmonary surfactant is a complex mixture that forms a film at the air-liquid interface of terminal bronchioles and alveoli. It consists of dipalmitoyl-phosphatidylcholine (which is responsible for much of the surface tension–lowering function) and other phospholipids, cholesterol, and surfactant proteins (SP-A, SP-B, SP-C, SP-D). Surfactant lipids are synthesized in type II pneumocytes; some are also produced by club cells. They are initially stored in lamellar bodies, then secreted onto the alveolar surface where they arrange in a functional surface-active form known as *tubular myelin* that adsorbs to the alveolar air-liquid interface. The main function of surfactant in the alveoli is to *lower surface tension in the alveolar space to prevent alveolar collapse during expiration*. The biology of the system is highly dynamic: with each breath, there is cycling between the subsurface surfactant reservoir and the bioactive surface film. Similarly, tubular myelin is constantly converted to a less functional vesicular form that must be recycled by type II pneumocytes or degraded by alveolar macrophages. SP-A, SP-B, and SP-C are important for secretion and recycling of the surfactant lipid, formation of tubular myelin, and the proper insertion of these lipids into the alveolar surface film. Beyond its role in regulating alveolar surface tension, SP-A and SP-D also have important immunoregulatory and pulmonary defense functions (see the Lung Defenses section). The biology of this system is highly relevant to the pathogenesis of interstitial lung diseases.

The proliferative capacity of type II pneumocytes is important in alveolar development, postnatal lung growth, and repair following injury. Type II cells can rapidly proliferate to repopulate denuded basement membrane following injury to type I pneumocytes. This process involves rapid migration of type II cells to cover the basement membrane, followed by proliferation, and later differentiation to membranous type I pneumocytes. The process is facilitated by the ability of the type II pneumocyte to modify the extracellular matrix. Type II cells synthesize a variety of matrix components, including fibronectin, type IV collagen, and proteoglycans, as well as matrix-degrading enzymes such as metalloproteases.

Fibroblasts are found within the alveolar wall associated with a network of extracellular matrix proteins, including collagen and elastin. This network is not uniformly distributed within the membrane, leading to regions of the wall that are "thick" and "thin," with gas exchange only occurring in the latter. The fibroblasts of the lung are heterogeneous in terms of morphology, functionality, and expression of surface markers. This heterogeneity is particularly well documented in experimental and human cases of pulmonary fibrosis. For example, different populations of lung fibroblasts vary in their adhesion to extracellular matrix, production of cytokines, and ability to produce extracellular matrix proteins including collagen. The array of matrix proteins potentially produced by lung fibroblasts includes collagen types I, III, IV, V, and VI, elastin, laminin, fibronectin, glycosaminoglycans, and proteoglycans.

Pulmonary macrophages are an important class of lung cells and are found in a variety of compartments within the organ. At least 6 separate populations have been recognized: *resident alveolar macrophages, recruited monocyte-derived macrophages, interstitial macrophages, pulmonary intravascular macrophages, dendritic cells*, and *pleural macrophages*.

Resident alveolar macrophages form a self-renewing pool of cells derived from progenitors in the yolk sac and fetal liver. They are minimally supplemented by, but not dependent on, renewal from marrow-derived circulating monocytes. Inflammation induces massive proliferation of these resident cells and also elicits monocytes from the circulation, and these cell types have differing functions. Resident alveolar macrophages are the lung's homeostatic housekeepers, phagocytosing debris and dead cells, and removing spent surfactant from the alveolus. Resident alveolar macrophages also function in surveillance, patrolling from one alveolus to another in search of threats, actively maintaining a noninflamed environment whenever possible, but recruiting inflammatory cells to the lung when needed. In contrast, **monocyte-derived macrophages** recruited to the lung from the blood are more proinflammatory, with greater capacity for cytokine production and tissue damage.

Dendritic cells are *ubiquitous immunoregulatory cells* found in all tissues. They are motile cells involved in surveillance for antigens at the epithelial and mesothelial surfaces of the respiratory tract. Various subpopulations can be distinguished by means of morphologic characteristics, primary location, and unique surface marker proteins. Morphologically, dendritic cells have numerous long processes and function as antigen-presenting cells, priming naive T cells and differentiating them into T-helper type 1 (Th1) or Th2 effector cells. The ability to present antigen to T cells requires that the dendritic cells themselves mature; this occurs within regional lymph nodes under the influence of appropriate proinflammatory signals. The numbers of dendritic cells can increase markedly in the respiratory tract given the proper stimuli, and they play an important role in allergic airway disease and asthma.

Lung macrophages and dendritic cells are *regulatory cells* that control inflammatory, immune, and repair processes through the release of a wide array of cytokines and other regulatory molecules. Inflammation and immunity are promoted by macrophage synthesis and release of cytokines such as interleukin (IL)1, tumor necrosis factor, and interferon-γ (IFNγ), as well as by release of inflammatory mediators such as leukotriene B4, C4, platelet-activating factor, and thromboxane A2. Repair processes are generally promoted or otherwise regulated by release of cytokines that include transforming growth factor–β and –α, fibroblast growth factor, insulin-like growth factor, and platelet-derived growth factor.

Interstitial macrophages are the least-understood class of pulmonary macrophages. Because of their location within the interstitium of the conducting airways and alveolar parenchyma, they are more difficult to isolate and characterize than other macrophage populations. In mice, interstitial macrophages have less phagocytic activity than alveolar macrophages, and instead are primarily immunomodulatory cells, expressing more major histocompatibility complex class II molecules and producing more cytokines, such as IL1 and IL6, than the alveolar macrophage.

Pulmonary intravascular macrophages are unique mononuclear phagocytes found within the alveolar capillaries of select species, including cattle, sheep, goats, horses, pigs, cats, and cetaceans (eFig. 5-2). These cells may be recruited into the lungs of rats and humans during inflammatory lung diseases. They form membrane-adhesive complexes with the capillary endothelium, which *keeps them localized to the vascular bed.* Pulmonary intravascular macrophages are highly phagocytic and play an important role in the clearance of circulating bacteria and particulates from the pulmonary circulation. They release an array of proinflammatory mediators following interaction with particulates and bacterial endotoxin. Because of their proinflammatory properties, they can increase the permeability of the blood-air barrier and contribute to the lung injury coincident with acute lung inflammation. Depleting these cells can attenuate lung injury following experimental bacterial infections or exposure to endotoxin.

Lung defenses

The necessary function of gas exchange requires that the lung remain exposed to the environment. Thus, the lung is continuously challenged by immense quantities of microorganisms and foreign material in inhaled air, and by opportunistic pathogens within droplets that are aspirated from the nonsterile upper respiratory tract. Despite this constant bombardment, the lung must maintain the balance of normal microbiota now documented to reside in the lung and prevent increases in the numbers of non-commensal organisms in the alveoli, as such increases can induce inflammation that impedes gas exchange in the lung. In addition, because of the tremendous blood flow through the lung, contamination of the lung by bacteria carries a significant risk of bacteremia. Thus, *the lung requires a multilayered system of defense against infectious agents*. This is accomplished by the following:

- *Mucus* lines the airways, entrapping particles and microbes, and is propelled by coughing or by ciliary beating to the pharynx where it is swallowed.
- *Antibody and innate defense proteins* kill microbes directly, prevent them from colonizing mucosal surfaces, and/or opsonize the microbes to make them more easily ingested by phagocytes.
- *Alveolar macrophages* recognize foreign invaders, particularly in the presence of opsonins, and engulf and kill these microbes without inducing inflammation.

If the infection cannot be contained by these mechanisms, inflammation is triggered in an attempt to control the threat. In these situations, macrophages and airway or alveolar epithelial cells produce cytokines and other mediators that recruit neutrophils and monocyte-derived macrophages. Inflammatory mediators also induce the production of antibacterial proteins by epithelial cells of the airway surface and tracheobronchial glands. But this response has the potential to do harm: *inflammatory exudates impair gas exchange, leukocyte-derived enzymes and oxygen radicals cause injury to lung tissue, and repair processes may result in organization of alveolar exudates or fibrosis of alveolar septa that permanently decreases lung compliance and thickens the blood-gas barrier*. The significance of these sequelae depends on the extent of lung involvement. The tremendous reserve capacity of the lung means that many animals have localized areas of pneumonia that are of no clinical significance, yet mild changes present throughout the lung can seriously compromise pulmonary function.

Inspired air carries a variety of particulates, including infectious agents, allergens, and inert particles. Particulate matter is classified by its aerodynamic diameter; for example, $PM_{2.5}$ particles settle in still air similar to spherical uncharged particles that are ≤2.5 μm diameter, but their physical size can be larger or smaller than 2.5 μm. *The aerodynamic diameter depends on the particle size, shape, density, hydrophobicity, and charge*. Particle size and aerodynamic diameter are relevant to transmission: particles ≤20-30 μm can form aerosols that can travel substantial distances by air; larger particles form droplets that settle to the ground within minutes. The aerodynamic diameter also predicts *the site of* **particle deposition** *in the respiratory tract*. Particles larger than ~10 μm are almost completely removed in the nasal cavity, mainly by impaction at sites in the nasal turbinates where the airflow changes direction. PM_{10} particles are more likely to impact the mucosa of the trachea and bronchi, where they can be cleared by the mucociliary apparatus. $PM_{2.5}$ particles have the greatest potential to reach the deep lung (terminal bronchioles and alveoli), and this is most common with smaller particles (PM_1). $PM_{0.1}$ tend not to be retained in the lung. However, the relationship of particle size and site of deposition is based on rodent and human studies and is assumed to be comparable for domestic species. The velocity of airflow declines precipitously in the terminal airways because the total cross-sectional area increases; as a result, particle deposition in the bronchioles and alveoli results from sedimentation, diffusion, and electrostatic charge.

Coughing and mucociliary clearance *are the major mechanisms for clearing particles that become entrapped in the airways*. Mucociliary clearance of particles from distal airways requires 2-6 hours, and innate defense proteins within the airway mucus (described in more detail below) probably serve to limit bacterial growth during this time. Mucociliary clearance may be as rapid as 10 mm/min in the trachea, with a more languid pace in the bronchioles. The airways are covered by a *periciliary liquid layer* and a superficial mucus layer. The mucus layer contains abundant glycoproteins that are sticky and trap a wide variety of particles that impact on the airway surfaces. The function of the periciliary liquid layer has long been considered to simply provide an aqueous medium in which the cilia can beat. However, evidence indicates that this layer forms a periciliary brush composed of mucins that transiently tether the cilia to the overlying mucus, trap water to maintain hydration, and prevent the mucus and other luminal substances from entering the periciliary layer. The quality of the periciliary liquid layer is also critical for clearance of entrapped particulates because the low viscosity of this fluid is needed for the cilia to beat effectively. In addition, clearance of sputum from the larger airways by coughing requires that the periciliary liquid layer be fluid and abundant, allowing the superficial mucus layer to be easily propelled. Finally, effective ciliary function is necessary for mucociliary clearance and requires coordinated unidirectional ciliary beating at an adequate frequency of around 15 beats per second. The regulation of this system is not well known. However, shear stress on the epithelium both increases the ciliary beating frequency and promotes epithelial secretion to maintain the quality of the liquid and mucous layer. Nitric oxide, cyclic adenosine monophosphate, and cyclic guanosine monophosphate are other regulators of ciliary beat frequency.

When entrapped particles reach the nasopharynx, they have the opportunity to interact with the well-developed lymphoid tissue in the tonsils and nasopharyngeal mucosa before they reach the pharynx and are swallowed. Although this clearance of inhaled particles is normally beneficial, it is a method for the spread of agents such as *Mycobacterium bovis* and *Rhodococcus equi* and is important in the migration of helminth eggs and larvae. Mucociliary clearance may be impaired by infection of the airway epithelium with viruses, mycoplasmas, or *Bordetella*, exposure to cold or dry air or ammonia, squamous metaplasia caused by chronic bacterial infection or toxin exposure (cigarette smoke and environmental pollutants being the best-characterized examples), inherited anomalies of ciliary structure or function, or abnormal mucus production in human cystic fibrosis.

The mucus covering the airway mucosa contains a rich spectrum of **antimicrobial factors**, which operate by several distinct mechanisms. Some cause *direct injury to pathogens*, such as the β-defensins, cathelicidins, lactoferrin, lysozyme, and lactoperoxidase, the complement membrane attack complex, and anionic antimicrobial peptides. *Lactoferrin binds iron* and makes it unavailable for use by many bacteria; neutrophil gelatinase-associated lipocalin—secreted by airway and alveolar epithelial cells and by neutrophils—binds the bacterial siderophores that otherwise allow pathogens to scavenge ferric iron. Other components, including immunoglobulin (Ig) A and polysaccharides within the mucus, *block the attachment of bacteria to mucosal surfaces. Infectious agents may be opsonized* by IgG, the complement component C3b, and surfactant proteins A and D. Two families of antimicrobial proteins, defensins and collectins, deserve particular mention. The **defensins** are a family of 3-5 kDa, cationic, arginine-rich peptides that are present in neutrophil granules, intestinal Paneth cells, and epithelial cells of the trachea and bronchi. Some defensins are constitutively expressed; others are rapidly induced by proinflammatory cytokines, lipopolysaccharide and other Toll-like receptor agonists, or cytokines secreted by Th17 cells. The defensins are able to kill bacteria, fungi, and enveloped viruses by forming pores within microbial membranes that are rich in anionic phospholipids, and they also have roles in leukocyte chemotaxis and wound healing. The **collectins** are a family of calcium-dependent carbohydrate-binding lectin proteins that include the surfactant proteins A and D. Both these proteins are produced by type II pneumocytes; SP-A is also secreted by club cells in the bronchioles. These pulmonary collectins agglutinate and opsonize bacteria, viruses, and fungi, and also maintain surfactant homeostasis, have antioxidant activity, and bind lipopolysaccharide to regulate inflammatory responses.

Alveolar macrophages *are critical for defending the lung against particles that are deposited in alveoli, and also play a key role in recycling and removal of surfactant.* Alveolar macrophages are decorated with cell surface receptors that recognize particles opsonized by antibody, complement, or collectins. In addition, CD14, Toll-like receptors, mannose receptors, and the scavenger receptor permit responses against bacteria that have not been previously encountered. Alveolar macrophages phagocytose most opsonized particles within 2-4 hours, although the ingestion of inert particles such as carbon and silicates is much slower. Alveolar macrophages kill bacteria using reactive oxygen and nitrogen species and enzymes within their lysosomes. In addition, these cells promote an inflammatory response by *secreting cytokines including chemokines* that recruit and activate neutrophils and macrophages. These newly recruited phagocytes are important in the clearance of more severe bacterial infections of the lung. Alveolar macrophages are integral to the immune response by presenting antigen, secreting cytokines that activate macrophages and modulate the immune response, and serving as effector cells in delayed hypersensitivity reactions. However, resident alveolar macrophages generally sequester or clear antigens and particulates from the alveoli without stimulating an immunoinflammatory response and without migration to regional lymph nodes. In contrast, when blood monocytes are recruited to the lung during inflammation and differentiate into macrophages, their phlogistic nature further stimulates local inflammation and immune responses.

The actual physical removal of particulates from alveoli is inefficient, in contrast to their removal when deposited on the mucociliary blanket. Most particles phagocytosed by macrophages are either inactivated or sequestered. Alveolar macrophages are mainly cleared through the bronchioles on the mucociliary blanket. As the particulate load increases, as occurs in pneumoconioses, some particles penetrate into the pulmonary interstitium by endocytosis across the type I pneumocytes, where they are phagocytosed by interstitial macrophages. Particle-laden macrophages often cluster around bronchioles and blood vessels, associated with local lymphatics (well illustrated by the common finding in dogs of carbon-laden particles in the walls of terminal bronchioles), with some entering the lymphatics and eventually finding their way to local lymph nodes. In addition to the alveolar and interstitial macrophages, *intravascular macrophages* are present in the lung of cats, horses, ruminants, and pigs. These cells remove infectious agents and other particles from the blood, and thus serve an analogous role to macrophages in hepatic and splenic sinusoids.

Pulmonary immune responses are initiated when inhaled antigens are taken up by *dendritic cells* that inhabit the airway epithelium and migrate to bronchial lymph nodes where the antigen is presented to lymphocytes. Although *bronchus-associated lymphoid tissue* (BALT) is often visible histologically, this structure is not present in germ-free animals of most species and may represent a consequence of inflammation and antigenic stimulation. Homing of lymphocytes to BALT depends on $\alpha_4\beta_1$-integrin/VCAM1 and CCR10/CCL28. In contrast, migration of lymphocytes into alveolar tissue is exceptional because it occurs in capillaries rather than venules, and the homing receptors differ from those in the airways. These mechanisms allow *T lymphocytes and natural killer cells* to constantly survey the respiratory tissues, where they are most useful in defense against viruses, intracellular bacterial pathogens, and fungi.

Thus, the lung is protected from inhaled bacteria by the filtering effect of the nasal cavity, innate and acquired humoral defenses, mucociliary clearance in the airways, resident alveolar macrophages, recruited neutrophils and elicited macrophages, and T lymphocytes and natural killer cells. These defenses can be considered in various layers, where most inhaled particles are removed in the nasal cavity or neutralized by innate defense proteins in the airway mucus prior to being cleared by the mucociliary apparatus. The small bronchioles seem to be a site of particular vulnerability, being poorly served by either mucociliary clearance or alveolar macrophages. Pathogens that reach the alveoli may be phagocytosed and killed by alveolar macrophages, particularly if the particles have been opsonized by complement or the surfactant proteins A and D, or by antibody if a previous encounter with the agent has resulted in an immune response. Still greater threats invoke a neutrophil inflammatory response, which may be essential to clear bacteria from the lung but also carries the risk of compromised lung function and damage to the pulmonary tissue.

NASAL CAVITY AND SINUSES

General considerations

The *upper respiratory tract* comprises the air-conducting structures from the external nares to the upper third of the trachea, including the specialized system of paranasal sinuses, the auditory tubes, and the guttural pouches of horses. The anatomy of the upper respiratory tract is described above. Functionally, this system conducts and conditions the air moving into and out of the lower respiratory tract during respiration. The upper airways, constantly exposed to materials from the external environment, play an important role in surveying the inspired air for pathogens and are exposed to a variety of potentially toxic particulates and gases.

The upper respiratory tract accounts for >50% of the airway resistance in the entire respiratory tract. This resistance leads to negative pressure during inspiration, shown to be greatest in the nasal cavity overlying the rostral aspect of the soft palate, the larynx, and the trachea; and indeed, these correspond to disease hot spots such as for dorsal displacement of the soft palate in racehorses and the tracheal edema and hemorrhage syndrome of cattle. The anatomy of the upper airways is also important in the generation of species-specific vocalization in animals, and abnormal vocal sounds (stertor, stridor) as well as inspiratory dyspnea are clinical indicators of diseases involving the upper airways.

Congenital anomalies

Congenital anomalies of the nasal cavity and sinuses are rare but occur in all species. They are usually part of more extensive craniofacial defects accompanied by various malformations of the mouth and eyes. Animals with absent, underdeveloped, or severely distorted nasal regions are usually stillborn or die immediately after birth because of the severity of the craniofacial defects.

Choanal atresia *is a failure of formation of one or both of the communications between the nasal cavity and nasopharynx.* The condition is relatively common in llamas and alpacas, well recorded in foals, and has been described in dogs, sheep, and cats. The obstruction at the junction of hard and soft palate may be membranous or bony and unilateral or bilateral. Affected animals have partial or complete obstruction of airflow, exercise intolerance, or respiratory distress, or develop aspiration pneumonia or malnutrition if mouth breathing interferes with suckling. The condition in llamas is often accompanied by other facial malformations. Related conditions in dogs and cats are imperforate nasopharynx and congenital nasopharyngeal stenosis caused by anomalous development of the soft palate.

Nasal amyloidosis

Deposits of amyloid sometimes occur in the nasal submucosa of horses. The deposition is not part of generalized amyloidosis, although there might be concurrent cutaneous amyloidosis. The amyloid usually forms one or more masses in the nasal vestibule and rostral portions of the nasal cavity and may obstruct airflow, but it can be located anywhere in the nasal cavity or form diffuse deposits. The amyloid forms multifocal deposits accompanied by numerous lymphocytes, macrophages, and giant cells (Fig. 5-3). There may be ulceration of the mucosa, especially overlying large nodular masses. Nasal amyloidosis in horses is of the *AL type*, composed of immunoglobulin light chains or light-chain fragments. Although AL amyloid results from plasmacytic neoplasms in other species, no such association has been established in horses.

Circulatory disturbances

Epistaxis *refers to hemorrhage from the nose, without regard to the source of the bleeding. Blood-stained foam* in the trachea and nasal cavity is often present in animals with pulmonary congestion and edema, but should not be confused with epistaxis in which larger amounts of blood are present. In epistaxis, the hemorrhage may arise from the nasopharynx, lungs, or elsewhere in the respiratory tract. Lesions within the nasal cavity often cause unilateral epistaxis; causes of such lesions include nasal trauma, severe rhinitis (lymphoplasmacytic, eosinophilic, or neutrophilic), mycotic infections of the nasal cavity or the guttural pouch, tooth root abscesses, and neoplasms. In contrast, bilateral epistaxis may indicate a severe manifestation of the above, hemorrhagic diatheses such as those causing thrombocytopenia, or lesions in or distal to the nasopharynx. The latter include pulmonary contusions, hemorrhagic purpura in horses, exercise-induced pulmonary hemorrhages in horses, rupture of embolic pulmonary abscesses in cattle, pulmonary neoplasia or granulomas, pulmonary hypertension, or vasculitis. Animals with epistaxis that swallow the blood may have considerable amounts in the stomach.

Immunology of the upper respiratory tract

As with other mucous membranes, the upper airway mucosa has an indigenous immune system, the *nasal-associated lymphoid tissue* (NALT). NALT is considered to be a component of the broader mucosal-associated lymphoid system present in a variety of mucous membranes. The nasopharyngeal lymphoid (Waldeyer) ring is a collection of lymphoid tissues that encircles the oropharynx and nasopharynx of animals. The degree of organization of this lymphoid tissue varies by species. In addition, there are lymphoid follicles and loose aggregates of mononuclear cells within the lamina propria. These lymphoid tissues induce a local immune response and also stimulate a systemic immune reaction to nasally delivered antigens. This tissue is particularly prominent in foals and gives a finely nodular appearance to the pharyngeal mucosa.

The organization of NALT is similar to mucosal lymphoid tissues at other sites. Specialized follicle-associated epithelium, with microfold (M) cells, covers the follicles and transfers antigen to the underlying lymphoid follicles. Within the follicles

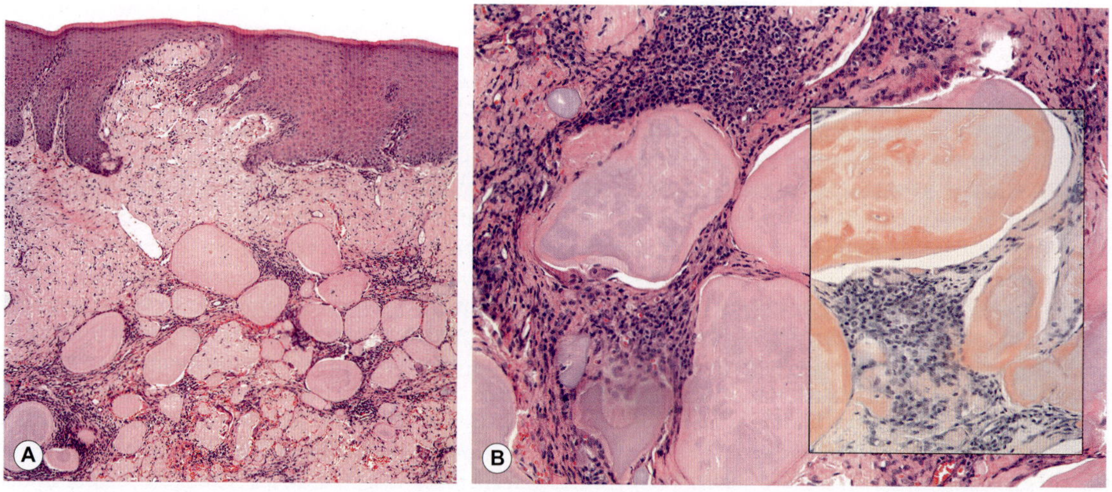

Figure 5-3 Amyloidosis of the nasal vestibule in a horse. **A.** The focal mass consists of amorphous eosinophilic aggregates of AL amyloid, separating a dense infiltrate of lymphocytes. **B.** Higher magnification. Inset: Congo red stain.

there are T cell– and B cell–rich regions, as well as dendritic cells and macrophages involved in antigen presentation. The formation of NALT is a postnatal event that is at least partly regulated by acquisition of commensal microbes in the nasopharynx. This resident microbial flora is often established by specific adherence of bacterial adhesins to carbohydrates on epithelial cells.

In addition to the role that nasopharyngeal commensals play in the formation of NALT, they can prevent colonization of the mucosa by more virulent organisms and modulate the immune response during infection. Injury to the nasal mucosa can allow infection of the underlying tissues by certain of the normal flora or, more importantly, affect surface binding sites so that adherence and colonization by pathogenic microorganisms can occur. Finally, disruption of the normal nasopharyngeal flora by prolonged antibiotic therapy may result in fungal or opportunistic bacterial infections of the nasal cavity, further illustrating the role of these commensals in mucosal defense.

Rhinitis

Rhinitis, inflammation of nasal tissue, can be localized or a manifestation of systemic disease. The main causes include viral, bacterial, fungal, and parasitic infections, allergens, inhalation of irritant gases, and particulate dusts (Box 5-1). Most cases of significant acute rhinitis begin with serous exudation, which changes in the course of the disease to become catarrhal, purulent, or hemorrhagic. **Fibrinonecrotic membranes** leave a raw ulcerated surface when removed and are most commonly caused by viral infection, inhalation of epitheliotoxic gases, or bacteria such as *Fusobacterium necrophorum*. Histologically, in acute rhinitis, the epithelial cells are normal or have hydropic degeneration, loss of cilia, or attenuation. Goblet cells may

Box • 5-1

Major causes of nasal and sinus disease in domestic animals

Dogs
- Foreign body
- Mycotic rhinitis
- Allergic rhinitis
- Idiopathic lymphoplasmacytic rhinitis
- Oronasal fistula
- Apical tooth infection
- Ciliary dyskinesia
- Neoplasms
- Other considerations
  1. *Bordetella bronchiseptica*
  2. Canine adenovirus 2
  3. Canine distemper virus
  4. Canine parainfluenza virus
  5. *Linguatula serrata*
  6. *Pneumonyssoides caninum*
  7. *Eucoleus boehmi*
  8. *Rhinosporidium seeberi*
  9. Systemic histiocytosis

Cats
- Felid alphaherpesvirus 1
- Feline calicivirus
- *Cryptococcus*
- Foreign body
- Nasopharyngeal stenosis
- Nasopharyngeal polyp
- Lymphoma
- Adenocarcinoma
- Other considerations
  1. *Bordetella bronchiseptica*
  2. *Chlamydia* sp.
  3. *Mycoplasma* spp.
  4. Mycotic rhinitis
  5. *Rhinosporidium*

Pigs
- Inclusion body rhinitis
- Atrophic rhinitis

Horses
- Equid alphaherpesvirus
- Equine influenza A virus
- Equine rhinitis virus
- *Streptococcus equi*
- *Streptococcus zooepidemicus*
- Bacterial sinusitis
- Ethmoid hematoma
- Sinonasal polyps
- Ethmoid and sinus cysts
- Neoplasms
- Maxillary bone tumors (fibrous dysplasia, ossifying fibroma, osteoma, fibrosarcoma)
- Other considerations
  1. Tooth root infection
  2. Nasal amyloidosis
  3. Glanders
  4. Mycotic rhinitis or sinusitis
  5. Phycomycosis
  6. *Schistosoma* spp.

Cattle
- Bovine alphaherpesvirus 1
- Bovine parainfluenza virus 3
- Mycotic nasal granuloma
- Allergic rhinitis
- Other considerations
  1. *Limnatis* spp.
  2. *Mammomonogamus* spp.

Sheep and goats
- *Salmonella diarizonae*
- *Oestrus ovis*
- Enzootic nasal tumor

be inapparent from having secreted their contents or may be hyperplastic. The lamina propria is edematous and contains inflammatory cells that often infiltrate the epithelium and may be visible in the surface exudate.

Chronic rhinitis may be classified by the nature of the leukocytic infiltrate, but caution should be exercised in equating this with a specific cause. For example, neutrophilic rhinitis can result from bacterial infection, aspergillosis, inhaled foreign body, tooth root infections, oronasal fistula, and perhaps gastric reflux, and is a common nonspecific response to mucosal injury. Eosinophils predominate in allergic rhinitis but may also be frequent adjacent to fungal plaques or carcinomas. Lymphoplasmacytic rhinitis is a common reaction pattern in chronic nasal disease of diverse etiology. The nasal epithelium in chronic rhinitis is often attenuated because of necrosis or may develop squamous metaplasia or dysplasia. Other features of chronic inflammation include hyperplasia of lymphoid tissue, fibrosis of the lamina propria with atrophy of the glands, and resorption of the conchae. Sessile or pedunculated polyps resulting from chronic inflammation or edema may be mistaken for neoplasms.

Nasal/nasopharyngeal stenosis or cicatrix formation occurs in cats and horses, probably as a result of previous erosive rhinitis with fibrous organization of exudates. *In pastured horses*, the typical lesion is circumferential weblike scarring of the mucosa in the laryngopharynx rostral to the epiglottis, but may be elsewhere in the pharynx, nasal cavity, or trachea. *In cats*, nasopharyngeal stenosis appears as more uniform membranous narrowing of the opening between the caudal nasal cavity and the nasopharynx. The histologic findings are chronic nonspecific rhinitis and/or granulation tissue with chronic hemorrhage. Clinical signs often include upper respiratory noise or respiratory distress in the absence of much discharge. Rarely, the inspiratory efforts resulting from bilateral nasal obstruction can lead to hiatal hernia and megaesophagus. Choanal atresia is described above.

Idiopathic lymphoplasmacytic rhinitis is an important condition in dogs, and to a lesser extent in cats. In dogs, the clinical disease may be either unilateral or bilateral, although histologic lesions are usually bilateral. Grossly, there is increased mucus production, mucosal inflammation, and turbinate destruction. Histologically, lymphocytes and plasma cells predominate, but neutrophils may be present. Chronic inflammation may lead to diffuse or polypoid thickening of the nasal mucosa and obstruction of nasal passages. The fibrotic stroma is heavily infiltrated by lymphocytes and plasma cells, and the surface epithelium may be hyperplastic, eroded, or undergo squamous metaplasia. The response of some cases to glucocorticoid therapy suggests an immune-mediated disease, but the above causes of chronic rhinitis must be ruled out.

Allergic rhinitis is observed sporadically in most domestic species. The diagnosis in *dogs* is based on chronic and often seasonal oculonasal discharge, sneezing, nose-rubbing, head-shaking, and perhaps epistaxis, and typically the *presence of eosinophils in nasal exudate* (eFig. 5-3). There is no definitive information on either the pathologic or immunologic basis of the condition but is assumed to be a type I hypersensitivity. *Cattle*, and occasionally *sheep*, develop a seasonal rhinitis that available evidence suggests is an allergic response to pollen antigens. A familial predisposition has been reported, and the disease occurs chiefly in the summertime when pastures are in bloom. Affected animals have nasal discharge, lacrimation, sneezing, and evidence of nasal itching. The nasal mucosa is pale and thick from edema, and mucosal erosions may be visible in the rostral nares. Eosinophils and mucus are a prominent component of the exudate. Histologically, *the surviving nasal epithelium is hyperplastic or eroded and is infiltrated by eosinophils*. The glandular epithelium can be hypertrophied, and mucus is produced in excess. In more severe cases, in which there is extensive superficial necrosis, many of the small mucosal vessels have fibrinoid necrosis.

Nasal "granuloma" in cattle *is generally considered to be a more chronic form of allergic rhinitis*. The affected mucosa is mainly in the caudal portion of the nasal vestibule and the rostral region of the ventral nasal cavity but may extend caudally even to the larynx and proximal trachea. Grossly, *the hyperplastic epithelium is granular or has nodular projections covered by intact epithelium*, and catarrhal exudate may be present. Histologically, the nodules typically consist of hyperplastic epithelium with areas of squamous metaplasia or ulceration, covering a superficial edematous lamina propria with a central core of inflamed granulation tissue. Goblet cell hyperplasia is more pronounced in the ducts of the nasal glands, at the lateral boundaries of the nodules. Eosinophils infiltrate the superficial lamina propria and epithelium, and lymphocytes, plasma cells, and mast cells are increased in number. Vascular proliferation, fibroplasia, and accumulation of mostly lymphocytes and plasma cells in the cores of nodules are features of chronicity. It is believed that the condition is an allergic reaction to plant pollens or fungal spores. Because there appears to be a familial predisposition in Jersey cattle, and to a limited extent in other cattle, the existence of susceptible "atopic" animals has been proposed. The condition is therefore sometimes referred to as *atopic rhinitis*.

Specific infectious causes of neutrophilic rhinitis deserve mention. *Salmonella enterica* ssp. *diarizonae* [specifically, serovar 61:k:1,5,(7)] causes flock problems in sheep, with mucoid nasal discharge, nasal obstruction, and granular swelling or sessile polyp formation in the ventral conchae. Histologically, there is polypoid hyperplasia of the mucosa with intraepithelial bacteria and infiltration of neutrophils. *Streptococcus canis* and *Streptococcus equi* ssp. *zooepidemicus* cause outbreaks or sporadic cases of rhinitis and sinusitis in dogs and cats, with extension through the cribriform plate leading to fatal meningitis. *Aspergillus fumigatus* commonly causes nasal disease in dogs and cats, with ulceration and neutrophilic or eosinophilic rhinitis in which the fungal hyphae are found mainly in plaques on the mucosal surface. However, neutrophilic rhinitis is also a nonspecific reaction to foreign bodies, neoplasms, bacterial infection, tooth root infections, oronasal fistula, and other causes.

Infectious causes of granulomatous rhinitis, with or without eosinophils, are diverse and are discussed in detail later (in the sections on infectious diseases). *Cryptococcus neoformans* and *Cryptococcus gatti* are readily recognized by their thick capsules; acapsular strains occur and incite more granulomatous inflammation but are recognized by their narrow-based budding. *Conidiobolus* spp. and *Basidiobolus haptosporus* cause granulomatous masses in the caudal nasal cavity of horses and ruminants that may invade surrounding tissues and disseminate to the lung or brain. Histologically, granulomas contain macrophages, many giant cells, eosinophils, central necrosis, and negatively stained fungal hyphae embedded in Splendore-Hoeppli material; silver stains reveal the hyphae to be 8-20 μm diameter, infrequently septate, with nonparallel walls and bulbous dilations. Although comparable, lesions caused by

Pythium insidiosum occlude mainly the rostral nasal cavity, induce eosinophilic inflammation, and have smaller hypha-like oomycetes that are 2-7 µm diameter and infrequently septate with thick nonparallel walls. *Rhinosporidium seeberi* causes inflamed polyps with sporangia that are 15-75 µm or greater and commonly have endosporulation. Granulomatous rhinitis caused by the yeast *Candida parapsilosis* is reported in an immunosuppressed cat. Nodular granulomatous rhinitis with eosinophils caused by *Pseudallescheria boydii* is described in dogs and cattle. *Besnoitia* spp. cause lesions in many organs, but the characteristic 150-450-µm-diameter thick-walled protozoan cysts are often found in the nares, nasal cavity, nasopharynx, or larynx. Finally, *Prototheca wickerhamii* and *Prototheca zopfii* affect the mucocutaneous junction of the nares in addition to the skin, with necrotizing pyogranulomatous lesions containing septated sporangia that are 3-15 µm and 7-30 µm diameter, respectively. Environmental mycobacteria rarely cause nasal granulomas.

A variety of toxic agents cause necrosis of nasal respiratory or olfactory epithelium. These may be direct-acting irritants or toxins. Furthermore, because of the cytochrome P450-dependent biotransformation activity of the nasal mucosa, systemic toxins such as acetaminophen, vincristine, coumarins, naphthalene, polychlorinated biphenyls, methimazole, and 3-methylindole target the nasal epithelium in some species. These are particularly well studied in rodents, but toxic nasal disease is not often investigated in domestic animals.

Diseases of the paranasal sinuses

Inflammation of the paranasal sinuses often goes undetected unless it has caused facial deformity or a fistula in the overlying skin. In acute catarrhal or purulent rhinitis, the mucosal swelling tends to occlude the orifices of the sinuses and impair drainage. The secretions and exudates then accumulate and predispose to bacterial infection and chronic purulent sinusitis. *The accumulation of seromucinous secretion is referred to as* **mucocele**, and *the accumulation of purulent exudate is known as* **empyema** *of the sinus* (eFig. 5-4). Sinusitis follows penetration of infection in dehorning wounds, fractures, and periodontitis. It is common in sheep infected with larvae of *Oestrus ovis*. Sinusitis is of most significance in the horse because of the size and complexity of its paranasal sinuses and the compounding effects of limited drainage and tendency for periodontitis to extend to the sinuses. In horses, primary sinusitis is most frequent in the maxillary sinus, but the exudates in the ventral conchal sinus are more likely to be inspissated and therefore respond more poorly to therapy. Other sinus diseases of horses include dental sinusitis from apical infection of a maxillary cheek tooth, oromaxillary fistula, mycosis, sinus cysts, trauma, or progressive ethmoid hematoma. Reported equine sinus neoplasms include cementoma, benign fibro-osseous tumor, myxoma, lymphoma, and carcinoma.

Non-neoplastic proliferative disorders of the nasal cavity and sinuses

Sialoceles and nasal glandular mucoceles occasionally expand into the nasal cavity or nasopharynx with similar morphology to those found elsewhere (eFigs. 5-5 and 5-6). *Polypoid thickening of the nasal mucosa* can form a discernible mass within the nasal cavity or sinuses. They are thought to be elicited by chronic mucosal edema, or from chronic rhinitis, and sometimes arise from the mucosa overlying tumors. Masses caused by infection and inflammation are described above.

Auditory polyps of cats *are non-neoplastic inflammatory masses arising within the middle ear or auditory tube* (Fig. 5-4). Clinical disease is seen primarily in young cats 1-3-years-old. The clinical signs are dependent on the location of the polyp; extension of the mass into the pharynx is associated with dyspnea, dysphagia, and gagging; involvement of the nasal cavity may cause sneezing, nasal discharge, and protrusion through the nares; involvement of the middle ear may result in ataxia, Horner syndrome, and/or facial nerve paralysis. The cause and pathogenesis are not known, although the appearance of the lesions suggests progressive fibroproliferation in response to localized chronic inflammation. Histologically, *feline nasopharyngeal polyps* consist of a loose fibrovascular core covered by ciliated respiratory or squamous epithelium. Even when the surface epithelium has undergone squamous metaplasia, ciliated cells are usually visible within nests of epithelial cells buried in the stroma. The stroma is infiltrated by a mixed chronic inflammatory infiltrate of lymphocytes, plasma cells, and macrophages; surface erosions, when present, elicit neutrophil infiltration of the stroma. Recurrence of the polyps is relatively common when removed by simple traction if the base of the mass is not excised. A second form of feline nasal polyps arises from nasal turbinates, consists of fibrous tissue, woven bone, and blood-filled spaces, and is covered by columnar ciliated epithelium. These have been termed *inflammatory polyps of the nasal turbinates of cats* or feline mesenchymal nasal hamartoma.

Respiratory epithelial adenomatoid hamartoma (REAH) is a polypoid or cystic mass containing glandular tissue lined by respiratory epithelium (eFig. 5-7). Those containing plates of cartilage or bone are termed chondro-osseous REAH.

Progressive ethmoid hematoma (**PEH**; hemorrhagic nasal polyp) **of horses** *is typically a unilateral hemorrhagic growth arising from the submucosa of the ethmoid turbinates.* These masses usually occur in older horses and may be more common in the Thoroughbred and Arabian breeds. The cause and pathogenesis of PEH are undetermined, although it is assumed that it represents an aberrant vasoproliferative response to submucosal hemorrhage. The lesions are progressive and may continue to enlarge until the cylindrical mass extends to the

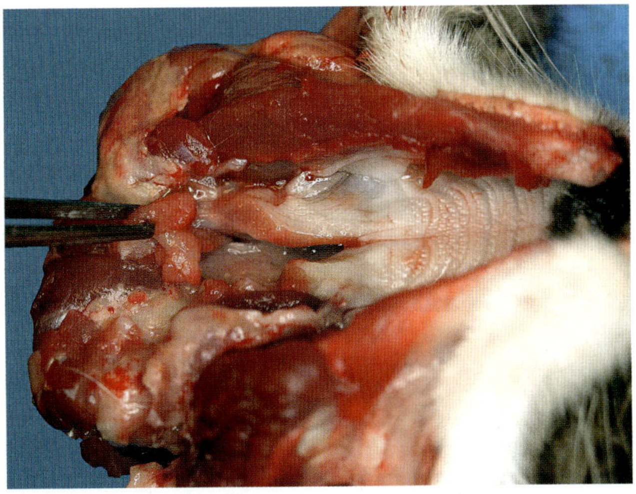

Figure 5-4 **Auditory polyp** in a cat. Forceps grasp the polyp in the nasopharynx, which has a stalk extending from the auditory tube. The soft palate has been incised.

external nares. Grossly, PEH is a mottled, hemorrhagic fibrovascular mass that can fill the ipsilateral nasal meatus, or occasionally grow into the maxillary sinus. Histologically, PEH consists mostly of organizing hemorrhages of various ages with extensive siderosis and mineralization of connective tissue fibers and vessel walls. The inflammatory response is variable, but multinucleate giant cells are usually present within the stroma. The surface is often covered by attenuated epithelium with underlying glands, or squamous metaplasia may occur. Ulceration of the surface epithelium is common.

Paranasal sinus cysts in foals or young-adult horses are within a maxillary or frontal sinus and have a thin bony wall lined by respiratory epithelium and filled with fluid. The masses can distort the profile of the maxillary bone sufficiently to cause obstruction of the ipsilateral nasal passage, destruction of the nasal turbinates, distortion of the teeth, and deviation of the nasal septum. **Cystic nasal conchae** are congenital lesions that cause progressive nasal obstruction with inspiratory and expiratory noise in cattle. They are bilateral or unilateral, and otherwise similar to those of horses. **Epidermal inclusion cysts** lined by stratified squamous epithelium are described in the nasal diverticulum (false nostril) of horses and have been seen in dogs. Other non-neoplastic nasal masses include branchial cyst, vascular hamartoma, and angiofibroma.

Neoplasms of the nasal cavity and sinuses

Although primary neoplastic disease of the nasal cavity and sinuses of domestic animals is not common, primary nasal neoplasia is most frequent in the dog and cat, with fewer reports in horses. Most nasal epithelial neoplasms in sheep and goats are of retroviral etiology (see the Infectious Respiratory Diseases of Sheep and Goats section). There is some epidemiologic evidence of a link between exposure to environmental tobacco smoke or coal-burning and kerosene heat sources, and the development of nasal neoplasms in dogs.

Origin from the nasal cavity is usual in dogs and cats, whereas tumors of the paranasal sinuses are most common in horses. Because of the inflexible osseous encasement, even benign growths can be associated with significant clinical disease. In general, *most neoplasms of the nasal cavity and sinuses are carcinomas*, followed in decreasing frequency by chondrosarcoma, fibrosarcoma, and osteosarcoma. **Nasal carcinomas** are most frequent in dogs and cats. They are classified as adenocarcinoma, nonkeratinizing squamous cell carcinoma, adenosquamous carcinoma, squamous cell carcinoma, neuroendocrine carcinoma, acinic cell carcinoma, adenoid cystic carcinoma, oncocytoma, and undifferentiated (solid) carcinoma. Regardless of the type, locally invasive growth is the usual reason for euthanasia. Stage 1 neoplasms have unilateral growth without bone invasion (other than into the conchae). Stage 2 neoplasms invade bone other than the conchae without progressing to form lesions described for stage 3. Stage 3 neoplasms involve the orbit or form a mass in the nasopharynx, subcutis, or oral mucosa. Stage 4 neoplasms invade the cribriform plate to cause seizures or depression. These consequences of invasive growth are the usual reason for euthanasia, and metastasis occurs relatively late in the course of disease.

Nasal adenocarcinoma is the most common type, and the diagnosis is based on identifying an invasive carcinoma with the formation of many or few acini, tubules, or papillary structures (Fig. 5-5). Occasional cases have prominent mucin production. **Adenoid cystic carcinomas** are rare and formed by nests and cords of neoplastic basal-like cells with scant cytoplasm and hyperchromatic nuclei; these cellular nests have a cribriform pattern with sharply demarcated "punched out" centers containing basophilic mucus. Lakes of this same material are present between the nests of cells. Nonkeratinizing squamous cell carcinoma (formerly transitional carcinoma) forms nodules or nests of stratified cuboidal epithelium that lacks keratinization; microcysts are sometimes present within the epithelial layers and must be distinguished from the acini seen in adenocarcinomas. **Adenosquamous carcinomas** have substantial amounts of both acinar components and squamous differentiation and may have more aggressive behavior. **Squamous cell carcinomas** are similar to those seen in other organs, with nodules or nests of epithelial cells that keratinize to form abundant glassy eosinophilic cytoplasm and occasional central aggregates of keratin. These are frequent tumors in the cat where most originate from the nasal vestibule, and in the horse where the maxillary sinus is a common site. **Acinic cell carcinomas** are rare and have a faintly packeted or acinar arrangement of cells that resemble salivary serous cells,

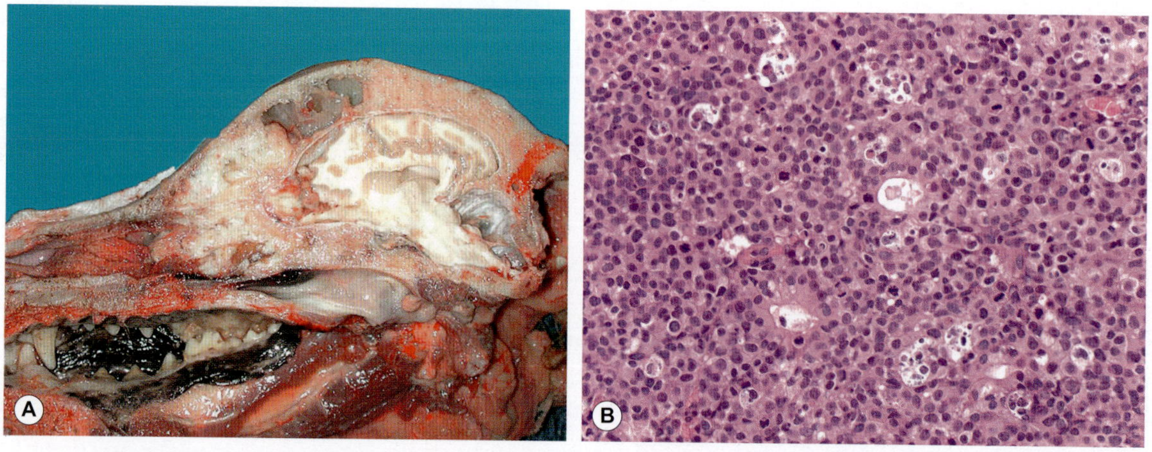

Figure 5-5 **Nasal adenocarcinoma** in a dog. **A.** Adenocarcinoma arising from the ethmoid conchae, with invasion of paranasal sinus and through the cribriform plate into the brain. **B.** The cells have a nearly solid arrangement, with a few acini formed by neoplastic cells.

with abundant pale cytoplasm containing fine basophilic PAS-positive diastase-resistant granules; this type is invasive but metastases are not expected. **Oncocytomas** form cords, nests, or acini of large epithelioid cytokeratin-positive cells with angular borders, and abundant eosinophilic cytoplasm containing numerous mitochondria that appear as fine eosinophilic granules that stain with phosphotungstic acid–hematoxylin. The few cases reported had either noninvasive or invasive growth habits. **Neuroendocrine carcinomas** have delicate septa of fibrous stroma separating nests or packets of neoplastic epithelial cells, most with fine cytoplasmic granules or others with clear cytoplasm (Fig. 5-6). In those forming rosettes, anatomic location, immunohistochemistry, or ultrastructure may differentiate them from olfactory neuroblastoma. Neuroendocrine carcinomas express chromogranin A, vasoactive intestinal polypeptide, neuron-specific enolase, and sometimes synaptophysin, S100, and other markers of neuroendocrine differentiation. Because these markers are also expressed by some adenocarcinomas, the morphologic features are essential for the diagnosis. **Undifferentiated carcinomas** are solid epithelial neoplasms that lack the patterns of differentiation mentioned above. **Benign epithelial neoplasms** are rare but include papilloma, adenoma, and basal cell tumor (of the vestibule).

Olfactory neuroblastoma (esthesioneuroblastoma) is a rare neoplasm derived from olfactory neuroepithelium and arising in the ethmoid conchae. The neoplastic cells form indistinct serpiginous ribbons, nests, or lobules with delicate fibrovascular stroma and are epithelioid but have indistinct borders and scant cytoplasm. *Rosette formation* is a characteristic feature (Fig. 5-7), more frequent in cats than in dogs, and includes pseudorosettes (neoplastic cells palisading around a blood vessel), Homer-Wright rosettes (neoplastic cells arranged around neurofibrillary material), and infrequent Flexner-Wintersteiner rosettes (neoplastic cells arranged around a mainly empty space). *Neurofibrillary material* often separates the cells, mineralization may be present, and necrosis is usually extensive in dogs and cats. Dense-core granules and neurofibrillary processes are diagnostically useful ultrastructural characteristics. Immunohistochemistry for chromogranin and neuron-specific enolase may be helpful, although nonspecific background staining can be problematic with NSE; synaptophysin is often negative; and neuron-specific markers such β-tubulin, MAP2, and NeuN are more specific but less widely available. Given that some are cytokeratin positive, this is not useful in distinguishing olfactory neuroblastoma from adenocarcinoma. A grading scheme is proposed, with higher grade tumors lacking lobular architecture, fibrillary matrix, or mineralization, few or no rosettes, and a greater degree of nuclear pleomorphism, necrosis, and mitotic activity. Penetration through the cribriform plate and into the cerebral cortex is commonly observed. **Olfactory ganglioneuroblastoma** contains clusters of ganglion cells and cords of neuroblastic cells.

Of the round-cell neoplasms, **lymphoma** is most frequent and is clinically important to distinguish from carcinoma. Lymphoma is the most common nasal/nasopharyngeal tumor in cats. It is usually primary, arising from the nasal cavity or uncommonly the nasopharynx, and not considered to be retroviral. Less often, nasal tissues can be secondarily affected in cases of multiorgan lymphoma. Feline nasal lymphoma is easily confused with carcinoma because the large neoplastic cells are often arranged as dense sheets, and faint packeting can result from delicate bands of stroma. Immunohistochemistry may be needed to resolve uncertainty. The vast majority are of diffuse large B-cell phenotype, but low-grade follicular B-cell lymphoma as well as T-cell lymphoma occurs. Epitheliotropism occurs with both B- and T-cell nasal lymphoma. Lymphoma can develop in other organs as the disease progresses (22-67% of cases, depending on the study), but nasal obstruction or invasion of local tissues including the brain is the more common clinical problem. Other round-cell tumors of the nasal cavity include mast cell tumor, melanoma, plasmacytoma, and transmissible venereal tumor.

Of the mesenchymal neoplasms, **chondrosarcoma** is most frequent, followed by **osteosarcoma and fibrosarcoma**. The appearance is typical of that in other tissues (eFig. 5-8). **Nasal perivascular wall tumors** in cats are polypoid noninvasive masses of uniform spindle cells and branching (staghorn) vessels. **Paranasal meningioma** occurs in dogs and horses, and in dogs appears similar to intracranial meningiomas but with

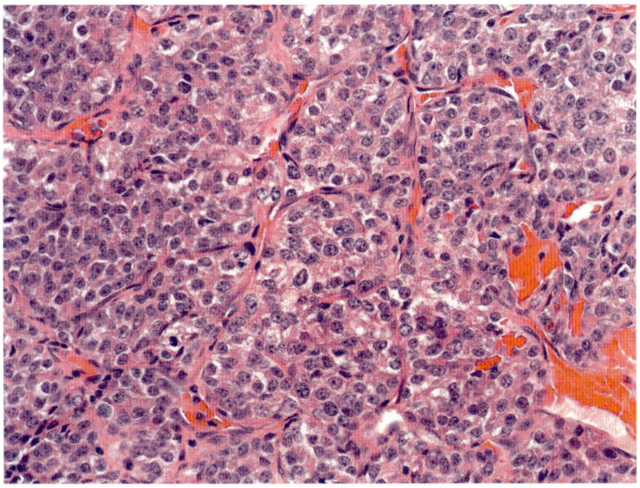

Figure 5-6 Nasal neuroendocrine carcinoma in a dog. Neoplastic epithelial cells are arranged in nests separated by delicate stroma. IHC was positive for synaptophysin.

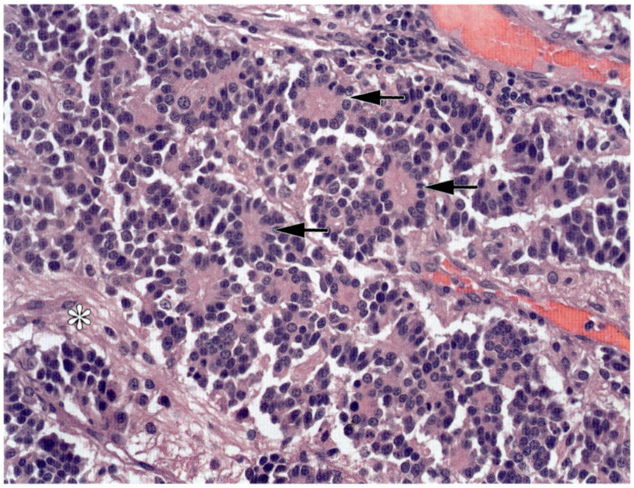

Figure 5-7 Olfactory neuroblastoma in a dog. The epithelioid cells form rosettes (arrows) with finely fibrillar material in the stroma (asterisk).

more invasive behavior. **Nasopharyngeal angiofibroma** in dogs forms a papillary mass composed of loose proliferative fibrous tissue with numerous tiny branching capillaries, and infiltrates of neutrophils and lymphocytes. Despite their benign histologic appearance, these masses have an aggressive locally invasive growth habit. **Nasomaxillary tumors of young horses**, including fibrosarcoma, ossifying fibroma, and fibrous dysplasia, are described elsewhere (see Vol. 1, Bones and Joints). Other mesenchymal tumors of the nasal cavity include **melanoma**, hemangiosarcoma, and fibroma.

PHARYNX, LARYNX, AND TRACHEA

Guttural pouch

The *guttural pouches* of equids are ventral diverticula of the auditory tubes. Neutrophilic inflammation leading to guttural pouch empyema occurs mostly after upper respiratory infections, particularly with *Streptococcus equi* or other streptococci. **Guttural pouch mycosis**, generally caused by *Aspergillus* spp., causes fibrinonecrotic inflammation that extends deeply to invade vessels and other structures (Fig. 5-8). Thus, severe complications are much more likely than for guttural pouch empyema. Guttural pouch inflammation can extend to involve nearby vessels, cranial nerves (VII, IX, X, XI, XII), and the cranial sympathetic trunk, or even spread to adjacent bones, middle ear, brain, or atlanto-occipital joint. Thus, erosion of the internal or external carotid artery or the maxillary artery causes epistaxis, damage to the glossopharyngeal or vagus nerves causes dysphagia, damage to the cranial sympathetic trunk or cranial cervical ganglion causes Horner syndrome, or damage to the facial nerve causes facial paralysis. Other complications include laryngeal hemiparesis, or permanent dorsal displacement of the soft palate. Guttural pouch hemorrhage can also result from fracture of the basisphenoid bone. A less common condition is *guttural pouch tympany*. This is mostly seen in young animals, and the accumulation of air is presumed to be the result of valvular action of the nasopharyngeal orifice of the auditory tube. *Tumors of the guttural pouches* are rare, but squamous cell carcinoma is most likely. Pharyngeal diseases are discussed elsewhere (see Vol. 2, Alimentary System).

Larynx

In young **horses**, it is common to find prominent lymphoid follicles in the pharyngeal mucosa near the larynx. This is usually an incidental finding; these follicles are part of the normal mucosal immune system (eFig. 5-9).

In the **horse**, *subepiglottic cysts* are believed to arise from thyroglossal duct remnants. *Entrapment of the epiglottis* below the aryepiglottic fold is usually associated with congenital hypoplasia or acquired shortening or distortion of the epiglottis. A short epiglottis also predisposes to *dorsal displacement of the soft palate*, and these conditions sometimes occur together. *Persistent frenulum of the epiglottis* has been reported in newborn foals, predisposing to oronasal reflux of milk after nursing and aspiration pneumonia. The persistent frenulum of the epiglottis leads to dorsal displacement of the soft palate, which can be assessed endoscopically.

Laryngeal paralysis

Laryngeal paralysis in horses is frequently subclinical but may cause abnormal respiratory noise *(roaring)* and poor performance. *The condition is almost always a left-sided hemiplegia caused by idiopathic degeneration of the left recurrent laryngeal nerve.* The resulting denervation atrophy affects the intrinsic laryngeal muscles supplied by this nerve, but the atrophy is not uniform; the lateral cricoarytenoid muscle is affected first and most severely, followed by the dorsal cricoarytenoid. Grossly, the affected muscles are pale and atrophic (Fig. 5-9). The cricothyroid muscle, which is supplied by the cranial laryngeal nerve, is the only intrinsic muscle not affected. Because the dorsal cricoarytenoid muscle is the main abductor of the larynx, denervation atrophy and dysfunction of this muscle allows the left arytenoid cartilage to sag into the lumen and obstruct airflow during inspiration.

Microscopic examination of affected nerve fibers reveals *severe loss of myelinated fibers in middle and distal portions of the left recurrent laryngeal nerve*. Ultrastructural features indicate progressive loss of fibers in the left recurrent nerve accompanied by chronic demyelination, remyelination, and abortive regenerative attempts. Similar but milder changes can be detected ultrastructurally in the distal right recurrent

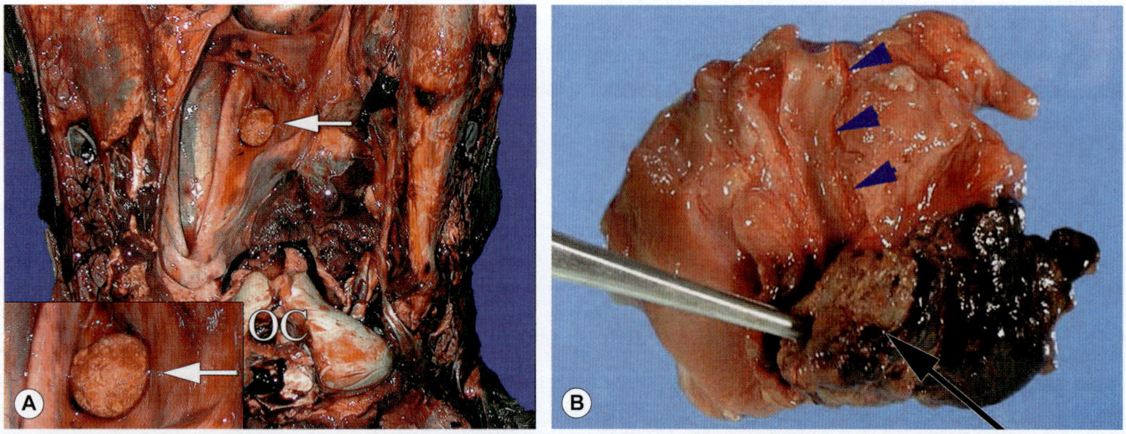

Figure 5-8 Guttural pouch mycosis in a horse. **A**. The fungal plaque (arrow; inset) is adjacent to the stylohyoid bone. Ventral view of the head. OC = occipital condyles. **B** (a different case). Within the guttural pouch, the carotid artery (arrowheads) is focally invaded by a fungal plaque (arrow). The pouch was filled with blood at the time of autopsy.

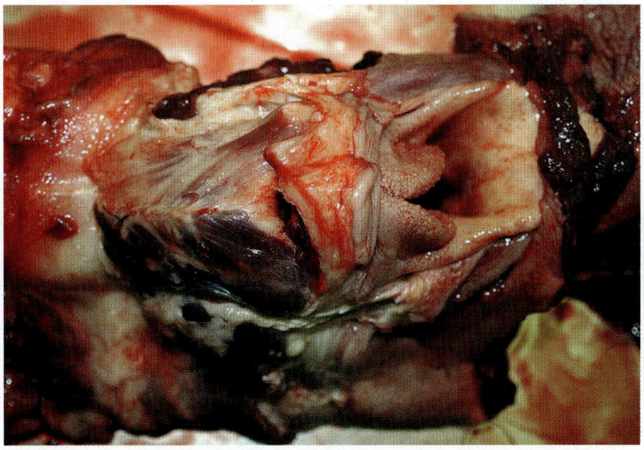

Figure 5-9 Equine laryngeal neuropathy. Pallor of left dorsal cricoarytenoid muscle from neurogenic atrophy. Dorsal view, tongue to the right. The transverse incision was made at autopsy.

nerve. The axons in the left recurrent laryngeal nerve are much longer than those in the right recurrent nerve, and this presumably makes them more susceptible to degeneration. Idiopathic laryngeal paralysis in horses—the most common form encountered—is unilateral, whereas bilateral paralysis is more typical of cases caused by hepatic encephalopathy and general anesthesia.

Laryngeal paralysis in dogs occurs most commonly in Labrador Retrievers and several other large breeds, and is most frequent in males. The condition is less common in cats. The disease is usually bilateral, in contrast to that in horses. It manifests as stridor, dysphonia and dysphagia, and predisposes to aspiration pneumonia. Although the cause is often not identified, the relationship between recurrent laryngeal axonopathy and denervation atrophy of the laryngeal muscles is usually as described in horses, except that dogs may have polyneuropathy with fewer myelinated fibers. *Congenital laryngeal paralysis* occurs in Bouvier des Flandres and Siberian Huskies associated with apparent hereditary degeneration of the nucleus ambiguus, Rottweilers as a manifestation of a polyneuropathy, white-coated German Shepherd dogs, and others. Occasionally, laryngeal paralysis occurs with hypothyroidism or following cervical trauma or general anesthesia with intubation.

In goats, laryngeal neuropathy and paralysis have been associated with copper deficiency.

Laryngitis

Laryngeal edema may be part of a local or systemic inflammatory process and can be caused by infections of the laryngeal mucosa or surrounding connective tissues, inhalation of irritant materials, local trauma, anaphylaxis, or hyperthermia. The amount of edema varies, but is most severe in the region of the epiglottis, the aryepiglottic folds, and the ventricles. Mild laryngeal edema is a common incidental finding in many species at autopsy.

Laryngitis accompanies inflammatory diseases of either the upper or lower respiratory tract or can occur without involvement of other tissues. **Necrotic laryngitis in cattle and pigs** is caused by *Fusobacterium necrophorum*, which colonizes previously damaged laryngeal mucosa. It differs from oral necrobacillosis in young calves, although both are known as calf diphtheria. The friable or purulent ulcerated lesions overlie the swollen arytenoid cartilages or affect the vocal folds and may invade the adjacent muscle and cartilage. Similar ulcers can result from septic phlebitis in calves with *Histophilus somni* septicemia and pneumonia. Inhalation or aspiration of *toxicants* is a rare cause of laryngeal and epithelial necrosis (eFig. 5-10). The nematode parasite *Mammomonogamus laryngeus* attaches to the laryngeal surface of cattle.

Laryngeal lesions in racing horses occur commonly. The simplest form is small mucosal ulcers in a variety of locations without deeper lesions, or a mass of granulation tissue on the medial face of the arytenoid cartilage. More severe is *arytenoid chondritis (laryngeal chondritis)*, with ulceration of mucosa at the rostral margin of the arytenoid cartilage immediately caudal to the attachment of the vocal fold, extending into and deforming the laryngeal cartilage (eFig. 5-11). The histologic lesions include cavitation from necrosis and loss of arytenoid cartilage, and granulation tissue and chronic neutrophilic or granulomatous inflammation that increases the size of the cartilage. The pathogenesis is not known, but may involve mucosal trauma as the larynx closes forcefully in rapidly breathing animals, with introduction of bacteria that stimulates inflammation and cartilage degradation.

Laryngeal chondritis in sheep, mainly affecting yearlings and lambs with possible breed predispositions, causes inflammation of laryngeal soft tissues that is often bilateral and invades the cartilage. The laryngeal orifice is partially occluded by pale swelling of the soft tissues around the arytenoid cartilages. Ulcers are often present, and foci or tracts of purulent exudate are adjacent to and within the cartilage. Histologic lesions are chronic purulent inflammation, granulation tissue, visible bacteria, and necrosis and excavation of the cartilage progressing from the edges to the center. Mixed bacteria can be isolated, including *Fusobacterium* spp., *Trueperella pyogenes*, and streptococci, and are thought to enter the tissue through mucosal damage from plant material, trauma, or toxic irritants. There is high mortality from airway obstruction and dyspnea, which can clinically resemble pneumonia and emphasizes the diagnostic importance of examining the upper respiratory tract.

Laryngeal neoplasia

Primary neoplasms of the larynx are rare in domestic species. **Papillomas** involving the larynx can be part of more widespread papillomatosis. **Chondromas**, some with myxomatous differentiation, are reported. **Squamous cell carcinoma** is the most common malignant tumor. The laryngeal epithelium has a florid hyperplastic response to underlying inflammation, so care should be taken in differentiating (non-neoplastic) pseudoepitheliomatous hyperplasia from laryngeal squamous cell carcinoma. **Plasmacytoma** is a round-cell tumor with eccentric nuclei, abundant glassy cytoplasm, and occasional karyomegaly or multinucleation. As for alimentary plasmacytoma, laryngeal plasmacytoma has a more aggressive course than those arising in the skin. Laryngeal neoplasms consisting of cells with abundant granular cytoplasm include rhabdomyoma, oncocytoma, and granular cell tumor. **Laryngeal rhabdomyoma or rhabdomyosarcoma** occurs in young dogs as a solitary raised nodule in or near the lateral ventricle of the larynx (eFig. 5-12). It consists of lobular masses of angular pleomorphic cells with abundant deeply eosinophilic granular or foamy cytoplasm (Fig. 5-10). Although this appearance has been interpreted as an oncocytoma, the diagnosis of

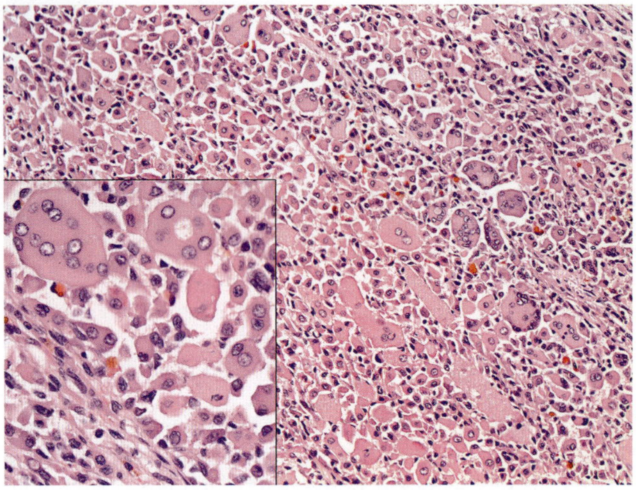

Figure 5-10 Laryngeal rhabdomyosarcoma in a dog. The neoplastic cells are round or spindle shaped, occasionally strap-like, pleomorphic, with abundant eosinophilic cytoplasm, and often multinucleate. Inset: higher magnification.

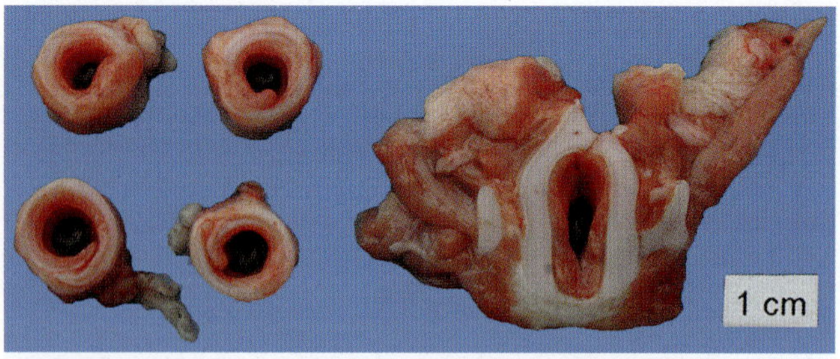

Figure 5-11 Brachycephalic obstructive airway syndrome in a bulldog. The larynx is hypoplastic with thickening of the mucosa and a narrow lumen. The trachea is collapsed from excessively negative inspiratory pressure, causing overlap of the cartilage rings.

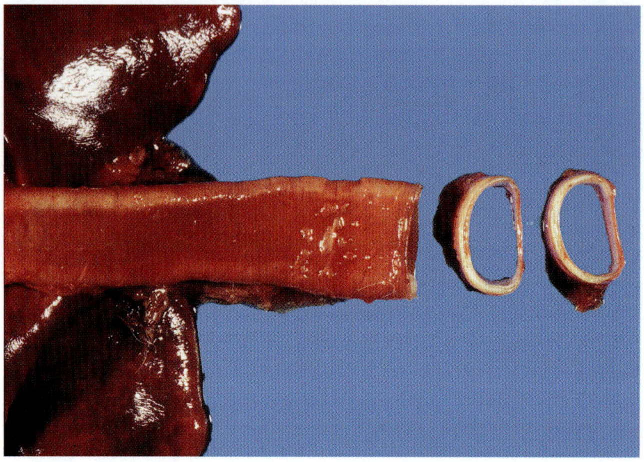

Figure 5-12 Tracheal collapse in a dog. The dorsal tracheal ligament is stretched and lax, with oblong flattening of the malacic cartilage rings. (Courtesy University of Guelph.)

rhabdomyoma is confirmed with immunohistochemistry for myogenin, MyoD1, *myosin, and muscle-specific actin*. **Granular cell tumor**, probably of Schwann cell origin, is less common in the larynx than in the tongue of dogs. The neoplastic cells have abundant cytoplasm with fine PAS-positive diastase-resistant granules (lysosomes and phagosomes) and are positive for S100 and vimentin. Various other neoplasms are described in the larynx.

Trachea

Brachycephalic obstructive airway syndrome is a constellation of lesions occurring in brachycephalic dogs and to a lesser extent in cats, resulting in exercise and heat intolerance, coughing and stertor, and can include inspiratory dyspnea, sleep-disordered breathing, cyanosis, and syncope. The primary and functionally significant changes are stenotic nares that form a vertical slit, insufficient pharyngeal space for the soft palate ("elongation" and thickening of the soft palate), tracheal hypoplasia with reduced luminal diameter (best measured from radiographs), small tracheal rings, and inapparent dorsal tracheal ligament. Other changes are abnormal morphology of nasal conchae and of hyoid bones, and a thick long tongue. Greater negative intraluminal pressures during forced inspiration secondarily cause eversion of laryngeal saccules, hypertrophied and folded pharyngeal mucosa, thickened nasopharyngeal mucosa, everted tonsils, laryngeal edema, collapse of the larynx, and/or collapse of the trachea and bronchi with overlapping ends of the cartilage rings (Fig. 5-11). These factors aggravate the problem by further obstructing airflow, as does mucosal thickening or exudates resulting from tracheitis or pneumonia. Gastroesophageal reflux, hiatal hernia, systemic hypertension, and hypercoagulability are additional consequences of excessive negative intrapleural pressure. Causes of death include suffocation, aspiration pneumonia, diffuse alveolar damage, and negative-pressure pulmonary edema. A comparable condition with narrowing of the larynx and excessive perilaryngeal soft tissue occurs in **Norwich Terriers**.

Tracheal collapse refers to *dorsoventral narrowing of the trachea* resulting in coughing and exercise intolerance. The disease is most common in middle-aged miniature breeds of dogs and is described in older donkeys and miniature horses. The cartilage rings are abnormally shaped and form shallow arcs, and the dorsal trachealis muscle (tracheal membrane) is widened and flaccid (Fig. 5-12). The condition is not limited to the trachea; bronchoscopy reveals bronchomalacia and bronchial collapse in many affected dogs. Earlier descriptions of the histologic and histochemical features associated with tracheal collapse describe foci of hypocellularity of the hyaline cartilage and areas where cartilage is replaced by fibrous and/or fibrocartilaginous tissue. It remains to be determined if these changes are causative or the result of biomechanical changes resulting from the tracheal collapse.

Tracheal edema and hemorrhage syndrome of feedlot cattle, in which the lumen is partially obstructed by mucosal and submucosal edema and hemorrhage of the dorsal region of the distal half of the trachea, occasionally causes death by asphyxiation in feedlot cattle (Fig. 5-13). The disease is known as "honker syndrome" for the resulting stertor. It is most frequent in heavy cattle during hot weather, and some have concurrent bronchopneumonia. The cause is not known but might involve trachealis muscle damage from heavy breathing or coughing, negative intratracheal pressures during forced inspiration, or tracheal trauma from feedbunks.

Tracheal disease in pigs occurs sporadically during respiratory disease outbreaks, affecting pigs of various ages that usually have concurrent lung disease. The obstructive lesions cause dyspnea and stridor. Lesions range from tracheal edema

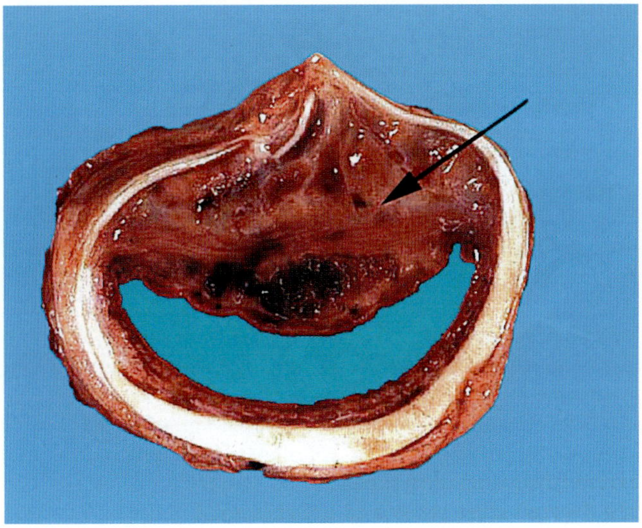

Figure 5-13 Tracheal edema and hemorrhage syndrome (honker syndrome) in a feedlot calf. Edema and focal hemorrhage asymmetrically thicken the dorsal tracheal mucosa (arrow) and partially obstruct airflow. (Courtesy E. G. Clark.)

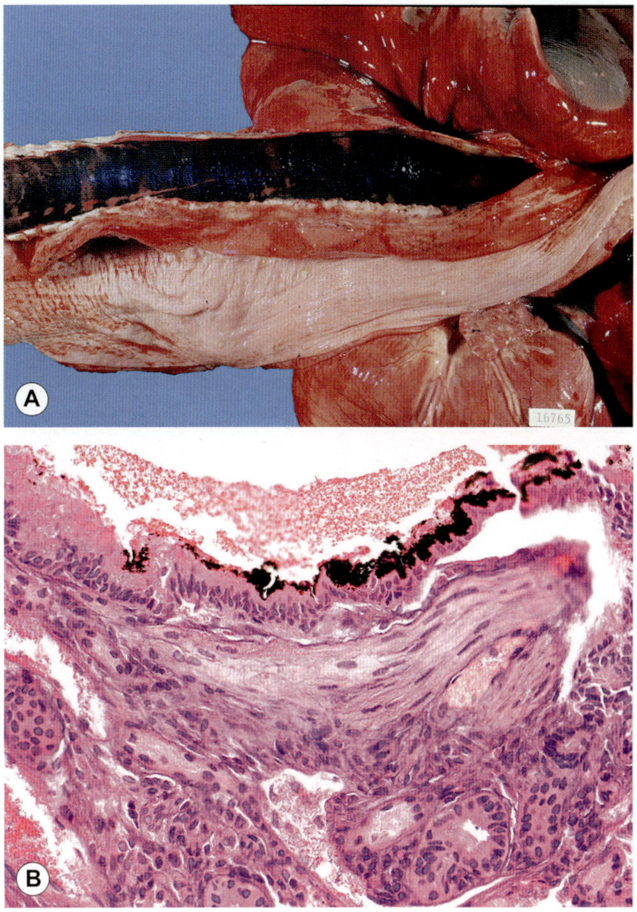

Figure 5-14 Smoke inhalation. A. Black soot covers the tracheal mucosa, confirming that the dog was alive during exposure. **B.** (a different case). Black soot on the mucosal surface (antemortem) and heat-induced coagulation of the tracheal tissue (probably developing after death). (Courtesy University of Guelph.)

and hemorrhage, to neutrophilic and lymphocytic tracheitis, to erosive or ulcerative tracheitis with a nonadherent fibrinonecrotic membrane. Various viral and bacterial pathogens may be present, but a consistent infectious cause has not been identified and might have a similar pathogenesis as described above for cattle.

Miscellaneous lesions occur uncommonly in the trachea. Foam is often present in the tracheal of normal sheep, horses, and dogs (eFig. 5-13) and may increase if there is pulmonary edema. *Malformations of the cross-sectional shape of the trachea* can be found as an incidental finding, especially in cattle. *Tracheal trauma*, such as during dystocia, can cause fracture or collapse of the cartilage. Necrosis of tracheal epithelium occurs after *endotracheal intubation*, as a result of transient ischemia from the inflated cuff; it is often subclinical and heals spontaneously, but rarely leads to a tracheal cast or fibrinous tracheal pseudomembrane that partially occludes the lumen. *Squamous metaplasia* of tracheal epithelium is a feature of vitamin A deficiency and severe iodide toxicosis. Black discoloration (soot) of the tracheobronchial mucosa is seen with smoke inhalation and is an indicator that the animal was alive at the time of the fire (Fig. 5-14). Coagulative necrosis of trachea and upper airways can occur from thermal injury in fires. Foci of chronic polypoid tracheitis, probably as a result of chronic inflammation, are occasionally observed in dogs and cats and may cause stenosis and dyspnea. *Pox viruses* (lumpy skin disease, sheeppox) cause hyperplastic nodules in the trachea. Tracheitis frequently accompanies bronchitis and bronchopneumonia. Small foci of *mineralization*, often with accompanying granulomatous inflammation, occur in the lamina propria of the dorsal trachea and ventral turbinates of adult pigs; the cause is not known. *Parasitic diseases* of the trachea of dogs, discussed later in the chapter, include infections by *Oslerus osleri*, *Eucoleus aerophilus*, and *Spirocerca lupi*.

Tracheal neoplasms are uncommon. *Osteochondromas* in the intrathoracic trachea of young dogs (<1-year-old) are cartilaginous masses having central ossification with marrow spaces and are considered dysplastic rather than neoplastic. In older dogs, chondrosarcoma and chondroma are rare; the latter has uniformly low cellularity, lacks nuclear atypia, and has no mitotic figures, necrosis, or invasive growth. In cats, *tracheal lymphoma* (mainly B cell) is more frequent and has longer median survival with therapy than for *adenocarcinoma and squamous cell carcinoma*, for which lung metastasis is frequently reported. Other neoplasms are also reported.

LUNG DEVELOPMENT AND ANOMALIES

Lung development and growth

The lungs develop early in gestation from a ventral diverticulum in the foregut endoderm. The 6 stages of lung development and growth are the embryonic, pseudoglandular, canalicular, saccular, alveolar, and vascular maturation stages. Important development continues postnatally in most mammalian species. In puppies, there is progressive reduction in thickness and cellularity of alveolar septa to resemble mature lung by about 60 days of age.

During the **embryonic** stage of lung growth (30-50 days of gestation in a bovine fetus), the primordial trachea and right and left primary bronchi develop, growing into the surrounding mesenchyme. The growth of the conducting airways occurs primarily in the **pseudoglandular** stage; in most species, the airways develop through a series of asymmetric dichotomous branching. Differentiation of conducting airway epithelial cells begins proximally and extends distally at this stage, with the development of ciliated cells, mucous cells, basal cells, and bronchial cartilage. At the end of the pseudoglandular period, all branches of conducting airways have developed and are embedded in mesenchymal stroma. Distal airway branches are lined by cuboidal-to-columnar epithelial cells that contain abundant cytoplasmic glycogen. During the **canalicular** stage of growth (120-180 days), "canalization" of the interstitium by blood vessels and airways occurs, with capillaries growing in apposition to the airway epithelium to form the developing air-blood interface. Also during the canalicular stage, there is development of the type II pneumocytes and type I pneumocytes within the newly formed terminal airspaces. Fetal lung development to the **saccular** stage (180-240 days) is important for survival outside the uterus. Lung volume and gas exchange surface increase, and there is further reduction in mesenchyme between airspaces. The terminal branches of the conducting airways extend through the nascent parenchyma, and conditions are set for alveolar development. Small accumulations of elastic fibers, the site of secondary alveolar septal development, are deposited during this stage. During the **alveolar** stage of lung growth (240-260 days), true alveoli form by ingrowth of septa from intersaccular crests at the sites of elastic fiber deposition. These secondary septa have a doubled capillary layer separated by mesenchymal tissue (eFig. 5-14). The acquisition of a mature air-blood interface, with a single capillary layer, occurs after birth in the final stage of lung development, the stage of **microvascular maturation**. The end result is a reduction of the interstitium and maturation of the alveolar septum. Further subdivision of alveolar septa results in continued increases in alveoli and alveolar surface area during a period of rapid postnatal growth. Airways increase in diameter and length through coordinated growth as overall lung volume and weight increase.

Movement of fetal lung fluid is important in directing normal lung development. Fetal respiration and spontaneous contraction of fetal conducting airways facilitate the movement of the fluid. Contraction of fetal airways occurs even in lung explants without central neurologic control because of the phasic contraction of the airway smooth muscle. Neural innervation of the lung occurs early in development, arising from neural tissue migrating through the fetal mesenchyme. Studies in the fetal pig show that both developing nerves and ganglia are present within the fetal bronchial tree as early as the pseudoglandular stage of development. This cholinergic neural innervation coordinates the fetal airway contractions mentioned above.

The coordination of intrauterine and extrauterine lung development and growth is complex and influenced by both local tissue factors and influences originating beyond the developing lung. Local epithelial-mesenchymal interactions, outlined above, are necessary for directing the distal expansion of the lungs; indeed, the formation of the diverticula from the foregut endoderm, branching morphogenesis, and cell differentiation are specifically coordinated by the adjacent lung-specific mesenchyme. In each stage of lung development, a number of diffusible mediators and transcription factors direct organogenesis. Examples include the fibroblast growth factor family, transforming growth factor β, and the sonic hedgehog signaling pathway.

Congenital anomalies

Congenital anomalies of the lung are rare and may reflect abnormal development of the lung bud, pulmonary circulation, or both. Major malformations such as pulmonary agenesis are incompatible with life and are often accompanied by malformations in other organs. **Pulmonary hypoplasia** *is defined as reduced lung weight and usually also has reduced numbers of alveoli* (eFig. 5-15). In contrast, the airways generally develop normally. Pulmonary hypoplasia may accompany malformations in other organs. Its development is closely linked to the lung liquid that is secreted by the pulmonary epithelium, fills the airspaces, and is required for growth of the lung mass. **Pulmonary hypoplasia and anasarca syndrome**, an inherited condition in several cattle breeds, involves these lesions along with generalized edema and body cavity effusions, with aplasia of lymphoid tissues and adrenal gland in some cases. **Pulmonary hyperplasia** is the result of overdistension of the lung, resulting from tracheal obstruction or laryngeal paralysis. In contrast, pulmonary hypoplasia ensues if the lung volume is not maintained. Pulmonary hypoplasia is caused by conditions that compress the lung, including congenital diaphragmatic hernia, intrathoracic masses, pleural effusions, or malformations of the thoracic cage; by oligohydramnios, in which the reduced uterine volume causes abnormal fetal positioning that compresses the chest and lungs; by impaired fetal breathing movements from abnormalities of the fetal nervous or musculoskeletal systems; by a tracheal fistula; and perhaps by reduced fluid secretion as a result of fetal hypoxemia or high levels of epinephrine.

When investigating congenital masses of lung-like tissue, key observations include the location of the lesion and whether it is contained within the pleura or not, the continuity of the trachea and primary bronchus with the bronchi within the mass, and the nature of the pulmonary and systemic arterial supplies. The classification evolves over time, and the nomenclature in animals and humans has not been well aligned.

Accessory lung is an extrapulmonary mass of lung tissue covered by its own pleura and with a bronchial attachment to the lung, trachea, or bronchi. It is well described in calves. **Pulmonary sequestration**, a term that has been used mainly in humans, is a mass of lung tissue with *no connection to the normal airways*, supplied by systemic but not pulmonary arteries, and named based on the location within or outside the pleural covering of the lung. *Extralobar pulmonary sequestration (**choristoma**) is a mass of pulmonary tissue completely separated from the lung* (with a separate pleural covering) and found in the pleural space, mediastinum, abdominal cavity, or skin. The reported pulmonary choristomas in ruminants vary from relatively normal bronchioles and alveoli with the absence of bronchi, to cartilaginous bronchi and underdeveloped (canalicular or saccular) bronchioles and alveoli. Those in humans often have anomalous microanatomy [see congenital pulmonary airway malformation (CPAM) type 2 later]. *Intralobar bronchopulmonary sequestration (**hamartoma**) is a tumorlike mass of pulmonary tissue within the lung*, enveloped by the normal pleura but cut off or sequestered from the normal airways. It may be supplied by anomalous branches of the aorta and drained by pulmonary veins but lacks communication with the bronchi or with the pulmonary arteries. Histologically, the development of bronchi, bronchioles, alveoli, and blood vessels is variable. Those formed by excessive amounts of alveolar tissue relative to bronchioles and vessels have been termed *polyalveolar lobe*; the differential diagnosis in humans includes CPAM type 4 and pleuropulmonary or pulmonary blastoma.

Congenital cystic pulmonary lesions include CPAM, congenital lobar emphysema, bronchogenic cyst, and extra- and intralobar sequestration. These should be distinguished from acquired nondevelopmental cystic lung diseases.

Congenital pulmonary airway malformation (CPAM) was formerly known as congenital cystic adenomatoid malformation or adenomatoid hamartoma. The various congenital cystic lesions are thought to result from errors at different times and/or locations in airway embryogenesis, with accumulation of secreted mucus in the isolated lung tissue distal to the defect inducing hyperplasia of bronchial, bronchiolar, or alveolar tissue. *Congenital acinar dysplasia* (**CPAM type 0**) is a small hypoplastic lung with abundant mesenchyme separating lobules that contain cartilaginous bronchi, branching and sometimes cystic bronchioles, and usually absent acini. **CPAM type 1** forms one or more large intrapulmonary cysts that compress adjacent tissues (eFig. 5-16). The cyst is lined by an undulating columnar or pseudostratified sometimes-ciliated epithelium and has smooth muscle in the wall but typically no cartilage. Some cases have bronchiole-like structures or mucin-secreting glandular structures adjacent to the cyst. **CPAM type 2** is a microcystic bronchiole-like lesion that forms poorly demarcated, small (often <2 cm) intrapulmonary foci that may not be grossly apparent. These are each formed by numerous irregularly shaped bronchiole-like structures with a cuboidal or columnar epithelium and often mucin in the lumen. Cartilaginous bronchi, bronchial glands, or pulmonary arteries are absent; a moderate amount of intervening connective tissue may contain skeletal muscle. **CPAM type 3** is a gland-like mass (usually non-cystic) as described above (pulmonary hamartoma, intrapulmonary sequestration). **CPAM type 4** forms a large cluster of cysts, usually within one lobe, that resemble expanded alveoli by their thin walls, barely discernable epithelium, and absence of bronchioles; pleuropulmonary blastoma is a differential diagnosis in humans. *Congenital lobar emphysema* appears as overinflation of a lobe and is described later (see the Pulmonary Emphysema section).

Bronchogenic cysts are extrapulmonary single unilocular cystic masses that do not communicate with the airways. They may be located anywhere in the thorax but are most frequent near the carina or in the mediastinum. Their walls contain cartilage plates, and the cystic cavity is lined by respiratory epithelium. *Enteric duplication cysts* are extrapulmonary cysts that have a wall resembling muscularis mucosae, are lined by intestinal, gastric, or stratified squamous epithelium, and may contain some respiratory epithelium.

In **anomalous pulmonary venous drainage**, the pulmonary veins drain into the right rather than the left atrium. Completely (total) or partially anomalous forms differ in whether all of the pulmonary veins are abnormal or not.

GENERAL PATHOLOGY OF THE LUNG

Artifacts and incidental findings

The color of the lungs at the time of postmortem examination is highly variable but may or may not reflect disease. Pooling of blood in the lung after death frequently causes diffuse or patchy purple-red discoloration, so *the color of the lung is often deceptive. Changes in lung texture are a more reliable indicator of underlying disease* and are best detected by deep and purposeful palpation of individual lobules, on a freshly cut surface instead of palpating through the pleura.

Common changes developing after death include gravitational pooling of blood in the lung closest to the ground (dependent congestion), redistribution of blood to the lung in a diffuse or patchy distribution (postmortem congestion), postmortem atelectasis in animals breathing supplemental oxygen, minor petechial hemorrhages reflecting the method of euthanasia, and histologic changes including sloughing of airway epithelium into the lumen, edema within 2-4 hours of death (attributed to altered pressure gradients and permeability of the air-blood barrier), edema and coagulation (lack of staining detail) after barbiturate overdose, and hemoglobin staining (hemolysis) from thawing frozen tissues. *Normal or incidental findings* include nodules of hyperplastic lymphoid tissue in the larynx and largyngopharynx of young animals, minor froth in the tracheobronchial lumen, opaque foci of pleural fibrosis, thick opaque pleura in dorsocaudal lung of cattle and horses, gritty deposits on pleura and epicardium of animals euthanized with intracardiac and/or intrapleural barbiturates, terminally aspirated feed material in the nasal cavity and bronchi of ruminants, bony foci of osseous metaplasia in dog lung, megakaryocytes in pulmonary capillaries especially in dogs, tiny black foci of carbon pigment adjacent to bronchioles, a few lymphocytes around vessels, foci of subpleural bronchioloalveolar epithelial hyperplasia and septal fibrosis, and alveolar macrophage aggregation (alveolar histiocytosis).

Atelectasis

Atelectasis *refers to incomplete expansion of the lung.* Atelectatic lung is homogeneously dark-red and sunken relative to aerated lung, and the texture is fleshy or firmer and nonspongy. Microscopically, simple atelectasis appears as slightly congested alveolar walls lying in close apposition with slit-like residual lumina having sharp angular ends (eFig. 5-17). Atelectasis is a common artifact in immersion-fixed lung tissue. In **congenital atelectasis**, the lungs appear as in the fetus but are dark red-blue because of dilation of alveolar capillaries, of fleshy consistency, and do not float (eFig. 5-18). **Obstructive atelectasis** *is caused by complete airway obstruction*. Whether airway obstruction causes atelectasis versus air trapping depends on the size of airway obstructed and the degree of collateral ventilation. *A lobular pattern of atelectasis suggests bronchial obstruction as the cause*, prompting a search for the offending exudates or tumors.

Compressive atelectasis *is caused by pleural or intrapulmonary space-occupying lesions*. Examples are hydrothorax, hemothorax, exudative pleuritis, and tumors. In large animals, the atelectasis caused by pleural effusions may occur below a sharply demarcated fluid line. Abdominal distension, as in severe ascites and ruminal tympany, may cause atelectasis, typically in the cranial regions. Large animals with prolonged recumbency, such as anesthesia, may develop atelectasis of the down side. Generalized and severe atelectasis is a consequence of *pneumothorax*.

Atelectasis develops after death in animals breathing 80-100% oxygen during anesthesia or intensive care. Because of the speed with which the oxygen is resorbed into tissues and the lack of nonabsorbable gas (especially nitrogen, which is present within atmospheric air), *the lungs are usually completely devoid of gas by the time they are examined after death.* Grossly, the lungs are markedly reduced in size, so the heart is especially prominent when the pluck is examined.

Pulmonary emphysema

Emphysema in its widest sense refers to tissue expansion by air or other gas. In the lung, there are 2 major forms:

1. **Alveolar emphysema**, which is rare in animals, refers to abnormal and permanent enlargement of airspaces resulting from destruction of alveolar septa, and an absence of obvious fibrosis. Emphysema thus differs from **overinflation of alveoli** caused by air trapping, which is a reversible lesion that is commonly encountered.
2. **Interstitial emphysema** is the presence of air within interlobular, subpleural, and other major interstitial zones of the lung. *"Emphysema," unless otherwise qualified, should only be used for alveolar emphysema.*

Emphysematous areas of the lung are grossly voluminous, pale, and puffy. The enlarged airspaces are often visible as small vesicles, and in severe cases coalescence of airspaces produces large air-filled bullae that can occasionally rupture to cause fatal pneumothorax.

Enlargement and coalescence of airspaces are apparent histologically and are most reliably assessed on lungs that have been infused with fixative to a volume approximating the in vivo state. *In true emphysema, fragments of alveolar wall should be obvious histologically*, in contrast to the more frequent lesion of alveolar overinflation from air trapping.

Knowledge of the **pathogenesis of emphysema** is based on investigations of the human disease and of animal models. Emphysema is an important condition in humans, where it frequently coexists with chronic obstructive pulmonary disease attributable to cigarette smoking and is the result of an imbalance between proteases and antiproteases. *Neutrophil-derived serine proteases (particularly elastase) and matrix metalloproteinases from a variety of sources are the likely culprits*, and their concentrations are enhanced by the neutrophil and macrophage activation induced by chronic bronchitis. Although antiproteases—α_1-antitrypsin, secretory leukoprotease inhibitor, and tissue inhibitors of matrix metalloproteinases—protect normal lung from proteolytic damage, their function may be reduced by genetic deficiency or by oxidative stress from cigarette smoke and the resulting inflammation. Unchecked proteases degrade elastin and other matrix proteins in the interstitium, and the weakened alveolar septa are vulnerable to stress-induced failure with the tensions generated by each ventilatory cycle.

The emphysematous lung is dysfunctional because the loss of alveolar septa reduces the alveolar surface area; although the affected portion of lung may be larger than normal, gas exchange is reduced. Loss of elastic recoil caused by degradation of elastin further compromises lung function. These factors make hyperpnea necessary to maintain lung function, which may exacerbate the disease by placing additional ventilatory stresses on the damaged lung.

Overinflation of alveoli is commonly encountered, although this does not qualify as alveolar emphysema unless it leads to destruction of alveolar septa. Overinflation is mostly the result of airway obstruction or constriction, with air trapping in alveoli and failure of the lung to deflate normally. Distended airspaces can be found at the apices of the lungs of dogs, cats, and horses with respiratory distress, or along the margin of a consolidated lung (secondary to bronchiolar obstruction by exudate). Lobar overinflation may result from bronchial mucus plugs or lung lobe torsion. Overinflated lobules are a common finding in horses with bronchiolar mucus plugging associated with severe equine asthma ("heaves").

Congenital lobar overdistension (congenital lobar emphysema, congenital large hyperlucent lobe) is rare in dogs and results from localized collapse or obstruction of a lobar bronchus, such as by hypoplasia or aplasia of the bronchial cartilage, leading to air trapping in the affected lobe or lobes. A right middle or cranial lung lobe is greatly enlarged by alveolar overinflation and/or bullous emphysema, sometimes with bronchiectasis. Pneumomediastinum, subcutaneous edema, or pneumothorax may occur. Affected dogs are typically <3-years-old and have slowly progressive dyspnea and coughing. Surgical excision is usually curative.

Interstitial emphysema is distinguished from alveolar emphysema by the presence of air in the connective tissues and lymphatics of the lung, including the interlobular septa, beneath the pleura, and around vessels and airways. Positive-pressure ventilation with excessively high tidal volume is an occasional cause in all species. Interstitial emphysema without alveolar emphysema occurs frequently in cattle, presumably because of their well-developed interlobular septa and lack of collateral ventilation of the alveoli (Fig. 5-15). It is an incidental finding in cattle at slaughter and is common in recumbent ("downer") cows with periparturient paresis or toxic mastitis, perhaps developing as cows forcibly exhale or grunt against a closed glottis. Thus, *the finding of interstitial emphysema in cattle does not necessarily imply primary lung disease*. Dramatic interstitial emphysema occurs in cattle with interstitial lung disease. Interstitial emphysema in such cases may result from abnormally high intra-alveolar pressures caused by increased expiratory effort or bronchiolar obstruction, or perhaps from altered permeability or strength of the barrier between airspaces and interstitium. In animals surviving a sufficient length of time with severe interstitial emphysema, the air can extend along lymphatics to the bronchial and mediastinal lymph nodes or along fascial planes of the mediastinum and into the subcutis.

Blebs and bullae are common causes of spontaneous pneumothorax in dogs. They occur mainly in large-breed or deep-chested dogs. The respiratory distress may be acute or worsen over a period of weeks and be continuous or intermittent. Surgical removal of the affected lobe is usually curative. These lesions appear as air-filled "bubbles" at the apices of the lung,

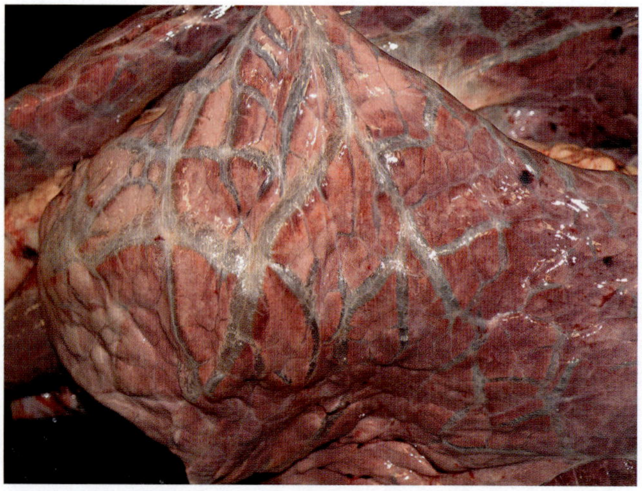

Figure 5-15 Interlobular emphysema in a "downer" dairy cow, with no respiratory distress and no other evidence of pulmonary disease. Pale bubbles of air distend the interlobular septa.

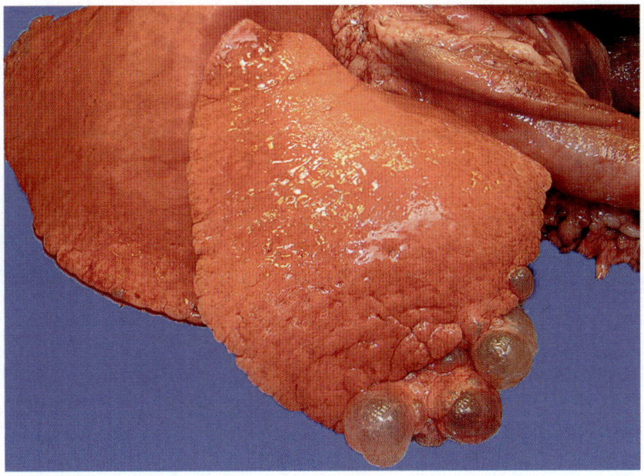

Figure 5-16 Bullae at the apices of the lung in a dog. Rupture of such bullae causes spontaneous pneumothorax.

usually in cranial or middle lobes, with more than one lobe affected in about half of cases (Fig. 5-16). Ruptured blebs and bullae are notoriously inconspicuous at autopsy, but holding the lungs under water and distending the lung by infusing air into the trachea or bronchus can usually identify the pleural leak. This should be done routinely in cases of anesthesia-associated death.

Histopathology distinguishes the 2 lesions: *air-filled spaces within the pleural connective tissue are termed **blebs*** (eFig. 5-19); *those arising in the lung parenchyma (by distension of alveoli or rupture of alveolar septa) and bulging into the pleura are termed **bullae*** (eFig. 5-20). Patchy subpleural areas of alveolar distension are often present within lobectomy samples, and some cases have prominent smooth muscle hypertrophy in alveolar ducts or bronchioles, or chronic bronchitis. Whether these airway lesions cause the air trapping and thereby bulla formation is uncertain. A differential diagnosis is congenital lobar overinflation caused by hypoplasia of bronchial cartilage.

Traumatic pulmonary pseudocyst is a cavitation within the lung parenchyma filled with air or fluid and lined by interstitial connective tissue. It is caused by blunt or sharp trauma, and there may be other evidence of chest trauma, such as pulmonary contusion, hematoma, laceration, pneumatocele, or bronchial fractures, as well as pneumothorax, hemothorax, rib fractures, or skin abrasions.

Pulmonary edema

Pulmonary edema is a frequent complication of many diseases and is therefore one of the most frequent and functionally significant lung lesions. If severe, it catastrophically compromises lung function by reducing pulmonary compliance, blocking ventilation of the alveoli, obstructing gas exchange across the alveolar septa, and reducing the surface area of the air-liquid interface in the alveoli. Furthermore, proteins in the edema fluid interfere with surfactant function, further reducing compliance and increasing the work of breathing. Edema of the lung is, in many respects, similar to edema of other tissues and is governed by the permeability of the vascular wall and by Starling forces—the balance of hydrostatic and osmotic pressures between the intravascular and interstitial compartments. Distinctive aspects of edema in the lung include the importance of type I pneumocytes as barriers to fluid movement, the role of type II pneumocytes and club cells in active transport of water from the alveolus, the effect of surface tension on fluid movement, and fluid exchanges between alveolar/bronchiolar airspace and pulmonary interstitium. It is useful to consider separately the means by which the alveoli are kept dry, and the ways in which excessive fluid is removed from the alveoli.

The alveoli are kept "dry" by several related mechanisms. Tight junctions between type I pneumocytes are relatively impermeable to fluid and proteins and confer >90% of the barrier to albumin flux across the blood-air barrier. In contrast, in the lung, capillary endothelium is relatively permeable to movement of fluid and small molecules into the interstitium, so that both type I pneumocytes and endothelial cells contribute to the air-water barrier in the alveolus. Complementing the barrier function of the type I pneumocyte are Na^+-K^+-ATPase channels (sodium pumps) on the basolateral surface and passive sodium channels on the apical surface of type II pneumocytes. The net effect is to actively transport sodium out of the distal airspaces into the interstitium, drawing water along the same pathways by osmosis, thus resulting in a slow but steady flow of liquid from the alveoli to the interstitium. Drainage of interstitial fluid from the interstitium to the lymphatics is facilitated by negative pressure in the lymphatic vessels. In addition, the surface tension in airways may draw fluid out of alveoli into distal bronchioles, where fluid resorption by club cells is driven by a variety of ion channels. The rate at which fluid is cleared from the distal airspaces varies by species, being slowest in dogs, intermediate in sheep, and fastest in rodents and rabbits.

Active transport of alveolar fluid is enhanced by catecholamines (through β_2-adrenergic receptors) and glucocorticoids; this is probably important in clearance of fluid from the lungs of neonates and is also used to advantage in the therapy of pulmonary edema. Conversely, active transport mechanisms are impaired by hypoxia, for example, as a result of high altitude, reactive oxygen and nitrogen species (as a result of inflammation), halogenated anesthetics, oleic acid, and perhaps lidocaine, suggesting that these factors—in addition to damage to pneumocytes or club cells—are additional contributors to development of pulmonary edema.

Mechanisms of pulmonary edema *include elevated hydrostatic pressure, increased permeability of the alveolar wall, excessive negative intra-alveolar pressure, impaired lymphatic drainage, and several miscellaneous causes* (Box 5-2). In contrast to other tissues, low oncotic pressure (hypoproteinemia) is not expected to cause pulmonary edema. *Elevated hydrostatic pressure* (increased pulmonary venous pressure) is commonly caused by left-sided heart failure *(cardiogenic edema,* see the Pulmonary Venous Hypertension and Consequences of Left Heart Failure section) or from hypervolemia resulting from excessive fluid administration. In these situations, fluid loss into the alveoli may occur from either the alveolar septa or the peribronchiolar or perivascular connective tissue. Other causes are considered clinically as "noncardiogenic pulmonary edema," a term that ignores the diversity of the underlying disease processes.

Increased permeability of the blood-alveolar barrier incites a rapid onset of high-protein edema. It develops in pneumonia of various causes, diffuse alveolar damage (see the Interstitial Lung Disease section), sepsis or endotoxemia, anaphylaxis or drug-induced histamine release, electrocution, near-drowning, tick paralysis (*Ixodes holocyclus*), and mechanical ventilation causing barotrauma or rapid re-expansion of collapsed alveoli. In the case of diffuse alveolar damage, edema may result

Box • 5-2

Mechanisms and causes of pulmonary edema

Increased venous hydrostatic pressure
- Left heart failure
- Increased blood volume (fluid overload)
- Occlusion of pulmonary veins

Increased permeability of the alveolar barrier
- Pneumonia
- Diffuse alveolar damage
- Sepsis/SIRS/endotoxemia
- Anaphylaxis
- Electrocution

Excessively negative intra-alveolar pressure
- Upper airway obstruction (e.g., strangulation, near-drowning, laryngeal collapse)
- Rapid removal of pleural fluid or air, lobectomy

Neurogenic pulmonary edema
- Brain trauma, seizures, hypoglycemia

Impaired active fluid transport from distal airspaces
- Damage to type II pneumocytes or club cells
- Hypoxia (high altitude)
- Oxygen and nitrogen radicals (increased by inflammation)
- Halogenated anesthetics
- Possibly lidocaine
- Malnutrition
- High alveolar protein content

Lymphatic obstruction
- Neoplastic emboli in lymphatics or lymph nodes (rare)

from more minor injury than is needed to cause formation of hyaline membranes. Fumonisin toxicity in pigs, African horsesickness virus and Hendra virus infection in horses, and blue tongue virus cause particularly spectacular pulmonary edema.

Negative-pressure pulmonary edema is caused by inspiratory effort in the face of upper airway obstruction from strangulation, choke, laryngeal or tracheal collapse, brachycephalic obstructive airway syndrome, or hanging, or alternatively from excessively rapid expansion of alveoli caused by rapid removal of pleural fluid, correction of pneumothorax, or lobectomy. The drop in intra-alveolar pressure increases the transmural pressure across the alveolar wall, thus encouraging fluid movement into the alveolus. Histologic lesions of negative-pressure pulmonary edema in dogs and cats are not described.

Several *additional causes of pulmonary edema* are uncommonly encountered. Obstruction of lymphatic vessels or lymph nodes by neoplastic cells is a rare cause of pulmonary edema. Increased intracranial pressure from trauma or damage to the central nervous system causes *"neurogenic pulmonary edema,"* probably related to catecholamine-induced pulmonary hypertension and increased vascular permeability. *Hypoxia at high altitude* induces pulmonary edema, an effect of both impaired alveolar active sodium transport and pulmonary hypertension. *Postanesthetic pulmonary edema* seems to involve various mechanisms.

On **gross examination**, edematous lungs are wet, heavy, and do not completely collapse when the thorax is opened. The ratio of lung weight to body weight (or to heart weight in ruminants) is a useful measure of pulmonary edema. Fluid or froth flows from the cut surface when gently compressed. Edema pools in the pleura and distends the interlobular septa of cattle, pigs, and horses (eFig. 5-21). Foam fills the trachea and bronchi (see eFig. 5-13) and may flow from the nostril, although this is a nonspecific finding in horses and sheep. The pleural cavity may contain excess fluid. It is important to understand that the above features occur in severe cases, but pulmonary edema may be functionally significant yet grossly inapparent.

Histologically, low-protein edema is often colorless fluid that distends alveoli and is accompanied by increased number and increased size of alveolar macrophages. With increased protein content, alveolar edema is eosinophilic. Histopathology is neither sensitive nor specific for detection of pulmonary edema: low-protein edema must be abundant before it is detected histologically, and the protein in edema fluid can leach from sections during processing and be quite inconspicuous. Conversely, pink material often fills the alveoli in autolyzed carcasses or those euthanized with barbiturates. Therefore, radiographs, lung weight, and gross appearance are important indicators of the presence and severity of edema.

Thrombosis, embolism, and infarction

Pulmonary thrombosis results from in situ thrombus formation within pulmonary veins or arteries, or embolism to the pulmonary arteries. Clinically, pulmonary thromboembolism often goes undetected, particularly in horses even with substantial thromboemboli. Reported clinical signs include dyspnea, tachypnea, coughing, lethargy, hemoptysis, cyanosis, or sudden death. Because the clinical features are nonspecific, the pulmonary arteries must be opened in all animals with respiratory disease for which gross lesions do not reveal a cause.

In situ development of pulmonary thrombi involves the Virchow triad of underlying mechanisms: increased blood coagulability, damage to endothelial cells or the vessel wall, or stasis of blood flow (Box 5-3). Hypercoagulability is of prime importance. Thrombi that develop in situ within the lung are usually microscopic (eFig. 5-22), whereas grossly visible thrombi are usually emboli (Fig. 5-17). Exceptions to this rule do occur. Microvascular thrombi dissolve rapidly after death if the fibrinolytic system has been activated, as is expected in disseminated intravascular coagulation; thus, the absence of thrombi does not rule out this condition. The lungs are strategically situated to catch **emboli** carried in venous blood (see Box 5-3).

The significance and sequelae of pulmonary thromboembolism depend on the extent of vascular obstruction, the rapidity of its development, and the occurrence of sepsis. Because the lung is supplied by both pulmonary and bronchial arteries and has extensive collateral vessels, *thromboembolism does not often cause infarction*. Ischemia and infarction are more likely if thrombosis or embolism occurs at the periphery of the lung (rather than affecting the large central vessels), or if the bronchial and systemic circulations are impaired, such as by concurrent heart failure. When infarcts occur, they form sharply demarcated wedge-shaped or polygonal raised firm

Box • 5-3

Causes of pulmonary thrombosis and embolism

Pulmonary thrombosis

- Glomerulonephritis and glomerular amyloidosis
- Immune-mediated hemolytic anemia
- Hyperadrenocorticism or corticosteroid therapy
- *Dirofilaria immitis, Angiostrongylus vasorum*
- Disseminated intravascular coagulation: SIRS/sepsis, neoplasia, pancreatitis, peritonitis, burns, massive trauma, bacterial pneumonia
- Heart disease
- Atherosclerosis, pulmonary vasculitis

Sources of emboli

- Valvular endocarditis (right heart)
- Jugular thrombi
- Hepatic abscess with thrombosis of the hepatic vein (cattle)
- Thrombosis of uterine and pelvic veins (cattle)
- Thrombi in deep veins of the limbs

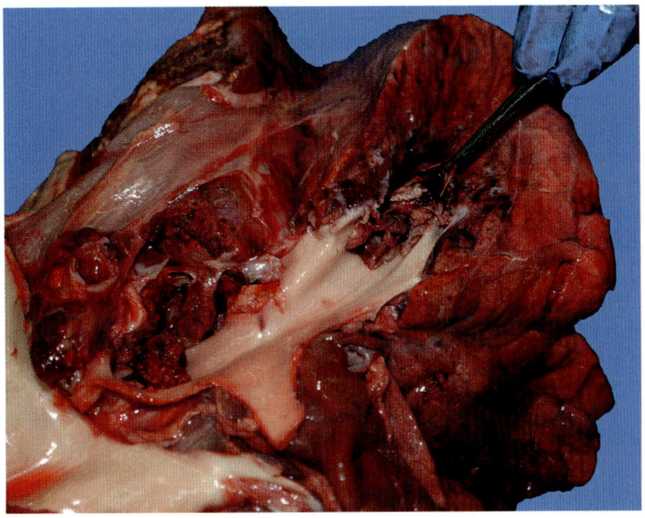

Figure 5-17 **Pulmonary embolus** in a caudal branch of a pulmonary artery (forceps), in a calf with endocarditis of the right atrioventricular valve. The affected lung tissue is grossly normal, and the embolus would have been overlooked had the pulmonary artery not been fully opened.

red-blue hemorrhagic lesions at the periphery of the lung lobes (eFig. 5-23); fibrin may give the pleural surface a dull granular appearance. Pulmonary hemorrhage and pleural effusion are frequent gross findings, even when infarcts are absent. Sublethal ischemia causes histologic lesions of diffuse alveolar damage. Infarcts can manifest as foci of coagulative necrosis, sometimes delineated by macrophages, fibroplasia, and inflammation of vessel walls. Emboli that obstruct large branches or several branches of the pulmonary artery may cause sudden death, or over time lead to cor pulmonale and right heart failure; right ventricular dilation may or may not be present. Large thrombi are detected by dissection of the terminal branches of the pulmonary arteries; these lesions are easily missed if only cross sections of the lung are examined.

Septic embolism with massive numbers of bacteria, as occurs when an abscess ruptures into a vein, induces acute pulmonary edema or interstitial lung disease. Chronic septic emboli produce widespread abscesses or neutrophilic embolic pneumonia. *Bone marrow emboli* result from fractures. *Fat embolism* is rarely important in animals. The fat can originate from bone marrow at sites of fracture, from severe hepatic lipidosis when the hepatocytes rupture, or from subcutaneous fat necrosis caused by pancreatitis, diabetes mellitus, or vitamin E deficiency. The emboli lodge in alveolar capillaries and produce sausage-shaped distensions that are empty in routine paraffin sections, but special stains of frozen sections reveal the fat. *Emboli of the brain or spinal cord* occur in cattle when improper use of captive bolt guns induces excessive increases in intracranial pressure. *Air emboli* are introduced into veins such as from an accidentally disconnected catheter, and can obstruct pulmonary blood flow leading to right heart failure, or enter systemic circulation and cause tissue infarction. *Other embolisms* to the lung include intravenously injected drugs or other compounds, ribbon-shaped hydrophilic polymers used to coat intravascular devices, multinucleate trophoblastic epithelial cells, brain or spinal cord resulting from captive bolt euthanasia, parasites, bacteria, neoplastic cells, and hairs.

Lung lobe torsion

Lung lobe torsion most often affects the right middle lobe of large deep-chested breeds of dogs as well as cats, presumably because of the narrow waist at the hilus; the left cranial lobe is more commonly affected in small-breed dogs. Underlying causes are not apparent in many cases, but some have pleural effusion, pneumothorax, pneumonia, neoplasia, or atelectasis of the affected lobe, congenital dysplasia or hypoplasia of the bronchial cartilage, or previous thoracic surgery. The clinical signs are variable and include respiratory distress, cough, and hemoptysis. The affected lobe is twisted at the hilus and deeply congested (Fig. 5-18). Pleural effusion is consistently present and may be transudative, chylous, exudative, or bloody. Pleural effusion could be either a cause of atelectasis and subsequent torsion or a consequence of venous and lymphatic obstruction by the torsion. Persistent chylothorax after lobectomy may suggest that this effusion causes torsion in some cases. Histologic lesions vary from simple congestion in acute or partial torsions, to diffuse alveolar damage with fibrinous alveolar exudates, to pulmonary infarction with coagulative necrosis of all tissue elements.

Pulmonary hemorrhage

Pulmonary hemorrhage varies from petechiae to extensive filling of large regions by blood. Hemorrhage and congestion can usually be grossly distinguished: *hemorrhages are typically multifocal or patchy splashes of blood; congestion is diffuse within the affected region of the lung.* Pulmonary hemorrhages occur frequently in hemorrhagic diatheses including thrombocytopenia, anticoagulant rodenticide toxicity, sepsis, disseminated intravascular coagulation, and with severe congestion. They can also be caused by vasculitis, pulmonary hypertension, infarction, ruptured aneurysms, trauma, migrating foreign bodies (eFig. 5-24), hemangiosarcoma, tumors that have undergone necrosis, bronchopneumonia, leptospirosis, drug

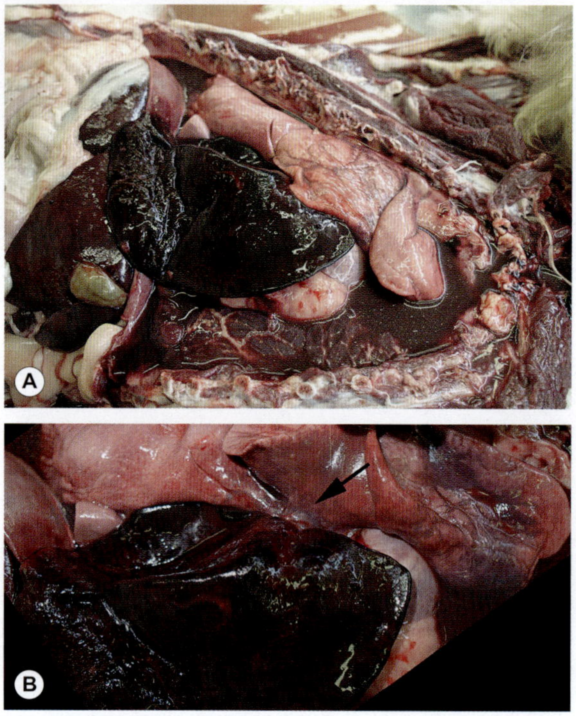

Figure 5-18 **Torsion** of the right middle lung lobe in a dog. The lobe is purple-red from venous obstruction, (**A**) there is abundant pleural fluid, and (**B**) the torsion is palpable and barely visible at the apex of the lobe (arrow).

reactions, and attempted resuscitation. Aspiration of blood is frequent at slaughter and has a characteristic pattern of multiple, small, bright-red foci with feathery borders (eFig. 5-25). In lung biopsies, hemosiderin-laden macrophages or distension of alveoli with blood suggests pre-existing hemorrhage; the hemorrhage of surgical trauma is more likely accompanied by alveolar collapse. Hemosiderin may be detected in alveolar macrophages by 24-72 hours after bleeding.

Abscesses *that erode large blood vessels cause massive hemorrhage*. Affected animals may develop hemoptysis or be found dead with blood flowing from the nares, and expectorated blood is often detected in the stomach. Liver abscesses in cattle may extend into hepatic veins, spreading to the lungs via the caudal vena cava to cause pulmonary thromboembolism, acute interstitial lung disease, or chronic lung abscesses. Such abscesses occasionally erode pulmonary vessels leading to epistaxis and death from exsanguination.

Equine exercise-induced pulmonary hemorrhage

Exercise-induced pulmonary hemorrhage (**EIPH**) is a common occurrence in strenuously exercising horses; ~75% of racehorses have endoscopically detectable blood in their airways at a single postrace examination, and this increases to 95% at a second examination. The severity of hemorrhage in EIPH-affected horses varies from mild to severe and may lead to epistaxis. Severe bleeding negatively impacts race performance and length of racing career, but beyond that there are few reported clinical signs in horses that experience EIPH.

EIPH lesions occur mainly in the caudodorsal lung, with dark-brown to blue-black discoloration of the caudodorsal pleura (eFig. 5-26). Pleural and interlobular septal fibrosis may be present, as well as patchy interstitial fibrosis and brown foci in the parenchyma reflecting hemosiderophage accumulation. In severe cases, discrete mass-like and curvilinear foci are noted in the caudodorsal lung that histologically consist of edema and fibrosis.

Histologic lesions of EIPH include pleural and interlobular septal fibrosis, pulmonary vein fibrosis, hemosiderophage accumulation, and interstitial fibrosis. The venous fibrosis especially affects the adventitia of small (100-200 µm) veins; in some, fibrosis also involves the intima and can narrow the vein lumen. In severe EIPH, discrete foci of interstitial edema and fibrosis may accompany the aforementioned lesions.

The pathogenesis of EIPH has been debated for years leading to diverse hypotheses, from bleeding occurring as a result of pre-existing airway inflammation to shock waves being transmitted into the lung from the forefeet striking the ground. The bleeding in EIPH has been postulated to arise from rupture of the alveolar capillary bed as a result of the high vascular pressures achieved within the lung during strenuous exercise. However, the distribution and features of the gross and histologic lesions of EIPH are not explained by simple pressure-induced capillary rupture. The data suggest that *the cause of EIPH is regional venous remodeling. This remodeling likely occurs as a result of the high vascular pressures and flow experienced by veins in the caudodorsal lung.* It is known that blood flow is preferentially distributed to the caudodorsal lung of horses at rest and increases further to this region during exercise. The high pressures and flow that must be achieved in the caudodorsal lung during strenuous exercise provide an explanation for the regional distribution of venous lesions present in the EIPH lung. Furthermore, hemosiderin accumulation and interstitial fibrosis do not occur without venous remodeling being present, suggesting that *venous remodeling is central to the pathogenesis of EIPH*. The proposed pathogenesis of EIPH can be summarized as follows: strenuous exercise in horses leads to extremely high vascular pressures and flow preferentially in the caudodorsal lung, leading to the characteristic remodeling of small veins of this region of lung; the venous remodeling reduces wall compliance, resulting in supraphysiologic upstream capillary pressures during exercise that cause capillary rupture and bleeding.

Equine exercise-associated fatal pulmonary hemorrhage

Massive diffuse pulmonary hemorrhage and edema is among the most common causes of sudden death in racing horses. Because these animals die during or shortly after strenuous exercise, often in the warmer months, there is often considerable autolysis by the time they are examined by the pathologist. Blood may be noted at the nares and often pours forth from the nose when the carcass is shifted. The *gross pathology* of exercise-associated fatal pulmonary hemorrhage (**EAFPH**) consists of widespread hemorrhage and edema in both lungs. Raised hemorrhagic foci, suggestive of acute infarcts, are occasionally found along the margins of the lung lobes. The degree of hemorrhage is usually more prominent within the caudodorsal regions but also extends into more cranial regions.

Histologically, hemorrhage is present throughout the alveoli, interlobular septa, and subpleural tissue and also surrounds airways and vasculature. In addition to the hemorrhage, the vasculature is markedly congested throughout the lung. Because of hemorrhage and autolysis, it is difficult to evaluate the integrity of the blood vessels and alveolar septa. Horses

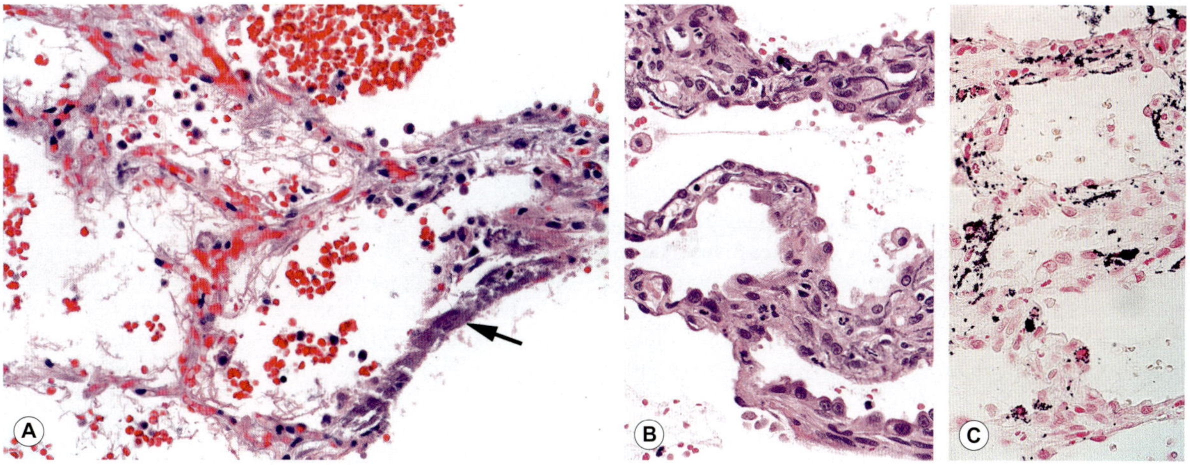

Figure 5-19 Uremic pneumonopathy caused by chronic renal failure. **A**. Acute lesion in a dog. Mineralization of alveolar septa (arrow), and lacy fibrin and hemorrhage in alveoli. **B**. Subacute lesion in a cat. Alveolar septa have basophilic mineralization of fibers (**C**: black with von Kossa stain), are thickened by fibrous tissue, and alveoli are lined by type II pneumocytes.

affected by EAFPH may or may not have obvious histologic lesions of antecedent EIPH.

The *pathogenesis* of EAFPH is not well understood. Acute cardiac failure has been suggested, but this seems unlikely, given that clinically apparent or fatal pulmonary edema would be expected before vascular pressures increased sufficiently to cause such widespread vascular rupture and hemorrhage. Because hemorrhage is the dominant feature of EAFPH, some refer to it as "fatal EIPH." Based on the limited descriptions and personal experiences, it is not clear that EIPH is consistently present in horses that die suddenly from EAFPH. Furthermore, the extent of lung involvement in horses dying from EAFPH is much greater than for EIPH, which is mostly a disease of the caudodorsal lung. It is speculated that if, during exercise, horses developed sudden widespread spasm of small postcapillary venules within the lungs, this could lead to a rapid rise in capillary pressures that might be sufficient to cause widespread acute rupture and hemorrhage as is seen in EAFPH. In rodents, there are smooth muscle sphincters in postcapillary veins that are capable of constricting and regulating local vascular perfusion and pressures through adrenergic receptors. If such structures are present in the equine lung, this might provide a mechanism for the sudden global edema and hemorrhage that occurs in EAFPH. This hypothesis remains to be tested.

Pulmonary mineralization

Mineralization of the pulmonary interstitium is caused by acute or chronic renal failure, hypercalcemia, hyperphosphatemia, vitamin D toxicosis, alkalosis, or hyperadrenocorticism. Dogs with pulmonary mineralization from renal disease (so-called uremic pneumonopathy) may have tachypnea and dyspnea. The magnitude of respiratory signs and lesions is often not related to the severity of renal dysfunction nor to the clinical outcome. Affected lung is edematous and may be diffusely reddened, with localized areas of firmness that correspond to more severe histologic lesions. Mineralization occurs within the smooth muscle and connective tissue fibers in alveolar septa, pulmonary veins, and the walls of bronchioles (Fig. 5-19). Alveoli are edematous and contain increased numbers of macrophages; giant cells occasionally engulf the mineralized material. Hemorrhage, thin strands of fibrin, and edema may be prominent in acute lesions (see Fig. 5-19). Mineral deposits in the lung can ossify with time. Alveolar septa and pulmonary veins, like the gastric mucosa, may be predisposed to mineralization because of their role in acid-base balance resulting from carbon dioxide excretion.

Multifocal osseous metaplasia (heterotopic ossification, "osteoma") of the pulmonary interstitium is frequently encountered as an incidental finding in dogs and other species (eFig. 5-27). Histologically, this appears as well-demarcated tiny nodules of bone within the lung parenchyma, sometimes containing marrow. **Mineralizing pulmonary elastosis** results from chronic pulmonary hemorrhage with yellow-brown-blue hyphae-like or staghorn-shaped mineral deposits in the connective tissue around vessels and bronchioles. The deposits—thought to be elastic fibers incrusted with iron and calcium—stain with Prussian blue and alizarin red but weakly with von Kossa and are accompanied by macrophages and giant cells. Basophilic streaks of mineral may also be present in airway and vascular walls. The appearance and pathogenesis resemble siderotic plaques in canine spleen.

ANATOMIC PATTERNS OF LUNG DISEASE

Damage to lung tissue varies according to the nature of the causative agents, their distribution (particularly the route by which they reach the lung), and their persistence. Pulmonary diseases can be classified in several ways:

- Morphologic pattern, according to the main anatomic target of the pathologic process: vascular disease, airway disease, bronchopneumonia, alveolar filling disorders, interstitial lung disease, granulomatous or eosinophilic pneumonia, embolic pneumonia, and pleural disease.
- *Histologic character:* fibrinous, neutrophilic, granulomatous, necrotizing, proliferative, fibrosing
- *Cause:* viral, bacterial, parasitic, toxic, allergic
- *Duration:* acute, subacute, chronic

- *Functional abnormality:* obstructive versus restrictive
- *Epidemiologic patterns:* shipping-fever pneumonia, enzootic pneumonia

The approach described here emphasizes morphologic patterns of pneumonia, for 2 reasons. First, gross and histologic examination is usually sufficient to classify a condition by this scheme, even if the cause cannot be identified. Second, knowledge of the pattern of pneumonia provides important clues as to the probable causes, route of exposure to the causative agent, pathogenesis of the lesions, effect on pulmonary function, and the sequelae and complications. Emphasizing the similarities between specific diseases, by grouping them based on morphologic patterns, often enhances our ability to recognize the sometimes subtle differences among these conditions.

Pulmonary vascular disease

The lung is a vascular organ comprising hundreds of billions of capillaries organized into hundreds of millions of alveoli whose surface area is estimated, in humans, to be 50-100 m^2. The entire output of the right ventricle is delivered to the lung with each heartbeat, delivering venous blood from the peripheral tissues through the alveolar septa for reoxygenation. Given the anatomy and physiology of the lung, it is not surprising that circulatory disturbances are important in many lung diseases. Thrombosis, embolism, infarction, and edema have been considered in the General Pathology of the Lung section.

Pulmonary arterial hypertension

The clinical diagnosis of **pulmonary arterial hypertension (PAH)** is based on documenting pulmonary arterial pressure >30 mm Hg. In veterinary medicine, this is usually estimated using echocardiography rather than direct catheterization of the right heart. PAH is often classified by the underlying cause (Box 5-4). Pulmonary hypertension can result from increased pulmonary blood flow (e.g., left-to-right cardiovascular shunts), increased resistance to flow through the pulmonary vasculature (precapillary hypertension, such as heartworm disease or high altitude), increased venous pressure (postcapillary hypertension with increased left atrial filling pressure, such as myxomatous mitral valve disease), or combined effects (such as left heart failure with subsequent remodeling of pulmonary vessels). The *pathogenesis* of PAH was historically considered to involve excessive vasoconstriction and thrombosis leading to vascular remodeling. PAH is now understood to be a *vasculopathy*, with dysregulation of vascular tone, abnormal vascular cell growth and apoptosis, along with inflammation. The vascular remodeling characteristic of PAH is a cause rather than a result of the hypertension. The dysregulation of vessel tone is caused by an imbalance in vasodilatory (e.g., prostacyclin, nitric oxide, cGMP) and vasoconstricting (e.g., endothelin, thromboxane A2, serotonin) molecules, whereas a number of growth factors and cytokines, (e.g., TGF-β, bone morphogenetic protein–2, platelet-derived growth factor, fibroblast growth factors) are implicated in the resulting vascular lesions.

Gross lesions are often not present within the lungs in cases of primary idiopathic pulmonary arterial hypertension. In secondary PAH, the gross lung lesions reflect the precipitating disease. Severe hypertension leads to right ventricular and sometimes right atrial dilation, and hypertrophy develops with time. Lesions of right heart failure may be present.

Irrespective of the cause, pulmonary arterial hypertension has a spectrum of characteristic histologic lesions that mainly reflect chronic remodeling of pulmonary arterioles, which can develop within 2 weeks. These include *thickening of the tunica intima by endothelial cell proliferation and later by fibrosis, hypertrophy of smooth muscle in the tunica media, and expansion of the adventitia by edema, fibroblasts, collagen, and elastic fibers* (Fig. 5-20). *Small arterioles at the level of the terminal airway that normally have a thin tunica muscularis become muscularized.* Various morphologic variants are recognized in human cases: intimal proliferation that may be concentric (in familial PAH), eccentric (as a result of thromboembolism and other causes), or obliterative; thrombosis and recanalization of the lumen; and plexiform lesions. The latter are weblike plexuses of vascular lumens within the arterial wall or in adjacent tissue, each surrounded by concentric rings of endothelial cells and matrix, which appear as a branching or outpouching of a larger artery, and are thought to represent chronic attempts to repair damage to the parent vessel wall and/or intrapulmonary anastomoses between bronchial and pulmonary arteries. *Severe acute PAH results in endothelial degeneration, vasoconstriction, fibrinoid necrosis of the vessel wall, vasculitis, and "onion skin" proliferation of intimal endothelial cells* (eFig. 5-28).

Box • 5-4

Causes of pulmonary hypertension

- Idiopathic (primary) pulmonary arterial hypertension
- Familial pulmonary arterial hypertension (humans)
- Systemic-to-pulmonary vascular shunts: ventricular septal defect, patent ductus arteriosus
- Disorders of pulmonary blood vessels: heartworm disease, pulmonary veno-occlusive disease, pulmonary vasculitis
- Chronic pulmonary thromboembolic disease
- Hypoxic vasoconstriction of pulmonary arterioles: high altitude (brisket disease), airway obstruction (severe equine asthma, tracheobronchial collapse)
- Chronic interstitial lung disease with fibrosis and occlusion of pulmonary vessels
- Left-sided heart failure causes pulmonary venous hypertension that may progress to pulmonary arterial hypertension
- Chronic liver disease: liver parasitism in New-World camelids

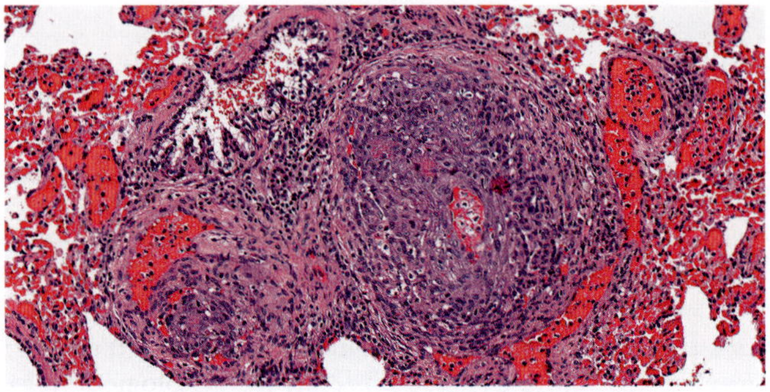

Figure 5-20 Cellular proliferation thickens the intima of 2 pulmonary arteries, as a consequence of **pulmonary hypertension** in a dog with patent ductus arteriosus.

Pulmonary venous hypertension and consequences of left heart failure

Pulmonary venous hypertension is commonly caused by left-sided heart failure and may lead to pulmonary arterial hypertension. Left heart failure causes pulmonary edema as a result of elevated pressure in the lung vascular bed and varies with the rapidity of onset of venous and capillary hypertension. In animals with longstanding left-sided failure (e.g., mitral valve insufficiency in small-breed dogs), the edema may be relatively modest compared with that occurring in an animal experiencing acute heart failure. This difference reflects the ability of the lymphatic system to clear the fluid. Pleural effusion is also common in acute heart failure, again reflecting the inability of pleural lymphatics to clear the sudden increase in pressure-driven pleural fluid formation.

Histologically, chronic left-sided heart failure results in Pulmonary edema, increased number and size of alveolar macrophages, and remodeling of pulmonary veins. The edema initially forms around airways and blood vessels (see the Pulmonary edema section), reflecting the location of the lymphatics that expand to clear the edema fluid. As fluid production increases and exceeds lymphatic clearance, fluid is more apparent within the alveoli. Alveolar macrophages are increased in number and usually have abundant cytoplasm with ruffled cell borders, a feature that is characteristic of alveolar edema. *Hemosiderin-laden alveolar macrophages*, the so-called "heart failure cells," are inconsistently present in chronic left heart failure and absent in acute heart failure (Fig. 5-21). Histochemical stains for iron are helpful for subtle lesions. This lesion affects alveolar macrophages more-or-less uniformly throughout the section; a single cell or a focal aggregate of hemosiderin-laden alveolar macrophages are not indicative of heart failure, nor are pigment-laden macrophages in the bronchiolar interstitium. Conversely, hemosiderin-laden alveolar macrophages are not pathognomonic of heart failure because pulmonary hemorrhage causes the same lesion. Hemosiderin-laden macrophages were first detected at 48-72 hours in vitro; at 2-5 days in lung lavage fluid after pulmonary hemorrhage in infants; and were absent on day 2 but detected at day 3, maximally at days 7-10, and still detected at 2 months after intrapulmonary instillation of blood in mice.

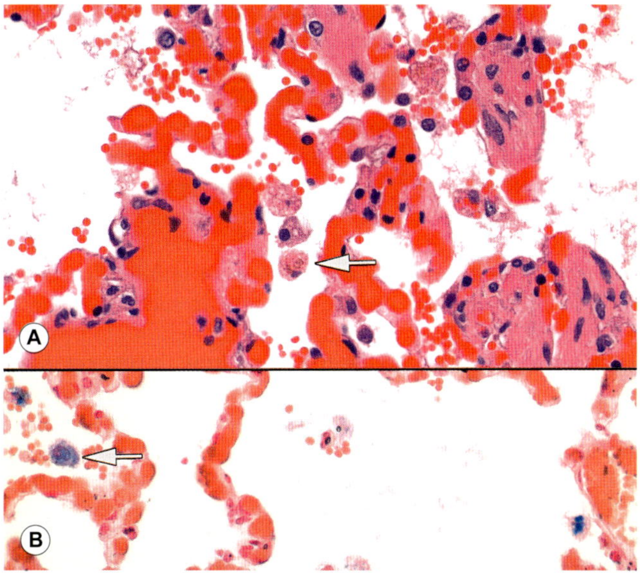

Figure 5-21 Heart failure cells in a cat with hypertrophic cardiomyopathy. **A**. Alveolar macrophages contain brown pigment (A, arrow) that stains blue with Perls Prussian blue (**B**, arrow) and is in the typically scant amount seen in animals with heart failure.

In chronic heart failure, careful evaluation of pulmonary veins, especially small to medium-sized vessels, often reveals increased amounts of collagen within the adventitia. In heart failure causing pulmonary hypertension, the media can be expanded by smooth muscle hyperplasia, as well as muscularization of normally nonmuscularized arteries, and occasional lymphocytes and macrophages. In acute heart failure, there is greater and more widespread edema, without heart failure cells or the aforementioned increases in adventitial collagen around pulmonary veins.

Pulmonary veno-occlusive disease and pulmonary capillary hemangiomatosis

Pulmonary veno-occlusive disease is a rare and serious cause of pulmonary hypertension in humans and adult dogs and cats that results from progressive remodeling of pulmonary veins. Clinically, affected dogs experience rapidly progressive respiratory signs that include coughing, tachypnea, dyspnea, and hypoxia; epistaxis and hemoptysis may be reported. *Grossly*, the lungs are diffusely firm and have widespread relatively well-demarcated foci of hemorrhage or congestion. *Histologically*, the lesions are patchy rather than diffuse. There is extensive remodeling of small to medium-sized pulmonary veins located in the alveolar interstitium (Fig. 5-22). The lumen of the most severely affected veins is obscured by plump spindle cells and collagen, sometimes with muscle hypertrophy of the media, or with many tiny capillaries within the wall of the vein. Many cases also have pulmonary capillary hemangiomatosis, which appears as areas of alveolar parenchyma in which alveolar capillaries have segmental lesions of marked congestion and extensive hypercellularity caused by endothelial proliferation. Some affected dogs also have pulmonary artery lesions of intimal hyperplasia and medial hypertrophy, probably secondary to pulmonary hypertension. The cause of the venous remodeling in dogs is not known.

Congestive heart failure in feedlot cattle

This condition mainly affects feedlot cattle at moderate elevations of 800-1,600 m; high-altitude disease typically affects cattle at elevations >2,000 m (or 1,600 m in Holstein calves). Gross lesions can include edema of the brisket, ventral body wall, intestine, and mesentery, with dilation and hypertrophy of the right ventricle, clear effusion in body cavities, and enlarged liver with chronic passive congestion. Many cases have concurrent lung disease. Histologic lung lesions suggest pulmonary hypertension: pulmonary arteries have expansion of the adventitia by fibrosis and edema, muscle hypertrophy of the media, and intimal hyperplasia and fibrosis, and consistently with muscularization of normally nonmuscular small pulmonary arteries. Proliferation of vessels in the arterial wall (vasa vasorum) is a notable finding. Some cases also have pulmonary vein lesions including hypertrophy of the muscular sphincters and of the media. It is proposed that formation of shunts from bronchial arteries to pulmonary veins promotes the venous muscular hypertrophy and vasa vasorum hyperplasia. Microscopic cardiac and hepatic lesions are described elsewhere. Some cases occur in heavy over-conditioned feedlot cattle as they near market weight, are considered obesity-related, and may result from myocardial adiposity and

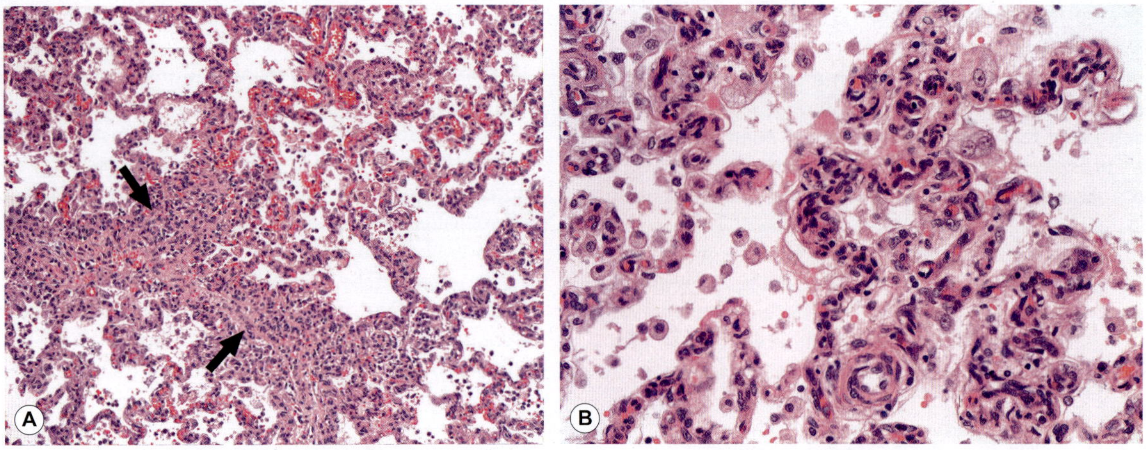

Figure 5-22 **Pulmonary veno-occlusive disease** in a dog. **A**. Remodeling of 2 branches of a pulmonary vein (arrows), along with segmental engorgement of alveolar capillaries, and hemosiderophages. **B**. Some alveolar septal capillaries have endothelial cell proliferation (pulmonary capillary hemangiomatosis) and others are normal. Alveoli contain hypertrophied macrophages. (Case courtesy S. Priestnall.)

fibrosis leading to left heart failure. Other cases occur earlier in the feeding period in lighter nonobese cattle, and perhaps represent primary pulmonary vascular disease exacerbated by altitude and in some cases by concurrent lung disease.

Pulmonary vasculitis

Pulmonary vasculitis is uncommon in domestic animals. *Septic pulmonary vasculitis* may be hematogenous or arise within lesions of bronchopneumonia. It results in numerous necrotic neutrophils in vessel walls, often with thrombi occluding the lumen, and necrosis of vessel walls. Specific infectious causes include feline infectious peritonitis virus (FIPV; *Coronaviridae, Alphacoronavirus 1*); *Dirofilaria immitis* in dogs; acute bovine viral diarrhea virus infection, malignant catarrhal fever, *Histophilus somni*, and *Aspergillus* in cattle; equine arteritis virus (EAV; *Arteriviridae, Alphaarterivirus equid*), equid alphaherpesvirus 1, African horse sickness virus, and Hendra virus in horses; and porcine circovirus 2 (PCV2; *Circoviridae, Circovirus porcine2*) and Nipah virus in pigs. Oral selenium supplementation of lambs causes subtle vasculitis affecting pulmonary alveolar septa, leading to edema and hemorrhage in addition to myocardial necrosis. Immune-complex vasculitis, other mechanisms of immune-mediated vascular injury, and drug-induced pulmonary vasculitis are well recognized in humans and probably occur in dogs.

Airway disease

Lesions that specifically target the airways include those that primarily cause epithelial necrosis and those that induce airway inflammation; combinations of necrosis, inflammation, and fibrosis may be present. Airway diseases may affect the bronchi, bronchioles, or both, and some damage both airway and alveolar epithelial cells. *The major consequences of airway diseases are coughing, airway obstruction, and impairment of lung defenses*. The flow of air can be obstructed by bronchoconstriction resulting from contraction of airway smooth muscle, by leukocytes or mucus within the lumen of the airway, and by thickening of the airway wall by edema and leukocytes. The consequence is failure of alveolar ventilation that may cause hypoxemia and hypercapnia. As a result of alveolar hypoxia–inducing reflex vasoconstriction, there is reduced perfusion of hypoventilated areas of the lung that, if widespread, may lead to pulmonary hypertension. Pulmonary compliance is reduced because of the higher transpleural pressure needed to ventilate the alveoli. Clinically important airway obstruction is particularly notable with bronchiolar disease, where it manifests as expiratory dyspnea because the airway obstruction is exacerbated from the slight collapse that occurs during exhalation.

Bronchitis *is relatively common in domestic animals* but receives little attention by pathologists because it is not usually fatal. Bronchitis and/or bronchial necrosis may be caused by viral or bacterial infection, parasitism, allergic disease, or exposure to irritants or toxins.

Morphologic manifestations of acute bronchitis include the same range of inflammation described for upper airways. The exudates may be catarrhal, mucopurulent, fibrinous, fibrinopurulent, or purulent. Ciliated epithelial cells are most sensitive to a wide array of injurious agents and are often the first to undergo necrosis and slough (Fig. 5-23). **Catarrhal bronchitis** is a relatively mild reaction in which the irritant induces both a mild neutrophil-dominated inflammatory response and secretion of mucus by goblet cells and bronchial glands. In **purulent bronchitis**, the exudate is yellow/white, opaque, and viscid. **Fibrinonecrotic bronchitis** resulting from viral or occasionally mycotic infection forms areas of epithelial necrosis with loosely adherent fibrinous exudate. In such cases, gentle removal of the exudate reveals a granular lesion of epithelial necrosis, which differentiates the lesion from the expectorated mucus that is often present in the large airways of animals with chronic bronchopneumonia. Animals with aspiration pneumonia may have extensive necrosis of the bronchial epithelium, with green-brown foul-smelling exudate.

Bronchial necrosis can resolve by epithelial regeneration if the offending stimulus is removed or neutralized. More severe or prolonged injury to epithelium results in fibrosis of the lamina propria, and accumulation of lymphocytes, macrophages, and plasma cells. Epithelial hyperplasia, mucous hyperplasia, and/or squamous metaplasia may also become prominent following mucosal injury of any cause. Chronic infection with

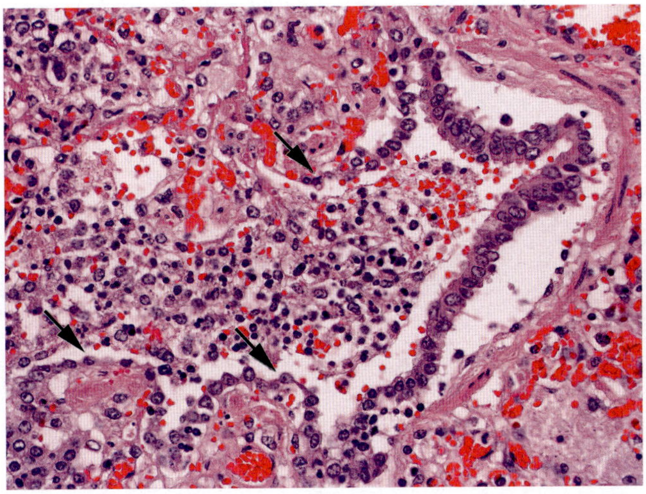

Figure 5-23 **Acute bronchiolar necrosis** caused by bovine coronavirus. Complete loss of some bronchiolar epithelium (upper left) and attenuation (arrows) of adjacent surviving epithelium. The bronchiolar lumen contains necrotic cells, leukocytes, and fibrin. Epithelial attenuation is a more reliable criterion for necrosis, as sloughed cells are a common artifact of autolysis. Coronaviral antigen was abundant in bronchiolar epithelium.

damage to the airway wall may result in bronchiectasis, discussed later. Fibrous polyps are a rare response to bronchial mucosal injury.

Common airway diseases in domestic animals include acute tracheobronchitis ("kennel cough") of dogs (discussed in the Infectious Respiratory Diseases of Dogs section), chronic bronchitis and eosinophilic bronchopneumopathy of dogs, feline asthma, severe equine asthma ("heaves") in horses, and *Dictyocaulus* spp. infection in cattle, sheep, goats, and horses. Bronchitis also results from inhalation of bacteria from the upper respiratory tract and, rarely, when the focal lesions of tuberculosis or caseous lymphadenitis erode into a large airway. Bronchitis causes coughing that may be paroxysmal, and airway obstruction manifests in wheezing. However, it is not expected to be fatal unless the lesion induces widespread bronchoconstriction, obstructs a large airway, or leads to secondary bronchopneumonia as a result of aspiration of infected material or impaired mucociliary clearance.

Bronchial diseases of dogs

Chronic bronchitis is common in older small and medium-sized dogs and manifests as chronic productive or nonproductive cough, exercise intolerance, expiratory or inspiratory wheezes, reduced expiratory airflow, and hypoxemia. The cause is rarely identified. Proposed causes include dry air, airborne pollutants including sulfur dioxide and particulates, environmental tobacco smoke, chronic gingivitis with aspiration of debris, immune-mediated inflammation, and viral infection. Opportunistic bacterial pathogens are occasionally isolated, but their significance as a primary cause is questionable. Similarly, viral and bacterial infections induce acute exacerbations in human patients with chronic bronchitis, even though infection is not the primary cause. Many dogs with chronic bronchitis also have chronic left heart failure.

The major gross finding in chronic bronchitis is excessive mucus or mucopurulent exudate in the trachea and bronchi. The bronchial mucosa in severe cases is hyperemic, thickened, edematous, and granular rather than glistening, and lymphoid nodules or hyperplastic polyps may project into the lumen. Microscopically, the bronchial mucosa is edematous and contains many lymphocytes, plasma cells, and occasional macrophages and neutrophils. Eosinophils may or may not be present. There is hyperplasia and hypertrophy of bronchial glands, hyperplasia of goblet cells, and variable hyperplasia, ulceration, or squamous metaplasia of the surface epithelium. Intraluminal mucus is commonly mixed with neutrophils. Many cases of uncomplicated bronchitis persist for years, but *sequelae* in severe cases include bronchiectasis, bronchopneumonia, or atelectasis leading to pulmonary hypertension. Emphysema is not an important sequel to chronic bronchitis in dogs, unlike in humans.

Eosinophilic bronchopneumopathy is an uncommon, usually steroid-responsive condition of young dogs. It causes chronic gagging, cough, dyspnea, nasal discharge, and variable blood eosinophilia and neutrophilia. The nodular or diffuse lung lesions include chronic eosinophilic bronchitis with epithelial hyperplasia, ulceration, or squamous metaplasia, which destroys the airway walls and leads to bronchiectasis (eFig. 5-29) in ~25% of cases. In addition to bronchial lesions, most cases have extensive involvement of lung parenchyma with diffuse eosinophilic and granulomatous infiltrates, focal eosinophilic granulomas centered on necrotic tissue and densely eosinophilic material (probably masses of eosinophil secretions), and large areas of necrosis and fibrosis (Fig. 5-24). Eosinophilic bronchopneumopathy overlaps with eosinophilic bronchitis, a nondestructive inflammatory disease of airways, and with eosinophilic pulmonary granulomatosis, a multinodular disease discussed below. Eosinophilic bronchopneumopathy is thought to be immune mediated, but specific causes should be ruled out: tracheobronchial and lung parasites, occult *Dirofilaria immitis* infection (causing eosinophilic granulomas in the lung), and pulmonary carcinoma, histiocytic sarcoma, lymphoma, and lymphomatoid granulomatosis. Allergic bronchopulmonary aspergillosis and drug reaction cause similar lesions in humans but have not been identified in dogs.

Aspergillus fumigatus and *A. flavus* rarely cause chronic destructive bronchitis in German Shepherd dogs, with erosion of epithelium, neutrophil infiltration, and formation of granulation tissue in the wall of small and large airways. The lesion can progress to form an aspergilloma or fungus ball, a cavitated mass in the lung composed mainly of fungal hyphae (eFig. 5-30). However, hyphae may be difficult to detect in the chronic bronchial lesions. Progression to invasive systemic aspergillosis is not described in dogs, and excision with antifungal therapy has been curative.

Bronchial collapse occurs in dogs, some with concurrent tracheal collapse, and manifests as chronic cough or dyspnea. Cases affecting primary or secondary bronchi are thought to arise from bronchomalacia of unknown cause, or as part of brachycephalic airway obstructive syndrome. Collapse of the left primary bronchus may result from left atrial enlargement as a result of myxomatous mitral valve disease.

Inflammatory airway diseases of cats

Feline airway diseases are considered as asthma or chronic bronchitis, although there is much overlap between these conditions. They manifest as cough and tachypnea, with or without sneezing, nasal discharge, wheezing, and dyspnea. Nearly half of cases have radiographically observed bronchiectasis,

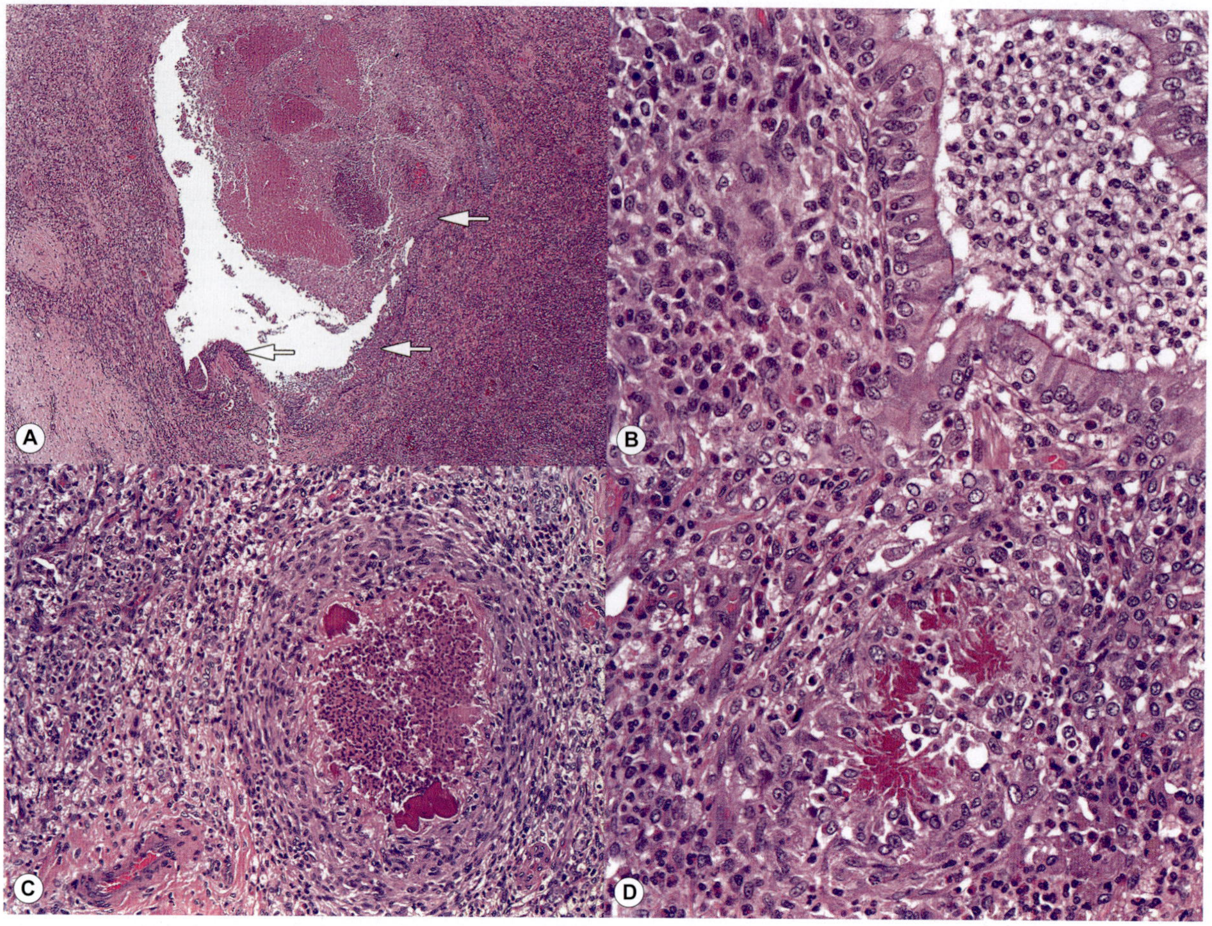

Figure 5-24 Eosinophilic bronchopneumopathy in a dog. **A**. A dense infiltrate of eosinophils, lymphocytes, and macrophages targets and effaces a bronchus. Remnants of bronchial epithelium (arrows) remain visible, with squamous metaplasia. **B**. Higher magnification of a more mildly affected bronchiole. **C, D**. Pulmonary parenchyma contains a diffuse leukocytic infiltrate with formation of granulomas around necrotic eosinophils (C) or deposits of brightly eosinophilic material (D).

and broncholithiasis may be present. Those cases with many *eosinophils* in bronchoalveolar lavage fluid are considered as **feline asthma**, which is relatively common, and characteristically manifests as acute onset or recurrent bouts of cough, dyspnea, or wheezing that respond to treatment with bronchodilators and corticosteroids, and are *mainly the result of airway inflammation, airway smooth muscle hyper-reactivity*, and bronchoconstriction. Feline asthma is thought to be immune mediated. Those cases with predominantly *neutrophils* in bronchoalveolar lavage fluid are considered as **chronic bronchitis**, which characteristically affects older cats and manifests as chronic cough. The cause of feline chronic bronchitis is not known; it is considered noninfectious, but parasitism, bacterial (including *Mycoplasma*) or fungal infections, and inhaled foreign bodies are differential diagnoses.

Cats parenterally sensitized then challenged with Bermuda grass allergens developed allergen-specific IgE, IgG, and IgA airway hyperreactivity, and the following histologic lesions in the bronchi: narrowing of the lumen, smooth muscle hypertrophy, infiltrates of eosinophils in the wall and lumen, hypertrophy and hyperplasia of goblet cells and bronchial glands, and hyperplasia and exfoliation of the surface epithelium. The histologic findings in natural cases are not as well characterized because mortality is uncommon. In addition to smooth muscle hyperplasia and eosinophil or neutrophil infiltration in airways, lymphoplasmacytic infiltrates with lymphoid follicles may develop in the adventitia of the bronchi and bronchioles.

Bronchiectasis

Bronchiectasis is defined as permanent dilation of bronchi as a result of chronic bronchial inflammation. Such bronchi become unable to clear the inflammatory exudate and are ineffective in ventilating the alveoli. Although most cases are a complication of bronchopneumonia or bacterial bronchitis, bronchiectasis may occur with immune-mediated bronchitis, or rarely as a congenital malformation. Bronchiectasis is relatively common in **cattle** with chronic bronchopneumonia because complete lobular septation and lack of collateral ventilation impair resolution of bronchopneumonia and lead to more extensive atelectasis because of airway blockage. Bronchiectasis is common in **dogs**. The lesions commonly affect the right cranial or middle lung lobes and are usually the result of eosinophilic bronchopneumopathy, bacterial infection, or occasionally tumors, bronchial foreign bodies, or ciliary dyskinesia. The condition in **cats** usually affects the caudal or middle lobes and is often a sequel to chronic bronchitis, bronchopneumonia, or pulmonary neoplasia. Endogenous lipid pneumonia and emphysema are sequelae in some cases. Bronchiectasis infrequently develops in **pigs, sheep**, and **goats** with severe parasitic bronchitis.

There are 3 anatomic forms of bronchiectasis: 1) *cylindrical bronchiectasis* causes relatively uniform dilation of the bronchus; 2) *saccular bronchiectasis* is probably a more advanced stage, in which there are circumscribed or fusiform cyst-like lesions at the end of progressively dilated airways; and 3) *varicose bronchiectasis*—rarely identified in animals—forms focal constrictions along dilated airways. The smaller distal bronchi are usually affected by bronchiectasis, and a similar lesion may involve the bronchioles.

Destruction of bronchial walls with luminal obstruction by exudate is the key to development of bronchiectasis and leads to their permanent dilation. In these situations, neutrophil- or eosinophil-derived proteases and oxygen radicals are thought to damage the bronchial wall. This results not only in weakening of the bronchial wall but also failure of mucociliary clearance that perpetuates the infection and pooling of exudates in the lumen. The exudates cause obstruction; as a result, the weakened airways are pulled outward with each inspiration and thus dilate over time.

Grossly, the dilated bronchi are filled with viscid yellow-green creamy exudate (Fig. 5-25), which may eventually form caseous or inspissated masses in the lumen. The intervening parenchyma may be atelectatic and fibrotic. The bronchi may be so dilated as to be visible from the pleural surface, but are best appreciated when sectioned transversely. *They may be confused with abscesses, but form cylindrical tracts, have remnants of cartilage, and are eventually continuous with recognizable bronchi.* In severe cases, the dilated bronchi give a honeycombed or cystic appearance to the lobe. Microscopically, the lumen is filled with mucus, cellular debris, leukocytes, and occasionally blood. The epithelium often has some combination of attenuation, ulceration, mucous or squamous metaplasia, and hyperplasia. The bronchial wall is infiltrated with leukocytes and may be obscured by granulation tissue, and this destructive and fibrotic lesion may extend to the deeper tissues and destroy cartilage and bronchial glands. Normal bronchi are dynamic structures that actively regulate airflow and defend the lung through mucociliary clearance; those crippled by bronchiectasis are forever dilated and unable to clear their burden of harmful pus and pathogens.

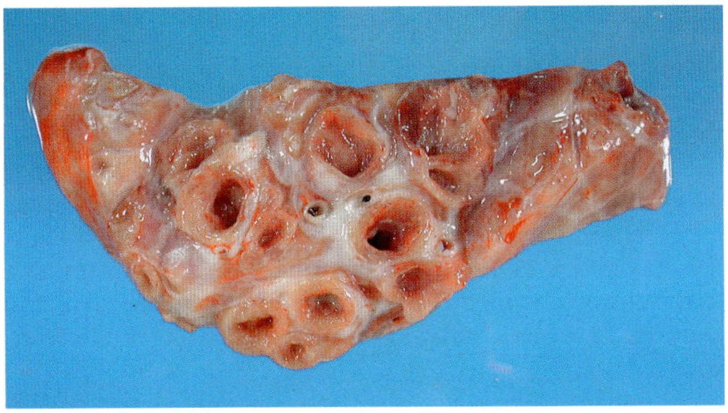

Figure 5-25 Bronchiectasis in a cow with chronic bronchopneumonia. The seemingly increased numbers of large airways result from dilation of smaller airways, resulting from degradation of their walls by the purulent exudate that had pooled within.

Primary ciliary dyskinesia

Cilia are complex structures: the "9 + 2" or "9 + 0" arrangement of microtubular doublets forms the basic structure, inner and outer dynein arms are the motors that force the cilium to bend, and nexin links and radial arms provide support. These structures contain hundreds of proteins, so it is not surprising that *primary ciliary dyskinesia is a diverse collection of disorders* involving mucus-propelling cilia in the nasal cavity and bronchi, sperm flagella, nodal cilia in the developing embryo, water-propelling cilia in the ependyma and epididymis, and cilia in the middle ear and retina. Primary ciliary dyskinesia or *immotile cilia syndrome* is an inherited condition reported infrequently in many dog breeds, which manifests as recurrent or persistent rhinitis and sinusitis, bronchiectasis, bacterial pneumonia, and/or male infertility as a result of reduced spermatozoal motility with abnormal tails. About half of affected humans and dogs have *Kartagener syndrome*, defined as the combination of sinusitis, bronchiectasis, and situs inversus. The latter is a left-right reversal of the thoracic and/or abdominal viscera resulting from dysfunction of cilia in the embryologic node. Otitis media or hydrocephalus may occasionally be present.

The *diagnosis* of ciliary dyskinesia can be considered if there is absence of histologically visible cilia (in the absence of squamous metaplasia), but requires confirmation based on abnormal ciliary motility in short-term cell cultures, in vivo imaging studies to measure movement of mucus, and/or detection of ultrastructural abnormalities in cilia. Because bacterial toxins or adhesion of *Bordetella* or perhaps *Mycoplasma* cause ciliary dysfunction, detection of dysfunction in cilia from more than one tissue is necessary. Ultrastructural studies are also useful in differentiating primary from acquired ciliary dyskinesia. Key ultrastructural lesions in primary ciliary dyskinesia are absence or reduced number of inner and/or outer dynein arms, of the radial spokes that extend from these arms, and/or of the central microtubules. Ultrastructural lesions in both primary and secondary ciliary dyskinesia can include ciliary disorientation, compound cilia, and others. The ultrastructural diagnosis depends heavily on the quality of the preparation, and some humans and dogs with the syndrome do not have ultrastructural changes in cilia.

Bronchiolar diseases

Bronchiolitis and/or bronchiolar necrosis are caused by viral infection, inhalation of toxic gases, toxins that are metabolized by cytochrome P450 in nonciliated club cells, inflammatory reactions to inhaled mineral dusts (see Pneumoconioses) or irritants, or hypersensitivity reactions. Autoimmune disorders, drug reactions, and reactions to mineral dusts are further causes of bronchiolar injury in humans. In addition to these primary bronchiolar disorders, bronchiolar lesions can occur with chronic bronchitis, asthma, parasitic bronchitis, bronchiectasis, or bacterial bronchopneumonia. Necrosis may target both the bronchiolar and the alveolar epithelium, such as in viral infections and toxic injury. Bronchiolar epithelial hyperplasia and lymphocytic bronchitis are common in chronic bronchiolar disease (eFig. 5-31).

Airway obstruction occurs more readily in bronchioles than in bronchi because their lack of cartilage rings and small luminal size readily permit collapse and occlusion by exudate. According to the Poiseuille law of frictional resistance, resistance to airflow varies with the fourth power of the radius, so narrowing of the airway by half will increase airway resistance

16-fold. Thus, if it is of diffuse distribution, even minor airway obstruction by bronchoconstriction, intraluminal exudates or mucus, or edema of the wall has profound effects on the work of breathing and on alveolar ventilation. These functional changes manifest as forced expiratory effort, hypoxemia, and hypercapnia in the later stages. *Complete airway obstruction causes atelectasis; partial obstruction leads to air trapping and overdistension of alveoli.* Both of these situations lead either to shunting of nonoxygenated blood past the perfused but hypoventilated alveoli, or arteriolar constriction that reduces perfusion of these hypoventilated alveoli but causes pulmonary hypertension if the airway obstruction is widespread.

Obliterative bronchiolitis or endobronchial polyp (bronchiolitis obliterans, also know as bronchiolitis fibrosa obliterans or organizing bronchiolitis) is a sequel to chronic bronchiolar damage. The term is used here to describe polyps of immature or mature fibrous tissue within the bronchiolar lumen (Fig. 5-26). Similar lesions affecting alveoli and bronchioles can be considered as organizing pneumonia. The lesion is distinct from **constrictive bronchiolitis,** a lesion not commonly identified in animals, in which fibrosis of the bronchiolar wall causes external compression that reduces the diameter of the lumen. *Obliterative bronchiolitis is wound healing gone awry.* Any agent that severely damages the bronchiolar epithelium—viral or mycoplasmal infection, neutrophil-mediated injury in bacterial pneumonia, toxic gases, toxins metabolized by club cells, lungworms, and rejection of transplanted lung—may lead to fibrin formation in the bronchiolar lumen (see Fig. 5-23). As in any wound, fibrinous exudates that are not rapidly removed heal by fibroblast infiltration, neovascularization, and migration and proliferation of epithelial cells across their surface. Organization of exudate into granulation tissue can take place in as little as 7-10 days after injury, and regeneration of epithelium over its surface can occur in a similar time period. *Fibrous polyps occluding the airways have disastrous and permanent effects on airflow and alveolar ventilation.*

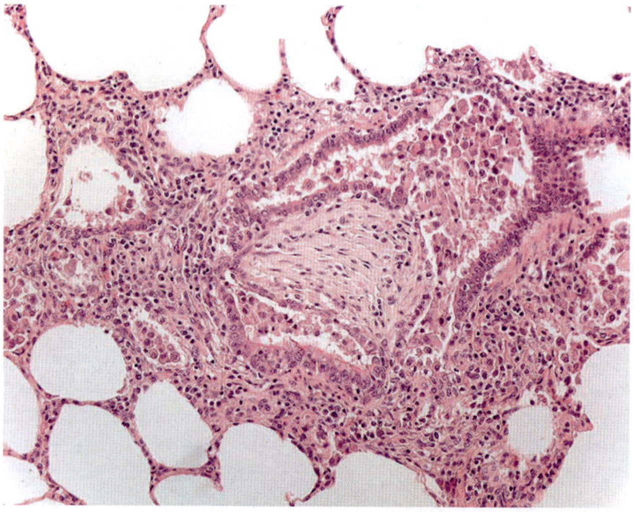

Figure 5-26 Obliterative bronchiolitis in a feedlot calf. A polyp of fibrous tissue, covered by epithelium, partially occludes the lumen of a bronchiole. Peribronchiolar leukocyte infiltration may reflect the viral or mycoplasmal infection presumed to have initiated the lesion. This calf had cor pulmonale with arterial medial hypertrophy, subcutaneous edema, and ascites.

Obliterative bronchiolitis is commonly identified within lesions of chronic bronchopneumonia in cattle, as a consequence of viral, mycoplasmal, or neutrophil-mediated epithelial damage. Histologic examination reveals epithelium-covered fibrous polyps that occlude the lumen of bronchioles (see Fig. 5-26). If widespread, it can cause cor pulmonale with right heart failure.

Hyaline scars are described in lambs with chronic viral or mycoplasmal pneumonia and appear as nodular masses of fibrillar eosinophilic matrix and fibroblasts within the wall of bronchioles that bluntly compress the lumen, but do not form the intraluminal polyps seen in obliterative bronchiolitis (eFig. 5-32). **Peribronchiolar metaplasia** (Lambertosis) is a non-neoplastic condition thought to result from bronchiolar injury, which involves hyperplasia but not dysplasia of the terminal bronchiolar epithelium, and extension of these bronchiolar club cells, goblet cells, or squamous cells from bronchioles into adjacent alveoli (eFig. 5-33). **Bronchomalacia** involves bronchial collapse from degeneration and softening of the cartilage of the larger bronchi. The pathologic findings have not been defined. In dogs, it affects a range of breeds, and comorbid conditions include tracheal collapse, bronchiectasis, and pulmonary hypertension, and less clear associations with brachycephalic obstructive airway syndrome, pneumonia, eosinophilic lung disease, chronic bronchitis, and interstitial lung disease. **Bronchial stenosis** is a bronchoscopic finding of localized narrowing of the bronchial lumen, which in cats with asthma, chronic bronchitis, or pneumonia mainly affects lobar bronchi of the left cranial, right middle, and accessory lobes; the histopathologic findings are not described. **Constrictive/obstructive bronchiolitis** involves inflammation and fibrosis of the bronchiolar tissue that reduces the luminal diameter and is described in cats that fail to respond to therapy for asthma. **Broncholithiasis** is mineralized or bony material in the bronchial lumen, which may be foreign material, mineralized exudate from chronic infection, or necrotic or mineralized material extruded from adjacent lung tissue or bronchial walls. Clinical signs can be minimal despite chronic lesions in many bronchi. **Foreign material** such as plant material may be aspirated into large airways and cause cough, purulent exudate, and focal swelling or erosions of bronchial mucosa.

Equine asthma

Asthma is a common condition of mature horses. The clinically significant condition—severe equine asthma—is known colloquially as *heaves* and was formerly named recurrent airway obstruction or chronic obstructive pulmonary disease. Severe equine asthma is usually induced or exacerbated by exposure to organic dusts (particularly dusty, poor quality hay) that may contain allergens, endotoxins, fungi, actinomycetes, and particulate irritants. Severe equine asthma *is a nonseptic inflammatory airway disease of adult horses in which airway hyper-responsiveness and episodes of reversible airway obstruction are caused by bronchospasm.* Other factors contributing to the airway obstruction include accumulation of mucus and neutrophils in bronchiolar lumina and thickening of the bronchiolar wall (Fig. 5-27).

Although severe equine asthma is undoubtedly an inflammatory disease, it remains controversial whether allergy (IgE- and mast cell–mediated type I hypersensitivity) is important to the pathogenesis. Evidence supporting a mast cell–dependent or allergic basis includes elevated levels of IgE and histamine in

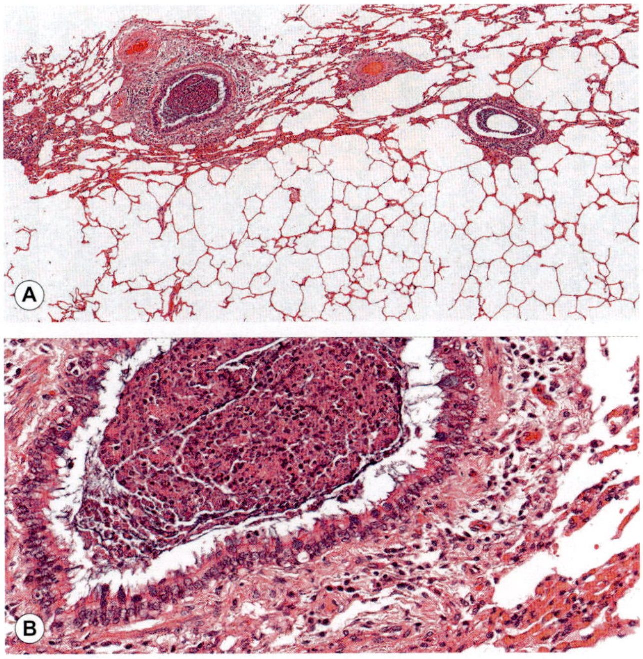

Figure 5-27 Severe equine asthma. Lesions target the bronchioles (**A**), with mucus, neutrophils, and sloughed epithelial cells filling the lumen, goblet cell metaplasia of the epithelium, and thickening of the adventitia by mononuclear cells and edema (**B**). The alveoli are overinflated because of air trapping but, in contrast to true emphysema, fragments of alveolar walls are not observed (A).

bronchoalveolar lavage fluid, and enhanced histamine release from pulmonary mast cells of horses with asthma. However, skin tests induce delayed rather than immediate reactions and are not correlated with airway reactivity, antigen-specific IgE levels are similar to controls, and stimulated bronchoalveolar lavage cells from affected horses produce both IL4 and IFNγ (in addition to tumor necrosis factor, IL1β, and IL8) mRNA, suggesting that a pure type 2 immune response is not characteristic of this disease. Alternatively, dysregulation of the normal anti-inflammatory functions of club cells may promote airway inflammation in affected horses. Challenge with molds, mold extracts, or endotoxin-containing dusts has induced airway neutrophilia and obstruction in asthma-susceptible horses but not in normal horses, implying that all these factors contribute to the airway responses.

The disease occurs in stabled horses in northern regions and as a summer pasture-associated form in warm wet climates. *Affected horses have chronic cough, increased expiratory effort, wheezing, variable nasal discharge, and exercise intolerance.* Increased pulmonary resistance and reduced dynamic compliance are typical functional changes, and the bronchioles are hyper-responsive to agonists. The signs wax and wane depending on exposure to dusts, and a seasonal effect is common, but many cases are slowly progressive over the course of months or years.

The lesions specifically target the small bronchioles, and alveolar changes are usually minor. Bronchioles contain mucus, neutrophils, and sloughed epithelial cells in their lumens, and lymphocytes, plasma cells, and mast cells in the lamina propria and adventitia. Some horses also have remodeling of bronchioles, which may include increased numbers of goblet cells in the epithelium (mucous metaplasia), hyperplasia of bronchiolar epithelium with thickened basement membrane, and hyperplasia of smooth muscle and inconsistent fibrosis of bronchiolar smooth muscle or adventitia (see Fig. 5-27). Of these, the mucus and neutrophils in bronchiolar lumens and hyperplasia of goblet cells are most characteristic; leukocyte infiltrates in the airway wall and smooth muscle hyperplasia can be seen in horses without the disease. Lesions are more severe in the caudodorsal lung. Eosinophils are usually infrequent but numerous in some cases; their presence perhaps reflects a different stage of the disease. Mucus spills into the adjacent alveoli in severe cases. Overinflation of alveoli can result from trapping of air distal to the obstructed bronchioles, but true emphysema with destruction of alveolar septa is not expected.

Mild-to-moderate equine asthma (formerly "inflammatory airway disease") affects all ages but is most recognized in 2-4-year-old performance horses; its relationship to severe equine asthma is uncertain. It causes no clinical signs at rest, but exercise induces excessive airway mucus production and coughing leading to exercise intolerance and poor performance. Bronchoalveolar lavage cytology reveals mild neutrophilia in some cases, eosinophilia in others, and some with increased numbers of mast cells. The histologic features are not described. Prior viral infection and exposure to airborne environmental allergens, dusts, and/or endotoxins are proposed causes.

Bronchopneumonia

The hallmark of bronchopneumonia is an exudative lesion originating at the bronchiolar-alveolar junction and an airborne route of entry of the causative agents. The lesions of bronchopneumonia most often affect the cranioventral regions of the lungs, with neutrophils, macrophages, edema, and sometimes fibrin, filling the airspaces of the bronchioles and alveoli (see Figs. 5-43 and 5-49).

The terminal bronchioles are the major site of deposition of 0.5-3.0-μm particles, yet they are particularly vulnerable to bacterial infection. In particular, the terminal bronchioles receive limited protection from the mucociliary clearance that is more active in the larger airways or from the alveolar macrophages that protect the more distal airspaces. This situation is worsened by the fact that clearance of large volumes of debris from the alveoli requires that this material transits the narrow lumen of the bronchiole, so inflammation of the bronchiole readily obstructs clearance of bacteria and exudates from the alveoli, especially in species that lack collateral alveolar ventilation.

The characteristic cranioventral distribution of bacterial bronchopneumonia in animals is perhaps partially explained by gravitational influences, which result in both increased deposition of inhaled particles and pooling of aspirated secretions in these regions. Intravenous administration of *Mannheimia haemolytica* also causes pneumonia in cranioventral regions, suggesting that this area of the lung might have less effective defenses, greater inflammatory responses, or is more favorable for bacterial growth.

Causes and predisposing factors

Bronchopneumonia is, in most cases, caused by opportunistic bacterial pathogens (Table 5-1), and development of disease requires increased exposure of the lung to bacteria, impairment of the pulmonary defenses, or an excessive

Table • 5-1

Major causes of bacterial bronchopneumonia in domestic animal species

CATTLE AND SHEEP	PIGS	HORSES	DOGS AND CATS
Mannheimia haemolytica	*Actinobacillus pleuropneumoniae*	*Streptococcus* spp.	*Bordetella bronchiseptica*
Histophilus somni	*Pasteurella multocida*	*Rhodococcus equi*	*Streptococcus* spp.
Pasteurella multocida	*Streptococcus suis*	*Actinobacillus* sp.	*Pasteurella* spp.
Mycoplasmopsis bovis	*Glaesserella parasuis*	*Klebsiella* sp.	*Staphylococcus* sp.
	Actinobacillus suis		*Escherichia*
	Bordetella bronchiseptica		Anaerobic bacteria

inflammatory response. The bacteria found in the lungs are generally similar to those in the upper respiratory tract of the same individual. *Aspiration pneumonia* (described below) is an obvious situation in which pulmonary challenge with massive numbers of bacteria overcomes the lung defenses. Similarly, in cattle, *stress* leads to increased numbers of *Mannheimia haemolytica* bacteria colonizing the nasal cavity so that more bacteria within inhaled droplets challenge the lung defenses. The *causes of impaired lung defenses* include stress, viral and mycoplasmal infection, unadapted exposure to cold, toxic gases, and inherited conditions. Agents or conditions that impair mucociliary clearance include exposure to cold, bovine alphaherpesvirus 1 (BoAHV1), bovine respiratory syncytial virus (BRSV), bovine parainfluenza virus 3 (BPIV3), *Mesomycoplasma (Mycoplasma) hyopneumoniae*, a variety of toxic gases, and ciliary dyskinesia. Corticosteroids (stress) and bovine viral diarrhea virus dampen the ability of airway epithelial cells to produce antimicrobial peptides. Alveolar macrophage function is reduced by BoAHV1, porcine reproductive and respiratory syndrome virus (PRRSV), stress, aflatoxin, and T2 mycotoxin. Conditions that reduce the number or function of circulating neutrophils may also predispose to opportunistic bacterial pneumonia, including parvoviral enteritis, acute bovine viral diarrhea virus infection, chemotherapy, stress, acidosis, uremia, and several mycotoxins. *Bovine leukocyte adhesion deficiency* is an autosomal recessive disease present in Holstein cattle. Neutrophils in affected animals have abnormal expression of the b2 integrin leukocyte adhesion molecule CD11a,b,c/CD18. Affected cattle have persistent marked neutrophilia and develop a variety of chronic bacterial infections, including severe chronic bronchopneumonia with bronchiectasis as a result of ineffective neutrophil function.

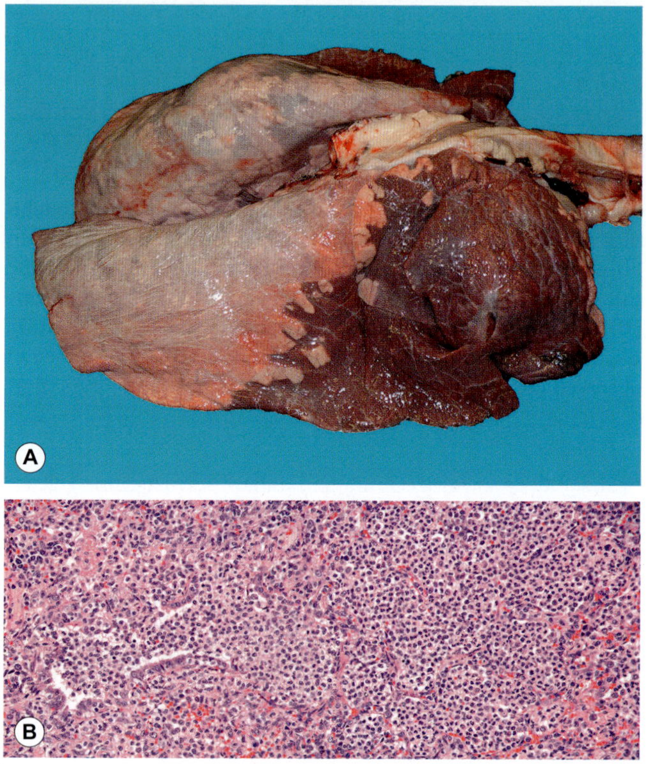

Figure 5-28 Bronchopneumonia. **A**. Subacute bronchopneumonia in a dairy calf, with red-tan discoloration and firmness of cranioventral areas of the lung. The lobular distribution is visible at the leading edge of the lesion, where completely consolidated lobules contrast with neighboring unaffected lobules. **B**. Neutrophils fill the alveoli (right) and a bronchiole (left) in a dog, *Bordetella bronchiseptica*.

Morphology

The typical gross appearance of bronchopneumonia is somewhat symmetrical consolidation in cranioventral regions (Fig. 5-28A), and most cranioventral lung lesions in domestic animals represent bronchopneumonia. There are, however, several exceptions to this rule. First, lesions of some viral infections, including BRSV and alphainfluenzaviruses of swine, are typically cranioventral and thus can easily be mistaken for bronchopneumonia. Second, the lesions of bronchopneumonia in pigs caused by *Actinobacillus pleuropneumoniae* and *A. suis* usually affect the caudal lung lobes. Third, although the lesions of bronchopneumonia in dogs and cats may be cranioventral, it is not unusual to find a patchy distribution throughout the lung.

Consolidation—*an increase in texture or induration—is best detected on a cut section to avoid the pleura, with deep and purposeful palpation of individual lobules*. The lesions are dark red-purple, maroon, or pink-gray depending on the age and nature of the process, but a color change without altered texture often represents congestion or hemorrhage rather than bronchopneumonia. The cut surface is usually edematous, and catarrhal or purulent material can be expressed from small airways in subacute cases. In contrast, there is no pus in fulminant cases because leukocytes are enmeshed in a tangle of fibrin, and the affected lung is discolored, dry, or edematous, and cuts crisply. Lesions of bronchopneumonia have a lobular or lobar distribution.

- **Lobular bronchopneumonia** *involves some lobules in their entirety, whereas adjacent lobules are unaffected*, most notably at the border of the lesions. It reflects the slow expansion of such lesions and is most apparent in species with well-developed interlobular septa, such as cattle and pigs.
- **Lobar pneumonia** *represents consolidation of an entire pulmonary lobe*. This is usually a fulminating bronchopneumonia, and typical causes are *Mannheimia haemolytica* in cattle, *Actinobacillus pleuropneumoniae* in pigs, and aspiration pneumonia. There may also be *pleuritis*, which varies from a dull granular appearance to a spectacular coating of fibrin with large pockets of fluid.

Histologically, the nidus of inflammation in bronchopneumonia is the bronchiolar-alveolar junction. Neutrophils begin to infiltrate these airspaces ~30 minutes after experimental infection. In early bronchopneumonia, bronchioles and adjacent alveoli are filled with neutrophils and sometimes cell debris, mucus, fibrin, and macrophages, and the wall of the bronchiole is edematous and infiltrated by neutrophils. By the time the bronchopneumonia is clinically apparent, the exudate has usually filled bronchioles and alveoli throughout the lobule (see Fig. 5-28B). The bronchiolar epithelium is usually normal; extensive bronchiolar necrosis may suggest underlying viral infection. However, bronchiolar necrosis can develop during experimental infection with *M. haemolytica* and probably with other bacteria and is thought to represent neutrophil-mediated damage to the epithelium. Neutrophilic or lymphoplasmacytic inflammation may be visible in the bronchi but, despite the term "*broncho*pneumonia," bronchitis is not always apparent and not a requirement of the diagnosis. Alveoli in mild or early lesions are atelectatic and edematous, but this is obscured by neutrophils in severe lesions.

Resolution and sequelae

Resolution of bronchopneumonia is possible if the infectious agent is destroyed by the immune response or antimicrobial therapy. Neutrophils undergo apoptosis within a day or 2, and fibrin may be removed by plasmin and/or phagocytosed by macrophages. Macrophages and extracellular debris are mostly cleared through the airways with the aid of coughing and collateral ventilation. If there is minimal damage to the alveolar septa and blood vessels, bronchopneumonia can begin to resolve within 7-10 days and return to normal within 3-4 weeks. In ruminants and pigs, the lack of collateral ventilation impedes clearance of alveolar exudates, and these species have a greater propensity to develop chronic neutrophilic bronchopneumonia.

Death from fulminant lobar bronchopneumonia may occur with only 20-40% of the lung affected. In such cases, the cause of death is not respiratory failure but rather *sepsis*, with or without bacteremia, and these animals are profoundly depressed and have grossly apparent petechiae on serosal surfaces and muscles throughout the body. *Bacteremia* is frequent in animals with severe peracute bronchopneumonia. In mouse models, both the bacterial pathogen and the genetic background of the mouse dictate the frequency of bacteremia and subsequent mortality. The extent of lung involvement in animals with chronic bronchopneumonia—up to 80% of the lung in some calves with chronic *Mycoplasmopsis (Mycoplasma) bovis* pneumonia—highlights the tremendous reserve capacity of the lung that must be consumed before bronchopneumonia causes death by simple filling of alveoli with exudate and emphasizes sepsis as a major mechanism of death in acute disease.

Reduced lung function does occur in bronchopneumonia. The obvious reason is the edema and neutrophils that fill alveoli and bronchioles, which impede ventilation of affected alveoli and block gas exchange in the alveolus. Furthermore, filling of airspaces and disruption of the surfactant system reduces the compliance of the lung and increases the work of breathing. Finally, pulmonary arterial vasoconstriction is the natural response to hypoxia in hypoventilated alveoli. However, prostaglandins and other inflammatory mediators cause vasodilation that can maintain perfusion of the pneumonic tissue, resulting in shunting of nonoxygenated blood past the hypoventilated alveoli into the systemic circulation; this ventilation-perfusion mismatching worsens the hypoxemia.

Chronic neutrophilic bronchopneumonia *develops if the infection remains active*. In many such cases, the lesions are colonized by secondary pathogens—such as *Trueperella pyogenes* in cattle—and the primary cause can no longer be identified. Chronic bronchopneumonia may manifest simply as filling of bronchioles and alveoli with neutrophils, as a result of persistent bacterial infection and ongoing recruitment of neutrophils. In other cases, the chronic infection causes *pulmonary fibrosis, bronchiectasis, abscessation, or sequestrum formation*. Extensive fibrinous exudate or injury to alveolar septa may heal by fibroplasia, which causes thickening of alveolar septa or locally extensive areas of fibrosis. Organization of fibrinous pleural exudate produces *pleural adhesions. Abscesses* develop within areas of chronic bacterial infection (eFig. 5-34).

A **sequestrum** is *a mass of necrotic lung parenchyma, often separated from viable lung tissue by purulent exudate, and usually encased in a fibrous capsule*. Sequestra commonly develop from the infarcted lung tissue in contagious bovine pleuropneumonia, and in pneumonia caused by *M. haemolytica* or *Mycoplasmopsis bovis* in cattle or *Actinobacillus pleuropneumoniae* in pigs. The lesions vary from several centimeters to large masses that occupy much of one lung (eFig. 5-35), and are firm, gray, or red, and may be friable or have a foul odor. *Sequestra are permanent and nonfunctional, and act as a nidus of persistent bacterial infection*. "Pulmonary sequestration" describes quite a different condition, a congenitally anomalous mass of lung tissue not connected to the bronchial tree (see Congenital anomalies, above).

Aspiration pneumonia

Aspiration pneumonia (lung inflammation caused by aspirated material) differs from *asphyxia* that results from airway obstruction by aspirated material (which can cause death before inflammation develops), and from "*terminal aspiration*" of regurgitated rumen content at the time of death. *Aspiration pneumonia refers to pneumonia caused by aspiration of material, often in liquid form, reaching the lungs through the airways*. This distinguishes it from most bronchopneumonias that are caused by inhalation of tiny droplets or particles. The response to the aspirated material depends on 3 factors: 1) the nature of the material, 2) the bacteria that are carried with it, and 3) the distribution of the material in the lungs.

Conditions that cause septic aspiration pneumonia in animals include force-feeding or inadvertent passing of a nasogastric tube into the lungs, vomiting and regurgitation (e.g., megaesophagus,

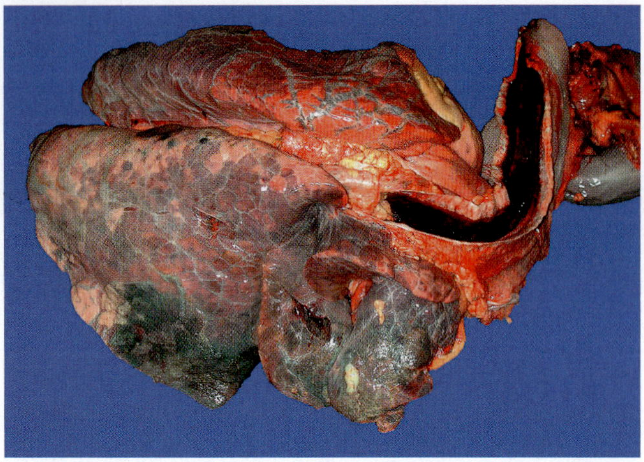

Figure 5-29 Aspiration pneumonia in a dairy cow. The unilateral distribution, green discoloration and necrosis, and foul smell are characteristic of pneumonia from aspiration of rumen content. The left lung has marked interlobular emphysema.

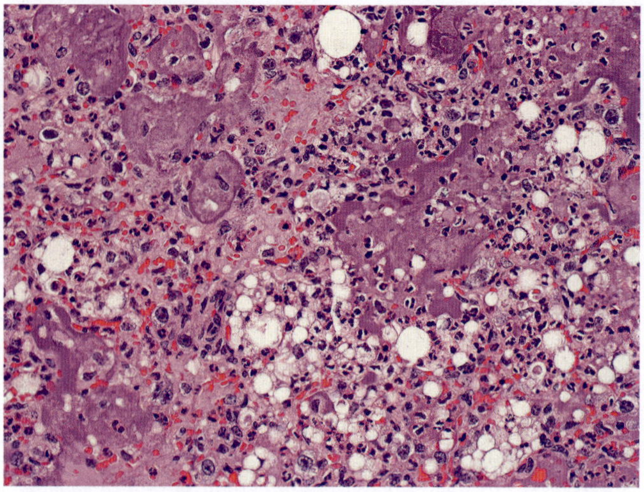

Figure 5-30 Milk aspiration in a dairy calf. Alveoli are flooded with densely amphophilic fluid (protein-rich milk), lightly eosinophilic proteinaceous edema, extracellular lipid droplets, and neutrophils.

myasthenia gravis, laryngeal paralysis and parvoviral enteritis in dogs; recumbency or white muscle disease in cattle), anesthesia, cleft palate, neurologic or laryngeal disease, brachycephalic obstructive airway syndrome, mouth breathing including choanal atresia, and bronchoesophageal fistula.

The lesions of septic aspiration pneumonia are similar to those described for other forms of bronchopneumonia, with some characteristic features (Fig. 5-29). First, they are usually localized or unilateral rather than bilaterally symmetrical. Second, aspiration of anaerobic bacteria incites extensive necrosis, liquefaction, foul smell, and green discoloration of the affected tissue. Third, in herbivores, plant material may be visible microscopically amid an inflammatory reaction. In contrast, grossly visible plant material is often absent by the time of death, and when present is of little diagnostic significance: ruminants frequently aspirate rumen content at the time of death, but this has no associated inflammatory reaction and is irrelevant to the cause of death. Finally, in cases of septic aspiration pneumonia, bacterial culture yields mixed flora of relatively low pathogenicity, whereas one or a few recognizable pathogens are isolated from cases of opportunistic bronchopneumonia.

The above conditions introduce large numbers of bacteria into the lung, in contrast to the aspiration of mostly sterile material such as milk, mineral oil, radiographic contrast material (eFig. 5-36), or drugs. *Widespread distribution of inhaled milk* is occasionally observed in pail-fed or tube-fed calves. The course of the disease in these cases can be as short as 1 day. The gross appearance is not characteristic. The lungs remain inflated; they are hyperemic, and excessive fluid may be present in the small bronchi. Histologically, there is acute bronchiolitis with various degrees of acute alveolitis, and the airspaces are filled with deep staining basophilic and eosinophilic material containing variably sized clear lipid droplets (Fig. 5-30).

Alternatively, in dogs, aspiration of relatively sterile gastric content causes acid-induced lung injury with diffuse alveolar damage including bronchiolar necrosis and infiltration of neutrophils. The aspiration of vomitus in a simple-stomached animal may be rapidly fatal as a result of laryngeal spasm or acute pulmonary edema, before there is time for much inflammation to develop. Disease resulting from aspiration of oil is discussed later (see Lipid pneumonia).

Alveolar filling disorders

Alveolar filling disorders *are a group of conditions in which abnormal material accumulates in alveoli*. In general, material accumulates in alveoli because its clearance is impeded by obstructed airways, it is produced in excess, or its removal is impaired. These conditions include exogenous and endogenous lipid pneumonia, alveolar proteinosis, alveolar phospholipidosis, pulmonary hyalinosis, alveolar microlithiasis, and alveolar histiocytosis. Bronchopneumonia and pulmonary edema could be included as alveolar filling disorder because their primary lesions are filling of alveoli (and bronchioles) with leukocytes and edema, respectively.

Lipid pneumonia *is a special form of aspiration pneumonia in which droplets of oil are aspirated into the lung*. Spectacular flooding of the lungs occurs when mineral oil is drenched through a stomach tube accidentally placed into the lung, or lesser amounts are aspirated if the oil is carelessly given per os. Oily droplets are noticed in the trachea and bronchi, or when lung slices are immersed in formalin (eFig. 5-37). The reaction is typically dominated by macrophages, but the appearance depends on the nature of the oil. In general, *vegetable oils* such as olive oil are not irritating and are eventually resorbed with little reaction or fibrosis. *Oils of animal origin* are irritants and provoke exudation of serofibrinous fluid and leukocytes. This is later replaced by foamy macrophages and giant cells that fill the alveoli; the alveolar septa are thickened by mononuclear cells and fibrosis. The oil is ultimately resorbed. The purest cellular response occurs to *mineral oil*, which is the usual offender in animals. Mineral oil can be identified by its permanence and by its failure to stain with osmic acid. The alveolar lipid is both extracellular and intracellular within macrophages. In time, lipid-laden macrophages accumulate in peribronchial and interlobular septal lymphatics, and there is fibrosis of these tissues and of alveolar septa. *Pneumonias caused by aspiration of exogenous lipid must be differentiated from endogenous lipid pneumonia described below*. The most important distinguishing feature is that, in lipid aspiration pneumonias, there are extracellular globules of lipid. In paraffin-embedded sections, these appear as clear spherical spaces with distinct borders. Lipid pneumonia caused by mycobacteria is a differential diagnosis.

Alveolar histiocytosis and **endogenous lipid pneumonia** (alveolar macrophage aggregation, foam-cell pneumonia, cholesterol pneumonia) *are opposite ends of a spectrum of focal accumulations of foamy macrophages in alveoli*, sometimes with cholesterol clefts and other leukocytes. The condition is most frequently encountered in laboratory rodents and mustelids but is also seen in cats. Minor lesions of alveolar histiocytosis are common in dogs. Many cases are idiopathic, but the same lesion can arise from obstruction of airways by exudates, bronchoconstriction, tumors, or anomalous bronchi, with the result that lipids such as surfactant accumulate within alveoli. The lesions should be distinguished from the foamy macrophages encountered in *Pneumocystis, Histoplasma, Leishmania*, or environmental mycobacterial infections. Drug-induced **alveolar phospholipidosis** in laboratory animals is a well-described sequel to administration of a group of cationic amphophilic drugs and is also seen with mutations in surfactant protein D. This causes lipid accumulation in lysosomes of macrophages, appearing as foam cells filling the alveoli. Lipid storage diseases and injury to type II pneumocytes by particulates and irritant gases are additional causes of endogenous lipid pneumonia described in humans.

Grossly, the lungs have irregularly distributed, often subpleural, yellow-white, firm foci that appear as sharply defined flecks or bulging nodules that rarely exceed 1 cm diameter (eFig. 5-38A). Histologically, *lesions of alveolar histiocytosis are often subpleural and multifocal, consisting of alveoli filled with foamy macrophages*, with only small amounts of interstitial fibrosis and accumulation of lymphocytes and plasma cells (see eFig. 5-38B). The lesion is considered *endogenous lipid pneumonia* if lipids can be demonstrated within the macrophages by Oil Red O or Sudan black stains on frozen sections. In severe cases, there are intracellular and extracellular cholesterol crystals (but no extracellular lipid droplets), more severe interstitial fibrosis, accumulation of neutrophils and mononuclear cells, and type II pneumocyte proliferation. The large cholesterol crystals stimulate development of giant cells and intra-alveolar fibroplasia.

Alveolar proteinosis (and *lipoproteinosis*) *is a rare disease with accumulations in alveoli of acellular granular eosinophilic or amphophilic material composed of surfactant proteins and surfactant phospholipids*. The material is strongly periodic acid-Schiff (PAS) positive and diastase resistant, particularly at the periphery, and ultrastructurally consists of lamellar and tubular myelin-like arrays. Alveoli may be lined by type II pneumocytes and foamy macrophages are present, but inflammation and fibrosis are usually minimal. The accumulation of surfactant lipids and proteins may result when they are produced in excess by type II pneumocytes, as occurs in rabbits and rats following inhalation of silica dust, surfactant protein (SP)-B–deficient humans, or SP-D knockout mice. Alternatively, degradation of these lipids and proteins by alveolar macrophages can be impaired, as occurs in granulocyte-macrophage colony-stimulating factor (GM-CSF) knockout mice, humans with autoantibodies to GM-CSF, IL10-induced inhibition of GM-CSF function, or inherited absence of the receptor. A similar lesion occurs in goats with pneumonia caused by caprine arthritis encephalitis virus (CAEV; *Retroviridae, Lentivirus capartenc*).

Pulmonary hyalinosis, *which consists of multifocal discrete accumulations of hyaline material*, is an incidental finding in the lungs of dogs. The material is thought to represent degraded surfactant based on ultrastructurally visible laminated membranes resembling surfactant lipids and immunohistochemically detectable surfactant protein A, as well as calcium salts. Histologically, alveoli contain discrete masses of acellular amorphous or faintly laminated hyaline material, which varies (sometimes within the same lesion) from amphophilic to basophilic, with or without birefringence, and is often PAS positive and diastase resistant (Fig. 5-31). The material is typically encircled by macrophages and giant cells, although their number varies greatly among cases. The deposits lack the obvious lamination of pulmonary alveolar microlithiasis.

In **pulmonary alveolar microlithiasis**, *concentrically laminated PAS-positive concretions* form extracellular deposits in alveoli and may be incorporated into alveolar septa (Fig. 5-32). This condition is rare in animals, but may be

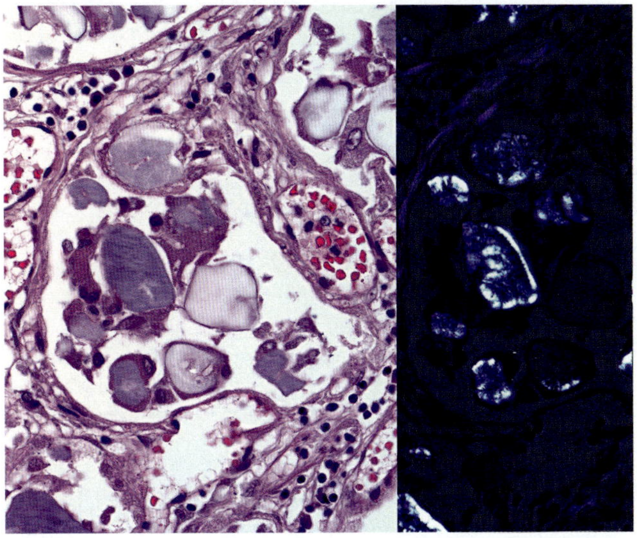

Figure 5-31 Pulmonary alveolar hyalinosis in a dog. An alveolus contains masses of amorphous noncellular material, partially encircled by multinucleate macrophages. The masses vary in their staining (left, H&E brightfield) and birefringence (right, polarized light of the same field).

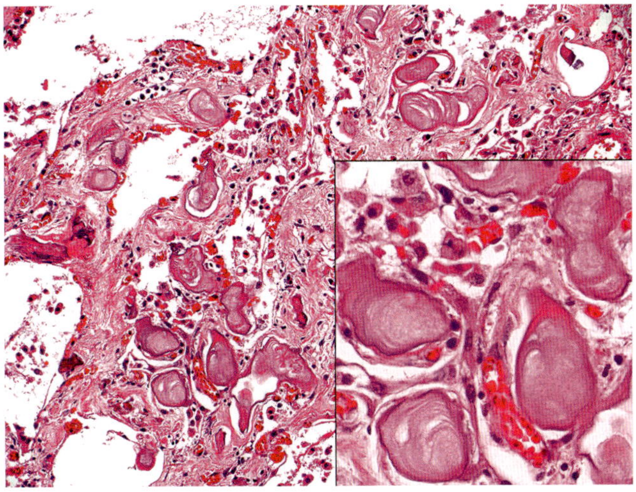

Figure 5-32 Alveolar microlithiasis. Eosinophilic concretions arise in alveoli and have a characteristic laminated appearance. This dog had progressive respiratory distress for 9 months. The central (hilar) area of the lung was hard and could not be incised without demineralization; peripheral areas were more normal. (Courtesy B. Stevens.)

associated with clinical signs of respiratory disease if the lesions are extensive. An analogous condition in humans has an apparently familial basis in some cases, whereas others are sequelae to heart failure. X-ray energy-dispersive spectroscopy of the microliths reveals phosphorus and calcium, reflecting their composition of calcium phosphate, calcium hydroxyapatite, or carboxyapatite.

Interstitial lung disease

Interstitial lung disease *is a broad term that describes damage to, or inflammation involving, the alveolar septa, which represent the interstitium of the lung.* Lesions often also affect the small bronchioles. This contrasts with *bronchitis and bronchiolitis* that involve the airways, and *bronchopneumonia*, which forms exudate in the airspaces of the alveoli and distal airways. The terminology used to classify the interstitial lung diseases suffers from a lack of consensus in veterinary pathology. We use the term interstitial lung disease to define a broad range of conditions affecting or arising from the pulmonary interstitium. It can be useful to consider the underlying disease mechanisms, including diseases that putatively 1) damage pneumocytes to cause diffuse alveolar damage (viruses, toxicants, or aspirated gastric acid); 2) recruit and activate macrophages and lymphocytes that incite inflammation and thicken alveolar septa ("interstitial pneumonia" such as from PRRSV or visna/maedi virus); 3) activate macrophages or lymphocytes to stimulate alveolar repair responses [epithelial hyperplasia and fibrosis, such as in equine multinodular pulmonary fibrosis or pneumoconioses]; or 4) represent responses of endothelial cells or intravascular macrophages in the alveolar wall to systemic inflammatory stimuli (such as increased alveolar wall permeability in sepsis and systemic inflammatory response syndrome). There are many histologic patterns of interstitial lung disease defined in humans, including diffuse alveolar damage, organizing diffuse alveolar damage, usual interstitial pneumonia, nonspecific interstitial pneumonia, organizing pneumonia, respiratory bronchiolitis, desquamative interstitial pneumonia, and lymphocytic interstitial pneumonia. Human organizing pneumonia is a bronchiolocentric condition with buds of immature fibroblastic tissue protruding into alveoli (and sometimes bronchioles) that requires temporal homogeneity and absence of significant fibrosis; this is not well recognized in domestic animals.

The term "**interstitial pneumonia**" sometimes describes a broad range of inflammatory (e.g., viral) or noninflammatory (e.g., toxic) diseases affecting the interstitium, but we prefer a restricted usage to describe thickening of alveolar septa by increased numbers of leukocytes, usually lymphocytes and macrophages [such as in porcine reproductive and respiratory syndrome (PRRS)]. The term **"atypical pneumonia"** has been used in the past to describe interstitial pneumonia; we suggest that its use be abandoned because it also denotes unusual forms of bronchopneumonia. Similarly, "bronchointerstitial pneumonia" is not used in this chapter because we have not found it useful for diagnosis or communication: most diseases with alveolar epithelial damage also affect bronchioles, and its meaning varies among different pathologists, and among pathologists, radiologists, and clinicians.

Diffuse alveolar damage

This form of interstitial lung disease represents diffuse injury to type I pneumocytes in the alveolar septa, and can result in pulmonary edema, formation of hyaline membranes, proliferation of type II pneumocytes, and interstitial fibrosis (Fig. 5-33). Lesions often also affect the bronchioles. *Acute respiratory distress syndrome* is a clinically defined condition with an acute onset of bilateral pulmonary disease with hypoxemia but no evidence of left atrial hypertension; diffuse alveolar damage is the histologic lesion in many cases.

Gross lesions *of diffuse alveolar damage (DAD) are widely distributed throughout the lungs, often with greater involvement of dorsocaudal regions* (see Fig. 5-33A). This pattern is a contrast to the cranioventral distribution of bronchopneumonia. The lesions can either be uniformly diffuse or lobular with a resulting checkerboard appearance throughout the lung. Histologically, most causes of DAD follow a stereotyped pattern of response, with an acute exudative phase, subacute proliferative phase, and chronic fibrosing phase. Because of the similar histologic appearance irrespective of etiology, identifying the specific cause is often based on clinical investigations and identifying lesions in other organs.

In the **acute exudative phase**, alveolar septa are congested and alveoli contain protein-rich edema fluid with flocculent material or delicate interlacing fibrin strands and variable numbers of neutrophils and macrophages. Although it may be histologically indistinct, alveolar edema is highly detrimental to lung function, and more readily detected by diagnostic imaging than by histopathology. *The characteristic pathologic finding is hyaline membranes*, which are aggregates of protein and cell debris (see Fig. 5-33B). These appear in alveoli, alveolar ducts, and/or terminal bronchioles as linear mats of discrete, densely eosinophilic material lining the junction between the airspace and the septum, and are often PAS positive. Given that type I pneumocytes are 10 times less permeable than endothelial cells, injury to type I pneumocytes causes loss of interstitial fluid into the alveolus. Alveolar type I and type II pneumocytes reabsorb alveolar fluid by active transport, so injury to these cells further promotes alveolar edema. Although type II pneumocytes cover only 10% of the alveolar surface, they are critical in production and recycling of surfactant lipids and proteins, and thus their damage can lead to abnormal intra-alveolar surface tensions that further damage the epithelium.

To repair the alveolar damage, **type II pneumocytes** *proliferate to repopulate the epithelium, secrete new basement membrane, and differentiate into membranous type I pneumocytes.* Single type II pneumocytes resemble alveolar macrophages on H&E-stained sections, but become recognizable when they form a single layer of cuboidal cells lining the alveolus (see Fig. 5-33C); cytokeratin or surfactant protein C immunohistochemistry can be used to confirm their identity. Proliferation of type II pneumocytes is initially observed at 2-3 days and is extensive by 6 days after insult. It is a dysfunctional stage of epithelial repair because these cuboidal cells block effective gas exchange. Type II pneumocytes are the major source of basement membrane if this structure has been previously damaged. If the injurious stimulus has been removed, then the type II cells differentiate into type I pneumocytes, and surplus cells undergo apoptosis. The cuboidal type II cells may no longer be visible histologically by 5-7 days after a single mild insult, but may remain for prolonged periods if the injurious stimulus persists or if interstitial fibrosis occurs. In some cases, the remarkable proliferation of type II pneumocytes may be mistaken for carcinoma.

Interstitial fibrosis develops in 2 ways. Alveolar exudates such as fibrin may be invaded by fibroblasts and organized into fibrous tissue that resembles granulation tissue in a skin wound; this fibrous tissue is later incorporated into the alveolar wall

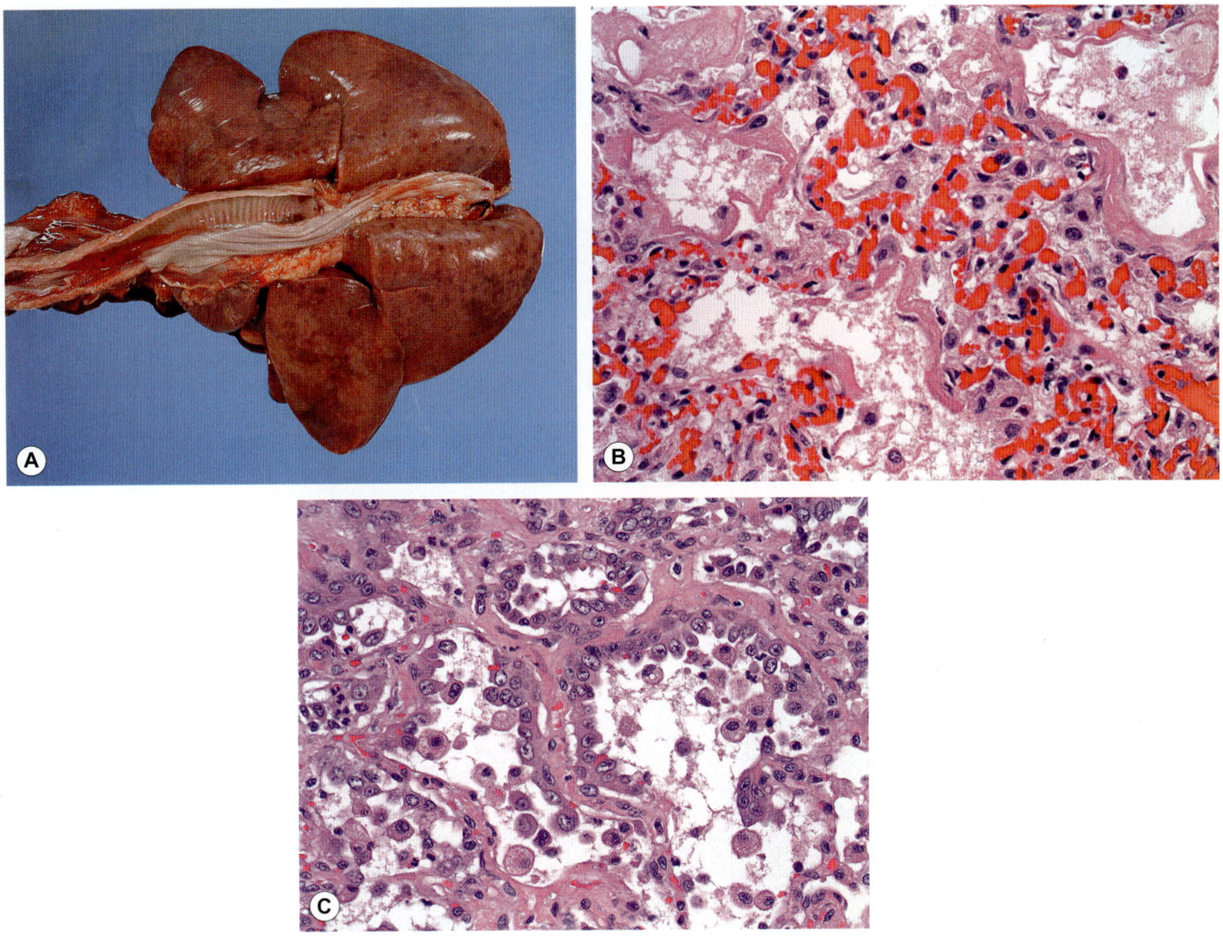

Figure 5-33 Interstitial lung disease. A. The lung is uniformly firmer than normal, with rubbery texture that lacks the sponginess of normal lung. Dog; cause not identified. **B**. Hyaline membranes line the alveoli, with protein-rich edema appearing as flocculent material in alveoli. Feedlot heifer, acute interstitial pneumonia. **C**. Alveolar septa have marked diffuse thickening by fibrous tissue, with extensive type II pneumocyte proliferation and increased numbers of foamy alveolar macrophages. Chronic interstitial lung disease in a West Highland White Terrier.

and covered by type II pneumocytes. Alternatively, fibrous tissue may develop within the alveolar septum itself as a consequence of repetitive, persistent, or severe damage to epithelial or endothelial cells, or induced by fibrogenic cytokines produced by macrophages (see Fig. 5-33C). Fibroblasts can appear within alveoli by 3-5 days after fibrin exudation, collagen fibers can be detected histologically by 5-7 days, and fibrosis may be well developed by 14 days. Myofibroblasts or smooth muscle cells are a prominent feature of some interstitial lung diseases, particularly in sheep (maedi) and cats (feline idiopathic pulmonary fibrosis).

The intimate encounters shared by alveolar epithelial cells, fibroblasts, and macrophages are key to understanding the chronic sequelae of diffuse alveolar damage. Normal type II pneumocytes limit fibroblast proliferation and the development of fibrosis, whereas repetitively injured type II pneumocytes and macrophages (or those experiencing endoplasmic reticulum stress) secrete transforming growth factor β and other growth factors that stimulate interstitial fibrosis. On the contrary, growth factors secreted by fibroblasts and macrophages promote type II pneumocyte proliferation and may preclude their differentiation to type I pneumocytes, and this possibly accounts for the observation that fibrotic alveolar septa are often covered by cuboidal epithelial cells. Alveolar fibrosis is not necessarily permanent, as fibrous tissue is remodeled and may be removed by matrix metalloproteases. However, because this process occurs over many months, and because the cause of chronic injury to the alveolar septa is often not identified or eliminated, *the finding of marked interstitial fibrosis confers a guarded prognosis*.

Diffuse alveolar damage causes hypoxemia that is refractory to oxygen supplementation, the difference between alveolar and arterial oxygen tension resulting from the barrier to diffusion of oxygen across the alveolar wall. Carbon dioxide diffuses more readily than oxygen, so hypercapnia is less frequent than hypoxemia in interstitial lung disease. Pulmonary elasticity is reduced, which reduces compliance (increases the work of breathing) and may reduce the functional lung volume. Cardiac function is expected to be normal.

The causes of diffuse alveolar damage are legion (Box 5-5), and most induce direct injury to alveolar epithelial cells or capillary endothelial cells in the alveolar septa. Many **infectious agents** infect type I pneumocytes, including respiratory syncytial viruses, parainfluenza viruses, herpesviruses, feline

Box • 5-5

Causes of acute or chronic diffuse alveolar damage, a form of interstitial lung disease

- Pulmonary infections: many viruses, *Toxoplasma gondii*, feline infectious peritonitis virus, ascarid larval migration, *Dictyocaulus*
- Systemic inflammatory response syndrome, sepsis
- Acid-induced injury from aspiration of sterile vomitus in monogastric animals
- Inhaled toxic gases: nitrogen dioxide, sulfur dioxide, chlorine, 100% oxygen, ammonia, phosgene, ozone
- Inhalation of smoke or toxic fire gases, in barn or house fires
- Ingested toxins: paraquat, kerosene, 3-methylindole, ipomeanol, perilla mint ketone, *Brassica*, Crofton weed
- Negative-pressure pulmonary edema: upper respiratory obstruction
- Neurogenic pulmonary edema: head injury, massive trauma
- Re-expansion pulmonary edema: rapid removal of pleural fluid, re-expansion of collapsed lung
- Ischemic lung injury: lung lobe torsion, reperfusion injury
- Surfactant dysfunction: prematurity (hyaline membrane disease), inherited defects in surfactant proteins B or C
- Ventilator-induced lung injury; pulmonary contusion; pancreatitis; uremia; irradiation
- Adverse drug reactions
- Acute hypersensitivity pneumonitis

calicivirus (FCV), adenoviruses, and *Toxoplasma gondii*. Many of these can also infect and damage airway epithelial cells.

Noninfectious causes of direct injury to type I pneumocytes include *physical forces* (as in surface tension in neonatal hyaline membrane disease, or ventilator-induced lung injury), *thermal and chemical injury* from inhalation of steam or smoke (as in barn or house fires), *acid-induced injury* from aspiration of sterile vomitus in monogastric animals (associated with vomiting, anesthesia, or seizures), and inhalation of *toxic gases* such as chlorine, nitrogen dioxide, sulfur dioxide, phosgene gas, or high concentrations of oxygen. Other xenobiotics must be *metabolized* by type II pneumocytes to reactive intermediates that damage the alveolar epithelium. These include 3-methylindole, ipomeanol, perilla mint, and nitrosourea chemotherapy, and are considered in the section on Toxic lung disease.

Ventilator-induced lung injury occurs when high tidal volumes cause injury to the alveolar septa and/or the small bronchioles. The most intuitive mechanism is overdistension of alveoli with damage to the septa, leading to interlobular emphysema, pneumomediastinum, or pneumothorax. Less obvious is the repetitive trauma suffered by alveoli and small bronchioles as they collapse at the end of expiration and are subjected to the high pressures required for reinflation. This mechanical strain and shear stress damages the type I pneumocytes and endothelial cells, with consequent alveolar edema, hyaline membranes, and neutrophil infiltration in alveoli or terminal bronchioles. Finally, ventilator-induced injury abnormally stretches and strains macrophages or epithelial cells, which can incite neutrophil influx and increased levels of proinflammatory cytokines in the alveolar lining fluid. The histologic lesions include hyaline membranes, bronchiolar necrosis, and/or neutrophil infiltration into alveoli, but it may be impossible to determine if these lesions are caused by mechanical ventilation or pre-existing lung disease. Pneumothorax, if present, is more suggestive of ventilator-induced injury if the clinical history is supportive.

Additional causes of diffuse alveolar damage *include sepsis, massive trauma, shock, disseminated intravascular coagulation, pancreatitis, multiorgan failure, postvaccinal reactions, and uremia*. Although these associations are established, the exact mechanisms are poorly described. Neutrophil-induced lung injury contributes to DAD in several experimental models, but the importance of this effect in natural disease is controversial.

Lung lesions of sepsis

Sepsis and endotoxemia *are well-recognized causes of interstitial lung lesions*. Sepsis induces an inflammatory cascade that affects the function of endothelial cells in the alveolar septa, by cytokine-induced retraction of endothelial cells leading to increased permeability, neutrophil-mediated damage to the endothelium or matrix proteins, and/or by promoting capillary thrombosis. Sepsis also causes surfactant dysfunction; in addition to direct injury to surfactant-producing type II pneumocytes, the serum proteins that flood the alveoli inhibit surfactant function. This in turn provokes atelectasis and abnormal surface tensions in alveoli that physically damage the vulnerable type I pneumocytes.

In lungs targeted by sepsis, lesions are typically of diffuse edema and congestion, with increased weight, slight firmness or loss of spongy texture, and separation of lobules by edema in ungulates; some cases have more severe edema and firmness of some lobules than others, giving a checkerboard appearance. There are various histologic manifestations (Fig. 5-34). One is interstitial pneumonia, in which the alveolar septa appear hypercellular as a result of hypertrophy of pulmonary intravascular macrophages and/or aggregation of neutrophils and mononuclear cells. A second manifestation is marked congestion and serofibrinous exudate in alveoli, which appears histologically as homogeneous, flocculent, or loosely fibrillar eosinophilic material. Finally, thrombi may be identified in small venules and capillaries in some cases of sepsis. Apart from severity and chronicity, the reasons for these differing manifestations are not apparent. Examples include *Salmonella* Dublin infection or acute toxic mastitis in cattle, and *Salmonella* Choleraesuis in pigs.

Anaphylaxis and hypersensitivity pneumonitis

Anaphylaxis affects the lungs in cattle, causing bronchoconstriction, pulmonary hypertension, and systemic hypotension. The lungs are congested and have alveolar and interlobular edema, and trachea and bronchi may contain froth. Emphysema may result from the marked dyspnea. Congestion or edema of the larynx is prominent and potentially fatal in some cases. Bronchoconstriction without marked alveolar changes is more typical of anaphylaxis in cats and horses. Less than half of dogs with anaphylaxis manifest respiratory signs.

Other reactions to injected materials result from administration of products contaminated by bacteria or their toxins, or inadvertent intravenous administration of vaccines or other drugs. These are not mediated by IgE and may result from activation of complement, coagulation, or macrophages. Such reactions are generally termed *anaphylactoid*. The onset of disease is typically 2-8 hours after vaccination, whereas IgE-mediated anaphylaxis usually occurs within 5-30 minutes. Histologic lesions include alveolar edema containing macrophages and neutrophils, congested alveolar septa with

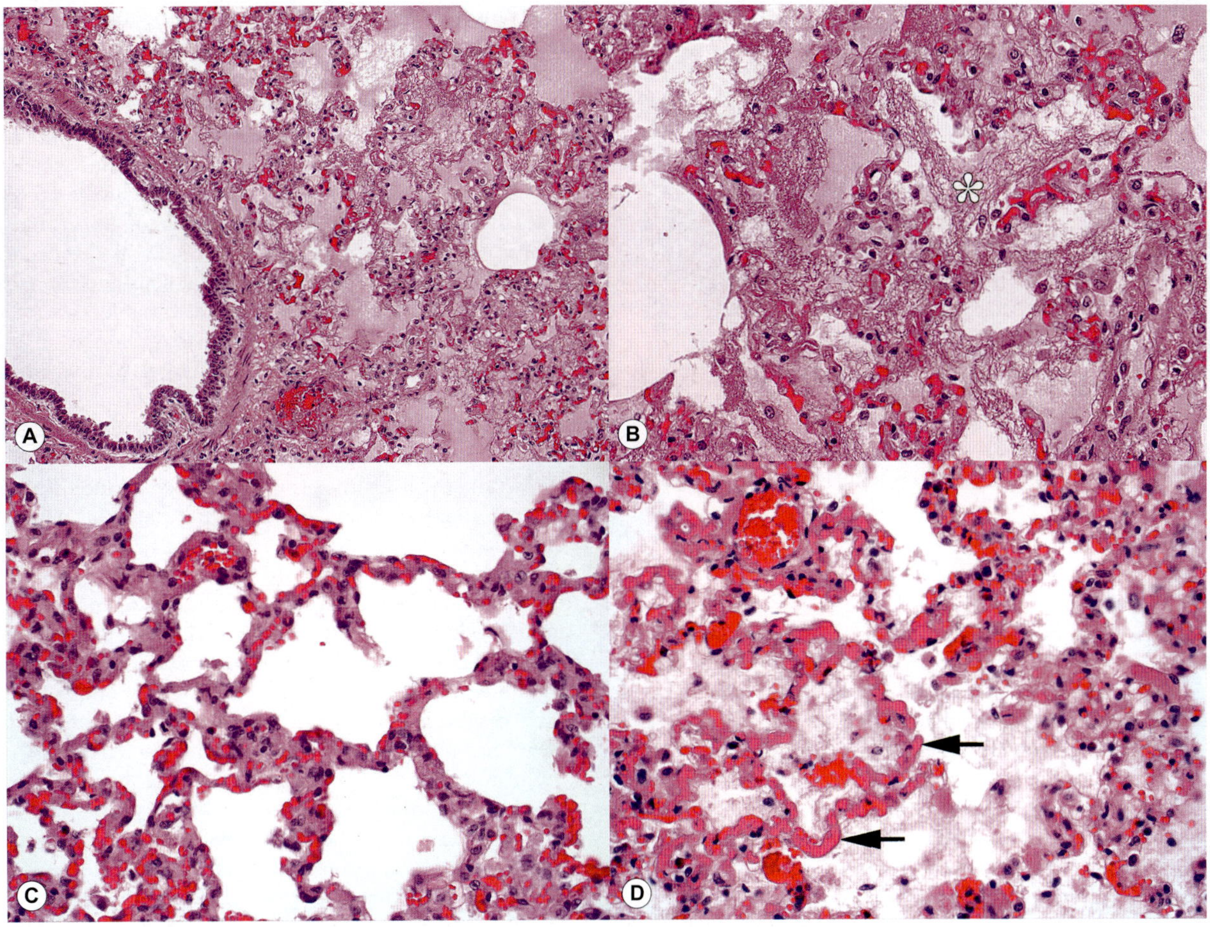

Figure 5-34 Pulmonary lesions of sepsis. A, B. Alveoli are flooded with protein-rich edema, which appears as lightly eosinophilic material containing delicate strands of fibrin (asterisk, image B), in a heifer with sepsis from necrotizing colitis. **C.** Hypercellularity of alveolar septa, probably corresponding to hypertrophied pulmonary intravascular macrophages, in a cow, with sepsis resulting from acute mastitis. **D.** Thrombosis of capillaries in alveolar septa (arrows), in a cow with sepsis caused by periparturient acute mastitis.

infiltrates of mononuclear cells and neutrophils, and periarterial hemorrhages. In diagnostic cases, additional testing of the offending material may be necessary to distinguish anaphylaxis, sepsis, and other mechanisms of postvaccinal reaction.

Hypersensitivity pneumonitis in animals occurs mainly in adult cattle reared in confinement, and rarely in horses, and can affect various animals in the group. It results from chronic inhalation of spores of thermophilic actinomycetes (especially *Saccharopolyspora rectivirgula*, formerly *Micropolyspora faeni)* in moldy hay, leading to inflammatory reactions that occur through several mechanisms concurrently. The bacteria directly activate complement by the alternative pathway, and there is solid evidence for immune complex (type III) reactions, even though the morphology suggests a delayed (type IV) hypersensitivity reaction. In cattle, tiny gray foci may be grossly visible throughout the lung. Lymphoplasmacytic or granulomatous infiltrates are consistently present in alveolar septa, often around the bronchi and bronchioles, and multinucleate macrophages are occasionally seen. During acute exacerbations, noncaseating granulomas are accompanied by edema and infiltration of eosinophils, neutrophils, and lymphocytes. Proliferation of alveolar type II pneumocytes, fibrosis of the alveolar septa and peribronchiolar tissue, and obliterative bronchiolitis occurs in chronic cases. Hyaline membranes are uncommon but may follow acute challenge. Similarly, the characteristic lesions in humans and in experimentally challenged dogs are airway-centered, with non-necrotizing poorly formed granulomas in the bronchiolar adventitia and extending into alveolar septa, mononuclear cell infiltrates in bronchioles and centrilobular alveolar septa, peribronchiolar fibrosis, and bronchiolar epithelial hyperplasia. The airway-centered distribution is a major diagnostic clue.

Interstitial lung diseases of cattle

Interstitial lung disease of feedlot cattle, known as "acute interstitial pneumonia", causes an acute onset of dyspnea and open-mouth breathing in feedlot beef cattle, particularly previously healthy cattle approaching slaughter weights, and is most prevalent in the summer. Heifers are disproportionately affected and the case fatality is high. The gross lesions are often variegated (checkerboard) due to a lobular distribution and are most prominent in the dorsocaudal lung. The red, rubbery, edematous, heavy lungs fail to collapse when the chest is opened, and interlobular and subpleural emphysema is frequent (Fig. 5-35). Histologically, alveoli contain *hyaline membranes, edema, and scattered hemorrhage*, with type II pneumocyte proliferation in

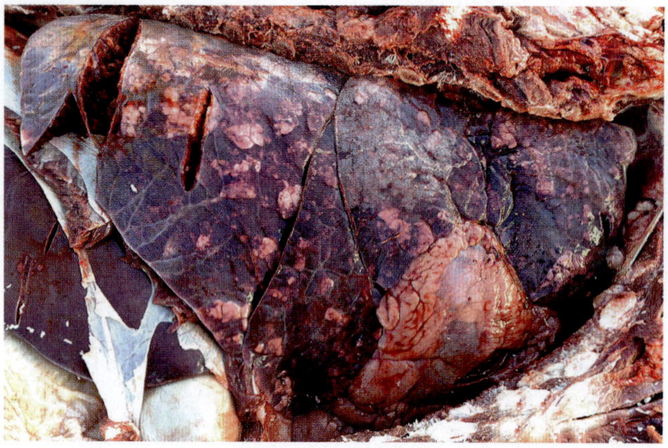

Figure 5-35 **Acute interstitial pneumonia** in a feedlot heifer. The lung fails to collapse, has a generalized lobular pattern of purple discoloration, is heavy, firm on palpation, lacks spongy texture, and has subpleural and interlobular emphysema.

some cases (see Fig. 5-33B). *Bronchioles have necrosis of epithelial cells* and sometimes of the entire wall. There can be few or numerous neutrophils in bronchioles and alveoli. The cause is uncertain. Epidemiologic evidence suggests 3-methylindole, high-energy diets, melengestrol acetate (fed to feedlot heifers to suppress estrus), dusty environment, and hot weather as potential causes or contributing factors.

Bronchopneumonia with interstitial pneumonia (BIP) of feedlot cattle is a common cause of sporadic mortality in feedlot steers and heifers, with bronchopneumonia in cranial areas and interstitial pneumonia in caudal areas of the lung. The cranial bronchopneumonia is usually chronic, affected calves often have had many prior episodes of pneumonia, and the lesions and microbes are typical of chronic bacterial pneumonia. The interstitial pneumonia is often acute and is the presumed cause of fatal respiratory distress, and resembles the lesions described above for "acute interstitial pneumonia" (AIP) of feedlot cattle. The cause of the interstitial lung disease is unknown, but inflammation-induced sensitivity to feed-related toxicants is proposed. In contrast to AIP, BIP affects both steers and heifers, causes death earlier in the feeding period and after more episodes of illness, and with highest occurrence in fall and winter.

Viruses including **BRSV** occasionally cause acute interstitial lung disease soon after arrival in feedlots, but they seem not to cause the above-described AIP that typically affects heifers late in the feeding period. Some more chronic cases of interstitial pneumonia in housed adult cattle, in which eosinophils and granulomas are present, may represent a hypersensitivity reaction. Other interstitial lung diseases of cattle include sepsis, such as from *Salmonella* Dublin, larval migration including *Dictyocaulus viviparus* or *Ascaris suum*, and toxicants such as 3-methylindole (fog fever) or ipomeanol, inhalation of toxic gases, and others.

Interstitial lung diseases of horses and donkeys

Interstitial (bronchointerstitial) pneumonia in 1-4-month-old foals has been recognized as a sporadic disease for many years, yet the cause remains a mystery. Affected foals may be found dead without premonitory signs or develop acute onset of severe dyspnea, tachypnea, and pyrexia, with profound hypoxemia and variable hypercapnia. Case fatality rates are high, and the foals respond poorly to therapy.

At autopsy, lesions are present throughout the lungs in a diffuse or lobular pattern. The lungs are firm, heavy, edematous, reddened, and fail to collapse (eFig. 5-39). Concurrent lesions of *Rhodococcus equi* pneumonia are present in up to 40% of cases, with cranioventral bronchopneumonia or scattered foci of liquefactive pyogranulomatous pneumonia. *Histologic lesions* include necrosis of bronchiolar epithelium, alveolar hyaline membranes, exudation of fibrin and a few neutrophils in alveoli, and syncytial cells in the bronchioles or alveoli. The prevalence of syncytial cells and the extent of bronchiolar versus alveolar lesions are variable.

A viral etiology is possible, given that the age of affected foals is correlated with waning maternal passive immunity, but attempts to identify viral agents in most cases have been unsuccessful. Metagenomic sequencing has identified parvoviruses and bocaparvovirus in the affected lung, but their causal role is unknown. Other proposed causes include an aberrant response to *Rhodococcus equi* or other bacterial pathogens, a complication of hyperthermia resulting from bacterial pneumonia or treatment with erythromycin, endotoxemia, and xenobiotics including 3-methylindole, pyrrolizidine alkaloids, and pentachlorophenol that are metabolized by club cells and type II pneumocytes. *Pneumocystis carinii* infection (see the Infectious Respiratory Diseases of Horses section) is a differential diagnosis for subacute lesions with extensive type II pneumocyte hyperplasia and foamy macrophages in alveoli.

Chronic interstitial lung diseases in horses (described elsewhere) include equine multinodular pulmonary fibrosis, Crofton weed or *Crotalaria* sp. toxicity, and silicate pneumoconiosis, as well as sporadic cases of unknown cause.

Donkey pulmonary fibrosis (DPF) is a common condition of aged donkeys. DPF may be an incidental finding at autopsy or, when there is more extensive lung involvement, may result in chronic respiratory disease and debilitation. *Grossly*, DPF is seen as *large coalescing foci of visceral pleural fibrosis* (without parietal pleural fibrosis) over the dorsal lungs (eFig. 5-40). *Histologically*, there is *pleural and subpleural fibrosis with subpleural intra-alveolar fibrosis* and occasional foci of septal and peribronchiolar fibrosis, as well as arterial and venous intimal fibrosis. In the most severely affected regions, fibrosis extends to the ventral lung. Elastic fibers are abundant within the regions of fibrosis and disruption of the pleural architecture. The lesions of DPF share features with pleuroparenchymal pulmonary fibrosis; a rare form of idiopathic interstitial pneumonia in humans. The causes of DPF remain unknown. Although asinine herpesviruses cause chronic interstitial pneumonia in donkeys (see the Infectious Respiratory Diseases of Horses section), they do not play a role in DPF.

Interstitial lung diseases of dogs

Diffuse alveolar damage describes a histologic lesion that can manifest clinically as **acute respiratory distress syndrome (ARDS)** and is occasionally encountered in dogs and infrequently in cats of various ages. It is important to separate the related concepts of diffuse alveolar damage (acute interstitial lung disease) as a disease process or histologic lesion in the lung, from ARDS as a clinically defined condition. Features of ARDS are severe hypoxemia, bilateral lung infiltrates on diagnostic imaging, and lack of evidence of left heart failure; some definitions additionally require a known risk factor and clinical evidence of pulmonary inflammation. Clinical signs can be present on admission or develop while in hospital and can include acute onset of tachypnea and dyspnea, cyanosis, variable coughing and lethargy, generalized or caudodorsal alveolar or interstitial pattern on radiographs, either resolution or worsening of signs over the next 1-3 days, and overall high mortality. Findings considered secondary to dyspnea include pneumothorax and subcutaneous emphysema, and gastroesophageal intussusception.

At autopsy, lungs with *diffuse alveolar damage* are diffusely firm, edematous, heavy, and mottled (eFig. 5-41). Histologic lesions include various combinations of neutrophil and macrophage infiltrates, protein-rich pulmonary edema, alveolar hemorrhage, *hyaline membranes* that often affect alveolar ducts, epithelial necrosis or attenuation in small bronchioles, and proliferation of type II pneumocytes in cases of more than several days of duration. Similar findings, but localized, may be identified in lung lobes that have undergone torsion, or in areas of ischemia resulting from thromboembolism.

Acute respiratory distress syndrome and diffuse alveolar damage can result from direct lung injury or from systemic diseases. Causes in dogs and cats include aspiration of sterile gastric acid (aspiration pneumonia), bacterial bronchopneumonia in other areas of lung, multiple transfusions, sepsis or systemic inflammatory response syndrome (such as from pancreatitis, cancer, acute kidney injury, or hemolytic anemia), hypovolemic or septic shock, disseminated intravascular coagulation, adverse drug reactions, massive trauma, smoke inhalation, oxygen toxicity, other inhaled or ingested toxins, and respiratory viral infection. Many cases are idiopathic. Upper airway obstruction, brain disease, electrocution, and near-drowning are additional causes of noncardiogenic pulmonary edema (discussed above).

West Highland White Terrier dogs and some other terrier breeds, *6-13-years-old, develop a syndrome of interstitial fibrosis* with chronic progressive exercise intolerance, or cough, or dyspnea. It is termed *idiopathic pulmonary fibrosis*, but this may be imprecise because it lacks the spatial heterogeneity, architectural distortion, and fibroblastic foci of the corresponding human disease. Histologic lesions include deposition of collagenous matrix in the alveolar septa and around small blood vessels (Fig. 5-36). The interstitial fibrosis is diffuse or patchy

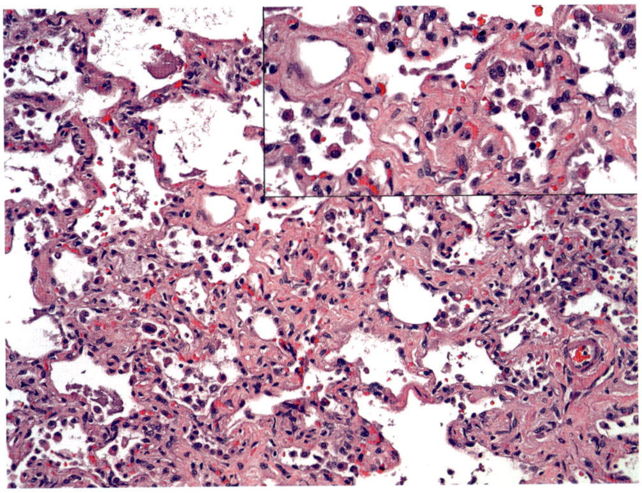

Figure 5-36 Chronic interstitial lung disease in a West Highland White Terrier. Irregular distribution within the lung of marked interstitial fibrosis, hyperplasia of type II pneumocytes, increased number of reactive alveolar macrophages, and a light infiltrate of lymphocytes. Inset: higher magnification of alveolar lesion.

in distribution but may be more severe near the pleura or bronchioles and is quite variable in severity between animals. Mildly affected cases have discontinuous deposition of matrix in alveolar septa that is most obvious when it forms concentric rings around small vessels in alveolar septa. Severe cases have distortion of alveoli with honeycombing, and proliferation of alveolar type II pneumocytes with atypia, cytomegaly, and occasional multinucleation may be present. Other findings can include intraluminal fibrous polyps (organizing pneumonia), smooth muscle in alveolar septa, proteinaceous material in alveoli, increased numbers of alveolar macrophages, hyaline membranes, or interstitial infiltrates of lymphocytes, plasma cells, and macrophages.

Chronic interstitial lung disease also occurs sporadically in adult dogs of a variety of other breeds. Histologically, the disease differs from what is seen in West Highland White Terriers. In these dogs, the fibrosis is not uniformly dense collagen as in usually seen in Westies, but rather consists of a mix of plump fibroblasts, immature collagen, and mild inflammation. The alveolar epithelial cells overlying the regions of fibrosis vary from plump and cuboidal in some cases to markedly attenuated with features of atypia in others. Causes of acute respiratory distress syndrome (described above) should be considered, as well as inhalation of inorganic dusts, chronic microaspiration, idiosyncratic drug reaction, chemotherapy, radiation injury, and immune-mediated or inherited conditions, although most cases are idiopathic.

Dalmatian dogs, *4-10-months-old, develop an apparently inherited condition with lesions of bronchiolar epithelial hyperplasia and dysplasia*. Affected dogs have a short course of tachypnea, increased respiratory noise, and dyspnea. The lungs are diffusely wet, heavy, firm, and purple-red with scattered hemorrhages. The microscopic findings are multifocal, peribronchiolar or subpleural, with bronchiolar epithelial cells affected by hyperplasia, atypia, and sometimes squamous metaplasia, as well as alveolar type II pneumocyte proliferation, fibrosis of alveolar septa, and mild infiltrates of mononuclear leukocytes. The adjacent lung tissue is edematous with hyaline membranes.

Bronchioloalveolar epithelial hyperplasia and fibrosis is a common incidental finding in dogs (eFig. 5-42). The lesions appear as subpleural wedges, sometimes at the apices of the lung, of alveolar septal fibrosis, mild inflammation, proliferation of alveolar and bronchiolar cuboidal epithelial cells that may be dysplastic or undergo squamous metaplasia, and increased macrophages in airspaces. The lesions can be distinguished from early pulmonary carcinoma by their multifocal subpleural distribution, involvement of bronchioles, and thickening of the alveolar septa by fibrosis.

Idiopathic pulmonary fibrosis in cats

Chronic interstitial lung disease is uncommon in cats and is usually seen as *chronic progressive tachypnea, respiratory distress, and cough in middle-aged to older cats*. The disease has been likened to idiopathic pulmonary fibrosis (cryptogenic fibrosing alveolitis) in humans, which does not merely mean lung fibrosis of unknown cause but is instead a specific clinical condition with characteristic histologic features known as usual interstitial pneumonia. Histologic lesions are often present throughout the lung, but must be patchy or multifocal rather than diffuse (i.e., spatial heterogeneity). In these, lung architecture is distorted by mature fibrosis, and alveolar septa are thickened by fibrosis or smooth muscle, with focal clusters of immature fibroblasts and myofibroblasts (fibroblastic foci;

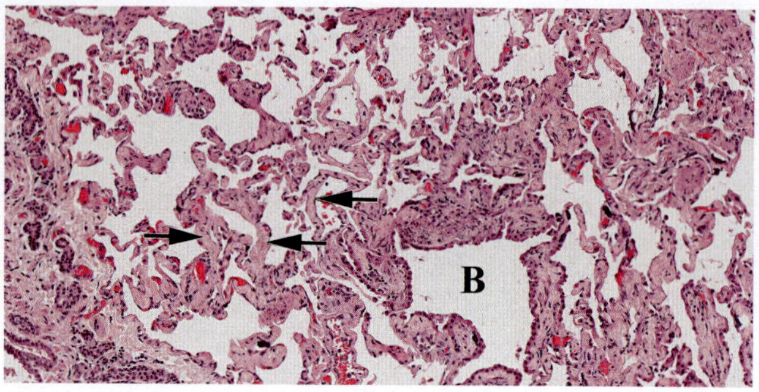

Figure 5-37 **Idiopathic pulmonary fibrosis** in a cat. Lung lesions have an irregular distribution, with interstitial fibrosis (arrows), mild type II pneumocyte proliferation and subtle attenuation of bronchiolar (B) epithelium. Other cases have smooth muscle metaplasia of alveolar septa, or more extensive type II pneumocyte proliferation.

i.e., temporal heterogeneity). Alveoli are lined by prominent cuboidal or columnar epithelial cells, which often contain mucus or occasionally undergo squamous metaplasia. There is variation in the relative prominence of the epithelial proliferation and matrix deposition (Fig. 5-37). Interstitial infiltration of lymphocytes is a variable finding, and concurrent pulmonary carcinomas are identified in some affected cats. The cause of idiopathic pulmonary fibrosis in cats and humans is unknown. Evidence in humans and animal models suggests that apoptosis of type II pneumocytes, as a result of shortened telomere length or to endoplasmic reticulum stress, leads to a failure to maintain and repair the alveolar epithelium. Subsequently, epithelial cell apoptosis is known to stimulate fibrosis in the underlying connective tissue. Thus, dysregulation of type II pneumocyte survival and function is a possible mechanism for development of the lung fibrosis.

Neonatal respiratory distress syndrome

Interstitial lung disease is common in neonatal foals and is occasionally encountered in other species. In foals, the causes include septicemia, alphaherpesvirus infection, hyaline membrane disease, and meconium aspiration. Other causes of respiratory disease in neonates include bronchopneumonia secondary to placentitis or aspiration of ingesta, and persistent pulmonary hypertension. *The biology of pulmonary surfactant* (see the Architecture and Cell Biology of the Lung section) is central to the pathogenesis of hyaline membrane disease.

Neonatal hyaline membrane disease is well recognized in premature or full-term foals and is occasionally seen in premature puppies, calves, lambs, and piglets. A similar condition is prevalent in cloned calves. The pathogenesis in domestic species is assumed to result from *a failure of the immature type II pneumocytes to secrete functional surfactant,* leading to elevations in surface tension that cause alveoli and small bronchioles to collapse with each exhalation. The tension and shear stress imparted on the lung during reinflation of these collapsed airspaces injures type I pneumocytes and club cells. As an alternative cause of abnormal surfactant, mutations of surfactant protein genes are described in cloned calves, humans, and mice. Fetal hypothyroidism and possibly hypoadrenocorticism can cause the condition in piglets because thyroid hormone is necessary for maturation of type II pneumocytes. Other contributing factors in all species are fetal asphyxia, aspiration of meconium from amniotic fluid, reduction in pulmonary arteriolar blood flow, and inhibition of surfactant by fibrinogen, other serum constituents in edema fluid, or by components in aspirated amniotic fluid.

Affected foals have respiratory distress from the time of birth, an expiratory grunt or "bark," hypoxemia, and in some cases heart failure and/or convulsions and opisthotonos. The lungs are diffusely atelectatic, plum-red, rubbery, and partially sink in formalin. Histologically, in addition to the thickened hypercellular alveolar septa expected in immature lung, hyaline membranes line the collapsed alveoli and sometimes the small bronchioles (eFig. 5-43). Alveoli are edematous, and cellular debris is occasionally noted.

Pulmonary hypertension results from pulmonary arterial vasoconstriction that may develop in neonatal hypoxia. The elevations in pulmonary arterial pressure can maintain patency of the ductus arteriosus and foramen ovale, with right-to-left shunting exacerbating the hypoxemia. Lesions of **bronchopulmonary dysplasia**, a chronic complication of prematurity, mechanical ventilation, and oxygen therapy in human infants, include alveolar hypoplasia, thickening of alveolar septa by type II pneumocyte proliferation and fibrosis, bronchiolar damage, medial hypertrophy of pulmonary arteries, and areas of alveolar emphysema; this complication is rare in domestic animals.

Meconium aspiration syndrome is described in human infants and neonatal calves, pigs, and dogs. The gross appearance varies from normal to mild bronchopneumonia to a mosaic pattern of alternating red atelectatic and paler normal or hyperinflated lobules. Affected lungs contain variable but usually low amounts of amorphous yellow-orange meconium, keratin, and/or squamous epithelial cells in bronchi, bronchioles, or alveoli, associated with atelectasis, hemorrhage, and a mild but diffuse alveolar infiltrate of neutrophils, macrophages, and occasional multinucleate cells. Hall stain for bile can highlight the meconium. When bacterial placentitis is present, pneumonia caused by aspiration of fluids before or during delivery can induce similar lesions and should be ruled out by bacterial culture. Meconium is aspirated under conditions of intrauterine hypoxia, and the aspirated meconium can obstruct large airways to cause immediate asphyxia and hypoxic pulmonary vasoconstriction, which leads to pulmonary hypertension and right-to-left shunting across the ductus arteriosus or foramen ovale. The meconium can also obstruct small airways to cause air trapping or atelectasis and induces inflammation and interferes with surfactant activity. This combination of changes leads to acidosis, hypoxemia, hypercapnia, and persistent pulmonary hypertension, which are the likely cause of death. In contrast, aspiration of squamous epithelial cells without other lesions is a common incidental finding and should be interpreted with caution (eFig. 5-44).

Familial forms of neonatal respiratory distress seem to occur but are rarely documented in domestic species. Interstitial lung disease caused by mutation of genes involved in surfactant function are described in humans and rodents, and their manifestations vary between genotypes and species: deficiency of the phospholipid transporter ABCA3 causes lymphocytic interstitial infiltrates and alveolar proteinosis; SP-A deficiency is associated with bronchopulmonary dysplasia and/or increased susceptibility to bacterial infection; SP-B mutations result in alveolar proteinosis, failure of formation of tubular myelin, and/or diffuse alveolar damage; SP-C mutations in humans cause fibrosis of the alveolar septa with infiltration of mononuclear cells, similar to that seen in idiopathic pulmonary fibrosis; and SP-D–deficient mice develop alveolar lipidosis with type II pneumocyte proliferation. A familial form of neonatal respiratory distress is described in pigs and may result from pulmonary dysmaturity caused by congenital hypothyroidism. Affected piglets have diffuse alveolar damage with hyaline membranes and bronchiolar necrosis, and features suggesting hypothyroidism, including mildly prolonged gestation, fine hair coat, generalized edema, and thyroid follicular hyperplasia with lack of colloid.

Granulomatous or eosinophilic pneumonia

Granulomatous pneumonia has diverse infectious causes including *Mycobacterium* (including *Mycobacterium fortuitum* located within extracellular lipid droplets); *Rhodococcus equi; Actinobacillus, Actinomyces,* and *Nocardia* (often with scattered aggregates of numerous bacteria); the fungal pathogens *Blastomyces, Cryptococcus, Coccidioides, Histoplasma,* and *Pneumocystis*; parasites including *Angiostrongylus* and *Spirocerca* in dogs, *Aelurostrongylus* in cats, *Dictyocaulus* in cattle, and *Muellerius* in small ruminants; a few viruses such as porcine circovirus, equine herpesvirus 5, and feline infectious peritonitis virus; and rarely protozoa such as *Balamuthia* or *Acanthamoeba*. Noninfectious conditions include silicosis and other pneumoconioses (in which crystalline material may be visible), inadvertent aspiration of barium-containing contrast materials or other foreign material, intravenous injection of Freund complete adjuvant or immunostimulants containing mycobacterial cell wall extracts, porcine dermatosis vegetans (giant cell pneumonia), hypersensitivity pneumonitis, endogenous lipid pneumonia, and alveolar histiocytosis. Some histiocytic disorders described elsewhere affect the lung: histiocytic sarcoma, systemic histiocytosis, Langerhans cell histiocytosis, and feline progressive histiocytosis.

Eosinophilic pneumonias are a compilation of pulmonary diseases. Some are caused by adult parasites residing in the lung or migrating larva. Other conditions probably represent hypersensitivity reactions.

Eosinophilic lung diseases in dogs include eosinophilic bronchitis, eosinophilic bronchopneumopathy, eosinophilic granulomatosis, angiotropic lymphoma (lymphomatoid granulomatosis), eosinophil infiltrates associated with parasitism, carcinoma, lymphoma, and fungal infection, and presumptive drug reactions. It is not clear how these conditions of dogs—eosinophilic bronchitis, eosinophilic bronchopneumopathy, and eosinophilic granulomatosis—are related in cause and pathogenesis. Whereas eosinophilic bronchitis affects only the airways, eosinophilic bronchopneumopathy (described elsewhere) has the morphology of eosinophilic bronchopneumonia with both airway destruction and parenchymal lesions (consolidation or granulomas), and eosinophilic granulomatosis forms eosinophilic granulomas in lung parenchyma (not specifically arising in airways) and more often has lymph node involvement and poor response to glucocorticoid therapy. Furthermore, there is uncertainty if idiopathic cases of these morphologically similar diseases should be considered as different diseases from those associated with *Dirofilaria immitis* infection or drug reaction.

Eosinophilic pulmonary granulomatosis is a rare condition in dogs that is seen as chronic cough, variable dyspnea, and blood eosinophilia. The granulomas arise within the lung parenchyma and are necrotizing lesions formed by eosinophils, epithelioid macrophages, lymphocytes, and variable fibrosis, with type II pneumocyte proliferation and eosinophil infiltrates in the surrounding alveoli. Similar granulomas are often present in lymph nodes and sometimes spleen and liver. A similar condition occurs in horses and should be distinguished from the eosinophilic granulomas of *equine multisystemic eosinophilic epitheliotropic disease*, which can affect the lung, with nodules near airways composed of eosinophils, macrophages, giant cells, lymphocytes, and plasma cells, and eosinophils within the airway epithelium.

Embolic pneumonia and lung abscesses

Embolic pneumonia results from hematogenous distribution of bacteria or fungi within the lung. The pattern of embolic pneumonia is multifocal and typically forms discrete variably sized round foci of necrosis and inflammation leading to abscess formation (eFig. 5-45). Widely distributed abscesses usually indicate hematogenous origin, especially if there are also abscesses in other organs or if a source of septic emboli is evident, such as from endocarditis of the right heart. Other causes in cattle are hepatic abscesses, udder cleft dermatitis, and hoof lesions. Few forms of embolic pneumonia have characteristic clinical presentations or lesions. An exception is in horses with colitis, wherein *Aspergillus* sp. can colonize the ulcerated colonic wall and disseminate via the blood to cause hemorrhagic and necrotizing embolic lesions in the lung. Other causes in horses include endocarditis and jugular thrombophlebitis.

In addition to blood-borne infections, *pulmonary abscesses can also arise in consolidated areas of cranioventral lung from chronic bronchopneumonia* (see eFig. 5-34). *Other causes* of pulmonary abscess include aspirated foreign bodies such as plant awns or bedding material, direct traumatic penetration of the lung, or multisystemic diseases, such as caseous lymphadenitis and melioidosis.

As abscesses expand, they may erode through the pleura to cause pleuritis, through blood vessels to cause massive blood loss into the lung and airways, or into a bronchus to cause neutrophilic bronchopneumonia.

Pleural disease

The relatively simple anatomy of the pleura belies the underlying complexity of the tissue. Mesothelial cells form a thin continuous layer and produce an underlying basal lamina. Although the pleural mesothelial lining is contiguous, it is subdivided into *parietal pleura* covering the thoracic wall, diaphragm, and mediastinum; and *visceral pleura*, covering the lungs.

Mesothelial cells are flat cells with surface microvilli on their apex; tight junctions between the cells have an important role in maintaining proper pleural fluid balance. Mesothelial cells sample materials within the pleural cavity by pinocytosis to take in pleural fluid as well as by phagocytosis to engulf particles such as bacteria. The cells participate in inflammation through production of cytokines and deposition of extracellular matrix and are capable of synthesizing large amounts of collagen and other extracellular matrix proteins. Both procoagulant and anticoagulant proteins are produced by the mesothelium, and an imbalance in these proteins, especially plasminogen-activator inhibitor, can promote pleural fibrin deposition.

Mesothelial cells normally have little baseline mitotic activity, and their ability to replace themselves following injury is not well understood. In response to pleural injury, mesothelial cells become cuboidal, and during long-standing stimulation often form villus projections into the pleural cavity covering a core of mesothelial-derived extracellular matrix and small capillaries.

The pleura has limited local defenses. *Kampmeier foci* can be seen as small white foci within the parietal pleura of the thoracic wall and mediastinum. They are aggregates of lymphocytes and macrophages covered by a layer of modified mesothelial cells that are assumed to function similarly to mucosal-associated lymphoid tissues in the surveillance of the pleural fluid.

Pleural fluid is present in very small amounts (1-2 mL) in health. It provides mechanical coupling between the lung and the chest wall in the negative-pressure environment of the pleural cavity and acts as a lubricant during respiration. Fluid enters the pleural cavity through stomata in the parietal pleura, following a hydrostatic gradient, and is pulled into the pleural space with the recoil of the lung during respiration. Pleural fluid is removed from visceral and parietal pleura through stoma, and to a lesser extent by transcellular means through mesothelial cells. **Pleural effusion** *occurs when filtration of fluid exceeds reabsorption*. When ascites is present, fluid can move into the pleural cavity through microscopic portals in the diaphragm.

Congenital anomalies of the pleura and mediastinum are of little significance. *Congenital cysts of branchial pouch origin* are rarely encountered, most often in brachycephalic dogs. They are found in the cranial mediastinum, often in close association with thymic tissues, and are lined by a single layer of cuboidal epithelium. *Bronchogenic cysts* are occasionally identified in the mediastinum. *Pleural cysts* lined by keratinizing squamous epithelium are described in horses, but their cause is uncertain. Tetrathyridia of the cestode *Mesocestoides* sp. cause cystic lesions on the pleural surface. **Degenerative** changes in the pleura occur in *uremia* in dogs, with mineralization of elastic and collagen fibers in the parietal pleura of the intercostal spaces; this change is grossly most consistently evident in the first 3-4 cranial intercostal spaces. Peritoneopericardial diaphragmatic hernia is rare in animals. Locally extensive areas with villus hyperplasia of pleural tissue are incidental findings in all species. Cattle commonly have depressed metaplastic foci of adipose, cartilage, and bone in the pleural connective tissue.

Pneumothorax

Pneumothorax *refers to air or gas in the pleural cavities and results in atelectasis because negative intrapleural pressure cannot be maintained*. At autopsy of normal animals, the diaphragm is concave but collapses when it is incised, with an in-rush of air reflecting the loss of negative intrapleural pressure. These features are absent in pneumothorax (but may also be lost with advanced autolysis). In small animals, in which detection of this diaphragmatic movement and in-rush of air in normal animals may be challenging, pneumothorax could be detected by opening the chest under water and observing the escape of air bubbles. Pneumothorax results in atelectasis, but in chronic cases there may also be hyperplasia or metaplasia of the pleural mesothelium as well as type II pneumocyte proliferation in the adjacent alveoli.

Pneumothorax can be spontaneous or traumatic. *Primary spontaneous pneumothorax* refers to rupture of blebs or bullae in the absence of apparent lung disease. Blebs and bullae are common causes of pneumothorax in dogs (see the Emphysema section). *Secondary spontaneous pneumothorax* is secondary to an underlying lung disease. The causes include rupture of lung tissue to form a communication between the airway and the pleural space, such as parasitic cysts (e.g., paragonimosis), abscesses, pyogranulomas, neoplasms, migrating foreign bodies, or infarcts. Other conditions causing emphysematous bullae, which may rupture and release air to the pleural space, include barotrauma (from forced ventilation during anesthesia), bronchopneumonia, asthma, chronic bronchitis, and thromboembolism. *Traumatic pneumothorax* is usually the result of accidental puncture of the thoracic wall and/or visceral pleura. Traumatic pneumothorax can also be a complication of cardiac resuscitation or biopsy of the lung. Air that tracks from ruptured alveoli through the pulmonary interstitium into the mediastinum *(pneumomediastinum)* does not usually cause pneumothorax unless there is also traumatic rupture of the mediastinum.

Noninflammatory pleural effusions

Hydrothorax *is the accumulation in the pleural space of transudate or modified transudate, which is clear, watery, colorless, or light-yellow, and has a low protein and cell content* (eFig. 5-46). Chronic hydrothorax causes pleural opacity because of reactive hyperplasia of mesothelial cells, which produce fibrous thickening of the underlying pleural connective tissue. Hydrothorax is caused by increased venous pressure (right-sided congestive heart failure, fluid overload, lung lobe torsion, heartworm, venous thrombosis), lymphatic obstruction, and rarely hypoproteinemia; or by extension from a peritoneal effusion. It is particularly common in cats with cardiomyopathy (with either left- or right-sided heart failure) and occasionally develops from heart failure in other species. Hydrothorax is also a feature of specific diseases such as lung lobe torsion, "mulberry heart disease" in pigs, black disease in sheep, African horsesickness, and α-naphthylthiourea poisoning. Unlike other species, cats (such as those with cardiomyopathy) often develop pleural effusion from left heart failure, and such cases have reduced left atrial function and increased right ventricle volume.

Chylothorax *is the accumulation in the pleural space of lymph, which appears milky and has a high triglyceride and lymphocyte content* (eFig. 5-47). The diagnosis is confirmed by measurement of a higher triglyceride concentration in the fluid than in serum, or a reduced cholesterol-to-triglyceride ratio. Chylothorax is seen in cats and occasionally dogs, and *many cases are idiopathic*. Recognized causes include cardiomyopathy and right-sided heart failure, wherein increased central venous pressure prevents emptying of lymph from the thoracic duct into the vena cava; vena caval thrombosis; thoracic masses such as lymphoma, thymoma, or granulomas that cause thoracic duct obstruction; or infrequently dirofilariosis, diaphragmatic hernia, or congenital anomalies in Afghan Hounds. Traumatic rupture of the thoracic duct is a well known but rarely identified cause. Chylothorax is frequent in dogs with lung lobe torsion. *Chylous effusion causes atelectasis and stimulates pleural fibrosis*. Repeated removal of the effusion may induce dehydration, electrolyte disturbance, depletion of lipids and fat-soluble vitamins, hypoproteinemia, and lymphopenia.

Hemothorax refers to *blood in the pleural cavity*. It is most often the result of traumatic rupture of blood vessels, but it can also be caused by coagulopathies such as anticoagulant rodenticide toxicity, rupture of highly vascularized tumors such as hemangiosarcoma, lung lobe torsion, or erosion of a vessel by an inflammatory or neoplastic process (eFigs. 5-48 and 5-49). Chronic hydrothorax or chylothorax may lead to the development of well-vascularized papillae on the pleura, and rupture of these may result in a blood-stained effusion.

Pleuritis

Noninfectious causes of pleuritis include uremia, pancreatitis, and neoplasms involving the pleura. Infectious agents can reach the pleura from the blood or from lesions of bronchopneumonia, aspiration pneumonia, or abscesses in the underlying lung. Other routes of infection include perforation of the chest wall or diaphragm, penetrating foreign bodies from the esophagus or reticulum, perforating esophageal ulcers, direct extension from the mediastinum or cervical soft tissues, or lymphatic permeation from the peritoneal cavity. *Pleural defenses against microorganisms are weaker than those of the lung,* and even a few organisms reaching the pleural surfaces are apt to have serious consequences. The appearance varies depending on the species affected, cause, magnitude of infection, and chronicity. Fibrinous or purulent exudates often form loosely adherent strands or veils of material on the pleural surface (eFig. 5-50), or voluminous serofibrinous exudate fills the pleural cavity (Fig. 5-38). Creamy white neutrophilic exudate fills the pleural space in cases of **pyothorax** or **pleural empyema**. Chronic lesions readily form adhesions between the parietal and visceral pleura, yet their functional impact on lung function is usually minimal. Swabs of the pleural exudate are the best sample for bacterial culture.

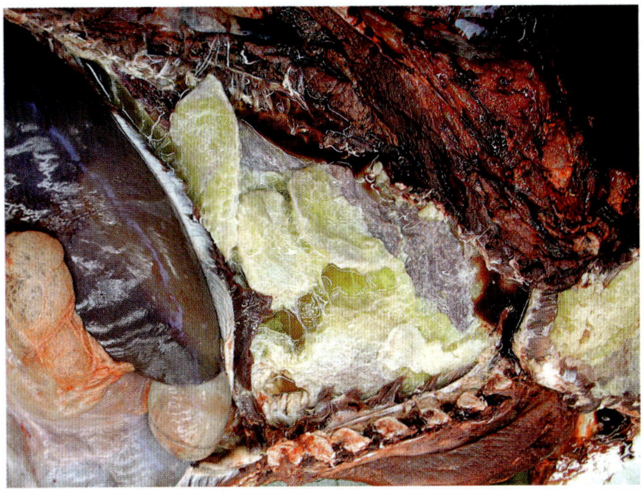

Figure 5-38 ***Histophilus somni*** **pleuritis** in a feedlot calf. Abundant yellow pleural fluid and thick mats of fibrin cover the pleural surface. The underlying lung tissue is otherwise normal.

Pleuritis in **pigs** may be an extension from obvious lesions of bronchopneumonia. *Streptococcus suis, Glaesserella* (formerly *Haemophilus*) *parasuis, Mesomycoplasma (Mycoplasma) hyorhinis,* and occasionally *Pasteurella multocida* are common causes of septicemia in pigs, and the fibrinous or fibrinopurulent pleuritis caused by these agents is usually accompanied by exudates on other serosal surfaces, joints, or meninges. The causes in **cattle** include bronchopneumonia, especially from *Mannheimia haemolytica* or *Histophilus somni,* direct extension from lesions of traumatic reticuloperitonitis, blood-borne *H. somni* infection (see Fig. 5-38), and *Pasteurella multocida* type B.

Pleuritis in mature **horses** often occurs with a history of travel and is described later (see the Infectious Respiratory Diseases of Horses section). The pleural exudate is unilateral or bilateral, and usually so florid that it masks the causative underlying lung lesion; but nearly all cases have either a focal area of consolidated lung that suggests aspiration pneumonia (eFig. 5-51) or a bilateral lesion of necrotizing bronchopneumonia. *Mycoplasmopsis (Mycoplasma) felis* is an uncommon cause of pleuritis in horses without underlying lung lesions. Pleuritis occurs in neonatal foals with septicemia caused by *Actinobacillus equuli* or other gram-negative bacteria.

In **dogs**, pyothorax occurs mostly in those with access to rural environments. The lesions are bilateral or occasionally unilateral, and pneumonia is absent or minor. The exudate is often bloody and opaque, resembling tomato soup, or creamy or darkly serofibrinous (eFig. 5-52). The pleural surfaces are usually thickened and velvety, red or gray-yellow, and fibrotic. *Actinomyces, Nocardia,* and *Bacteroides* spp. are the most frequently recovered organisms, and these are commonly associated with yellow "sulfur" granules amid the pus. Histologically, there is chronic neutrophilic or pyogranulomatous inflammation, hyperplasia of the pleura, and infrequent aggregates of filamentous bacteria (Fig. 5-39). Inhaled or ingested grass awns or florets that migrate into the pleural space are thought to be the source of infection in most cases, although they are usually impossible to find in the copious pleural exudate.

Other causes of pleuritis in dogs include bite wounds, esophageal perforation, or bacteremia. *Sparginosis,* caused by larval cestodes of the genus *Spirometra,* result in pleural

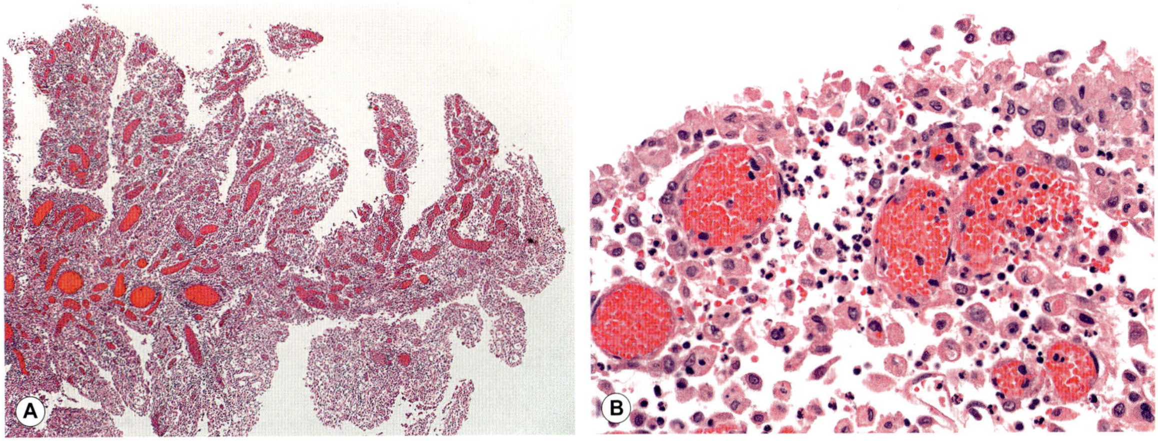

Figure 5-39 Chronic pleuritis in a dog. **A.** Papillary hyperplasia of the pleural tissue. **B.** The pleura is covered by hypertrophied mesothelial cells and infiltrated by neutrophils and macrophages.

thickening from chronic inflammation, with 6-mm-long rice grain–like structures (plerocercoids or spargana). The latter have numerous invaginations of the tegument, subtegmental muscle, loose stroma of low cellularity that contains clear "osmoregulatory canals," no coelomic cavity, and no reproductive or digestive tracts.

In **cats**, feline infectious peritonitis is a common cause of pleuritis, with numerous pyogranulomas visible on the pleural surface; identifying substantial numbers of plasma cells favors this diagnosis over bacterial pleuritis. Pyothorax is fairly common in cats, and *Pasteurella multocida*, *Actinomyces* sp., various gram-negative enteric bacteria, streptococci, staphylococci, and anaerobes are commonly isolated, often in mixed infection. Penetrating bite wounds, migrating awns, penetration of an esophageal foreign body, and extension from bacterial pneumonia are likely causes.

Pleural neoplasia

Mesothelioma arises from the pleura, as well as from the pericardium or peritoneum. Histologically, *epithelioid, sarcomatous, and biphasic patterns* are described. The epithelioid cells form nests, ribbons, acini, or papillary protrusions that resemble carcinoma, and the mesenchymal component may resemble fibrosarcoma. Distinguishing mesothelioma from mesothelial hyperplasia, carcinoma, and pleuritis with fibroplasia is a diagnostic challenge because of overlapping cytomorphology. Mesothelioma fully invades collagenous connective tissue within the pleura and extends beyond the elastic layer of the pleura into underlying lung tissue (along interlobular or alveolar septa) or into the chest wall and usually incites a desmoplastic stromal reaction. In humans, features suggesting a reactive lesion include abundant pleural inflammation or fibrin, multinucleate mesothelial cells in the fibrin, capillaries growing perpendicular to the pleural surface into the fibrin, and parallel rather than storiform arrangement of collagen. *Malignant and normal mesothelial cells typically express vimentin and cytokeratin and contain acid mucins that are stained with Alcian blue*. However, pulmonary adenocarcinomas also frequently coexpress cytokeratin and vimentin. Positive thyroid transcription factor 1 labeling may be useful for differentiation from epithelioid mesothelioma. Calretinin and HBME1 are used as markers of mesothelioma in humans but have been inconsistent or negative in domestic animals, and other markers used in humans have not been validated in domestic animals. Nonetheless, *demonstration of substantial invasive growth is key to the diagnosis of mesothelioma*. Caution is also warranted with mesothelial or epithelial cells in lymph nodes because reactive non-neoplastic mesothelial cells from cavitary effusions can form cohesive clusters within lymphatics and subscapsular and trabecular sinuses of draining lymph nodes (reportedly, with little nuclear pleomorphism), as can type II pneumocytes in cases of interstitial lung disease. Pleural mesothelioma spreads and implants within the pleural cavity to cause persistent pleural effusion, invades the underlying tissue, and may reach the abdominal cavity via lymphatics.

Metastatic neoplasms localizing to the pleura are more common than mesothelioma. Transpleural dissemination of carcinomas and sarcomas may occur by extension from the lungs, chest wall, or mediastinum, and carcinomas from the abdominal cavity can reach the pleura by pleuroperitoneal migration of fluid through the diaphragm.

PULMONARY NEOPLASIA

Primary pulmonary neoplasms are encountered most often in dogs and cats and are rare in most other domestic animals. A variety of mechanisms explain the clinical effects of lung tumors. Respiratory failure may ensue if tumors occupy a large proportion of lung parenchyma. Effects on specific anatomic structures explain other clinical signs: coughing resulting from compression of a bronchus, pleural effusion and dyspnea from pleural invasion, hemoptysis from erosion of blood vessels, or rarely regurgitation caused by esophageal obstruction. Other sequelae include cytokine production leading to malaise, anorexia, and cachexia; the distant effects of metastasis; and paraneoplastic syndromes including hypertrophic osteopathy, hypercalcemia, fever, and malaise, or adrenocorticotropic hormone secretion. About 30% of cases have no associated clinical signs on presentation.

Epithelial neoplasms: general

Epithelial tumors are the most frequently encountered type (Box 5-6). For primary epithelial lung tumors, hilar or central neoplasms are more likely of bronchial origin, whereas peripheral tumors—which are far more common—are more likely to have arisen from distal bronchiolar or alveolar epithelium. The causes are generally unknown. In dogs and cats, pulmonary neoplasia is slightly more frequent in areas with higher levels of radon gas. Dogs are reported to develop pulmonary carcinoma associated with cystic airspaces, similar to those arising in areas of bullous emphysema, and pulmonary adenocarcinoma sometimes develops in cats with idiopathic pulmonary fibrosis.

Because the lung is a frequent site for metastatic neoplasms, it is essential to differentiate metastases of a distant tumor from primary lung neoplasms. *Features supporting the diagnosis of a primary lung neoplasm* include the absence of a primary tumor in a distant organ, and a single large lung mass with or without smaller metastases (eFig. 5-53). Mucus production can occur in adenocarcinomas of lung or other origin. Ciliated

Box • 5-6

Classification of epithelial lung tumors in domestic mammals

Benign epithelial lung tumors

- Papilloma
- Adenoma

Malignant epithelial lung tumors

- Adenocarcinoma: see Table 5-2
- Squamous cell carcinoma
- Adenosquamous carcinoma
- Large-cell carcinoma
- Small-cell carcinoma (human)
- Neuroendocrine tumor
- Pulmonary blastoma
- Combined carcinoma
- Carcinosarcoma

From Dungworth DL, et al. Histological Classification of Tumors of the Respiratory System of Domestic Animals. 2nd series. Vol. VI. Armed Forces Institute of Pathology, 1999.

cells are usually absent but if present suggest a respiratory origin. Given that pulmonary carcinomas often form intrapulmonary metastases, finding tumor emboli within vessels is not helpful in distinguishing those of the lung versus distant origin. Immunohistochemistry is of value. Surfactant protein A is considered specific for carcinomas of pulmonary origin and reportedly labels 97% of them. Napsin A and thyroid transcription factor 1 (TTF1) label 93% and 64-95% (depending on the study) of pulmonary carcinomas of various subtypes, although both are also expressed by thyroid carcinomas that can metastasize to lung (and renal carcinomas may express napsin), and more undifferentiated carcinomas are more often negative for TTF1. Pulmonary adenocarcinomas are consistently labeled for pancytokeratins (AE1/AE3), and vimentin is coexpressed in less-differentiated tumors (Table 5-2).

Pulmonary adenocarcinoma

Epithelial lung tumors are classified as in Box 5-6. **Histologic subtypes of pulmonary adenocarcinoma** in humans are described in Table 5-2. This represents a major revision

Table • 5-2

Classification of human pulmonary adenocarcinoma

General points:

1. The term "bronchoalveolar carcinoma" has been abandoned.
2. The *lepidic pattern of growth* is an important feature of several neoplasms described below in which septa of pre-existing alveoli are lined by a single layer of neoplastic epithelial cells that do not invade into the connective tissue (see Fig. 5-39A; eFig. 5-21). Simple fingerlike ingrowths may occur, but secondary or tertiary branching indicates a papillary rather than lepidic pattern. The name lepidic refers to the resemblance to a row of butterflies perched on a branch. In addition to lepidic, other patterns of growth are papillary (see Fig. 5-39B; eFig. 5-22), acinar, micropapillary (see Fig. 5-40), and solid.
3. *Invasion* does not refer to extension of neoplastic cells into lung tissue adjacent to the neoplasm, but instead indicates invasion of neoplastic cells into the tumor stroma (see Fig. 5-39C; eFig. 5-23), blood or lymphatic vessels, or pleura. Invasion of stroma is recognized by areas of fibroblastic or myofibroblastic stroma (desmoplastic reaction) containing neoplastic cells. In addition, any papillary, acinar, micropapillary, or solid growth pattern is considered invasive growth.
4. Invasive adenocarcinomas often have more than one morphologic pattern in a single mass, and the classification is based on the predominant pattern across the entire tumor. It is recommended to state the percentage of the mass comprised by each of the various pattens, in 5% increments.

Atypical adenomatous hyperplasia	Not well-characterized in animals. Small (≤0.5 cm) solitary lesions in which alveoli are lined by cuboidal bronchioloalveolar epithelial cells with gaps between the peg-like cells (lepidic noninvasive). In contrast to carcinoma in situ, crowding or stratification of cells is not present, and there is gradual transition with normal adjacent alveoli. In contrast to alveolar injury, septal thickening or inflammation is minimal.
Adenocarcinoma in situ	Small lesion (≤3 cm) with neoplastic cells continuously (without gaps) lining the surface of pre-existing alveoli; anisokaryosis and nuclear atypia are absent or minimal. Septa may be thickened, sclerotic, or inflamed. There is no necrosis, papillary or acinar growth, no neoplastic cells growing in alveolar lumens, and no invasion into tumor stroma, blood or lymphatic vessels, or pleura (any of these features indicate invasive adenocarcinoma). These tumors do not cause clinical disease in humans.
Minimally invasive adenocarcinoma	Small (≤3 cm) solitary lesion, similar to adenocarcinoma in situ, but with small foci (≤0.5 cm diameter in humans) of invasion into the tumor stroma or pleura.
Lepidic-predominant adenocarcinoma	Similar to adenocarcinoma in situ, with lepidic growth along pre-existing alveoli (see Fig. 5-39A; eFig. 5-21), but may have invasive growth into tumor stroma forming an area >0.5 cm diameter.
Papillary-predominant adenocarcinoma	Growth of neoplastic cells on stalks containing fibrovascular connective tissue that project into spaces within the tumor. Note that the aforementioned patterns involve growth of neoplastic cells along pre-existing alveoli, whereas the alveolar architecture is lost in papillary adenocarcinoma and the cells grow upon stroma of newly formed papilla (see Fig. 5-39B; eFig. 5-22).
Acinar-predominant adenocarcinoma	Neoplastic cells arranged around clearly visible glandular spaces within tumor stroma.
Solid adenocarcinoma	Sheets of neoplastic cells lacking papillary or acinar growth.
Micropapillary-predominant adenocarcinoma	Neoplastic cells form tiny fingerlike protrusions into spaces within the mass but, unlike true papillae, these protrusions lack fibrovascular cores (see Fig. 5-40). The micropapillae often have clear cystic centers surrounded by rings of neoplastic cells. This pattern has a highly aggressive growth habit in humans and seemingly in dogs and cats. It must be distinguished from autolysis with sloughed epithelial cells, and sections through the tips of papillae.
Other patterns	Mucinous variants of each subtype (cells contain abundant mucin in the cytoplasm, correlating with molecular changes and neoplastic behavior in humans), as well as colloid adenocarcinoma (abundant mucin distends the airspaces within the tumor).

Data from Travis WD, et al. International association for the study of lung cancer/American Thoracic Society/European Respiratory Society international multidisciplinary classification of lung adenocarcinoma. J Thorac Oncol 2011;6:244–285.

since the last consensus on classification of these tumors in domestic animals, yet it seems desirable to use the same nomenclature in animals for consistency with humans and because their tumors follow similar morphologic patterns, even though the prior literature on tumors of animals cannot be directly translated to this current system. Caution is necessary because the prognostic relevance of histologic subtyping seems less relevant for dogs and cats than for humans based on available data. *Atypical adenomatous hyperplasia* and *adenocarcinoma in situ* do not cause clinical disease in humans; their occurrence in domestic animals has not been well defined. *Papillary-predominant adenocarcinoma* is the most frequent lung tumor in dogs, and lepidic, acinar, micropapillary, and solid types also occur (see Table 5-2; Figs. 5-40 and 5-41; eFigs. 5-54 through 5-57). In dogs, lung adenocarcinomas appear to progress in a stepwise manner from solitary tumor to involvement of other lobes, ipsilateral and contralateral spread, and then nodal involvement, spread through the pleural cavity, and distant metastasis. The common sites of metastasis are elsewhere in the lung, throughout the pleural cavity, and less frequently to distant sites including the mediastinum, bone, muscle, skin, or eye. Spread within the lung can be blood-borne with histologically visible tumor emboli, or via the airways in a pattern known as "spread through alveolar spaces" with histologically visible clusters of neoplastic cells in alveoli near the tumor that (in humans) increase the risk of recurrence following excision without lobectomy.

Lepidic-predominant and papillary-predominant adenocarcinoma are characteristic of ovine pulmonary adenocarcinoma (jaagsiekte), the retroviral lung tumor discussed in the Infectious Respiratory Diseases of Sheep and Goats section.

Staging of adenocarcinoma (using the system of Lee, 2020) is based on invasive growth, solitary verus separate tumors and their location, and nodal and distant metastases. *Indicators of survival* in dogs include tumor grade, tumor size, features of the lung tumor (i.e., invasion of pleura, bronchi, or extrapulmonary tissues; and solitary vs. separate nodules involving the same vs. ipsilateral vs. contralateral lobe), incomplete surgical margins, lymph node status, and malignant pleural effusion or distant metastasis. Tumor type (papillary vs. other) was not predictive. In human pathology, *key elements of staging* include the size and location of masses, invasion along a bronchus (rare in animals), careful examination of pleural puckers to detect invasion through the elastic layer of the pleura or through the pleural surface, invasion across an interlobar fissure into a different lobe, formation of physically separate additional grossly visible tumor nodules of the same histologic subtype in the same or different lobes, and micrometastases of neoplastic cells in lymph nodes (cell clusters, but not isolated neoplastic cells).

In dogs, grading of pulmonary carcinomas (using the system of McNiel, 1997; including squamous cell, adenocarcinoma, and others) is based on overall differentiation, degree of nuclear pleomorphism, mitotic count, nucleolar size, tumor necrosis, fibrosis, and demarcation of the mass. Grades were assigned from the sums of the above scores. Factors most predictive of survival were overall differentiation, nuclear pleomorphism, mitotic count, tumor necrosis, and nucleolar size. Histologic type was not correlated with survival.

In **cats**, pulmonary adenocarcinoma is a relatively common and aggressive neoplasm of older animals. The tumors may be single, multiple, lobar, or diffuse (see eFig. 5-57) and often affect the caudal lobes. Thyroid transcription factor 1 labels 58-87% of cases in cats including some adenosquamous carcinomas, although less-differentiated carcinomas have weak or no labeling. All pulmonary carcinomas label for cytokeratin, and ~20% are vimentin positive. Adenosquamous carcinomas label with p40.

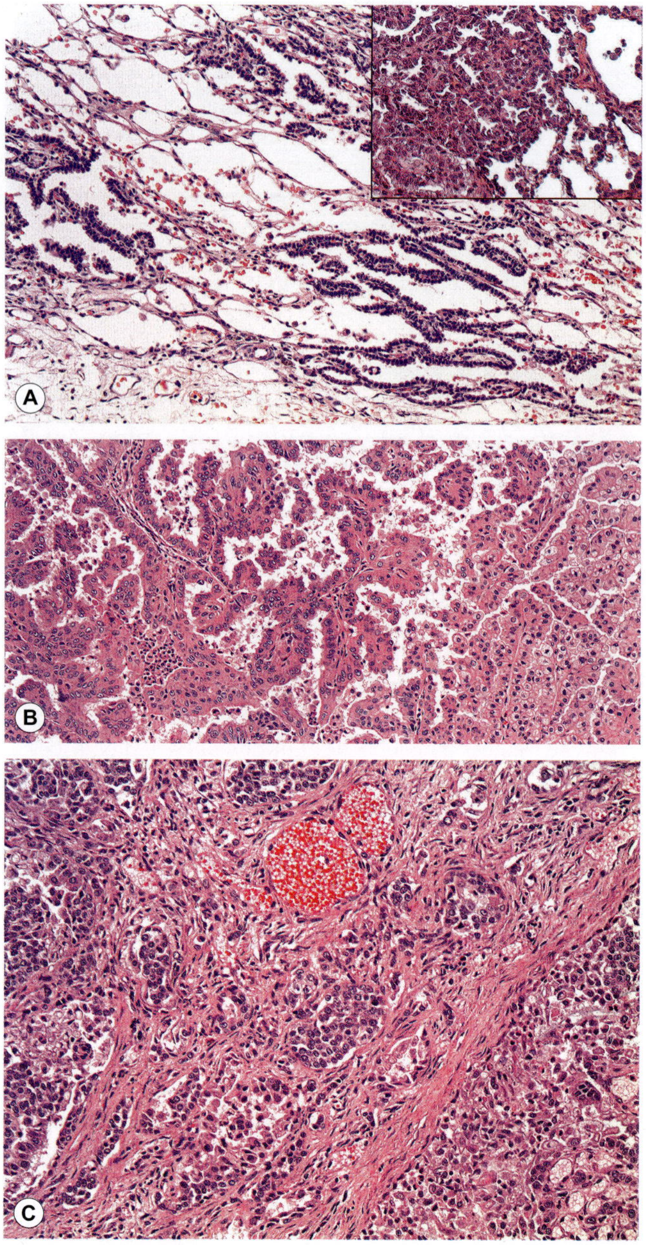

Figure 5-40 Pulmonary adenocarcinoma. **A**. Lepidic growth of neoplastic cells in pulmonary adenocarcinoma in a dog. Pre-existing alveoli adjacent to the main mass are lined by a continuous layer of cuboidal neoplastic epithelial cells that do not invade the stroma. Because the neoplastic cells spread along pre-existing septa, alveoli with and without neoplastic cells have a similar size and shape. Inset: ovine pulmonary adenocarcinoma (jaagsiekte) with lepidic growth of neoplastic cells. **B**. Papillary-predominant pulmonary adenocarcinoma in a cat. A stalk of vascularized fibrovascular tissue covered by neoplastic epithelial cells protrudes into a space within the tumor. Lack of the stromal core at the tips of the papilla could be confused with a micropapillary pattern. **C**. Invasive growth of pulmonary adenocarcinoma into fibroblastic stroma within the tumor, in a dog. Invasion is defined by growth of neoplastic cells into tumor stroma, blood vessels, or pleura. The invasive focus shown is bordered above and below by a papillary pattern of tumor growth (not visible).

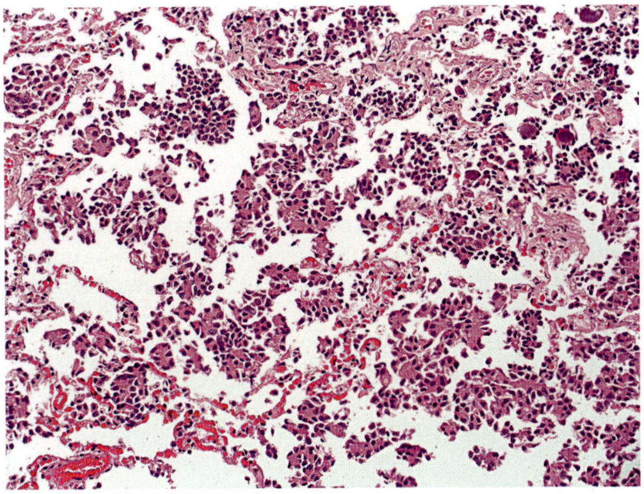

Figure 5-41 **Pulmonary adenocarcinoma, micropapillary pattern,** in a dog. Alveoli contain tufts and clusters of neoplastic epithelial cells, but, in contrast to true papillae, these do not contain a core of fibrous tissue.

Lung adenocarcinomas in cats follow the above-mentioned lepidic, papillary, acinar, solid, and micropapillary patterns; most are papillary or acinar; adenosquamous and, uncommonly, squamous cell carcinomas also occur (see Box 5-6 and Table 5-2). The histologic pattern has not been shown to be correlated with clinical outcome; in fact, frequent metastasis is reported for large lepidic tumors. Affected cats develop progressive dyspnea and coughing from the invasive tumor. In addition, most feline pulmonary adenocarcinomas metastasize within the lung and often form myriad intrapleural metastases (carcinomatosis) causing pleural effusion (eFig. 5-58). Other cats often exhibit no evidence of respiratory disease, and the clinical signs result from metastasis to the muscle, eye, bone, skin, aorta, or other viscera. *A peculiar feature of this tumor is the propensity to cause lameness by metastasizing to the digits* (especially to the dermis on the dorsum of a distal phalanx and beneath the footpad epidermis; eFig. 5-59), skeletal muscle, and eye. Factors most predictive of shorter survival are greater tumor size, poor differentiation (i.e., marked cellular pleomorphism, disorganized infiltrative growth, and vascular invasion, microscopic tumor emboli, or widely separated tumors), nodal or distant metastasis, and pleural effusion.

Occasionally, the epithelial hyperplasia associated with feline idiopathic pulmonary fibrosis (IPF) is mistaken for an adenocarcinoma. Unlike true epithelial neoplasms, which have features consistent with their clonal origin, feline IPF is a heterogeneous lesion with smooth muscle proliferation, fibrosis, and honeycomb lung formation. Conversely, some affected cats can have coincident primary lung carcinomas.

Other epithelial neoplasms

Nonadenocarcinomatous epithelial neoplasms are less frequent in animals (see Box 5-6). **Papillary adenomas** are solitary circumscribed tumors of well-differentiated epithelial cells in the bronchi or lung parenchyma. **Squamous cell carcinoma** is histologically similar to that in other tissues, with a usual mix of small basaloid cells and larger differentiated cells that are polygonal with abundant glassy eosinophilic cytoplasm. Basaloid squamous cell carcinoma is a variant with a dense arrangement of small basophilic epithelial cells. **Adenosquamous carcinoma** forms both acinar/tubular and squamous patterns of differentiation (each forming ≥10% of the tumor), with prominent atypia of neoplastic cells, higher grade, and a particularly aggressive growth habit. Squamous and adenosquamous patterns reflect the pattern of differentiation and do not imply an origin from squamous epithelium. **Large cell carcinoma** is a rare and anaplastic variant of pulmonary carcinoma, in which the individual neoplastic cells are large, polyhedral, sometimes separated from one another, and have abundant often-vacuolated cytoplasm, pleomorphic nuclei with anisokaryosis and multinucleation, but lack keratinization, intercellular bridges, acini, or mucin. Histiocytic sarcoma and large cell neuroendocrine tumor are important differential diagnoses in cases of large cell carcinoma. **Carcinosarcoma** is a primary pulmonary tumor with both adenocarcinomatous and sarcomatous components, rarely seen in animals, which is thought to represent epithelial-mesenchymal transition of carcinomatous cells. **Mesothelioma** is described elsewhere.

Neuroendocrine tumors in humans are classified as low-grade carcinoid, intermediate-grade atypical carcinoid, high-grade small cell carcinoma, and high-grade large cell neuroendocrine carcinoma. All are rare in domestic animals and mainly affect the young. ***Pulmonary neuroendocrine tumor*** *is the preferred term because the validity of subclassifying these tumors in animals is unknown. Carcinoids* in humans are thought to arise from bronchial neuroendocrine tissue and exhibit the characteristic features of neuroendocrine tumors: arrangement in nests, palisades, or pseudorosettes; expression of chromogranin and serotonin (synaptophysin is weak; neuron-specific enolase is considered nonspecific); and dense-core granules may be visible by electron microscopy. The few cases of pulmonary neoplasms in dogs that resemble carcinoids have developed adjacent to a bronchus and have a neuroendocrine pattern of nests or ribbons of cells separated by delicate vascularized stroma. The cells are uniform, round-to-polygonal, with abundant pale eosinophilic cytoplasm and relatively small nuclei. Features in humans indicative of an intermediate grade (i.e., atypical rather than typical carcinoid) are mitotic rate >2 per 10 high-power fields, and punctate coagulative necrosis of the tumor. *Large-cell neuroendocrine carcinoma* has >1 mitosis per high-power field with comedo-like necrosis. In dogs, increasing tumor grade has been correlated with progression from well-demarcated nodules to infiltrative or metastatic neoplasms. The diagnosis is based firmly on morphology, and immunohistochemical findings alone do not justify the diagnosis. **Small-cell carcinoma** is an important neuroendocrine tumor in humans but rare and poorly characterized in dogs and cows. It has a hilar location and consists of loosely arranged packets of small cells (~10 μm diameter) separated by a thin stroma. The neoplastic cells have scant basophilic cytoplasm and may be round (resembling lymphocytes), fusiform ("oat cells"), or polygonal. The immunohistochemical staining patterns in domestic animals are not characterized.

Pulmonary blastoma, rarely described in animals, is a multinodular lesion that implants in the pleural cavity, metastasizes to lymph node, and invades extrapulmonary structures. Blastoma consists, by definition, of both *malignant epithelial and mesenchymal components*, although there is much variation in the relative amount of each component between tumors and within different areas of the same neoplasm. The cuboidal epithelial cells are arranged in nests or branching tubules. The mesenchymal component appears embryonal, with loose matrix separating spindle-shaped, stellate, or angular cells with vesicular or hyperchromatic nuclei. Pleuropulmonary blastoma is of similar morphology and is located in pleura, lung, or mediastinum, but the epithelial component is well differentiated rather than atypical. The differential diagnoses include pulmonary hamartoma and mesothelioma.

Mesenchymal and round-cell neoplasms

Granular cell tumor *is the most common primary lung tumor in horses and is thought to originate from neurolemmocytes (Schwann cells) in the peribronchial tissue*. It is often discovered as an incidental finding in older horses, but can cause coughing or rarely dyspnea. Metastasis is not described. Grossly, the mass is white-to-beige, usually multinodular, and unilateral. Granular cell tumors are associated with large bronchi and often bulge into the bronchial lumen to cause variable degrees of obstruction. Histologically, the neoplasm is composed of sheets or lobular aggregates of large, round, or angular cells with abundant cytoplasm containing innumerable tiny acidophilic granules (Fig. 5-42). There is minimal variation in cell size, and few mitotic figures. The granules usually stain with Luxol fast blue and more variably with PAS. Immunohistochemical markers for pulmonary granular cell tumors in horses are expressed in a variety of other cell types, and so are not pathognomonic for this neoplasm; S100 and vimentin are consistently present, with inconsistent expression of neuron-specific enolase and glial fibrillary acidic protein.

Histiocytic sarcoma *is a malignant neoplasm of myeloid interstitial dendritic cell phenotype* (see Vol. 3, Hematolymphoid System). Histiocytic sarcoma can arise in the lung and spread to thoracic lymph nodes, or histiocytic sarcoma of splenic or other origin (disseminated histiocytic sarcoma) may secondarily involve the lung. Primary pulmonary histiocytic sarcoma affects dogs of a wide age range, with over-representation of Bernese Mountain Dogs, Miniature Schnauzers, and Labrador Retrievers. Some cases have no clinical signs at diagnosis. The neoplasm may form a single mass or invade to fill an entire lobe, and many have intrapulmonary or nodal metastases at the time of diagnosis. The morphology varies from individualized round cells with scant-to-abundant eosinophilic cytoplasm, to spindle-shaped or dendritic cells with indistinct borders (Fig. 5-43). The nuclei are round or cleaved with marked anisokaryosis. Most cases have significant numbers of multinucleate cells, lymphocytes, and plasma cells intermingled with the neoplastic cells. Definitive diagnosis requires immunohistochemistry on frozen sections to demonstrate expression of CD1, CD11c, major histocompatibility complex class II, and intercellular adhesion molecule (ICAM)1. However, in formalin-fixed specimens, demonstration of a typical morphology along with expression of IBA1, CD204, or CD18 but absence of CD3, PAX5, and MUM1 is sufficient for routine diagnosis. Dogs with splenic hemophagic histiocytic sarcoma (of macrophage phenotype) may have neoplastic cells within pulmonary blood vessels.

Feline pulmonary Langerhans cell histiocytosis is a rare condition of old cats causing coalescing masses or diffuse infiltrates within the lung and may affect the pancreas, kidney, liver, and local or distant lymph nodes. The infiltrate targets the wall and lumen of bronchioles and may extend to adjacent alveoli. The histiocytic cells are pleomorphic with a moderate amount of homogeneous or finely vacuolated eosinophilic cytoplasm, anisokaryosis, poikilokaryosis, and nuclear hyperchromasia. These cells express CD18 and E-cadherin and have ultrastructurally visible Birbeck granules, consistent with a Langerhans cell phenotype. In addition to this disease, cats with **progressive histiocytosis** and dogs with **cutaneous Langerhans cell histiocytosis** or **systemic histiocytosis**, described elsewhere, may have lung involvement.

Angiocentric large cell lymphoma (lymphomatoid granulomatosis) is a rare and poorly understood disease of dogs, and very rarely of cats. In humans, lymphomatoid granulomatosis is a B-cell proliferation associated with Epstein-Barr virus infection. Although the disease is discussed here as a pulmonary neoplasm, there is considerable debate as to whether the analogous condition in humans represents a neoplasm or a non-neoplastic lymphoproliferative disorder. The clonality of the lymphoid cells has not been evaluated in case series in domestic animals, so the biology of this disease remains enigmatic. Most cases affect young dogs (4-9 years) with some as young as 9 weeks. The masses are multiple and usually found within the caudal lung lobes. They are poorly demarcated and pale, or can occur as a diffuse infiltrate within the

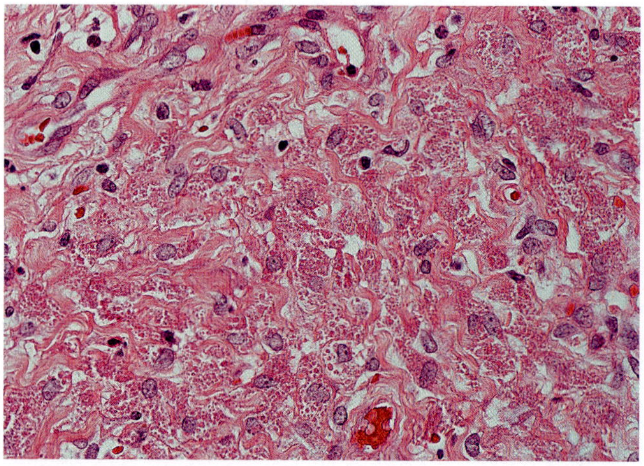

Figure 5-42 Pulmonary granular cell tumor in a horse. The neoplastic cells have indistinct borders and innumerable eosinophilic granules in the cytoplasm; the collagenous matrix is abundant.

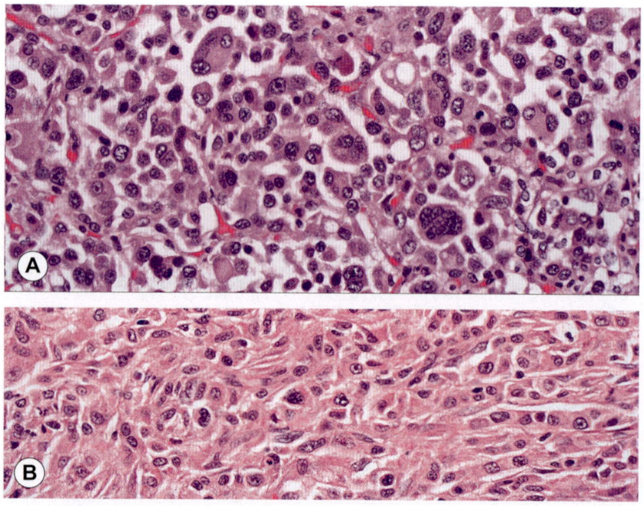

Figure 5-43 Pulmonary histiocytic sarcoma in a dog. Within the same mass, the phenotype varies from pleomorphic round cells with abundant cytoplasm and frequent multinucleation (**A**), to spindle cells with less obvious histiocytic differentiation (**B**).

affected lobes. Histologically, angiocentric lymphoma *is an angioinvasive, angiodestructive, pleocellular infiltrate* (Fig. 5-44). A requirement for the diagnosis is large atypical cells accompanied by a mixed infiltrate of small lymphocytes (mainly T cells) and often plasma cells and eosinophils. The atypical cells are round with distinct borders, large but variably sized, occasionally binucleate, and often have a high mitotic count. The immunophenotype of the atypical cells is inconsistent in the current literature and requires further study. *Destructive invasion of the pleomorphic cells into the walls of blood vessels is the characteristic feature of the disease*, and infarction of adjacent tissue may be present. The infiltrates frequently involve local and distant lymph nodes and occasionally the liver and other viscera, but it is the progressive involvement of the lung that causes death in most cases. The differential diagnosis includes eosinophilic granulomatosis, pyogranulomatous inflammation, anaplastic carcinoma, and round cell tumors such as histiocytic sarcoma, lymphoma, and mast cell tumor. Other than angiocentric lymphoma, primary pulmonary lymphoma is not recognized in domestic animals.

Diffuse pulmonary meningotheliomatosis with sarcomatous transformation is described in a dog, having disseminated nodules of polygonal or spindle cells with abundant cytoplasm and indistinct cell borders; the diagnosis was based on immunohistochemistry and ultrastructural features.

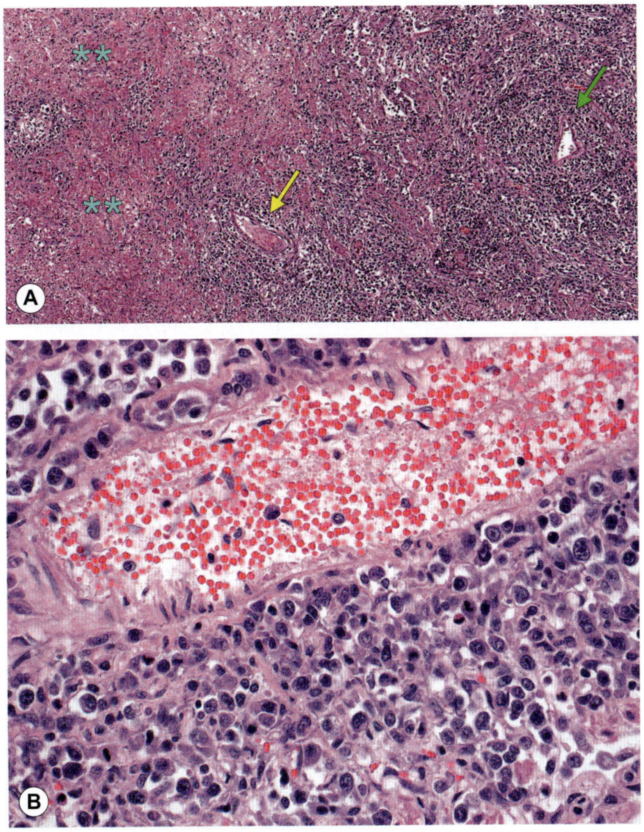

Figure 5-44 Angiocentric lymphoma in a dog. **A.** Angioinvasive growth of neoplastic cells (white arrow), angiodestructive behavior with effacement of a vessel wall (black arrow), and coagulative necrosis (*) from infarction of adjacent neoplastic tissue. **B.** Pleomorphic large neoplastic round cells and small non-neoplastic lymphocytes infiltrate a vessel wall.

Metastatic tumors commonly arise within the lung because of the organ's rich capillary and lymphatic network. Criteria for differentiating metastases of nonpulmonary neoplasms from intrapulmonary spread of a primary lung neoplasm are described above. Before diagnosing a primary lung tumor, it is important to exclude nonpulmonary sites of primary neoplasia by a thorough examination of the body. Metastatic carcinomas may form acini, solid sheets, lepidic growth along pre-existing alveolar septa, and/or clusters within blood vessels. Some of the most common metastatic neoplasms include lymphoma in all species; uterine adenocarcinoma in cows and sows; malignant melanoma in horses; and osteosarcoma, hemangiosarcoma, oral melanoma, mast cell tumor, urothelial carcinoma, and adenocarcinomas of mammary, biliary, pancreatic, intestinal, anal sac, or thyroid origin in dogs and cats (eFigs. 5-60 and 5-61).

TOXIC LUNG DISEASE

The lung is the target of toxic injury by several mechanisms: inhalation of gases or fumes that are directly toxic to epithelial or endothelial cells, ingestion or inhalation of toxins that are metabolized to reactive intermediates mainly by club cells or type II pneumocytes, hypersensitivity reactions, effects of inhaled persistent material such as asbestos or fiberglass, and xenobiotic-induced carcinogenicity. Typical lesions include epithelial cell necrosis, hyperplasia, dysplasia, squamous metaplasia, or neoplastic transformation; alveolar histiocytosis; or fibrosis. Inhaled or ingested xenobiotics causing nasal lesions are well studied in animal models, but are rarely encountered in diagnostic veterinary pathology.

Severe lung injury from **inhalation of toxic gases** is rarely encountered in domestic animals because they do not have the occupational exposures that are usually responsible in humans. The anatomic location of injury by inhaled toxins depends on the dose, chemical reactivity, aqueous solubility, and particle size. Water-soluble gases such as sulfur dioxide and ammonia usually cause upper respiratory injury; less-soluble gases, such as nitrogen dioxide, are more widely distributed and may cause bronchiolar or alveolar injury. Poisoning of cattle, pigs, and chickens by **nitrogen dioxide (silo gas)** can cause massive mortality with lesions of pulmonary edema and congestion, necrosis of bronchial and bronchiolar epithelium, and alveolar hemorrhage and/or fibrin exudation. Acute pulmonary injury caused by inhalation or **smoke and toxic fire gases** is seen in animals trapped in burning buildings (see Fig. 5-14). Evidence that animals were alive during the fire includes grossly or microscopically observed soot in the lumen of airways, esophagus, and stomach; and increased carboxyhemoglobin concentrations in blood (from reaction of carbon monoxide and hemoglobin). Edema and vesicles may also be noted in the upper respiratory and alimentary tracts. When asphyxia is not immediate, the combined chemical and heat effects of smoke can cause widespread epithelial necrosis and exudation, and death within a few days. Exposure to **copper-containing drenches**, perhaps by aspiration, causes bronchiolar necrosis in sheep, with elevated copper levels in the lung but not in the liver. **Hydrocarbon waterproofing sprays** are reported to cause lung disease in dogs, but the lesions or mechanisms are not defined.

Exposure to 85-100% **oxygen** (or perhaps lower levels, in animals with pre-existing lung disease) damages capillary endothelium and type I pneumocytes and causes alveolar edema or diffuse alveolar damage. In intensive care patients, it may be impossible to determine if diffuse alveolar damage was caused by the underlying disease, or hyperoxic or ventilator-induced lung injury. *Reactive oxygen species* (superoxide, hydroxyl radicals, and hydrogen peroxide) are currently favored as the injurious metabolites, causing cellular injury by lipid peroxidation, protein oxidation, and DNA strand breaks. Neutrophil-dependent lung injury and dysfunction of surfactant are additional proposed mechanisms of hyperoxic lung injury.

The toxicity of other compounds depends on their *conversion to reactive intermediate metabolites* by phase I enzymes that include several cytochrome P450 (CYP) isozymes. These isozymes have a species-dependent distribution in nasal tissue, club cells, type II pneumocytes, and to a lesser extent in ciliated epithelial cells, type I pneumocytes, endothelial cells, and pulmonary macrophages. Reactive intermediates generated by CYP isozymes are further detoxified by phase II enzymes, including glutathione-S-transferases and glucuronyltransferases, to form water-soluble metabolites that are excreted. However, toxicity may develop when the phase II systems are inadequate (e.g., when glutathione is depleted or glutathione-S-transferase activity is impaired or absent) or overwhelmed by high concentrations of the reactive metabolite. In these situations, the electrophilic metabolite binds to essential proteins or nucleic acids, or leads to the formation of oxygen radicals that damage cell membrane lipids. Thus, *the cellular susceptibility to toxic injury depends not only on cell-specific expression of the appropriate CYP isozymes but also on the adequacy of the antioxidants (glutathione, vitamin E, superoxide dismutase, and others) and phase II enzymes that protect the cell from injury*. Inherited polymorphisms in CYP genes and induction of these enzymes by glucocorticoids or other drugs may also influence the susceptibility of individual animals to pulmonary toxins.

3-Methylindole (3MI) toxicity *causes acute bovine pulmonary emphysema and edema, or fog fever, in cattle.* L-Tryptophan in grazed pastures is metabolized in the rumen (or the large colon of nonruminants) to 3MI, which travels via blood to lung and is converted primarily by CYP to an electrophilic intermediate that alkylates cellular macromolecules, resulting in lipid peroxidation and membrane damage. The early ultrastructural changes are necrosis of nonciliated and ciliated bronchiolar epithelial cells and type I pneumocytes, and transient swelling of endothelial cells. Although type II pneumocytes have high CYP activity, the high levels of glutathione and phase II enzymes are thought to spare these cells from injury.

3-Methylindole toxicity affects adult cattle in the autumn, 4-10 days after they are moved from dry to lush pastures; younger animals are resistant to the toxic effects of 3MI. Affected animals have acute onset of dyspnea with expiratory effort, tachypnea, open-mouth breathing, and froth in the mouth. The trachea is filled with foam, and the lungs contain striking alveolar and interlobular edema, resulting in heavy wet lungs that fail to collapse. Interlobular or bullous emphysema is prominent in the caudal lobes in less fulminant cases. Histologically, hyaline membranes line the edematous alveoli and alveolar ducts, and type II pneumocyte proliferation is extensive in the subacute stages. The alveolar septa are distended by edema and may contain eosinophils and/or neutrophils in natural cases. Although bronchiolar lesions are often absent in natural cases, bronchiolar necrosis is described following intentional administration of 3MI.

The *differential diagnoses* for this histologic picture includes other toxins listed below as well as the disease "AIP of feedlot cattle"; post-patent forms of *Dictyocaulus viviparus* infection, for which the histologic lesions are similar but recent access to lush pasture would favor fog fever; acute infection with *Dictyocaulus* or *Ascaris suum* larvae, which generally occur in younger calves and have many eosinophils with at least a few histologically visible larvae; viral pneumonia, which may be difficult to distinguish without laboratory testing unless viral syncytia or inclusion bodies are present; anaphylaxis, which causes pulmonary edema, congestion, emphysema, and rarely eosinophil infiltration, but not hyaline membranes; and extrinsic allergic alveolitis, in which lymphocytes and granulomas form beside bronchioles and within alveolar septa. In contrast to the predominantly alveolar damage in ruminants, experimental 3MI toxicity in horses causes necrosis of club cells in the bronchioles, probably reflecting the species-dependent distribution of CYP.

4-Ipomeanol from moldy sweet potatoes induces a comparable condition in calves, of alveolar damage with or without bronchiolar injury following CYP-induced formation of a reactive intermediate. **Perilla ketone** toxicity (from perilla mint, *Perilla frutescens)* in cattle and horses follows a similar pattern, ascribed to the toxin 1-(3-furyl)4-methylpentatone. Other toxins causing alveolar damage in cattle include stinkwood *(Zieria arborescens*, a small tree in southeastern Australia), moldy garden beans, *Brassica* (turnip tops or kale), and rape. **Crofton weed** *[Ageratina (Eupatorium) adenophora]*—specifically the flowering plant—causes generalized multinodular chronic interstitial lung disease in horses; pulmonary edema, proliferation of alveolar epithelial cells, and fibroplasia are the prominent features. Similarly, horses chronically ingesting ***Crotalaria* spp. containing pyrrolizidine alkaloids** develop interstitial fibrosis with hyperplasia and dysplasia of bronchiolar and alveolar duct epithelium, with or without alveolar type II pneumocyte proliferation. **Carbolic dips**, used to prepare sheep for showing, are also reported to cause fatal pulmonary disease 1-3 days later, probably by absorption through the skin, with pulmonary lesions of hyperemia, edema, and type II pneumocyte proliferation.

Paraquat *is a highly toxic herbicide that can cause acute alveolar damage* if ingested. In veterinary medicine, acute lung injury has been reported in cattle, sheep, pigs, and dogs following ingestion of foodstuffs contaminated with the herbicide. Paraquat is taken up by type I and II pneumocytes and club cells and induces alveolar injury through reduction-oxidation (redox) cycling, depleting the cells of NADPH and glutathione, which results in uncontrolled generation of superoxide anion and oxidant injury. Cases of malicious poisoning are more likely to cause fulminant pulmonary edema and hemorrhage because of the high dosage; in accidental poisonings, there is more often time for hyperplasia of alveolar type II cells and fibroplasia to be superimposed on the earlier exudative changes. In the acute intoxication with survival up to 2-3 days, the lungs are heavy, dark, and rubbery, and the alveolar spaces are filled with fluid and blood with much fluid in the hilar connective tissue. Hyaline membranes are present in alveolar ducts, and bronchiolar necrosis in some reports. With longer survival, profuse fibroplasia and type II pneumocyte proliferation thicken the alveolar septa. Extrapulmonary lesions are often present and include patchy necrosis of the adrenal zona glomerulosa and of renal tubular epithelium.

Other toxins cause pulmonary vascular disease. **Fumonisin B1**, a mycotoxin usually associated with corn, causes massive interlobular pulmonary edema and hydrothorax as well as pancreatic necrosis in pigs. The toxin causes damage to alveolar endothelial cells associated with altered sphingolipid metabolism. Similarly, poisoning by the rodenticide **α-naphthylthiourea** causes respiratory distress resulting from pulmonary edema and pleural effusion. Pulmonary vascular lesions are also produced in horses, pigs, sheep, and cattle by **pyrrolizidine alkaloids** *(Crotalaria, Trichodesma, Senecio)*; the resulting vascular lesions are described in the Pulmonary Vascular Disease section. ***Pimelea* sp.** (St. George disease), which contains simplexin and dihydroxycoumarin glycoside toxins, is another toxic cause of pulmonary hypertension in cattle and horses in Australia. Sodium selenite and selenomethionine, found in **selenium-accumulator plants** ingested by lambs, cause mainly myocardial necrosis but also pulmonary edema and hemorrhage resulting from vasculitis of the alveolar septa.

Drug reactions are important causes of acute or chronic pulmonary injury in humans, manifesting as pulmonary edema, asthma-like disease, bronchiolar necrosis, diffuse alveolar damage, eosinophilic pneumonia, pulmonary vascular disease with hemorrhage, or pleural effusion. Pulmonary drug reactions are poorly described and apparently rare in domestic animals. ***CCNU, a nitrosourea chemotherapeutic*** used for treatment of lymphoma, causes chronic lung injury with interstitial fibrosis, smooth muscle hyperplasia, and type II pneumocyte hyperplasia.

Pneumoconiosis—*lung disease ensuing from inhalation and retention of inorganic dusts*—is uncommon in animals because they lack occupational exposures that are the basis for most human cases. In general, inorganic dusts are engulfed by and persist within macrophages, which secrete mediators that induce the *characteristic fibrosis and granulomatous inflammation*. Mild pulmonary **anthracosis** is a common incidental finding in city-dwelling animals or those cohabiting with cigarette smokers, in which carbon particles accrue within macrophages adjacent to airway bifurcations including the wall of terminal bronchioles. In **asbestosis**, *asbestos (ferruginous) bodies* (i.e., asbestos fibers coated with ferritin and hemosiderin that are linear with a beaded appearance and globose ends) are present within granulomatous and fibrosing lung lesions. The ability to form ferruginous bodies varies by species, thus asbestos-related lung disease in some animals can be difficult to diagnose. Sheep have been used as an experimental model of the disease, but natural cases are rare. Asbestos-associated mesothelioma seems not to occur in domestic animals.

Silicosis is caused by inhalation of crystalline silica particles ($Si0_2$ tetrahedra) that are largely derived from quartz and thus most common in people who work with quartz-bearing stone or rocks. **Silicate pneumoconiosis** in horses and rarely dogs results from inhalation of silicates, formed when silicon dioxide combines with magnesium, calcium, aluminum, or other cations. Silica and silicates are common minerals from the earth's crust. In horses, silicate pneumoconiosis causes weight loss, exercise intolerance, and dyspnea and has been associated with an osteoporosis-like bone fragility syndrome. Miliary firm or gritty lesions are distributed throughout the lung. Microscopically, the lesions are mainly centered on bronchioles or less frequently target the interlobular septa and consist of multifocal fibrosis with granulomatous inflammation, often with necrosis and mineralization in the centers. Clear, brown or black birefringent crystals are indistinctly visible in the cytoplasm of the macrophages. These are sometimes birefringent, can usually be highlighted by acid-fast stains, and are identified by X-ray spectroscopy. The association of silicate particles with the characteristic granulomatous inflammation suggests a causal relationship.

INFECTIOUS RESPIRATORY DISEASES OF PIGS

Viral diseases

Porcine reproductive and respiratory syndrome

PRRS was first identified in the late 1980s. It is an *important cause of reproductive failure and interstitial pneumonia*, and a predisposing factor for bacterial pneumonia and septicemia. The disease varies greatly in severity and clinicopathologic presentation depending on the strain of the PRRSV, the age of pigs affected, the level and distribution of immunity within the herd, and the presence of other pathogens.

On initial exposure, infection spreads slowly through a naive herd and causes a variety of clinical presentations: anorexia and lethargy of all age groups; reproductive failure, such as late-term abortion, stillbirth, mummified fetuses, or weak-born piglets; interstitial pneumonia causing fatal hyperpnea, dyspnea, and lethargy in suckling pigs infected in utero or in the neonatal period; and respiratory disease in weaned and grower-finisher pigs.

Viral infection often persists and circulates within the herd indefinitely, the result of prolonged viral shedding from individual animals and continuous entry of naive animals. The disease in endemically infected herds is highly variable. Some herds have endemic respiratory disease or a failure to thrive in nursery and grower-finisher pigs, or a PRRSV-induced increase in susceptibility to bacterial pneumonia and septicemia, or continuing losses as a result of abortion in gilts or dyspnea in neonatal or weaned pigs. Many herds have stable infections in which virus continues to circulate but does not cause clinical disease, and there is persistent absence of viremia in weaning-age pigs. PRRS in these herds can become unstable from a decline in immunity or incursion of a new strain of PRRSV.

PRRSV (*Arteriviridae*, Species *Betaarterivirus europensis* and *Betaarterivirus americense*, the Euopean and North American genotypes) is an enveloped, 50-65 nm diameter, positive-sense, single-stranded RNA virus. The viral genome includes 8 open-reading frames (ORFs): ORF 1a and 1b encode proteins necessary for replication and transcription, ORFs 2-4 encode structural glycoproteins of uncertain function, ORF 5 encodes an envelope glycoprotein, ORF 6 encodes the integral membrane protein M, and ORF 7 encodes the nucleocapsid protein N.

Genomic variability is an important feature of PRRSV and may be attributed to the high mutation rate associated with the error-prone RNA polymerase and perhaps recombination between viral strains in coinfections. As a result, PRRSV isolates can be considered as low virulence verus virulent or high virulent. In general, virulent or high-virulent strains cause >20% mortality, disease in various age groups, prolonged high fever, severe clinical signs, extensive interstitial pneumonia and often concurrent bacterial bronchopneumonia or septicemia, higher diversity of virus-infected cells (e.g., brain, liver, heart, intestine; rather than only lung and lymphoid tissues), greater replication of virus within tissues, higher levels of viremia, and higher levels of inflammatory cytokines including IFNγ, increased regulated cell death in lymphoid tissues, and increased susceptibility to secondary bacterial infections. Mortality is not the only factor defining virulent strains because coinfections and other herd factors contribute to disease severity in a herd. Differences in virulence have not been shown to be correlated with simple alterations in specific genes; rather, the virulence of particular strains is apparently determined by a combined effect of many genetic differences. Differences between virulent and high-virulent strains are not well defined.

Modified-live virus vaccine strains may rarely cause disease. Vaccine strains of the virus can infect in-contact animals and persist in herds, but do not commonly cause clinical disease. However, as these vaccine strains circulate in swine herds, *mutation to a less attenuated form of the virus may result in disease caused by vaccine-derived strains*. Extralabel intranasal administration of modified-live PRRSV vaccine has induced clinical signs and lesions typical of PRRS.

The common mode of *transmission* of PRRSV is direct nasal, oral, or coital contact with saliva, oropharyngeal mucus, urine, semen, serum, mammary secretions, or perhaps feces of infected pigs. Transmission of PRRSV by artificial insemination has been documented, and transmission by contamination of pharmaceutical preparations or needles with infected serum is a potential risk. Transmission by fomites may occur, but because the enveloped virus is rapidly inactivated in most environmental conditions, disinfection procedures should be effective. Aerosol transmission is apparently of limited importance, but can occur at low frequency over short distances.

The pathogenesis of PRRS centers on infection of macrophages at the site of nasal, tonsillar, or pulmonary infection, extension to associated lymphoid tissue, rapid viremia, and infection of macrophages throughout the body. Following experimental intranasal challenge, viral antigen is expressed within 12 hours of infection in nasal and tonsillar macrophages and epithelium, pulmonary alveolar, intravascular, and interstitial macrophages, bronchiolar epithelium, and endothelial cells of pulmonary arterioles. Viremia occurs rapidly, in some cases within 12 hours of infection, and leads to widespread infection of monocytes and tissue macrophages. Viral antigen may be detected in pulmonary alveolar macrophages, myocardial macrophages and endothelium, follicular macrophages and dendritic cells in lymph nodes, interdigitating cells in the thymus, macrophages and dendritic cells in the spleen and intestinal lymphoid follicles, and macrophages in hepatic sinusoids, adrenal gland, interstitium of the kidney, and choroid plexus.

Persistent infection is a key feature of PRRSV. Virus has been detected in serum for at least 4 weeks; in nasal mucosa, pulmonary macrophages, and spleen for 4 weeks; and in oropharyngeal mucosa for up to 22 weeks after infection. Animals remain infectious for in-contact naive pigs for at least 22 weeks after infection. Persistent infections are of epidemiologic importance in the maintenance of PRRSV infection in endemically infected herds. Suppression of type I interferon responses by several of the viral nonstructural proteins is a proposed mechanism of viral persistence, as well as manipulation of cellular cytokine responses, induction of autophagy, activation of unfolded protein responses, and genomic recombination of viral RNA. Following experimental PRRSV infection, serum antibody detectable by ELISA and virus-neutralizing antibody are first detectable at 7-14 days and 9-28 days after infection, peak at 5 weeks and 10 weeks, and remain detectable for 46 weeks and over 1 year, respectively. Antibody responses are directed against all proteins encoded by ORFs 2-7; the products of ORF 3, 4, and 5 may represent protective epitopes.

Infection with PRRSV impairs host defenses and increases susceptibility to infection with *Streptococcus suis, Glaesserella parasuis. Salmonella* Choleraesuis, and other opportunistic pathogens. Experiments to investigate this effect have been conflicting, and the ability of PRRSV to predispose to other agents is probably dependent on the viral and bacterial strains examined and on the specific experimental conditions. The ability of PRRSV to infect and reduce the function of pulmonary intravascular macrophages is one mechanism whereby PRRSV predisposes to septicemia; a similar impairment of alveolar macrophage functions—including phagocytosis, oxidative burst, and cytokine secretion—may reduce lung defenses against bacterial bronchopneumonia. Subclinical or clinical infection with *Mesomycoplasma hyopneumoniae* exacerbates the clinical signs and lesions of PRRS, possibly because mycoplasma-induced proliferation and activation of macrophages enhances the replication or persistence of PRRSV. In contrast, infection with PRRSV has little effect on the severity of mycoplasmal lesions. This finding is of clinical importance because control of *M. hyopneumoniae* is one strategy for minimizing the effect of PRRSV in endemically infected herds. The effect of PRRSV infection on immune responses to other pathogens has not been fully addressed, but a state of generalized immunosuppression is not a likely feature of PRRS.

The major **lesions** *of the postnatal form of PRRS include interstitial pneumonia, generalized lymphadenopathy, and lymphocytic infiltrates in various organs*. Gross lung lesions vary from undetectable to affecting the entire lung and tend to be most striking in younger age groups. The lungs fail to collapse when the diaphragm is incised, occasionally retain impressions of the ribs, and have generalized, patchy, lobular, or diffuse distribution of lesions. Affected areas of the lung are discolored tan or red and have a firm texture reminiscent of thymus, which contrasts with the crisp consolidation of bacterial pneumonia (Fig. 5-45). A cut section reveals separation of lobules and oozing of edema fluid. In pigs that develop bacterial bronchopneumonia secondary to PRRS, lesions of cranioventral consolidation may be superimposed on the diffuse interstitial pneumonia. In these cases, the lesions of PRRS may be subtle, yet play a critical role in the development of pneumonia in the herd. Lymph nodes throughout the body—most notably the bronchial, mediastinal, cervical, and inguinal nodes—are enlarged, white or tan, solid, and rarely contain clear cavitations on cut section. Periocular and subcutaneous edema, pulmonary infarcts, myocardial necrosis, renal petechiae, and serous effusions into body cavities are variable findings. Characteristic lesions of virulent (vs. low-virulence) PRRSV strains include pleuritis, widespread petechiae, thymic atrophy, lymphadenopathy, intestinal ulcers, and body cavity effusions (in addition to the interstitial pneumonia found with all strains), some of which reflect the more frequent bronchopneumonia, pleuropneumonia, and septicemia from secondary bacterial pathogens.

Histologic *lung lesions are of interstitial pneumonia*. Alveolar septa are thickened by infiltrates of lymphocytes and macrophages (see Fig. 5-45). This feature is easily obscured by atelectasis in routinely prepared samples, but can usually be confirmed by searching for areas of lung in which alveoli are not collapsed. Alveoli contain a cellular infiltrate of macrophages, lymphocytes, and fewer neutrophils, and scattered clusters of alveoli are filled with cells with pyknotic nuclei or

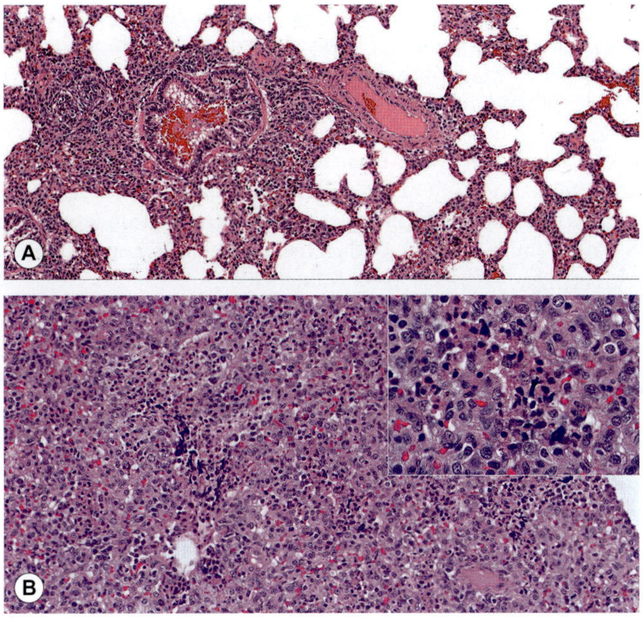

Figure 5-45 Porcine reproductive and respiratory syndrome. A. Diffuse thickening of alveolar septa by mononuclear cells, and a normal bronchiole. Porcine circovirus 2 or septicemia can cause similar lesions. **B.** Characteristic clusters of apoptotic macrophages (inset) in alveoli, in an area of atelectasis.

free chromatin. *Clusters of dead/apoptotic alveolar macrophages and free chromatin are highly suggestive of PRRS.* In addition to alveolar macrophages, PRRSV also causes apoptosis of mononuclear cells in alveolar septa. Type II pneumocytes are increased in number, but may or may not form a continuous layer of cuboidal epithelium lining the alveolus. Bronchiolar epithelium is not affected by PRRSV, and a finding of bronchiolar necrosis should incite a search for an alternative or additional diagnosis.

Histologic examination of lymph nodes, tonsils, and spleens of pigs with PRRS may reveal *follicular and paracortical hyperplasia, and apoptosis of follicular lymphocytes.* Multinucleate cells, probably of histiocytic origin, may be present. Although this lesion is also common in porcine circovirus 2 infection, it has been described in PRRSV-infected pigs that have no evidence of PCV2 infection.

Perivascular infiltrates of lymphocytes, macrophages, and plasma cells form in many organs in PRRS. Commonly affected sites include the nasal mucosa, heart, kidney, and brain. Severe neurologic disease occasionally occurs in association with other manifestations of PRRS, possibly related to the infecting viral strain, and lesions in the central nervous system include lymphocytic meningoencephalitis, lymphocytic perivascular cuffs, and focal gliosis. PRRSV may cause *vasculitis* in the lung and other organs, manifesting as necrosis of the walls of large and small blood vessels in addition to perivascular and mural infiltrates of lymphocytes and plasma cells.

Aborted fetuses usually lack gross or histologic lesions, and, when present, the lesions are often not specific for PRRSV. Infection may progress from one fetus to another, resulting in live, stillborn, and mummified fetuses in the same litter. Fetal lesions that suggest PRRS include segmental or diffuse hemorrhage of the umbilical cord caused by fibrinoid necrosis and neutrophilic inflammation of the umbilical artery, mild interstitial pneumonia, pulmonary arteritis, lymphocytic myocarditis and encephalitis, and retroperitoneal and mesocolonic edema.

Diffusely firm lungs and histologic lesions of interstitial pneumonia are common findings at autopsy. In addition to PRRS, *a major differential diagnosis is septicemia.* Lesions of lymphadenopathy and mild proliferation of type II pneumocytes favor a diagnosis of PRRS, but differentiation requires ancillary testing. PCV2 may cause similar interstitial pneumonia, but granulomatous infiltrates and inclusion bodies may also be present in lymph nodes and intestinal lymphoid follicles. Proliferative and necrotizing pneumonia causes an alveolar lesion similar to PRRS, but bronchiolar necrosis is a feature of this disease that is absent in PRRS.

PCR and immunohistochemistry are mainstays for the **detection** of PRRSV in tissue specimens. In addition to tissue samples, PCR assays are performed on serum, oral fluids obtained with cotton ropes, or semen. Serology is useful on a herd level to identify prior exposure to PRRSV in unvaccinated herds. Immunohistochemistry on formalin-fixed paraffin-embedded sections of the lung and tonsil is an economical approach to diagnosis, but because these assays are less sensitive than PCR, various sections should be examined. Virus isolation on chilled or frozen samples of lung, lymphoid tissues, serum, EDTA-treated blood, or pulmonary alveolar macrophages is a highly sensitive but slow method of diagnosis.

Results of detection assays must be interpreted with caution in herds vaccinated with modified-live viruses because vaccine strains of PRRSV may circulate and persist in these herds and cause positive tests. Molecular analyses assist in differentiating field and vaccine strains of virus in vaccinated herds. Sequence variation in ORF 5 and 7 genes is commonly used to monitor patterns of PRRSV infection in large herds and to differentiate vaccine strains from some field strains. However, these gene sequences in vaccine strains may change to an intermediate pattern as they circulate in herds.

Obtaining a diagnosis of PRRS in aborted fetuses can be frustrating because lesions are usually absent or nonspecific and the agent often cannot be identified. PCR assays on fetal lung and lymphoid tissue and identification of antibody to PRRSV in precolostral sera can be used, but the low diagnostic rate remains a problem considering the importance of reproductive failure in infected swine herds.

Influenza

Orthomyxoviruses are pleomorphic, spherical to filamentous, 80-120 nm viruses containing negative-sense single-stranded RNA. Transcription of viral genes occurs in the nucleus, viral proteins are produced in the cytoplasm, and virions bud from the plasma membrane. Three genera of orthomyxoviruses are described based on variation of the nucleocapsid proteins: 1) *Alphainfluenzavirus* (formerly influenza A) causes influenza in humans, aquatic and domestic birds, pigs, horses, and other species; 2) *Betainfluenzavirus* (influenza B) is isolated from humans and seals; 3) *Deltainfluenzavirus* (influenza D) infects cattle, pigs, and others; and 4) *Gammainfluenzavirus* (influenza C) is rare and infects humans, pigs, cattle, and dogs. Orthomyxoviruses readily develop genomic variants, as a result of *genetic drift* caused by point mutations and *genetic shift* caused by recombination of genomic segments. *Identification of viral strains is based on antigenic variation of the 15 hemagglutinin (H) and 9 neuraminidase (N) envelope glycoproteins,* which mediate virus entry into cells and release of virus from infected cells, respectively. Analysis of viral strains is of practical importance in epidemiologic tracking of outbreaks and changing disease patterns, and to ensure that vaccine strains are representative of those in the field to ensure protective immunity.

Influenza viruses are usually host specific, and although several strains are known to cross species barriers, transmission rates are generally low and most foreign strains are not maintained in the population. In general, alphainfluenza viruses of pigs rarely infect humans, and those that do are termed variant influenza viruses (e.g., H1N2v). Although the direct zoonotic potential is of only moderate consequence, this phenomenon is important in the evolution of new viral strains. *Given that pigs possess cell-surface receptors for both avian and human viral strains, pigs may act as hosts for reassortment among avian, porcine, and human strains of influenza viruses, with the potential for human pandemics resulting from the introduction of novel pathogenic strains into immunologically naive human populations*. It is now recognized that such reassortment can also occur in other species.

Influenza viruses are transmitted by aerosol or by contact with secretions. Infection is usually restricted to the respiratory tract, although myocarditis, myositis, and encephalitis are more frequent in carnivores and occasionally seen in horses and humans. Such nonrespiratory lesions may be a consequence of viremia, or an effect of a "cytokine storm" with dysregulation of cytokine production in the respiratory tissues.

Influenza is an important respiratory disease of pigs, manifesting as rapidly spreading outbreaks of severe nonfatal disease or endemically as part of the porcine respiratory disease complex. Outbreaks are most common in the winter in cool climates, or late summer in warm climates. Disease severity may be enhanced by stresses, seasonal change in climate, PRRSV infection, or concurrent disease. Vaccination may enhance the disease that results from subsequent challenge with heterologous strains of the virus. Outbreaks have a characteristic clinical presentation: the disease appears acutely and spreads rapidly to affect all ages of pigs, and despite severe clinical signs of coughing, fever, and stiffness, most pigs recover in 5-14 days and the mortality rate is low. Endemic disease is also common, in which pigs develop bacterial bronchopneumonia secondary to subclinical infection with influenza virus, but this clinical picture is not specific for influenza and differentiation from other causes of porcine respiratory disease complex requires laboratory testing.

Identification of alphainfluenzavirus subtypes is important because there is limited cross-protection between subtypes; vaccines must be representative of circulating field strains. Subtypes H1N1, H3N2, and H1N2 are the common alphainfluenzaviruses of swine in North America, but infection of pigs is documented with many other subtypes, including reassortants of swine, avian, and human viruses. SIV is transmitted by infected droplets, aerosol, or contact with infected secretions. After experimental infection, serum antibody titers are detectable in many pigs by 7 days and peak 2-3 weeks after infection, and mucosal IgA and IgG are maximal at 1 and 4 weeks after infection, respectively. Pigs shed virus for 5-7 days after infection, although viral antigen is often cleared from the lung in as little as 72 hours after infection. Virus infection is probably maintained in swine populations by continuous infection of naive pigs, given that there is no evidence of a long-term carrier state or significant wildlife vector.

The **gross lesions** of influenza in pigs include a *cranioventral lobular distribution of atelectasis*, which is often sharply demarcated from normal lung tissue (eFig. 5-62). Affected lobules are red, firm, and collapsed. Adjacent lobules are occasionally emphysematous. Generalized pulmonary edema may occur. Mediastinal and bronchial lymph nodes are enlarged and edematous, but usually not congested. The mucosa of the trachea and bronchi is often hyperemic and edematous. In most fatal cases, secondary bacterial bronchopneumonia obscures the gross lesions of influenza.

The **histologic lesions** reflect *necrosis of airway epithelium* and, to a lesser extent, alveolar epithelium, and include attenuation of bronchiolar epithelial cells, necrotic debris and neutrophils in bronchiolar lumens, atelectasis, and peribronchiolar, perivascular, and interstitial infiltrates of lymphocytes and plasma cells (Fig. 5-46). Vacuolation of bronchial and bronchiolar epithelial cells with loss of cilia occurs by 8 hours after experimental infection. By 24 hours, there is necrosis of bronchiolar and bronchial epithelial cells, and accumulation of sloughed necrotic cells in the lumen. Airway lumens—and to a lesser extent alveoli—contain neutrophils, and alveoli are atelectatic and edematous. Mononuclear cell infiltration occurs by 48 hours after infection. Alveolar injury, manifesting as exudation of neutrophils and scant fibrin with thickening of alveolar septa, is described in experimental cases at 48 hours after infection, but is often inapparent in pigs experiencing natural disease, or obscured by bacterial pneumonia. Later lesions include hyperplasia of airway epithelium as regeneration occurs, and peribronchiolar and perivascular aggregation of lymphocytes and plasma cells as immune responses develop. Infection is, in most cases, restricted to the respiratory tract and associated lymph nodes, although viremia has been described infrequently in neonates.

The **diagnosis** of influenza is suggested by the characteristic clinical signs of severe rapidly spreading disease with high morbidity and low mortality and by the histologic lesions of necrotizing bronchiolitis with targeting of larger rather than terminal bronchioles by the neutrophil infiltrate (see Fig. 5-46). *Differential diagnoses* for bronchiolar necrosis include porcine circovirus 2 infection, proliferative and necrotizing pneumonia, pseudorabies, Nipah virus infection, and

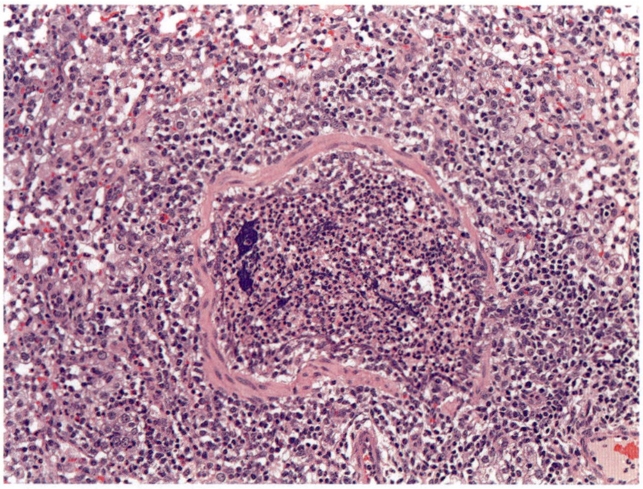

Figure 5-46 Influenza in a pig. A large bronchiole has attenuation of bronchiolar epithelium, with neutrophils and chromatin debris in the lumen, and is surrounded by lymphocytes.

airway injury caused by inhaled toxic gases. The diagnosis is confirmed by PCR testing of fresh lung tissue, antigen-detection ELISA on nasal or bronchial swabs, or immunohistochemistry on fixed tissues using monoclonal antibodies to conserved type A nucleoproteins. Initial PCR testing can target the conserved matrix gene, followed by subtype-specific testing or sequencing of the hemagglutinin and neuraminidase genes, or whole-genome sequencing. Virus isolation using embryonated eggs or cell lines can be useful for full characterization. Sample selection is critical for the diagnosis of influenza. Viral titers are highest 24 hours after infection, before gross lesions are obvious, and virus often cannot be identified by 72 hours after infection. Consequently, *selecting tissue from the cranioventral areas of the lung, from many pigs early in the course of the disease, is critical for both histologic and virologic diagnosis*. Pigs with a high fever and clear nasal discharge are the most suitable subjects for diagnostic investigation. The transient nature of the infection may complicate an investigation of the role of influenza in swine herds with endemic respiratory disease. In these cases, herd-level serology may be useful. Herd-level PCR testing is of value, using nasal swabs or oral fluids collected with cotton ropes.

Porcine circovirus

Porcine circoviruses (*Circoviridae, Circovirus*) are 17-nm, nonenveloped viruses that contain circular single-stranded DNA. Porcine circovirus 1 (PCV1) is a nonpathogenic virus that was discovered as a cell culture contaminant. Porcine circovirus 2 is pathogenic and was first isolated in 1997 from pigs with a novel disease, *postweaning multisystemic wasting syndrome*. This and other PCV2-associated diseases can be considered as *PCV2 systemic disease* (**PCV2-SD**) or *PVC2 lung disease* (**PCV2-LD**). Reasons that some pigs develop only lung disease versus systemic disease are unknown. Three genogroups—2a, 2b, and 2c—are recognized. Since its original identification in 2004, PCV2b has become the predominant genogroup, but the associated spectrum of lesions appears comparable among the 3 genogroups.

PCV2-disease was originally described in high-health herds, but it occurs now in herds infected with PRRSV or other pathogens. *Serum antibody to PCV2 is widespread in swine herds, and PCV2 infection is common in herds with no clinical evidence of PCV2-disease*. PCV2-disease usually progresses slowly within the herd, with most cases developing in 5-12-week-old pigs. Morbidity is typically 5-10% but may be up to 20%, and most affected animals die or are euthanized. Pigs with PCV2-disease lose weight or gain poorly and have a variable combination of tachypnea, respiratory distress, diarrhea, pallor, and jaundice. Although uncommon, the finding of jaundice in pigs should suggest a diagnosis of PCV2-SD.

Porcine circoviral antigen and nucleic acid are most consistently present in the cytoplasm of monocytes, macrophages, and dendritic cells throughout the body, and less often in the nuclei and cytoplasm of epithelial cells in bronchioles, pulmonary alveoli, liver, renal tubules, intestine, stomach, and pancreas. Vascular smooth muscle and endothelial cells occasionally express circoviral antigen. Transmission is poorly characterized.

Experimental infection of gnotobiotic or cesarean-derived colostrum-deprived pigs induces mild clinical signs and lesions of PCV2-disease in the absence of other demonstrable pathogens. However, coinfection with PCV2 and other pathogens, including parvovirus or PRRSV, results in more severe disease. Immunostimulation itself, either as a consequence of viral infection or vaccination, precipitates more severe disease. Thus, *activation of the immune response may encourage replication of PCV2, resulting in more severe manifestations of PCV2* disease.

PCV2-LD affects only the lung; PCV2-SD affects lymphoid tissues and often other organs including the lung. The role of PCV2 in other swine diseases remains less certain, in part because the virus can be isolated from many healthy pigs. These PCV-associated diseases include dermatitis-nephropathy syndrome, proliferative and necrotizing pneumonia, enteric disease, reproductive disease, sow abortion and mortality syndrome, acute pulmonary edema, congenital hypomyelination, and abortion with fetal myocarditis.

The spectrum of **gross lesions** and their severity are highly variable. Pigs with PCV2-SD are often thin, pale, and may be jaundiced. Lymph nodes throughout the body—particularly the inguinal, mesenteric, and bronchial nodes—are enlarged, soft, and white or gray-tan. Lung lesions, which are common, consist of interstitial pneumonia with generalized firm or rubbery texture, failure to collapse, and mottled color (Fig. 5-47A). Cranioventral bronchopneumonia is a frequent concurrent lesion. The liver may be atrophic and discolored yellow-orange. Kidneys may contain patchy pallor or obvious

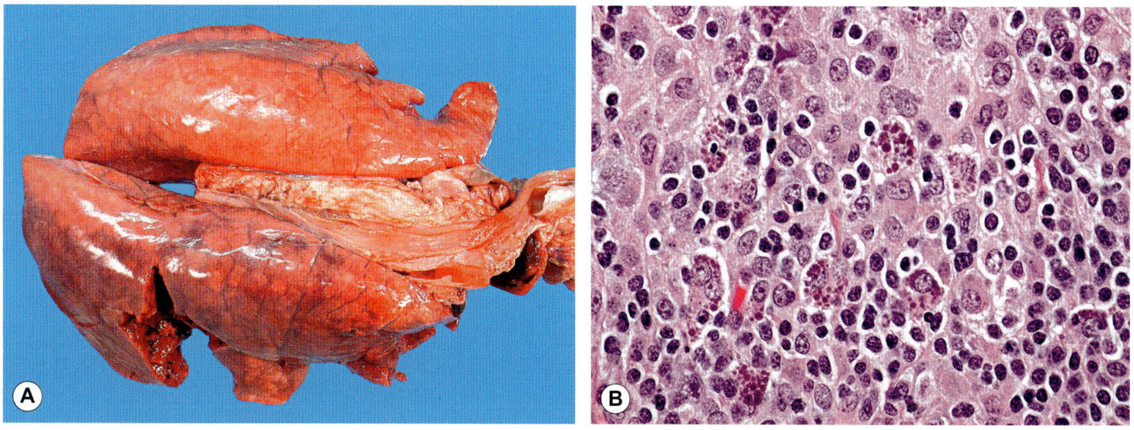

Figure 5-47 **Postweaning multisystemic wasting syndrome** caused by porcine circovirus 2. **A.** The lungs fail to collapse, are diffusely firm and heavy, and have interlobular edema. **B.** Basophilic botryoid cytoplasmic inclusion bodies in macrophages of an ileal lymphoid follicle.

white foci. Lesions resembling dermatitis-nephropathy syndrome may also occur, including swelling and edema of the kidneys, and cutaneous hemorrhages and necrosis. Infrequent lesions include splenic and cutaneous infarcts, cerebellar hemorrhages, renomegaly, and pallor, or necrotizing colitis.

The **histologic lesions** of PCV2-disease include *lymphoid depletion and granulomatous lymphadenitis, necrotizing lymphadenitis, interstitial pneumonia, enteritis, interstitial nephritis, myocarditis, meningoencephalitis, and vasculitis*. Inclusion bodies were commonly observed when the disease initially emerged in the 1990s but are inconsistent in contemporary cases. The inclusions are in macrophages, intracytoplasmic, usually multiple in a single cell, and basophilic. Inclusion bodies are most numerous and obvious in lymphoid tissues, including lymph nodes, intestinal lymphoid follicles, tonsil, splenic periarteriolar lymphoid sheaths, and thymus (see Fig. 5-47B). In these tissues, there is depletion of lymphocytes from B-cell follicles, with striking infiltration of macrophages into follicles and, to a lesser extent, T cell–rich paracortical areas. Multinucleate histiocytes may be present amid the granulomatous infiltrates. Widespread necrosis of lymphocytes in follicles is described but rare.

Histologic examination of the lungs of pigs with PCV2-SD or PCV2-LD reveals diffuse or patchy *granulomatous interstitial pneumonia*. Epithelioid macrophages, multinucleate macrophages, lymphocytes, and fewer eosinophils or neutrophils infiltrate alveolar septa and may fill the alveoli. Lymphocytes and macrophages often encircle bronchioles and blood vessels. Bronchiolar necrosis is a variable finding and may progress to obliterative bronchiolitis in chronically affected pigs. Peribronchiolar fibroplasia with relatively mild lymphocytic inflammation is suggestive of PCV2 infection.

Liver lesions are highly variable, progressing from mild aggregates of lymphocytes in portal tracts, to single-cell necrosis of hepatocytes, periacinar necrosis, or widespread hepatocellular loss with condensation of hepatic stroma. Granulomatous enteritis with multinucleate cells may be prominent in the ileum, or infrequently in the colon. Perivascular infiltrates of lymphocytes and macrophages may be present in other organs, including the kidney, myocardium, leptomeninges, pancreas, adrenal, stomach, and intestine. These lesions may be associated with renal tubular necrosis, interstitial nephritis, or necrosis of cardiac myocytes. Vasculitis, with necrosis of tunica muscularis accompanied by lymphohistiocytic infiltrates, and exudative glomerulonephritis are less common lesions. Lymphohistiocytic meningoencephalitis, with or without vasculitis, is reported.

Infection with PCV2 is usually identified using *immunohistochemistry, in situ hybridization, or PCR*. Assessing the viral load by PCR may be of value, given that the load is higher in wasting than in subclinically infected pigs. The virus may be isolated in PK15 cells, but this finds more use in research than as a diagnostic technique. Serologic assays, including indirect immunofluorescence and immunoperoxidase tests, have been developed, but the high prevalence of antibodies to PCV2 in healthy pigs limits the diagnostic usefulness of this test.

It is critical to recognize that simple detection of PCV2 infection does not in itself indicate a diagnosis of PCV2-associated disease. A **diagnosis** of PCV2-SD or PCV2-LD is mainly based on the demonstration of consistent clinical findings and gross and histologic lesions and confirmed by the demonstration of active PCV2 infection by moderate to abundant viral antigen by immunohistochemistry or nucleic acid by in situ hybridization (or for PCV2-SD, detection by $\geq 10^6$ copies per mL serum, or per 500 ng total RNA in fetal tissue by PCR). PRRS is the major differential diagnosis for lesions of interstitial pneumonia and lymphadenopathy in pigs. The following are helpful differentiating features, but *the lesions of PCV2-disease and PRRS may be difficult to distinguish, and many pigs are coinfected with PCV2 and PRRSV:*

- Numerous basophilic inclusion bodies in macrophages are a diagnostic feature of PCV2 infection and support the diagnosis of PCV2-disease.
- Clusters within alveoli of apoptotic macrophages and streaming extracellular chromatin suggest PRRSV infection.
- Bronchiolar necrosis is present in some cases of PCV2-disease (and influenza), but is not a lesion of PRRS.
- Lung lesions of PCV2-disease tend to be dominated by macrophages; lesions in PRRS are more lymphocytic, although there is much overlap in the morphology of these diseases.
- Granulomatous infiltrates and multinucleate macrophages in lymphoid organs are more typical of PCV2-disease than of PRRS, although both lesions may be present in PRRS.

PCV3 and PCV4 are genomically distinct viruses that have had an uncertain association with disease because they are also detected in healthy pigs, coinfections may be present, and experimental infections have not fully replicated the associated diseases. They have been mainly associated with presentations comparable to PCV2, including stillbirths and mummification, perinatal mortality, or failure to thrive, and with histologic lesions of myocarditis or myocardial fibrosis, epicarditis, interstitial pneumonia, encephalitis, infiltrates of perivascular lymphocytes and plasma cells in the kidney, liver, spleen, and lymph node, porcine dermatitis nephropathy syndrome, granulomatous lymphadenitis, and systemic vasculitis.

Proliferative and necrotizing pneumonia

Proliferative and necrotizing pneumonia is a severe acute disease of weaner and grower pigs. Affected animals have acute onset of severe dyspnea, tachypnea, and fever. Gross lesions usually affect the entire lung, but may be restricted to the cranial and middle lobes. Lung lesions include remarkably increased firmness, failure to collapse, reddening, and edema. Generalized lymphadenopathy is usually present. Histologically, alveoli are edematous, contain macrophages and abundant necrotic cellular debris, and are lined by cuboidal type II pneumocytes. Alveolar septa are thickened by mononuclear cell infiltrates (see eFig. 5-54). Although many of these lesions may be present in severe cases of PRRS, *bronchiolar necrosis is often present in proliferative and necrotizing pneumonia but absent in PRRS*.

The understanding of the cause of this lesion is made difficult by the presence of various viruses. When the lesion was first reported in the early 1990s, it was associated with an H1N1 influenza virus that was genetically and antigenically distinct from common North American alphainfluenzavirus isolates of swine. Later publications associated proliferative and necrotizing pneumonia with PRRSV infection, porcine circovirus 2, and H3N2 influenza virus. It remains uncertain whether this lesion is caused by particular strains of PRRSV or by combined infection with several agents, or if it represents a pattern of reaction shared by more than one pathogen.

Porcine respiratory coronavirus

Porcine respiratory coronavirus (PRCoV; *Coronaviridae, Alphacoronavirus suis*) is a minimally pathogenic virus that arose in the mid-1980s by deletion and point mutation of the transmissible gastroenteritis virus genome. European and American isolates of PRCoV differ, and apparently developed independently from TGEV. Following experimental challenge, neonatal pigs develop viremia and respiratory infection, whereas in 5-week-old pigs, viral antigen is limited to the respiratory tract, particularly alveolar and bronchiolar epithelial cells and alveolar macrophages. Lesions in naturally infected pigs are not described. In experimental cases, there is necrosis of bronchiolar epithelium, mild proliferation of type II pneumocytes, mononuclear cell infiltrates in alveolar septa, and lymphocytes and macrophages in alveoli. Most field cases are subclinical, although coinfection with *Bordetella* or PRRSV appears to exacerbate the disease. The major importance is that *antibodies to PRCoV cross-react with those to TGEV, leading to false-positive serologic tests in swine herds that are expected to be free of TGEV*. Diagnosis is based on isolation of the virus or indirect fluorescent antibody tests. Virus neutralization tests and some ELISAs do not differentiate PRCoV from TGEV antibodies, but newer blocking ELISAs do differentiate these coronaviruses.

Inclusion body rhinitis

Suid betaherpesvirus 2 (porcine cytomegalovirus; **SuBHV2**, PCMV; *Orthoherpesviridae, Roseolovirus suidbeta2*) infections are ubiquitous and occur throughout the world, but clinical disease is much less frequent. *Inclusion body rhinitis is typically an acute-to-subacute disease of 3-5-week-old suckling piglets*. Piglets have fever, sneezing, catarrhal nasal exudate, shivering, and occasional dyspnea. Morbidity is high and mortality is low unless secondary bacterial infections develop. *Systemic* cytomegalovirus infections usually affect piglets <3-weeks-old. Such animals may be found dead without premonitory signs or exhibit sneezing, lethargy, and anorexia, subcutaneous edema of the jaw and tarsal joints, and dyspnea. Infection of naive pregnant sows induces mild lethargy, anorexia, and delivery of stillborn or weak piglets.

Piglets commonly shed the virus soon after weaning at 3 weeks of age, suggesting that infection is usually acquired by contact with nasal secretions of infected cohorts. Other pigs, particularly those that develop generalized disease, are probably infected from the sow in the neonatal period. SuBHV2 replicates in nasal submucosal and lacrimal glands. Viremia develops 5-14 days after infection, depending on the age of the pig, and leads to infection of epithelial cells in renal tubules, liver, duodenum, and elsewhere. Pulmonary alveolar and splenic macrophages may be additional sites of viral replication. Virus is shed in nasal and ocular secretions, in the urine, and in vaginal secretions of sows.

Gross lesions in pigs infected with cytomegalovirus are usually only seen in piglets <3-weeks-old with generalized disease, and may include catarrhal rhinitis, hydrothorax, hydropericardium, pulmonary and subcutaneous edema, and renal petechiae. **Histologically**, *large 8-12 μm basophilic intranuclear inclusion bodies* (INIBs) are numerous in the epithelial cells of the nasal mucosal glands and their ducts (Fig. 5-48). Affected glands are not diffusely distributed but tend to occur in irregular clusters. As the inclusion forms, cytomegaly and karyomegaly develop. The nuclear membrane becomes indistinct, the inclusions appear as blue-gray smears, and the necrotic epithelium sloughs into the lumen. The developing immune response incites a lymphocytic

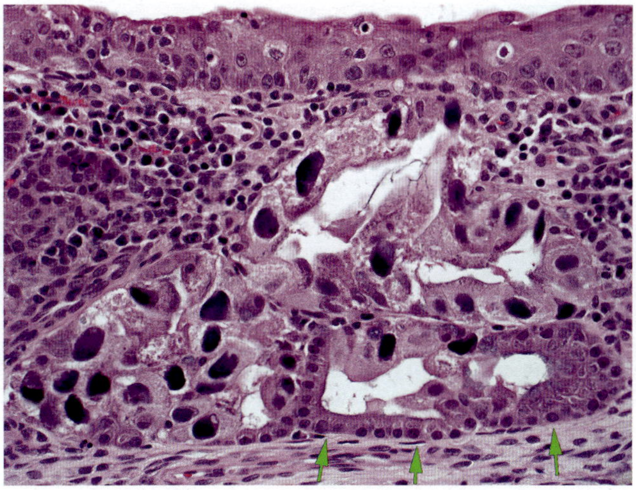

Figure 5-48 Inclusion body rhinitis in a pig. Cytomegaly of affected epithelial cells in nasal glands with large homogeneous smudgy basophilic inclusions that completely fill the nucleus. Contrast to the normal glandular epithelium (arrows). The lamina propria is diffusely infiltrated by lymphocytes, and the surface epithelium (top) is disordered.

infiltrate in the lamina propria, macrophages and lymphocytes cluster within degenerating glands, and there is squamous metaplasia of the surface epithelium.

Systemic lesions develop following viremia, with INIBs in epithelial cells of renal tubules and glomeruli; lacrimal and salivary glands; and less commonly in hepatocytes and sinusoidal lining cells, adrenal gland, esophageal glands, lymph nodes, spleen, renal medulla, lung, and elsewhere. *Inclusions are most numerous in epithelium but also occur in macrophages and endothelial cells;* this vascular disease accounts for the petechiation and edema. Inclusion bodies are often accompanied by cytomegaly, lymphocytic infiltrates, and occasionally focal necrosis. Focal gliosis with INIBs in scattered glial cells occurs throughout the central nervous system. The viremic phase may last for 2-3 weeks, and is followed by persistent infection in pulmonary macrophages.

Inclusion bodies, cytomegaly, and karyomegaly are pathognomonic when present. Adenovirus is the only viral agent likely to cause similarly large basophilic INIBs, but adenovirus does not induce cytomegaly and is usually restricted to the intestinal epithelium in pigs. The intranuclear inclusions of pseudorabies are eosinophilic, less obvious than those of cytomegalovirus, focal necrosis is more prominent, and lesions are most prominent in the brain, respiratory tract, and lymphoid tissue. Confirmation of cytomegalovirus infection may be achieved by electron microscopy to search for herpesviral particles, or by virus isolation, immunofluorescence, or PCR on nasal scrapings, lung wash cells, or kidney homogenates.

Pseudorabies

Pseudorabies (Aujeszky disease), caused by suid alphaherpesvirus 1 (**SuAHV1**; *Orthoherpesviridae, Varicellovirus suidalpha1*), is described in more detail in Vol. 1, Nervous System, because neurologic signs predominate in most cases of pseudorabies in young pigs. However, *certain strains of SuAHV1 tend to cause respiratory disease*, particularly following aerosol exposure of older pigs. The respiratory form is typified by high morbidity and low mortality, unless secondary bacterial pneumonia develops. Affected pigs are depressed, febrile, and have episodes of sneezing, coughing, and dyspnea. Gross lesions in the upper respiratory tract are most common and include necrotizing rhinitis and laryngotracheitis, with foci of necrosis in the tonsils. Lung lesions are less consistent, but patchy areas of reddening and consolidation may be scattered throughout the lung, or target the cranioventral lung. Histologically, there is necrosis and sloughing of bronchial and bronchiolar epithelium, *with frequent intranuclear eosinophilic or faintly basophilic inclusions* in the early stages of disease. Alveolar lesions include multifocal necrosis, sloughing of necrotic alveolar epithelium, fibrinous exudate in alveoli, hemorrhage, infrequent inclusion bodies, and infiltration of lymphocytes, macrophages, and fewer plasma cells and neutrophils. Experimentally, necrotizing lesions develop within 3-6 days of infection, infiltration of lymphocytes is prominent by days 5-8, and repair occurs during days 6-10.

Nipah virus

Nipah virus emerged as an epidemic cause of nervous and respiratory disease in pigs and humans in Malaysia in 1998 and 1999 and in humans in Bangladesh in 2004. The disease also affects dogs and cats; horses and goats develop an antibody response. Nipah and Hendra viruses are the lone members of the genus *Henipavirus* (*Paramyxoviridae*). *Pteropus* fruit bats (flying foxes) are the reservoir and major source of infection; pigs are considered a major source of infection for humans and other pigs; human-to-human transmission appears to be rare.

Gross lesions are nonspecific, but *the characteristic histologic findings are lymphocytic and/or fibrinoid vasculitis; lymphoid necrosis; syncytial cells within lymphoid tissues, endothelium, and perivascular cells; and eosinophilic intracytoplasmic inclusion bodies*. The lesions include lymphocytic meningitis and, to a lesser extent, encephalitis that is present throughout the brain but most severe in the olfactory bulb; necrotizing, lymphocytic, and/or hyperplastic rhinitis, tracheitis, bronchitis, and bronchiolitis; lymphohistiocytic interstitial pneumonia; necrosis of lymphoid tissues, particularly tonsil and submandibular and bronchial lymph node; and lymphocytic infiltrates in various organs.

Nipah virus is readily isolated from blood, tonsil, nasal mucosa, lung, and other lymphoid tissues. Viral antigen is demonstrated by immunohistochemistry in epithelial cells in tonsil, trachea, bronchioles, and alveoli; alveolar macrophages; meningeal connective tissue and possibly astrocytes; endothelium and muscularis of inflamed blood vessels; and areas of lymphoid necrosis.

Other viral diseases

Porcine respirovirus 1 (porcine parainfluenza virus 1; PPIV1, *Paramyxoviridae, Respirovirus suis*) has been isolated from cases of porcine respiratory disease, but its role in causing disease is unknown.

Porcine orthorubulavirus (La Piedad Michoacán Mexico virus; (*Paramyxoviridae*, ***Orthorubulavirus suis***) caused "blue-eye disease" of pigs in Mexico. Clinical manifestations include neurologic disease, respiratory disease, and less frequent corneal opacity or reproductive failure. Lesions in experimentally infected pigs were lymphocytic interstitial pneumonia with cuffs around bronchioles.

Torque teno sus virus 1 (*Anelloviridae, Iotatorquevirus suida1a*) is not considered important as a primary pathogen, but it may exacerbate other infections such as with PCV2. Challenge of gnotobiotic pigs induced interstitial pneumonia, thymic atrophy, glomerulopathy, and lymphocytic hepatitis.

Bacterial diseases

Actinobacillus pleuropneumoniae

Actinobacillus pleuropneumoniae (APP) causes contagious pleuropneumonia, an important cause of severe, often fatal, pneumonia in growing pigs. The disease is most common in 6-week to 6-month-old hogs. Disease severity is highly variable, but case fatality rates of 20-80% are common in acute outbreaks. Clinical signs in severely affected pigs include fever, lethargy, severe dyspnea, cyanosis, bloody discharge from the nose, and occasionally vomiting or diarrhea. Convalescent pigs with chronic pneumonia may fail to thrive and display exercise intolerance and coughing.

APP is a gram-negative coccobacillus of the family *Pasteurellaceae*. Twelve serotypes are defined by antigenic variation in capsular polysaccharide and cell wall lipopolysaccharide. Serotypes 1, 5, and 7 are most common in North America, serotypes 2 and 9 are prevalent in Europe, and serotypes 1, 7, and 12 are frequent in Australia. Serotypes 1, 5, 9, and 11 secrete both Apx I and II toxins and tend to cause more severe disease than other serotypes. Immunity to heterologous serotypes is only partially protective.

APP has a rich spectrum of *virulence factors* important in pathogenesis. Three cytotoxins, named Apx I, II, and III, are members of the RTX (repeats in toxin) family of secreted toxins that includes *Mannheimia haemolytica* leukotoxin and *Escherichia coli* hemolysin. A fourth *Apx* toxin gene expressed in vivo but not in vitro is of uncertain significance. The Apx toxins are potent inducers of cytolysis in porcine neutrophils, alveolar macrophages, erythrocytes, and epithelial cells. Low concentrations induce an oxidative burst in porcine neutrophils. These toxins appear critical to development of disease; Apx toxin-deficient mutants have reduced virulence that is restored when the toxin genes are reintroduced. Lipopolysaccharide induces macrophage activation and secretion of neutrophil chemoattractants, procoagulant activity, and complement activation, similar to that described for *M. haemolytica*. The capsule impairs phagocytosis by macrophages and may prevent complement activation. Isolates with thin capsules may be less pathogenic. APP produces superoxide dismutase, catalase, and hydroperoxide reductase, which may protect against oxidative killing by neutrophils and macrophages. Other virulence factors include fimbrial adhesins, outer-membrane proteins, iron-binding proteins, metalloproteinase, and urease.

Infection is acquired by direct contact with infected pigs or by spread of aerosol droplets over short distances. The bacteria may be carried in the nasopharynx of apparently healthy animals, and these carriers are the principal method of introduction onto a naive farm. In contrast to *Pasteurella multocida* and *Bordetella bronchiseptica* in pigs and *Mannheimia haemolytica* of cattle, APP often causes disease in the absence of predisposing factors. Nevertheless, disease severity is enhanced by *Mesomycoplasma hyopneumoniae* or pseudorabies infections, and by factors that cause ciliary stasis.

Following inhalation, APP rapidly binds to the epithelium lining terminal bronchioles and alveoli. Neutrophil infiltration and alveolar exudate develop as early as 90 minutes after infection. Neutrophil recruitment is primarily the result of secretion of neutrophil chemoattractants by macrophages in response to infection; bacterial products themselves do not directly induce neutrophil chemotaxis. *Leukocyte necrosis is a prominent feature of the histologic lesions*, presumably mediated by the Apx cytotoxins.

Immunity to APP is conferred by mucosal IgA and serum IgG antibody responses, particularly to the Apx cytotoxins. However, heterologous infections impart only partial immunity, and this effect is not dependent on patterns of Apx toxin expression, implying that antibody against other bacterial antigens also contributes to protection. Antibody against surface components such as capsular polysaccharide greatly enhances phagocytosis of APP by neutrophils and macrophages, and neutrophils but not macrophages effectively kill these opsonized bacteria in vitro. In endemically infected herds, maternal antibody declines over the first 12 weeks of life, and active immune responses contribute to increasing titers thereafter. In experimental infections, serum antibody titers are detectable at 2 weeks and maximal at about 5 weeks after infection.

Gross findings in pigs that die of contagious pleuropneumonia are typified by *fibrinosuppurative, hemorrhagic, and necrotizing lobar pneumonia or pleuropneumonia*. The lesions commonly affect the *middle or caudal lung lobes* and may be unilateral or bilateral (Fig. 5-49). Lesions are deep-red, firm-to-hard, protrude above the surrounding lung, and cut crisply. The cut surface often exhibits sharply demarcated, irregularly shaped, 1-10 cm foci of coagulative necrosis that are friable and pale. In peracute cases, interlobular septa are expanded by fibrin and edema, and fibrinous exudate on the pleural surface ranges in appearance from a haze resembling ground glass to mats of fibrin. The bronchi may contain frothy or bloody fluid, and blood may ooze from the nostrils. Bronchial and mediastinal lymph nodes are enlarged, edematous, and congested. The pericardial and peritoneal cavities can contain scant serosanguineous fluid. Lesions in chronically affected pigs include fibrous pleural adhesions, sequestra, and locally extensive pulmonary fibrosis or abscess formation. Acutely affected pigs occasionally develop hyaline thrombi and fibrinoid necrosis of glomerular capillaries, afferent arterioles, and interlobular renal arteries, perhaps mediated by endotoxemia.

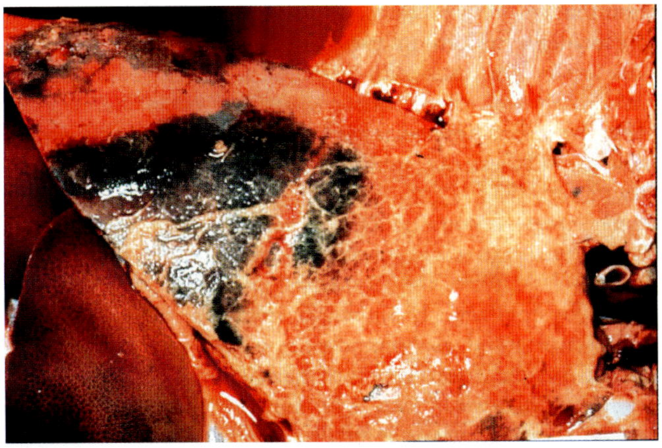

Figure 5-49 Contagious pleuropneumonia in a pig caused by *Actinobacillus pleuropneumoniae*. Hemorrhage and fibrinosuppurative pneumonia in the caudal lobe, covered by fibrin. (Courtesy University of Guelph.)

Microscopically, alveoli and terminal bronchioles are filled with fibrin, neutrophils, fewer macrophages, and many necrotic leukocytes (probably neutrophils). The foci of necrosis, which are often centered on alveolar septa, are delineated by a basophilic band of intense neutrophil infiltration and extensive neutrophil necrosis. In the center of the necrotic areas, the exudate varies from protein-rich edema, to fibrin, to leukocytes. Many leukocytes contain streaming, lightly basophilic, homogeneous chromatin similar to the "oat cells" of bovine shipping fever pneumonia. These neutrophils are in an apparent state of activation and express tumor necrosis factor, IL1, and IL8 mRNA.

The mucosa of bronchi and bronchioles may be infiltrated by neutrophils with fewer macrophages, and bronchiolar epithelium can be necrotic or sloughed. This aspect of the lesions can resemble those of influenza. Thrombi may develop in small venules and capillaries in the alveolar and interlobular septa, and fibrinoid vasculitis has been described infrequently. Lymphatics in the alveolar septa are distended by serofibrinous exudate with variable numbers of neutrophils. Extrapulmonary lesions are uncommon, but include renal glomerular thrombosis, renal vasculitis, or osteomyelitis.

Lesions of localized or locally extensive fibrinous and necrotizing pneumonia suggest APP, *A. suis*, *Glaesserella australis*, or *Salmonella* Choleraesuis. *Definitive* **diagnosis** *depends on isolation of the agent, and microscopic identification of neutrophilic bronchopneumonia with neutrophil necrosis*. Isolation on blood agar requires a *Staphylococcus* streak or supplemented medium containing a source of nicotinamide adenine dinucleotide. Alternatively, bacteria in lung smears or primary cultures can be identified using antigen detection techniques such as ELISA or latex agglutination. Serologic identification of APP is particularly useful in the maintenance of minimal-disease herds.

Bronchopneumonia caused by opportunistic bacterial pathogens

The porcine respiratory disease complex is an exemplar of multifactorial disease causation. Although bacterial pneumonia is the final cause of death in many cases of porcine respiratory disease, its development is highly dependent on host factors, environmental influences, and other infectious agents. Important contributing environmental factors include elevated levels of dust and ammonia, temperature fluctuations, and extremes of temperature and humidity. In temperate climates, the incidence of swine pneumonia is maximal in the autumn and early winter, in part caused by fluctuating temperatures and the impact of cold weather on barn ventilation and air quality. Immunity to respiratory pathogens is dependent on patterns of pig flow through production units, vaccination practices, and alterations in innate resistance resulting from social and environmental stresses, nutrition, and management practices. Against this background of host and environmental factors, interactions among various pathogens are commonly identified in swine pneumonia. Thus, *effective control of disease requires that diagnostic investigations identify not only the immediate causes of fatal disease but also the underlying infectious and noninfectious factors*.

PRRSV, *Mesomycoplasma hyopneumoniae*, alphainfluenzaviruses, and PCV2 all cause primary lung disease. In addition, each of these agents impairs the pulmonary defenses against inhaled bacterial pathogens by, among other mechanisms, impairing mucociliary clearance and suppressing alveolar macrophage function. Pigs are commonly exposed to the **opportunistic pathogens** *Pasteurella multocida, Streptococcus suis, Bordetella bronchiseptica, Glaesserella parasuis,* and *G. australis,* and failure of lung defenses resulting from viral or mycoplasmal infection, poor air quality, and stresses are key factors in development of disease caused by these bacterial pathogens.

P. multocida serotypes A and D are important causes of fatal pneumonia in weaner and grower-finisher pigs. The massive doses of *P. multocida* needed for experimental induction of disease suggest that the predisposing causes listed above are necessary components of the natural disease. *Bordetella* is particularly noteworthy as a cause of fatal pneumonia in piglets <3-weeks-old, and causes nonprogressive atrophic rhinitis (described below), but may also cause bronchopneumonia in older pigs. The pathogenesis of bordetellosis is described in the Infectious Respiratory Diseases of Dogs section.

Gross lesions of bronchopneumonia, in which cranioventral areas of lung are swollen, consolidated, reddened, and sharply demarcated from more normal lung, are typical of infection with these opportunistic bacterial pathogens. In many but not all cases, mucopurulent exudate may be expressed from airways on cut section. Fibrinous pleuritis may be present but is usually minor. Bronchial lymph nodes are often enlarged and mottled red and white. The predominant **histologic findings** are of numerous neutrophils and macrophages filling alveoli and bronchioles. Fibrin exudation may occur but is usually minor. These lesions contrast with those of *A. pleuropneumoniae* and *A. suis,* where fibrinous exudate in airspaces and on the pleural surface is often prominent, most of the neutrophils are necrotic and have streaming basophilic chromatin, and focally extensive coagulative necrosis is often present. In cases of bronchopneumonia, the bronchiolar epithelium is generally normal or mildly hyperplastic, but bronchiolar necrosis is usually absent unless there is underlying influenza or PCV2 infection. *M. hyopneumoniae* also causes a cranioventral pattern of bronchopneumonia, but in contrast to the red swollen lung of bacterial bronchopneumonia, the acute lesions of mycoplasmosis are red and atelectatic, whereas the subacute lesions are gray-to-tan and only mildly swollen to firm. Cranioventral bronchopneumonia superimposed on generalized or patchy lesions of interstitial pneumonia suggests underlying PRRSV or PCV2 infection, or septicemia.

Although bacterial bronchopneumonia may be the immediate cause of death, viral or mycoplasmal pathogens should be considered as underlying causes. Microbiologic testing is commonly employed to identify the spectrum of pathogens causing pneumonia, but the plethora of currently available tests does not diminish the importance of morphologic examination of the lung. Determining the patterns of gross and histologic lesions allows the pathologist to narrow the list of differential diagnoses to select a panel of ancillary tests efficiently, to provide a tentative diagnosis when rapid therapeutic intervention is required or when ancillary microbiologic tests are negative, and to evaluate critically the contribution of particular pathogens, many of which are commonly present in healthy pigs, to the case being investigated.

Atrophic rhinitis

Nonprogressive atrophic rhinitis (**NPAR**), caused by *Bordetella bronchiseptica,* viral infections, and high concentrations of dusts and ammonia, causes mild transient sneezing and nasal discharge and is *not usually of herd significance*. In contrast, **progressive atrophic rhinitis** (**PAR**) is caused by *Pasteurella multocida* strains that produce *P. multocida* toxin encoded by the *toxA* gene, often in concert with *B. bronchiseptica* or other bacterial pathogens, and causes production loss. PAR affects pigs of at least 6-12 weeks of age, causing sneezing, mucopurulent nasal discharge, unilateral epistaxis, nasal deformity, failure to thrive, and secondary bacterial bronchopneumonia. Freedom from PAR is a frequent requirement in minimal-disease herds, so *differentiation of PAR and NPAR is of substantial significance. Toxigenic P. multocida* infects rodents, cats, dogs, and ruminants and may be of zoonotic concern.

Both NPAR and PAR are multifactorial conditions for which air quality and other pathogens influence the severity of disease. **NPAR** is primarily caused by strains of *B. bronchiseptica* that adhere to nasal cilia and tonsillar epithelium and produce a toxin that causes mucosal edema, loss of cilia, and resorption of turbinate bone. Infection is acquired by inhalation of infected aerosol droplets.

PAR *is caused by cytotoxin-producing strains of P. multocida type D or, less commonly, type A.* Infection is acquired by inhalation following direct contact with infected pigs. Colonization of the nasal mucosa and tonsil is inefficient, but augmented by factors that harm the nasal mucosa, including *B. bronchiseptica* infection, ammonia, and dusts. The *cytotoxin,* also referred to as *dermonecrotic toxin,* is a secreted, heat-labile toxin encoded by the *tox*A gene. Intranasal or intramuscular administration of *P. multocida* cytotoxin has similar effects on the nasal turbinates, including epithelial hyperplasia, glandular atrophy, resorption of turbinate bone by osteoclasts, reduced formation of bone by osteoblasts, and fibroblast proliferation. The cytotoxin does not directly affect osteoclast function; rather, hyperplasia and increased function of these cells are apparently stimulated by soluble mediators secreted from nearby stromal cells in response to the cytotoxin.

Atrophy and malformation of the nasal turbinates are the principal lesions of atrophic rhinitis and are more severe in the ventral than the dorsal conchae. To assess the integrity of the nasal turbinates, cross sections of the snout should be made at the level of the first or second upper premolar teeth; in affected pigs the normally scroll-like turbinates are misshapen and blunted. Turbinate atrophy may be partial or complete, leaving a hollow nasal cavity with an often-deformed nasal septum.

Distortion of the snout is a prominent external finding in pigs with chronic atrophic rhinitis. Brachygnathia superior occurs when the maxillary bones of the snout fail to grow. Lateral deviation toward the most severely affected side is common.

Histologic lesions in the nasal turbinates include *osteoclast hyperplasia, osteoclast-mediated resorption of bone, and replacement with fibrous tissue containing many plump fibroblasts.* Lymphocytes and fewer neutrophils infiltrate the nasal mucosa, and there may be squamous metaplasia of the ciliated epithelium.

The gross lesions of NPAR and PAR are qualitatively similar, although those of NPAR are generally less severe. Nevertheless, given the significance of a diagnosis of PAR caused by toxigenic *P. multocida,* definitive identification is usually warranted. *B. bronchiseptica* and *P. multocida* can be readily isolated from swabs of nasal mucosa or tonsil, but *definitive* ***diagnosis*** *of PAR depends on demonstrating P. multocida cytotoxin production using PCR or ELISA.* Various grading systems have been described to assess the severity of nasal turbinate atrophy. These grading systems are not intended to differentiate NPAR from PAR, but are useful in monitoring the herd response to management or therapeutic interventions.

Mycoplasmal diseases

General features of mycoplasmas

Mycoplasmas, which are members of the class *Mollicutes*, are the smallest self-replicating organisms, lack a cell wall, and have a protein- and lipid-rich plasma membrane. They are obligate parasites, and several species lack the ability to synthesize required amino acids, cholesterol, and fatty acids. The success of culturing mycoplasmas in vitro is highly dependent on the particular species: some mycoplasmas grow so readily that they commonly contaminate cell cultures, yet many of the pathogenic mycoplasmas grow slowly, have frustratingly fastidious growth requirements, and are easily overgrown by other agents. Mycoplasmas have a relatively small genome, 580-1,380 kb, which contains many repetitive elements and a propensity for genomic rearrangement through homologous recombination. Many mycoplasmas have highly specific host and tissue tropism, are commonly commensals on mucosal surfaces, and adhere to ciliated epithelium. Several are capable of surviving within host cells. Spread of infection through the blood with subsequent localization in joints or serosal surfaces is a feature of some mycoplasmoses.

High-frequency variation of surface antigens allows some mycoplasmas to evade the humoral immune response by changing their surface lipoprotein antigens when antibodies against these structures are formed. The mechanisms by which *Mycoplasma* infections result in disease remain poorly characterized. Mycoplasmas have not been shown to secrete exotoxins. *Pathogenic mechanisms* of respiratory disease include ciliostasis caused by membrane alterations, induction of inflammation by membrane lipoproteins, induction of apoptosis in lymphocytes or other host cells, and biofilm formation to aid bacterial survival.

Mesomycoplasma (Mycoplasma) hyopneumoniae

Mesomycoplasma hyopneumoniae is the cause of *mycoplasmal pneumonia of swine*, often known as **enzootic pneumonia**. It is a common, chronic, usually nonfatal disease of young pigs. The disease may be endemic, or spread slowly through a facility over the course of weeks, and morbidity may be as high as 70-100%. Although pigs as young as 5 weeks of age may develop disease, it is *most important in grower-finisher pigs* and is a key component of fatal multifactorial pneumonia in 4-6-month-old hogs. Clinical expressions of the uncomplicated disease are coughing, unthriftiness, poor weight gain, and reduced feed conversion. Because there is usually low mortality associated with mycoplasmal pneumonia, the lesions are generally seen in slaughtered animals or those dying from other diseases. When deaths do occur, they are mainly from superimposed infections with other bacteria.

Like other mycoplasmal pathogens, *M. hyopneumoniae* is a tiny bacterium that lacks a cell wall. The agent adheres to ciliated epithelium of the large airways and bronchioles, using 97 and 145 kDa outer-membrane proteins. Adherent organisms are closely associated with the cilia, often with extensive ciliary loss, and they may survive within epithelial cells. Membrane proteins of many mycoplasmas, presumably including *M. hyopneumoniae*, induce proliferation of lymphocytes and result in the characteristic aggregates of lymphocytes around airways and blood vessels. Infection with *M. hyopneumoniae* is mainly transmitted by direct contact with nasal secretions from infected pigs, although aerosol transmission over short distances can occur. A common clinical scenario involves infection of a few young pigs by contact with an infected sow, followed by slow spread to in-contact pigs when groups are assembled in weaner or grower-finisher units.

Clinical disease is not an inevitable consequence of infection with *M. hyopneumoniae*. Rather, its development is highly dependent on other predisposing factors, including crowding, poor air quality, fluctuations in temperature or humidity, and the presence of other pathogens. Many infections are subclinical, and carrier animals are important sources of infection of naive herds. Primary *M. hyopneumoniae* infection is not fatal, but reduced mucociliary clearance and possibly impaired macrophage function may lead to fatal bacterial pneumonia from opportunistic pathogens such as *Pasteurella multocida*, *Streptococcus suis*, *Bordetella bronchiseptica*, or *Glaesserella parasuis*. The interaction of PRRSV with *M. hyopneumoniae* is particularly noteworthy: mycoplasmal infection exacerbates the severity and the duration of PRRS, although the effect of PRRSV infection on mycoplasmal pneumonia is apparently minor. As a result, new infections with *M. hyopneumoniae* may cause outbreaks of PRRS in herds with previously subclinical PRSSV infections.

The characteristic **gross feature** *of mycoplasmal pneumonia is red-tan-gray discoloration, collapse, and rubbery firmness affecting cranioventral regions of the lungs in a lobular pattern* (Fig. 5-50). Lesions often affect cranial and middle lung lobes, accessory

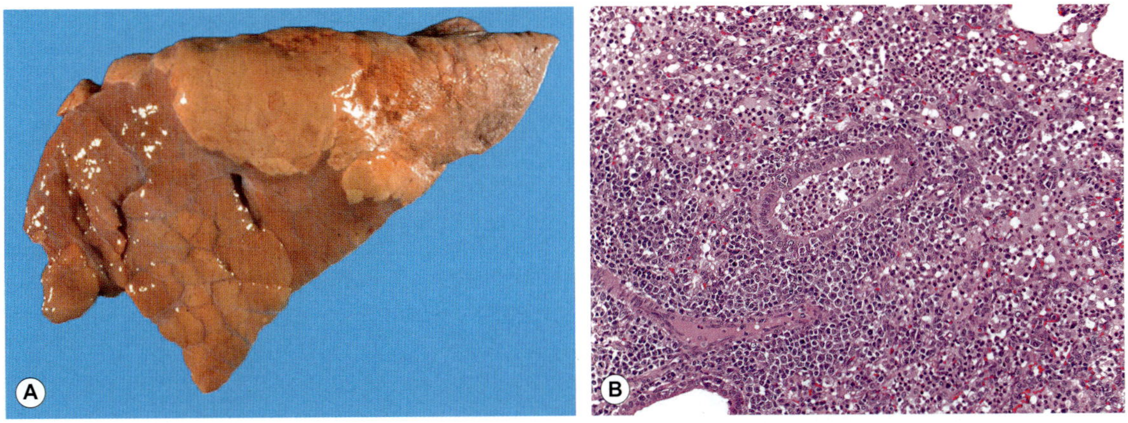

Figure 5-50 ***Mesomycoplasmaa hyopneumoniae*** infection in a pig. **A**. Cranioventral lung (to the left) is collapsed, gray-brown, with firm-rubbery or fleshy texture. **B**. Lymphocytes encircle a bronchiole and blood vessels. The bronchiole and alveoli contain edema, mononuclear cells, and aggregates of neutrophils.

lobe, and cranioventral portions of the caudal lobes. The mildest lesions resemble atelectasis, with a lobular pattern of reddening and collapse. More severe lesions evolve from dark-red through gray-pink to more homogeneous gray as the lesion ages. The rubbery or thymus-like texture of the lung contrasts with the more firm or hard consistency of *Pasteurella* pneumonia, although this is often present concurrently. The cut surface of affected lung is edematous, and catarrhal exudate can be squeezed from bronchi. The bronchiolar orientation of the inflammation often gives a regular pattern of tiny gray foci against a red background. *M. hyopneumoniae* rarely causes serofibrinous pleuritis or polyserositis, but this is more commonly caused by opportunistic bacteria or *Mesomycoplasma hyorhinis*. Pulmonary lymph nodes are enlarged and on cut surface are moist, usually bulging and sometimes hyperemic.

Histologically, subacute-to-chronic mycoplasmal pneumonia in pigs is typified by lymphocytic infiltrates around airways, increased numbers of alveolar macrophages, and alveolar edema. In the fully developed mycoplasmal pneumonia, there is *extensive lymphoid hyperplasia* around bronchi, bronchioles, and their associated vessels; and lymphocytes infiltrate the lamina propria of the airway mucosa (see Fig. 5-50). The epithelium can be histologically normal or hyperplastic. Although ciliary loss and exfoliation of ciliated epithelium may occur, this is difficult to detect by light microscopy. Goblet cells in the airway mucosa are increased in number and the bronchial glands are hyperplastic, reflecting the excessive mucus secretions seen grossly. The alveolar exudate consists predominantly of macrophages and protein-rich edema, but variable numbers of plasma cells, lymphocytes, and neutrophils are present. The alveolar septa are mildly thickened by lymphocytes and a few plasma cells.

Experimental studies of the pathogenesis of mycoplasmal pneumonia indicate that typical gross lesions do not occur until 2-4 weeks after infection. The rate of development of lesions is dependent on the dose and strain of *M. hyopneumoniae*, method of administration, and susceptibility of the pigs exposed. Young pigs naturally exposed to infectious aerosols soon after birth can develop lesions by the time they are 3-5-weeks-old. In the first week after experimental infection, neutrophils are present in airway lumens and, to a lesser extent, in alveoli. The numbers of neutrophils diminish, and lymphoid cells increase over the subsequent several weeks to reach the fully developed stage of consolidation. After it has reached its peak some 5-6 weeks after infection, lesions of uncomplicated mycoplasmal pneumonia may either persist or completely resolve within 2 months.

The gross lesions of gray-tan discoloration and thymus-like texture are quite characteristic. However, many fatal cases are secondarily infected by opportunistic bacteria, resulting in red, firm or hard, cranioventral consolidation that appears identical to the bacterial pneumonia that complicates PRRSV, PCV2, or SIV infections. Similarly, the well-developed histologic lesions with thick peribronchial cuffs of lymphocytes are highly suggestive, yet lymphoplasmacytic peribronchiolitis—usually milder—is also often present in chronic PRRSV, SIV, or PCV2 pneumonia. In these cases, other histologic features can suggest a *tentative diagnosis: M. hyopneumoniae* also induces alveolar edema and increased numbers of plump alveolar macrophages, PRRSV results in diffuse lymphocytic infiltrates in alveolar septa, SIV and some PCV2 infections are accompanied in the acute stages by bronchiolar necrosis and neutrophils, and granulomatous infiltrates in lymph nodes suggest PCV2 infection.

Establishing a definitive **diagnosis** in swine herds with pneumonia often requires laboratory support. *M. hyopneumoniae* is fastidious in its growth requirements, and isolation in culture is not a useful method of diagnosis. More sensitive confirmation of a morphologic diagnosis can be obtained by identifying antigen in lesional lung tissue by immunohistochemistry, or detection of *M. hyopneumoniae* DNA by PCR using lung tissue, nasal swabs, or transtracheal washes. Detection of serum antibody by ELISA is a useful method of confirming prior exposure, or validating the *M. hyopneumoniae*-free status of minimal disease herds.

Parasitic diseases

Metastrongylus apri *(elongatus)*, *Metastrongylus pudendotectus*, and *Metastrongylus salmi* (*Protostrongylidae*) are all parasitic in the bronchi and bronchioles of pigs. Because the intermediate host is the earthworm, pulmonary metastrongylosis is now rare in housed pigs, but it is common in wild boar. They are believed to occasionally transmit swine influenza virus and rarely infect humans. The adult worms are white, threadlike, and 14-60 mm long (eFig. 5-63A). In heavy infections, which are mostly in young pigs, they may be found in all lobes of the lung. When there are fewer worms, particularly as occurs in older animals, the worms may be restricted to airways along the caudoventral borders of the caudal lobes. In histologic sections, the adults have polymyarian coelomyarian musculature, cuboidal multinucleate intestinal epithelium with an indistinct microvillus layer, and thick-shelled eggs or embryonated eggs in the uterus (see eFig. 5-63B). Eggs are laid in the bronchi and a few of them hatch there, but most hatch after passing to the exterior in the feces. First-stage larvae are inactive and are capable of prolonged survival in moist conditions. Their further development depends on ingestion by earthworms, which are the intermediate hosts. The larvae develop to the third, infective stage in about 10 days, and then remain quiescent unless the earthworm is eaten by a pig. The larvae may survive for as long as 18 months in the earthworms and, by that time, thousands may be accumulated by a single worm. Migration within the pig is through the lymphatics from the intestine to the lungs. Some larvae pass through the liver and produce focal hepatitis.

Even with heavy adult infestations, gross lesions are inconspicuous. The worms live in the smallest airways, and on superficial examination the parasites are frequently only suggested by gray-pink, 1-3 mm nodules and by hyperinflated lobules along the caudoventral margins of the caudal lobes. Histologically, the lesions are similar to those produced by *Dictyocaulus* spp. The initial lesions are foci of intense accumulations of eosinophils surrounding larvae in alveoli. Subsequently, when reproduction is active, an eosinophilic and granulomatous response occurs to the eggs and larvae in the alveoli. The prepatent period for *Metastrongylus* spp. is ~25 days, after which the rate of egg production rapidly reaches a peak and then subsides to a low level. At this later stage, the adults persist mainly in the bronchioles and small bronchi and provoke goblet cell hyperplasia and exudation of mucus, eosinophils, neutrophils, and mononuclear cells. The bronchiolar epithelium is hyperplastic, and eosinophils, lymphocytes, and plasma cells permeate the lamina propria.

Ascaris suum is an intestinal nematode in pigs. The female worms have tremendous biotic potential, producing numerous eggs that are passed in the feces. Consumption of large numbers of embryonated eggs or ingestion of infected paratenic hosts (usually earthworms) results in the synchronous migration of huge numbers of larvae that can be fatal. The lesion is acute, diffuse, eosinophilic, interstitial lung disease associated with large numbers of larvae. Characteristic morphologic features of the larvae are the lateral alae, prominent lateral chords, and uninucleate intestinal epithelial cells (eFig. 5-64).

Paragonimus spp. and **hydatid disease** are rare parasitisms of the respiratory tract of pigs.

INFECTIOUS RESPIRATORY DISEASES OF CATTLE

Viral diseases

General features of herpesviruses

Herpesviruses (family *Orthoherpesviridae*) are 120-200 nm diameter and composed of an icosahedral nucleocapsid surrounded by a proteinaceous tegument and an outer envelope. Herpesviruses have large genomes composed of double-stranded DNA. Viral infection of cells induces a highly regulated cascade of viral gene expression: preformed tegument proteins and the products of immediate-early and early genes regulate the host transcriptional machinery and viral gene expression, and late genes encode structural proteins of the virus. Viral glycoproteins form peplomers that project from the surface of the envelope; in addition to being key targets of protective immune responses, these envelope glycoproteins mediate viral entry into target cells, cellular fusion to form syncytia, and spread of virus between cells without exposure to extracellular antibody. Some envelope glycoproteins act as complement C3b or immunoglobulin Fc receptors, and several herpesviruses encode chemokine or chemokine receptor homologues that modulate the immunoinflammatory response. Viral replication occurs in the nucleus, and virions acquire an envelope by budding through the nuclear membrane. Lysis of the cell releases the mature virions to the extracellular space.

Herpesviruses are classified into *Alpha-*, *Beta-*, and *Gammaherpesvirinae* subfamilies. Characteristics of the **alphaherpesviruses** are rapid growth in cell culture, lytic infection of cells, necrotizing lesions, latent infections, and in some instances the formation of syncytia and eosinophilic intranuclear inclusion bodies (INIBs). They can have narrow or broad host ranges. Most alphaherpesviruses establish *latent infections* in neurons of the trigeminal ganglia and other sensory ganglia, as well as other sites such as olfactory bulb, optic nerve, nasal turbinates, and cornea. During latent infection, the so-called latency-associated transcripts are the only evidence of viral gene expression; these have been utilized as markers of latent infection. Alphaherpesviruses (and their associated diseases) affecting the lung of domestic mammals include bovine alphaherpesvirus 1 [**BoAHV1**, infectious bovine rhinotracheitis (IBR)], caprine alphaherpesvirus 1 (**CpAHV1**; *Varicellovirus caprinealpha1*), **SuAHV1** (pseudorabies), equid alphaherpesviruses 1 and 4 (**EqAHV1**, **EqAHV4**; aborton, equine viral rhinopneumonitis), canid alphaherpesvirus 1 (**CaAHV1**; *Varicellovirus canidalpha1*), and felid alphaherpesvirus 1 (**FeAHV1**, feline viral rhinotracheitis; *Varicellovirus felidalpha1*).

The **betaherpesviruses**, including SuBHV2 (PCMV), have a limited host range, and these cytomegaloviruses induce pathologic enlargement of infected cells and prominent basophilic INIBs. Replication of cytomegaloviruses is slower than that of alphaherpesviruses, and disease is more chronic. As the immune response is generally effective, disease caused by cytomegalovirus occurs principally in immunodeficient or immunosuppressed animals.

Infectious bovine rhinotracheitis

Infection with bovine alphaherpesvirus 1 (**BoAHV1**; *Orthoherpesviridae, Varicellovirus bovinealpha1*) is widespread in cattle populations, but the disease infectious bovine rhinotracheitis (IBR) is uncommon in areas where vaccination is practiced. IBR causes an abrupt onset of fever, anorexia, tachypnea, mucopurulent nasal discharge, and dyspnea or open-mouth breathing. The nasal mucosa and muzzle are often hyperemic, suggesting the epithet "red nose," and white, loosely adherent plaques may peel from the surface. The mortality rate is low unless secondary bacterial pneumonia develops.

BoAHV1 infections cause IBR, keratoconjunctivitis, interstitial lung disease, abortion, encephalitis, systemic herpesviral infection in young calves, and pustular vulvovaginitis or balanoposthitis. The factors that determine the manifestation are not fully understood, but include the following: route of infection (genital infection usually manifests as vulvovaginitis or balanoposthitis); strain of the virus (a distinct virus type, BoAHV5, is the usual cause of herpesviral encephalitis in calves); and degree of immunity (systemic herpesviral infection develops in young calves with low serum antibody titers to the virus).

BoAHV1 has a large 136 kb genome encoding 67 proteins. Twelve envelope glycoproteins have been described. The glycoproteins gC and gD bind cell surface receptors, allowing virus entry into the cell by gB, gH, and gL. Fusion of cells, mediated by gB and gD, allows intercellular spread of virus and evasion of the immune response, and is the molecular basis of the epithelial syncytia that are occasionally noted histologically. The gC glycoprotein binds C3 component of complement and prevents complement activation; gI and gE are Fc receptors for immunoglobulin that impair antibody-mediated neutralization of the virus.

BoAHV1 infects a wide range of animals, including cattle, sheep, goats, llamas, pigs, water buffalo, mustelids, and rabbits, but *primary viral respiratory disease is described only in cattle.* Sources of BoAHV1 infection include clinically or subclinically infected cattle, and reactivation of latent infections. Wild ruminants may be subclinical reservoirs. Infection is transmitted by aerosol; direct contact with nasal, ocular, or vaginal secretions; or by indirect contact with fomites, semen, feed, or water. Systemic spread of the virus is a feature of the syndromes of systemic infection, abortion, and encephalitis. Viremia is not usually evident in cases of IBR, keratoconjunctivitis, vulvovaginitis, or balanoposthitis, although monocyte- or lymphocyte-associated viremia may occur at a low level. In these conditions, virus spreads along mucosal epithelia, nerves, and lymphatics. *Latent infection of trigeminal or other sensory ganglia is common* and follows axonal spread of infection rather than viremia. In latently infected neurons, viral DNA is present but, with the exception of a few "latency-associated transcripts," viral RNA or protein cannot be detected. Stress, administration of glucocorticoid or epinephrine, hyperthermia, or hypothermia trigger reactivation of the latent infection, and virus reaches the mucosal surface by retrograde axonal transport where mucosal replication leads to shedding of infectious virus. Reactivated infections are usually subclinical but may infect naive, in-contact animals.

Infection of the respiratory tract induces *clinical disease* after an incubation period of 2-6 days, and virus is shed in nasal secretions for at least 10-16 days. Clinical IBR results from lytic infection of nasal and airway epithelial cells. Functional abnormalities such as serotonin- or dopamine-induced bronchoconstriction may also contribute to clinical signs. Secondary bacterial pneumonia in calves with IBR is a consequence of the destruction of ciliated epithelium by lytic viral infection, and impairment of the ability of alveolar macrophages to phagocytose bacteria and secrete neutrophil chemotactic factors. These impairments of lung defenses are maximal at 4-5 days after viral infection.

Interferon-α and -β secretion is detectable within 5 hours of BoAHV1 infections and peaks at 36-72 hours. These interferons mediate innate resistance to spread of the infection, in part by recruiting macrophages and natural killer cells to the sites of viral infection. Cell-mediated immune responses are detectable in the respiratory tract within 5 days of infection and mediate lysis of virus-infected cells. Neutralizing IgG is first detected at 10 days after infection, and IgA responses develop later. Antibody prevents disease in calves exposed to the virus. In infected calves, antibody neutralizes free virus and may prevent mucosal shedding of virus following reactivation of latent infection. However, because the virus evades the humoral immune response by spreading locally from cell to cell, a combination of cellular and humoral immunity is probably necessary for recovery from infection.

Gross lesions of IBR are usually restricted to the *nasal cavity, larynx, and trachea*. Pustules erupt early after infection, but are fragile and rarely observed. Petechiae, a granular appearance of the mucosa, and serous exudate may be present in acute lesions. More commonly, there is intense hyperemia of the mucosal tissue, multifocal-to-coalescing erosions with loosely adherent plaques of white debris, or diffuse ulceration covered by a fibrinonecrotic membrane (Fig. 5-51). When the exudate is peeled from the surface of the trachea or nasal cavity, dull granular eroded tissue remains. In contrast, in cases of bacterial pneumonia in which expectorated material accumulates on the tracheal or nasal mucosa, gentle removal of the exudate reveals a shiny intact mucosal surface. In severe cases, obstruction of the laryngeal or tracheal lumen by abundant exudate may prove fatal. Emphysema is a sequel to dyspnea in severely affected calves.

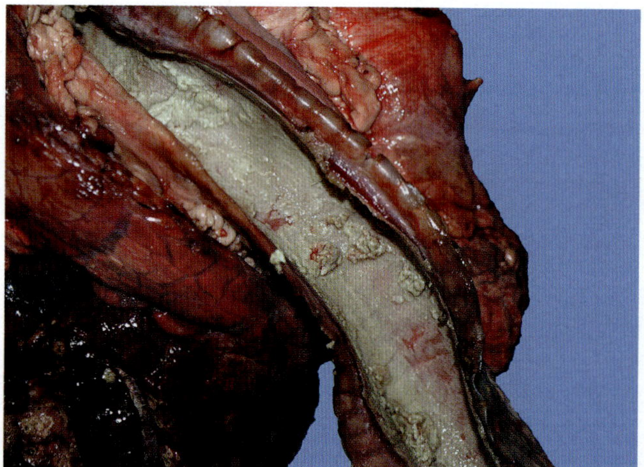

Figure 5-51 Infectious bovine rhinotracheitis. Necrosis of tracheal epithelium forms a fibrinonecrotic membrane that cannot be removed.

The earliest **histologic lesions**, in the first 2 days after infection, include cytoplasmic vacuolation and pallor, and nuclear pyknosis or karyolysis. Eosinophilic INIBs are present in the epithelium of the nasal turbinates, tracheobronchial glands, and bronchial epithelium, but are rare in the tracheal surface epithelium. *Inclusions are absent in most diagnostic cases*, and the lesions at these later times include erosion or ulceration of nasal and tracheal mucosa, with necrosis and exfoliation of infected epithelial cells and exudation of neutrophils and fibrin. Neutrophils and mononuclear cells infiltrate the lamina propria. Mild perivascular infiltrates of lymphocytes may be detected in the trigeminal ganglion and brainstem.

Viral pneumonia includes erosion of bronchiolar epithelium and proliferation of type II pneumocytes. *Primary viral pneumonia occurs in young calves*, sometimes without significant upper respiratory lesions. These calves may have epithelial syncytia in alveoli, and eosinophilic INIBs are more common than is seen in IBR.

Systemic lesions of BoAHV1 infection in young calves, usually <2-months-old, include coalescing, sharply demarcated, 1-7-mm foci of necrosis in the upper digestive tract, including the oral cavity, esophagus, and rumen. Necrotic foci are often covered by adherent debris and ingesta, which appears as caseous clumps of curdled milk. Multifocal, pinpoint to 1 mm, white foci of necrosis are often present in the liver, and occasionally in the kidney and spleen. The nasopharynx and larynx may contain erosive and exudative lesions, but tracheal and pulmonary lesions are not typical. Histologically, eosinophilic INIBs are usually apparent at the margins of the necrotic lesions. The lesions of herpesviral abortion are described in Vol. 3, Female Genital System.

The gross appearance of IBR is highly suggestive. A casual observer may mistake loosely adherent expectorated material for the tracheal ulceration of IBR. BPIV3 can cause nasal erosions, but aspiration or inhalation of chemical irritants—which is rarely encountered—is the only process likely to be confused with florid lesions of IBR. However, as subclinical BoAHV1 infection impairs pulmonary defenses, laboratory investigation to demonstrate this pathogen may be warranted in calves with acute bacterial pneumonia. PCR tests and immunohistochemistry are effective detection methods if samples can be obtained early in the disease. Otherwise, measuring antibodies in acute and convalescent sera may be the only option for etiologic diagnosis. An important caveat is warranted when diagnosing BoAHV1 infection in the absence of characteristic lesions: *cattle with other diseases experience stress-induced reactivation of latent herpesviral infections, leading to identification of the reactivated virus in any of these assays*.

Bovine respiratory syncytial virus

Infection with bovine respiratory syncytial virus (**BRSV**; *Pneumoviridae, Orthopneumovirus bovis*) is common in North American and European beef and dairy herds. Seroprevalence studies suggest that about half of range calves in North America are exposed to BRSV, and most nonexposed calves seroconvert within a month of entering feedlots. The seroprevalence of BRSV in adult cattle varies from 40 to 95%. *BRSV is an important cause of acute outbreaks of respiratory disease and of "enzootic pneumonia"* in 2-week to 5-month-old dairy and beef calves, with a peak incidence at 1-3 months of age. BRSV certainly causes *fatal bronchiolar and alveolar damage* soon after arrival in beef feedlots, but rarely causes acute interstitial lung disease in the late feeding period. Finally, *BRSV predisposes to* *bacterial pneumonia* in feedlot beef cattle by impairing lung defenses and occasionally causes respiratory disease in naive adult dairy cows.

The disease is most prevalent in the autumn or early winter. *Clinical signs* in calves and cows are similar and include high fever, coughing, tachypnea, and variable nasal discharge and conjunctivitis. Some animals develop dyspnea with open-mouth breathing and increased abdominal effort. Calves often maintain a reasonable appetite in the face of severe respiratory distress, in contrast to the consistent depression of cattle with bacterial pneumonia. A biphasic clinical course is not present in all cases; when present, transient pyrexia and mild respiratory disease is followed by temporary improvement for days to weeks, and then rapid onset of severe respiratory distress.

BRSV is pleomorphic, spherical or irregularly shaped, enveloped, 80-450 nm diameter, and contains negative-sense single-stranded RNA. The viral genome encodes 10 proteins, including the G glycoprotein (in membrane-anchored and secreted forms), which mediates attachment of viral particles to host cells; the F protein, which induces fusion of infected cells; matrix proteins (M, M2 or 22 K), nucleocapsid protein (N), phosphoprotein (P), polymerase (L), small hydrophobic protein (SH), and nonstructural proteins [NS1(1 C) and NS2(1B)]. A high mutation rate confers much genetic and antigenic diversity, with 4 antigenic groups and variation in the G and F proteins, but their clinical significance is uncertain.

An understanding of the **pathogenesis** of BRSV pneumonia has been hindered by the difficulty of establishing experimental infections that are representative of naturally occurring disease. In general, experimentally infected calves develop less-severe clinical disease and less-extensive lesions than natural cases, in part because in vitro passage of the virus in cell culture attenuates virulence. As a result, descriptions of the pathogenesis of experimental infections are not necessarily representative of natural disease. *Airborne spread, probably by aerosol, is the common route of infection.* Clinical signs are observed from 2 to 7 days after experimental infection. In natural cases, viral infection is restricted to the respiratory tract, and viral antigen is most abundant in bronchiolar epithelium of the cranioventral areas of lung. Alveolar type II pneumocytes and macrophages express lesser amounts of viral antigen, and infrequent virus-infected cells are present in nasal, tracheal, and bronchial epithelium. The virus infects but does not replicate in lymphocytes in vitro. Following experimental infection of naive calves, viral shedding was first detected on the second day, maximal at about 4 days, and absent by 7-10 days after infection (although viral nucleic acid can be detected for at least 2-4 weeks). This transient infection is consistent with the difficulty experienced in demonstrating virus in naturally occurring subacute or chronic cases.

Interactions with other agents contribute to the severity of disease. Experimental BRSV infections result in more severe disease if calves are also infected with bovine viral diarrhea virus or exposed to 3-methylindole. BRSV is an important predisposing factor in the development of bacterial bronchopneumonia in cattle because the virus impairs alveolar macrophage function, reduces mucociliary clearance, and may enhance proteolysis to facilitate bacterial invasion of the blood.

Calves with BRSV develop specific serum and mucosal antibody responses; however, most antibody is directed to the F and N proteins and is non-neutralizing, and serum titers are poorly correlated with protection from disease. Similarly, passively acquired colostral antibodies do not prevent disease. Although virus-neutralizing antibody is produced during infection, the role of humoral immunity in protection from disease requires further investigation. As for many viral infections, CD8+ T-lymphocyte responses may be important in recovery of calves following BRSV infection.

The role of the immune response in enhancing disease is controversial. It has been proposed that vaccination with inactive virus promotes a type 2 immune response in which antiviral IgE exacerbates the disease. Furthermore, the biphasic clinical course, noted in some but not all natural cases, has been interpreted to represent a worsening of the disease as an immune response develops. Such comparisons have been used as a model to study human RSV infection, where children vaccinated with a formalin-inactivated vaccine developed more severe and prolonged disease course than nonvaccinates. However, attempts to reproduce this phenomenon in cattle have given conflicting results, and vaccinated calves developed milder disease than nonvaccinates in several studies. Similarly, it has been proposed that virus- or immune-complex–induced activation of complement or production of IgE may contribute to bronchoconstriction or pulmonary lesions in calves infected with BRSV, but the significance of complement activation and IgE responses in infected calves remains uncertain.

Gross lesions *in the lungs of calves with naturally occurring BRSV pneumonia often differ in cranioventral and caudodorsal areas of the lung.* The cranioventral lung is atelectatic, deep-red or mottled, and rubbery (Fig. 5-52). In contrast, the caudodorsal areas are voluminous because they fail to collapse, and are edematous, heavy, and firmer than normal. *Variations in these gross lesions occur commonly:* first, occasional cases have a generalized rubbery texture and red discoloration, with no difference between cranial and caudal lung; second, calves that die in respiratory distress may develop marked subpleural and interlobular emphysema with formation of bullae; and third, the raised, consolidated, firm-to-hard lesions of bronchopneumonia may obscure the aforementioned viral lesions in cases with secondary bacterial infection. Apart from hypertrophy and edema of bronchial and mediastinal lymph nodes, lesions are usually absent from other organs.

The **histologic hallmarks** of pneumonia caused by BRSV are *bronchiolar and alveolar epithelial necrosis with the formation of epithelial syncytia.* The lesions and viral antigen are mainly in the cranioventral areas of the lung. In the acute lesions, from 1 to 8 days after infection, bronchioles are lined by flattened epithelium, bronchiolar lumens contain necrotic epithelial cells and modest numbers of neutrophils, and lymphocytes infiltrate around bronchioles. Alveoli contain neutrophils and macrophages, and alveolar septa may be mildly thickened by mononuclear cells, but hyaline membranes are infrequent. Syncytia are prominent in the early stage and appear as multinucleate cells closely associated with the bronchiolar or alveoli epithelium (see Fig. 5-52). Sloughed multinucleate cells with pyknotic nuclei are often more numerous than those within the epithelial layer. *Eosinophilic intracytoplasmic inclusion bodies (ICIBs)* are occasionally present in syncytial cells and uncommonly in bronchiolar and alveolar epithelium (eFig. 5-65).

The *subacute lesions* of BRSV infection—beginning at about 8 days after infection—represent *early repair of the above lesions following lymphocyte-mediated lysis of virus-infected cells.* The bronchiolar epithelium becomes hyperplastic (see Fig. 5-52), and there is disappearance of syncytial cells as viral antigen is cleared. Proliferation of type II pneumocytes

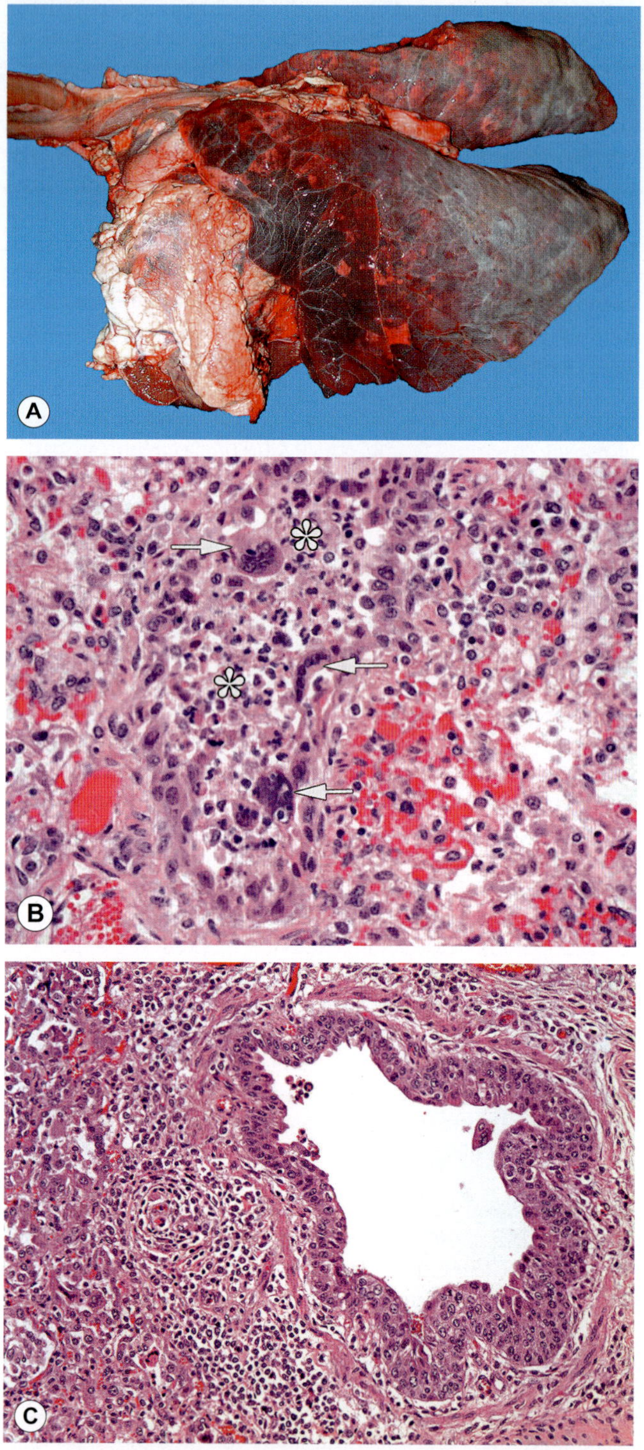

Figure 5-52 Bovine respiratory syncytial virus infection. **A**. Grossly, individual lobules throughout the lung have firm-rubbery texture. Cranioventral areas are reddened and collapsed because of atelectasis; caudodorsal areas are expanded by overinflation or emphysema. The white opacity of the caudal pleura is normal in cattle. **B**. Bronchiole with syncytial epithelial cells (arrows). There is attenuation of remaining epithelium, and cellular debris and leukocytes in the lumen (asterisk). **C**. At a later stage, syncytial cells are absent but bronchiolar epithelium is hyperplastic and multilayered, and lymphocytes and plasma cells surround bronchioles and blood vessels. Alveoli (at the left) are lined by cuboidal type II pneumocytes.

appears as scattered "tombstone-like" cells or complete cuboidal epithelialization of the alveoli. Lymphocytes and plasma cells encircle bronchioles and blood vessels and thicken alveolar septa, and are most numerous 10 days after infection. Obliterative bronchiolitis may occur as early as 10 days after infection, forming polyps of fibrous tissue covered by epithelium that partially occlude bronchiolar lumens.

The histologic lesions of necrotizing bronchiolitis with syncytial cells should be highly suggestive of BRSV infection, but 2 caveats should be considered. First, BPIV3 infection may also induce the formation of syncytia with ICIBs. Second, alveolar and sometimes bronchiolar multinucleate macrophage giant cells are common in subacute or chronic fibrinous bronchopneumonia, and probably represent an attempt to remove the fibrinous alveolar exudate (see eFig. 5-65B). This can present a diagnostic dilemma, given that many calves with BRSV develop secondary bacterial pneumonia, and these multinucleate macrophages must be distinguished from viral syncytia. Viral epithelial syncytia tend to affect alveoli and bronchioles, some have pyknotic nuclei or other features of necrosis, some have centrally arranged nuclei, and ICIBs are helpful when present. In contrast, multinucleate macrophage giant cells tend to be alveolar and less frequently bronchiolar, viable rather than necrotic, and some cells have peripheral nuclei. Finally, when syncytia are absent, the lesions resemble those caused by other viruses, and laboratory testing is needed for diagnosis.

Various assays are available to confirm BRSV infection. Lung tissue from the lesional cranioventral areas of the lung are the most profitable to detect virus; viral antigen or nucleic acid is less frequent in caudodorsal lung tissue. Virus isolation is not recommended for routine diagnostic use, given that the development of an immune response interferes with virus isolation and the virus is easily inactivated by transport conditions. *Quantitative RT-PCR assays are ideal and more sensitive than immunohistochemistry.* Nevertheless, identification of viral antigen by immunohistochemistry or antigen detection by ELISA is also useful and cost-effective. *Cattle vaccinated with intranasal modified-live virus vaccines have detectable viral nucleic acid for 14 days, and up to 28 days in some calves. Thus, positive RT-PCR tests in this time interval may not indicate the true cause of the respiratory disease.*

Bovine parainfluenza virus 3

Infection with bovine parainfluenza virus 3 (BPIV3; *Paramyxoviridae, Respirovirus bovis*) is widespread in 2-8-month-old beef and dairy cattle, but *clinically significant disease caused by primary BPIV3 infection is rare.* Clinical findings in uncomplicated primary BPIV3 infection include transient fever, nasal discharge, sporadic cough, mild depression, and hyperpnea. The virus causes occasional outbreaks of nasal disease in mature cows, with nasal erosions, fibrinous casts, epistaxis, and submandibular edema. Seroconversion to BPIV3 commonly occurs during periods of temperature fluctuations in the autumn, in association with shipping fever of feedlot calves and with enzootic pneumonia of dairy calves. The prevalence of positive serum titers to BPIV3 is 2-67% on arrival in feedlots, but 23-91% of animals seroconvert within a month after arrival. There is a variable association between seroconversion to BPIV3 and development of pneumonia, and BPIV3 is one of the viruses that predisposes to shipping fever.

Paramyxoviruses are pleomorphic, 150-200 nm diameter, and contain negative-sense single-stranded RNA. Structural proteins include hemagglutinin-neuraminidase glycoprotein (HN), fusion glycoprotein (F), high–molecular-weight protein (L), phosphoprotein (P), nucleocapsid protein (NP), and matrix protein (M). The HN protein mediates viral attachment to and release from infected cells, and the F protein allows penetration and spread of the virus between infected cells. Both the HN and F proteins are necessary for formation of syncytia and virulence. Variation in the M protein is the basis for classification of genotypes a, b, and c.

BPIV3 infects ciliated and nonciliated epithelial cells of the upper and lower respiratory tract, alveolar macrophages, type II pneumocytes, and lymphocytes. The *virus reduces pulmonary defenses* by several mechanisms: injury to ciliated epithelium results in functional and structural impairment of mucociliary clearance, alveolar macrophages from infected calves have reduced capacity for phagocytosis and oxidative killing of bacteria, and infected alveolar macrophages induce contact-mediated suppression of lymphocyte responses.

The HN and F proteins are immunodominant antigens, and serum antibody titers to these antigens are correlated with disease resistance. Serum antibody responses develop at 8 days after experimental infection, peak at about 12 days, and a strong anamnestic response occurs after subsequent infections. Cytotoxic cell-mediated immune responses, which are probably important for clearance of virus-infected cells, are maximal at 6-9 days after infection.

The **gross lesions** in natural cases of primary BPIV3 pneumonia are usually mild and consist of a *cranioventral or generalized, lobular pattern of gray-red discoloration, firm, or rubbery texture, and mild swelling or atelectasis of lung tissue*. In calves that die in respiratory distress, there may be emphysema of the caudal lung lobes. *Bronchiolitis and mild bronchitis are the major* **histologic lesions** in natural cases of primary uncomplicated BPIV3 pneumonia. Epithelial cells lining small bronchioles are rounded, occasionally vacuolated, and slough into the lumen, and the epithelial layer may be discontinuous, attenuated, or hyperplastic. In the acute stages, many bronchial, bronchiolar, and alveolar epithelial cells and alveolar macrophages contain prominent *eosinophilic intracytoplasmic inclusion bodies*. In experimentally infected calves, inclusions are most numerous from 2 to 4 days after infection, and less common from 5 to 12 days. *Epithelial syncytial cells may be present in alveoli*, but are fewer than in BRSV infection. Airways contain low numbers of neutrophils, and lymphocytes infiltrate the mildly edematous bronchiolar walls. Alveoli are atelectatic, edematous, contain increased numbers of macrophages and neutrophils, and may have proliferation of alveolar type II pneumocytes. Fibroblasts and macrophages begin to organize the bronchiolar exudate at 7-12 days after experimental infections, and obliterative bronchiolitis may develop thereafter.

BPIV3 infection should be considered in calves with necrotizing bronchiolitis. Confirmation of the **diagnosis** is based on *detection of nucleic acid by RT-PCR or of viral antigen by immunohistochemistry*. These detection methods are effective in acute cases (<9-12 days after infection), but may be unrewarding in the more common presentation of chronic bacterial pneumonia with concurrent bronchiolar necrosis or obliterative bronchiolitis. *Definitive diagnosis in these cases may be impossible* because viral antigen and nucleic acid may be cleared before the bacterial pneumonia proves fatal. As for BRSV, PCR tests may be positive in animals recently administered a modified-live virus vaccine. If acute and convalescent sera are available, then demonstration of a *rising antibody titer* using the hemagglutination inhibition assay supports the histologic diagnosis.

Bovine coronavirus

Bovine coronavirus (**BCoV**; *Coronaviridae, Betacoronavirus) is an important cause of enteric disease in young calves, winter dysentery in adults, and may induce respiratory disease in <1-8-month-old calves*. Nonetheless, it is difficult to determine the causal role of BCoV in individual cases because BoCV is frequently detected in healthy calves, the lesions resemble those of other viruses that may have been cleared by the time of death, and experimental BCoV infections induce only mild and inconsistent disease. Tropism for both the digestive and respiratory tracts is shared by some other betacoronaviruses including severe acute respiratory syndrome coronavirus-2 (SARS-CoV-2). BCoV isolates from occurrences of respiratory and diarrheic diseases have similar genotypes, and a single outbreak may include both forms of disease. Respiratory signs include fever, serous nasal discharge, sneezing, and coughing. The virus replicates primarily in the nasal and tracheal epithelium and occasionally in the lung within the bronchiolar epithelium.

Bronchiolar necrosis is the typical lesion seen in BCoV-infected calves (see Fig. 5-23). Bronchiolar syncytia have been described in feedlot calves with concurrent BCoV infection and bacterial pneumonia, but the contribution of other viruses such as BRSV to these lesions is uncertain. BCoV may be demonstrated using immunohistochemistry or RT-PCR, or isolated using specific rectal tumor cell lines.

Bovine viral diarrhea virus

The contribution of bovine viral diarrhea virus (BVDV) to pneumonia in cattle is a long-standing source of controversy. Virus can be isolated from the lung in primary (acute) infections and in persistently infected calves. *Epidemiologic and experimental studies show that BVDV-infected calves do indeed have heightened susceptibility to bacterial pneumonia*, and respiratory signs may be the chief clinical complaint resulting from acute BVDV infections. Mechanisms by which BVDV predisposes to bacterial pneumonia include reduced antimicrobial protein production by virus-infected airway epithelial cells, reduced function of alveolar macrophages, and virus-induced neutropenia. BVDV has also been shown to exacerbate BRSV and bovine herpesvirus 1 infections in experimental situations, but not *Mycoplasmopsis bovis*.

It has been proposed that some isolates of BVDV induce primary respiratory disease, independent of opportunistic bacterial pathogens. During primary BVDV infection, viral antigen is present in pulmonary alveolar macrophages and in airway epithelium (see eFig. 5-56). In addition, viral antigen may be demonstrated in the tunica muscularis of arterioles in the lung, heart, and occasionally in other tissues, often in association with lesions of lymphocytic arteritis. Calves or lambs challenged with certain isolates of BVDV develop fever and hyperpnea or, in other studies, nasal discharge and coughing. The lesions described are mild, consisting of peribronchiolar, perivascular, or interstitial aggregates of lymphocytes and macrophages, and/or mild neutrophilic exudate in bronchioles. However, other studies have found no lung lesions in calves infected with BVDV, and *the importance of BVDV as a cause of primary lung disease is probably minimal*.

Bovine adenovirus

Bovine adenoviruses are a recognized cause of hemorrhagic colitis, but their role in respiratory disease is more controversial. Epitheliotropic bovine adenoviruses are occasionally isolated from feedlot calves with bacterial pneumonia, and many calves seroconvert to a range of bovine adenovirus (**BAdV**, *Adenoviridae, Mastadenovirus*) serotypes within 5 weeks of entering feedlots. Adenoviruses may predispose to bacterial pneumonia by injuring ciliated epithelium and, for some strains, by impairing alveolar macrophages. However, compared with the roles of stress and other viral infections, *adenoviruses are probably minor contributors to bacterial pneumonia in cattle.*

Calves experimentally infected with BAdV generally develop only mild respiratory disease; the severity of primary adenoviral pneumonia is probably dependent on both the strain of the BAdV and the immune status of the calf. Experimentally infected calves developed lobular or patchy areas of atelectasis and reddening. *Histologic lesions* include proliferation of bronchial and bronchiolar epithelium, lymphocytic infiltration of airway epithelium, formation of *large basophilic intranuclear inclusions* in airway epithelial cells, and exfoliation or necrosis of virus-infected cells. In well-developed cases, there is extensive bronchiolar necrosis, occlusion of bronchiolar lumens by sloughed epithelium, and inclusions in intact or sloughed epithelial cells. Thickening of alveolar septa by mononuclear cells may occur, but proliferation of type II pneumocytes is uncommon.

Other viral diseases

Other viruses can be detected in cattle with respiratory disease, but it is uncertain if they cause disease. Methods to identify novel viruses are now easily accessible, but it is more laborious to build evidence that the infection causes disease. Bovine respiratory disease often occurs after co-mingling animals from different sources, and these are times when nonpathogenic viruses are expected to be circulating even if the disease outbreaks are caused by other pathogens and risk factors. Principles for critically evaluating evidence that a newly identified virus directly causes disease (Bradford Hill criteria for causation) can include: identifying the virus (but not other plausible causes) in various unrelated cases of a similar disease, a higher frequency and/or load of infection in diseased versus healthy animals that are otherwise comparable, evidence that new infection consistently precedes the onset of disease, consistently identifying the virus in animals with a unique type of lesion or clinical presentation, colocalization of the virus within the lesion, a plausible pathogenesis of how infection causes the lesion, reduction of disease by virus-specific control such as vaccination, and induction of disease in sufficient numbers of experimentally infected animals but not in controls. For the following viruses, few of these criteria have been met, and more work is needed to determine their relevance to disease.

Cattle are the reservoir of **deltainfluenzavirus (influenza D virus)**, which also infects pigs and other species including humans. Many studies have identified deltainfluenzaviruses in cattle with respiratory disease. Some evidence supports deltainfluenzaviruses as a predisposing cause or cofactor in bovine respiratory disease, including higher frequency in cases versus controls, an association of viral load with more severe clinical disease (albeit sometimes complicated by a higher frequency of other viruses), but no reduction in clinical disease or lesions in vaccinated calves. Experimentally infected calves have had mild respiratory signs, viral antigen in nasal epithelium and minimally in lower airway epithelium, and grossly visible fibrinopurulent tracheal exudate and mild lung consolidation in a few animals. The histologic lesions were mainly present in the upper respiratory tract, with nasal or tracheal ciliary loss and erosions with mononuclear cells and neutrophils; some calves had lung lesions of mild bronchitis/bronchiolitis or infiltrates of mononuclear cells in alveolar septa. There is limited evidence of more severe disease when coinfected with *Mycoplasmopsis bovis* or *Mannheimia haemolytica*. Thus, *current evidence suggests that deltainfluenzavirus mainly infects the upper respiratory tract of cattle and by itself causes only mild clinical disease and lesions*, but it remains as a possible cofactor in development of bovine respiratory disease.

Alpha- and gamma-influenzaviruses (influenza A and C viruses) have been found in cattle with pneumonia, but there is no evidence that they cause disease. An H5N1 highly pathogenic avian influenza strain infects the mammary gland of cattle; although virus has been detected in lungs of some cattle by PCR, respiratory disease is not reported at the time of this writing (2024).

HoBi-like pestivirus (Pestivirus H, **HoBiPeV**; *Flaviviridae, Pestivirus brazilense*) was identified in cattle dying of necrotizing rhinotracheitis, interstitial pneumonia, and enteritis, with other reports describing tracheitis and bronchopneumonia with leukopenia, or ulcerative lesions of upper and lower alimentary tract, or infertility and abortion. Its prevalence in healthy animals is not known, and experimental infections have induced only mild respiratory signs (hyperthermia and nasal discharge). Thus, it remains uncertain if (and under which circumstances) this pestivirus causes respiratory disease in cattle.

Bovine rhinitis A and B viruses (**BRAV**, **BRBV**; *Picornaviridae, Aphthovirus bogeli, Aphthovirus reedi*) are widespread in cattle populations. *They are generally believed to be of little importance as a cause of respiratory disease in cattle.* Virus isolation and serologic responses occasionally provide circumstantial evidence that BRAV/BVs are involved in causing upper respiratory disease. Experimental infection has inconsistently induced interstitial pneumonia.

Bacterial diseases

Bacterial bronchopneumonia caused by Pasteurellaceae: Mannheimia haemolytica, Histophilus somni, and Pasteurella multocida

Bacterial bronchopneumonia is a common and economically important disease of cattle, particularly in temperate climates, and is mainly caused by bacteria of the family *Pasteurellaceae*. The *most important clinical entities are enzootic pneumonia of young calves and shipping fever of feedlot cattle*, but bacterial pneumonia may occur in any age group, often as a complication of stress, viral infection, or inclement weather.

Shipping-fever pneumonia has long been considered the most economically important disease of beef cattle in temperate climates. The *classic presentation* of shipping fever is of pneumonia affecting many calves, 3 days to 3 weeks after being shipped from their farm of origin to a feedlot. Affected animals have acute onset of depression, pyrexia, anorexia, rapid and shallow respiration, and mucopurulent nasal discharge. Coughing is variably present and dyspnea develops in later stages. Most cattle respond rapidly to appropriate antibiotic therapy if given early in the course of disease, but relapses are common. Most reports of shipping fever describe 15-45%

morbidity, 1-5% mortality, and case fatality rates of 5-10% depending on the rapidity with which treatment is initiated. *Risk factors* for shipping fever include those associated with: 1) increased exposure of naive calves to animals shedding viral pathogens, such as mixing of calves from various sources; 2) stress, such as weaning, transport, crowding, disruption of social groups, deprivation of feed and water, handling, vaccination, dehorning, and pregnancy checking; 3) metabolic acidosis, such as rapid introduction to grain or corn silage; and 4) exposure of calves to adverse environmental conditions, such as changes in temperature and humidity, cool weather in the autumn months, snow or rain, or dusty environment.

Bacterial pneumonia is also common in 1-4-month-old dairy and veal calves and less common in suckling beef calves. Although commonly referred to as *"enzootic pneumonia,"* cases may be sporadic, enzootic, or occur in outbreaks. Affected calves are febrile, hyperpneic, variably dyspneic, depressed, and anorexic. *Risk factors* include: 1) reduced air quality, such as indoor housing, poor ventilation, high stocking density, high levels of airborne particulates, ammonia, and humidity; 2) failure of adequate passive transfer of immunoglobulin; 3) factors exposing calves to viral or mycoplasmal pathogens, such as co-mingling animals from different sources, housing younger calves with older calves or adults, and unsanitary feeding equipment; and 4) stressors such as concurrent diseases.

Outbreaks or sporadic cases of bacterial pneumonia occur in lactating dairy cows. The disease is otherwise similar to *M. haemolytica* pneumonia in other age classes, is more frequent in the winter, and is associated with the entry of new animals to the group, recent calving, adverse weather, concurrent diseases, and poor barn ventilation.

Pasteurellaceae are gram-negative coccobacilli; several members of the family are common causes of pneumonia or septicemia in domestic animals. *Many species of Pasturellaceae inhabit the upper respiratory tract of healthy animals*, but cause pneumonia when pulmonary defenses are impaired, or there is excessive inflammation in the respiratory tract. These pathogens can also cause septicemia in naive animals or those with reduced systemic defenses. In general, the defense against many *Pasteurellaceae* depends on a combination of innate resistance mechanisms and acquired humoral immunity. The most common pathogenic *Pasteurellaceae* of domestic animals include *Pasteurella multocida* of pigs, ruminants, and cats; *Mannheimia haemolytica* and *Bibersteinia trehalosi* of ruminants; *Actinobacillus pleuropneumoniae* and *A. suis* of pigs; *A. equuli* of horses; *Histophilus somni* of cattle and sheep; and *Glaesserella parasuis* of pigs.

Mannheimia haemolytica and ***Bibersteinia trehalosi***: 12 serotypes of *M. haemolytica* are discerned based on soluble capsular polysaccharide antigens. Serotype names were maintained when the species *Pasteurella haemolytica* biotypes A and T were reclassified as *M. haemolytica* and *B. trehalosi*, respectively; as a result, serotypes 3, 4, 10, and 15 are represented only by *B. trehalosi* (discussed in the Infectious Respiratory Diseases of Sheep and Goats section). Serotype 2, and, to a lesser extent, serotype 1, is a sporadic isolate from the nasopharynx of healthy calves. Serotypes 1 and 6 are the most common isolates from pneumonic lung, but other serotypes in addition to many untypeable isolates regularly cause bovine pneumonia. Conversely, genotype 1 is mainly isolated from healthy calves and genotype 2 more commonly causes pneumonia.

Virulence factors of *M. haemolytica* include leukotoxin, lipopolysaccharide, a polysaccharide capsule, transferrin-binding proteins A and B, O-sialoglycoprotease, neuraminidase, IgG1-specific protease, outer-membrane proteins, adhesins, and fimbriae. All serotypes secrete *leukotoxin*, a member of the RTX family of bacterial toxins, during the log phase of growth. The products of *lkt*A and *lkt*C genes represent the active leukotoxin; *lkt*B and *lkt*D are necessary for toxin secretion. At high concentrations, leukotoxin lyses ruminant leukocytes and platelets, mediated by binding to CD18 on the leukocyte surface and formation of pores in the cell membrane. At lower concentrations, leukotoxin activates leukocytes and platelets. Although leukotoxin clearly plays a role in the pathogenesis of pneumonia, some disease can develop in calves vaccinated against leukotoxin and in those challenged with *M. haemolytica* constructs that do not secrete leukotoxin.

Lipopolysaccharide is a major component of the cell wall; O-polysaccharide side chains confer a smooth phenotype to most serotypes. Lipopolysaccharide from *M. haemolytica* stimulates alveolar macrophages to secrete inflammatory mediators, including tumor necrosis factor, IL1, and the chemokines IL8, ENA, and GROα. Other effects of *M. haemolytica* lipopolysaccharide on alveolar macrophages include triggering of oxidative burst, an important bactericidal mechanism that may also lead to oxidative tissue injury; expression of tissue factor, a mediator of the thrombosis characteristic of the disease; and secretion of nitric oxide, which may augment lung defenses but is also a potent mediator of vasodilation and thus ventilation-perfusion mismatching. Other effects of lipopolysaccharide include activation of the extrinsic coagulation pathway, and complement activation. The mannose-rich polysaccharide capsule confers resistance of *M. haemolytica* to phagocytosis by macrophages and neutrophils, and may also block complement-dependent killing. Neuraminidase enhances adhesion of bacteria to mucosal epithelium by cleaving sialic acid from the surface of epithelial cells, and may reduce mucus viscosity to prevent mucociliary clearance.

Low numbers of M. haemolytica colonize the nasopharynx of normal calves, and there are several potential explanations for the shift from a commensal to a pathogenic relationship. First, stress or exposure to cold results in greater numbers of nasopharyngeal *M. haemolytica* bacteria, so inhalation of droplets containing increased numbers of bacteria may overwhelm pulmonary defenses. The mechanisms whereby stress or exposure to cold induces expansion of the bacterial population, and whether these factors also alter expression of bacterial virulence factors, have not been defined. Second, stress and cold exposure induce a shift from serotype 2 to the more pathogenic serotype 1. Third, viral infections, inhaled particulates, and perhaps stress create a proinflammatory state that promotes harmful inflammatory responses to infection. Fourth, viral infections or stress impair lung defenses. The lung is normally exposed to low numbers of aspirated *M. haemolytica*, but a combination of mucociliary clearance, antimicrobial function of secreted mucosal proteins, and phagocytosis by alveolar macrophages controls this infection without inciting an inflammatory response. BoAHV1, BRSV, and BPIV3 infect ciliated epithelium and reduce mucociliary clearance, and BoAHV1 and BRSV infect and impair the function of alveolar macrophages. In addition, BoAHV1 infection upregulates CD18 on the surface of bovine neutrophils. Since CD18 is a receptor of *M. haemolytica* leukotoxin, these activated neutrophils are more susceptible to the leukotoxin. Viral infections may also impair secretion of antimicrobial proteins by airway or alveolar epithelium. The mechanisms whereby stress impairs innate pulmonary defenses are poorly defined. As a result of these processes, exposure of the lung to increased numbers of virulent *M. haemolytica* coincides with a reduction in pulmonary defenses and a tendency for excessive inflammation. The finding that outbreaks are often polymicrobial (with isolates of multiple *Pasteurellaceae* bacteria including diverse genotypes of *M. haemolytica*) supports the notion that this disease results from failure of lung defenses, with colonization by opportunistic pathogens that are well equipped to evade the remaining defenses and incite disease.

Clinical disease is principally a consequence of the host response to infection of the lung with *M. haemolytica*, rather than a direct effect of bacterial toxins on lung tissue. Massive exudation of fibrin into alveoli is a prominent feature of severe pneumonia in cattle and is mediated in part by a direct effect of lipopolysaccharide on endothelial cells, but also by macrophage-derived inflammatory mediators such as tumor necrosis factor. Phagocytosis of *M. haemolytica* by alveolar macrophages is limited unless the bacteria are opsonized by antibody or complement; the significance of other opsonins such as the collectins remains speculative. Alveolar macrophages that have ingested *M. haemolytica* or been exposed to bacterial products secrete an array of neutrophil chemoattractants, including IL8, ENA, GRO, platelet-activating factor, and leukotriene B4. Neutrophils migrate to the alveoli and terminal bronchioles within 3 hours of experimental challenge with *M. haemolytica*. Neutrophil migration to alveoli employs a β_2 integrin-independent mechanism, whereas neutrophil recruitment to airways is dependent on interactions between β_2 integrin and ICAM1. In contrast to most bacterial infections, in which neutrophils and macrophages phagocytose and kill the offending bacteria, neutrophils and macrophages recruited to the sites of established infection with *M. haemolytica* are lysed by leukotoxin. *There is massive recruitment of neutrophils and macrophages; these are ineffective in killing bacteria, but nonetheless exacerbate the severity of clinical disease*. Infiltration of neutrophils and monocyte-derived macrophages into alveoli is harmful in several ways: the physical presence of these cells precludes normal ventilation and gas exchange; oxygen radicals, nitric oxide derivatives, and proteinases secreted by leukocytes injure lung cells and the interstitial stroma; expression of tissue factor by activated alveolar or intravascular macrophages promotes fibrin formation in the alveolus and thrombosis of blood vessels in the alveolar septa; and both macrophages and neutrophils secrete chemoattractants that perpetuate the recruitment of additional leukocytes.

Focal areas of coagulative necrosis are a characteristic feature of infection with M. haemolytica. Some represent infarcts caused by thrombosis of intralobular blood vessels, but leukocyte secretions might also cause direct lung injury. The foci are encircled by a dense band of leukocytes, many of which are necrotic, and these leukocytes are in a state of intense activation featuring prominent gene expression of IL8 and inducible nitric oxide synthetase. Profound depression and "toxemia" are constant features of acute infection with *M. haemolytica;* although the basis for this systemic illness is unknown, tumor necrosis factor in the plasma of some cases may be responsible.

Immune responses to *M. haemolytica* occur rapidly following exposure, with alveolar IgM detectable by 48 hours after experimental infection, and detectable serum IgM and IgG by 5 and 7 days after infection, respectively. Animals that recover from disease or are vaccinated with live bacteria are immune to subsequent challenge, and serum antibody titers to leukotoxin, outer-membrane proteins, and capsule are all correlated with resistance to naturally occurring disease. However, it is likely that an immune response to several antigens is necessary for protection, as antibody to individual antigens—including leukotoxin, capsular polysaccharide, lipopolysaccharide, or outer-membrane proteins—does not confer complete protection.

Histophilus somni causes bronchopneumonia, pleuritis (see Fig. 5-38) or pericarditis, polyarthritis, and infectious thrombotic meningoencephalitis, although an individual animal is usually affected by only one of these conditions. The importance of *H. somni* as a cause of bovine pneumonia varies considerably between geographic regions. As with *M. haemolytica*, this pathogen possesses a broad array of virulence factors. Resistance to serum- and complement-mediated killing is mediated by proteins that bind the Fc component of immunoglobulin, making these Fc receptors unavailable for complement activation. Lipooligosaccharide has many proinflammatory effects, analogous to lipopolysaccharide in other gram-negative bacteria. The lipooligosaccharide of disease-associated, but not commensal, isolates of *H. somni* undergoes structural and antigenic variation during the course of an experimental infection, and this variation may serve as a mechanism of immune evasion and resistance to complement-mediated killing. Transferrin- and hemoglobin-binding proteins enable the bacteria to acquire iron for growth. *H. somni* binds to and induces apoptosis in endothelial cells in vitro, and this may contribute to the vasculitis that is characteristic of *H. somni* septicemia. Deposition of immune complexes is apparently not the cause of vasculitis. *H. somni* is considered a facultative intracellular pathogen given that it survives within monocytes, yet both intra- and extracellular bacteria are numerous in acute pneumonia, and biofilm formation is described. The bacterium persuades macrophages to release tissue factor in microparticles, which may contribute to the thrombosis and florid fibrinous exudates typical of this disease. Finally, *H. somni* impairs the phagocytic function of neutrophils and macrophages and induces degeneration of macrophages and apoptosis of neutrophils. Vasculitis is a characteristic feature of *H. somni* infection, from diverse mechanisms including induction of an inflammatory response, apoptosis of endothelial cells, activation of platelets, and histamine production by the bacteria.

Pasteurella multocida is an important cause of pneumonia in cattle. Serotypes A-F are based on capsular antigens, and somatic serogroups 1-8 based on lipopolysaccharide; these can be categorized by PCR assays. Serotypes A:3 and A:6 are most commonly isolated from cases of pneumonia. As for *M. haemolytica*, the bacteria are carried in the nasopharynx of many clinically normal calves. Adhesins, an antiphagocytic capsule, neuraminidase, iron-binding proteins, and lipopolysaccharide are among the described virulence factors.

The **gross lesions** of acute fulminant "shipping-fever" pneumonia caused by *M. haemolytica*, *H. somni*, or *P. multocida* are not reliably distinguished and include *cranioventral lobar or lobular fibrinous bronchopneumonia and sometimes fibrinous pleuritis* (Fig. 5-53). Lesions are most severe in the cranial and middle lung lobes, but may also affect the caudal lung. Acute fulminant cases often exhibit lobar fibrinous pneumonia and pleuritis and may die with as little as 30% of the lung affected, because of systemic effects of the lung infection rather than failure of lung function. Lesions are often sharply demarcated from less affected areas of lung, are discolored purple-red and later tan-gray, and the filling of alveoli with fibrin bestows a firm or hard texture to the affected lung.

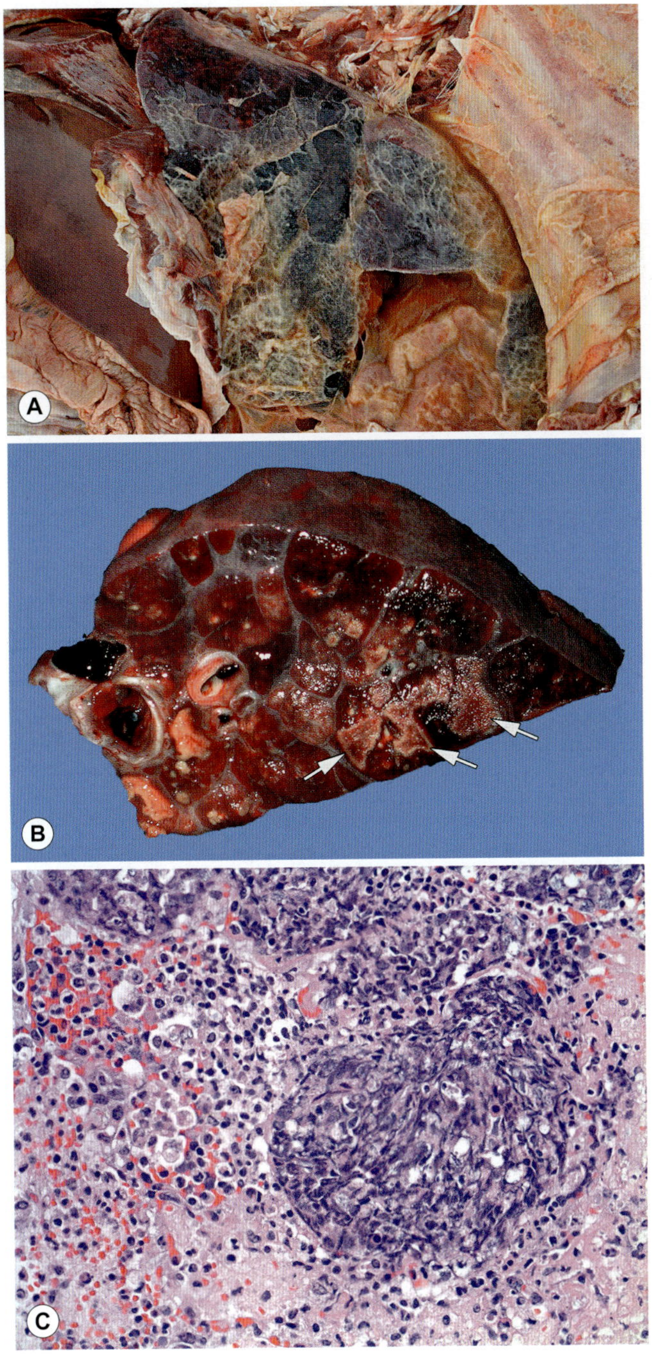

Figure 5-53 Peracute fibrinous bronchopneumonia in a feedlot calf. **A.** Characteristic lesions of peracute bronchopneumonia: mats of loosely adherent fibrin on visceral and parietal pleurae (see the reflected ribs at the right), red-purple discoloration and crisp texture of affected lung tissue. A thin line of ventilated pink tissue remains along the dorsal border of the lung. **B.** The cut surface reveals irregular foci of coagulative necrosis with a white rim of leukocytes (arrows), typical of *Mannheimia haemolytica* infection. **C.** Alveoli contain fibrin and viable leukocytes (at the left) and necrotic leukocytes with streaming chromatin characteristic of "oat cells" (at the right).

The cut section of the lung is purple-red, firm or hard, and moist. It is often not possible to express exudate from the transected airway because the leukocytes are enmeshed in polymerized fibrin. Sharply demarcated, irregularly shaped, 0.5-5-cm, pale, dry foci of coagulative necrosis are frequent in fulminant cases of *M. haemolytica* infection (see Fig. 5-53). Bronchi may contain catarrhal or neutrophilic material or hemorrhage or may be free of exudate. Interlobular septa are distended with fibrinous or serofibrinous exudate, and this lends a marbled appearance to the cut surface. Bacterial emigration from lung to the pleural space elicits fibrinous pleuritis, with a lattice or mat over the pleural surface of affected lung lobes, and serofibrinous yellow pleural fluid that clots when the chest is opened. Fibrinous pericarditis may accompany the pleuritis.

Necrosis of laryngeal epithelium at the point of contact of the vocal folds may occur in cattle with severe pneumonia, as a result of mucosal trauma induced by abrupt laryngeal closure in a dyspneic animal. Vasculitis resulting from *H. somni* bacteremia can cause a similar lesion.

Differentiation of acute from subacute lesions is challenging but important to determine whether early clinical recognition of ill animals was adequate. Indicators of peracute pneumonia include red-purple hemorrhagic and infarcted lobules, crisp texture of the cut section, abundant and loosely adherent pleural fibrin, and systemic petechiae (see Fig. 5-53). Characteristics of subacute bronchopneumonia may include a lobular distribution of lesions (see Fig. 5-28), mottled tan-gray as well as red appearance, neutrophilic exudate that oozes from small bronchi when a cut section is compressed, purulent or catarrhal exudate on the mucosal surface of the large airways, and pleural adhesions. Mild subacute cases with atelectasis and rubbery consolidation may be difficult to distinguish from lesions of viral pneumonia.

Sequelae indicative of chronic disease include *sequestra, bronchiectasis, abscesses, and fibrous pleural adhesions*. Sequestra consist of a necrotic core of firm but friable tissue, sometimes surrounded by fluid or caseous exudate, enveloped in a capsule of fibrous tissue. Bronchiectasis manifests as dilated airways that are filled with purulent exudate and thickened by fibrous tissue (see Fig. 5-25). The surrounding lung tissue is invariably atelectatic and may be swollen due to persistent bronchopneumonia. Ectatic bronchi appear similar to abscesses, but bronchiectasis has cylindrical tracts filled with pus, remnants of bronchial cartilage, and communication with a bronchus. Lesions of bronchiectasis and abscesses are often secondarily colonized by *Trueperella pyogenes* or other opportunistic pathogens.

The **histologic lesion** of *acute fulminant "shipping-fever" pneumonia is fibrinous and neutrophilic bronchopneumonia*. Alveoli and small bronchioles are filled with variable proportions of neutrophils and macrophages, fibrin, edema fluid, erythrocytes, necrotic cellular debris, and aggregates of bacteria. Larger airways may contain neutrophilic exudate, but neutrophil infiltration of the mucosa is often absent. Necrosis and attenuation of bronchiolar epithelium, when present, may prompt a search for underlying viral or *Mycoplasmopsis bovis* infection. However, this lesion is present in some calves experimentally infected with *H. somni* or *M. haemolytica*, and may represent neutrophil-induced damage to the epithelium or a direct effect of *H. somni*. In acute cases, thrombi commonly occlude arterioles, venules, and alveolar septal capillaries, and interlobular septa are distended with serofibrinous exudate and have fibrin or fluid in the septal lymphatic vessels.

A characteristic feature of *M. haemolytica* and *B. trehalosi* is necrosis of intra-alveolar leukocytes (neutrophils and macrophages) with a fusiform streaming pattern of pale basophilic chromatin (termed "oat *cells*" for their resemblance to grains of oats) (see Fig. 5-53), where leukotoxin is the likely cause of the neutrophil cell death. Leukocyte necrosis may also be present in *H. somni* and *Trueperella pyogenes* infections, but in such cases the dead cells are rounded or pyknotic and lack the characteristic fusiform streaming chromatin of oat cells. With *M. haemolytica* and *B. trehalosi*, sharply demarcated, irregularly shaped areas of coagulative necrosis are often apparent. In these, alveolar and bronchiolar lesions are as described above, but all cells within the lesions are necrotic, and karyolysis or karyorrhexis is prominent. A dense band of necrotic leukocytes encircles these foci of necrosis, and thrombi occasionally fill blood vessels at the edge of or within the lesions. Lesions of *H. somni* can include neutrophilic phlebitis with fibrinoid necrosis in acute fulminant cases.

The appearance of these lesions changes in later stages. Macrophages and multinucleate histiocytic cells encompass the alveolar masses of polymerized fibrin; removal of fibrin by these macrophages and by fibrinolysis presumably occurs in some nonfatal cases. Otherwise, alveolar fibrin is infiltrated by fibroblasts and replaced by connective tissue, visible by 5 days after infection, with 2 possible sequelae: incorporation of the re-epithelialized alveolar fibrous tissue into the alveolar septum to form a thickened alveolar septum and a "recanalized" alveolar lumen, or large expanses of pulmonary fibrosis. Chronic neutrophilic or lymphoplasmacytic bronchitis occurs regularly in calves with chronic pneumonia.

Less fulminant cases tend to lack the fibrinous alveolar exudate, thrombosis, and interlobular fibrin that are typical of fulminant shipping-fever pneumonia. Rather these lesions are dominated by exudation of neutrophils in alveoli and bronchioles, congestion of pulmonary vessels, but little other morphologic change in lung tissue.

The gross lesions of cranioventral bronchopneumonia are usually **diagnostic**. The swollen and hard nature of bacterial pneumonia aids in the differentiation from the atelectatic cranioventral lesions of BRSV pneumonia. A histologic finding of neutrophilic bronchopneumonia implies a diagnosis of bacterial pneumonia; the clinical challenge is to identify the underlying causes. Lesions of aspiration pneumonia may closely resemble bacterial pneumonia; however, focal or unilateral, necrotizing, and foul-smelling lesions containing histologically recognizable foreign material with an associated inflammatory reaction are indicators of aspiration, and foci of coagulative necrosis with oat cells do not occur in aspiration pneumonia. Differentiation of the foci of coagulative necrosis from the caseous necrosis of *Mycoplasmopsis bovis* pneumonia is discussed in the section on mycoplasmal disease.

B. trehalosi and *M. haemolytica* serotype 2 also cause outbreaks of septicemia in neonatal calves, similar to that described in lambs. Affected calves are obtunded and tachypneic, and have fibrinous exudate in pleural and other body cavities, fibrinous polyarthritis, and fibrinous pneumonia of ventral regions of lung mainly affecting the interlobular septa.

The use of *aerobic and microaerophilic culture* to identify the specific cause is usually successful unless animals have been medicated with antimicrobials. It is helpful to genotype or serotype *M. haemolytica* isolates using MALDI-TOF MS or multiplex PCR, respectively, because genotype 2 or serotype 1 isolates are generally considered more virulent. Subacute or chronic cases are often colonized by opportunistic bacteria and the primary bacterial cause may no longer be present. Immunohistochemistry to identify *M. haemolytica* and *H. somni* has been described, and may be of use in antimicrobial-treated, autolyzed, or archival tissues, or if fresh tissue is not available. Detection of serum antibody to *M. haemolytica* is a research tool but of limited value in field investigations.

Hemorrhagic septicemia

Hemorrhagic septicemia is caused by ***Pasteurella multocida****, and usually* ***serotypes B:2 or E:2***. It is now limited largely to tropical countries of Asia and Africa, and in these regions is primarily a disease of buffalo and to a lesser extent cattle. Outbreaks in tropical climates occur particularly during the rainy season. In intervening periods, the organism is apparently maintained in the nasopharynx of carriers. The start of an outbreak depends on some stress disturbing the balance in a carrier animal. This results in extensive proliferation and dissemination of the organisms to susceptible contact animals.

Approximately 10% of animals survive subclinical infections and become immune, but once clinical signs are apparent, the mortality is almost 100%, even with appropriate antimicrobial therapy. This, together with the immense proliferation of organisms in the clinical disease, suggests that bacterial toxins (particularly endotoxin) are important in causing death.

Hemorrhagic septicemia is a peracute disease and many animals die without clinical signs. Less fulminant cases have high fever and rapid prostration, with profuse drooling. Petechial hemorrhages are present on the serous membranes and in various organs, especially the lungs and muscles. Severe endotoxemia may cause *acute, fibrinohemorrhagic interstitial lung disease*. Lymph nodes are swollen and hemorrhagic, and there may be blood-stained fluid in the serous cavities. Acute gastroenteritis, which can be hemorrhagic, is often present. The spleen is not greatly enlarged, which is a point of differentiation from anthrax.

There is a *subacute edematous form of hemorrhagic septicemia*, in which edema of the throat is unusually pronounced. The whole head, tongue, brisket, or a limb may also be affected. The swellings are produced by copious, clotted, straw-colored exudate. Death results from asphyxiation.

Cilia-associated respiratory bacillus

Filobacterium rodentium [formerly, cilia-associated respiratory (CAR) bacillus] causes chronic respiratory disease in rats, mice, and rabbits. The filamentous bacilli interdigitate between cilia and induce lymphocytic bronchitis and bronchiolitis, bronchiectasis, and lung abscesses. The filamentous bacteria among the cilia are visualized with Warthin-Starry silver stains. Morphologically similar bacteria have been observed in the tracheal epithelium of cattle, deer, pigs, and cats. In *calves*, CAR bacilli are suggested to induce lymphoid follicles in the airway wall. *Porcine* CAR bacilli are apparently nonpathogenic, for they are present in pigs with and without respiratory disease, and experimentally infected pigs have not developed clinical signs or lesions. *Filobacterium* sp. have been identified in cats with chronic neutrophilic bronchitis, but additional work is needed to infer causality. The major differential diagnosis agent is *Bordetella bronchiseptica*, which is rod-shaped rather than filamentous.

Tuberculosis

Bovine tuberculosis, caused by ***Mycobacterium bovis****, is a chronic disease with caseating granulomas in lung, lymph nodes,* *and other organs*. Control programs have minimized the occurrence of bovine tuberculosis in many developed countries.

Success of tuberculosis eradication schemes is complicated by *wildlife reservoirs*, which maintain infection and transmit disease to cattle. Wildlife reservoirs of *Mycobacterium bovis* include European badgers *(Meles meles)* in Ireland and the United Kingdom, brush-tailed possum *(Trichosurus vulpecula)* in New Zealand, feral pigs in Spain, swamp buffalo *(Bubalus bubalis)* in Australia's Northern Territory, Cape buffalo *(Syncerus caffer)* and lechwe antelope (*Kobus leche*) in southern Africa, bison *(Bison bison)* in Wood Buffalo National Park in western Canada, and various species of deer in the United States and New Zealand. In contrast, dead-end or spillover hosts, including goats, wart hogs, cats, mustelids, and humans, may be infected with *Mycobacterium bovis* but do not maintain infection in an area and rarely transmit *M. bovis* to cattle.

Many mycobacteria persist in soil for prolonged periods, and the infectivity of *M. bovis* is likely maintained for several weeks in the environment. However, because oral infections require high doses of bacilli, the importance of environmental survival in the epidemiology of disease is likely limited.

Tuberculosis is caused by the classical tubercle bacilli that are members of the *Mycobacterium tuberculosis* complex including *Mycobacterium tuberculosis*, *M. bovis*, *M. africanum*, *M. canetti*, *M. microti*, *M. caprae*, *M. pinnipedii*, and *M. mungi*. Disease conditions caused by other "nontuberculous" mycobacteria (such as the *Mycobacterium avium* complex, *M. fortuitum*, and *M. smegmatis*) are referred to as **mycobacterioses**. Nontuberculous mycobacteria are widespread in soil and water and typically cause disease in immunocompromised hosts. The manifestations are pulmonary lesions similar to tuberculosis, cervical lymphadenitis or abdominal visceral infection from ingested mycobacteria, or cutaneous lesions associated with their local penetration through wounds.

M. tuberculosis, *M. bovis*, and *M. avium* occur most frequently in their respective hosts, but cross-infections do occur, and various other species of animals are affected.

- **Bovine tuberculosis** refers mainly to disease in cattle caused by ***Mycobacterium bovis***, but the term is also used to describe the pathogenic effects of this bacterium in other hosts. The host range of *M. bovis* is broad, including cattle, deer, elk, bison, buffalo, goats, camels, llamas, pigs, elephants, rhinoceros, dogs, foxes, cats, mink, badgers, nonhuman primates, and humans. Natural disease is most common in cattle and cervids.
- ***M. avium*** causes mycobacteriosis chiefly in birds and is occasionally found in cattle, pigs, horses, sheep, and monkeys.
- ***M. tuberculosis*** is the main cause of tuberculosis in humans, and humans can transmit infection to dogs, cattle, pigs, and horses; cats are thought to be relatively resistant although cases do occur. Lesions in dogs affect lung and bronchial lymph nodes or may be disseminated, with caseous necrosis with or without mineralization and surrounded by epithelioid macrophages.
- **Human infections** with *M. bovis* are well documented, but are less common than *M. tuberculosis*. Immunosuppressed individuals, such as those with the acquired immunodeficiency syndrome, are at particular risk. *Ingestion of milk from cows with mammary tuberculosis is a major route of infection in humans*, typically inducing cervical lymphadenitis or other nonpulmonary forms of disease. This pattern of disease is of great historical importance as the impetus for identification of the tubercle bacillus and the subsequent *pasteurization of milk*, but *infection from raw milk continues to occur in regions where bovine tuberculosis is common*. Transmission from cattle to humans by aerosol or by contamination of cutaneous wounds also occurs, mainly in those in close contact with infected cattle.

Mycobacteria are nonmotile, non–spore-forming pleomorphic coccobacilli. They are gram-positive but almost unstainable by the simpler bacterial stains because of their high content of lipids. They are routinely stained with carbol-fuchsin and then resist decoloration by inorganic acids. This property of acid-fastness of the stained bacilli depends on the amount and spatial arrangement of mycolic acids and their esters in the bacterial wall. They are also demonstrable by fluorescent dyes such as auramine. In cultures or in old lesions, the organisms can have a beaded or granulated appearance. This beading is partly caused by lipid droplets within the bacteria and is an indication of an unfavorable environment for organisms in the postexponential growth phase.

In addition to the cell membrane and peptidoglycan layers found in other bacteria, *the mycobacterial cell wall contains a large hydrophobic layer of mycolic acids, which bestows hydrophobicity of the cell wall, conferring environmental and antimicrobial resistance*. The waxes and cell wall glycolipids are important inducers of the initial macrophage response and, together with peptidoglycan (muramyl dipeptide), are responsible for most of the adjuvant activity of mycobacteria that facilitates recruitment of antigen-presenting cells. Increased glycolipid content of mycobacterial cell walls, acid-fastness, and the amount of trehalose dimycolate (cord factor) in the cell wall are associated with increased virulence. Other glycolipids (mycosides) form a barrier against lysosomal digestion and partly explain the ability of the organisms to survive after phagocytosis by macrophages; intracellular survival is also facilitated by preventing fusion of phagosomes and lysosomes. The differing effectiveness of such mechanisms determines the relative ability of various mycobacteria to resist intracellular degradation.

Tuberculoproteins are the other major category of immunoreactive substances in mycobacteria. They provide most of the antigenic determinants, but the adjuvant activity of the lipids and polysaccharides in the mycobacterial cell wall is needed for an animal to produce an immunologic response to these tuberculoproteins. *Purified protein derivatives (PPDs)* from mycobacteria are capable of eliciting delayed-type hypersensitivity once the animal is sensitized, however, and this is the basis of *PPD intradermal skin testing*. Both tuberculoproteins and the adjuvant lipids are present in infection, and the result is the development of both humoral and cell-mediated immune responses. Humoral antibodies can be demonstrated by serologic techniques, but do not participate in the development of lesions or in the production of immunity. Cell-mediated responses are responsible for both aspects of the disease.

The *method of transmission* influences the spectrum of lesions of bovine tuberculosis. Inhalation of droplets containing *M. bovis* is the most common route of infection and leads to infection of the upper and lower airways. Oral infection requires a greater dose of bacilli than airborne infection to cause disease and elicits lesions in the gut and associated lymph nodes, or in lymph nodes draining the oral cavity. Transplacental transmission is a sequel of endometrial tuberculosis and leads to fetal lesions in hepatic and portal lymph nodes. Percutaneous inoculation causes lesions in the skin and associated lymph nodes. Genital transmission is described.

Disseminated lesions can occur with most routes of infection. In cats, *M. microti, M. bovis, and M. avium* cause lesions in the skin of the head and submandibular lymph nodes, thought to originate from wounds induced by infected prey species, and typically without lung lesions; whereas *M. bovis* causes lesions in retropharyngeal or abdominal lymph nodes from ingestion of contaminated milk or raw diets. Previously described differences in the distribution and nature of tuberculous lesions in different species may be partially explained by differences in route of infection, mycobacterial species or strains, and host resistance.

Important concepts in the ***pathogenesis*** *of tuberculosis include the ability of mycobacteria to survive within macrophages, and the role of cellular immune responses in inciting granulomatous inflammation and enhancing the ability of macrophages to kill bacilli.* Most animals that are infected with *M. bovis* do not develop clinical disease. The outcome of infection depends on bacterial factors, including the dose and virulence of infecting bacteria, but also on host factors, including the state of immune competence and heritable resistance to tuberculosis. Heritable variation in disease susceptibility has been identified in cattle and in deer. In humans and mice, mycobacterial resistance is partly related to allelic variation in the natural resistance-associated macrophage protein (*Nramp*) genes 1 and 2, which affect intracellular survival of pathogens by modifying lysosomal transport of divalent cations, including iron and manganese. Other forms of heritable resistance to *M. bovis* are unrelated to variation in *Nramp* genes.

There are several facets to immune-mediated control of tuberculosis, and most of this understanding is based on the study of *M. tuberculosis* infections in humans and laboratory animals. In the early phases of infection, bacilli are phagocytosed by macrophages and may be eliminated. Alternatively, infected macrophages may remain at the site of primary infection for prolonged periods before the disease progresses. An initial innate immune response develops at this site of primary infection, as macrophages secrete cytokines—particularly tumor necrosis factor and the C-C chemokines—that recruit additional macrophages and lymphocytes to the site. Macrophages stimulated by exposure to mycobacteria secrete IL12, which skews the immune response to favor secretion of interferon-γ (IFNγ) and IL2 by CD4+ Th1 lymphocytes. These IFNγ-producing T-helper lymphocytes signal the development of **cell-mediated immunity**, first detected at 14-28 days after infection by positive tuberculin skin test reactions. The arrival of these antigen-specific lymphocytes is crucial for host defense, activating macrophages and thus allowing them to overcome the block in phagosome maturation, and upregulate production of bactericidal products, including reactive nitrogen and oxygen intermediates and lysosomal enzymes that kill intracellular bacilli. Activated macrophages appear epithelioid, with abundant cytoplasm and indistinct cell borders, or form multinucleate giant cells.

The cytokines tumor necrosis factor and IFNγ act synergistically to promote formation of the **tuberculoid granuloma**, a dynamic structure that prevents spread of infection to other sites in the lung, as well as animal-to-animal transmission, and represents a localized target for the immune response. An excessive tissue-damaging cell-mediated immune response is thought to kill heavily infected macrophages and form the caseous center of the granuloma. Matrix metalloproteinases released from activated macrophages are a likely cause of the characteristic cell necrosis and liquefaction of tissues in some granulomas. Bacilli within the caseous center may remain dormant for years, until immunosuppression caused by diseases, drugs, hormones, malnutrition, or other unidentified factors disturb the balance between host and agent, allowing proliferation of the pathogen and reactivation of the disease.

Whether the delayed-type hypersensitivity reaction is beneficial or harmful to the host depends on the circumstances. On the one hand, the reaction to relatively small numbers of bacilli causes accelerated tubercle formation that enhances the killing of the organisms and helps prevent reinfection or dissemination from the initial site of infection. On the other hand, the delayed-type hypersensitivity response to large amounts of mycobacterial antigen causes extensive cell necrosis and tissue destruction, which is seriously detrimental. Liquefaction, brought about by hydrolytic enzymes of macrophages and possibly neutrophils, is the most harmful response. The bacilli multiply extracellularly in the liquefied material and are available in large numbers for dissemination through cavities, vessels, and airways. In summary, *the final determinants of the nature and intensity of lesions are the magnitude of the bacterial infection, the intensity and appropriateness of the immune response, and the modifying influences of the structure of the tissue involved.*

Gross or histologic lesions are absent in most cattle that react to tuberculin skin tests, and although *M. bovis* cannot be isolated from many of these cases, they are generally considered to be infected for the purposes of epidemiology and control. Thorough examination of lymph nodes throughout the body is necessary before declaring a carcass free of visible lesions, as *gross lesions may be absent, few, or multiple*. The distribution of lesions of bovine tuberculosis depends on the mode of transmission. In most cases, gross lesions are restricted to the respiratory tract and associated lymphoid tissues and suggest inhalation as the route of infection. Tubercles or craterous ulcers in gut or mesenteric lymph nodes suggest an oral route of infection, or ingestion of infected sputum that has been coughed up from the lung. Generalized disease is less common but well described.

In **respiratory infections**, *lesions are most common in retropharyngeal, tracheobronchial, and mediastinal lymph nodes*, and less frequent in palatine tonsils and mandibular, parotid, and mesenteric lymph nodes. Lung lesions are detected in only 10-30% of cattle with gross lesions and often affect the caudal lobes. Thus, secondary lesions in lymph nodes may be easier to detect than primary lesions in the lung. *The classic gross lesion is the tubercle: a circumscribed, often encapsulated, pale-yellow or white focus of granulomatous inflammation, often with central caseous necrosis and/or mineralization* (Fig. 5-54). Larger lesions may contain liquefied or neutrophilic exudate and be mistaken for abscesses caused by pyogenic bacteria. Bacilli are released from expanding tubercles into the airways, and coughing up of infected sputum may spread the infection by ingestion to cause lesions in the intestine or mesenteric lymph nodes, by adhesion to laryngeal or tracheal mucosa to incite ulcers or ulcerating tubercles, or by aspiration to seed secondary sites in the lung. Numerous, raised, yellow, 1-3-mm plaques on the mucosal surface of the nasal cavity and nasopharynx are early lesions following experimental intranasal infection. Erosion of pulmonary tubercles through the pleura may implant bacilli throughout the pleural cavity, with development of granulomas on pleural surfaces. Lymphatic spread has been suggested as an alternative route of pleural infection.

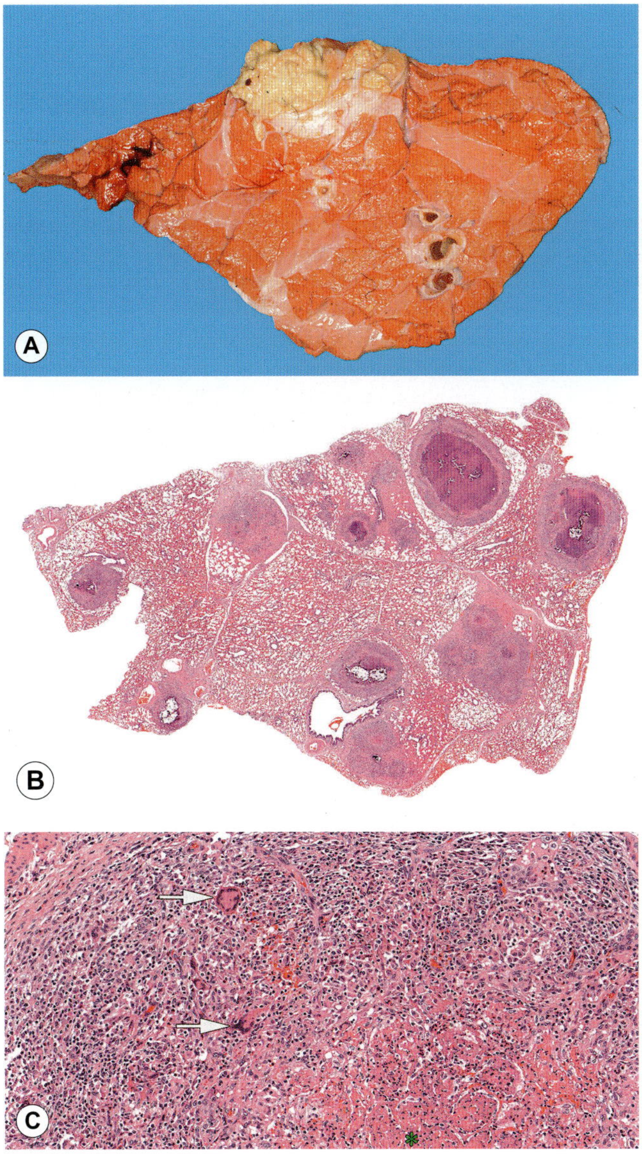

Figure 5-54 Bovine tuberculosis. A. A granuloma forms a pale homogeneous bulging mass in the lung of a cow. **B, C.** Numerous granulomas (B), each with (C) central caseous necrosis (asterisk), a wall of macrophages, giant cells (arrows) and lymphocytes, and a peripheral fibrous capsule (top left), in an elk.

Generalized lesions are reported in about 1% of animals with gross lesions of tuberculosis, and probably result from hematogenous dissemination of bacilli following erosion of the wall of a blood vessel by an expanding tubercle. Embolic lesions are most common in lung and may involve the lymph nodes, bone, liver, kidney, mammary gland, uterus, pleura, peritoneum, pericardium, and meninges. Lesions are rare in the salivary gland, pancreas, spleen, brain, myocardium, or muscle. In some instances, presumably following substantial release of bacilli into the blood, the innumerable tiny white foci justify the term *"miliary tuberculosis."* In contrast, other carcasses display generalized lesions that are variable in size and degree of caseation or fibrosis and imply a less catastrophic but more prolonged bacteremia. Erosion through serosal or mucosal surfaces by expanding tubercles spreads the infection by implantation on pleural, peritoneal, pericardial, or meningeal surfaces or along the airways, intestine, or urinary tract.

Histologic features of the tubercle include: 1) a central coagulum of caseous necrosis, consisting of eosinophilic homogeneous material with scant nuclear debris and sometimes mineralization; 2) a mantle of macrophages and Langhans-type multinucleate giant cells; 3) a capsule containing lymphocytes, clusters of neutrophils in some cases, and a rim of collagenous connective tissue in chronic lesions; and 4) acid-fast bacteria—often in very low number—within macrophages and giant cells of the mantle zone or extracellularly in the caseous core (see Fig. 5-54). In experimentally infected cattle, with some variability of timing among studies, the early lesions at 7-15 days after infection consist of intra-alveolar clusters of macrophages, CD4-, CD8- and δγ-T cells, and acid-fast bacteria. At 14-30 days after infection, corresponding to the onset of lymphocyte proliferative responses, tubercles contain central aggregates of neutrophils surrounded by epithelioid macrophages and giant cells. Necrosis in the center of the tubercles and presence of extracellular acid-fast bacteria develops later, at 21-42 days after infection, and the first mineralized lesions are at 35-60 days. However, this progression is variable among granulomas, with significant heterogeneity in a single animal. The amount of fibrosis increases with time and tends to be more prominent in individuals and species with greater resistance. The presence of neutrophils is highly variable, and large numbers are most common in cases with rapid multiplication of bacteria, numerous reactive lymphocytes, and easily distensible tissues.

In **cervids**, *M. bovis* causes a similar spectrum of lesions as in cattle, with several notable features. As in cattle, lesions are most common in retropharyngeal lymph nodes, lungs, thoracic lymph nodes, and mesenteric lymph nodes. However, deer may develop superficial lymphadenitis and abscesses that drain to the skin surface. Disease progression may be more rapid in cervids than cattle; deer shed larger numbers of bacilli, and the disease may be more likely to remain subclinical. These features suggest that deer are less able to contain *M. bovis* infections than cattle, although limited evidence indicates that they are not more susceptible to infection. In elk (*Cervus elaphus* nelsoni), red deer (*C. elaphus* elaphus), and fallow deer (*Dama dama*), fibrosis and giant cells are less evident than in cattle, mineralization is more variable, and—importantly—*neutrophilic inflammation may be prominent*. Multifocal lesions of caseous necrosis or neutrophilic inflammation in the lungs and lymph nodes of cervids are commonly caused by *Fusobacterium necrophorum* infection, and *these lesions should be carefully examined for acid-fast bacteria as a routine procedure*. Occasional cases of tuberculosis in these species may have concentrically laminated caseous abscesses reminiscent of caseous lymphadenitis in sheep and goats. The lesions of tuberculosis in sika deer (*Cervus nippon*) are distinctive, consisting of nonencapsulated invasive accumulations of epithelioid macrophages and numerous irregularly shaped giant cells, a few neutrophils, and minimal necrosis or mineralization.

A detailed laboratory postmortem examination is the most sensitive method of detecting M. bovis *infection (96% sensitivity), even compared with antemortem tests, because the likelihood of isolating M. bovis in culture is low if gross lesions are not detected*. Sensitivity of slaughterhouse inspection is lower (71%), reflecting the importance of a detailed gross examination. The differential diagnosis for granulomas of lung or lymph nodes includes cestode cysts; pyogranulomas caused by fungi, bacteria, or inhaled foreign material; bacterial abscesses;

and neoplasms. Thus, the presence of many eosinophils, lymphoid hyperplasia, or bacterial colonies makes tuberculosis less likely.

Gross findings of focal caseous lesions in the lymph nodes or lung, or histologic detection of granulomas, particularly with central areas of necrosis and/or mineralization, should prompt an extensive and thorough search for the *low numbers of acid-fast bacilli* that are typically present. *Bacterial culture and PCR-based assays are necessary for definitive diagnosis and identifying the mycobacterial species*. Immunohistochemical identification of *M. bovis* has been described. This procedure is more sensitive than examining acid-fast–stained sections in terms of number of animals detected, staining intensity, and ease of detection, but the antibodies in current use cross-react with other mycobacteria as well as some gram-positive bacteria and fungi.

Chlamydia psittaci

Chlamydia psittaci infections, usually subclinical, have occasionally been identified in cattle. Experimentally challenged calves had *C. psittaci* DNA detected in exhaled breath, blood, and lung tissue. The challenged calves had fever, tachypnea, cough, conjunctival hyperemia, and blood neutrophilia. Histologic lesions were of fibrinous and neutrophilic bronchopneumonia with multifocal necrosis, and chlamydial inclusion bodies in alveolar epithelial cells, neutrophils, and macrophages.

Mycoplasmal diseases

Contagious bovine pleuropneumonia

Contagious bovine pleuropneumonia (**CBPP**), a World Organisation for Animal Health (WOAH) list A disease, is a production-limiting disease in Africa and an important barrier to global trade. The disease is endemic in some regions of sub-Saharan Africa, causes epizootics in other regions, and may occur in Asia. CBPP caused devastating epidemics in cattle populations in the 19th century, but sporadic disease is now more common in endemically infected countries practicing vaccination. When the agent is introduced into naive populations, the effects vary from insidiously spreading disease to spectacular mortality affecting up to 50% of the animals.

CBPP is caused by ***Mycoplasma mycoides*** **subspecies** ***mycoides*** (the older "small colony" designation is obsolete) with low diversity among isolates. There is strain-dependent variation in virulence. Galactan in the mucus capsule is correlated with virulence and induces necrosis, thrombosis, and inflammation. The bacteria produce hydrogen peroxide, but peroxide from leukocytes is thought to contribute more to tissue damage. The host range includes cattle *(Bos taurus)*, zebu *(B. indicus)*, water buffalo *(B. bubalis)*, bison, and yak, although ***cattle*** *are most commonly affected by clinical disease*. *M. mycoides* is an obligate pathogen that survives poorly in the environment; hence, transmission usually depends on repeated close contact with acutely infected animals. Transmission across the placenta or via semen may occur. The transmission risk from chronically infected animals is considered low. *The respiratory tract is the site of primary infection*, and bacteremia develops secondarily. The incubation period varies from 5 to 200 days, but is typically 20-40 days.

Clinical signs and mortality rates are highly variable, depending on the strain of the pathogen, the age of the animal (adults are more susceptible than young), comorbidities, crowding, or stressors. Peracute cases die without clinical signs. Acutely ill animals are febrile, anorexic, and depressed, with profound loss of milk production, open-mouth rapid breathing, mucoid nasal discharge, and occasional coughing. Chronically affected animals may be clinically normal or have an intermittent cough and fever. Calves <6-months-old commonly develop polyarthritis affecting carpal and tarsal joints, rather than pneumonia.

Gross lesions are often *unilateral* and mainly affect the *caudal lung lobes*. In the acute stages, there is abundant fibrin and fluid exudate in the pleural cavity. Interlobular septa are remarkably distended with serous fluid, and the lobules vary from normal to consolidated and red or yellow-gray. The pattern of interlobular edema and consolidation of lung lobules lends a *characteristic marbled appearance* to the lung. Focal areas of necrosis increase in size over time, and eventually develop into sequestra. Sequestrum formation and fibrous thickening of the pleura with adhesions to the ribs are typical of chronic CBPP. Regional lymph nodes are enlarged. Serofibrinous arthritis or tenosynovitis is common in young calves.

Histologic examination of bronchioles and alveoli reveals serofibrinous or neutrophilic exudates with necrosis of neutrophils, mononuclear leukocyte infiltrates around bronchioles, and multifocal coagulative necrosis in the lung parenchyma. Interlobular septa are expanded by edema and fibrin, and interlobular lymphatics contain fibrin. Thrombosis of arteries, veins, and lymphatics is common, and arteritis may be evident. *Vasculitis* is central to the development of the necrotic lesions and sequestration of lung tissue. In the kidney, cortical infarcts are thought to result from immune-complex reactions.

The **differential diagnosis** includes *Mannheimia haemolytica* and *Mycoplasmopsis bovis*. The unilateral lesions, caudal lobe involvement, prominent inflammation in interlobular septa, and frequent development of sequestra should suggest a diagnosis of CBPP, although the latter 2 features do occur in shipping fever caused by *M. haemolytica*. The lesions of *M. bovis* lack the extensive fibrinous exudates in interlobular septa and on the pleural surface seen in CBPP.

Definitive **diagnosis** is based on *culture with special media*, which may take several weeks. Frozen samples of lesional lung, pleural fluids, and lymph nodes are optimal for isolation of the agent. PCR is a more rapid method of diagnosis. Serologic assays are useful for herd screening but do not detect all infected animals; a complement fixation test for IgM antibodies detects acutely infected animals, whereas ELISA for IgG detects all disease stages but may be less sensitive for very early infections.

Mycoplasmopsis bovis

Mycoplasmopsis (*Mycoplasma*) *bovis causes various combinations of chronic pneumonia, arthritis, and otitis media in young dairy and veal calves and in feedlot cattle; Mycoplasmopsis bovis mastitis* is discussed elsewhere. In contrast to the appearance of shipping fever, feedlot calves with *M. bovis* pneumonia or polyarthritis usually die or are euthanized in the second or third month after arrival. These calves have often had prolonged antimicrobial therapy for nonresponsive or relapsing respiratory disease, which is indistinguishable from shipping fever in the early stages. Calves may be lame and have swelling of one or more joints, and many have both respiratory disease and lameness.

The prevalence of chronic pneumonia and polyarthritis is often low, although up to 30% of calves may be affected in exceptional cases. Nevertheless, given that the diagnosis is only made on fatal cases, the true prevalence of the disease is unknown. In contrast, the prevalence of infection with *M. bovis* has been reported to vary from 20 to 70%, and most calves seroconvert to *M. bovis* during the first month in the feedlot. Prior or concurrent respiratory tract inflammation, BoAHV1, and bovine viral diarrhea virus are suggested to predispose to severe mycoplasmal disease.

Mycoplasmopsis bovis may be carried and shed in secretions of the respiratory tract, the genital tract, and the mammary gland. Infection of the respiratory tract probably occurs by direct contact with nasal secretions, or perhaps by inhalation of infected droplets. Contact with genital secretions or ingestion of infected milk may cause infection in neonatal calves. Infection can remain confined to the respiratory tract for many months. Lung infections often lead to bacteremia (at about 9 days after experimental infection), with subsequent infection of joints and other tissues. Alternatively, *Mycop. bovis* in the nasopharynx often ascends the auditory tube to reach the middle ear, where it infrequently traverses the vestibulocochlear nerve to incite meningitis of the brainstem.

Mycoplasmopsis bovis is seemingly well equipped to evade the immune response. The bacterium induces apoptosis of bovine lymphocytes, suppresses the proliferative response of lymphocytes to mitogens, and impairs neutrophil activation. The bacterial surface is decorated with a family of highly immunogenic variable-surface lipoproteins, encoded by at least 13 *vsp* genes containing multiple repeat sequences, which undergo high-frequency phase variation (turning expression on and off) and size variation. *M. bovis* seems to alter surface lipoprotein expression in response to binding of specific antibody, suggesting that rapid change in surface antigen expression is a mechanism of evading the humoral immune response. In support of this hypothesis, although antibody titers develop 2-3 weeks after experimental infections, the cellular and humoral immune responses are not protective.

Many isolates of *M. bovis* are resistant to antimicrobials commonly used in feedlot medicine, including β-lactam antibiotics, florfenicol, tilmicosin, oxytetracycline, and spectinomycin. The pathogenetic implications of this antimicrobial resistance are uncertain. However, one theory suggests that *M. bovis* may be one of several pathogens infecting calves as they enter the feedlot, but the ability of this bacterium to resist antimicrobials and evade the immune response leads to chronic disease that fails to respond to therapy.

Many calves with lesions of *Mycoplasmopsis bovis* pneumonia are also infected with *Mannheimia haemolytica or Pasteurella multocida*, and there is epidemiologic, morphologic, and experimental evidence that inflammation triggered by these infections or by respiratory viruses may be important for development of *M. bovis* caseonecrotic lesions. Many cases have concurrent infection with *Mycoplasmopsis (Mycoplasma) arginini*, but there is no evidence that it contributes to disease. Conversely, *M. bovis* is not thought to predispose to other bacterial lung infections, given that *M. bovis* is reportedly less effective than *Mesomycoplasma (Mycoplasma) dispar* at impairing ciliary function.

The **gross appearance** of *Mycoplasmopsis bovis* pneumonia may be indistinguishable from neutrophilic bronchopneumonia of other causes: there is cranioventral reddening and consolidation, and bronchial lymph nodes are enlarged and diffusely white. However, *the characteristic lesion is of caseonecrotic bronchopneumonia, in which the consolidated cranioventral lung contains raised, white, sharply demarcated, friable foci of caseous necrosis* (Fig. 5-55). These are often 2-10 mm in diameter, but occasionally enlarge to many centimeters diameter. The largest lesions may contain fluid pus rather than caseous exudate, presumably as a result of secondary or concurrent bacterial infection. These foci of necrosis form sequestra in some cases (see eFig. 5-35). Uncommonly, foci of necrosis and inflammation may be present in bronchial lymph nodes, and similar nodular masses are rarely encountered in the tracheal submucosa, along the dorsal tracheal ligament, or in other tissues.

Joint lesions are present in ~50% of calves with *M. bovis* pneumonia, and the lesions may vary considerably within the same animal. *Pneumonia is found in nearly all calves with* M. bovis *arthritis*. Acute lesions consist of serofibrinous exudate within joint cavities and tendon sheaths, and the synovium is reddened and hyperplastic. Cartilage erosion is reported in experimental cases but is often absent in clinical material. Purulent or fibrinopurulent exudate is often florid in more established lesions. Foci of caseous necrosis, similar to those described in the lung, may be present in the synovium or joint capsule, or in the tendon sheaths or peri-articular soft tissues.

Other manifestations of *M. bovis* infection include fibrinous, purulent, or caseating *otitis media* in young calves, from feeding of contaminated milk; decubital abscesses; endocarditis; and necrotizing myocarditis of the papillary muscle that resembles *Histophilus somni* myocarditis.

The **histologic lesions** of neutrophilic bronchopneumonia are nonspecific, but the foci of caseous necrosis are characteristic. The lesions originate in small bronchioles, alveoli, or interlobular septa. The mildest, and probably earliest, lesion consists of neutrophils within small bronchioles, which develop a characteristic appearance—they become necrotic but retain their cellular outlines, and have hypereosinophilic cytoplasm and inapparent or fragmented nuclei (see Fig. 5-55). As the lesion progresses, there is erosion of bronchiolar epithelium, with expansion of the necrotic foci to incorporate peribronchiolar alveoli. Plump macrophages and lymphocytes infiltrate the margins, infrequent giant cells may be present, and immature fibrous tissue develops at the outermost edge of the lesion. Mineralization of the necrotic tissue is frequent. Lesions affecting bronchi often progress to bronchiectasis. In animals coinfected with *Mannheimia haemolytica*, large lesions may contain coagulative necrosis in their centers with retention of the alveolar and bronchiolar architecture of the dead parenchyma, and caseous necrosis from *M. bovis* at the periphery.

Using immunohistochemistry, mycoplasmal antigen is most abundant in necrotic debris and within alveolar macrophages and neutrophils at the periphery of the foci of necrosis. Lesser amounts of antigen are present at the apical surfaces of bronchiolar and bronchial epithelial cells. Foci of necrosis or lymphoplasmacytic inflammation may be present in the liver, kidney, or other viscera.

The gross and histologic appearance of caseonecrotic bronchopneumonia is distinctive. The foci of necrosis caused by *Mannheimia haemolytica* or *Histophilus somni* are irregular in shape, nonfriable, delineated by a white rim (see Fig. 5-53B), retain the histologically visible tissue architecture (coagulative necrosis), and contain streaming necrotic leukocytes. In

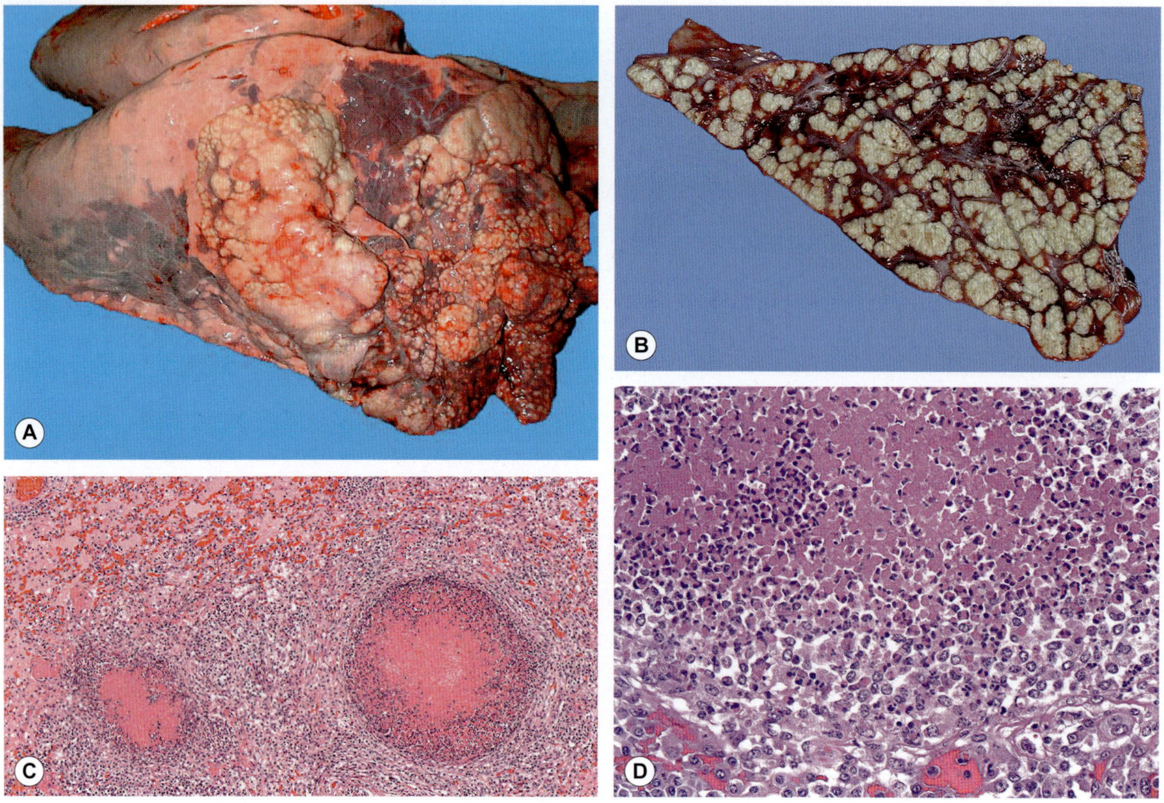

Figure 5-55 Caseonecrotic bronchopneumonia caused by ***Mycoplasmopsis bovis*** in a feedlot calf. **A**. Cranioventral consolidation containing pale raised nodules. **B**. On section, the nodules are pale, round, dry, and friable. **C**. Caseous necrosis arising in a bronchiole, with remnants of bronchiolar epithelium remaining at the left. **D**. The caseonecrotic lesion has an eosinophilic core with ghostlike remnants of macrophages and neutrophils (top), a thin outer layer of viable macrophages and a few neutrophils, and a periphery of fibrous tissue with mononuclear cells.

contrast, the lesions of *M. bovis* are usually circular and white throughout and appear histologically as an eosinophilic coagulum with the ghostlike outlines of eosinophilic necrotic leukocytes (see Fig. 5-55B and D). Larger foci with fluid pus rather than crumbly content may be abscesses and contain both *M. bovis* and *Trueperella pyogenes* or other bacterial pathogens.

Various techniques are available to confirm the tentative **diagnosis** of *M. bovis* infection. It grows readily on Mycoplasma enrichment media and is occasionally isolated on blood agar. PCR and culture have similar diagnostic sensitivity. Immunohistochemistry is also advantageous for correlating the location of mycoplasmal antigen with the characteristic lesions. It is important to note that many calves without apparent pneumonia are infected with *M. bovis*. Thus, *the diagnosis rests on identifying both infection with this agent and on the characteristic lesions*. Seroconversion occurs in many healthy calves in the first month after entering feedlots, making this assay of no value for diagnosis of disease; serology is mainly used in epidemiologic studies and to identify noninfected herds.

Mycoplasmopsis bovis causes particularly severe disease in farmed bison with high morbidity and mortality. The lesions are of caseonecrotic bronchopneumonia that may be unilateral. Other manifestations are pleuropneumonia, polyarthritis, necrotic pharyngitis, endometritis and placentitis with vasculitis, or disseminated abscesses in multiple viscera and lymphoid tissues.

Other mycoplasmas of cattle

Mycoplasmas are regularly isolated from the lungs of calves with pneumonia, but their importance in disease is often difficult to interpret. Only *Mycoplasmopsis bovis* is likely to cause severe primary disease. Infection with ***Mesomycoplasma dispar, Ureaplasma diversum***, and perhaps ***Mycoplasmopsis bovirhinis*** causes bronchiolitis and may contribute to development of acute or chronic enzootic pneumonia in young calves by predisposing to bacterial pneumonia. Experimental infections with ***Mycoplasmopsis bovigenitalium, Mycoplasmopsis arginini****, and* ***Mycoplasmopsis canis*** induce mild lesions and no clinical signs.

Some of these mycoplasmas attach to ciliated epithelial cells, on and between microvilli and covering the base of the cilia. *The typical lesion is chronic catarrhal bronchitis and bronchiolitis with prominent lymphocytic cuffs around airways*. Affected lungs contain patchy, cranioventral, purple-red foci of atelectasis. When secondarily infected by opportunistic bacterial pathogens, more confluent, meaty consolidation may also occur. Microscopically, accumulations of neutrophils and mucus are present in airway lumens, and there is increased prominence of goblet cells. Moderate infiltrates of lymphocytes and fewer plasma cells encircle the airways and accompanying blood vessels. Inflammation of alveoli adjacent to terminal bronchioles occurs in experimental infections in colostrum-deprived, specific-pathogen-free calves and can probably occur in heavy natural infection. Alveolar lesions are not specific and include atelectasis, accumulation of neutrophils and alveolar macrophages with occasional lymphocytes and plasma cells, and mild hypercellularity of alveolar septa. As the infection becomes chronic, lymphocytic peribronchiolar cuffs thicken, develop germinal centers, and extend to the lamina propria of the bronchiole. At this stage, the epithelium may be hyperplastic with goblet cell hyperplasia and hypertrophy of bronchial glands.

Ureaplasma diversum causes abortion, and lung lesions include interstitial pneumonia and cuffs of lymphocytes around bronchioles. In feedlot cattle, *U. diversum* is infrequent on arrival but common at later stages in the hospital pen, suggesting contagious spread of unknown relevance to disease.

Fungal diseases

Mortierellosis

Acute fatal mycotic pneumonia is a sequel to placental infection with ***Mortierella wolfii***, *the most important cause of mycotic abortion of cattle in New Zealand*. It is rarely reported elsewhere. Acute fibrinonecrotic pneumonia occurs in infected cows within a few days of abortion or parturition, as a result of extensive hematogenous dissemination of fungi when the placenta detaches. In the acute disease, the lung is diffusely firm, edematous, and red-yellow. Histologic lesions include serofibrinous and neutrophilic exudate in alveoli, with vascular necrosis, thrombosis, and coagulative ischemic necrosis of lung parenchyma. In the subacute and chronic disease, there is an embolic pattern of multifocal fibrinous and neutrophilic inflammation. Similar lesions may occur in the spleen. Fungal hyphae are present within the lesions, but may be inconspicuous in chronic lesions. The hyphae are PAS positive, nonseptate, branching, and 2-12 μm in diameter.

Other fungi such as ***Aspergillus***, ***Mucor***, and *Rhizopus* are occasional opportunistic invaders of lung and cause nodules of caseous necrosis or granulomatous inflammation.

Parasitic diseases

Dictyocaulus viviparus

D. viviparus is a common and important cause of respiratory disease in cool, wet, seasonal climates. **Primary infections**, sometimes known as "husk" or "hoose," cause disease in calves during their first grazing season, and occasionally affect mature animals that have not had sufficient exposure to develop immunity. Although clinical disease may develop within 3 weeks of access to infected pastures, it is most common late in the grazing season when calves have been at pasture for 3-5 months. Affected herds usually have high disease prevalence, and mortality rates are variable depending on the degree of pasture contamination. A second manifestation, **reinfection syndrome**, occurs when partially immune adult cattle on endemically infected farms have access to pastures that are contaminated with large numbers of infective larvae. In these herds, there is a high prevalence of coughing, tachypnea, and depression about 2 weeks after exposure. Some animals develop fatal dyspnea without coughing.

D. viviparus (superfamily *Trichostrongyloidea*, family *Dictyocaulidae*) is the only adult nematode of bovine lung. *Adult lungworms inhabit the large bronchi*. The eggs are embryonated when laid and hatch rapidly. First-stage larvae are expelled from the lung by coughing, are swallowed, and then passed in the feces. Further development to infective third-stage larvae occurs on the ground over the next 5-7 days. Larval development is optimal in moist cool conditions; the larvae can develop at temperatures as low as 5°C, and their viability is prolonged at these temperatures. The third-stage larvae are ingested by cattle, penetrate the wall of the intestine, and migrate via the lymphatics to the mesenteric lymph nodes. In the lymph nodes, they molt to form fourth-stage larvae and then go by way of lymph and blood to enter the lungs about 7 days after infection. Some larvae accidentally take the portal route and are destroyed in the liver, or rarely enter the systemic circulation to cause intrauterine infections in the fetus. The final molt to the fifth-stage larvae occurs in the bronchioles, and adults develop in the larger airways. Eggs are first detectable in feces at 21-30 days after infection; the infection is usually patent for another 1-3 months. However, a few egg-laying adults may persist in some animals over the winter months and serve as a source of pasture contamination in the following grazing season.

The clinical and pathologic manifestations of *Dictyocaulus* infestation are dependent on the stage of infection, the level of immunity of the host, and the number of invading larvae. *The following description pertains to primary infections of naive animals;* reinfection of partially immune cattle is discussed subsequently. *Lesions differ in the prepatent period, the patent period, and the period of recovery*. During the **prepatent period**, 7-25 days after infection, the principal lesions are eosinophilic bronchiolitis and/or alveolitis with pulmonary edema and fibrin, in response to the larvae in the alveoli and bronchioles. Clinical signs include coughing and tachypnea, and calves infected with many larvae may die at this stage. Where the larvae emerge from pulmonary capillaries, they cause microscopic foci of necrosis and fibrin exudation, with an alveolar infiltrate of eosinophils and fewer neutrophils, macrophages, and giant cells. Mononuclear cells thicken the alveolar walls, and hyaline membranes or hyperplasia of alveolar type II epithelial cells may occur. The larvae, some of them dead, can be found in the alveoli. When the number of larvae is large, the foci of acute interstitial pneumonia may be visible grossly as lobular or smaller foci that are slightly depressed, purple, and widely distributed throughout the lungs.

By about the 10th day, many of the larvae have reached the terminal bronchioles. Frothy fluid is present in the bronchi and, in very heavy infestations, there is edema, atelectasis, and/or emphysema. Eosinophils invade the septal tissues in large numbers and pursue the larvae into the bronchioles. Most of the bronchioles contain plugs of exudate composed largely of eosinophils with fewer neutrophils, lymphocytes, and macrophages. The early bronchiolar epithelial response is of necrosis, sloughing and flattening of remaining cells, with subsequent hyperplasia and metaplasia. At this stage, adult worms are not yet present in the airways, but larvae are detectable histologically or in a smear of exudate harvested from the smallest airways.

During the **patent period**, beginning 25 days after infection, the inflammatory response targets adult worms in the bronchi, and eggs and recently hatched first-stage larvae that have been aspirated into the alveoli. At this stage, calves may have chronic cough, increased respiratory rate, and weight loss, or develop severe dyspnea and death. Adult worms, which are slender, white, and up to 8 cm long, are most numerous in the caudodorsal bronchi of the caudal lobes (Fig. 5-56). Infections may be missed if only the trachea and

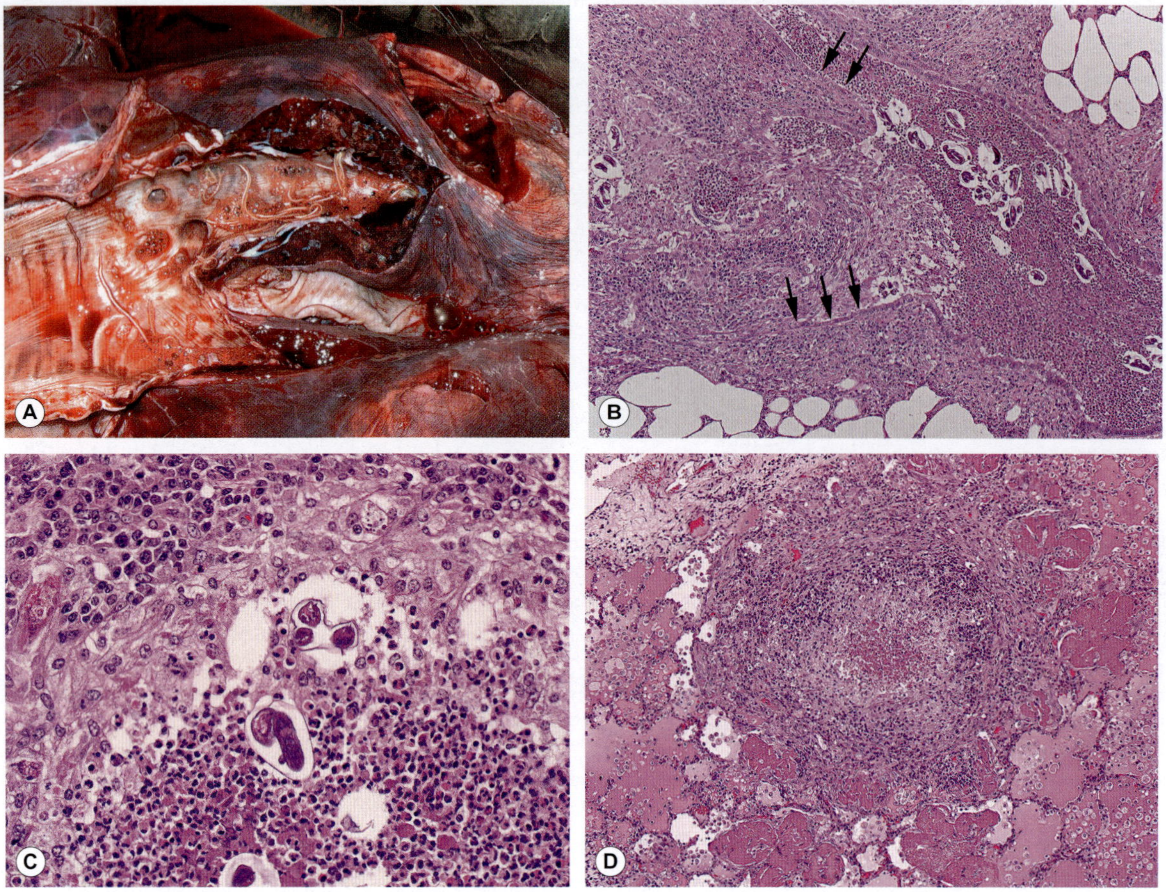

Figure 5-56 *Dictyocaulus viviparus*. **A**. Grossly visible adult nematodes in the caudal bronchi, with frothy exudate, in an elk. (Courtesy D. Campbell.) **B**. Effacement of a bronchus with attenuation of remaining epithelium (arrows), fibrosis, an intense infiltrate of eosinophils and mononuclear cells, and numerous nematode larvae and ova, in a cow. **C**. Embryonated eggs and associated granulomatous inflammation in a bronchiole. **D**. Granuloma formation in lung parenchyma in response to aspirated eggs and larvae.

large cranial bronchi are examined, as *many infestations are restricted to the small branches of the caudal bronchi*. Patchy lobular atelectasis may be the only other gross finding in mild infestations. In more severe cases, there are wedge-shaped, red-gray, firm, depressed areas of consolidation at the caudal border of the caudal lung. Examination of a cut section may reveal similar areas of consolidation in much of the pulmonary tissue surrounding larger bronchi.

Histologic lesions in patent infections include eosinophilic and necrotizing catarrhal bronchitis and bronchiolitis, and eosinophilic granulomatous alveolitis (see Fig. 5-56). The bronchi and large bronchioles contain adult worms, eggs, and larvae mixed with mucus and numerous eosinophils. In histologic sections, adult worms have thick intestinal epithelium composed of a few multinucleate cells with indistinct microvilli, prominent lateral chords, coelomyarian-polymyarian musculature, and the uterus may contain larvae or embryonated eggs. The airway mucosa contains infiltrates of eosinophils and mononuclear cells, the epithelium is necrotic or hyperplastic and contains increased numbers of goblet cells, and the peribronchial lymphoid tissue is expanded (see eFig. 5-55). The accompanying alveolar lesions consist of atelectasis secondary to the obstructive bronchiolitis, and macrophages, giant cells, and lymphocytes encircling fragments of cuticle, aspirated eggs, or newly hatched larvae. It is complicated in some cases by bacterial bronchopneumonia. Alveolar septa are thickened by cellular infiltration, slight fibroplasia, and inconsistent proliferation of type II pneumocytes. At this stage, the infection may be diagnosed by gross observation of adult worms in the bronchi, examination of histologic sections of bronchi and alveoli, identification of all stages in wet mounts of airway mucus, identifying larvae in feces by the Baermann technique, and/or detection of antibodies in serum or milk by ELISA.

During the **period of recovery**, *adult worms are eliminated*. However, gross lesions of consolidation may persist, and there is obliterative bronchiolitis, lymphocytic cuffs around bronchi, hyperplasia of type II pneumocytes, and fibrosis of peribronchiolar alveoli. Establishing a firm diagnosis at this stage may be impossible, given that adults are not present and the feces no longer contain larvae. The distribution of lesions in the caudal lung helps to differentiate chronic parasitism from bacterial pneumonia, which usually affects the cranioventral areas of lung. Acutely fatal exacerbations of the disease during the period of recovery, when larvae and adults are no longer present, have been described. These cases may be impossible to differentiate from toxic interstitial lung disease, but acute exacerbation of a chronic illness is not typical of pulmonary toxicity.

Emphysema may be a prominent gross lesion in severe cases of *Dictyocaulus* infection and is probably a consequence of forced expiration, the result of severe dyspnea, in the presence of bronchiolar obstruction by exudate and bronchoconstriction. Cases in which emphysema is the major lesion may be mistaken for acute interstitial lung disease of toxic cause. This is particularly likely when the pulmonary damage is caused by massive invasion of larvae, and mature worms are not yet present for gross detection. Microscopic detection of larvae and immature worms usually provides the diagnosis.

The typical lesion in the **reinfection syndrome**—in which partially immune adult cattle are infected with numerous larvae—is scattered, 2-4-mm, gray nodules that often contain a green caseous center. The nodules are dense accumulations of lymphocytes and plasma cells, encircling an eosinophilic and granulomatous response to a degenerating larva. As a result of this robust immunoinflammatory response, the larvae do not reach the large airways or develop into adults, and the infection does not usually achieve patency.

Miscellaneous parasites

Ascaris suum larvae are an occasional cause of severe interstitial lung disease in calves housed where pigs were previously kept. In these situations, infective eggs are ingested, larvae hatch within 18 hours, and migrate to the lungs 5-13 days after infection. The lesions are of severe acute interstitial lung disease, in which the lungs are diffusely rubbery, wet, and heavy, and interlobular septa are distended with clear fluid. Migration of larvae through the liver may cause white streaks. Histologically, there is attenuation or hyperplasia of bronchiolar epithelium, alveolar edema and hyaline membranes or type II pneumocyte proliferation, numerous eosinophils in alveoli, and lymphocytes and plasma cells around airways and thickening alveolar septa. Larvae are readily identified in bronchioles and alveoli of cases that die about a week after infection, but a diligent search may be required in calves that survive for 2-3 weeks after infection. Larvae cannot be consistently recovered from lung digests. The histologic appearance of the larvae is characteristic: they have thick triangular lateral alae that are nearly as wide as their height, large lateral chords, and an intestine (the only internal organ present) composed of uninucleate cells (see eFig. 5-64).

The trematodes ***Fasciola gigantica*** and ***Fasciola hepatica*** occasionally invade the lungs accidentally from the liver. Since they are large parasites that wander extensively, a small number in the lungs can produce extensive cavitations. ***Schistosoma nasalis*** causes nasal granulomas in India. In cattle, the lung is less common than the liver as a site of hydatid cysts caused by ***Echinococcus granulosus***. The leeches ***Limnatis nilotica*** and ***Limnatis africana*** are taken in while drinking and attach to the mucosa of the pharynx and nasopharynx. They suck large quantities of blood, and their presence induces localized edema that leads to dyspnea or asphyxiation. The nematodes ***Mammomonogamus (Syngamus) nasicola*** and ***M. ierei*** are found in the nasal passages of ruminants in tropical countries, and ***M. laryngeus*** causes lymphocytic polypoid hyperplasia in the pharynx and larynx of cattle in tropical Asia and South America.

INFECTIOUS RESPIRATORY DISEASES OF SHEEP AND GOATS

Viral diseases

Ovine respiratory syncytial and parainfluenza viruses

Many aspects of the pathogenesis, lesions, and role of these viruses in predisposing to bacterial pneumonia are similar to those described for the bovine viruses. Ruminant respiratory syncytial viruses have been divided into bovine and ovine subgroups based on nucleotide and antigenic differences in the G protein. Sheep are susceptible to infection and disease with both ovine and bovine subgroups, and ovine strains infect cattle and deer.

Adenovirus

Adenoviral infections are common in sheep, but primary adenoviral pneumonia is rare. Ovine adenovirus can exacerbate disease caused by experimentally inoculated *Mannheimia haemolytica*, and adenoviruses are occasionally isolated from outbreaks of bacterial pneumonia in lambs. These findings suggest that adenoviral infection may predispose to the development of bacterial pneumonia in some groups of lambs. Lesions in experimentally infected lambs are similar to those described for calves. A noteworthy feature of the lesions caused by at least one strain of ovine adenovirus is the enlargement of both nucleus and cytoplasm of inclusion-bearing bronchiolar and alveolar epithelial cells, which could be mistaken for cytomegalovirus infection. Adenoviruses have been isolated from goats, but their role in causing disease appears minor.

Peste des petits ruminants

Peste-des-petits-ruminants virus (PPRV; *Paramyxoviridae, Morbillivirus caprinae*) (see Vol. 2, Alimentary System) is closely related to rinderpest virus in the genus *Morbillivirus*. Sheep and goats with PPR commonly have clinical signs and lesions affecting the respiratory and alimentary systems, which resemble those of canine distemper and rinderpest, respectively. The gross lung lesions usually affect the cranioventral lobes, which are firm, reddened, and may have fibrinous exudate on the pleural surface. Nasal and tracheal erosions with a fibrinonecrotic membrane may be present. Histologically, there is necrosis and attenuation of epithelial cells lining the trachea, bronchi, and bronchioles, proliferation of alveolar type II pneumocytes, and formation of epithelial syncytia in the alveoli. Infected epithelial cells often contain eosinophilic inclusion bodies in the cytoplasm or the nucleus. As PPRV is difficult to isolate in culture, definitive diagnosis depends on PCR or serology.

Sheeppox and goatpox

Sheeppox and goatpox (*Poxviridae, Capripoxvirus*; see Vol. 1, Integumentary System), WOAH list A diseases, cause disseminated white nodules in the lung and trachea in addition to cutaneous lesions. Histologically, these are hyperplastic virus-containing type II pneumocytes and tracheal and bronchiolar epithelial cells, variable numbers of neutrophils and lymphocytes, flocculent eosinophilic extracellular material, and foci of caseous necrosis. "Sheeppox cells" in these lesions are enlarged angular or stellate cells with vacuolated nuclei and intracytoplasmic inclusion bodies.

Small ruminant lentiviruses: maedi-visna, ovine progressive pneumonia, and caprine arthritis encephalitis

Small ruminant lentiviral infections are common in sheep and goats worldwide, with the exceptions of Iceland, where the disease was eradicated in 1965, and Australia and New Zealand, where ovine lentiviral disease has not been recorded. The seroprevalence varies greatly, for example from 1 to 70% in various areas of the United States. Most infected animals are not clinically ill, and infection may become widespread before diseased animals are noticed. *Lentiviruses cause slowly progressive pneumonia, encephalomyelitis, arthritis, and mastitis; the various syndromes may occur independently or concurrently.*

The descriptive terminology of the ovine disease is a colorful consequence of the history of the disease. The respiratory form in sheep, which is termed **maedi** ("labored breathing" in Icelandic) in much of the world and **ovine progressive pneumonia** in the United States, is the most common presentation, and manifests as inexorably progressive dyspnea, hyperpnea, and weight loss in sheep >1-2-years-old. Other outcomes in sheep include encephalitis, arthritis, and mastitis. Encephalitis—**visna** ("fading away" in Icelandic)—results in ataxia, weakness, tremors, hypermetria, and profound weight loss. Mastitis manifests as agalactia and a hard udder. Less common in sheep is arthritis, with lameness and swollen joints (particularly carpal joints), respectively.

Goats with **caprine arthritis encephalitis** (**CAE**) develop one or more of arthritis, encephalitis, and pneumonia. *Arthritis affects adult goats*, resulting in acute or chronic lameness and swelling of carpal or tarsal joints. *Neurologic disease*, occurring in 2-4-month-old kids, or less commonly in older animals, manifests as progressive ataxia and weakness beginning in the hindlimbs. *Pneumonia* may occasionally be the major presenting complaint in kids or adults, or occur concurrently with arthritis or neurologic disease.

Maedi-visna and CAE are caused by closely related lentiviruses in the family *Retroviridae*, genus *Lentivirus*. The extreme genetic diversity created by replicative infidelity of the lentiviruses has blurred the concept of distinct viral species: some strains infect only sheep or only goats, while others are capable of cross-species infection, so *the term **small ruminant lentiviruses** may be more appropriate than visna-maedi virus or caprine arthritis encephalitis virus*. These viruses are enveloped, 100 nm diameter, and contain a dense nucleoid and a positive-sense single-stranded RNA genome. Viral genes include *gag*, which encodes group-specific nucleocapsid and matrix glycoproteins that are detected by antibody-based detection tests; *pol*, which encodes reverse transcriptase and other enzymes; *env*, encoding the surface glycoprotein that mediates receptor binding and virus entry into cells, and is the target for neutralizing antibody; and the regulatory proteins encoded by *vif, rev*, and *vpr-like*. Long terminal repeats that flank the encoding regions of the genome bind transcription factors and are necessary for replication.

Lentiviral diseases in sheep and goats are marked by their variability. Viral strains or quasispecies may differ in their rapidity of replication, cytopathic effects, tropism for particular cell types, and their propensity to cause pulmonary, nervous, joint, or mammary disease. Disease manifestation is also influenced by host genetics, as certain breeds of sheep are more susceptible than others. Finally, the local tissue microenvironment affects viral replication and development of disease; for example, proinflammatory cytokines generated in response to concurrent infection with other pathogens augment lentiviral replication and hasten disease onset.

Transmission of small ruminant lentiviruses through colostrum or milk is the major method of disease spread. Inhalation of nasal secretions following prolonged close contact, as occurs in confined animals in the winter months, is a recognized mode of horizontal transmission. In utero transmission occurs infrequently in sheep. The virus is shed in semen, but infection by coitus or artificial insemination has not been documented. Mucosal dendritic cells are thought to deliver virus to lymph nodes, where the mannose receptor is the likely route of entry into macrophages. Ovine lentivirus infects a variety of cell types, including choroid plexus and mammary epithelium, fibroblasts, endothelial cells, and monocytes. However, viral replication is restricted in these cells, and complete viral replication and assembly occur in mature macrophages. Viral antigen is widespread, having been detected in the lung, bone marrow, mammary gland, lymph node, spleen, synovium, brain, and spinal cord of sheep with maedi, and is most abundant in areas of lymphocytic inflammation. Similarly, viral nucleic acid is demonstrable in the lung, liver, spleen, lymph nodes, brain, synovium, intestine, kidney, and thyroid gland of goats with CAE. Infected pulmonary alveolar macrophages produce cytokines that recruit and activate leukocytes in the area of infection and may also incite fibrosis and smooth muscle metaplasia. Cytokine-dependent activation of macrophages stimulates lentiviral replication, which may in turn stimulate additional leukocyte recruitment. Altered organ function is a result of the immunoinflammatory response, rather than a direct effect of the lentiviral infection.

In contrast to primate and feline lentiviruses, *immunosuppression is not a feature of small ruminant lentiviral infection. Infection and shedding of the virus persist for life*, but the disease in sheep develops slowly and the incubation period usually exceeds 2 years. The mechanisms of persistent lentiviral infection may include proviral integration, lack of avidity of neutralizing antibody, or decoy viral antigens that are immunodominant but non-neutralizing. Integration of provirus into the host genome is necessary for viral replication, occurs increasingly as the disease progresses, and may facilitate persistence of the virus. The development of serum neutralizing antibody responses during persistent infection is perplexing; the higher affinity of virus for macrophage receptors than for antibody has been suggested as a reason for failure of these antibodies to prevent cell-to-cell spread of infection in vivo.

The lungs of **sheep** with maedi fail to collapse when the chest is opened, and are heavy, firm, and diffusely pale gray or tan with ~1-mm gray foci (Fig. 5-57). The lesions are generalized but most obvious in the caudal lobes. Mediastinal and bronchial lymph nodes are enlarged, white, and edematous. Lesions of cranioventral bronchopneumonia caused by *Pasteurella multocida* or *Trueperella pyogenes* are commonly superimposed on the lesions of maedi. Lungworms—*Dictyocaulus* or *Protostrongylus*—are common in sheep with maedi, and an association between maedi and retroviral pulmonary adenomatosis has been described.

*The **histologic** pulmonary lesion of maedi-visna is interstitial pneumonia* (see Fig. 5-57). Infiltrates of lymphocytes, macrophages, and plasma cells thicken alveolar septa and form cuffs around blood vessels and airways. The cellular infiltrates often form *lymphoid nodules with germinal centers*, a characteristic feature of maedi although not always present. In addition to

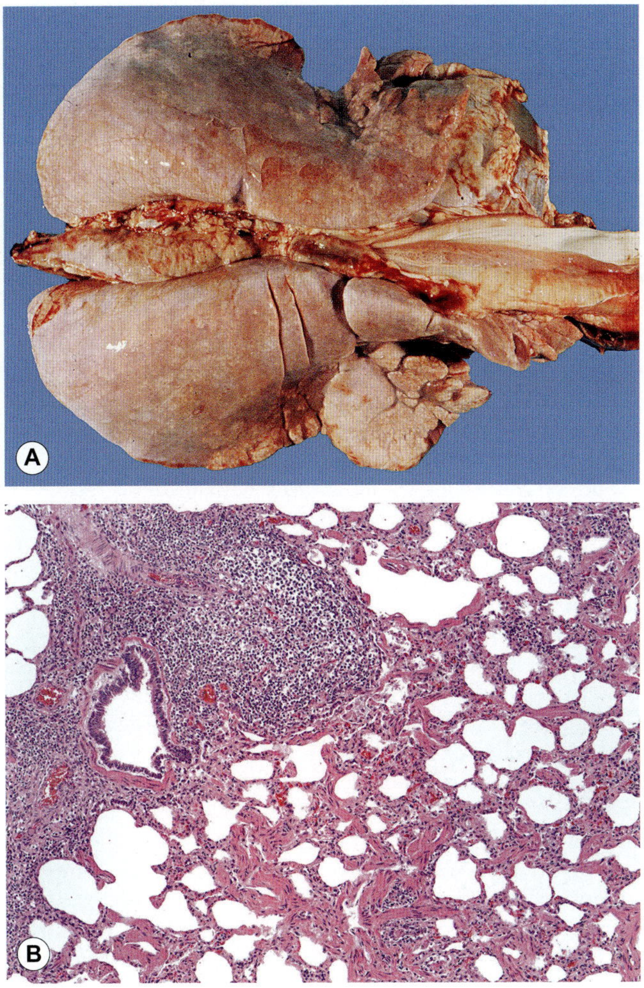

Figure 5-57 **Maedi-visna** in a ewe. **A**. Interstitial lung disease with diffuse pallor, failure to collapse, and firm-rubbery texture. (Courtesy University of Guelph.) **B**. A dense cuff of lymphocytes around a bronchiole, with follicle formation. Alveolar septa are thickened by metaplasia of smooth muscle and interstitial lymphocytes.

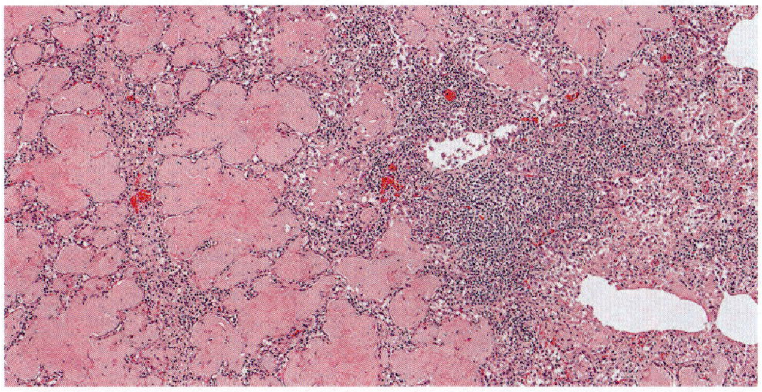

Figure 5-58 **Caprine arthritis encephalitis virus** infection in a goat kid. Dense infiltrates of lymphocytes are present diffusely and congregate around blood vessels. Densely eosinophilic fluid fills alveoli in affected areas, and there is hyperplasia of type II pneumocytes.

the cellular infiltrate, alveolar septa are thickened by *hypertrophy of smooth muscle* and by *mild interstitial fibrosis, and giant cells may be present*. Proliferation of type II pneumocytes is not prominent, in contrast to CAE viral pneumonia and pulmonary adenocarcinoma. Mild hyperplasia of bronchiolar epithelium is occasionally present.

Mastitis is frequent, and histologic lesions include diffuse infiltrates or follicular aggregates of lymphocytes, plasma cells, and macrophages in the mammary interstitium. Mesangial or proliferative glomerulonephritis is an uncommon lesion in lentivirus-infected sheep.

Brain and spinal cord lesions of sheep with maedi-visna are mainly periventricular in the brain, affect white matter of the spinal cord, and may be perivascular or infiltrative. The lesions consist of lymphocytic and/or histiocytic leukoencephalomyelitis, gliosis, demyelination leading to malacia, and meningitis, with mononuclear infiltrates forming lymphoid follicles in choroid plexus.

In **goats**, the *lung lesions* of caprine arthritis encephalitis virus (**CAEV**) infection are distinctive. The gross appearance is of diffuse or multifocal pale firm lesions throughout the lung. Histologically, these foci are abruptly demarcated from relatively unaffected areas of lung. In the lesional areas, alveoli are filled with densely eosinophilic fluid (resembling pulmonary alveolar proteinosis) containing foamy macrophages and lined by a continuous or patchy layer of cuboidal type II pneumocytes, and alveolar septa are thickened by lymphocytes and fibrosis (Fig. 5-58).

Arthritis due to CAEV is unilateral or bilateral, affects the carpal joints, or less commonly the tarsal, fetlock, stifle, and atlanto-occipital joints. Histologic lesions include striking villus hyperplasia of the synovium, with lymphocytes, plasma cells, and macrophages. Fibrosis, mineralization, and necrosis of synovium and joint capsule develop in chronically affected animals. The brain and mammary lesions of CAE are similar to those of sheep with maedi.

Serology (agar gel immunodiffusion assays or ELISAs) is useful to detect infected flocks but of less value for individual-animal diagnosis. For both serologic and molecular detection tests, false-positives can occur in preweaned lambs caused by uptake of antibody and provirus from infected colostrum and milk. False-negative serologic tests can result from the delayed development of antibodies after infection, or transient periods of seronegativity. *Quantitative PCR assays* to detect proviral DNA or viral RNA in blood mononuclear cells or lung tissue may be positive earlier in the disease course than serologic assays. PCR assays are considered less sensitive than serology, but may be positive before development of an antibody titer. Depending on the specific PCR assay, genetic variability of the virus can cause false-negative tests. *Immunohistochemistry*, such as for detection of the p27 or gp130 viral proteins, has the advantage of associating viral antigen with the histologic lesion. Antigen is usually in macrophages within the inflammatory lesions.

Enzootic nasal tumor

Viral adenomas and carcinomas of the nasal cavity that affect sheep and goats often affect various animals in a flock over long periods. Clinical disease typically arises in adults, but lambs as young as 6 months have been affected. Clinical signs are insidious, progressive, and include stertor, inspiratory dyspnea, open-mouth breathing, nasal discharge, nasal deformity, and weight loss.

Enzootic nasal tumor virus (ENTV; *Retroviridae, Betaretrovirus*) includes ENTV1 from sheep and ENTV2 from goats, which are related to jaagsiekte sheep retrovirus (JSRV). Long terminal repeat promoters in the viral genome are

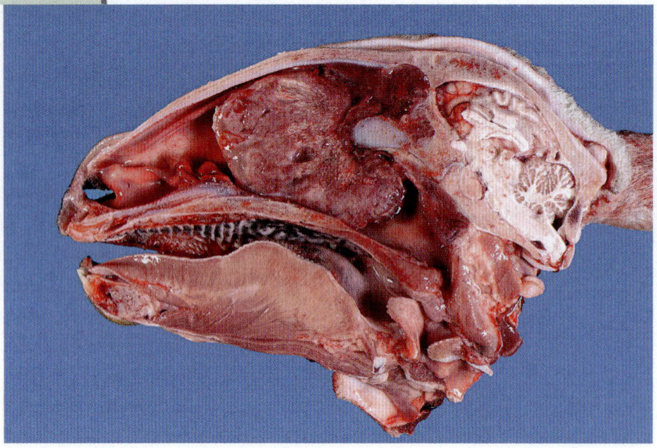

Figure 5-59 **Enzootic nasal tumor** in a ewe. An expansile mass arises from ethmoid conchae and fills the nasal cavity.

proposed determinants of whether these retroviruses infect the nasal or lung epithelium. The viral envelope glycoprotein is responsible for tumor development and is detectable within neoplastic epithelial cells but not in the adjacent normal tissue. The disease has been transmitted to sheep and goats using cell-free nasal fluids or tumor filtrates. Incubation periods after experimental infection are as little as 3 months, although those in the natural disease are considered to be 1-3 years. Transmission is thought to be by contact with nasal secretions. However, subclinical infection is common, and most experimentally challenged animals do not develop tumors.

Tumors may be unilateral or bilateral and *usually originate from the ethmoid turbinates*, but expand to fill much of the caudal nasal cavity before severe clinical signs develop (Fig. 5-59). In protracted unilateral cases, the entire nasal cavity is occluded by tumor, there is deviation of the nasal septum, and tumor may protrude from the nostril. Most tumors grow by expansion into sinuses, contralateral nasal cavity, or pharynx, without cellular invasion of adjacent tissues; the term adenocarcinoma may be justified in those cases with demonstrable invasion of bone. Metastasis does not occur. The neoplastic tissue is white, firm, and multinodular, or may contain brown-red areas of hemorrhage and necrosis.

The **histologic** appearance is of adenoma or low-grade adenocarcinoma. The cuboidal or pseudostratified nonciliated epithelial cells form orderly tubular, papillary, or acinar arrangements; squamous differentiation is described but rare. Neoplastic cells have basal round nuclei and typically a low mitotic count. Mucus secretion is occasionally abundant, and the fibrovascular stroma is usually scant. Neoplastic tissue and adjacent non-neoplastic tissues often contain numerous lymphocytes, and glandular hyperplasia or polyps may be present.

The diagnosis is usually based on gross and histologic findings. However, morphologic features do not differentiate viral neoplasms from the sporadic (nonviral) nasal tumors that occasionally develop in small ruminants. Immunohistochemistry, a PCR assay, or electron microscopy can detect ENTV in tumors. An ELISA may be of value for identifying infected animals in flocks.

Ovine pulmonary adenocarcinoma (jaagsiekte)

Ovine pulmonary adenocarcinoma (**OPA**), *also known as jaagsiekte, is a contagious retroviral pulmonary carcinoma of sheep, and rarely of goats*. The disease is common in South America, South Africa, and Scotland, where 5-20% of infected animals have pulmonary tumors. OPA occurs regularly in the rest of Europe, Africa, and Asia, but is rare in North America and not reported in Australia. Mortality rates tend to increase gradually for several years following introduction of infection, and subsequently decline gradually. Clinical disease is most common in 2-4-year-old sheep, but 3-month-old lambs have been affected. Clinical signs include progressive dyspnea, tachypnea, exercise intolerance, nasal discharge, coughing, and weight loss; fever and anorexia are unusual unless secondary infections occur. Drainage of lung fluids from the nose following elevation of the hindlimbs is seen in some sheep.

Jaagsiekte sheep retrovirus (JSRV; *Retroviridae, Betaretrovirus ovijaa*), the agent of OPA, is a 100-nm, enveloped betaretrovirus. Infection is thought to be acquired by direct contact of young animals with nasal secretions of infected animals. Most naturally infected animals do not have tumors. In those that do, the typical incubation period has been estimated to be 2 years, but is age and dose dependent; tumors may develop in 10-20 days if high doses are administered experimentally to neonatal lambs. The increased propensity for tumor development in neonatally infected lambs may be related to the greater frequency of proliferating type II pneumocytes during postnatal lung development. In contrast, lung cells from adult sheep or goat kids are restrictive for JRSV replication. Disease is more common in certain breeds of sheep, but the reasons for this familial predisposition are unknown.

The JSRV envelope glycoprotein induces similar tumors in immunodeficient mice and is the likely mechanism of tumor formation in sheep. It is exceptional that a retroviral structural protein should induce neoplasia, but oncogenes have not been identified in JSRV. Weak cellular and humoral immune responses in infected sheep, probably resulting from the presence of related endogenous retroviruses, may permit the persistent infection that typifies the disease.

Lungs of sheep with OPA contain locally extensive lesions that are firm, gray, and exude fluid from the cut section (Fig. 5-60). Affected lungs are heavy, up to 3 times their normal weight, and airways are filled with foamy secretion from the neoplastic cells. The tumors are expansile, and often have satellite nodules adjacent to the main lesion, with normal intervening lung tissue. Metastases to regional lymph nodes are present in about 10% of cases. Metastases to other tissues are reported but rare. Maedi and/or bacterial pneumonia are often also present, and the diffuse lymphocytic interstitial pneumonia or cranioventral neutrophilic bronchopneumonia induced by these diseases may complicate the gross and histologic appearance of the tumors.

The **histologic** appearance is of a well-differentiated pulmonary carcinoma (see Fig. 5-60). The neoplastic masses usually have a lepidic or papillary pattern. Others have acinar or solid patterns, a myxomatous variant is described, and polypoid lesions may arise from bronchioles. The neoplastic cells variably express immunohistochemical markers of type II pneumocytes and bronchiolar club cells, suggesting an origin from multipotent lung epithelial progenitor cells. Alveoli adjacent to the tumors are atelectatic and contain many macrophages, and interstitial fibrosis may be present in advanced cases.

In the most frequent or classical form, tumors are poorly demarcated and extend into adjacent alveoli or form satellite nodules. An atypical form of the disease is subclinical and

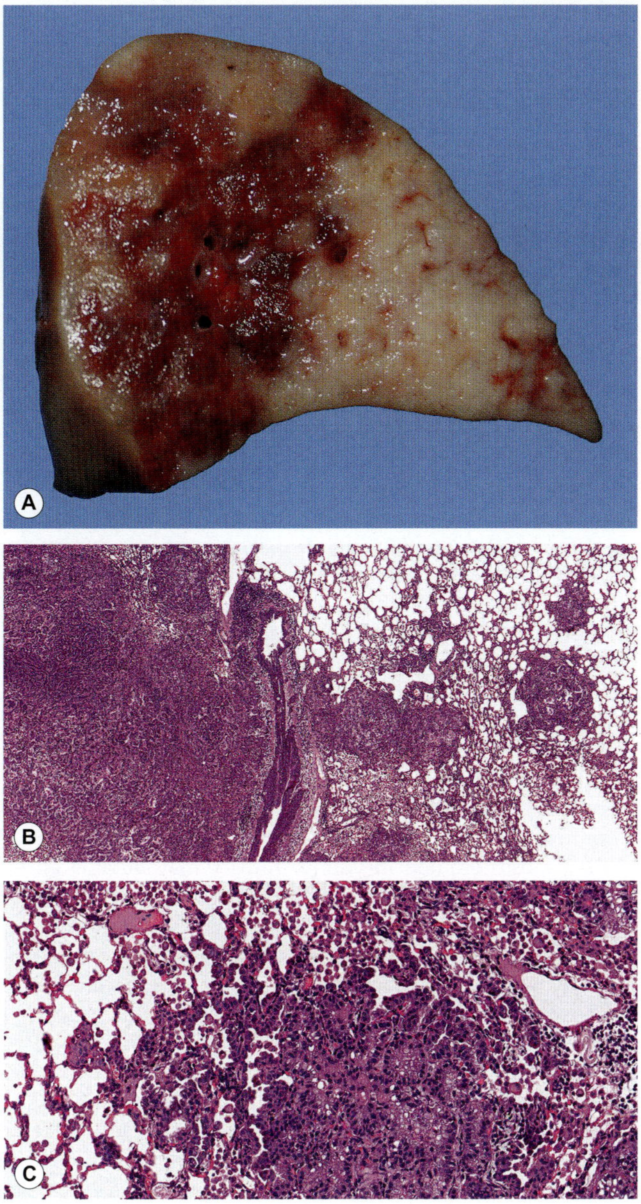

Figure 5-60 Ovine pulmonary adenocarcinoma caused by jaagsiekte sheep retrovirus in a sheep. **A.** Coalescing white nodules solidify the lung. **B.** Larger tumor at the left and satellite tumors in the adjacent lung tissue. **C.** Lepidic and papillary patterns, and increased number of reactive alveolar macrophages. (Courtesy B. Cloak, J. Cassidy.)

probably nonprogressive, and the tumors are isolated or well demarcated, dry, and firmer than the classical form, and surrounded by a more prominent infiltrate of lymphocytes and plasma cells. It is suggested that the classical progressive form reflects abundant JSRV replication in proliferating alveolar epithelial cells, promoting infection of the surrounding lung tissue with ensuing expansion of the tumors. In contrast, the atypical form may reflect infection of lungs that have less alveolar epithelial cell proliferation, with well-demarcated nonprogressive tumors arising from expression of the tumor-causing envelope glycoprotein but minimal viral replication.

The pulmonary lesions of OPA are characteristic. Grossly, intrapulmonary masses adjacent to the main tumor help distinguish OPA from maedi with concurrent bronchopneumonia. Immunohistochemistry for the JSRV envelope glycoprotein is useful for confirmation of the viral origin of the tumors. A PCR assay is able to differentiate JSRV from endogenous sheep retroviral sequences and ENTV, although the low JSRV loads in blood leukocytes limit its sensitivity for analysis of blood samples.

Bacterial diseases

The bacteria causing pneumonia in sheep and goats include *Mannheimia haemolytica, Bibersteinia trehalosi, Pasteurella multocida, Histophilus somni, Helcococcus ovis*, hemolytic streptococci, and *Staphylococcus aureus*; *Trueperella pyogenes* is a common secondary pathogen. The important role of mycoplasmas is discussed later. Caseous lymphadenitis (eFig. 5-66) is described elsewhere (see Vol. 3, Hematolymphoid System). Pneumonia caused by *M. haemolytica* is comparable to the disease in cattle, except that serotype 2 is isolated from most cases.

Chronic nonprogressive pneumonia ("atypical pneumonia") is primarily attributed to *Mesomycoplasma (Mycoplasma) ovipneumoniae* or a more slowly progressive *M. haemolytica* infection, in contrast to "typical" pneumonia caused by more fulminant infection with *M. haemolytica* or other bacteria listed above. Chronic nonprogressive pneumonia is described below with *M. ovipneumoniae*. Predisposing factors include failure of passive transfer, starvation or negative energy balance, sudden climatic changes, poor air quality, overcrowding, and predisposing infection with *Mycoplasma* spp., parainfluenzavirus, ovine or bovine respiratory syncytial virus, or adenovirus. The *Pasteurellaceae* bacteria listed above cause hemorrhagic or fibrinonecrotic, lobar or lobular bronchopneumonia and serofibrinous pleuritis in acute cases, and neutrophilic bronchopneumonia leading to abscess formation and fibrous pleural adhesions in subacute-to-chronic cases. *M. haemolytica* causes sporadic cases or outbreaks of acute pneumonia and pleuritis in goat kids, often in late autumn and winter. At autopsy, a sheet of yellow fibrin adheres loosely to the pleural surfaces. The cranial lobes of the lungs are firm and dark-red with a transition to less-firm tissue with mottled gray-pink discoloration in the caudal lobes. Acute diffuse bronchopneumonia is characterized microscopically by neutrophils, protein-rich exudate, and numerous bacteria filling bronchioles and alveoli. There is usually little evidence of necrosis. In the caudal lobes, neutrophils fill the bronchioles and extend into the alveoli.

H. ovis causes chronic neutrophilic bronchopneumonia, lung abscesses, and pleuritis in sheep and goats. The gram-positive bacterial cocci are visible histologically amid necrotic debris in the abscesses or on the pleural surface.

Aspiration pneumonia occurs in sheep as a result of tube feeding, cleft palate, neurologic or laryngeal disease, white muscle disease, or anesthesia.

Septicemic pasteurellosis

Mannheimia haemolytica can cause septicemia with or without pneumonia in lambs <3-months-old. The lesions are fibrinous polyserositis and widespread petechiae. Septicemia caused by *Bibersteinia trehalosi* occurs mainly in weaned lambs during the fall months, but it can occur in other age groups and at other times of the year. Deaths can be sporadic or multiple and usually follow within a few days of changes in pasture, feed, or other management practices.

Signs of illness are vague, and the usual course is short, or lambs may be found dead. At autopsy, *petechial and ecchymotic hemorrhages* are usually present in subcutaneous tissues, particularly of the neck and thorax, in intermuscular fascia, and in the pleura, epicardium, and mesentery (Fig. 5-61). Retropharyngeal and mesenteric lymph nodes are hemorrhagic and edematous. *Ulcerative lesions* covered by yellow plaques of fibrin and necrotic debris are common on the tongue, pharynx in the area of tonsillar crypts, larynx, and esophagus, and are considered an entry point to the systemic circulation. The abomasal, intestinal, and colonic mucosae occasionally have shallow ulcers. The lungs are diffusely congested, edematous, and contain *widespread foci of hemorrhagic necrosis*. The liver may contain pinpoint to 1-cm yellow necrotic foci. There is occasionally inflammation of joints, pericardium, meninges, and choroid plexus, but these lesions are absent in peracute cases.

Microscopic examination of tissues reveals *widespread bacterial embolism* (see Fig. 5-61). The pulmonary lesions consist of masses of bacteria filling capillaries, accompanied by hemorrhagic and fibrinous exudate into alveoli. A peripheral zone of necrotic leukocytes may be present. The pale hepatic foci consist of colonies of bacteria with a surrounding zone of necrosis. There may be thrombosis of the adjacent tributaries of the portal vein and small amounts of parenchymal necrosis, but the leukocyte response is generally slight. This is probably related to the short course of the disease and perhaps to the effects of bacterial toxin on leukocytes. Bacterial emboli are regularly found in the spleen and adrenals, occasionally in the kidney, but are rare in other organs. Masses of bacteria adhere to the surface of the pharyngeal ulcers and occlude underlying blood vessels and lymphatics, and probably represent the *principal site of bacterial proliferation and systemic invasion*.

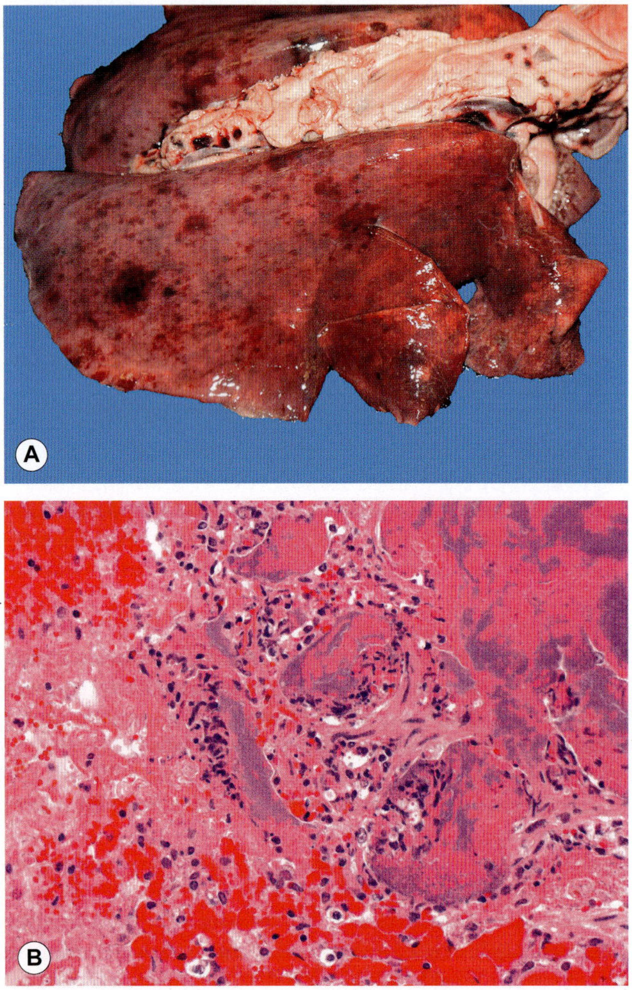

Figure 5-61 ***Bibersteinia trehalosi*** **septicemia** in a weaned lamb. **A**. Petechiae and ecchymoses throughout the lung. **B**. The lung is deeply congested and edematous. Myriad tiny bacteria fill blood vessels with only a minimal reaction by leukocytes. (Courtesy M. J. Hazlett.)

Melioidosis

Melioidosis is a systemic infectious disease affecting a wide range of animal species in tropical climates. The disease is endemic in Southeast Asia and northern Australia, is probably common in the Indian subcontinent and the Caribbean, and also occurs in southern Africa and the Middle East. The prevalence is highest in wet seasons and causes acute outbreaks or chronic endemic disease. Clinical signs are variable and reflect the range of organs affected; case fatality rates are high. Melioidosis is most common in goats, sheep, pigs, and rodents and is an emerging tropical disease of humans. Horses, deer, camels, and laboratory animals are less commonly affected; dogs, cats, cattle, water buffalo, and fowl are resistant to the disease unless they are immunosuppressed.

Melioidosis is caused by ***Burkholderia pseudomallei***, a facultatively anaerobic gram-negative bipolar-staining bacillus. Infection is acquired from contaminated soil or water, by inhalation, ingestion, or inoculation of cutaneous wounds. *Acute disease*, most common in young animals, may initially affect the lungs with later spread to other organs, or be primarily septicemic from the site of inoculation. *Chronic disease* is the more frequent manifestation, in which abscesses in various organs cause chronic nonspecific illness or are an incidental finding of public health importance at slaughter.

Virulence factors of *B. pseudomallei* include the iron-scavenging protein malleobactin, secreted proteases that degrade host tissues, a polysaccharide capsule that confers resistance to killing by phagocytes, lipopolysaccharides, and Burkholderia lethal factor 1, a protein toxin that inhibits translation and causes cell death. The bacterium survives within macrophage phagolysosomes and in epithelial cells, and elicits a granulomatous and neutrophilic tissue reaction.

Melioidosis causes abscesses in various organs. The lungs are most consistently affected, with disseminated coalescing nodules, or locally extensive areas of consolidation. Abscesses also affect the spleen, liver, lymph nodes, subcutis, kidney, or joints and may occur in any visceral tissue. Lesions are particularly widespread in goats and may include mastitis or aortic aneurysm. Neurologic disease is most common in goats, with multifocal aggregates of neutrophils and lymphocytic perivascular cuffs in the brainstem and spinal cord. Nodular lesions in the nasal mucosa may be mistaken for glanders. Endometritis and placentitis are important manifestations in cattle.

The abscesses of melioidosis are not distinctive in their appearance. *The chronic lesions are encapsulated nodular masses, up to 5 cm diameter, with creamy or caseous yellow centers*. Aggregates of neutrophils form within 12 hours of infection. Granulomas, present by 3 days, form as nodular aggregates of epithelioid macrophages and lymphocytes, and these develop central areas of caseous necrosis and neutrophil infiltration.

The gross and histologic appearance of melioidosis is not pathognomonic. Caseous lymphadenitis, glanders, and abscesses caused by other bacteria may have a similar appearance, and the brain lesions may be mistaken for listeriosis. A tentative diagnosis may be based on identifying gram-negative bipolar-staining bacilli in sections or tissue smears, but *definitive diagnosis requires culture*. Because of its zoonotic potential, great care should be taken when dealing with suspect cases during autopsy and subsequent tissue handling and testing.

Chlamydia abortus

Intratracheal challenge of lambs with ***Chlamydia abortus*** (*C. psittaci*) induces mild infiltration of neutrophils and macrophages into alveoli and alveolar septa, and mild proliferative alveolitis. Lesions were most prominent adjacent to terminal bronchioles. Moderately sized cuffs of lymphocytes are present around bronchioles and small blood vessels at the height of the lesion. The chlamydiae are mostly destroyed during the acute phase of inflammation, which then subsides. Resolution can be complete within 3-4 weeks of experimental infection. Chlamydiae may contribute to some cases of enzootic pneumonia in lambs and calves, in combination with other agents, but are probably of *limited importance as primary pulmonary pathogens*.

Mycoplasmal diseases

Contagious caprine pleuropneumonia

Contagious caprine pleuropneumonia (CCPP) was first described in Africa in the late 1800s and remains an important disease in northern and western Africa, the Middle East, and the Indian subcontinent. The difficulty in isolating the causative agent in culture caused much confusion in the early literature, but the cause of CCPP is now known to be ***Mycoplasma capricolum* ssp. *capripneumoniae***. Although other mycoplasmas may cause similar lesions, these are not considered CCPP. Classical CCPP caused massive outbreaks with high morbidity and mortality in naive goats of all ages. *Currently, CCPP, a WOAH list B disease, causes endemic sporadic disease in some countries and intermittent epizootics in others*. Affected goats are lethargic, dyspneic, and febrile and have bouts of coughing.

M. capricolum ssp. *capripneumoniae* (formerly *Mycoplasma* F38) is phylogenetically related to, but distinct from, *M. mycoides*. Virulence factors have not been well defined. Subclinical carriers are important sources of infection and are the usual source of introduction of the disease into naive herds. Stress may trigger shedding of organisms from subclinically infected animals. Individual goats are infected by inhalation of droplets through close contact with coughing goats. The infection is restricted to the respiratory tract. It mainly affects goats, although infection has been detected in wildlife.

Pulmonary lesions are often unilateral but may be bilateral. The pleura is covered by a thick layer of fibrin, and serous fluid fills the pleural cavity. Consolidation and purple-gray discoloration are present in the lung, either diffusely or forming focal lesions, and these can contain extensive areas of necrosis or have a dry granular texture. Fibrinous pericarditis is common. Chronic cases develop nodules of necrosis and mineralization with a fibrous capsule, or lung abscesses if secondary bacterial infection develops. However, in contrast to contagious bovine pleuropneumonia, *sequestra and interlobular edema are not features of the caprine disease*. Histologically, the exudate in alveoli and interlobular septa varies from serofibrinous to fibrinopurulent. Thrombosis and vasculitis are often present. With time, the fibrinous exudates organize to form a mass of fibrous tissue.

Gross lesions are suggestive, but not diagnostic. Other mycoplasmas—particularly *M. mycoides* subsp. *capri*—may cause epidemics with similar lung lesions. Features that suggest CCPP rather than other mycoplasmas include both pneumonia and pleuritis, the absence of interlobular edema and inflammation, and the absence of mastitis, arthritis, or keratitis. Laboratory examination is required for definitive diagnosis.

M. capricolum ssp. *capripneumoniae* is difficult to isolate in culture, although it can often be recovered from the pleural fluid and consolidated lung of acutely ill animals. Detecting mycoplasmal nucleic acid using a PCR assay on samples of pleural fluid is a more rapid and sensitive method of detection. Complement fixation and latex agglutination tests are effective methods of serodetection.

Mesomycoplasma (Mycoplasma) ovipneumoniae

Chronic bronchopneumonia in lambs and kids <12-months-old is common, often subclinical, but reduces growth rates. It is often known as *chronic nonprogressive or atypical pneumonia*, in contrast to fatal ovine progressive pneumonia (maedi), and the "typical" acutely progressive pneumonia caused by *Mannheimia or Pasteurella*. Numerous causes of **chronic nonprogressive pneumonia** are implicated including *Mesomycoplasma ovipneumoniae, Mannheimia haemolytica, Pasteurella multocida, Bordetella parapertussis*, parainfluenza-3 virus, and respiratory syncytial virus, and fatal cases are typically polymicrobial. Of these agents, *M. ovipneumoniae* is particularly frequent and most important. *Mycoplasmopsis arginini* is often isolated but is not considered a primary pathogen. Failure of passive transfer, negative energy balance, inadequate ventilation, commingling animals from different sources, and adverse weather conditions contribute to development of disease.

Lesions of *M. ovipneumoniae* infection are typically pink-gray lobular consolidation and/or atelectasis in cranioventral lung, with microscopic lesions of neutrophils and macrophages in alveoli and bronchioles, bronchiolar hyperplasia and mucous metaplasia, peribronchiolar cuffs of lymphocytes, interstitial infiltrates of leukocytes in alveolar septa, and variable type II pneumocyte proliferation and interstitial fibrosis. A characteristic and unique lesion of hyaline scars consists of nodular masses of collagen and fibroblasts within the wall of bronchioles that bluntly compress the lumen but do not form the intrabronchiolar polyps seen in obliterative bronchiolitis. **Diagnosis** is based on PCR, culture, or immunohistochemistry of lesional lung tissue. The mycoplasmal lesions have cranioventral distribution, more neutrophil infiltration, thicker peribronchiolar cuffs, and more minimal interstitial changes compared with maedi-visna (which affects adult sheep). More acute lesions with necrotic lysed leukocytes (oat cells) and fibrin suggest *Mannheimia* or *Pasteurella*; abscesses suggest secondary pathogens such as *Trueperella*.

Other mycoplasmas of sheep and goats

Many mycoplasmas cause respiratory or systemic disease in sheep and goats throughout the world, including *M. ovipneumoniae, M. mycoides* ssp. *capri, M. capricolum* ssp. *capricolum*, and *Mycoplasmopsis agalactiae. Mycoplasma capricolum* ssp. *capripneumoniae*, the cause of contagious caprine pleuropneumonia, is discussed above. *M. agalactiae* causes contagious agalactia of sheep and goats, but can also induce respiratory disease. Non- or minimally pathogenic mycoplasmas in small ruminants include *M. arginini, Metamycoplasma auris, Mycoplasma cottewii*, and *Mycoplasma yeatsii*. Transmission requires close contact with infected animals. Young animals are often infected by ingestion or inhalation of contaminated milk.

These agents cause a diverse spectrum of clinical signs and lesions. *Mastitis and agalactia are common in adults and may be accompanied by arthritis or keratitis. Kids and lambs more commonly develop pneumonia or pleuropneumonia, fibrinopurulent polyarthritis, or septicemia with fibrinous polyserositis and interstitial pneumonia.* The lung lesions may resemble those described above for CCPP, but thickening of interlobular septa by edema and fibrin exudation is not typically present in CCPP. *M. mycoides* ssp. *capri* (including strains formerly named *M. mycoides* ssp. *mycoides* large-colony type) is particularly capable of causing pleuropneumonia, polyarthritis, septicemia, and rarely meningitis in goat kids, and to a lesser extent in lambs. *M. capricolum* principally causes fibrinopurulent polyarthritis in kids, but may also cause septicemia in kids and mastitis in does.

Parasitic diseases

Oestrus ovis

Oestrus ovis (sheep bot fly) adult flies deposit first-stage larvae on the nares. The larvae molt twice as they *migrate through the nasal passages*. Larvae may be incarcerated in sinuses or recesses of turbinates as they grow, and eventually die there (eFig. 5-67). Development in the nasal passages can take up to 10 months, although larvae deposited early in summer are able to mature in that season. The full-grown larvae are ~3 cm long, with black oral hooks, dorsal dark transverse bands, and ventral rows of small spines. Pupation occurs on the ground.

The larvae attach by their mouthparts to the mucous membrane where they produce mucosal defects, and their spinous cuticle causes irritation as they wander. An immune response against excreted or secreted larval antigens, and the ensuing eosinophil and mast cell response, may also contribute to nasal inflammation and irritation. Affected sheep develop catarrhal rhinitis and sinusitis. Apart from persistent annoyance and the debility that this may cause, *there are seldom untoward effects of parasitism*. Rarely, larvae penetrate the cranial cavity, or secondary bacterial infections spread from the olfactory mucosa to the meninges. Mild infestations of *O. ovis* occur in goats and dogs, as well as conjunctival infections in humans.

Muellerius capillaris

Muellerius capillaris is the most common and ubiquitous lungworm of sheep and goats (Table 5-3). There are usually no clinical signs in sheep, whereas goats are more likely to develop disease.

Muellerius capillaris is a nematode of the superfamily *Metastrongyloidea*, family *Protostrongylidae*. Adults, which are 12-24 mm long and threadlike, are not grossly visible but live within nodular lesions in the alveoli and rarely in bronchioles. Eggs are laid and rapidly hatch, and first-stage larvae are coughed up, swallowed, and passed in the feces. In some cases, each nodule in the lung may contain adult worms of only one sex. The infection in such cases is sterile, and larvae will not be detected in feces. The intermediate hosts are various slugs and snails. The infective stage is reached after 2 molts in the intermediate host, and the life cycle is completed when sheep and goats swallow the intermediate hosts. The larvae migrate to the lungs, presumably via the lymphatics, and break out into the alveoli. As a consequence of this type of life cycle, infections are gradually acquired, and large worm burdens are seldom observed in animals <6-weeks-old. On the contrary, heavy infections are not common in old sheep and goats, as repeatedly infected animals become resistant.

The characteristic finding is multiple subpleural nodules in the dorsal regions of the caudal lobes (Fig. 5-62). However, they may occur anywhere in the lung, and occasionally in the regional lymph nodes. The nodules are soft and hemorrhagic in the acute stages, corresponding to histologic lesions of hemorrhage and eosinophil infiltration. However, most cases represent chronic infestations with raised gray-pink or yellow nodules that may mineralize.

The nodules contain masses of adult worms, embryonated eggs, and coiled larvae (see Fig. 5-62). The adults have polymyarian-coelomyarian musculature, the intestine is composed of a few multinucleate cells with an indistinct brush border, and the uteri often contain thick-shelled embryonated eggs and larvae. The inflammatory response is often minimal, although alveolar septa may be thickened by fibrous tissue, lymphocytes, and smooth muscle hyperplasia (see Fig. 5-62). In older animals or chronic infestations, presumably associated with developing resistance, the cellular reaction is more marked and targets the first-stage larvae and adults. Eosinophils aggregate around the larvae; the alveolar spaces contain macrophages, eosinophils, and giant cells. Larvae that escape into small bronchioles are enclosed in plugs of mucus and cellular debris. When larvae leave the nodules, the cellular reaction subsides, but thickening of the alveolar septa persists because of patchy or diffuse fibrosis.

Table • 5-3

Major lungworms of sheep and goats

LUNGWORM	GROSS FEATURES	HISTOLOGIC FEATURES
Muellerius capillaris	Pale nodules Worms are microscopic	Adults and larvae mainly in alveoli Alveolar fibrosis ± granulomatous inflammation
Cystocaulus ocreatus	Dark nodules Hairlike worms	Adults and larvae in alveoli and *small* bronchioles
Dictyocaulus filaria	Focal atelectasis or consolidation ± emphysema Threadlike worms in bronchi	Bronchi and *large* bronchioles contain adult worms. Lymphoplasmacytic or eosinophilic inflammation, and smooth muscle and epithelial hyperplasia
Protostrongylus rufescens and *Neostrongylus linearis*	Angular nodules Adults grossly visible in parenchyma and smallest bronchi	Adults in *terminal* bronchioles Granulomatous and/or eosinophilic bronchiolitis, with prominent peribronchiolar lymphofollicular cuffs

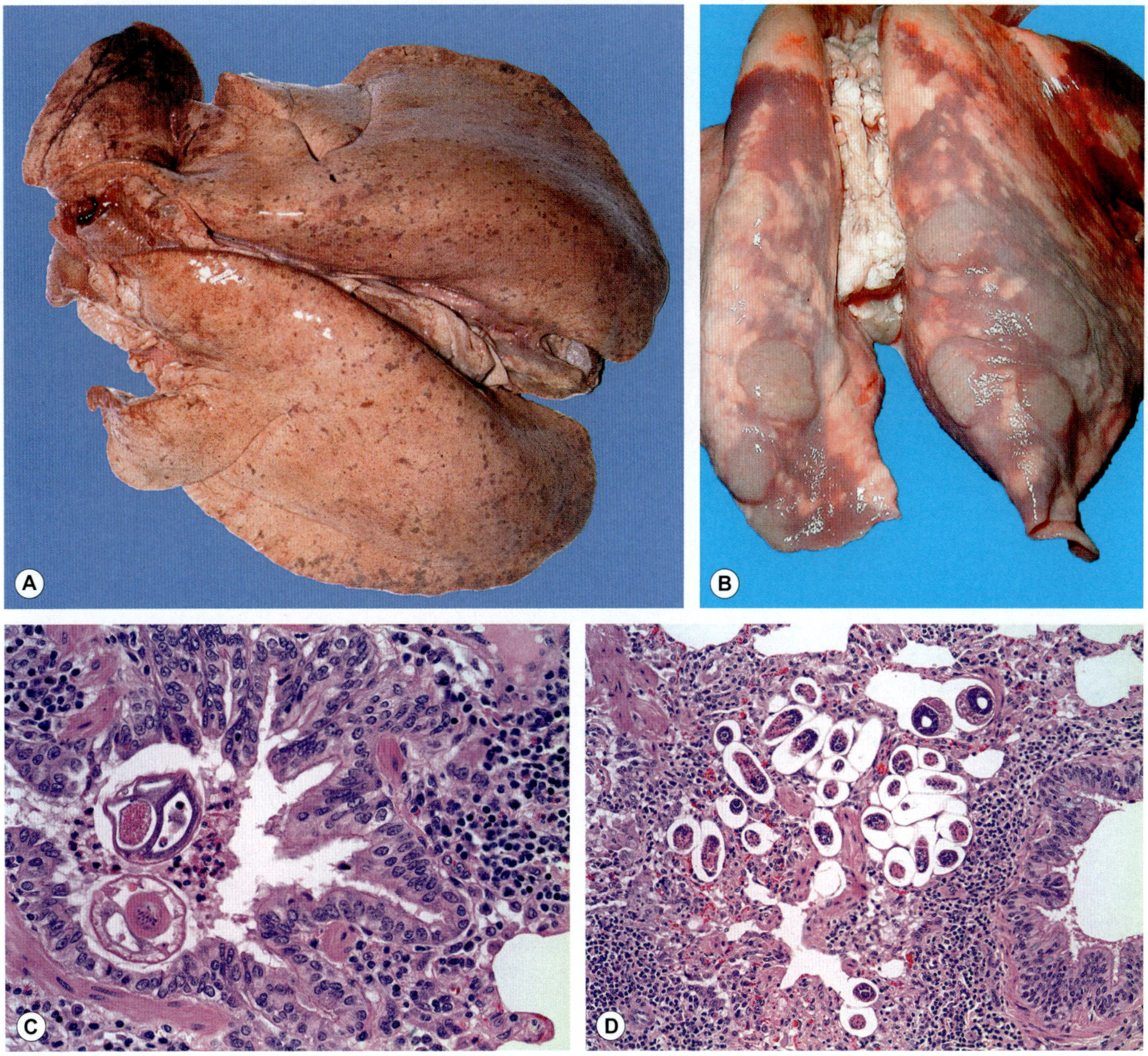

Figure 5-62 *Muellerius capillaris* pneumonia. **A**. Small nodules mainly in the dorsocaudal areas of lung of a sheep. **B**. Larger nodules with similar distribution in a goat. **C**. Tiny adult nematodes in a bronchiole. **D**. Nodules are formed by numerous embryonated eggs and larva, with lymphocytic or granulomatous inflammation and smooth muscle metaplasia in alveolar septa.

Adult worms incite a similar reaction of eosinophils, macrophages, and giant cells. *The cellular debris becomes mineralized, particularly when the worms die, and these mineralized nodules persist indefinitely as spherical mineralized masses surrounded by a fibrous capsule*.

The gross appearance of *Muellerius* infestation can closely resemble that of ***Cystocaulus***. However, the nodules of *Cystocaulus* are darker and may be larger than those of *Muellerius*, the adult worms may be grossly visible, and bronchial epithelial hyperplasia is more likely in *Cystocaulus* infestation. In ***Dictyocaulus*** and ***Protostrongylus*** infections, the adult worms are located in large bronchioles/bronchi and the terminal bronchioles, respectively.

Muellerius infestation in **goats** has been associated with severe diffuse interstitial pneumonia in the absence of nodular lesions. Histologic lesions included diffuse thickening of alveolar septa with mononuclear cells, and fibromuscular hyperplasia in alveolar septa; but the possibility that these lesions might have been caused by caprine arthritis encephalitis virus or *Mycoplasma* infection cannot be ruled out.

Protostrongylus rufescens

Protostrongylus rufescens is a nematode of the superfamily *Metastrongyloidea*, family *Protostrongylidae* that infects sheep, goats, and deer. The adults are 16-35 mm long, red, and mainly inhabit the terminal bronchioles. Eggs hatch to first-stage larvae in the lung and are passed in the feces. They enter intermediate hosts, which are various genera of terrestrial snails, by boring through the foot. Two molts occur in the snail, and the infective third-stage larvae develop in 46-49 days. Sheep and goats eating the snails are infected by the larvae, which pass by way of the mesenteric lymphatics to the lungs.

Lesions consist of 2-4 cm diameter, angular, tan, nodules distributed throughout the lungs. The nodules are usually soft, in contrast to the firm texture of *Muellerius* nodules. Cross sections may reveal fine white worms exuding from the parenchyma or occasionally leading to a small bronchus. Histologically, an eosinophilic inflammatory reaction targets adult worms, larvae, and eggs in the terminal bronchioles. Prominent lymphofollicular aggregates surround these airways. Smooth muscle hyperplasia is not a feature of *Protostrongylus* infestation.

Dictyocaulus filaria

Dictyocaulus filaria is a slender, white, 3-10 cm long nematode that inhabits mainly the small bronchi of sheep and goats. The life cycle and lesions are similar to those described for *D. viviparus*. The lesions are localized, 3-4 cm diameter areas of atelectasis or consolidation that are most common in the dorsal parts of the caudal lobes. Bronchi are thickened by smooth muscle and cuffs of lymphocytes and granulocytes, and often contain adult threadlike worms. Alveoli may contain granulomatous inflammation amid aspirated eggs.

Other parasitic diseases

Neostrongylus linearis, a nematode comparable to *P. rufescens*, is common in western Europe, the Middle East, and probably elsewhere. The adults are 5-15 mm long, and terrestrial gastropods are the intermediate hosts. The worms are contained within 1-4 mm diameter, red-violet or gray-pink nodules that are most numerous in the caudal lobes.

Cystocaulus ocreatus *(C. nigrescens)* reside in 5-20-mm, dark, firm nodules in the dorsocaudal lung. Cross sections reveal brown-black hairlike worms. The life cycle resembles that of *Muellerius*.

Mammomonogamus *(Syngamus)* ***nasicola*** and *M. laryngeus* are nematodes of the nasal cavity and larynx. ***Schistosoma nasalis*** causes nasal granuloma in India. ***Habronema*** spp. is a rare cause of fibrotic nodules adjacent to bronchioles. In sheep, the lung is a common site of hydatid cysts caused by ***Echinococcus granulosus***; the cysts have multiple protoscolices within brood capsules (but these are apparent only in fertile cysts) surrounded by a thin layer of germinal epithelium, an eosinophilic PAS-positive noncellular laminated layer, and an outer adventitial layer that contains macrophages, lymphocytes, giant cells, and remnants of bronchiolar epithelium.

INFECTIOUS RESPIRATORY DISEASES OF HORSES

Viral diseases

Equine influenza

General features of influenza viruses are discussed above (see the Infectious Respiratory Diseases of Pigs section). Infection with equine influenza virus (EIV; *Orthomyxoviridae*, *Alphainfluenzavirus influenzae*) is widespread in most intensively managed horse populations. Outbreaks occur most commonly in the autumn and winter months in young immunologically naive horses. *Risk factors* for infection and disease include close confinement, transportation, training, and mixing of animals. These factors increase the chance of contact between naive and subclinically infected animals. Antigenic drift is a feature of influenza viruses, thus epizootics of influenza may occur even in vaccinated horses, when new antigenic variants of influenza viruses emerge.

All currently circulating EIV belong to the **H3N8 subtype**. H7N7 influenza virus was an important cause of equine respiratory disease in the 1950s, but has been considered extinct since 1978.

Surface hemagglutinin is the immunodominant antigen, and inactivated vaccines induce short-lived protection that is correlated with induction of antibody to this antigen. Vaccinated horses may be infected and shed virus, but have a milder and shorter clinical course. Horses that recover from natural infection have more prolonged resistance to disease, for at least 1 year, but in this case, resistance is not closely correlated to antihemagglutinin antibody titers.

As with influenza in pigs and humans, *the disease in horses and donkeys usually has high morbidity and low mortality, unless secondary bacterial pneumonia develops*. Most outbreaks spread rapidly through groups of horses, with acute onset of fever of <4 days of duration, severe nonproductive cough, mucopurulent nasal discharge, lethargy, anorexia, and occasionally dependent edema. Although most clinical signs resolve within 1-2 weeks, coughing may persist for weeks or months. Rarely, introduction of certain strains of influenza virus into naive populations has caused outbreaks with nearly 100% morbidity and high mortality.

Infection with EIV is usually acquired by inhalation of infected aerosols. Viral replication is most extensive in epithelial cells of the upper respiratory tract and trachea, where infective viral particles bud from the plasma membrane within 2-4 days after infection. Influenza reduces mucociliary clearance both by impairing ciliary beating and by inducing necrosis of infected cells, and can also impair alveolar macrophage function; the ensuing bacterial pneumonia is responsible for many of the fatal cases. Epithelial repair following influenza may take up to 3 weeks and affected horses may continue to cough well past the point of complete repair.

Gross and histologic lesions of uncomplicated EIV are not commonly seen given that horses rarely die of from such infections. *Grossly*, coalescent angular foci of atelectasis or consolidation are separated by unaffected or hyperinflated lung; less commonly, diffuse consolidation is reported. Both foals and adult horses develop secondary bacterial bronchopneumonia. Histologically, tracheitis is common, and foals may develop bronchiolar epithelial necrosis and later hyperplasia, with neutrophils in the lumen and lymphocytes, plasma cells, and neutrophils in the airway wall. Alveoli can have hyaline membranes and/or type II pneumocyte hyperplasia. Rarely, severe EIV infection affects the brain, heart, gastrointestinal tract, kidneys, and other parenchymal organs.

The major differential diagnoses for nonfatal cases of upper respiratory infection include equid herpesviruses 1 and 4 and equine rhinitis A virus. In such cases, clinical diagnosis is most commonly based on detection of virus by RT-PCR from nasal swabs. In the fatal cases, virus is detected in lung by RT-PCR, ELISA, or immunohistochemistry. Serology is mainly used to follow animal exposure during EIV outbreaks but is also of value in routine diagnosis.

Equid alphaherpesviruses

General features of herpesviruses are described above (see the Infectious Respiratory Diseases of Cattle section). Equid alphaherpesviruses (EqAHV; *Orthoherpesviridae*) cause upper respiratory infections, abortion, systemic disease of neonates, and neurologic disease. The latter 3 manifestations are described in more detail elsewhere. Systemic disease of yearling horses or adults is rare, but notable for the high mortality rates that may occur.

Upper respiratory infections of juvenile and adult horses are caused by EqAHV1 or EqAHV4. Uncomplicated rhinitis elicited by these 2 viruses is clinically indistinguishable, with disease most common in foals <1-year-old. Affected animals are febrile with serous or mucopurulent nasal discharge. Both viruses readily infect nasal respiratory epithelial cells causing local epithelial necrosis and inflammation, which results in the aforementioned clinical signs. Less commonly, viral infection extends into the trachea, resulting in coughing. Infection is rarely fatal, unless secondary bacterial pneumonia develops.

Viral replication occurs in the nasopharynx and associated lymphoid tissue, and the development of viremia is dependent on the strain of the virus and prior exposure of the host. Virus is shed from nasal secretions starting 2-10 days after infection. Viral shedding commonly occurs only during the phase of pyrexia, but is occasionally prolonged up to 3 weeks after infection. Latency for EqAHV1 and EqAHV4 is established within neuronal cells (e.g., trigeminal ganglion) and lymphocytes, as well as lung epithelial cells in the case of EqAHV4. Seroconversion to both viruses is common, with nearly 100% of horses surveyed having seroconverted to EqAHV4. Because of this, as well as the prevalence of vaccination for the viruses, serology is of limited use in diagnosing infection with these 2 viruses. Definitive diagnosis of EqAHV1 or EqAHV4 infection of the upper respiratory tract can be done using *virus-specific PCR* on material collected from nasal swabs.

EqAHV1 causes systemic disease in live-born neonates. Lesions are similar to those in aborted foals (see Vol. 3, Female Reproductive System) and include interstitial pneumonia, multifocal necrosis in the liver, spleen, adrenal, and other tissues, prominent intranuclear inclusion bodies, and sometimes syncytial cells. The lungs are heavy with a diffuse rubbery-firm texture, white foci of necrosis may be present but inconspicuous (eFig. 5-68), and the trachea and bronchi may contain a fibrin cast. EqAHV1 occasionally causes systemic disease in yearling or adult horses. Lesions include pulmonary or systemic necrotizing vasculitis, pulmonary edema and hemorrhage, lymphoid necrosis, and encephalomyelitis with vasculitis.

Equid gammaherpesviruses

Members of the subfamily *Gammaherpesvirinae* known to infect the respiratory tract of equids include ***EqGHV2** and **EqGHV5** in horses and 2 asinine herpesviruses (**AHV4**, **AHV5**, unclassified gammaherpesviruses) in donkeys*. PCR-based detection of EqGHV2 and EqGHV5 is reportedly more common in surveys of nasal swabs and tracheal washes from horses with respiratory disease, but their role in the pathogenesis of upper respiratory tract disease in horses remains uncertain. Lower respiratory tract disease is reported in horses and donkeys in association with infection with *EqGHV5*, AHV4, and AHV5.

Equine multinodular pulmonary fibrosis** is a progressive fibrosing interstitial lung disease associated with lung infection with **EqGHV5. It is largely a disease of adult horses with clinical signs of low-grade fever, weight loss, and progressive exercise intolerance. *Gross lesions* are restricted to the lungs and tracheobronchial lymph nodes. Within the lungs there are variably sized nodules of fibrosis (Fig. 5-63). These vary from individual discrete nodules separated by relatively normal lung parenchyma to coalescent foci with little unaffected lung present. The tracheobronchial lymph nodes are often markedly enlarged. *Histologically*, the nodules comprise abundant interstitial collagen and cuboidal epithelial cells lining alveoli. The alveoli contain neutrophils and macrophages, and occasional large macrophages contain an eosinophilic INIB (see Fig. 5-63). The *diagnosis* is based on the characteristic lesions and detection of EqGHV5 in the lung by PCR.

The evidence for a link between lung infection with EqGHV5 and the development of equine multinodular pulmonary fibrosis has been based on detection of virus by PCR as well as virus isolation, colocalization of the virus with the lesions, and development in horses experimentally infected with EqGHV5 of nodular lung fibrosis with features similar to the natural disease.

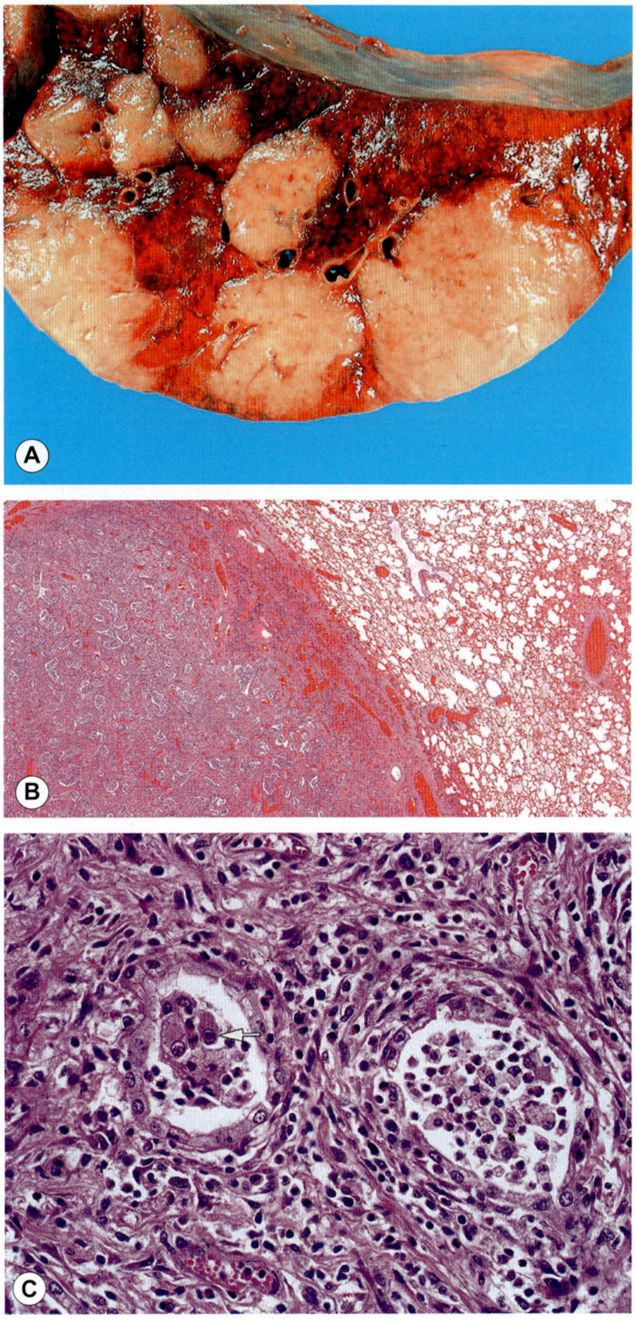

Figure 5-63 Equine multinodular pulmonary fibrosis. **A**. Pale well-demarcated nodules throughout the lung. **B, C**. The nodules have marked expansion of the interstitium by connective tissue, and alveoli are lined by type II pneumocytes and contain macrophages and neutrophils. A macrophage has an intranuclear inclusion (arrow).

***AHV4** and **AHV5** cause interstitial pneumonia in donkeys.* *Grossly*, the lungs fail to collapse and have patchy or multifocal firm lesions, most commonly in the cranioventral areas. *Histologically*, affected animals have a mix of bronchiolitis and interstitial pneumonia with the consistent presence of large multinucleate *syncytial cells*. Viral inclusion bodies are not present. Lesions include combinations of mononuclear cell and neutrophil infiltrates around bronchioles and in alveolar septa, necrosis of bronchiolar epithelium, alveolar type II pneumocyte proliferation, and interstitial fibrosis. *Diagnosis* is based on PCR to detect AHV4 or AHV5 in association with the characteristic histologic lesions. This condition differs from donkey pulmonary fibrosis, which mainly affects the pleura and subpleural lung tissue.

Adenovirus

Equine adenovirus 1 (**EAdV1**; *Adenoviridae, Mastadenovirus equi*) infection is widespread in horses and is mainly associated with upper respiratory tract infections. Adenoviral pneumonia is a well-described complication of inherited combined immunodeficiency in young Arabian foals. This severe disease has become rare as the genetic immunodeficiency is now less common. The *gross lesions* are lobular or confluent atelectasis and/or consolidation primarily, but not exclusively, within cranioventral lung. In the early stage of severe infection, there is extensive necrosis and sloughing of bronchiolar epithelium. Later, bronchiolar epithelium is hyperplastic, and swollen superficial epithelial cells contain amphophilic intranuclear inclusion bodies. Occasionally, there are inclusions in alveolar epithelial cells and increased numbers of macrophages and neutrophils. Secondary bacterial pneumonia or *Pneumocystis* pneumonia may also be present in these immunocompromised foals.

Hendra virus

Hendra virus was first described as a cause of fatal pulmonary disease of horses in 1994 in Australia. Natural infections and disease have been reported in humans and horses and experimentally induced in cats and guinea pigs. Fruit bats (flying foxes) in the genus *Pteropus* are the reservoir host for the virus, carrying the virus subclinically and serving as the source of infection for horses. Most human infections have occurred following contact with clinically ill horses. Hendra virus and the related Nipah virus are members of the genus *Henipavirus*, family *Paramyxoviridae*. *Hendra virus has tropism for endothelial cells, and many of the lesions arise from vascular injury*. Viral particles are detectable in the cytoplasm of endothelial cells. *Gross lesions* in horses reflect the viral vascular tropism and include prominent *pulmonary edema and congestion* with dilation of subpleural lymphatic vessels, petechial hemorrhages, and abundant tracheal froth. The most prominent *histologic lesion* is serofibrinous fluid and increased numbers of macrophages in alveoli. Closer inspection reveals subtle vascular lesions in the lung, heart, glomeruli, and stomach, consisting of thrombi in capillaries and/or necrotic debris and hemorrhage in the walls of arterioles. The presence of syncytial cells in small vessels is a unique but inconsistent lesion. The *differential diagnosis* for massive pulmonary edema includes African horse sickness, heart failure, and anaphylaxis.

Bacterial diseases

Rhodococcus equi

Rhodococcus equi is an important cause of pneumonia and occasionally enteric disease in 1-8-month-old foals. The prevalence is highly variable among farms and probably reflects the bacterial load within airborne dust, given that soil is the important source of infection. Environmental factors favoring the disease include hot seasonal temperatures in temperate climates, neutral soil pH, and repetitive high-density stocking of dry paddocks. The clinical presentation may be acute or insidiously progressive, although the infection and lesions are invariably chronic by the time clinical signs are noted. Thoracic ultrasound shows that most foals with lung abscesses do not develop clinical disease, and many recover without therapy. When clinical disease occurs, it is most frequent in the summer, with pyrexia, tachypnea, dyspnea, cough, and mucopurulent nasal discharge. *Because of the chronic nature of the disease, case fatality rates can be high in untreated foals*. Animals with the *colonic form* of disease may have diarrhea, weight loss, ascites resulting from hypoproteinemia, and occasionally colic.

Foals with interstitial pneumonia, described above, frequently have concurrent *R. equi* infection, yet the relationship between these conditions remains obscure. Foals with *R. equi* pneumonia occasionally have histologic evidence of *Pneumocystis carinii* infection of the lung.

R. equi is a gram-positive facultative intracellular pathogen, distantly related to mycobacteria, which grows well in soil and in horse manure. Neonatal foals have the greatest susceptibility to infection, compared with those 6-weeks-old. *Pulmonary infection results from inhalation of soilborne bacteria*, and inhalation of greater numbers of bacteria is facilitated by a dusty, contaminated environment. Enteric infections may result from ingestion of soil-contaminated feed, or swallowing expectorated material from the lungs. Experimental studies indicate that hematogenous spread from enteric lesions is not a common route of pulmonary infection.

The bacterium is engulfed by equine macrophages but survives this encounter by preventing maturation of the phagosome and its fusion with the lysosome. Nevertheless, macrophages are able to kill *R. equi* when the bacteria are opsonized or when the macrophages are activated by lymphocyte-derived IFNγ. Infection elicits a pyogranulomatous inflammatory response, presumably as a result of cytokines secreted by infected macrophages or responding lymphocytes.

The *virulence* of *R. equi* varies between isolates and is associated with an 80-90 kb virulence-associated plasmid. Species-specificity for horses, pigs, or ruminants is conferred by the various host-adapted plasmids: pVAPA in equids, pVAPB in swine, or pVAPN in ruminants. The plasmid carries a pathogenicity island that contains the variety of genes needed by the bacteria to survive within macrophages following phagocytosis. The macrophage is the preferred cell type for replication of the bacterium, and central to the pathogenesis. Other virulence factors of *R. equi* include glycolipids containing long-chain mycolic acids, capsular polysaccharide, the "equi factors" cholesterol oxidase and choline phosphohydrolase, and the iron-binding protein rhequichelin.

Immune responses to *R. equi* have been intensively investigated because of the interest in developing vaccines against this important disease of foals. The finding that passive immunization with hyperimmune plasma is effective in preventing disease indicates that humoral immunity is protective, probably because antibody-mediated opsonization augments phagocytosis and killing of *R. equi* by macrophages and neutrophils. In contrast to the role of humoral immunity in prevention of disease, Th1 cellular immune responses are probably necessary for recovery from established infection. Both CD4+ and CD8+ T cells are important in clearing *P. equi* in mouse models of disease. CD4+ T cells produce IFNγ, which activates macrophages to produce more bactericidal nitric oxide, oxygen radicals, and peroxynitrite; CD8+ T cells induce lysis of infected macrophages.

The *pulmonary lesions* caused by *R. equi* are most constant in the cranioventral lung, but much of the lung may

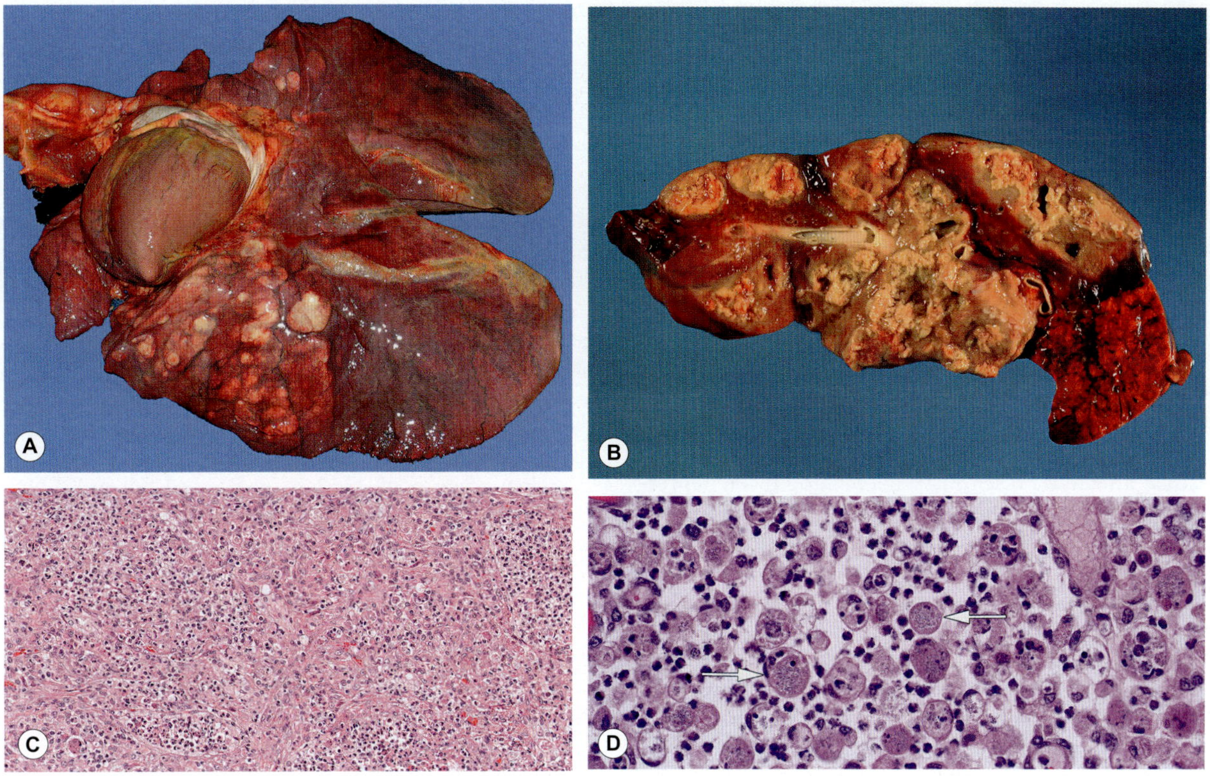

Figure 5-64 ***Rhodococcus equi*** **pneumonia** in a foal. **A.** Ventral view of the lungs, with cranioventral consolidation containing numerous pale bulging nodules. **B.** On section (a different case), the consolidated lung contains liquefying foci of pyogranulomatous inflammation. **C.** Macrophages and neutrophils fill alveoli. **D.** Some enlarged macrophages contain bacteria in their cytoplasm (arrows).

be affected in severe cases. *The most consistent lesion is pyogranulomatous bronchopneumonia*, forming 1-10-cm, white-tan, firm, coalescing nodules (Fig. 5-64). Intervening areas of the lung are reddened and firmer than normal. With time, the centers of the pyogranulomas become friable and caseous or liquefying. These may appear as abscesses, but they have many macrophages and generally lack a fibrous capsule. Pleuritis is uncommon. Bronchial lymph nodes are enlarged and may contain focal caseous necrosis.

Intestinal lesions are present in about half of foals with pulmonary lesions; 5% of cases have lesions restricted to the intestine. The colon, cecum, and associated lymph nodes are most commonly affected, but small intestinal lesions may occur. Colonic lesions begin as focal mucosal ulcers that are centered on lymphoid follicles. The ulcer bed is reddened and covered with fibrin, and the borders of the ulcers are raised and pale because of pyogranulomatous infiltrates. Pyogranulomas or foci of caseous necrosis may extend through the wall of the intestine. The colonic lymph nodes are often enlarged, pale, and contain necrotic foci. The colonic pyogranulomas enlarge over time and develop central areas of caseation or liquefaction. Large abdominal abscesses may be the sole lesion in some cases and should be distinguished from bastard strangles.

The earliest histologic lesion following *R. equi* infection is neutrophilic bronchopneumonia. By 4 days after infection, alveoli and bronchioles are filled with macrophages, neutrophils, and fewer lymphocytes and plasma cells. *Macrophages are numerous in the well-developed lesions, but neutrophils may also be plentiful. Gram-positive bacteria are present in the cytoplasm of plump uni- or multinucleate macrophages in this exudate* and are particularly numerous within degenerating macrophages that have hypereosinophilic cytoplasm and nuclear pyknosis (see Fig. 5-64). Areas of caseous necrosis, when present, usually contain cellular debris, many neutrophils and macrophages, fibrin, and edema.

In the intestine, the dome epithelium overlying lymphoid follicles is the primary route of infection. Macrophages underlying the dome epithelium contain intracytoplasmic bacilli, and neutrophils infiltrate the epithelium and exude into the lumen. With time, the lymphoid follicles are invaded by macrophages and neutrophils, and central areas of caseous necrosis eventually extend to the mucosal surface. In the developed lesions of ulcerative colitis, ulcers are filled with fibrinonecrotic debris and encompassed by neutrophils and macrophages, many of which contain bacteria.

About 1/3 of affected foals have *polyarthritis*. This may cause severe lameness, neutrophilic synovitis, and positive joint cultures, as a result of hematogenous spread of infection. In contrast, other foals have milder, probably *immune-mediated polyarthritis*, with sterile joints, lymphoplasmacytic synovitis, mononuclear cells in joint fluid, and immunoglobulin deposits in synovium.

More widespread dissemination of infection in foals can occasionally give rise to abscesses in the mesenteric or mediastinal lymph nodes, liver, spleen, or skin; osteomyelitis affecting the vertebrae or metaphyses of long bones; and uveitis with hypopyon. *R. equi* may also cause ulcerative lymphangitis and has been associated with metritis and abortion in mares. Disease is uncommon in cattle and pigs and typically involves granulomatous lesions in submandibular or thoracic lymph nodes that resemble tuberculosis or caseous lymphadenitis. Infected goats may have disseminated granulomas or abscesses in the lung, liver, other viscera, skin, and bones.

Lesions of cranioventral pyogranulomatous pneumonia or multifocal ulcerative colitis in foals are highly suggestive of *R. equi* infection. In most cases, the *diagnosis is easily confirmed by culture* or by identifying intracytoplasmic gram-positive bacilli in macrophages on impression smears or tissue sections.

Bacterial pneumonia and pleuropneumonia in mature horses

Pleuropneumonia is common in 2-4-year-olds, and older horses may also be affected. Presenting signs include fever, depression, respiratory distress, and colic. Evidence of pleural pain may be apparent at rest, with grunting respiration or abduction of the elbows, or be elicited by thoracic percussion. Horses with bacterial pneumonia develop fever, tachypnea, and cough. Risk factors for pneumonia or pleuropneumonia include recent transportation, general anesthesia (probably leading to aspiration pneumonia), other stressful events, and viral infection.

Numerous opportunistic bacterial pathogens have been isolated from lesions of pleuropneumonia in horses, and *mixed infections are often present*. Attempts to isolate bacteria may fail in cases that have been treated with antibiotics. *Streptococcus equi* ssp. *zooepidemicus* is the most common isolate; others include *Streptococcus equisimilis*, *S. equi* ssp. *equi*, other streptococci, *Actinobacillus equuli* ssp. *haemolyticus*, *Klebsiella pneumoniae*, *Pasteurella* spp., *Bordetella bronchiseptica*, *E. coli*, *Bacteroides*, and *Fusobacterium*. *Mycoplasmopsis felis* is an infrequent cause of pleuritis without pneumonia in horses.

Many cases result from aspiration pneumonia, particularly those with unilateral or asymmetric distribution of lesions. The equine trachea at the thoracic inlet contains a pool of secretions contaminated by bacteria—the so-called "*tracheal puddle*." Transport of horses with the head held in an elevated position predisposes to aspiration of these contaminated secretions into the lung. Thus, aspiration pneumonia in horses can be caused by respiratory pathogens such as *Streptococcus zooepidemicus*, or by mixed bacterial infections as for aspiration pneumonia in other species.

The gross lesions of well-developed cases of pleuropneumonia are spectacular, and the lesions are often more chronic than suggested by the clinical history (perhaps reflecting a subclinical pneumonia with development of clinical signs when bacteria reach the pleural cavity). Massive amounts of fibrin and malodorous serofibrinous exudate fill the pleural space and may form cavitating masses encased in maturing fibrous tissue. Most cases of pleuritis in horses arise from underlying pulmonary lesions, although the lesions of pneumonia are overshadowed by the pleural exudate. Although often described as lung abscesses, the lung lesions are more usually localized areas of consolidation. Lesions in the lung are often unilateral and most frequent in the cranial part of the caudal lobe. Occasionally, pleuritis extends from bilateral lesions of bronchopneumonia, which may include localized areas of thrombosis and infarction.

Opportunistic bacterial pathogens in foals

Pneumonia caused by opportunistic bacterial pathogens is common in 1-8-month-old foals and appears to be of similar pathogenesis as in other species. *Streptococcus zooepidemicus* is the most prevalent cause; others are α-hemolytic streptococci, *Klebsiella pneumoniae*, *Actinobacillus equuli*, *Bordetella bronchiseptica*, *Staphylococcus epidermidis*, and others. Pneumonia in neonates is commonly caused by bacteria that cause septicemia and the 2 processes may be concurrent; *E. coli*, *Streptococcus* spp., *A. equuli*, and *K. pneumoniae* are the most common isolates.

Strangles and Streptococcus equi

Strangles is an acute contagious disease of horses with inflammation of the upper respiratory tract and abscessation of the regional lymph nodes. The disease typically occurs in young horses following exposure to carriers or diseased horses. Clinical signs can include fever, dysphagia, purulent nasal discharge, inappetence, depression, unilateral or bilateral swelling of the throat region, and stertor.

Strangles is caused by *Streptococcus equi* **ssp**. *equi*, a Lancefield group C streptococcus. Unlike *S. equi* ssp. *zooepidemicus*, which may infect a variety of species, *S. equi* is mainly restricted to horses, although human disease thought to be acquired from horses is described. A range of virulence factors is described. The hyaluronic acid capsule is necessary for virulence, mediates binding of the bacterium to host cells, and confers resistance to phagocytosis. The M protein and a factor-H-binding protein bind fibrinogen and prevent deposition of complement factor C3b, thereby blocking recognition and phagocytosis by macrophages. Two endopeptidases cleave IgG. Peptidoglycan activates complement by the alternative pathway, inciting recruitment of neutrophils to sites of infection. The fact that many of the recruited neutrophils rapidly undergo necrosis may be an effect of streptolysin-S and another cytotoxin.

S. equi in exudates are thought to survive for months in the external environment and may be transmitted through contaminated drinking water or by fomites. The initial source of infection, however, is usually a carrier animal or one with active but not necessarily obvious clinical disease. The incubation period of strangles is 3-4 days, although it may be as short as 2 or as long as 15 days. The pathogenesis involves rapid transport of bacteria from the tonsil to local lymph nodes, within 3 hours after experimental infection. *S. equi* only transiently colonizes nasopharyngeal epithelial cells, so attempts to culture the bacteria from nasopharyngeal samples can be fruitless in the face of an active infection. Following the entry of the bacteria into regional lymph nodes, there is chemotaxis of neutrophils to the infected lymph nodes. The organism resists phagocytosis leading to further increases in the number of neutrophils, neutrophil lysis, and formation of lymph node abscesses. Recovery from strangles confers immunity in ~75% of horses, associated with IgA and IgG antibody produced locally in the nasopharynx. Although antibodies to M protein confer partial immunity, other protective antigens are not yet fully defined.

The submandibular and retropharyngeal nodes are the first and usually the most severely affected. The swollen lymph nodes are initially firm, but this swelling becomes fluctuant as the neutrophilic exudate liquefies. The typical and most favorable clinical outcome of the lymphadenitis is for the abscesses to rupture onto the skin 1-3 weeks after the onset of infection, releasing pus containing numerous infective bacteria. Infection also often extends from retropharyngeal lymph nodes to involve the guttural pouches, and purulent exudates within these structures can inspissate to form the so-called *chondroids*. Drainage from the guttural pouch into the nasal cavity is a major reason for neutrophilic nasal discharge.

Most cases of strangles recover quickly unless the enlarging lymph nodes obstruct the upper respiratory tract, but complications develop in 20% of clinically affected animals. This may involve extension of infection to adjacent structures, resulting in purulent sinusitis, guttural pouch empyema, periorbital abscess formation, facial cellulitis, or local damage to cranial nerves resulting in laryngeal paralysis (roaring), facial nerve paralysis, or Horner syndrome. Horses with guttural pouch empyema may remain infected, intermittently shed bacteria, and be an important source of infection for at least 8 months after resolution of the acute disease.

More serious ***complications*** *include pneumonia or pleuropneumonia, myocarditis, mesenteric lymph node abscesses, and hemorrhagic purpura.* Retropharyngeal abscesses may discharge into the pharynx, allowing pus to be aspirated into the lungs where localized areas of necrotizing pneumonia develop. Metastatic abscesses ("*bastard strangles*") occasionally form in the liver, kidneys, synovium, and brain, but are most common in mediastinal and mesenteric lymph nodes. Abscesses in these lymph nodes tend to be very large and, although rupture is unusual, the neutrophilic process can extend to adjacent serous membranes and cause purulent pleuritis or peritonitis. Hemorrhagic purpura is a systemic leukocytoclastic vasculitis and follows deposition of immune complexes of IgA or IgG with bacterial M protein in small blood vessels and glomeruli. Hemorrhagic purpura develops in 1-2% of cases, 2-4 weeks after the acute infection. There is edema of the head and limbs, petechial hemorrhages on mucosal and serosal surfaces and in muscles, and occasionally glomerulonephritis.

Because similar, but usually milder, lesions may be caused by *S. zooepidemicus* or other bacteria, *definitive diagnosis relies on isolation of S. equi from purulent exudate*. PCR assays are also available and are particularly useful in detecting chronically infected horses.

Glanders

Glanders is caused by ***Burkholderia mallei*** and typically causes acute disease in donkeys and mules, and chronic disease in horses. It is now mostly of historic importance, having flourished when horses played a larger role in human transport and military campaigns and has disappeared from many countries, but still exists in Eastern Europe, Asia, and South America. Natural disease occurs in carnivores, sheep, and goats; cattle and pigs are considered more resistant. Humans are susceptible, and it has been used as a biological weapon. *B. mallei* is sensitive to the external environment, and infection is acquired directly or indirectly from excretions and discharges of affected animals. In the absence of definitive information, it is assumed that the organisms traverse the pharyngeal mucosa, and perhaps the intestinal mucosa, and are conveyed to the lungs where lesions almost always occur. From there, hematogenous spread is believed to result in nasal, cutaneous, and lymph node lesions.

Lesions in glanders include pulmonary nodules, and ulcerative and nodular lesions of the skin and respiratory mucosa. Lung lesions are often present as generalized pinpoint to 2-cm *pyogranulomatous nodules throughout the lung*, often with central areas of liquefactive necrosis. Histologically, the nodules are composed of a central core of neutrophils, often with necrosis of neutrophils and liquefaction of the tissue, and a peripheral rim of epithelioid macrophages, giant cells, and fibrosis. The relative proportions of neutrophils, macrophages, fibrosis, and mineralization are variable.

Nasal lesions are often unilateral, with copious, purulent, green-yellow exudate. Small nodules in the submucosa each consist of an inner core of neutrophils and a periphery of macrophages. The core liquefies and the overlying mucosa may slough, leaving a crateriform ulcer that heals to form a white stellate scar. Similar pyogranulomatous ulcerative lesions line the pharynx, larynx, and trachea. Hematogenous metastases are common in the spleen and less common in other tissues. Enteric lesions are rare. *The cutaneous lesions of glanders are termed "farcy."* These consist of chains of nodules or ulcers that follow lymphatic vessels and represent purulent lymphangitis with extensive leukocyte necrosis.

Mycoplasmal diseases

Although several mycoplasmas have been isolated from the respiratory tract of horses, particularly *Metamycoplasma (Mycoplasma) equirhinis* and *Mycoplasmopsis felis*, there have been no studies to determine whether they are capable of causing pneumonia. *M. felis* is an uncommon cause of fibrinous pleuritis without pneumonia, and lesions were reproduced by intrapleural inoculation of *M. felis*. *M. felis* has also been associated with outbreaks of lower respiratory tract disease in horses, based on seroconversion and isolation of the organism.

Fungal diseases

Coccidioidomycosis, cryptococcosis, and **pneumocystosis** are described elsewhere. **Pulmonary aspergillosis** is an uncommon disease of horses and usually represents hematogenous spread of fungal hyphae from colitis, as a consequence both of neutropenia and disruption of the mucosal barrier. Lesions are multifocal embolic pneumonia, often centered on pulmonary vessels, and include neutrophil and fibrin exudate in alveoli, hemorrhage, necrosis, and leukocytoclastic vasculitis. Septate branching hyphae are most common at the periphery of foci of necrosis (Fig. 5-65).

Entomophthoromycosis (phycomycosis) is a chronic nasal or cutaneous disease of horses, dogs, sheep, and rarely of cattle, caused by *Conidiobolus coronatus*, *Conidiobolus lamprauges*, and *Basidiobolus haptosporus* (class *Zygomycetes*, order *Entomophthorales*), which are saprophytic fungi limited to tropical and subtropical climates. The nasal lesions may affect the nostril, or form masses in the ethmoid conchae that obstruct the nasal cavity and invade adjacent tissues including the sinuses, retro-orbital space, or brain, and may spread to the lung, brain, and other tissues. The masses consist of ulcerating and cavitating granulomas containing coral-shaped granules. Histologic evaluation reveals eosinophils, neutrophils, macrophages, and giant cells. Fungal hyphae of *C. coronatus* and *B. haptosporus* appear with H&E stain as unstained filaments mainly within the brightly eosinophilic amorphous material (the Splendore-Hoeppli phenomenon); a silver stain reveals the hyphae to be nonpigmented, commonly septate, irregular in contour, 5-13 μm or 5-20 μm diameter, respectively, and irregularly branched. PAS stains are not considered useful.

Pythium insidiosum (an aquatic fungus-like oomycete pathogen) induces a lesion in horses, cattle, and sheep that is similar to entomophthoromycosis, but eosinophils are numerous, and

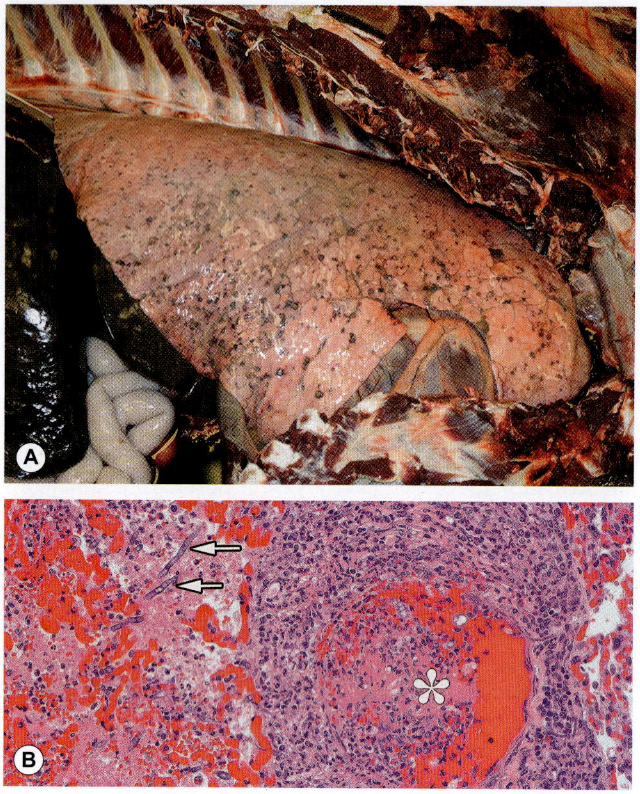

Figure 5-65 Embolic aspergillosis in a horse with necrotizing colitis. **A.** Dark nodules in an embolic pattern throughout the lung. **B.** A blood vessel in the lung (asterisk) contains a fibrin thrombus, neutrophils, and other leukocytes that extend to adjacent tissue, and fungal hyphae (arrows).

the hyphae are 2-7 μm diameter, thick-walled, and infrequently septate. However, pythiosis and entomophthoromycosis are difficult to differentiate histologically, and definitive diagnosis requires culture, PCR testing, or immunohistochemistry. The differential diagnoses for eosinophilic cutaneous or nasal masses in horses include habronemosis and mast cell tumor.

Parasitic diseases

Dictyocaulus arnfieldi is mainly a lungworm of donkeys, in which it survives for long periods with few clinical signs. *D. arnfieldi* is an occasional cause of chronic coughing in horses. Infection of adult horses often results in failure of the worm to develop to sexual maturity, and larvae cannot be detected in the feces of these animals. The worms can mature if horses or ponies are infected as young foals. The gross lesions are scattered wedge-shaped foci of overinflation, mostly in caudal lobes. In the center of the lesions are *small bronchi packed with coiled adult worms*. Histologically, the worms are associated with goblet cell hyperplasia and lymphocytic infiltrates. Adult worms cause relatively little luminal response, whereas first-stage larvae stimulate an intense mucopurulent reaction, or chronic catarrhal and eosinophilic bronchiolitis.

Parascaris equorum larval migration causes *nodular lesions in the lung*. The acute lesions are distinctive by virtue of the mass of eosinophils present and occasional ascarid larvae in bronchioles or alveoli. However, the chronic nodules consist of aggregates of lymphoid tissue with fibrosis and mineralization, which resemble residual lesions of small abscesses or granulomas.

Echinococcus equinus causes cysts in the lung of horses in western Europe. The cysts have a characteristic histologic appearance, with an inner germinal membrane containing brood capsules, protoscolices, and mineralized corpuscles; a noncellular laminated middle layer; and an outer adventitial layer of fibrosis and chronic inflammation (eFig. 5-69).

Infection with **amebae** rarely causes encephalitis in horses. Multifocal granulomatous pneumonia with necrosis and thrombosis, with histologically visible trophozoites and cysts, are reported in those cases caused by ***Acanthamoeba***.

Miscellaneous parasitisms include ***Schistosoma nasalis***, a cause of nasal granuloma in India; hydatid cysts; and ***Habronema*** spp., a rare cause of fibrotic nodules adjacent to bronchioles.

INFECTIOUS RESPIRATORY DISEASES OF DOGS

Canine infectious respiratory disease (CIRD) complex is important and common in dogs. The disease is most prevalent in dogs that have been brought into close contact with others at shelters, pet stores, kennels, and dog shows. The name recognizes that, as in cattle and pigs, highly contagious respiratory disease occurs in dogs as a result of complex interactions among host factors and a variety of viruses and bacteria. The bacterial causes include *Bordetella bronchiseptica*, *Streptococcus zooepidemicus*, and *Mycoplasmopsis (Mycoplasma) cynos*. Canine parainfluenza virus (CPIV), canine adenovirus 2 (CAdV2), canine distemper virus (CDV), and canine herpesvirus have been important in the past and still occur, but frequent viral causes now include CPIV, canine respiratory coronavirus, and canine influenza virus. Other viruses of less certain significance include canine pneumovirus, pantropic canine coronavirus, canine bocavirus, canine bufavirus, and canine hepacivirus.

Viral diseases

Canine distemper

Canine distemper continues to be a frequent and serious disease in many parts of the world, although it is now uncommon in countries with well-vaccinated dog populations. **Canine distemper virus (CDV**; *Paramyxoviridae, Morbillivirus canis) infects a wide range of terrestrial carnivores*, including *Canidae* (wild and domestic dogs), *Mustelidae* (ferrets, mink), and *Procyonidae* (raccoons); ferrets are particularly susceptible. Some species of seals are vulnerable to CDV infection, and distinct closely related phocid morbilliviruses are also important causes of distemper-like disease in these species.

As with the closely related morbilliviruses causing human measles and bovine rinderpest, CDV is a large, 150-250-nm, irregularly shaped virus with an outer lipoprotein envelope, an inner matrix, and a nucleocapsid containing single-strand negative-sense RNA. The envelope is studded with hemagglutinin glycoproteins that mediate viral attachment to host cells, and fusion glycoproteins that allow penetration of host cells and fusion of infected with uninfected cells.

Virus is shed in secretions of the respiratory tract, and to a lesser extent in other secretions. Infection is usually acquired by inhaling aerosols or by close contact with infected dogs. The virus infects macrophages of the upper respiratory tract or lungs, which convey it to local lymph nodes and tonsils during the first 24 hours. The virus replicates further in local lymphoid tissues, and by 2-5 days after exposure is present in lymphoid tissues throughout the body, including the bone marrow, thymus, spleen, and intestinal lymphoid tissue.

Clinical signs of fever, depression, and anorexia develop about 5 days after infection. At this stage of viremia, virus particles are free in the plasma as well as within blood mononuclear cells. *Further development of the disease is highly dependent on the immune status of the host, the titer of antibodies to envelope glycoproteins, the age of the host, and the strain of virus.* Dogs with adequate humoral and cellular immunity can neutralize the virus and clear the infection by 14 days and may not shed virus from mucosal surfaces. In dogs with intermediate levels of cellular and humoral immunity, viremia leads to infection of mucosal epithelium and brain. Virus is shed in secretions, but clinical signs attributable to epithelial infection may be minor or absent, although neurologic disease can develop in these partially immune dogs. Dogs that fail to mount an adequate immune response develop systemic infection of epithelial tissues that evokes clinical signs of respiratory and enteric disease, infection of the central nervous system, and shedding of virus in respiratory secretions, feces, and urine.

Clinical disease in dogs is most common at 12-16 weeks of age, as puppies with waning passive immunity are exposed to subclinically infected dogs. *The infection is systemic, and clinical signs are often referable to the respiratory, gastrointestinal, and nervous systems.* Ocular disease, pustular and/or hyperkeratotic cutaneous lesions, dental defects, and abortion are other manifestations. In some cases, clinical signs are primarily the result of secondary infections that are a consequence of *virus-induced immunosuppression*, probably an effect of viral infection of lymphocytes and macrophages. Secondary diseases include *Bordetella*, adenovirus, and *Pneumocystis* infections of the lung; toxoplasmosis, Tyzzer disease, sarcocystosis, and encephalitozoonosis; and enteric infections with *Cryptosporidium* or attaching-effacing *E. coli*.

The systemic form of the disease often begins with fever and conjunctivitis, and rapid progression to coughing, depression, anorexia, vomiting, and diarrhea. Affected dogs may die at this stage, fully recover, or develop neurologic disease 1-4 weeks later. Neurologic disease may also be the primary clinical manifestation, particularly in animals with partial immunity. Neurologic manifestations are quite variable depending on the anatomic location of the lesions and include seizures, cerebellar or vestibular ataxia, paraparesis or paraplegia, and myoclonus.

The **histologic lesions** of canine distemper are fairly specific when the disease is well developed and if inclusion bodies are apparent. However, *lesions in mild cases are nonspecific*, particularly in dogs with clinical signs limited to the upper respiratory tract. *Inclusion bodies are most numerous 10-14 days after infection*, but their numbers diminish by 5-6 weeks. *Inclusions are most obvious in the brain and epithelial tissues*, and less easily identified in lymphoid tissues. Inclusion bodies can be found in the central nervous system before changes of encephalomyelitis are present, and they often persist in the neural tissue when they have disappeared from other sites. The inclusion bodies are eosinophilic and often intranuclear in nervous tissue, and intracytoplasmic or intranuclear in other tissues.

Lymphopenia and lesions in lymphoid organs are regularly present. *Lymphoid lesions* may be inapparent on gross examination, or there may be either atrophy or edematous swelling. Thymic atrophy is particularly common in CDV-infected puppies. The earliest lesions following experimental infection with CDV are depletion of lymphocytes in the cortical zone of the lymph nodes within 6 days of infection. By day 9, the lymph nodes and spleen have lymphocytic necrosis and depletion, and infiltration of neutrophils. Syncytial cells may form in the lymph nodes, and these often contain inclusion bodies. Approximately 2 weeks after exposure, hyperplasia of histiocytic cells develops, but repopulation of the node by lymphocytes may be delayed for weeks or months. Thymic atrophy results from both loss of cortical thymocytes and reduction in the medulla.

Respiratory tract lesions are common. Grossly, serous, catarrhal, or mucopurulent exudate covers the nasopharynx. The lungs are edematous, and secondary bronchopneumonia is often present, particularly in subacute or chronic cases. *The lesions of canine distemper* usually appear as patchy, generalized, red-tan, rubbery lesions beneath the pleura and at the margins of the lung. Generalized diffuse reddening and consolidation is a less-common manifestation. Histologically, bronchioles contain scant neutrophilic exudate, there is patchy necrosis and attenuation of bronchiolar epithelium, and lymphocytes are present around bronchioles. *Inclusion bodies are often most obvious in the cytoplasm or nucleus of bronchial and bronchiolar epithelial cells* (eFig. 5-70). Alveoli contain protein-rich edema, scant fibrin, mononuclear cells, and necrotic epithelial cells. Alveolar septa are thickened by mononuclear cells. Type II pneumocytes may form a complete cuboidal lining in scattered groups of alveoli. Inclusion bodies are common in type II pneumocytes and alveolar macrophages, and *alveolar epithelial syncytial cells are a characteristic feature when present.* Chronic lesions in subpleural and peribronchiolar alveoli include macrophage accumulation, type II pneumocyte proliferation, and alveolar septal fibrosis. Inclusion bodies tend to persist in the bronchiolar and alveolar epithelium longer than in other non-neural tissues.

Intracytoplasmic and rarely intranuclear inclusion bodies are regularly found within swollen urothelial cells of the *urinary bladder and renal pelvis* in the acute systemic disease. Inclusion bodies, mild degenerative changes, and mononuclear cell infiltrates may be present in a variety of other epithelia, including the gastric surface epithelium, chief and parietal cells of the stomach, cholangiolar epithelium in the liver, pancreatic ductular epithelium, epididymis, and testis.

In the *central nervous system*, the virus appears first in perivascular astrocytes and macrophages, but infection of the choroid plexus epithelium occurs early, and the cerebrospinal fluid contains large amounts of virus. Lesions in the white matter and gray matter differ histologically; these may occur concurrently or one may predominate. *Demyelination in white matter tracts* is most severe in the cerebellum, rostral medullary velum, optic tracts, spinal cord, and surrounding the fourth ventricle, and probably arises from distribution of virus through the cerebrospinal fluid. The lesions are multifocal or patchy in distribution, with vacuolation of the neuropil, loss of myelin (particularly notable with Luxol fast blue stain), and, in the early stages, preservation of axons. Astrocytes usually contain nuclear and less frequently cytoplasmic inclusions, and astrocyte-derived syncytia are present in a minority of cases. As the lesion progresses, gliosis and axonal degeneration may occur and mononuclear cells infiltrate the lesion in low numbers; however, the early lesion is noninflammatory. Animals that survive may be left with sclerotic astrocytic foci and myelin loss.

Gray matter lesions, which are less frequent than those in the white matter, often target the cerebral cortex, cerebellum, brainstem, and spinal cord. In early stages, inclusion bodies are usually present in the nucleus or occasionally in the cytoplasm of neurons; these neurons undergo necrosis and mononuclear cells congregate around the dying neurons. With time, a mononuclear inflammatory response develops, and mononuclear cells aggregate around blood vessels and infiltrate the neuropil. Mononuclear meningitis is usually mild.

Old dog encephalitis is a rare variant, possibly caused by infection with replication-defective CDV. This syndrome is a chronic progressive neurologic disease, with widely distributed perivascular infiltrates of lymphocytes and plasma cells, and intranuclear inclusions in astrocytes and neurons. Viral antigen may be demonstrated by immunohistochemistry, but virus cannot be isolated from the brain. Canine distemper may occasionally result from administration of modified-live CDV vaccines. Neurologic disease is the usual manifestation in these cases, and lesions in the gray matter include neuronal necrosis, intranuclear inclusions, and lymphocytic encephalitis.

Dental lesions follow infection of young animals with CDV. Necrosis and cystic degeneration of ameloblastic epithelium of the developing tooth, associated with syncytia and cytoplasmic inclusions, give rise to the *defective enamel* seen in animals that have recovered from infection. The defects vary from focal depressions to large, sharply demarcated areas of enamel hypoplasia.

Ocular lesions include conjunctivitis, keratitis, retinitis, and optic neuritis. Conjunctivitis is very common in the early stages of disease and occasionally extends to the cornea to cause ulcerative keratitis. Retinal lesions, which are common following systemic infection, include intranuclear inclusions in ganglion cells and glia, degeneration of ganglion cells, photoreceptor loss, retinal edema, and perivascular cuffs of mononuclear cells. These lesions progress to neuronal loss, retinal scarring, and proliferation of retinal pigment epithelium in the chronic stages. Lesions in the optic nerve are inconstant, but papilledema may be observed in acute cases, and gliosis or demyelinating neuritis in chronic ones.

Cutaneous lesions of hyperkeratosis and parakeratosis may affect the footpads and nose, and rarely the haired skin. The epidermis may contain syncytial cells, and nuclear and cytoplasmic inclusion bodies. Pustular dermatitis due to secondary pyoderma may be present. Experimentally infected dogs commonly develop *bone lesions*, with necrosis of osteoclasts and consequent persistence of the primary spongiosa. Pale streaks in the heart caused by multifocal *myocardial necrosis and mineralization* are described.

The histologic findings are characteristic if a spectrum of lesions is present and inclusion bodies are discovered. Rabies and poxviruses are the other causes of intracytoplasmic inclusions in dogs, but the clinical and pathologic findings in these diseases are usually distinct from canine distemper. Other viruses causing inclusion bodies in bronchiolar or airway epithelial cells include CAdV2, canid herpesvirus 1, and canine minute virus (canine parvovirus 1). Confirmation of the diagnosis benefits from a diversity of detection options, including PCR tests, immunohistochemistry, indirect immunofluorescence, in situ hybridization, and virus isolation.

Canine parainfluenza

Canine parainfluenza virus (CPIV; *Paramyxoviridae, Orthorubulavirus mammalis*) causes clinical signs 3-10 days after experimental infection, mainly of fever and hacking cough typical of infectious tracheobronchitis. Virus is shed in nasal secretions for about 8 days after infection. Lesions are of *tracheobronchitis and bronchiolitis*, with epithelial vacuolation and necrosis, mixed cellular inflammatory infiltrates, and submucosal edema. Subacute and chronic lesions include bronchitis and bronchiolitis with epithelial hyperplasia and occasionally obliterative bronchiolitis. The virus does not replicate in macrophages and does not induce significant pneumonia in immunocompetent dogs. CPIV can act as a primary pathogen, but mainly causes disease in conjunction with *Bordetella* infection. In addition, CPIV predisposes to bacterial pneumonia by impairing mucociliary clearance and increases the bronchoconstrictive response to agonists such as histamine. Infection has been shown to impair olfaction in the absence of nasal lesions; the clinical significance of this intriguing phenomenon is unknown.

Canine respiratory coronavirus

Canine respiratory coronavirus (CRCoV; *Coronaviridae, Betacoronavirus gravedinis*) infection was first identified as a cause of CIRD in 2003 and occurs mostly in situations of frequent contact with other dogs. The causative virus is a betacoronavirus and is thus related to bovine coronavirus. In contrast, enteric or pantropic canine coronavirus is an alphacoronavirus. CRCoV infections cause mild upper respiratory tract disease, leading to nonspecific clinical signs of coughing and nasal discharge. Following experimental infection with CRCoV, viral shedding from the oropharynx has been detected for up to 10 days using RT-PCR and by virus isolation for up to 6 days postinfection.

CRCoV preferentially infects respiratory epithelial cells, including ciliated cells and goblet cells in the trachea, bronchi, and bronchioles. The reported lesions include shortening or loss of cilia on ciliated cells and a modest inflammatory response, mainly in the upper respiratory tract with only minor lesions in the lung. Diagnosis of CRCoV infection can be made using ELISA and immunofluorescence. Serology, using paired sera 2-3 weeks apart, is valuable to follow animals during an outbreak of CIRD.

Influenza

H3N8 and H3N2 influenza viruses cause respiratory disease in dogs. The H3N8 virus has homology to and is thought to have arisen from EIV. These viruses spread readily among dogs, and thus are most common in animals involved in racing, shows, or frequent commingling with others. Dogs may be infected with other influenza viruses, but their ability to spread among dogs and cause disease are less studied.

Clinically, *canine influenza is usually a self-limiting upper respiratory tract disease* that manifests as anorexia, oculonasal discharge, and coughing. Histologically, influenza virus infection causes tracheobronchial epithelial cell necrosis, hyperplasia, and infiltration of neutrophils, and a unique lesion that similarly affects the bronchial glands. Less frequent is involvement of the distal airways, with bronchiolar erosion or hyperplasia with neutrophil exudates in the lumen, and alveolar infection with neutrophils in alveoli and subtle proliferation of type II pneumocytes. Influenza can cause peracute disease and death related to hemorrhagic pneumonia associated with bacterial infection; hemorrhage into the pleural cavity and mediastinum may also be present. Diagnosis of canine influenza is based on RT-PCR assays using samples collected from the lung or upper airways of typically affected dogs.

Other respiratory viruses

Pantropic canine coronavirus, an *Alphacoronavirus* (related to feline coronaviruses and transmissible gastroenteritis virus, but distant from betacoronaviruses including canine respiratory coronavirus) mainly causes enteric and neurologic disease but has been associated with necrotizing bronchiolitis and pulmonary vascular necrosis.

Canine adenovirus 2 (**CAdV2**; *Adenoviridae, Mastadenovirus canidae*) is serologically related to, but genetically distinct from, CAdV1, the cause of infectious canine hepatitis. The contribution of CAdV2 to CIRD complex is assumed to be similar to CPIV2 discussed above. Naturally occurring adenoviral pneumonia is rare in dogs and is often a consequence of immunosuppression. Gross lesions may be cranioventral or disseminated, lobular or confluent, and consist of atelectasis, reddening, edema, and mild firmness. *Amphophilic intranuclear inclusions* are present in alveolar macrophages, type II pneumocytes, and airway epithelium. Bronchioles contain necrotic epithelial cells and neutrophilic exudate, and macrophages, neutrophils, and fibrin are present in alveoli. Peribronchiolar and interstitial infiltrates of lymphocytes occur but are not prominent.

Canid alphaherpesvirus 1 (**CaAHV1**; *Orthoherpesviridae, Varicellovirus canidalpha1*) is occasionally isolated from dogs with *acute respiratory disease*, although systemic disease in neonatal puppies is a more common manifestation. Aerosol challenge of 12-week-old dogs caused necrotizing rhinitis, and multifocal bronchiolar and alveolar necrosis with infrequent eosinophilic intranuclear inclusion bodies. Intraperitoneal inoculation of neonatal puppies with the same viral strain caused necrosis and hemorrhages in many organs, supporting the contention that the manifestation of disease is dependent on the route of exposure and the age of the host. Herpesviruses are infrequently isolated from dogs with kennel cough, either alone or with other infectious agents. The respiratory lesions are those to be expected from herpesviruses, namely necrotizing rhinotracheitis and possibly bronchopneumonia. Eosinophilic intranuclear inclusions can sometimes be found in epithelial cells in early lesions, particularly in nasal mucosa.

Several other viruses have been identified in respiratory tissues of dogs with respiratory disease, including **canine pneumovirus, canine hepacivirus, canine bocavirus, canine polyomavirus**, and **feline morbillivirus**. Their causal role in canine respiratory disease is thus far inconclusive.

Bacterial diseases

Pneumonia caused by opportunistic bacterial pathogens is moderately common in dogs. Because most of the pathogens involved are commonly isolated from healthy dogs, a diagnosis of bacterial pneumonia should prompt a search for predisposing causes. *Aspiration pneumonia* is frequent in dogs and may result from anesthesia, megaesophagus, myasthenia gravis, neurologic disease, laryngeal paralysis, or other causes of regurgitation or vomiting, as well as brachycephalic obstructive airway syndrome, and cleft palate. Alternatively, bacterial pneumonia may follow from *impaired respiratory defenses*. These include respiratory viral infections (reviewed above); drugs that induce immunosuppression or neutropenia; concurrent disease conditions that impair immune responses or neutrophil function including uremia, hyperadrenocorticism, diabetes mellitus, parvoviral enteritis, systemic mycoses, or primary immunodeficiencies; ciliary dyskinesia; and environmental and social stresses. Recurrent episodes of bacterial pneumonia may suggest underlying bronchiectasis, laryngeal paralysis or abnormal esophageal function, or very rarely ciliary dyskinesia or primary immunodeficiencies.

Bordetella bronchiseptica, Streptococcus spp., *Staphylococcus* spp., *Pasteurella* spp. (including *P. canis, P. dagmatis, and P. multocida*), *E. coli, Klebsiella pneumoniae, Pseudomonas aeruginosa, Acinetobacter* spp., and *Mycoplasmopsis cynos* are the most common isolates from transtracheal aspirates of dogs with pneumonia. *Bordetella, Streptococcus*, and extraintestinal pathogenic *E. coli* are discussed more fully below. Other strains of *E. coli* are frequently associated with aspiration pneumonia. ***Yersinia pestis***, of public health significance as the cause of *plague*, can cause hemorrhagic, necrotizing, and neutrophilic pneumonia in dogs, typically with numerous gram-negative bacteria.

Leptospirosis, discussed elsewhere, frequently causes dyspnea and hemoptysis associated with thrombocytopenia. Microscopic lesions are pulmonary hemorrhage and edema, necrosis of alveolar septa, thin hyaline membranes and fibrin within alveoli, thrombosis, and occasional lymphocytic interstitial pneumonia. Leptospires were not identified in the lung.

The morphology of bacterial pneumonia in dogs does not usually suggest a specific infectious agent (see the Bronchopneumonia section). Lesions may affect entire lobes or follow a lobular distribution. Unilateral or lobar pneumonia may suggest aspiration as the cause.

Streptococcus zooepidemicus

Streptococcus equi **ssp.** ***zooepidemicus*** (β-hemolytic, group C) is an opportunistic pathogen causing bronchopneumonia as described above. It is also notable for causing outbreaks of fatal hemorrhagic pneumonia in dogs in kennels or shelters. Affected dogs have fever, depression, and dyspnea, with a rapidly progressive fatal course. The typical pathologic findings are acute fibrinous neutrophilic necrotizing hemorrhagic pneumonia, in some cases with bloody pleural and mediastinal fluid. Gram-positive cocci are histologically visible, and thrombosis and fibrin exudation may be present. Neutrophils can be few or many, presumably dependent on the rapidity of disease progression. Clusters of bacteria may also be observed in the spleen and renal glomeruli. Exotoxins, perhaps acting as superantigens, are thought to play a role in development of disease, and the degree of host cytokine production may also be important.

Extraintestinal pathogenic Escherichia coli

Extraintestinal pathogenic ***Escherichia coli*** (ExPEC) strains that produce cytotoxic necrotizing factor 1 and 2, α-hemolysin, and other toxins cause a rapidly progressive necrohemorrhagic pneumonia and sepsis in dogs and cats that leads to death in 24-48 hours. In laboratory dogs, an association with recent arrival at the facility is described. Infection is thought to reach the lung by inhalation or via the blood, and does not apparently result from aspiration of gastrointestinal content. The gross distribution of ExPEC pneumonia may be cranioventral or generalized, bilateral or unilateral, and multifocal, diffuse, or patchy. The characteristic features are *extensive hemorrhage, coagulative necrosis, thrombosis, and many or few aggregates of tiny coccobacilli* (eFig. 5-71). The absence of histologically visible bacteria should not rule out the diagnosis. Some lesions have very few leukocytes despite the presence of many bacteria, whereas others have more typical infiltration of neutrophils. Necrotizing lesions may be present in the liver and other organs. Definitive diagnosis is based on identification of toxin genes in the bacterial isolate.

Bordetella bronchiseptica

Bordetella bronchiseptica is a gram-negative coccobacillus that is commonly carried in the upper respiratory tract—but not the lungs—of healthy dogs, cats, and many other domestic animals. It can act as a primary pathogen, causing *tracheobronchitis* and occasionally *pneumonia*, but causes more frequent and more severe disease in polymicrobial infections with viruses, mycoplasmas, and other bacteria. Some animals affected by tracheobronchitis develop persistent, harsh, nonproductive or productive coughing, but are otherwise clinically normal. Most of these cases recover spontaneously, although signs can persist for 3 weeks or longer. Others develop bacterial pneumonia with lethargy and dyspnea; only half of affected dogs have fever or leukocytosis. The gross and histologic findings are similar to bronchopneumonia caused by other bacteria, with the unique finding of cilia-adherent bacteria in the large airways of some cases. These appear as a densely fibrillar layer covering the respiratory epithelium and are highlighted by Warthin-Starry silver stain or Gram stain (Fig. 5-66).

There is considerable genetic diversity among strains of *B. bronchiseptica*. The expression of virulence factors of *Bordetella* is dependent on environmental conditions, regulated by the *Bordetella virulence gene (bvg) operon*. In vitro, such virulence genes are repressed at 25°C or in the presence of sulfate or nicotinic acid, and activated at 37°C. After entering the host, a first wave of *bvg*-regulated genes is expressed including those encoding the adhesive proteins filamentous hemagglutinin (FHA) and pertactin, and fimbriae that allow *B. bronchiseptica* to attach to ciliated epithelial cells. Following attachment of bacteria to the mucosal surface, a second wave of *bvg*-regulated genes is expressed that mediate motility, iron scavenging, and urease and phosphatase activity.

Secreted toxins are important contributors to bordetellosis. The adenylate cyclase toxin (hemolysin) is an RTX toxin, like *Mannheimia haemolytica* leukotoxin and the Apx toxins of *Actinobacillus pleuropneumoniae*. The RTX domain of the toxin forms pores in target cell membranes that permit transfer of the adenylate cyclase component. Entry of this toxin into leukocytes causes increased cyclic AMP production that impairs phagocytosis and oxidative burst. Other virulence factors that are not regulated by the *bvg* operon include a lipooligosaccharide with endotoxin activity and a soluble peptidoglycan-derived tracheal cytotoxin. The latter is not directly toxic to tracheal epithelium, but stimulates host cells to produce nitric oxide that in turn induces ciliostasis and apoptosis of ciliated epithelial cells.

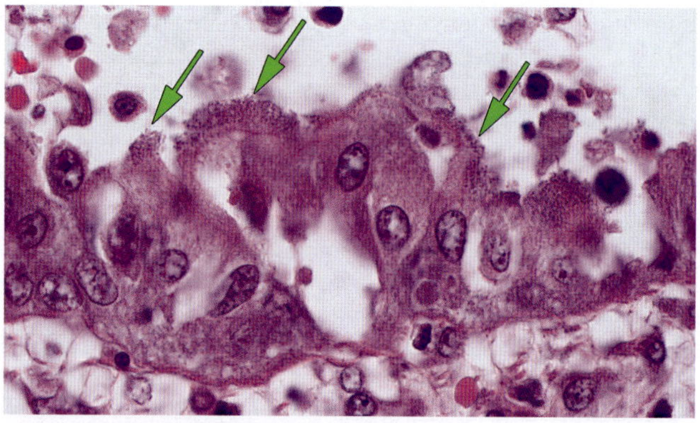

Figure 5-66 ***Bordetella bronchiseptica*** **pneumonia** in a dog. The lung had lesions of bronchopneumonia, with the unique feature of cilia-adherent bacteria (arrows) on the mucosal surface of large airways.

B. bronchiseptica can adhere to macrophages and neutrophils, probably by binding of FHA to complement receptors on macrophages. Following adhesion, the bacteria are internalized and survive within macrophages without inciting an oxidative burst and may induce apoptosis of these cells through secretion of the adenylate cyclase toxin. In addition, *Bordetella* can form a biofilm and is also able to enter and survive within nonphagocytic cells, presumably affording protection from host defenses and a ready supply of nutrients.

Although mucosal antibody responses are detectable within 4 days of infection and the duration of clinical illness is usually only 2-3 weeks, *Bordetella* infections often persist for 2-3 months and infected dogs may remain a source of infection for others in the kennel. Immune responses to *B. bronchiseptica* confer partial protection against subsequent challenge. FHA and pertactin are immunodominant antigens, and mucosal antibody responses to these antigens are partially protective.

Mycoplasmal diseases

Mycoplasmas that infect the respiratory tract of dogs include *Mycoplasmopsis cynos, M. canis, M. bovigenitalium, Metamycoplasma (Mycoplasma) spumans, Mycoplasmopsis (Mycoplasma) edwardii, Metamycoplasma (Mycoplasma) gateae, Mycoplasma feliminutum*, and several unclassified species of *Mycoplasma, Ureaplasma*, and *Acholeplasma*. Mycoplasmas are present in the nasopharynx of most normal dogs and can be isolated from tracheobronchial washes from ~30% of normal adult dogs and a similar percentage of those with pneumonia.

Of the mycoplasmas, ***M. cynos*** is the most pathogenic. Experimental infection with *M. cynos* did not result in clinical signs of disease, but induced peribronchial infiltration of lymphocytes and plasma cells, exfoliation and hyperplasia of bronchiolar epithelium, and neutrophil exudation into bronchioles and alveoli. Its presence seems to contribute to the polymicrobial respiratory disease that develops in animal shelters.

Other mycoplasmas appear to be minimally or nonpathogenic. Experimental infection with *M. bovigenitalium* resulted in mild neutrophilic and lymphocytic bronchiolitis, but no clinical signs. Pathologic or clinical changes were not apparent in dogs challenged with *M. spumans, M. canis*, or *M. gatae*, although *M. canis* was more frequent in affected versus healthy dogs. Unclassified mycoplasmas have been associated with similar lesions and with chronic bronchitis and bronchiectasis in dogs.

Fungal diseases

Mycotic rhinitis

Mycotic rhinitis is common in dogs and occasionally diagnosed in other species. It causes chronic sneezing, stertor, unilateral or bilateral mucopurulent nasal discharge, nasal hemorrhage, or nasal pain. Nasal bones can become distorted, and infection can extend to adjacent structures and rarely induce exophthalmos or neurologic signs.

Aspergillus fumigatus is the usual cause of mycotic rhinitis in dogs, but other fungi can cause similar disease. These are opportunistic pathogens, common in the environment, that reach the nasal cavity by inhalation. It is not known whether disease results from exposure to higher numbers of inhaled fungi or from suppression of the normal nasal defenses, but immunosuppression or other predisposing causes are rarely identified in dogs with nasal aspergillosis.

Lesions are often focal within the nasal cavity or paranasal sinuses and consist of yellow, green, or black plaques of fungal growth. The surrounding mucosa is hyperemic and edematous, and there is often purulent exudate, caseous debris, or hemorrhage. Destruction of conchae and remodeling of the nasal septum or nasal bones may occur. *Histologic diagnosis requires that the fungal plaques are specifically sampled*, which may be very localized despite the widespread exudate. The plaques consist entirely of fungal hyphae, occasionally with conidia (eFig. 5-72). *Aspergillus* spp. hyphae are 5-7 µm diameter and have parallel sides, frequent septa, and branch dichotomously at 45 degrees. The infection is noninvasive, and hyphae are very rarely observed in biopsies of inflamed nasal tissue biopsies, but these tissues do have nonspecific lesions of neutrophilic or eosinophilic rhinitis.

Pneumocystis carinii

P. carinii is a sporadic cause of acute or chronic dyspnea, usually without fever, in dogs, foals, pigs, and other domestic animals. *Clinical disease caused by* Pneumocystis *is thought to be unlikely without underlying immunodeficiency;* identified causes include corticosteroid or other immunosuppressive therapy; severe combined immunodeficiency in foals, sometimes in association with adenovirus or *Rhodococcus* infection; common variable immunodeficiency of Miniature Dachshunds (and Cavalier King Charles Spaniels are also overrepresented for unknown reasons), demodicosis, or canine distemper in dogs; and perhaps PRRSV or PCV2 infection in pigs. Outbreaks of respiratory disease in pigs have been associated with *Pneumocystis* infection, but it is uncertain whether *Pneumocystis* was the primary cause.

Pneumocystis is an ascomycete fungus. Isolates from different host species are special forms (e.g., *P. carinii* f. sp. *canis* or *P. carinii* f. sp. *suis*) that do not infect other species, a host adaptation that is unusual for fungal pathogens. *Pneumocystis* has a reduced genome and limited biosynthesis that confers high dependence on the host. The life cycle involves a 2-10-µm, thin-walled, uninucleate, *trophic form* that is most numerous, replicates by binary fission, and clusters or attaches to pneumocytes; and a 5-8-µm, thick-walled, multinucleate *cyst form* that develops 8 intracystic bodies that each develop into trophic forms when the cyst is transmitted to a new host. The cell wall is composed of mannose-rich polysaccharides and the major surface glycoprotein. This glycoprotein A is the immunodominant antigen and mediates binding of *Pneumocystis* to type I pneumocytes and macrophages, surfactant proteins, and fibronectin. Macrophages and cell-mediated immune responses are essential for controlling *Pneumocystis;* hence, clinical disease implies that there has been impairment of macrophage function or cell-mediated immune responses. In addition to the space-occupying effect of the fungus, *Pneumocystis* may alter lung function by interfering with surfactant homeostasis.

Gross lesions of *Pneumocystis* pneumonia are diffuse, patchy or miliary, red to yellow-brown regions of rubbery firmness or consolidation. The characteristic **histologic** finding is *foamy or "honeycomb" material filling alveoli*, with numerous intra- and extracellular, 5-µm, round or crescent-shaped, clear fungal bodies, each containing a central, 0.5-µm, lightly basophilic dot (Fig. 5-67). Foamy macrophages are present and contain the organisms, but the presence of lymphocytes, plasma cells, type II pneumocytes, and interstitial fibrosis is variable. Most cases involve only the lung, but spread to eye and systemic disease are reported. *The* ***diagnosis*** *is made by identifying the fungi in histologic sections*. They are easily overlooked on H&E-stained sections, but the wall of the cyst form (but not the more numerous trophic form) stains with methenamine silver, which is more reportedly sensitive than PAS. *Pneumocystis* cannot be cultured using conventional techniques. PCR and immunohistochemistry are more sensitive in rats and humans but not widely available for domestic animals.

It is notable that immunodeficient rats and humans develop a similar lesion with many cysts, whereas immunocompetent rats develop lymphohistiocytic interstitial pneumonia with perivascular cuffs of lymphocytes (or necrotizing granulomas in immunocompetent humans) but few *Pneumocystis* cysts; this manifestation is not recognized in domestic animals.

Rhinosporidiosis

Rhinosporidiosis affects humans, dogs, and occasionally other domestic mammals and fowl. The disease is endemic in wet tropical and subtropical environments. The causative agent, ***Rhinosporidium seeberi***, is not a fungus but in the class *Ichthyosporea* (*Mesomycetozoa* or "DRIP" clade) of aquatic protistan parasites. The agent can be cultured only with specialized

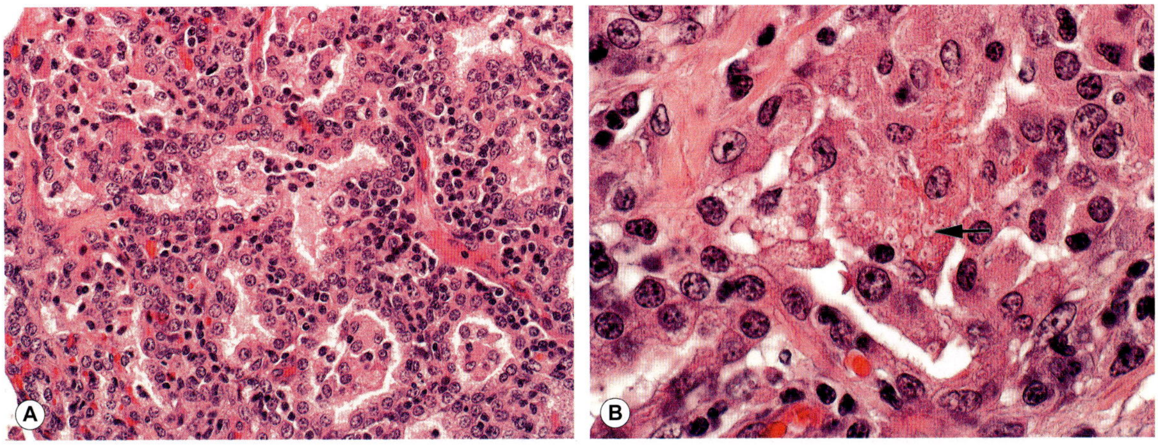

Figure 5-67 ***Pneumocystis carinii***, in a foal with no evidence of immunosuppression. **A.** Extensive type II pneumocyte proliferation with interstitial lymphocytes. **B.** In a few areas, alveoli contain foamy material with fungal cysts (arrow). Note the type II pneumocyte hyperplasia (bottom center).

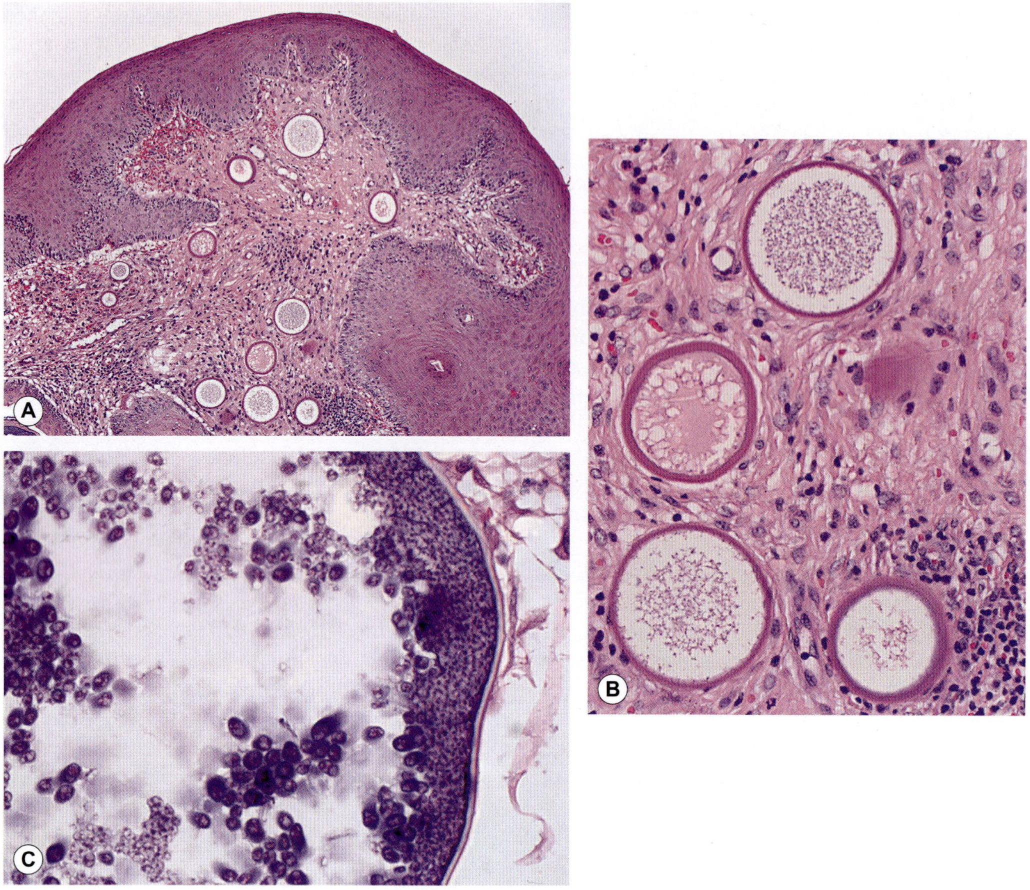

Figure 5-68 ***Rhinosporidium seeberi*** laryngeal polyp in a horse. **A, B.** The mass contains juvenile sporangia, up to 100 µm diameter. **C.** A mature sporangium with numerous endospores. (Courtesy H. Burgess.)

techniques. Infection results from exposure of nasal mucosa to contaminated water.

The typical lesion is a *single unilateral nasal polyp*, which is soft, pink, up to 3 cm diameter, and bleeds easily. Histologically, the polyp consists of epithelial hyperplasia, loose fibrous tissue, lymphoplasmacytic inflammation, and sporangia of *R. seeberi* (Fig. 5-68). Juvenile sporangia are 15-75 µm diameter, contain a single nucleus, and have a unilamellar PAS-positive wall. Mature sporangia, which may be visible grossly as pinpoint white foci, are 100-500 µm diameter with a bilamellar wall, and contain numerous 5-10-µm endospores. The large size of the sporangia with endospores might only be mistaken for *Coccidioides*, and finding such structures in a nasal polyp is considered diagnostic.

Blastomycosis

Blastomycosis is an infectious noncontagious disease primarily of dogs and humans, and sometimes cats, horses, and other species. It occurs primarily in North America, and occasionally in Africa, Europe, Asia, and Central America. Endemically infected areas in North America include the Mississippi, Ohio, and St. Lawrence River valleys, northern Ontario and Manitoba in Canada, and the mid-Atlantic States in the United States.

Blastomyces spp. are dimorphic ascomycete fungi, of which ***Blastomyces dermatitidis*** is best recognized. At environmental temperatures, it grows as a mycelial form (teleomorph; *Ajellomyces dermatitidis*) and undergoes sexual reproduction to form fruiting bodies and conidia that are infectious to animals. The ecologic source of the mycelial form is uncertain, but is associated with acidic sandy soils. *Recently disturbed soil* is a recognized factor in some outbreaks, and geographic clustering of cases is well documented. *At body temperatures, the fungus grows as a yeast (asexual; anamorph) form that is not contagious by inhalation.* Although the potential exists for mycelial forms to grow in cooled tissue specimens, reports of infection acquired at autopsy are rare and have been caused by accidental penetrating wounds rather than inhalation.

Infection is usually acquired by inhalation of spores into the lung, where they rapidly transform to the yeast form. Local inoculation may be the cause of the rare lesions that are restricted to the skin. Experimentally infected dogs develop a much higher prevalence of lesions than for other systemic mycoses, although in most the disease is mild and resolves without treatment. Subclinically infected dogs are apparently rare. Yeast forms proliferate in the lungs and disseminate via the blood and lymphatic vessels.

Virulence factors of *B. dermatitidis* are poorly described. BAD1 is a surface protein that mediates adhesion to host cells, may modulate the inflammatory response, and is an immunodominant antigen. The cell wall polysaccharide α-glucan is associated with virulence and may protect against killing by macrophages.

Antibody responses to BAD1 reduce disease severity but are not completely protective. Th1 immune responses have been associated with protection in mouse models, and immune responses target cell wall components including BAD1. Naturally infected animals may have suppression of humoral and cellular immune responses but, as for other systemic mycoses, this probably represents an effect rather than a cause of the disease. Most animals do not have pre-existing immunosuppressive conditions.

The lung is the most consistently affected site. **Grossly**, there is generalized distribution of 3 mm to several centimeter diameter coalescing gray-white nodules of granulomatous inflammation (Fig. 5-69). Most pulmonary nodules are firm throughout, but some undergo central caseation and resemble abscesses. Such foci may fistulate into a bronchus or onto the pleura. Mineralization is minimal or absent. **Microscopically**, coalescing granulomas are formed by epithelioid macrophages, histiocytic giant cells and variable numbers of neutrophils, an outer layer of lymphocytes and less reactive macrophages, and often a peripheral rim of fibrous tissue (see Fig. 5-69). In some cases, there is extensive caseous necrosis in the centers of the granulomas, with merely a thin rim of macrophages. *Yeast bodies are quite variable in number and may be overlooked if only H&E-stained sections are examined*; in cases treated with antifungal drugs or with partial immunity, a diligent search of sections stained by PAS or methenamine silver may be required to reveal the fungi. The yeast forms are 8-15 μm diameter (or occasionally up to 30 μm), round, nonencapsulated, with a thick (~1 μm) refractile wall, and multiple indistinct nuclei completely or partly filling the center (see Fig. 5-69). A double-contour wall is well described in cytologic preparations but is typically inapparent histologically. Occasional yeast display *broad-based budding* of a single daughter cell. Filamentous or pseudohyphal forms and conidia are infrequently found in tissues and are usually accompanied by yeast forms.

Disseminated lesions are common in lymph nodes, eyes, skin and subcutaneous tissues, bones, and joints. Testes, prostate, brain, heart, liver, spleen, kidneys, intestines, and other organs are less commonly affected. The lesions are either granulomas with numerous epithelioid and giant cells, or pyogranulomatous foci with central accumulation and necrosis of neutrophils and macrophages.

The **differential diagnosis** for multinodular lesions in lung and other organs includes other systemic mycoses and metastatic neoplasia. *Demonstration of the yeast bodies in tissue section or in cytologic preparations is the usual method of postmortem diagnosis*. Morphologic features are often adequate to differentiate *B. dermatitidis* from other yeast-like fungi: *Cryptococcus* spp. (4-10 μm) usually has a thick capsule, narrow-based budding, and only a mild inflammatory response (Fig. 5-70); *Histoplasma capsulatum* and *Blastomyces helicus* at 2-4 μm are much smaller and form clusters in the cytoplasm of macrophages; *Coccidioides immitis* at 10-200 μm is much larger and often contains endospores (Fig. 5-71); and *Candida* yeast are 3-5 μm and usually with pseudohyphae. Variants of *Cryptococcus* can have a thin capsule that resembles *Blastomyces* and incites a similar granulomatous response, but narrow-based budding contrasts with the broad-based budding of *Blastomyces*. Nonetheless, other fungi can rarely

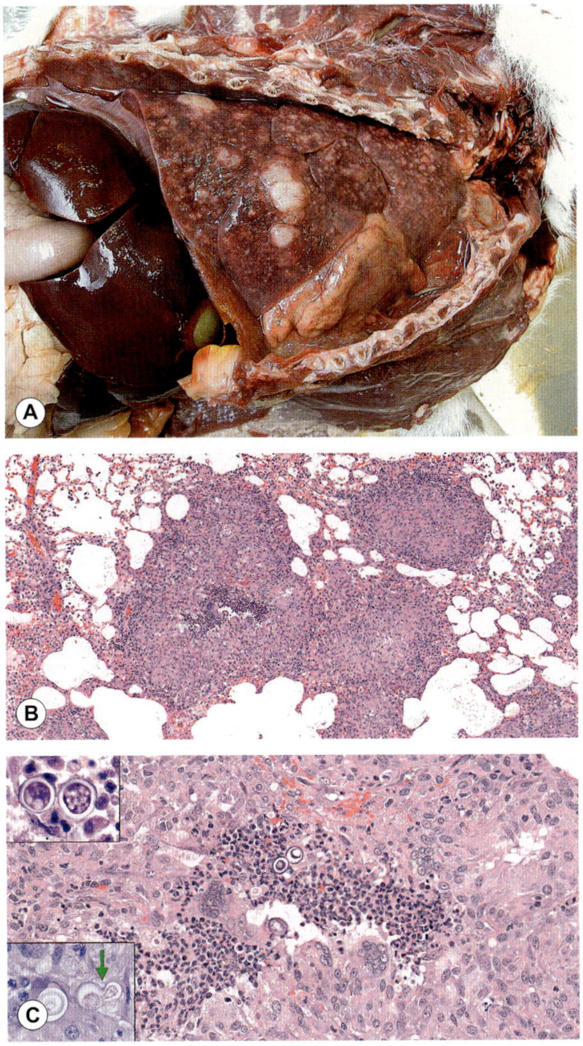

Figure 5-69 Blastomycosis in a dog. **A.** The lung contains coalescing nodules. (Courtesy Michigan State University.) **B, C.** Coalescing granulomas formed by epithelioid macrophages and giant cells, some with centrally located neutrophils and thick-walled yeast (C; top inset) with broad-based budding (C; bottom inset, arrow).

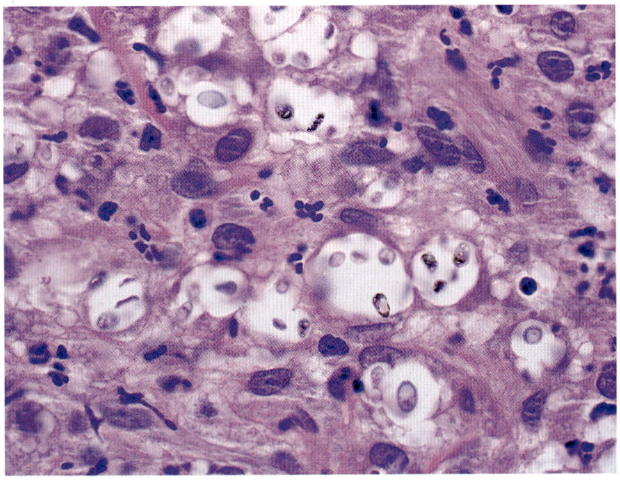

Figure 5-70 *Cryptococcus neoformans* in the lung of a dog. Yeast have a thick mucoid capsule, small cell bodies, melanization, and minimal inflammatory response.

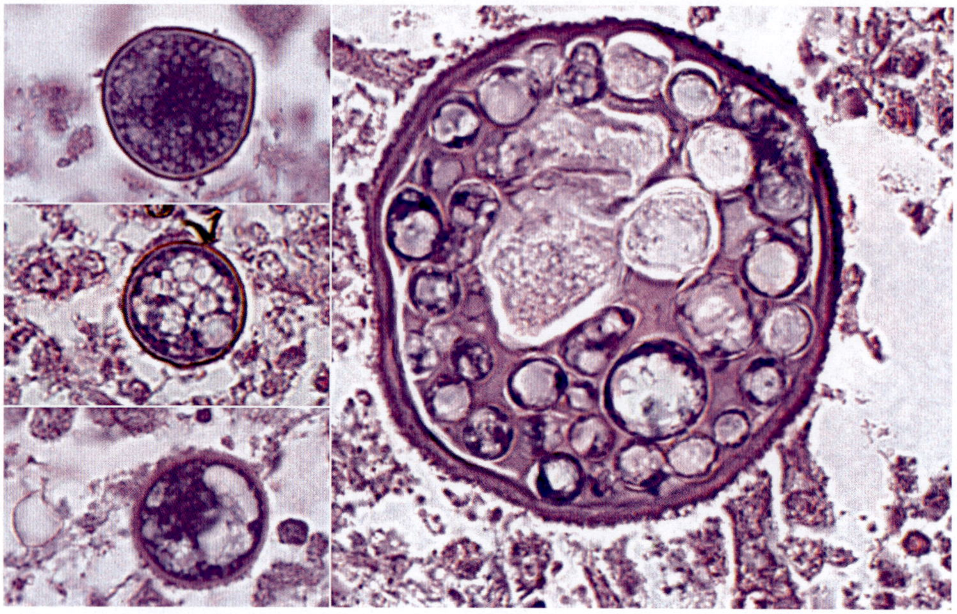

Figure 5-71 ***Coccidioides immitis*** in the lung of a dog. An area of caseous necrosis in the lung has ~15-μm uninucleate spherules and a 200-μm mature spherule (sporangium) with numerous endospores. (Courtesy D. Wilson.)

be 8-15 μm with broad-based budding; as for other fungal pathogens, definitive diagnosis requires confirmation by other methods. *Blastomyces* is differentiated from other fungi in culture, but safety precautions must be in place because infection of laboratory personnel by the cultured mycelia is well documented. An immunoassay to detect *B. dermatitidis* galactomannan is widely used for clinical diagnosis; the sensitivity to detect the fungal antigen was 94% and 87% for urine and serum, respectively. Serologic tests are available, but false negatives are common.

Cryptococcosis

Cryptococcosis is caused by numerous species considered as ***Cryptococcus neoformans*** or ***C. gatti*** complexes. Cryptococcosis is the most common systemic mycosis of cats and also affects dogs, sheep, goats, horses, cattle, humans, and many other species. Disease is sporadic and, as is generally true for the systemic mycoses, the infection is apparently *neither contagious nor zoonotic. Many cases have chronic nasal disease,* with sneezing and serous or mucopurulent discharge. Other common manifestations include ulcerating cutaneous nodules, encephalitis, chorioretinitis or panophthalmitis, and pneumonia.

Cryptococcus spp. *are* basidiomycete yeast-like fungi. Unlike the dimorphic fungi *Blastomyces* and *Coccidioides*, the sexual mycelial phase of *Cryptococcus* does not occur under normal laboratory conditions. *C. neoformans*, the usual cause of disease in temperate climates, is a saprophyte found in soil, pigeon or other avian guano, and decaying organic matter. *C. gatti* historically was found mainly in tropical climates but is now considered to have a global distribution and is an important cause of disease in humans and dogs, especially in the Pacific Northwest of North America. *C. neoformans* and *C. gatti* exist in these environments in a filamentous form (teleomorph). Based on genome sequence information, *C. neoformans* is subdivided into types VNI, VNII, VNIII, and VNIV, and *C. gatti* is divided into VGI, VGII, VGIII, and VGIV, and these vary in pathogenicity and response to therapy.

Most infected animals do not develop clinical disease. *C. neoformans* and especially *C. gatti* can act as primary pathogens, but many cases have underlying immune deficiencies such as from immunosuppressive therapy or pre-existing infections. Infection is usually acquired by inhalation of yeast from contaminated dust. These small forms are inhaled into nasal tissues, or to pulmonary alveoli where replication can occur with subsequent spread hematogenously or locally to other organs such as the brain, eyes, lymph nodes, skin, and other organs. Occasional cases of cutaneous cryptococcosis are probably the result of local inoculation, and *cryptococcal mastitis* in cows is an ascending rather than hematogenous infection.

The major virulence factors of Cryptococcus are the capsule and the production of melanin. The thick capsule, composed of glucuronoxylomannan and other mannose-rich polysaccharides, impairs phagocytosis, activates complement, and may suppress T-cell responses. The role of the capsule in concealing the fungus from the immune response is highlighted by uncommon strains of *Cryptococcus* that lack a capsule; these are readily phagocytosed, incite a strong granulomatous response, and are generally minimally pathogenic. Most strains consistently produce a capsule in tissues, but its thickness is variable in cultures. The ability to synthesize melanin when grown on specific substrates is associated with virulence, and attributed in part to the enzyme phenoloxidase (laccase). Melanin and/or phenoloxidase may scavenge oxygen radicals produced by activated macrophages and modulate the host immunoinflammatory response. Other potential virulence factors include secretion of eicosanoids and mannose protein that modulate immune and inflammatory responses, and production of superoxide dismutase and laccase that augment resistance to oxidative killing.

Immunity to *Cryptococcus* is dependent on delayed type hypersensitivity reactions, in which IFNγ and other cytokines elicit and activate macrophages and perhaps neutrophils to kill the fungus using reactive nitrogen and oxygen intermediates. In addition, cytotoxic T-cell responses may directly limit viability or proliferation of this pathogen.

Lesions take the form of gelatinous masses, granulomas, or ulcerating nodules. Facial swelling is a common feature of cryptococcal rhinitis of cats. Infection may spread locally from the nasal cavity to involve the skin, oral mucosa, eyes, or brain, and occasionally there is wider dissemination to local lymph nodes, lung, and other viscera. Skin lesions are often nodular and ulcerative. Visceral lesions are multifocal, discrete, white, and gelatinous. Gross lesions in the brain are often subtle, but may include gelatinous material in meninges and ventricles.

The prominent histologic lesion is a mass of yeast, and the abundant nonstaining capsular material lends a "soap bubble" appearance to the lesion. In contrast to other mycotic infections, the granulomatous reaction is often minimal because the capsule masks the yeast from recognition by phagocytes. C. *neoformans* yeast are 4-10 μm diameter, plus a capsule that is 1-30 μm thick (see Fig. 5-70). Occasional yeast have single buds that are attached by a thin stalk and may appear separated from the mother cell by the capsule. A few yeast within lung are up to 100 μm diameter and are thought to resist phagocytosis and modulate the immune response.

The **diagnosis** is usually based on identifying the yeast in histologic sections or cytologic smears. The yeast can be highlighted with PAS or methenamine silver stain. *The thick capsule is characteristic*—C. *neoformans* is the only pathogenic fungus with a thick capsule—and it can be further identified with mucicarmine or Alcian blue. Melanin production can be demonstrated with the Masson-Fontana stain. In wet mounts, the capsule can be identified by negative staining with India ink. Occasional strains have only a thin capsule and are identified by the narrow-based budding. Culture is required for definitive diagnosis. Detection of antibodies to capsular antigen in serum or cerebrospinal fluid is a useful method of clinical diagnosis, but may be negative with poorly encapsulated strains.

Coccidioidomycosis

Coccidioidomycosis, caused by the dimorphic ascomycete fungi ***C. immitis*** or ***Coccidioides posadasii***, is endemic in the semi-arid Lower Sonoran life zone of the southwestern United States, northern Mexico, and parts of Central and South America. The fungus can apparently infect all mammals, with disease reported in many terrestrial and aquatic mammals. It is a persistent and serious health issue in humans living in these areas. Of domestic animals, the disease is most common in dogs, llamas, and alpacas, less common in horses and cats, and may cause incidental pulmonary lesions in cattle and pigs. Clinical manifestations in dogs include fever; chronic respiratory disease with coughing, weight loss, and eventual respiratory distress; visceral disease causing anorexia, weight loss, and malaise; draining cutaneous nodules; lameness resulting from osteomyelitis; ocular disease; and heart failure caused by myocardial or pericardial lesions. Nodular skin disease is the most common presenting sign in cats. Clinical findings in horses include chronic weight loss, pulmonary disease, and lameness resulting from osteomyelitis.

Coccidioides is a geophilic dimorphic fungus. The mycelial form survives well in dry hot conditions, grows after periods of intense rainfall in soil containing fecal or other organic matter, and releases arthroconidia that are disseminated widely in wind-blown dust after the soil desiccates. *Inhalation of airborne arthroconidia is the usual route of infection*; local inoculation occasionally causes a cutaneous lesion that does not usually progress to systemic infection. *Although most animals in endemic areas probably become infected during their life, relatively few develop disease*. Following deposition in the lung, the arthroconidia transform into the yeast form. Immature *spherules* are 10-20 μm diameter; as they mature, the spherules (or sporangia) enlarge up to 200 μm diameter and develop numerous 2-5 μm *endospores* (see Fig. 5-71). Mature spherules rupture, and the released endospores form either new spherules in tissue or mycelia if released to the environment. Infection of autopsy personnel has been attributed to inhalation of aerosolized tissue endospores, although the paucity of such cases suggests that the risk is limited.

Lesions may be limited to the *lungs*, where they vary from nodular to miliary. Nasal mucosa may also be affected. The *pyogranulomas or granulomas* are gray-white nodules that often contain a caseous or liquefying center. Large nodules may be formed by a collection of small discrete granulomas separated by fibrous tissue. The initial reaction to the infectious forms is primarily neutrophilic but forms a pyogranuloma or granuloma as it matures, with epithelioid macrophages, a few giant cells, lymphocytes, and neutrophils. In diagnostic cases, the lesions mainly appear as multifocal areas of necrosis with a few spherules, and granulomatous or pyogranulomatous inflammation in the adjacent tissue. Formation of discrete granulomas is less frequent. When spherules rupture, the released endospores can resemble other yeast species. In cattle, spherules are often enmeshed in eosinophilic material resembling the Splendore-Hoeppli phenomenon; this may reflect the higher level of resistance of this species.

Systemic lesions develop from hematogenous spread from the lung. Cases with systemic lesions that lack pulmonary involvement are thought to reflect resolution of the lung disease rather than an extrapulmonary route of infection. Tracheobronchial lymph nodes are often enlarged and reactive, but generalized lymphadenopathy is uncommon. Nodular lesions in the skin develop draining tracts or form fluctuating abscesses. Osteomyelitis often occurs late in the disease, with osteolytic granulomatous or cavitating masses surrounded by proliferating new bone tissue. Granulomatous lesions may be present in the pericardium or the heart and cause right-sided heart failure. Granulomas in the central nervous system are most common in the cerebrum and midbrain. Ocular lesions include chorioretinitis, retinal detachment, anterior uveitis, and keratitis. Other organs affected include the liver, spleen, kidney, and testes. Abortion and mastitis are described in horses.

The **diagnosis** is usually established by identifying the spherules in tissue sections, although they are usually few. *The large size and endosporulation of the mature spherules are characteristic*, and can only be confused with *R. seeberi*. Culture is a useful method of definitive identification; safety precautions are essential because arthroconidia are easily detached from the mycelial form and are infectious for laboratory personnel. Serum antibodies to C. *immitis* can be detected in most cases, particularly in the acute stages of disease, and high titers suggest active disease.

Other fungal diseases

Adiaspiromycosis is primarily a disease of wild rodents, but rarely affects domestic animals and humans. The causative agents, ***Emmonsia parva*** and ***Emmonsia crescens*** (formerly *Chrysosporium* spp.), are dimorphic fungi related to *Blastomyces*. Lesions are most common in the *lung* but occasionally

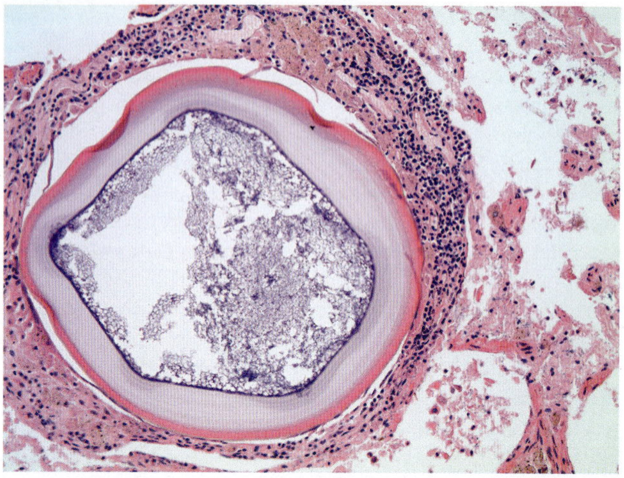

Figure 5-72 **Adiaspiromycosis** in the lung of a badger. Adiaspores of *Emmonsia* sp. are uninucleate and thick walled. (Courtesy D. Ni Bhuachalla.)

involve local lymph nodes, and consist of *nodules of granulomatous inflammation*. The diagnosis is based on finding adiaspores—large, spherical, uninucleate conidia—in the nodules (Fig. 5-72). The adiaspores of *E. parva* are often 10-20 µm diameter; those of *E. crescens* may be up to 300 µm diameter (but 7-60-µm adiaspores are reported for *E. crescens* in mice). Both have a thick (5-µm) PAS- and GMS-positive wall and can be empty or contain internal granules. Their large size and thick wall might be mistaken for *Coccidioides*, but endosporulation is not a feature of *Emmonsia* or *Besnoitia*, and the strongly PAS- and GMS-positive cell wall supports adiaspiromycosis.

Lycoperdon spp. (puffball mushrooms) release large numbers of spores to the environment, and inhalation of these spores by dogs incites a multifocal pyogranulomatous reaction throughout the lung. Intra- and extracellular 3-5-µm spores are visible within the pyogranulomas and are highlighted by silver stains.

Parasitic diseases

Pneumonyssoides caninum *is a parasitic mite of the nasal cavity and paranasal sinuses of dogs*. The female adult mite is motile, oval, light-yellow, and 1-1.5 mm long. The mites are presumably transmitted by direct contact. They are usually an incidental finding, but clinical signs include sneezing, head-shaking, and impaired olfaction. The mites induce catarrhal rhinitis and sinusitis with goblet cell hyperplasia, hyperemia, and infiltration of neutrophils, eosinophils, and lymphocytes. *Pneumonyssoides* is, in addition to allergic rhinitis, a consideration in cases of eosinophil-rich inflammation in the nasal mucosa.

Linguatula serrata—*pentastomiasis*

Linguatula serrata is a pentastome, related to annelids and arthropods, of wide geographic distribution. Adult pentastomes are large, long-lived, specialized hematophagous parasites of the respiratory tracts of reptiles, amphibians, and carnivorous mammals. The adults of *L. serrata* are transversely striated and tongue shaped (hence the name). Males are ~2 cm long and females 1.0-1.2 cm. The definitive hosts are carnivores, but in aberrant parasitisms herbivores and humans may be host to the final stage. Herbivorous animals are the intermediate hosts. Carnivores are infected by eating the infected viscera of herbivores, and the nymphs migrate to the nasal passages where they mature. The parasites may be found anywhere in the nasal cavity, and occasionally, they find their way into the paranasal sinuses or pass via the auditory tube to the inner ear. They lie on the surface of the nasal mucosa and induce nasal irritation and catarrhal to lightly blood-stained exudate. The gravid females discharge large numbers of eggs that infect herbivore intermediate hosts.

The larvae of *Linguatula*, or pentastomids of other species, develop in the alimentary tract of the intermediate host and migrate to the mesenteric lymph nodes and other organs where they develop into infective nymphs within cysts that are encircled by eosinophilic and granulomatous inflammation and fibrous tissue. The nymphs have histologic features of arthropods: pseudosegmented body, a chitinous cuticle with sclerotized openings, striated muscle, and a body cavity, as well as numerous brightly eosinophilic glands, and cuboidal intestinal epithelial cells with prominent villi.

Eucoleus aerophilus

Eucoleus aerophilus (Capillaria aerophila) is a trichurid nematode (order *Enoplida*, superfamily *Trichuroidea*, family *Trichuridae*) that *parasitizes the trachea and bronchi of wild canids, domestic dogs, and occasionally cats*. The worms are slender, 2-3 cm long, and embedded in the airway mucosa. Histologic examination reveals characteristic features: bacillary bands, which are segmental thickenings of the hypodermis; a stichosome, which is a deeply basophilic gland encircling the esophagus; and the possible presence of embryonated eggs. The eggs are laid in the airways, move with mucus to the pharynx, are swallowed, and passed in the feces. The eggs are oval with characteristic bipolar plugs and closely resemble those of *Trichuris vulpis* of the intestine or *Pearsonema (Capillaria) plica* of the urinary bladder. The larvae undergo initial development in the egg and then progress to the infective stage within earthworms, which are a required intermediate host. Eggs also hatch in ~40 days under suitable environmental conditions, but the resulting larvae are apparently not infective. After ingestion of the earthworm, the larvae reach the lungs in ~1 week and are mature in the trachea in ~25 days. Most infestations of *E. aerophilus* are inapparent and provoke only mild catarrhal inflammation. Heavy infestations cause more severe irritation that may result in obstruction of the lumen of the airways. Chronic coughing and intermittent dyspnea may then be observed, and secondary bacterial bronchopneumonia can occur.

A related trichurid, ***Eucoleus*** *(Capillaria)* ***boehmi***, is reported occasionally in the mucosal surface of nasal cavity and sinuses of wild canids and rarely in domestic dogs. Infection can cause sneezing, nasal discharge, and impaired olfaction.

Oslerus osleri

Oslerus (Filaroides) osleri is of wide geographic distribution and is common in wild canids. The tracheal nodules are uncommonly encountered during bronchoscopy or autopsy of domestic dogs; they rarely cause clinical signs of chronic coughing or dyspnea. Most infestations occur in dogs <1-year-old and are acquired from the dam through grooming or regurgitative feeding.

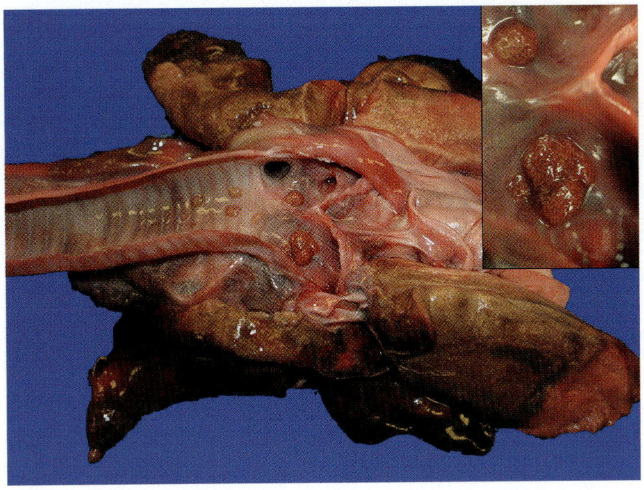

Figure 5-73 ***Oslerus osleri*** in a wolf. Tightly coiled adult nematodes (inset) dwell in nodules near the tracheal bifurcation. (Courtesy D. G. Campbell.)

O. osleri (superfamily *Metastrongyloidea*, family *Filaroididae*) is a 5-15 mm long nematode. The thin-walled embryonated eggs are coughed up and swallowed and many hatch before being passed as infective larvae in the feces. Unlike other metastrongyles, the *Filaroididae* do not require an intermediate host. The first-stage larvae of *O. osleri* are immediately infective, and pups are infected by ingestion of larvae in the saliva, tracheobronchial secretions, or feces of their dams. Larvae migrate from the gut through the blood to the lung. They develop into fifth-stage larvae by 5 weeks after infection, and the tracheal nodules are detectable at 10 weeks and well developed by 18 weeks. The caudal end of the gravid female protrudes through the epithelium, and the eggs are laid onto the tracheal surface.

The typical lesions are single or multiple, 1-10-mm, firm, gray-pink, sessile or polypoid, subepithelial nodules in the trachea and bronchi, often in the region of the tracheal bifurcation (Fig. 5-73). The larger masses are oval with the long axis parallel to that of the trachea. On careful inspection, coiled worms are visible through the intact overlying mucosa.

The nodules are formed by coiled adult or fifth-stage larval nematodes lying in tissue spaces in the lamina propria, often encircled by fibrous tissue. The adults have coelomyarian musculature, a gut formed by a few multinucleate cells with indistinct microvilli, and larvae or embryonated eggs within the uterus. The live worms provoke little reaction apart from a few lymphocytes and plasma cells. Dead worms incite a foreign-body reaction with neutrophils and giant cells. Immature worms, probably still migrating towards the trachea, may be found in the pulmonary lymphatics and occasionally in the alveoli without significant tissue reaction. The **diagnosis** is based on identifying the adults in histologic or crush preparations of the tracheal nodules, or discovering larvae in smears of tracheal mucus or Baermann preparations of feces.

Crenosoma vulpis

Crenosoma vulpis (superfamily *Metastrongyloidea*, family *Crenosomatidae*) is a common lungworm of foxes, but also occurs in other canids, including domestic dogs, perhaps in mustelids, but not in cats. Snails and slugs are intermediate hosts. *Adult worms reside in bronchioles and small bronchi.* After a prepatent period of 18-21 days, adults produce larvae that are coughed up, swallowed, and passed in the feces. The usual gross lesions in dogs are gray consolidation of the dorsocaudal lung. Histologically, the adult worms cause catarrhal eosinophilic bronchitis and bronchiolitis. Aspirated larvae may induce a granulomatous reaction in alveoli.

Angiostrongylus vasorum

Angiostrongylus vasorum occurs in endemic foci in parts of Western Europe and is also reported in Uganda, South America, Eastern Asia, and Atlantic Canada; reports suggest that the prevalence is increasing in Europe. Clinical expression of angiostrongylosis varies from mild-to-severe respiratory disease; cor pulmonale may develop in response to chronic pulmonary vascular disease and lung fibrosis. Other less common clinical signs include neurologic signs referable to cerebral hemorrhage as a result of disseminated intravascular coagulation, as well as miscellaneous signs that reflect aberrant larval migration in a variety of organs.

A. vasorum is a nematode (superfamily *Metastrongyloidea*, family *Angiostrongylidae*). *Adults inhabit the pulmonary arteries and right ventricle of dogs and foxes*. Eggs pass via the blood to the lungs, where the larvae hatch, penetrate into alveoli, are coughed up and passed in the feces. The prepatent period is 38-57 days. Snails and slugs are intermediate hosts, and frogs can be paratenic hosts.

Lesions during the prepatent period are mild. *Adult worms are 14-21 mm long and present in the pulmonary arteries*; the lungs contain a few 1-2-mm red nodules, consisting of aggregates of eosinophils and mononuclear cells. The females have a "barber-pole" appearance because of the helically arranged red gut and white ovaries. *Angiostrongylus* can be differentiated from *Dirofilaria* by examination of intact adults, or by histologic examination. *Angiostrongylus* adults are 270-350 µm diameter with thin coelomyarian musculature, a large strongylid intestine composed of a few tall multinucleate cells, and eggs in the uterus. In contrast, *Dirofilaria* has well-developed coelomyarian musculature, a smaller intestine, and a uterus containing microfilariae.

More severe lesions develop at the time of patency, including proliferative endoarteritis in response to the adult worms in the pulmonary arteries, and eosinophilic and granulomatous pneumonia from the embolized eggs and larvae. Arterial lesions include thrombosis, thickening of the tunica intima by fibromuscular tissue and numerous eosinophils, medial hypertrophy, and lymphoplasmacytic aggregates in the adventitia. Pulmonary lesions consist of red or golden-brown, nodular or confluent areas of hemorrhage, edema, and firmness at the periphery of the lung. Histologically, *coalescing granulomas* are formed by macrophages, eosinophils, neutrophils, and giant cells and are sometimes centered on parasite eggs and larvae. The larvae are ~10 µm wide; the eggs are ~100 µm diameter and contain either basophilic and eosinophilic granular material or embryos (larvae). There is mild proliferation of type II pneumocytes, alveolar hemorrhage, hemosiderin-laden macrophages, and arteriolar thrombosis. Fibrosis and recanalization of arterial thrombi develop as the lesion ages. Similar granulomas are reported in the brain, kidney, and other tissues.

Coagulation abnormalities are the second most common clinical manifestation associated with angiostrongylosis. The abnormalities are suggestive of disseminated intravascular coagulation, with prolonged activated partial thromboplastin time or prothrombin time, thrombocytopenia, and increases in circulating D-dimer and fibrin degradation products in affected dogs. The pathogenesis of the coagulopathy is not well understood, but may represent thrombosis triggered by parasite proteins or endothelial damage from the adult and larval nematodes. Petechiae and ecchymoses may develop in tissues of such dogs, and some develop severe neurologic signs from intracerebral hemorrhage.

Other parasitic diseases

Toxocara canis larvae infect puppies transplacentally or by ingestion of milk, and migrate via the liver to pulmonary alveoli, then to the trachea and oropharynx, and are swallowed to establish intestinal infection. This can cause loss of vigor, dull mentation, and death in neonatal puppies, or coughing in older puppies. Histologically, the lungs contain patchy alveolar inflammatory lesions with macrophages, eosinophils, neutrophils, multinucleate giant cells, hemorrhage, cellular debris, fibrinoid necrosis of vessels, and ascarid larvae in alveoli and airways.

Filaroides hirthi infection is mostly reported in colonies of laboratory Beagles, but cases are described in pet dogs. Adult *F. hirthi* are 6-10 mm long and contain larvae or embryonated eggs in the uterus. *The adults live in alveoli and respiratory bronchioles.* Like other *Filaroididae*, *F. hirthi* has a direct life cycle, and infective first-stage larvae are passed in the feces. Many infections are probably acquired from the dam.

The lesions in most cases are incidental at autopsy, with gray-tan or black-green, 1-5-mm nodules scattered widely in subpleural regions of the lung. Nodules may have clear cystic centers, or be white and firm. The lesions in fatal cases, which may occur in immunosuppressed dogs, are of severe generalized diffuse or miliary *granulomatous pneumonia*. Histologically, there is little response to living adult worms, but a severe granulomatous response with many eosinophils around dead or degenerating worms. Anthelmintic treatment may incite a severe response. Larvae stimulate an acute neutrophilic reaction. Foci of granulomatous interstitial pneumonia can often be found without any visible worm remnants. The **diagnosis** is based on discovery of larvae in smears of bronchial exudate, or identifying the adults in histologic sections of lung. Definitive diagnosis requires extraction of intact adults from the lungs, as the histologic appearance is similar to *Andersonstrongylus milksi*.

Andersonstrongylus milksi (*Angiostrongylus milksi*, *Filaroides milksi*) is a metastrongylid nematode (superfamily *Metastrongyloidea*, family *Angiostrongylidae*). The literature related to this parasite is uncertain because the diagnosis in many reports is exclusively based on histologic lesions, yet examination of intact worms—which are difficult to tease from the lung—is required to differentiate *A. milksi* and *F. hirthi*. A molluscan intermediate host is proposed, but the life cycle is unknown. *Adults inhabit bronchioles and alveoli*, and the gross and histologic lesions are similar to those caused by *F. hirthi*. Larvae may also be found in the brain, abdominal viscera, and other organs.

Dirofilaria immitis is described elsewhere (see Vol. 3, Cardiovascular System). The microfilaria can be encountered incidentally in pulmonary vessels or elicit thrombosis (eFig. 5-73) or eosinophilic and granulomatous pneumonia.

Babesia microti infection can cause increased number of macrophages and lymphocytes in alveolar septa, alveolar edema with fibrin, and acute respiratory distress.

INFECTIOUS RESPIRATORY DISEASES OF CATS

Viral diseases

Feline viral rhinotracheitis

Felid alphaherpesvirus 1 (FeAHV1, *Orthoherpesviridae*, *Varicellovirus felidalpha1*; feline viral rhinotracheitis virus) *infection is widespread in most cat populations and is an important cause of acute and chronic upper respiratory tract disease.* Clinical signs are most common in kittens but occur regularly in adult cats, probably as a result of recrudescence of latent infections. Morbidity may be high in naive populations of kittens, but mortality is generally low and most recover in 10-14 days. Clinical signs include fever, oculonasal discharge, sneezing, coughing, and anorexia. *Chronic rhinitis and sinusitis* are frequent and serious sequelae resulting from intermittent reactivation of latent infections, loss of respiratory defenses caused by excavation of nasal conchae, or failure of drainage of sites of secondary bacterial infection in the sinuses.

General features of *Herpesviridae* are described in the Infectious Bovine Rhinotracheitis section. FeAHV1, like other alphaherpesviruses, *causes cytolytic infections of mucosal epithelial cells and establishment of latency in the trigeminal ganglion, optic nerve, olfactory bulb, and cornea.* The virus replicates optimally at temperatures <37°C; thus, most infections are limited to the upper respiratory tract and conjunctiva.

FeAHV1 is transmitted by contact with infected nasal or ocular secretions, or by aerosol. Transmission by fomites may occur, but the virus survives for <18 hours under most environmental conditions. The host range is limited to cats including various nondomestic felids. The incubation period is short, typically just 2-4 days. In most cases, infection is restricted to the nasal mucosa, nasopharynx, sinuses, and tonsils, with lesser viral replication in the conjunctiva and upper trachea. Viremia may occur in neonates but is not common in older kittens. Instead, in cats with herpesviral pneumonia, cell-to-cell spread of the virus is responsible for infection of epithelial cells in the lower airways and lung. It is likely that most cats recovering from the disease remain latently infected, and perhaps 20-40% of these cats intermittently shed infective virus during periods of stress, such as following a change in housing, parturition, or during lactation; recrudescence may also be triggered by corticosteroid therapy or stressors.

The distribution of **gross lesions** corresponds to the predilection sites for viral replication—the epithelium of nasal passages, pharynx, soft palate, conjunctivae, tonsils, and to a lesser extent trachea and lung. The initial serous inflammation becomes mucopurulent or fibrinous within a few days, and crusting is often present around the eyes and nares. Multifocal erosions of the nasal mucosa are covered by mucoid or mucopurulent exudate. The trachea may contain hemorrhage or fibrinous exudate. Tonsils are enlarged and contain petechiae or rare foci of necrosis. The regional lymph nodes are usually enlarged, reddened, and edematous. *Ulceration of the tongue is uncommon* but does occur, whereas vesicular-to-ulcerative lesions on tongue, hard palate, or nostrils are frequent with feline calicivirus infection. Ocular involvement from FeAHV1 is usually limited to conjunctivitis, but it can progress to ulcerative keratitis.

Microscopically, *large eosinophilic* intranuclear inclusion bodies (INIBs) are present in many virus-infected cells during the period of active viral replication from 2 to 7 days after infection (eFig. 5-74). They may be found in lesions from cats dying of the disease but are rarely detected beyond 7 days after infection. Infected cells undergo hydropic change with cytoplasmic swelling and pallor. There is loss of epithelial organization, and the disrupted epithelium is soon eroded or ulcerated. An acute inflammatory reaction develops with exudation of fibrin and many neutrophils. Repair may be delayed for up to 17 days after infection, and the epithelium undergoes squamous metaplasia as it repairs.

Resorption of nasal turbinate bones along with new bone formation and fibroplasia occur in natural and experimental infections, mainly in cats <6-months-old, and may lead to chronic nasal disease by impairing clearance of opportunistic pathogens. Focal necrosis accompanied by acute inflammation may be found in tonsils and local lymph nodes. Erosive lesions can occur in stratified squamous epithelium of the nares or the tongue.

Pulmonary involvement is uncommon except in fatal cases. In fulminant FeAHV1 infections, lesions are multifocal and characteristically centered on affected airways. There is widespread necrotizing tracheitis, bronchitis, and bronchiolitis, with serofibrinous flooding of airspaces along with neutrophils and fewer macrophages and lymphocytes. INIBs are identified in airway epithelial cells. Necrosis or thrombosis of pulmonary blood vessels may occur, with viral antigen in the vessel wall. Secondary bacterial bronchopneumonia is a more common complication of FeAHV1 infection than is primary viral pneumonia.

Systemic disease is uncommon in FeAHV1 infection, in contrast to the analogous alphaherpesviral infections of young calves and puppies. Ocular lesions are described elsewhere. Experimental infection of pregnant female cats produces abortion and generalized neonatal disease, but this has been difficult to identify in natural outbreaks. Multifocal hepatic, pancreatic, and adrenocortical necrosis are the expected features of systemic disease. A syndrome of nasofacial ulcerative dermatitis and stomatitis with histologic lesions of eosinophilic inflammation and infrequent epithelial INIBs may be associated with corticosteroid therapy or crowding. After intravenous inoculation of kittens, bones can have necrosis accompanied by INIBs in sites of osteogenesis. Degeneration of olfactory nerve fibers and focal lymphocytic infiltration of the olfactory bulbs have occurred in experimentally infected, germ-free cats.

The major **differential diagnosis** for upper respiratory disease in cats is feline calicivirus infection, but the progression from upper airways to bronchioles and finally alveoli differs from lesions of calicivirus that are focused on the alveoli. PCR assay is a sensitive means of detection of FeAHV1 nucleic acid in tissues; other methods include immunohistochemistry, in situ hybridization, indirect immunofluorescence assays, and virus isolation. Finding eosinophilic INIBs amid necrotizing lesions of respiratory epithelium is usually sufficient for diagnosis in postmortem samples, but viral inclusions are inapparent at later stages.

Feline calicivirus

*Feline calicivirus (*FCV*; Caliciviridae, Vesivirus felis) is a common cause of upper respiratory tract disease that can also cause oral ulcers, chronic stomatitis, pneumonia, systemic disease, or lameness*. Infection with FCV is widespread; *15-25% of cats are subclinical carriers*. Morbidity can be high in kittens, but most cats recover from clinical disease. Clinical signs are variable and include serous or mucopurulent nasal and ocular discharge, *oral ulcers*, conjunctivitis, sneezing and coughing, anorexia, and fever. FCV is a nonenveloped, 35-40 nm, positive-sense, single-stranded RNA virus. ORFs 1, 2, and 3 encode a helicase, a protease, and polymerase; the single capsid protein; and an RNA-associated structural protein, respectively. The capsid protein is the target of protective immune responses, but hypervariable regions in this gene confer antigenic variability that allows viral persistence in the face of a developing immune response.

Transmission is by direct contact with infected oronasal secretions, and fomites are a potential source of infection. The clinical manifestations likely depend on virus strain, host immune status, and route of infection. The incubation period varies from 2 to 14 days, and many cats recover in 7-14 days after the onset of illness. However, *viral infection persists despite resolution of clinical signs*, and 25% of infected cats continue to shed virus for months or years. These cats are important sources of infective virus for naive cats or those with immunity to other strains of FCV. Occasionally, these persistently infected cats develop chronic lymphoplasmacytic and/or ulcerative stomatitis that is refractory to therapy.

In addition to upper respiratory infections, *ulcerative stomatitis may occur*. The oral ulcers, which begin as vesicles that rapidly rupture, are most often on the dorsal surface or lateral margins of the tongue and on the hard palate. *The finding of oral ulcers with nasal disease is suggestive of calicivirus infection*, although FeAHV1 can cause similar lesions. Cutaneous ulcers may occur on the nares and muzzle.

Caliciviral pneumonia is uncommon, and many cases also have FeAHV1 infection. Pneumonia is more likely following aerosol rather than oronasal exposure, and specific strains of FCV may have tropism for the lungs. It is thought that the virus reaches the distal airspaces directly by aerosol inhalation, as opposed to herpesvirus, which spreads from cell to cell into the deeper parts of the lung. FCV mainly replicates in alveolar macrophages, but type II pneumocytes are also infected, and the virus is thought to induce apoptosis of both cell types.

Gross lesions are irregularly distributed but often include the margins of the cranioventral lung. Histologic lesions affect alveoli and are diffuse (panlobular, rather than centrilobular for FeAHV1). Alveoli contain numerous activated macrophages that are large, round, and often vacuolated, with fibrin and sloughed type II pneumocytes and fewer neutrophils. Bronchiolar necrosis may be present but is not a prominent feature unless there is concurrent FeAHV1 infection. In the later stages, alveoli are lined by type II pneumocytes, and alveolar septa are thickened by lymphocytes, plasma cells, and fibrous tissue.

Virulent systemic feline calicivirus (VS-FCV) infection is a rare manifestation, occurring in individual cats or as a localized epizootic. The disease is highly contagious and rapidly fatal, affecting both kittens and adult cats—even those previously vaccinated. Cats develop edema and ulcers, mainly on the head, limbs, footpads, and inguinal region. Subcutaneous edema with foci of fat necrosis, pancreatitis with peripancreatic fat necrosis, disseminated intravascular coagulation, intestinal crypt necrosis, single-cell necrosis of hepatocytes, and lung lesions as described above are all reported in VS-FCV infections. The disease has been experimentally reproduced, suggesting that viral factors are at least partly responsible for increased virulence.

Whereas the lesions of FeAHV1 are airway-focused and necrotizing, those of FCV are alveolar and desquamative and airway lesions are usually not present. Influenza, SARS-CoV-2,

Toxoplasma, sepsis, and aspiration of gastric acid are additional causes of interstitial lung disease in cats. The lesions are, in most cases, not etiologically specific, and *definitive diagnosis requires laboratory support*. IHC, PCR, and virus isolation can be used to detect FCV in tissues.

Other viral diseases

Influenza viruses adapted to cats have not been described, but cats are susceptible to disease arising from human H1N1, avian H5N1, H5N6, H7N2, and H7N7, and canine H3N2 viruses, and cat-to-human transmission is reported. Inhalation results in similar lesions as in other species, with lesions mainly affecting the alveolar epithelium with interstitial pneumonia and fibrinoid vasculitis. With systemic H5N1, vasculitis and necrotizing inflammatory lesions may be present in the lung, brain, liver, adrenal gland, and pancreas. Ingestion of H5N1-infected chicken liver induced systemic infection with targeting of endothelial cells, widespread hemorrhages, and multifocal necrosis in lymphoid tissues and many other organs.

SARS coronavirus-1 or -2 infects mink, white-tailed deer, cats, dogs, and many others in experimental studies. Dogs, pigs, and cattle were inoculated but had minimal or no disease. During the COVID-19 epidemic, cats became infected by exposure to diseased humans. Natural disease in cats was infrequent and often mild, although cat-to-cat and cat-to-human transmission was documented. Cats infected with SARS-CoV-2 develop various degrees of rhinitis, tracheobronchitis, necrosis, and inflammation of tracheobronchial glands, bronchiolar epithelial necrosis, histiocytic bronchiolitis, and diffuse alveolar damage with alveolar edema and fibrin, hyaline membranes, type II pneumocytes, intra-alveolar syncytial cells, interstitial and alveolar hemorrhages, perivascular aggregates of lymphocytes and plasma cells, fibrinoid vasculitis, and thrombosis.

Cowpox virus mainly causes skin lesions in cats, with uncommon cranial lung lesions with necrosis, epithelial hyperplasia, syncytial cells, and intracytoplasmic inclusion bodies. **Bufavirus** and **chaphamaparvovirus** infect the feline respiratory tract with little evidence of associated respiratory disease.

Bacterial diseases

Bacterial pneumonia is common in cats and affects all ages. The most frequent isolates are *Bordetella bronchiseptica*, *Pasteurella multocida*, *Staphylococcus*, *Streptococcus*, and *Mycoplasmopsis felis*. These agents (described with diseases of dogs) are carried in the nasopharynx of some healthy cats, and the likelihood of disease is increased by associated factors such as stressors, antecedent viral infections such as FeAHV1 or feline coronavirus, or concurrent illness such as immunosuppressive diseases or treatments, malnutrition, diabetes mellitus, or chronic kidney disease. ***B. bronchiseptica*** is a minor zoonotic pathogen with several reported cases of cat-to-human transmission. ***Streptococcus equi* ssp. *zooepidemicus*** causes neutrophilic or necrosuppurative bronchopneumonia. **Extraintestinal pathogenic *E. coli*** is associated with hemorrhagic and necrotizing pneumonia and fibrinous pleuritis. Aspiration pneumonia results from similar risk factors as described for dogs.

Chlamydia felis (*C. psittaci*) causes *persistent conjunctivitis in cats*. PCR-based surveys of the feline upper respiratory tract suggest that *C. felis* is a minor contributor to upper respiratory disease in cats and, despite the disease name "feline pneumonitis," does not apparently cause pulmonary infection or disease. ***C. felis*** was associated with interstitial pneumonia in cats with multifocal hepatic necrosis and visible bacteria in hepatocyte cytoplasm.

Mycoplasmal diseases

Mycoplasmopsis felis reportedly causes pneumonia in kittens after experimental inoculation, has been identified more frequently in diseased than healthy animals, and immunolabeling was identified in bronchiolar epithelium, fibrinonecrotic exudate, and alveoli of cats with pneumonia. However, it can be identified in many healthy cats, so determining its causal role in individual cases is difficult. *Mycoplasmopsis felis, M. gatae, M. arginini*, and *Acholeplasma laidlawii* often colonize the upper respiratory passages of cats. With the exception of *M. felis*, mycoplasmas are not considered important primary causes of respiratory disease in cats. Mycoplasmas can be isolated from tracheobronchial washes of 20% of cats with pulmonary disease, but from few normal cats. As in dogs, the significance of this finding is complicated by the potential for mycoplasmas to secondarily colonize lungs that are diseased for other reasons. Kittens experimentally infected with *M. felis, M. gatae, and M. arginini* did not develop clinical signs of respiratory disease. Unclassified *Mycoplasma* spp. have been isolated from pulmonary abscesses and lesions of neutrophilic pleuritis in cats.

Fungal diseases

Fungal diseases of cats are described with those of dogs (see the Infectious Respiratory Diseases of Dogs section). *Aspergillus spp*. rarely causes bronchitis and pneumonia in diabetic cats.

Parasitic diseases

Toxoplasmosis

Toxoplasmosis is described more fully in the chapter on the alimentary system. Gross lung lesions are *pinpoint white foci scattered throughout the lung or diffuse interstitial pneumonia* (Fig. 5-74), either alone or as a component of multisystemic disease. Histologically, there are multifocal-to-diffuse alveolar lesions with hyaline membranes, fibrinonecrotic debris, or proliferation of type II pneumocytes, necrosis of bronchiolar

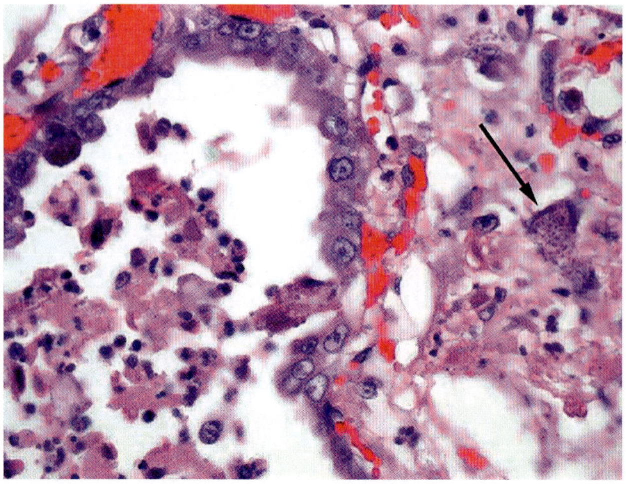

Figure 5-74 Toxoplasmosis in the lung of a cat. Alveoli are lined by cuboidal type II pneumocytes with necrotic debris in the lumen, and *Toxoplasma* cysts are present in alveolar epithelial cells and the interstitium (arrow).

epithelium, and infiltration of neutrophils, mononuclear cells, variable numbers of eosinophils, and protozoal cysts (see Fig. 5-74). *Diagnosis* can be made using PCR or immunohistochemistry to identify cysts within the lung.

Aelurostrongylus abstrusus

Aelurostrongylus abstrusus is a moderately common lungworm of cats. Cats may be infected subclinically and display no clinical signs, but heavy infections cause coughing or increased respiratory rate.

Adult *A. abstrusus* (nematode, *Metastrongyloidea, Angiostrongylidae*) are slender, up to 1 cm long, and live in the alveolar ducts and respiratory bronchioles. The eggs form nodular deposits in alveoli, where they embryonate and hatch to release first-stage larvae. The larvae move to the airways, are coughed up and swallowed, and passed in the feces. Snails and slugs are intermediate hosts; birds, rodents, frogs, and lizards are paratenic (transport) hosts. The life cycle is completed when a cat eats either an intermediate host or a paratenic host. Infective larvae migrate to the lungs and reach maturity 4-6 weeks after ingestion of the third-stage larvae.

Heavy infections in the prepatent period cause randomly distributed hemorrhages or white foci, which are an eosinophilic and granulomatous reaction to the migrating larvae. *In the patent period, there are 1-10 mm diameter, firm, off-white to pale-yellow, slightly raised nodules scattered throughout the lungs.* In severe infections, nodules may coalesce to form confluent areas of consolidation.

Microscopically, *the nodules are formed by masses of eggs and larvae in the alveoli and terminal bronchioles, with fewer adult worms* (eFig. 5-75). Eosinophils and neutrophils infiltrate the early lesions, but most cases are dominated by mononuclear cells and giant cells in the alveoli and around degenerating eggs and larvae. Alveoli are dilated and alveolar septa may be disrupted. Necrosis and mineralization seldom occur. Lymphocytic nodules form around vessels and airways, and there is hypertrophy and hyperplasia of smooth muscle in the walls of the bronchioles and alveolar ducts. Adult worms, eggs, or larvae in the bronchioles are associated with chronic catarrhal and eosinophilic bronchiolitis; similar inflammation may be present within the tracheal mucosa, presumably in response to larvae moving up the trachea to be swallowed. In older lesions from which eggs and larvae have disappeared, alveoli remain epithelialized and septa are persistently thickened by fibrous tissue and smooth muscle. Bronchial glands and smooth muscle in the media of small pulmonary arteries and arterioles may be quite prominent in cats infected with *Aelurostrongylus*, but these changes are also common in clinically healthy cats that have no evidence of parasitism.

Paragonimus kellicotti

Of the *trematodes*, the only genus that has its final habitat in the lungs is *Paragonimus*. *Paragonimus kellicotti* occurs in America, and ***Paragonimus westermani*** in Asia. Mink and other fish-eating carnivores are the usual hosts of *P. kellicotti*, but it infects many other species. Among domestic animals, it is *most common in cats* and occasionally in dogs. Most infected animals have no clinical signs.

The life cycle is typical of trematodes. The first intermediate hosts are small aquatic snails. The second intermediate host is a freshwater crab or crayfish. When the crayfish is eaten by the definitive host, the metacercariae are liberated in the intestine and migrate across the peritoneal and pleural cavities to the lungs. Their passage through the pleura is marked by many small hemorrhages and foci of eosinophilic and fibrinous pleuritis that heal as small umbilicated scars. Adult flukes are ovoid, red-brown, and up to 17 mm long. They are often found in pairs in inflammatory cavitations in the pulmonary parenchyma and occasionally in the bronchi. The cavitations frequently communicate with bronchioles, permitting release of eggs into the airways, expulsion to the nasopharynx, and passage in the feces.

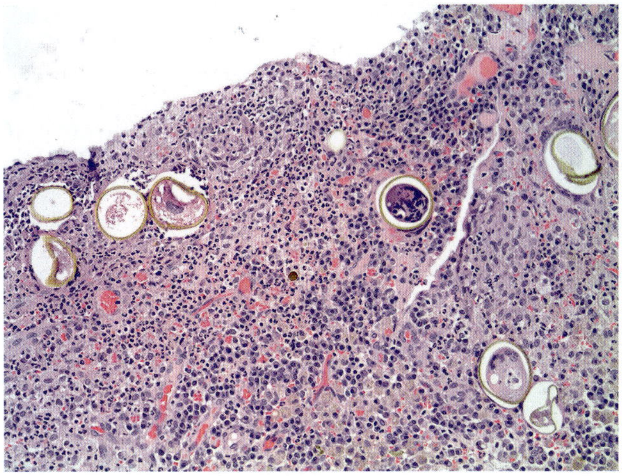

Figure 5-75 ***Paragonimus kellicotti*** in a cat. Parietal pleura with pyogranulomatous inflammation and pigmented ova. The cat died of respiratory distress, presumably from pneumothorax caused by rupture of the bronchus-associated cyst. The chronic inflammatory reaction in the parietal pleura suggests prior leakage of cyst contents.

The cavitations, which are more common in the caudal lobes, are spherical, 1-3 cm diameter, soft, and dark red-brown (eFig. 5-76). The cavitations contain intense eosinophilic and granulomatous inflammation, hemorrhage with numerous hemosiderin-laden macrophages, a fibrous capsule, and adult flukes. The adults exhibit characteristic features of trematodes: the body is filled with loose parenchyma but there is no body cavity, paired ceca contain dark pigment, oral suckers are present in some sections, the tegument has surface spines, and vitellaria beneath the tegument contain eosinophilic globular yolk material. In patent infections, there are numerous 80-100 µm long, yellow-brown, operculate eggs, which persist as fractured shells in chronic lesions (Fig. 5-75; see eFig. 5-76). As cavitations mature and establish connections with bronchioles, they become partially lined by cuboidal epithelium to form *true cysts*. At this stage, bronchioles contain eggs and eosinophilic exudate, with hyperplasia of peribronchiolar glands and smooth muscle. Other lesions include chronic catarrhal eosinophilic bronchiolitis, granulomatous pleuritis, and pleural lymphangitis associated with the eggs and fluke-derived pigment. Rupture of the cysts causes pneumothorax, which may lead to acute respiratory distress and distribution of eggs and pigmented debris throughout the pleural cavity.

Other parasitic diseases

Troglostrongylus brevior and ***Troglostrongylus subcrenatus*** are metastrongyloid (*Crenosomatidae*) nematodes, ~0.4 x 14 mm, that reside in the trachea and bronchi of cats. In heavily infected cats, clinical signs consist of dyspnea, tachypnea, and coughing. Catarrhal inflammation within the airways and bronchopneumonia may develop in response to the parasites. The life cycle of this parasite is not completely known, but likely involves L1 larvae being passed in cat feces to infect terrestrial mollusks, where they develop into L3 larvae to be consumed by cats or a variety of paratenic hosts.

Mammomonogamus ierei, a strongylid nematode, infects the nasal sinuses, larynx, and trachea of cats, whereas ***Mammomonogamus** auris* infects the middle ear. ***Eucoleus aerophilus*** is as described for dogs. ***Oslerus rostratus*** is a viviparous parasite of cats that causes sinuous thickenings of the submucosa of large bronchi, formed by adult worms within cystic spaces. When the adults die, they provoke intense infiltration of neutrophils, with eventual mineralization and fibrosis. ***Angiostrongylus chabaudi*** resides within small (muscular) pulmonary arteries and causes intimal proliferation and thrombosis.

Visit Elsevier eBooks+ (eBooks.Health.Elsevier.com) for eFigures and further readings.

INDEX

Page numbers followed by "*f*" indicate figures, "*t*" indicate tables, and "*b*" indicate boxes.

B

C

H

M

O

P

T